Integrated Biomaterials Science

Integrated Biomaterials Science

Edited by

ROLANDO BARBUCCI

Interuniversity Research Center for Advanced Medical Systems (C.R.I.S.M.A.)
and
Department of Chemical and Biosystem Sciences and Technologies
University of Siena
Siena, Italy

Kluwer Academic / Plenum Publishers
New York, Boston, Dordrecht, London, Moscow

Library of Congress Cataloging-in-Publication Data

Barbucci, Rolando.
Integrated biomaterials science/Rolando Barbucci.
p. ; cm.
Includes bibliographical references and index.
ISBN 0-306-46678-3
1. Biomaterials. 2. Medical instruments and apparatus. 3. Artificial organs. 4. Transplantation of organs, tissues, etc. I. Title.
[DNLM: 1. Biocompatible Materials. 2. Transplantation. QT 37 B24li 2001]
R856. .B374 2001
610′.28—dc21

2001038949

ISBN 0-306-46678-3

233 Spring Street, New York, N.Y. 10013

http://www.wkap.nl/

10 9 8 7 6 5 4 3 2 1

A C.I.P. record for this book is available from the Library of Congress

Printed in the United States of America

To my wife, Gloria
Rolando Barbucci

Contributors

Giovanni Abatangelo
Institute of Histology and Embryology
Faculty of Medicine
University of Padova
35121 Padova, Italy

Ron Alkalay
Orthopaedic Biomechanics Laboratory
Beth Israel Deaconess Medical Centre
Boston, Massachusetts 02215, United States

Luigi Ambrosio
Institute of Composite Materials Technology C.N.R., and C.R.I.B.
University of Naples "Federico II"
80125 Naples, Italy

Emma Angelini
Dipartimento di Scienza dei Materiali ed Ingegneria Chimica
Politecnico di Torino
10129 Torino, Italy

Marcus K. H. Auth
Universitätskinderklinik, Abteilung Allgemeine Kinderheilkunde mit Schwerpunkt, Neuropädiatrie, Klinikum der Universitäts-Gesamthochschule
Essen, Germany

Alfonso Barbarisi
Istituto di Biochimica delle Proteine ed Enzimologia
Consiglio Nazionale delle Richerche
0072 Arco Felice, Napoli, Italy

Marc Bolla
Laboratoire de biomatériaux dentaires
UFR Odontologie
Université de Nice Sophia Antipolis
04537 Nice Cedex 05, France

Paola Brun
Institute of Histology and Embryology
Faculty of Medicine
University of Padova
35121 Padova, Italy

Paolo Caliceti
Department of Pharmaceutical Sciences
University of Padova
35131 Padova, Italy

Angelo Caputo
Advanced Prosthodontics, Biomimetics and Hospital Dentistry Department
UCLA School of Dentistry
Los Angeles, California 90095-1668, United States

Marie-Paule Carreno
Laboratoire d'Immunopathologie Humaine
INSERM U430, Hôpital Broussais
75014 Paris, France

Gerardo Catapano
Department of Chemical and Materials Engineering
University of Calabria
87036 Arcavacata di Rende (CS), Italy

Luigi Celli
Clinica Ortopedica e Traumatologica
Università degli Studi di Modena e Reggio Emilia
Departimento delle Discipline Chirurgiche e delle Emergenze
41100 Modena, Italy

Elisabetta Cenni
Laboratorio di Fisiopatologia degli Impianti Ortopedici
Istituti Ortopedici Rizzoli
40136 Bologna, Italy

Roberto Chiesa
Dipartimento di Chimica Fisica Applicata
Politecnico di Milano
20131 Milano, Italy

Krishnan K. Chittur
Chemical and Materials Engineering Department
University of Alabama at Huntsville
Huntsville, Alabama 35899, United States

Gabriela Ciapetti
Laboratorio di Fisiopatologia degli Impianti Ortopedici
Istituti Ortopedici Rizzoli
40136 Bologna, Italy

Alberto Cigada
Dipartimento di Chimica Fisica Applicata
Politecnico di Milano
20131 Milano, Italy

Roberta Cortiro
Institute of Histology and Embryology
Faculty of Medicine
University of Padova
35121 Padova, Italy

Stephen P. Denyer
School of Pharmacy and Biomolecular Sciences
University of Brighton
Brighton, BN2 4GJ, United Kingdom

Alfredo De Rosa
Istituo di Biochimica delle Proteine ed Enzimologia
Consiglio Nazionale delle Ricerche
0072 Arco Felice, Napoli, Italy

Roberto De Santis
Institute of Composite Materials Technology C.N.R., and C.R.I.B.
University of Naples "Federico II"
80125 Naples, Italy

Luca Fambri
Department of Materials Engineering
University of Trento
38050 Trento, Italy

Antonietta M. Gatti
INFM, Laboratorio dei Biomateriali
Dipartimento di Discipline Chirurgiche e delle Emergenze
Università di Modena e Reggio Emilia
41100 Modena, Italy

Roberto Giardino
Experimental Surgery Department
Codivilla-Putti I.O.R. Research Institute
40136 Bologna, Italy

Francisco-Javier Gil
CREB (Biomedical Engineering Research Center)
Department of Materials Science and Metallurgical Engineering
Universitat Politècnica de Catalunya
08028 Barcelona, Spain

Maria-Pau Ginebra
CREB (Biomedical Engineering Research Center)
Department of Materials Science and Metallurgical Engineering
Universitat Politècnica de Catalunya
08028 Barcelona, Spain

Donatella Granchi
Laboratorio di Fisiopatologia degli Impianti Ortopedici
Istituti Ortopedici Rizzoli
40136 Bologna, Italy

Giuseppe Guida
Istituto di Clinica Ortopedica
Università di Napoli
80138 Napoli, Italy

Franck J. Hagege
Laboratoire de biomatériaux dentaires
UFR Odontologie
Université de Nice Sophia Antipolis
04537 Nice Cedex 05, France

Richard T. Hart
Department of Biomedical Engineering
Tulane University
New Orleans, Louisiana 70118, United States

Kunihiro Hisatsune
Department of Dental Materials Science
Nagasaki University School of Dentistry
Nagasaki 852, Japan

Yoshito Ikada
Research Center for Biomedical Engineering
Kyoto University
Sakyo-ku
Kyoto 606, Japan
Present address:
Department of Medical Electronics
Faculty of Medical Engineering
Suzuka University of Medical Science
Suzuka City, Mie 510-0293, Japan

Kemal Kesenci
Chemical Engineering Department and Bioengineering Division
Hacettepe University, Beytepe
06530 Ankara, Turkey

Jonathan C. Knowles
Department of Biomaterials-Eastman Dental Institute
University College London
London WC1X8LD, United Kingdom

Adriano Krajewski
Research Institute for Ceramic Technology of the Italian National Research Council
48018 Faenza (Ravena), Italy

Denis Labarre
Laboratoire de Biomatériaux et Polymères
UMR CNRS 8612
Université Paris-Sud XI
92290 Châtenay-Malabry, France

Domenico Lepore
Department of Ophthalmology
Catholic University of the Sacred Heart
00168 Rome, Italy

Andrew W. Lloyd
School of Pharmacy and Biomolecular Sciences
University of Brighton
Brighton, BN2 4GJ, United Kingdom

Patrizia Loria
Department of Biophysical Medical and Odontostomatological Sciences and Technologies
University of Genova
16132 Genoa, Italy

Donald Lyman
Department of Materials Science and Engineering and Department of Bioengineering
University of Utah
Salt Lake City, Utah 84122, United States

Agnese Magnani
Dipartimento di Scienze e Tecnologie Chimiche e dei Biosistemi
Università degli Studi di Siena
53100 Siena, Italy

Walter Marconi
Department of Chemistry
University of Rome "La Sapienza"
00185 Rome, Italy

Sabrina Margarucci
Istituto di Biochimica delle Proteine ed Enzimologia
Consiglio Nazionale delle Ricerche
0072 Arco Felice, Napoli, Italy

Claudio Migliaresi
Department of Materials Engineering
University of Trento
38050 Trento, Italy

Arturo N. Natali
Centre of Mechanics of Biological Materials
Dipartimento di Costruzioni e Trasporti
University of Padova
35131 Padova, Italy

Paolo A. Netti
Institute of Composite Materials Technology C.N.R., and C.R.I.B.
University of Naples "Federico II"
80125 Naples, Italy

Luigi Nicolais
Institute of Composite Materials Technology C.N.R., and C.R.I.B.
University of Naples "Federico II"
80125 Naples, Italy

Nicolò Nicoli Aldini
Experimental Surgery Department
Codivilla-Putti I.O.R. Research Institute
40136 Bologna, Italy

Sandro Paci
ENEA
00100 Roma, Italy

Alessandro Pegoretti
Department of Materials Engineering
University of Trento
38050 Trento, Italy

Gianfranco Peluso
Istituto di Biochimica delle Proteine ed Enzimologia
Consiglio Nazionale delle Ricerche
0072 Arco Felice, Napoli, Italy

Orsolina Petillo
Istituto di Biochimica delle Proteine ed Enzimologia
Consiglio Nazionale delle Ricerche
0072 Arco Felice, Napoli, Italy

Maria Rosa Pinasco
Dipartimento di Chimica e Chimica Industriale
Università degli Studi di Genova
16146 Genova, Italy

Antonella Piozzi
Department of Chemistry
University of Rome "La Sapienza"
00185 Rome, Italy

Erhan Piskin
Chemical Engineering Department and Bioengineering Division
Hacettepe University, Beytepe
06530, Ankara, Turkey

Arturo Pizzoferrato
Laboratorio di Fisiopatologia degli Impianti Ortopedici
Istituti Ortopedici Rizzoli
40136 Bologna, Italy

Josep-Anton Planell
CREB (Biomedical Engineering Research Center)
Department of Materials Science and Metallurgical Engineering
Universitat Politècnica de Catalunya
08028 Barcelona, Spain

Maria Vittoria Primiceri
Notarbartolo & Gervasi SpA
00198 Roma, Italy

Marco Radice
Institute of Histology and Embryology
Faculty of Medicine
University of Padova
35121 Padova, Italy

Antonio Ravaglioli
Research Institute for Ceramic Technology of the Italian National Research Council
48018 Faenza (Ravenna), Italy

Peter A. Revell
Department of Histopathology
Royal Free and University College Medical School
Royal Free Campus
London NW3 2PF, United Kingdom

Dante Ronca
Istituto di Clinica Ortopedica
Università di Napoli
80138 Napoli, Italy

Matteo Santin
School of Pharmacy and Biomolecular Sciences
University of Brighton
Brighton, BN2 4GJ, United Kingdom

Lucia Savarino
Laboratorio di Fisiopatologia degli Impianti Ortopedici
Istituti Ortopedici Rizzoli
40136 Bologna, Italy

Luigi Scullica
Department of Ophthalmology
Catholic University of the Sacred Heart
00168 Rome, Italy

Susanna Stea
Laboratorio di Fisiopatologia degli Impianti Ortopedici
Istituti Ortopedici Rizzoli
40136 Bologna, Italy

Francesco M. Veronese
Department of Pharmaceutical Sciences
University of Padova
35131 Padova, Italy

Libero Vitiello
Department of Biology
University of Padova
35121 Padova, Italy

Fabrizio Zucchi
Centro Studi Corrosione A. Daccò
Università di Ferrara
44100 Ferrara, Italy

Preface

Progress in medical science has led to an extension of the average human lifetime, which has brought a rising demand for materials for tissue and organ replacement. These materials are called biomaterials and the discipline involved is called Biomaterials Science.

Biomaterials Science was born to fulfill the demands of patients and physicians for more efficient as well as new products. These products are designed and, first, tested *in vitro* in research laboratories; they then must pass through *in vivo* and clinical experimentation before being introduced into the market. *Integrated Biomaterials Science* provides an intriguing insight into that world, exploring the materials and the technology that has brought us new biomaterials. The book covers knowledge in chemistry, engineering, biology, and medicine that has had a significant impact on biomaterials. In particular, it highlights the way in which modern biology and medicine is inextricably linked to the other scientific disciplines, all contributing to the process of discovery and helping us to understand the complex world of biomaterials.

Biomaterials Science is multidisciplinary because it needs the support of many classical disciplines, including Physics, Chemistry, Biology, Engineering, and Medicine. Indeed, the special feature of this science is the interdiscipline among the different areas involved; this means that there must be perfect integration among the several disciplines in order to develop and advance Biomaterials Science. This is its main characteristic and the greatest difficulty that a researcher faces when studying or simply trying to understand Biomaterials Science. None of the disciplines involved in Biomaterials Science can be considered the most important; researchers know perfectly well that no one discipline takes precedence over another, but that there is only good research and bad research.

Although the chapters of this book can be read independently of one another, they are arranged in a logical sequence.

The book starts with the study of properties and characteristics of materials used to produce biomaterials. Before dealing with the use of these biomaterials as implants, the nature and characteristics of tissues to be replaced are explained. The interactions occurring between the material and the biological environment, and thus the tests necessary to prove their biocompatibility, are treated starting from the intended applications. Some chapters deal with tissue engineering and gene therapy, too. We have also included aspects less often covered in other biomaterials books, such as patents and regulations as well as standards on biomaterials, with a view toward covering interactions with the industrial world and its needs.

One huge area that we have been unable to include is physicochemical characterization. This subject is so large that it would easily fill a volume on its own. We do, of course, fully recognize that analytical techniques designed to solve the structures, both in the bulk and on the surface of biomaterials, have revolutionized research in biomaterials science, but the techniques utilized are extremely sophisticated and continuously being upgraded, so there is a risk that they will be obsolete by the time the book is published.

This book is a good guide to understanding the subject. Admittedly, there are still large areas of ignorance in biomaterials and many facts that cannot yet be explained. However, these unsolved problems provide much of the excitement, and we have tried to point them out in a way that will stimulate readers to join in the enterprise of discovery.

While previous books have supplied extensive information on all subjects concerning biomaterials, this one is not just informative but is designed to provide all the researchers involved in the biomaterials field with an opportunity to probe further: researchers using biomaterials and studying their properties as well as those involved in their industrial production. The book will be extremely useful for students of biomaterials courses and can be used as a textbook.

Rolando Barbucci

Contents

3. Fundamentals of Polymeric Composite Materials

Claudio Migliaresi and Alessandro Pegoretti

4. Biodegradable Polymers

Luca Fambri, Claudio Migliaresi, Kernal Kesenci, and Erhan Piskin

7. Degradation Processes on Metallic Surfaces

Emma Angelini, Angelo Caputo, and Fabrizio Zucchi

14. Soft Tissue Replacement

Matteo Santin, Luigi Ambrosio, Andrew W. Lloyd, and Stephen P. Denyer

15. Mechanics of Hard Tissues

Arturo N. Natali and Richard T. Hart

16. Hip Joint Replacements

Giuseppe Guida and Dante Ronca

17. Knee Joint Replacements

Dante Ronca and Giuseppe Guida

18. Biomaterial Applications: Elbow Prosthesis

Luigi Celli

19. Biomaterial Applications: Shoulder Prosthesis

Luigi Celli

20. Acrylic Bone Cements

Maria-Pau Ginebra, Francisco-Javier Gil, and Josep-Anton Planell

21. Mechanical Properties of Tooth Structures

Roberto De Santis, Luigi Ambrosio, and Luigi Nicolais

22. Dental Materials and Implants

Maria Rosa Pinasco, Arturo Natali, Patrizia Loria, Marc Bolla, and Franck J. Hagege

23. Materials/Biological Environment Interactions

Orsolina Petillo, Alfonso Barbarisi, Sabrina Margarucci, Alfredo De Rosa, and Gianfranco Peluso

24. Protein Adsorption and Cellular/Tissue Interactions

Agnese Magnani, Gianfranco Peluso, Sabrina Margarucci, and Krishnan K. Chittur

25. Inflammatory Response to Polymeric Materials

Denis Labarre and Marie-Paule Carreno

26. Inflammatory Response to Metals and Ceramics

Arturo Pizzoferrato, Elisabetta Cenni, Gabriela Ciapetti, Donatella Granchi, Lucia Savarino, and Susanna Stea

27. Biocompatibility and Biological Tests

Antonietta M. Gatti and Jonathan C. Knowles

28. Infection and Sterilization

Roberto Giardino and Nicolò Nicoli Aldini

29. Drug Delivery Systems

Francesco M. Veronese and Paolo Caliceti

30. Gene Delivery as a New Therapeutic Approach

Libero Vitiello and Francesco M. Veronese

31. Tissue Engineering

Giovanni Abatangelo, Paola Brun, Marco Radice, Roberta Cortiro, and Marcus K. H. Auth

32. Assist Devices

Gerardo Catapano

Integrated Biomaterials Science

1

Biological Materials

Yoshito Ikada

1.1. Introduction

Currently used biomaterials can be divided into two categories: biological and synthetic. The biological materials are composed of polypeptides (proteins), polysaccharides, nucleic acids, polyesters, hydroxyapatites, or their composites. Table 1.1 gives representatives of biological materials. Nucleic acids have not yet found application as biomaterials owing to their poor mechanical properties even after cross-linking. Remarkable advantages of biological materials over synthetics are their excellent physiological activities such as selective cell adhesion (e.g., collagen and fibrin), similar mechanical properties to natural tissues (e.g., animal heart valves and blood vessels), and biodegradability (e.g., gelatin and chitin). However, similar to synthetics, biological materials have several deficiencies including risk of viral infection, antigenicity, unstable material supply, and deterioration which accompanies long-term implantation. The biodegradability of biological materials can be both advantageous and disadvantageous depending on their biomedical applications, as will be shown later.

Application of biological materials in medicine has a longer history than synthetic biomaterials, but the demand for biological biomaterials has recently decreased because they have unavoidable deficiencies, as mentioned above. However, it seems probable that some biological materials will continue to play an important role as biomaterials, since they possess unique properties that synthetic biomaterials lack.

This chapter describes basic properties of biological materials listed in Table 1.1 and examines prospects for their application in medicine.

Yoshito Ikada • Research Center for Biomedical Engineering, Kyoto University, 53 Kawahara cho, Shogoin, Sakyo-ku, Kyoto 606, Japan. *Present address:* Department of Medical Electronics, Faculty of Medical Engineering, Suzuka University of Medical Science, 1001-1 Kishioka, Suzuka City, Mie 510-0293, Japan.

Integrated Biomaterials Science, edited by R. Barbucci. Kluwer Academic/Plenum Publishers, New York, 2002.

Table 1.1. Components of Biological Materials

Organic materials (polymers)			Inorganic materials	
Polypeptides	Polysaccharides	Polyesters	Phosphates	Carbonate
Collagen Gelatin Fibrin Albumin Silk fibroin	Cellulose Starch Dextran Chitin Chitosan Hyaluronate Alginate Agarose	Poly(2-hydroxy butyrate) (PHB)	Hydroxyapatite $[Ca_{10}(PO_4)_6(OH)_2]$ Tricalcium phosphate $[Ca_3(PO_4)_2]$	Calcium-carbonate $[CaCO_3]$

1.2. Fundamentals of Biological Materials

1.2.1. Polypeptides

A mammalian body has different kinds of polypeptide including plasma, structural, and functional proteins. The majority of proteins used as biomaterials originate from blood plasmas and structural skeletons. Functional proteins such as enzymes, cell growth factors, and interleukins are also used, but mostly incorporated in biomaterials as ingredients.

1.2.1.1. Plasma Proteins (Serum Albumin and Fibrinogen)

The plasma protein which is present in blood in the largest amount is serum albumin. This globular protein is unable to form tough film or sponge, but only microbead through its denaturation or chemical cross-linking. In contrast, fibrinogen is readily polymerized into hydrogel when partially hydrolyzed by thrombin. This fibrin hydrogel can be further cross-linked chemically by factor XIII.

1.2.1.2. Collagen and Gelatin

Approximately one-third of the proteins present in the human body is collagen, which forms a family of different kinds from Type I to Type XIII. The collagen most widely used as biomaterial is of Type I, which is distributed in the skin, bone, tendon, and intestinal gut. The regenerated collagen obtainable by extraction from animal tissues under mild conditions keeping triple-helical collagen molecules are also employed as biomaterials. The native collagen chain has a molecular weight around 1×10^5 and a tello portion at the chain end which is responsible for high antigenicity. The collagen from which the tello portion has been eliminated is called *atellocollagen* and is generally used as biomaterial. The triple-helical collagen in the monodispersed state can exist only in acidic solution and quickly undergoes fibrous aggregation when the solution pH is adjusted to 7. This aggregation ability of collagen molecules in neutral aqueous solution enables them to form films and porous sheets (sponge) from the solution. Although collagen films and sheets are insoluble in water of pH 7, they are quickly degraded and absorbed in the body when implanted. Delay in collagen absorption can be realized if chemical cross-linking is introduced into collagen molecules. Figure 1.1 shows how chemical cross-linking retards hydrolysis of a collagen film when immersed in collagenase solution (Tomihata *et al.*, 1994). Collagen cross-linking can be performed through a variety of chemical reactions, as shown in Figure 1.2. Formaldehyde is no longer used as the cross-linking agent of proteins because of its possible neoplastic formation. The most widely used agent for cross-linking of commercial proteinous products is glutaraldehyde.

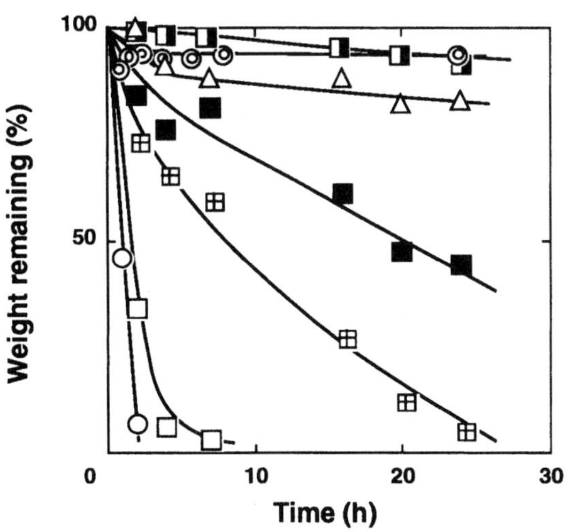

Figure 1.1. *In vitro* degradation of various gelatin films cross-linked with glutaraldehyde (GA), epoxide (EX-810), water-soluble carbodiimide (WSC), and dehydration treatment (DHT) upon hydrolysis in 40 units/ml collagenase solution at 37 °C and pH 7.4. (□) GA 5 mM, (■) GA 20 mM, (◨) GA 100 mM, (△) WSC 50 mM, (⊞) DHT (150 °C, 24 h), (○) EX-810 0.2 mM, and (◎) EX-810 2.0 mM

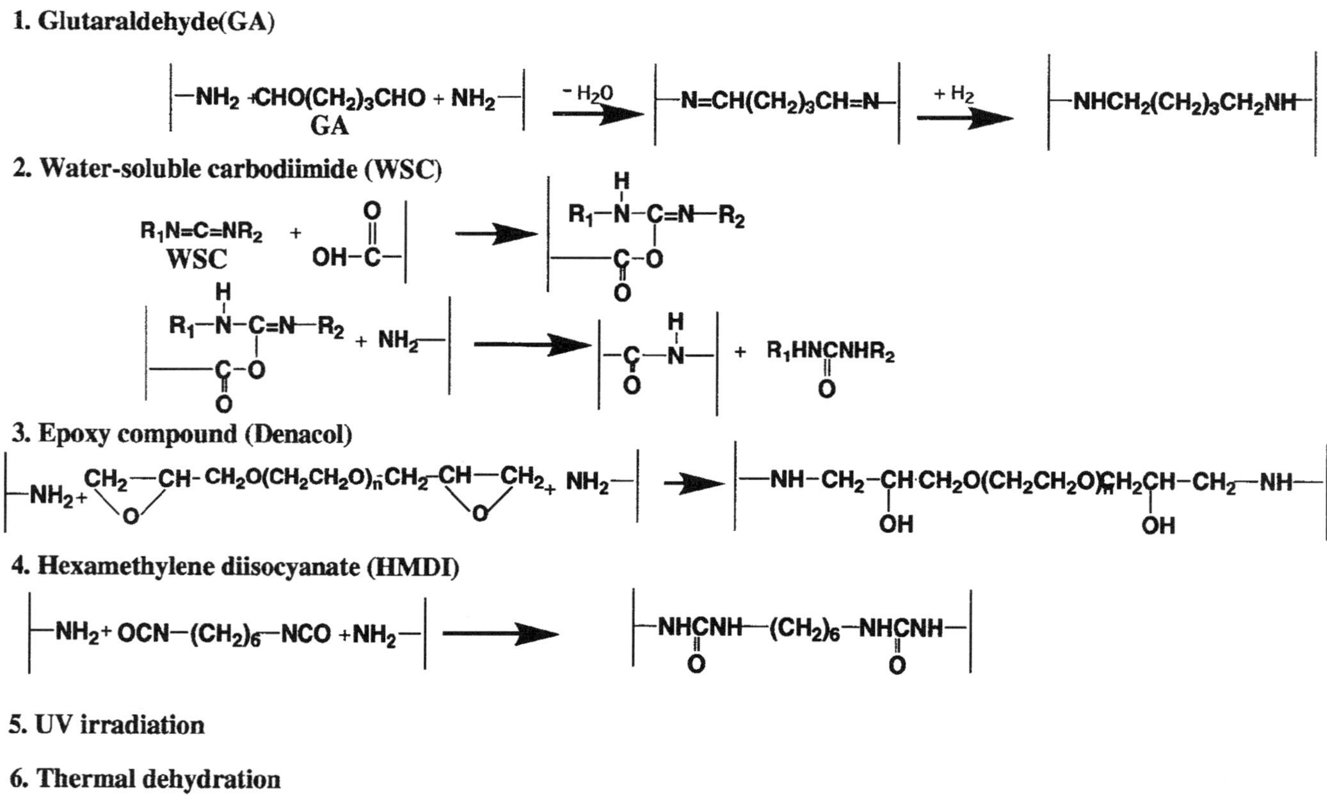

Figure 1.2. Various methods for protein cross-linking.

Gelatin is a denatured form of collagen consisting of random chains without triple helix. Extraction of animal collagenous tissues with lime or acids yields gelatin, as illustrated in Figure 1.3. Gelatin is readily soluble in water over a wide pH range, unless the temperature is lower than *ca* 25 °C. This sol–gel transition is reversible for aqueous gelatin solution. To avoid very rapid absorption of gelatin films or sponges implanted in the body, they should be cross-linked chemically with similar methods employed for collagen. It is noteworthy that cross-linked gelatin generally possesses more excellent mechanical properties than cross-linked collagen. *In vivo* biodegradation of gelatin films cross-linked to various extents is demonstrated in Figure 1.4.

1.2.2. Polysaccharides

In animals, polysaccharides are important as components of extracellular matrix while these biomacromolecules, especially cellulose and chitin, are the major elements of the skeleton of plants, crustacea, and insects. Figure 1.5 shows the chemical structure of polysaccharides, which have been used as biomaterials or have potential for medical application. Cellulose has the largest production among the whole natural and synthetic macromolecules existing on the earth, while the macromolecule of the second largest production is chitin.

1.2.2.1. Cellulose

Cellulose is not used as implanted biomaterials at all but is a very important material for production of hollow fibers used for hemodialyzers (Ikada, 1996). They are fabricated also from cellulose diacetate and triacetate, which activate the complement system to a lesser extent than cellulose. The cellulose hollow fibers for hemodialysis are regenerated from cuprammonium solution of refined cotton linters with high purity, which has higher molecular weight than the pulp, leading to higher-tenacity fibers. The superiority of regenerated cellulose is due to: (1) high chemical stability, (2) low price, (3) high tenacity in the wet state, allowing the preparation of a thin membrane, (4) ease of the control of pore size, ranging from 1 to 100 nm in diameter, and (5) controllable porosity.

Cellulose can be oxidized with NO_2 in the fibrous state without altering the original shape (Olson *et al.*, 1982). The oxidized cellulose is absorbed into the body upon implantation as a result of physical dissolution (not biodegradation).

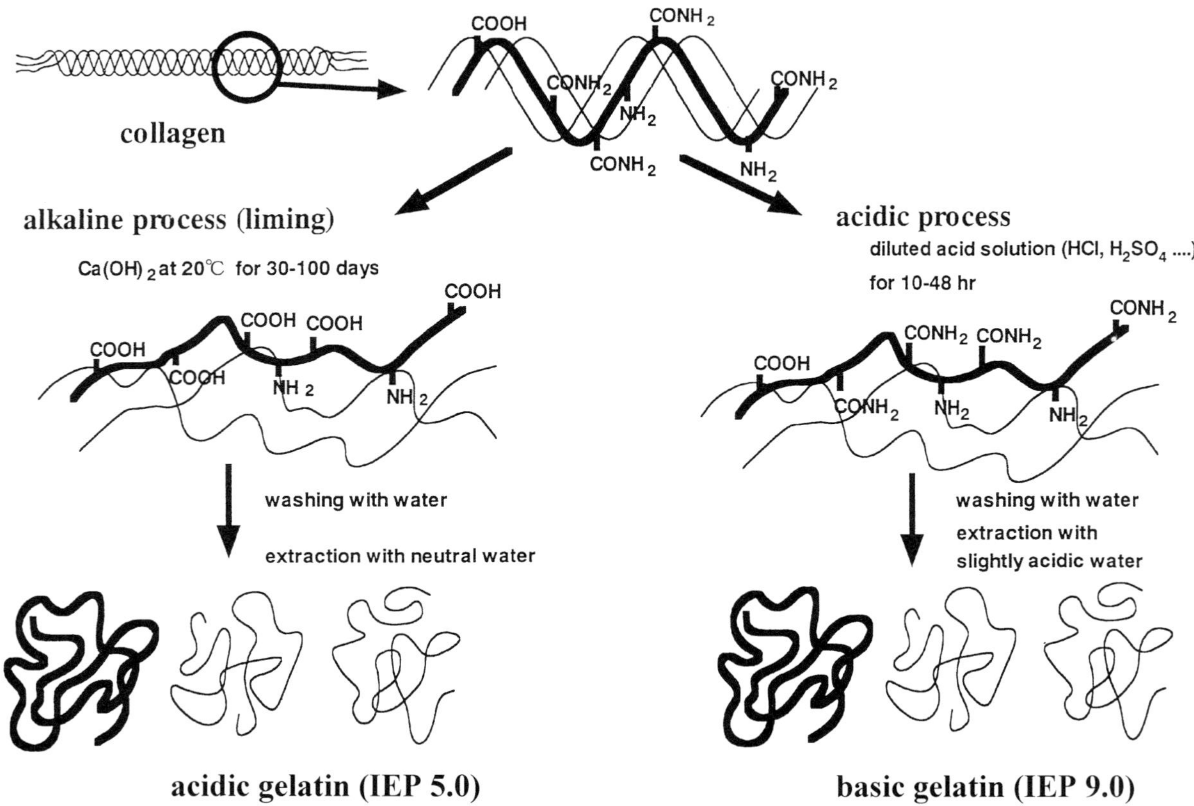

Figure 1.3. Two methods for gelatin extraction from tissues containing collagen.

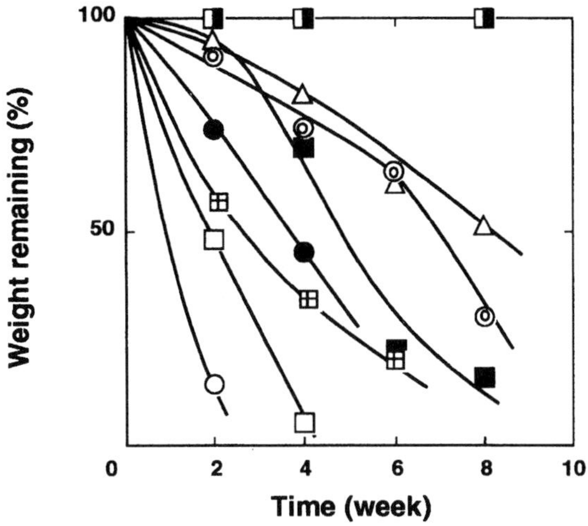

Figure 1.4. *In vivo* degradation of various cross-linked gelatin films after subcutaneous implantation in rats. (□) GA 5 mM, (■) GA 20 mM, (◨) GA 100 mM, (△) WSC 50 mM, (⊞) DHT (150 °C, 24 h), (○) EX-810 0.2 mM, (◎) EX-810 2.0 mM, and (●) EX-830 2.0 mM.

1.2.2.2. Starch

Starch is a mixture of amylose and amylopectin, both of which undergo enzymatic degradation in the body. To delay the rapid clearance of starch from the body, it is derivatized, for instance, by hydroxyethylation and chemical cross-linking. Hydroxyethyl starch (HES) was widely used previously as a plasma expander, but derivatized starches are currently used in most cases as drug carriers.

1.2.2.3. Dextran

In contrast to starch, dextran is practically not biodegraded although it is readily soluble in water over a wide pH range. The major medical application of dextran is its use as a plasma expander. Once dextran is chemically cross-linked, it no longer becomes absorbable in the body. This is the reason why cross-linking is not required for medical application of dextran.

1.2.2.4. Hyaluronate

The characteristics of hyaluronate as a biomaterial are high biodegradability and extremely high viscosity of its dilute aqueous solution.

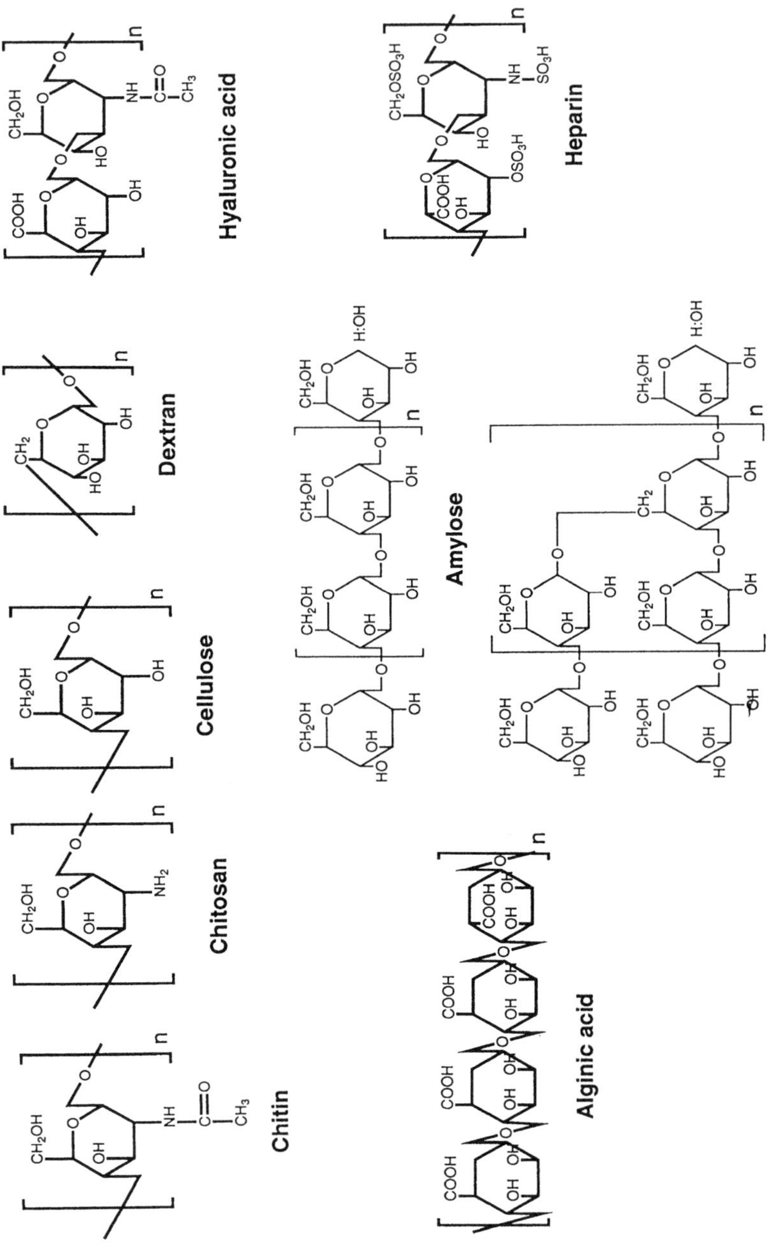

Figure 1.5. Chemical structure of polysaccharides of high potentials for medical applications.

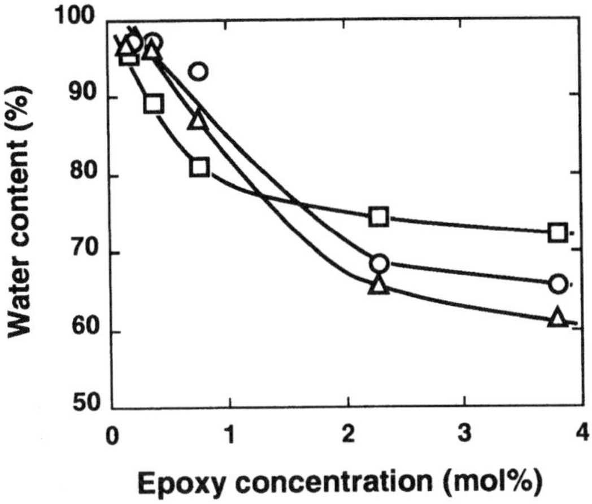

Figure 1.6. The water content of hyaluronate (HA) films cross-linked with different concentrations of epoxide (EX-810) at pH 4.7, 6.1, and 8.0 for 120 hs. (○) pH 4.7, (△) pH 6.1, and (□) pH 8.0.

Therefore, this polysaccharide is used clinically in a dilute viscous solution as a viscoelastic material in ophthalmology. Dilute solutions of hyaluronate have also been used to prevent tissue adhesion by covering the tissue with the solution for its protection. In order to prolong the time period of effective covering with the hyaluronate solution, an attempt was made to modify this biopolymer by esterification and crosslinking (Ghezzo *et al.*, 1992). Figure 1.6 demonstrates the effect of cross-linking with diepoxide on the equilibrated water content of hyaluronate (Tomihata and Ikada, 1997a). It is evident that cross-linking greatly reduces the water content of the hyaluronate film. Biodegradation of hyaluronate could be also reduced by cross-linking (Tomihata and Ikada, 1997a). Films prepared from derivatized hyaluronates are used clinically to prevent tissue adhesion.

1.2.2.5. Chitin and Chitosan

All the polysaccharides described above are hydrophilic and noncrystallizable except for cellulose and its acetates. On the contrary, chitin, which is an entirely naturally-occurring polymer, is hydrophobic and crystallizable (Proceedings, 1996). Therefore, chitin films and fibers fabricated from organic solutions of chitin have mechanical properties typical of synthetic fibers and films. In addition, chitin undergoes enzymatic degradation at least in rat (Tomihata and Ikada, 1997b). These unique properties of chitin appear to provide high potential for medical applications. However, current applications of chitin in medicine are quite limited. In Japan, wound covering is the only medical application of chitin approved by the Japanese government (Okashima *et al.*, 1991). The major reason for few medical applications of this polymer is not due to its toxicity [chitin seems to be nontoxic (Tomihata and Ikada, 1997b)], but may be ascribed to its lack of superiority to synthetic biodegradable polymers such as glycolide and lactide polymers. These aliphatic polyesters can be readily synthesized on a large scale by polymerization or copolymerization to various molecular weights and chemical compositions.

Chitosan can be obtained by deacetylation of chitin and is soluble in acidic media, in contrast to chitin. At the neutral pH, chitosan is no longer soluble in water. This indicates that chitin and chitosan do not require any chemical cross-linking, which is a common means to render water-soluble polymers water-insoluble. Partial deacetylation of chitin or partial acetylation of chitosan yields chitin derivatives with different degrees of acetylamino group. Figure 1.7 shows the water content of chitin derivatives as a function of the degree of deacetylation (Tomihata and Ikada, 1997b) (100% deacetylation gives chitosan while 0% deacetylation gives chitin). It is interesting to note that chitin and chitosan films have the lowest water content among the chitin derivatives. When these films were subcutaneously implanted in rat, chitosan exhibited no significant biodegradation while the chitin film was absorbed in the body, leaving no trace of film pieces (Tomihata and Ikada, 1997b). The biodegradation rate is plotted against the degree of deacetylation in Figure 1.8. Histological studies showed that both

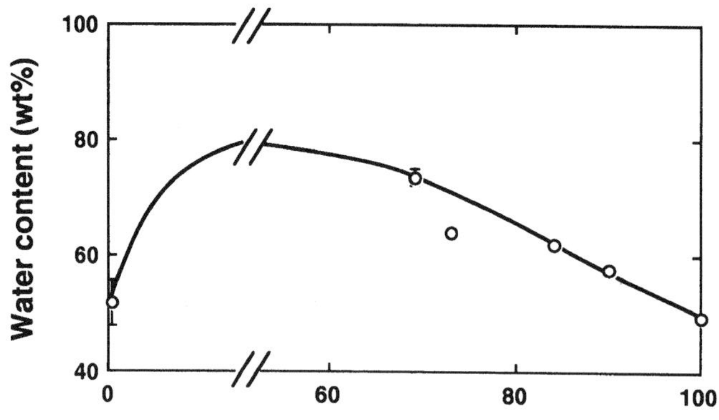

Figure 1.7. The water content of films of chitin and its deacetylated derivatives swollen with PBS at 37 °C as a function of the degree of deacetylation.

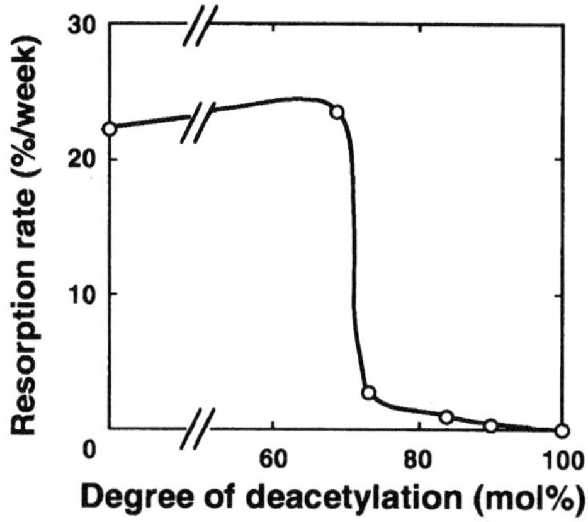

Figure 1.8. Dependence of the initial resorption rate of films of chitin and its deacetylated derivatives on the degree of deacetylation.

chitin and chitosan films did not evoke any severe inflammation and induced only a mild response from the host to an extent almost similar to cross-linked collagen (Tomihata and Ikada, 1997b). The zeta potential of chitosan film at pH 7 was not positive but near zero.

1.2.2.6. Miscellaneous

Heparin is the most well-known material among the polysaccharides used in medicine, but this water-soluble polysaccharide is not used as a biomaterial but as a drug in solution to prevent blood coagulation. Agar gel has also been used for cell culture in biology but not as a biomaterial. However, it has been attempted to apply agarose, a derivative of agar, as a membrane to encapsulate islets of Langerhans (Iwata, 1996). In other words, agarose has high potential as an encapsulating membrane for bioartificial pancreas. Similar to agarose, alginate has been used as an immunosuppressive membrane for bioartificial pancreas along with poly(L-lysin). Agarose undergoes physical cross-linking through hydrogen bonding at room temperature, while alginate requires divalent cationic ions for its salt cross-linking through the Coulombic forces.

1.2.3. Polyesters

Some microorganisms biosynthesize aliphatic polyesters. Among them are poly(2-hydroxyalkanoate)s. The most well-known natural polyester is poly(2-hydroxybutyrate) (PHB). This polyester is hydrophobic and crystallizable, similar to chitin, but can be molded by injection and extrusion because it melts at high temperature without oxidation. This is in contrast to chitin. The largest drawback of this natural polyester is its very low biodegradability when used as a biomaterial. Therefore, in an attempt to increase the biodegradability and reduce the Young's modulus, various copoly(2-hydroxyalkanoate)s have been synthesized using microorganisms.

1.2.4. Inorganic Materials

The major component of the skeleton of mammals comprises hydroxyapatite, a calcium phosphate, while calcium carbonate is the main structural body of corals. Both can be used as biomaterials, but synthetic hydroxyapatite and calcium carbonate are also commercially available and used in medicine much more than the natural biomaterials.

1.2.5. Composites

Most biological tissues are composite materials consisting of proteins, polysaccharides, and hydroxyapatite. Some are harvested from cadaverous bodies, preserved in the native state as much as possible, and delivered to hospitals. This is the tissue bank system. On the other hand, the biological tissues which have been used as biomaterials undergo processing mostly to minimize the antigenicity, to optimize the mechanical properties, and to prolong the biodegradation.

Human tissues used as biomaterials include bone (after deproteination), umbilical cord (after eliminating endothelial cells and cross-linking), amnion (after cross-linking), and dura mater (after freeze-drying and cross-linking). As an example, Figures 1.9 and 1.10 show the effect of cross-linking of amnion with glutaraldehyde on its mechanical strength and *in vitro* biodegradation, respectively (Tomihata *et al.*, 1999). Cross-linking is seen to have no effect on the tensile strength, but greatly suppresses the enzymatic degradation with collagenase.

Biological tissues of animal origins have also been used as biomaterials after processing, similar to human tissues. They include heart valves (porcine), pericardium (bovine), arteries (porcine), skin (porcine), and intestinal gut (goat). The major component of these animal tissues is the textured collagen, which is very biocompatible in terms of mechanical properties. Most of the tissues are preprocessed prior to implantation, generally using glutaraldehyde for the purpose of killing cells, reducting antigenicity, retarding biodegradation, and increasing mechanical properties.

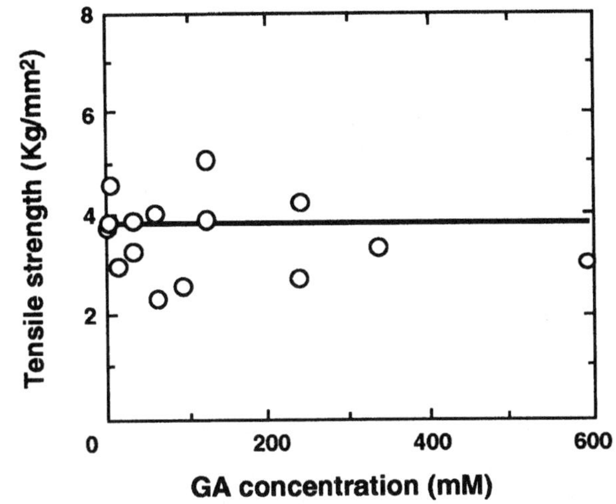

Figure 1.9. Glutaraldehyde (GA) concentration dependence of the tensile strength of GA-cross-linked amniotic membrane.

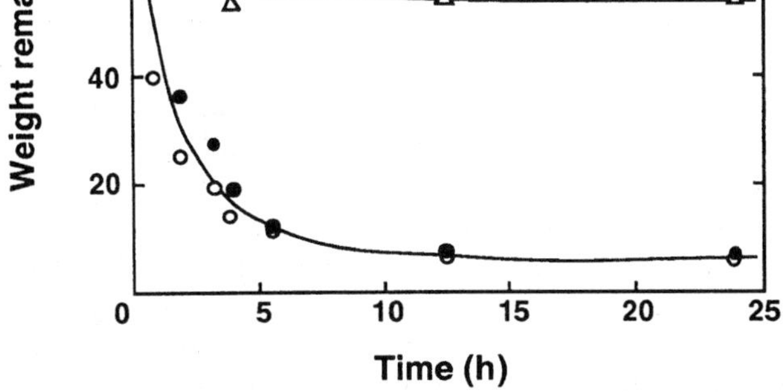

Figure 1.10. Weight remaining after treatment with 1 U ml^{-1} collagenase solution at 37°C for the native (○) and amniotic membranes cross-linked with 0.1 (●), 0.5 (△), 1.0 (▲), 2.5 (□), and 5.0 mM of GA (■).

1.3. Medical Application of Biological Materials

Synthetic materials have a much shorter history in biomedical application than biological ones, which have been used to assist the treatment of defective tissues such as tooth and skin in the BC era. The following overview is confined only to current clinical application of biological materials as biomaterials.

1.3.1. General Surgery

1.3.1.1. Sutures

Suturing is very important in surgery, because almost all surgical treatments need suturing. Before the advent of synthetic sutures, collagen and silk were most popular as suturing materials (Chu *et al.*, 1997). These biological sutures are still widely used in surgery, but are not regenerated from the biomacromolecules extracted from the mother natural tissues or products. Currently used collagenous sutures are fabricated mostly from the goat's gut, followed by chrome treatment. Silk sutures are prepared from cocoons, similar to silk fibers for apparel use.

1.3.1.2. Hemostats, Sealants, and Adhesives

There has been a great demand from surgeons for excellent hemostats, sealants, and adhesives because these biomaterials are very often needed in surgery (Sierra and Saltz, 1996). However, biomaterials that exhibit strong adhesion to tissues and are absorbed after wound healing have not yet been developed. These biomaterials should be delivered to surgeons in the form of flowable sol, viscous solution, or very pliable material and must set to a gel as quickly as possible when the sol or solution is applied to a wound tissue site. Currently used biomaterials that nearly meet such stringent requirements include fibrin glue, microfibrillar collagen, and gelatin. All of them are of natural origin. Fibrin glue is most widely employed as surgical adhesives and sealants outside the U.S. and Canada. This glue before curing consists of two aqueous solutions: fibrinogen and thrombin. Mixing of these two solutions yields a gel within ten seconds. The major problems of fibrin glue yet to be solved are possible viral infection and poor tissue adhesion. The topical hemostatic agent currently used most extensively throughout the world is probably sponge-type or microfibrillar collagen. Table 1.2 compares the ranking of currently applied hemostats including gelatin sponge and oxidized regenerated cellulose (Wagner *et al.*, 1996). As can be

Table 1.2. Ranking of Collagenous Hemostatic Agents[a]

Test	Actifoam	Avitene	Helistat	Gelfoam	Instat	Surgicel
Material	Collagen sponge	Microfibrillar collagen	Collagen sponge	Gelatin sponge	Collagen sponge	Oxidized regenerated cellulose
Platelet aggregation	4	3.5	2	3	2	2
Platelet aggregation w/thrombin	4	NA[b]	3	3	3	NA
Platelet deposition w/perfusion	2	4	3	0	1	NA
Platelet ATP secretion (5 min)	4	2.5	3.5	1.5	0.5	0
Lee–White clotting time	4	4	4	3.5	3.5	3.5
Overall average	3.6	3.5	3.1	2.2	2	1.8

[a] For each test the statistically highest hemostatic agent or group of agent was given 4 points, the second highest 3, etc. In the event that groups overlapped, as was the case for Avitene being statistically no different from Actifoam or Gelfoam for platelet aggregation, the agent was ranked between the other two.

[b] NA, not applicable; the test was not utilized in determining the overall average score.

seen, a collagen sponge has the highest ranking as a hemostatic agent according to this evaluation study.

1.3.1.3. Adhesion Prevention Materials

It is well known that a defective tissue often adheres to the surrounding tissue after surgical operation, causing trouble, especially in gynecology and in abdominal and cardiovascular surgery. A viscous solution of hyaluronate is often coated on the tissue to be protected, but is not always effective in preventing tissue adhesion because of rapid elimination (Benedetti *et al.*, 1993; Campoccia *et al.*, 1996). As alternatives, sheets of oxidized cellulose and derivatized hyaluronate have been applied to the damaged tissues, but tend to move from the proper site earlier than required.

The human amniotic membrane was also studied in an attempt to prevent tissue adhesion after cross-linking, but results of animal experiments were not so promising as to encourage its clinical application (Arora *et al.*, 1994).

1.3.2. Replacement of Diseased Tissues

In contrast to the biological materials regenerated from natural tissues, a variety of natural tissues themselves have been used to replace diseased tissues. Table 1.3 gives the representative biological tissues being used clinically for tissue replacements. Especially, biological heart valves and freeze-dried skins are widely used among the biological tissues listed in Table 1.3.

Also, for small-caliber blood vessels of about 4-mm diameter, substitutes made from natural tissues show higher patency rates than synthetic

Table 1.3. Natural Tissues Being Used as Biomaterials

Animal	Tissues	Application
Human	Demineralized bone	Bone substitutes
	Umbilical cord	Artery substitutes
	Amnion	Adhesion prevention
	Dura mater	Dura mater substitutes
Porcine	Heart valve	Heart valve substitutes
	Arteries	Artery substitutes
	Freeze-dried skin	Skin regeneration
Bovine	Pericardium	Heart valve substitutes, Staple line reinforcement
Goat	Intestine sera	Suture

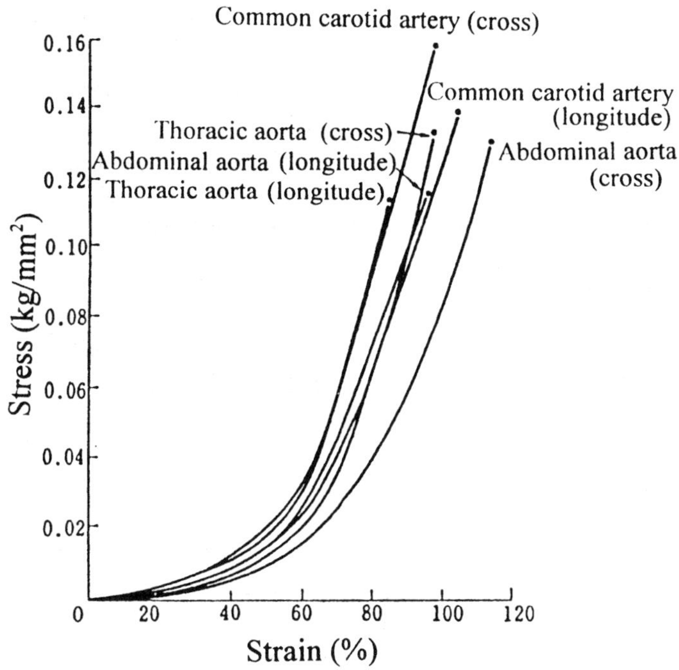

Figure 1.11. Stress–strain curves of human arteries.

ones. Four chemically processed biological tissues used as infrarenal arterial substitutes in dogs were evaluated in terms of patency rates, healing characteristics, and biostability by Marois *et al.* (1989). It should be pointed out that natural arteries exhibit unique stress–strain curves, as demonstrated in Figure 1.11, which are quite different from those of synthetic elastomers.

The use of human dura mater obtained from volunteers in neurosurgery was discontinued due to a WHO recommendation which issued a warning about a risk of prion contamination. As an alternative, neurosurgeons are currently using polytetrafluoroethylene membranes, which remain, however, permanently in the body. To avoid the foreign-body reaction eventually induced by this synthetic membrane, we have developed a bioabsorbable, synthetic membrane which meets most of the requirements as a dura mater substitute (Yamada *et al.*, 1997). The fabrication procedure of this new membrane is depicted schematically in Figure 1.12.

An attempt was made to replace a tendon tissue by regenerated collagen, as shown in Figure 1.13, but the regenerated collagen fiber was not

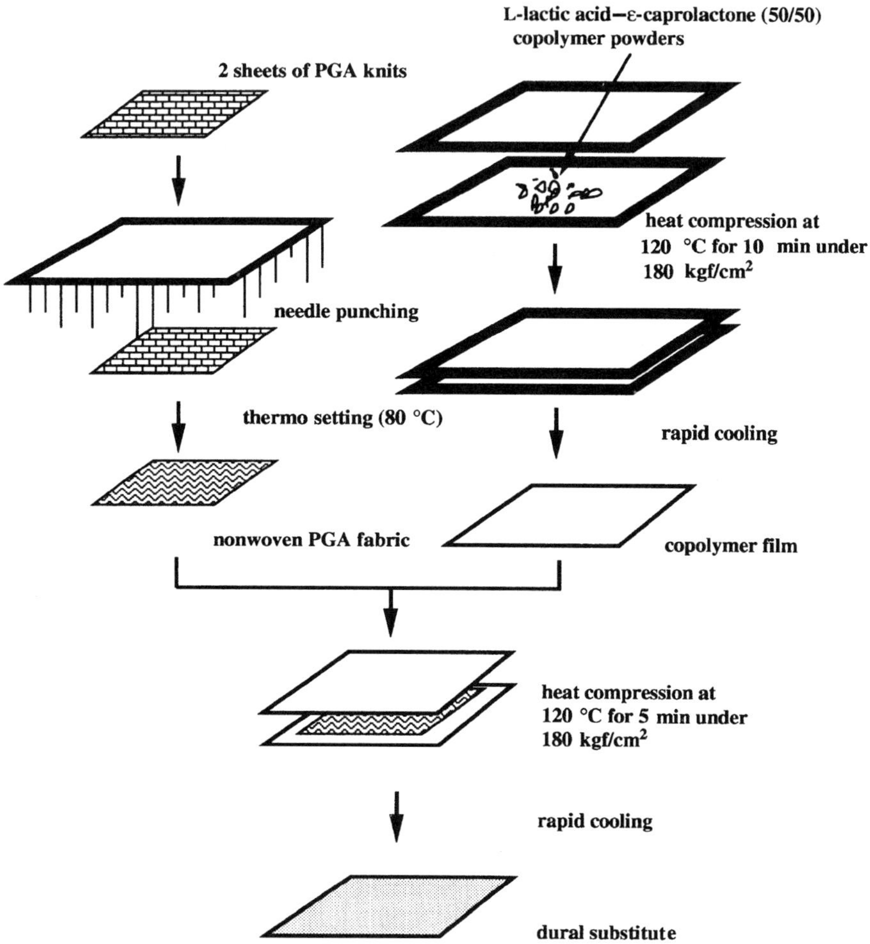

Figure 1.12. Fabrication of the composite sheet made of an L-lactic acid–ε-caprolactone (50% L-lactic acid, 50% ε-caprolactone) copolymer and poly(glycolide) (PGA).

as strong as the natural tendon (Kato *et al.*, 1991). In general, native connective tissues have highly oriented textures of triple-helical collagen fibers, which account for the superior mechanical properties of biological tissues. Figure 1.14 shows three examples of collagen orientation in soft connective tissues (Prizek *et al.*, 1989).

Regenerated chitin and collagen molecules have been used clinically as skin wound covers, after being fabricated into a sponge or nonwoven fabric form, since skin application does not require high-strength materials.

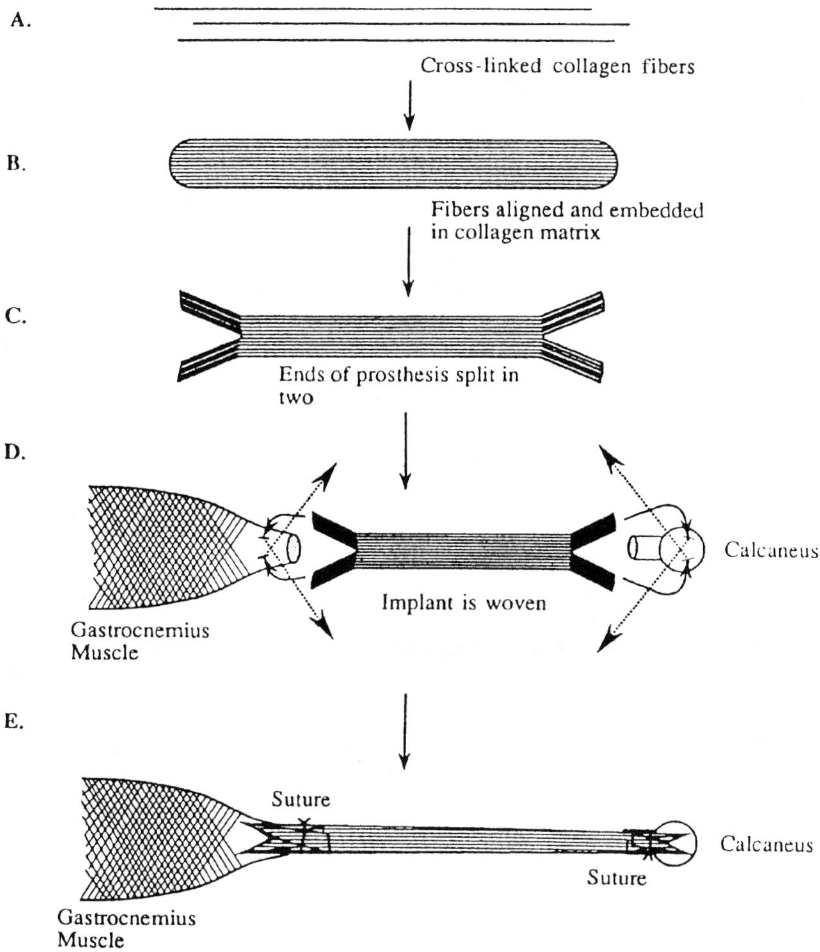

Figure 1.13. Schematic diagram illustrating the experimental steps that were used in preparing reconstituted collagen-fiber prostheses and in subsequent implantation. Cross-linked collagen fibers (A) are aligned and embedded in a non-cross-linked collagen matrix (B). After air-drying, the ends are split (C). They are woven with sutures into the gastrocnemius muscle at one end and are wrapped around the calcaneus at the other end (D and E).

1.3.3. Drug Delivery Systems (DDS)

In some DDS, drug carriers made of polymers are needed for controlled release of drugs. In addition to synthetic polymers, biological materials have been explored extensively as candidates for drug carriers in the water-soluble or water-insoluble state. They include collagen, gelatin, serum

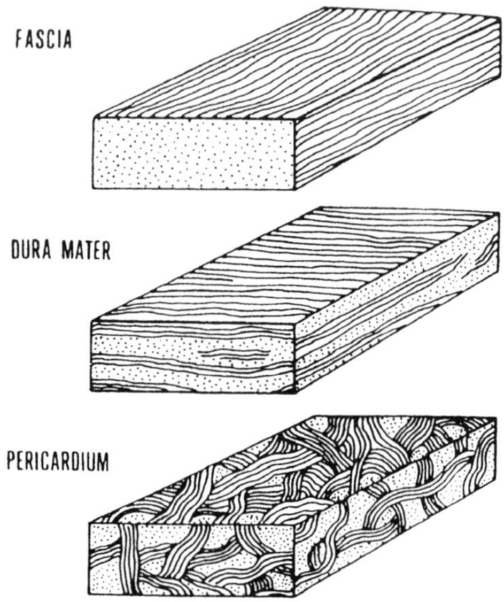

Figure 1.14. Diagram showing the basic organization of collagen fibers in natural tissues. The collagen fibers run parallel in the fascia (upper), form laminae with crossing layers in the dura mater (center), and have a felt-like orientation in the pericardium (lower).

albumin, fibrin, starch, cellulose derivatives, dextran, pullulan, hydroxyapatite, and calcium carbonate. Although drug carriers do not require high mechanical strength, appropriate absorbability is necessary. Most biological materials satisfy this requirement. Gelatin is the most important material for soft and hard capsulation of drugs for oral administration, while acidic cellulose derivatives are used for enteric coating of drugs.

1.3.4. Tissue Engineering

Tissue engineering is an emerging, interdisciplinary field in biomedical engineering and aims at regenerating new biological tissues for replacing diseased or devastated tissues using cells (Patrick *et al.*, 1998). Another important objective of tissue engineering is to substitute damaged tissues and organs with biological tissues and organs newly constructed using cells. Formation of new biological tissues by tissue engineering can be achieved both *in vitro* and *in vivo*, as illustrated schematically in Figure 1.15. It is seen that an artificial extracellular matrix is generally required for tissue regeneration by tissue engineering, because cell proliferation and differentiation, resulting in tissue regeneration, would be difficult unless such a matrix

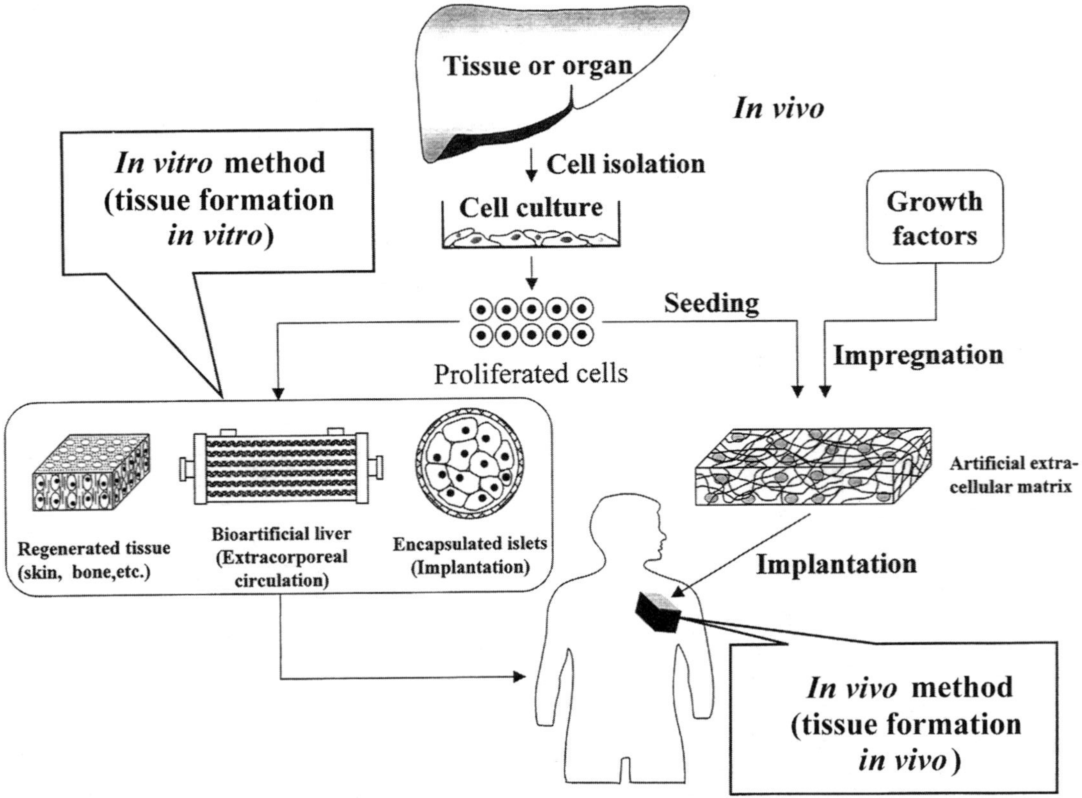

Figure 1.15. Schematic representation of the current tissue engineering.

that functions as a cell scaffold is provided. Since this artificial extracellular matrix should disappear through absorption into the body when a new tissue is regenerated, materials for the matrix should be prepared from biodegradable polymers. This requirement as well as adequate cell adhesion onto the matrix surface make biological materials attractive in tissue engineering. In fact, collagenous, porous materials have been widely used for scaffolding of cells (Atala and Mooney, 1997).

If a biological tissue is to be constructed from allo- or xenogeneic cells, the newly constructed tissue should be immunologically protected from the host self-defensing system because the constructed tissue is used in direct contact with the blood or tissues of patients. An effective method for this immunological protection is to separate the heterogeneous cells from the host immune system using a membrane. This material has to supply oxygen and nutrients to the cells but prevent the attack of immunological proteins of the host against the heterogeneous cells. This membrane is termed "immunoisolation membrane" and is currently prepared mostly from biological materials such as agarose and a combination of alginate with poly(L-lysin).

1.4. Conclusions

Governmental regulations of biomaterials intended to be used clinically have become increasingly strict in recent years. Even if biological materials are of natural origin, they are not always biosafe and biocompatible. The major reason for this is a possibility of antigenicity and viral (or prion) infection. If biological materials are entirely free of this risk, they will find more medical applications because biological response to these natural materials has been studied in more detail than that to synthetic ones. As mentioned above, the unique mechanical properties of biological tissues that differ from those of synthetic materials are also one reason for the advantage of biological over synthetic materials.

References

Arora, M., Jaroudi, K.A., Hamilton, C.J., Dayel, F. (1994). *Eur. J. Obstet. Gynecol. Reprod. Biol.* **55**, 179.

Atala, A., Mooney, D.J. (eds.). 1997. *Synthetic Biodegradable Polymer Scaffolds*, Birkhäuser, Boston.

Benedetti, L., Cortivo, R., Berti, T., Berti, A., Pea, F., Mazzo, M., Moras, M., Abatangelo, G. 1993. *Biomaterials* **14**, 1154.

Campoccia, D., Hunt, J.A., Doherty, P.J., Zhong, S.P., O'Regan, M., Benedetti, L., Williams, D.F. 1996. *Biomaterials* **17**, 963.

Chu, C.C., von Fraunhofer, A. J., Greisler, H. (eds.), 1997. *Wound Closure Biomaterials and Devices*, CRC Press, Florida.

Ghezzo, E., Benedetti, L., Rochira, M., Biviano, F., Callegaro, L. 1992. *Int. J. Pharmacol.* **87**, 21.

Ikada, Y. 1996. In: *Polysaccharides in Medicinal Applications* (S. Dumitriu, ed.), p. 663, Marcel Dekker, New York.

Iwata, H. 1996. In: *Polysaccharides in Medicinal Applications* (S. Dumitiu, ed.), p. 603, Marcel Dekker, New York.

Kato, Y.P., Dumn, M.G., Zawadsky, J.P., Tria, A.J., Silver, F.H., 1991. *J. Bone J. Surg.* **73A**, 561.

Marois, Y., Boyer, D., Guidoin, R., Donville, Y., Marois, M., Teijeira, F.-J., Roy, P.-E. 1989. *R. Biomaterials* **10**, 369.

Okashima, Y., Nishino, K., Okuda, R., Minami, A., Kifune, K. 1991. *Eur. J. Plast. Surg.* **14**, 207.

Olson, R.A.J., Roberts, D.L., Osbon, D.B. 1982. *Oral Surg.* **53**, 441.

Patrick, C.W., Mikos, A.G., McIntire, L.V. (eds.), 1998. *Frontiers in Tissue Engineering*, Pergamon, Oxford.

Prizek, J., Mericka, P., Spacek, J., Nemecek, S., Elias, P., Sercl, M. 1989. *J. Neurosurg.* **70**, 905.

Proceedings of the Second Asia Pacific Symposium: *Chitin and Chitosan*, 21–23 November 1996. Bangkok, Thailand.

Sierra, D., Saltz, R. (Eds.), 1996. *Surgical Adhesives and Sealants*, Technomic Publ., Pennsylvania.

Tomihata, K., Ikada, Y. 1997a. *J. Biomed. Mater. Res.* **37**, 243.

Tomihata, K., Ikada, Y. 1997b. *Biomaterials* **18**, 567.

Tomihata, K., Burczak, K., Shiraki, K., Ikada, Y. 1994. *Polymers of Biological and Biomedical Significance*, ACS Symp. Ser. 540.

Tomihata, K., Fujisato, T., Tomihata, K., Tabata, Y., Iwamoto, Y., Burczak, K., Ikada, Y., 1999. *J. Biomater. Sci. Polymer Edn.* **11**, 1171.

Wagner, W.R., Pachence, J.M., Ristich, J., Johnson, P.C. 1996. *J. Surg. Res.* **66**, 100.

Yamada, K., Miyamoto, S., Nagata, I., Kikuchi, H., Ikada, Y., Iwata, H., Yamamoto, K. 1997. *J. Neurosurg.* **86**, 1012.

2

Structure and Properties of Polymeric Materials

Walter Marconi and Antonella Piozzi

2.1. Introduction

A biomaterial can be defined as a substance (with the exception of drugs), or a combination of substances (both synthetic and natural), employed for the treatment, improvement, or substitution of organism tissues, organs, or function. Since interaction with the biological system is involved, biocompatibility implies the capability of the material to exhibit in the host the appropriate functional and "biomimetic" qualifications. In recent years, interest in biomedical applications of natural and synthetic polymers has grown steadily, with a substantial contribution to the quality and duration of human life.

Their applications are very numerous and can be of either intracorporeal or extracorporeal type. Intracorporeal applications include short-term devices (like sutures and adhesives) or long-term cardiac valves, artificial tendons, contact lenses, etc. Also, complex systems aimed at substituting the function of a corporeal organ (like an artificial kidney, or heart, or pancreas) must be included in this class. Among extracorporeal applications, the most important are catheters, filters for hemodialysis, extracorporeal oxygenators, and detoxification circuits.

Recent achievements obtained through intensive and interdisciplinary research on biomaterials have made it possible to obtain polymers intrinsically provided with fairly good hemocompatibility, further improved by grafting on their surface biologically active molecules. Biocompatibility is the essential requisite for the employment of a material in the biomedical

---

Walter Marconi and Antonella Piozzi • Department of Chemistry, University of Rome "La Sapienza," P.le Aldo Moro 5, 00185, Rome, Italy.

Integrated Biomaterials Science, edited by R. Barbucci. Kluwer Academic/Plenum Publishers, New York, 2002.

field, is strictly related to the specific application and location of the biomedical device, and can be defined as its substantial inertia with respect to the surrounding physiological environment. Since at the present time no absolutely inert material exists, it is probably more correct to define it as "biotolerability." For this reason research is now oriented not only toward the invention of new intrinsically biocompatible materials, but also to find suitable surface modifications able to realize specific interactions with the mechanisms of the biological reaction.

In general, any foreign material in contact with body tissues or fluids generates thereby a specific reaction. The type and level of this reaction will depend on the particular body organ where this reaction originates and will consist of a complex and integrated defensive system. In particular, a reaction of inflammatory type can occur, involving the progressive intervention of macrophages and leukocytes and subsequent secretion of mucopolysaccharides and procollagen, which will finally give rise to a fibrous tissue coating the foreign body. A further reaction can be of immune type, due to the antigenic activity exerted by the material or by its release products. Other adverse reactions can be the activation of the complement system and the creation of carcinogenesis or mutagenesis phenomena.

In order to minimize or inhibit these negative responses, the ideal biomaterial must further possess the following special properties:

- constant surface properties under operational conditions, in order to avoid phenomena of adsorption and modification of proteins or modification of the composition of the biological fluids;
- constancy of the bulk properties, in order to maintain the functional properties of the device, and to avoid the release of potentially toxic substances like monomers, additives, or degradation products;
- good hemocompatibility, i.e., absence of the activation of clotting mechanisms leading to the eventual formation of thrombi.

This latter is the most complex and potentially ominous phenomenon taking place when blood contacts a foreign body, and involves several interconnecting biochemical pathways aimed at protecting the organism from hemorrhagic risks. As a general statement, the long-term success of a prosthetic implant depends on several factors, such as type of material employed; design of the prosthesis; techniques of fabrication, sterilization, and employment; the physiological (and pathological) conditions of the patient. For this reason, in order to attain clinical success in this extremely interdisciplinary field, it is necessary to obtain the collaboration of skilled chemists, polymer technologists, often engineers, surgeons, hematologists, and specialists in the various branches of clinical medicine.

2.2. Polymers

2.2.1. General Properties

A polymer may be defined as a large molecule (*macromolecule*) built up by the repetition of small, simple chemical units (*monomers*). In the case of most existing thermoplastics, there is in fact only one species of unit involved. For example, the polyethylene molecule consists essentially of a long chain of repeating —(CH_2)— groups. In addition to plastic materials, many fibers, surface coatings, and rubbers are also basically high polymers, and in nature too there is an abundance of polymeric materials. Proteins, starch, cellulose, lignin, and rubber are high polymers.

The arrangements of these units, the various types of chains that can be synthesized, and the shapes that these chains can assume, result in a class of materials characterized by a very broad range of properties.

The simplest type of polymer is a linear *homopolymer*, i.e., a chain made up of identical units arranged in a linear sequence. An example of a polymer synthesized in the form of a linear chain is polyethylene (PE), which, however, can be produced also as a branched polymer (by a high pressure process). The term *copolymer* is usually used to describe a polymer derived from two or more monomers, as in the case of ethylene-propylene. The sequence of repeating units along the polymer chain can form different structures, in particular copolymers can be classified as *statistical* copolymers, *alternating* copolymers, and *block* copolymers. For example, if only two types of repeating units (A and B) are present, the sequential distribution of these units in statistical copolymers is random, while in alternating copolymers the repeating units are arranged alternately along the polymer chain and in block copolymers the repeating units only exist in long sequences, or blocks, of the same type. Furthermore, *graft* copolymers are branched polymers in which the branches have a different chemical structure with respect to that of the main chain. Figure 2.1 illustrates some possible ways in which two monomers can combine together in one chain. The properties of statistical and alternating copolymers are generally intermediate to those of the corresponding homopolymers while, to the contrary, block and graft copolymers show properties characteristic of each of the constituent homopolymers.

Differences in the chemical structure between linear and branched macromolecules can affect remarkably the physical and mechanical properties. In fact, linear chains can pack in a three-dimensional lattice to form a crystalline continuous phase, while a highly branched polymer is unable to do this. However, at low degrees of branching, there is a lower degree of crystallinity than that found in a linear polymer, and properties such as

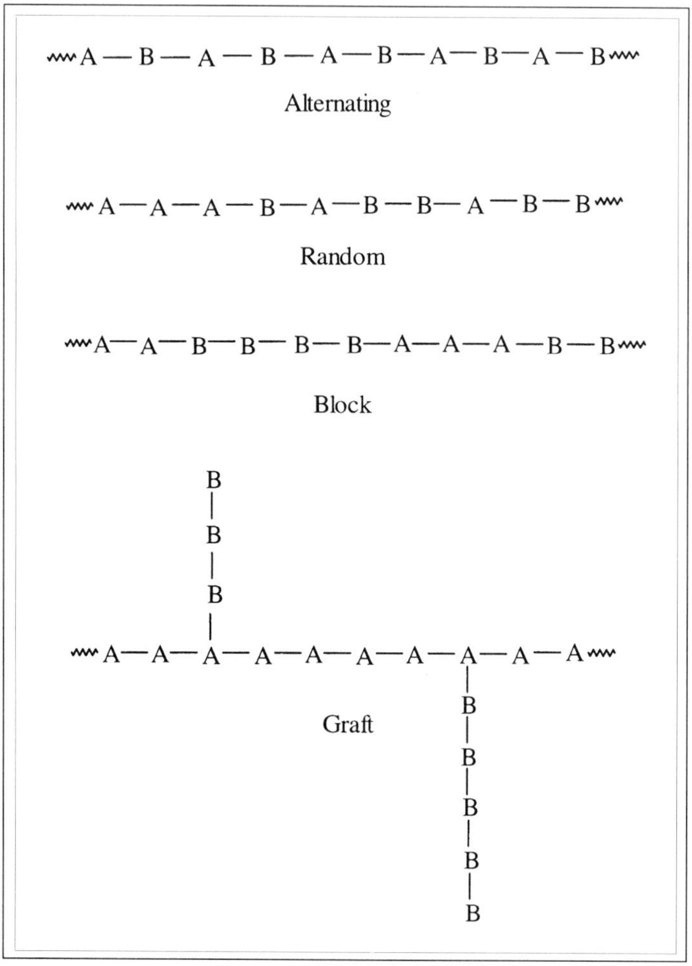

Figure 2.1. Some possible arrangements of two monomers (A, B) in polymer materials.

tensile strength, stiffness, density, clarity, solubility, etc. are deeply affected. Certain types of monomer (trifunctional or tetrafunctional molecules) can polymerize to form a very complex three-dimensional structure known as a *network*. Networks can also be formed by taking linear polymer chains and linking them together chemically. This cross-linking process, typical of elastomeric materials, is called *vulcanization*.

As structural materials, polymers can be classified according to their characteristics of processability and final employment. Plastomers form the most important class and can be divided in two subclasses: thermoplastic and thermosetting materials. The first, whose backbone consists of linear or branched chains, are fusible and can be molded by various techniques (injection, blow or rotational molding, etc.); the second are obtained (directly or in a two-step process) by polyfunctional monomers. Thermosetting polymers possess a three-dimensional structure, i.e., consist of an infinite network that cannot be modified by molding or solubilization procedures after the fabrication of the manufactured article.

2.2.2. Synthesis

There are basically three ways by which polymers may be produced synthetically from simple starting materials. These techniques are referred to as *addition polymerization*, *condensation polymerization*, and *rearrangement polymerization*.

In addition, polymerization (chain reaction) of a low molecular weight molecule which possesses a double bond is induced to break the double bond and join up to other similar molecules (as for polyethylene, polystyrene, polymethyl methacrylate, and many others). The polymerization takes place by opening a carbon–carbon double or triple bond, carbonyl carbon–oxygen double bond, carbon–oxygen epoxy bond, etc. Furthermore, it is possible, by polymerization of conjugated dienes, to generate long-chain molecules with residual double bonds in the chain (polybutadiene, polyisoprene). In all these syntheses the monomer is converted through the stages of initiation, propagation, and termination into the polymer, and no side products are formed. The polymerization must be initiated in fact by a molecule (free radical, cation, anion, or anionic coordinated catalyst) which generates an active site on the monomer. Successively, the chain propagates, i.e., the active site is transferred simultaneously to the newly added monomer. At last, the polymerization terminates due to destruction of the active site. Sometimes, a chain transfer process can occur in which the active site is transferred to another molecule (monomer, solvent, a specially added reagent, etc.). Therefore, this chain reaction process produces high molecular weight polymers with broad molecular weight distribution because of the chain transfer reactions.

Polymerization condensation (stepwise growth) is a synthetic process that generally produces polymers containing heteroatoms in the main chain. For this type of synthesis monomers containing at least two distinct functional groups able to react with each other must be employed. Monomers combine to give dimers; dimers and trimers can also combine to give higher oligomers, and so on. As a result of this stepwise growth process, high molecular weight polymers are only produced as a result of the polymerization.

One example of condensation polymerization is given by the synthesis of nylon 6,6 obtained by reaction of adipic acid and hexamethylenediamine (Figure 2.2). Condensation polymerization differs from addition polymerization in that some small molecules are eliminated during the reaction (in case of the formation of nylon 6,6 the small molecule eliminated is water).

The use of bifunctional monomers gives rise to linear polymers, while multifunctional monomers may be used to form network or thermosetting polymers.

Finally, another process used to synthesize polymers is rearrangement polymerization or *polyaddition*. This process is intermediate between addition and condensation polymerization. In fact, no small molecule is eliminated (as in the former technique) while the kinetics is similar to the latter. An example is the preparation of polyurethanes by reaction of diols with diisocyanate (Figure 2.3).

2.2.3. Molecular Weight

A peculiarity of macromolecular products, strongly affecting their physical properties and mechanical behavior, is the molecular weight, depending on the degree of polymerization, i.e., on the average number of monomer units bonded in the polymer chain. Also important is the molecular weight distribution, i.e., the statistical distribution (broader or narrower) of the molecular weights of the single chains present in the overall polymer mass (Figure 2.4).

All polymerization processes give chains of different length due to either casual or promoted events. Therefore, polymers will consist of macromolecules containing a different number of structural units with different degrees of polymerization and molecular weight. In order to verify these differences, the molecular weight of polymers is expressed by average values. Two of the most commonly used averages are the number-average molecular weight ($\bar{M}_n$) and the weight-average molecular weight ($\bar{M}_w$) defined respectively by

$$\bar{M}_n = \sum \frac{M_i N_i}{N_i} \qquad \text{and} \qquad \bar{M}_w = \sum \frac{N_i M_i^2}{N_i M_i}$$

where N_i is the number of moles of molecule i and M_i is the molecular weight of molecule i. The ratio of the weight-average to the number-average molecular weight is generally used as a measure of the distribution breadth. This ratio is called the polydispersity (P) of the polymer:

$$P = \frac{\bar{M}_w}{\bar{M}_n} \geqslant 1$$

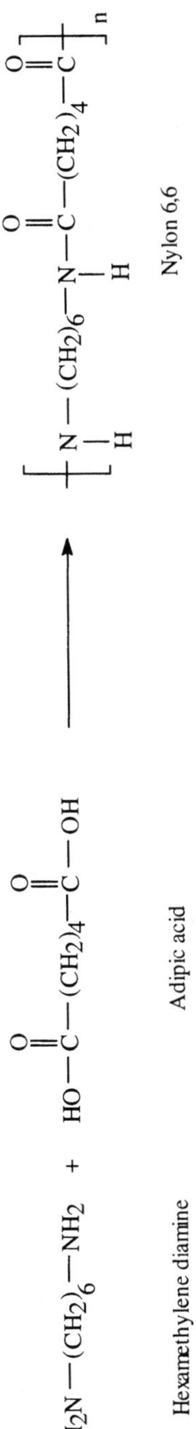

Figure 2.2. Synthesis of nylon 6,6.

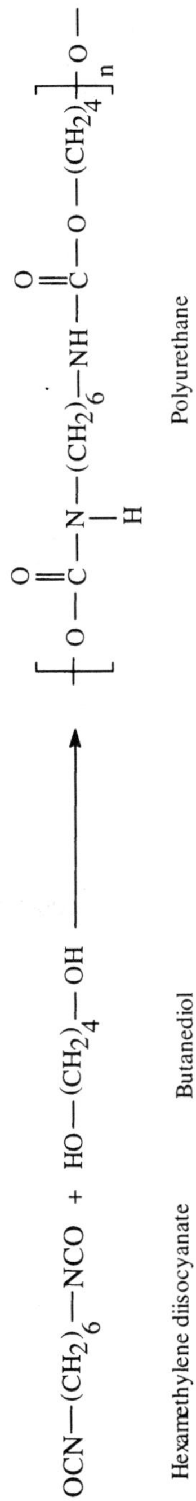

Figure 2.3. Synthesis of a polyurethane.

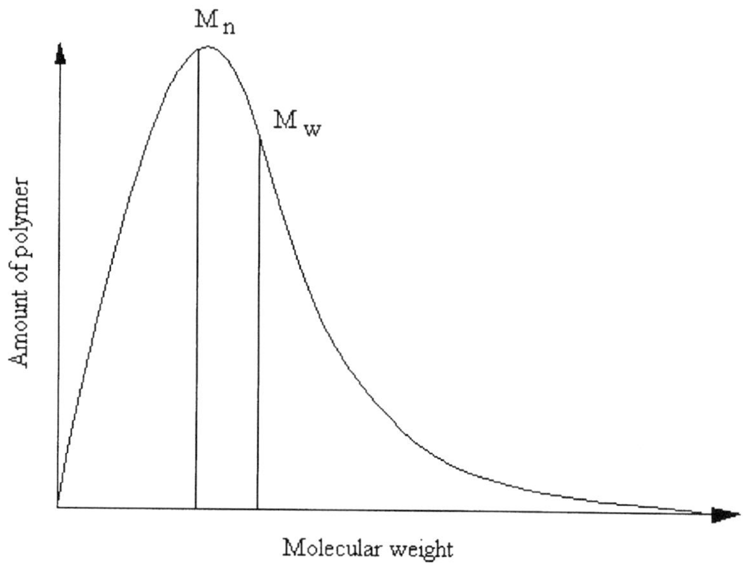

Figure 2.4. Typical molecular weight distribution of a synthetic polymer.

For a homogeneous sample in which the polymer chains all have the same length (a monodispersive sample), $\bar{M}_n = \bar{M}_w$ and the polydispersity is equal to 1. Most commercial polymers have distributions in the order of 5–10. An increase in molecular weight brings about an increase in the physical properties and a decrease in the polymer processability.

2.2.4. Isomerism

If a polymer is synthesized starting from an asymmetric monomer (in particular, a monomer containing an asymmetric carbon atom), we can obtain different types of isomerisms of which the most important are *sequence isomerisms*, *stereoisomerisms*, and *structural isomerisms*.

A monomer unit can add to a growing chain in three different ways: head-to-tail, head-to-head, and tail-to-tail. Generally, most polymers add head-to-tail, while only some polymers have a significant number of head-to-head and tail-to-tail units. This type of structure is called a *sequence isomerism* (Figure 2.5).

Polymerization of a vinyl monomer of general structure $CH_2{=}CXY$, where X and Y are two different substituent groups (in this case the carbon atom is asymmetric), leads to polymers with microstructures that are described in terms of *tacticity* (Figure 2.6). The substituents have two

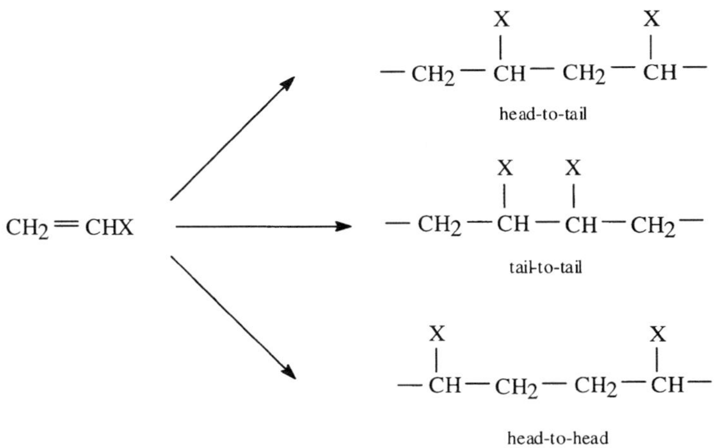

Figure 2.5. Possible sequential additions of monomer to the growing polymer chain.

possible arrangements along the polymer chain: above and below the plane of the sheet (producing two stereoisomers). In case they are on the same side of the extended chain the structure is known as *isotactic*, while if the substituents are on opposite sides of the main chain the structure is called *syndiotactic*. Atactic polymers have random placement of the substituent groups. Since the structures are dissimilar, it is to be expected that the bulk properties of the polymer will differ. The regular syndiotactic and isotactic structures are capable of crystallization, while the atactic polymer is not normally capable of crystallization.

Furthermore, there is the possibility of *cis,trans* isomerism (structural isomerism) that derives from the polymerization of a monomer such as butadiene, isoprene, or other conjugate dienes. For example, the molecule of natural rubber is a 1,4-*cis*-polyisoprene while that of gutta-percha is the *trans* isomer; consequently, the bulk properties of polymers are very different (gutta-percha is no longer a rubber).

2.2.5. Crystallinity

The ability of a material to crystallize is determined by the regularity of its molecular structure. A regular structure is potentially capable of crystallinity while an irregular structure will tend to give amorphous polymers. Generally, the crystallization is limited to linear or slightly branched polymers with high structural regularity.

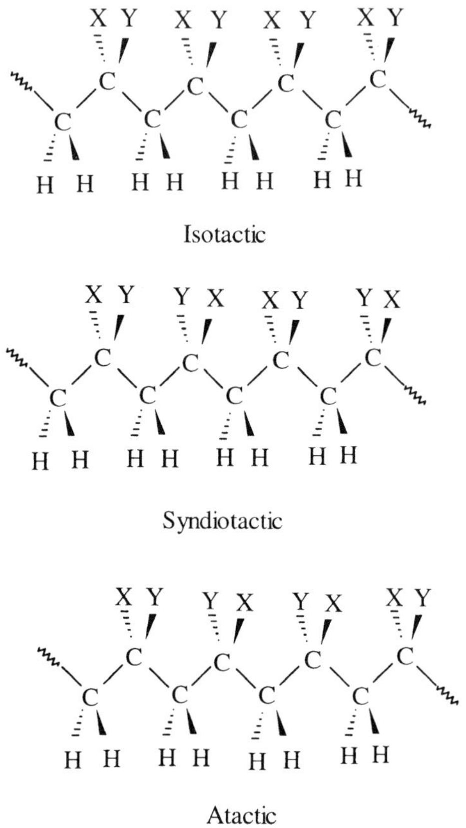

Figure 2.6. Configuration of the various isomeric chains, derived from monomers of the type $CH_2{=}CXY$.

The organizational level of the macromolecules and the conformation induced in material by interactions among atoms or functional groups determine the crystalline or amorphous nature of the polymer. An increase in crystallinity brings about an increase in physical and mechanical properties like tenacity, hardness, and stress resistance. Side groups in the main polymer chain or cross-links joining two or more chains decrease the overall polymer crystallinity, since the structural irregularity so introduced disturbs the packing of the macromolecules into the polymeric lattice. Knowledge of the crystallinity percent of a polymeric material hence enables one to forecast the following functional characteristics:

- how forces distribute in the different parts of the structure,
- the type of structural modifications that occur under the action of both plastic and elastic deformations,
- how breaks could propagate.

An important property of polymers, relevant to their amorphous portion, is the glass transition temperature (T_g), which can be defined as the temperature at which the polymer chains not aligned in a crystalline lattice turn from a stiff, glassy state to a flexible structure. Since all polymers (including crystalline ones) usually contain a not negligible amount of amorphous phase, it is important to determine both the melting temperature T_m (typical of the crystalline phase) and T_g to obtain a good knowledge of the thermal properties of the material and the temperature range for its processability.

2.2.6. Mechanical Properties

In order to understand the mechanical behavior of a polymeric material, it is necessary to consider the type of *strain* that can take place when a *stress* (which, for the sake of simplicity, we suppose to be of the tensile type) is applied (Figure 2.7). The above-mentioned behavior can be of the following types:

- Instantaneous elasticity, i.e., strain involving bond length and angle, with very small shifts. In this case the modulus (which is an index of the material stiffness) is elevated.

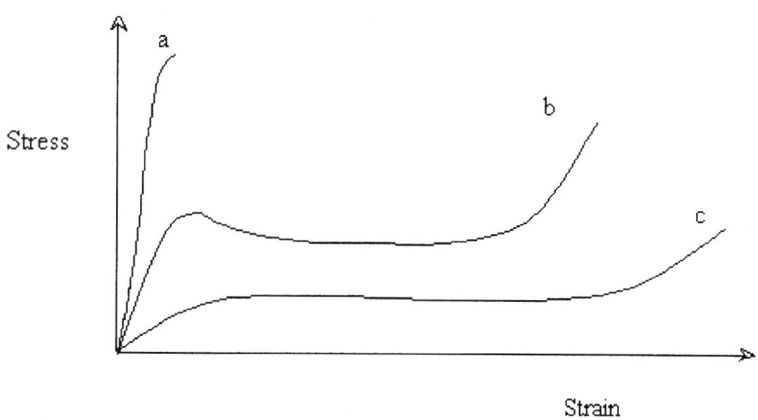

Figure 2.7. Tensile behavior of polymeric material: (a) glassy polymer, (b) semicrystalline polymer, (c) rubber.

- Delayed elasticity: the strain takes place in the same direction as the applied stress, with conformational modifications of the whole macromolecule or of some of its segments. In this case the modulus decreases progressively with time up to a minimum value, when the system reaches the new equilibrium status.
- Shear of the polymer chains over each other: this situation implies overcoming attrition forces due to secondary bonds.

All these mechanisms are always operating while, according to the situation, one of them can prevail. The experimental evaluation of the mechanical behavior of a synthetic polymer or of a natural tissue is made by a series of tests of both static and/or dynamic type.

In static tests, carried out in such a way that stress or strain increases at a constant rate, the following important parameters can be obtained:

- elasticity modulus,
- maximum values of stress and strain,
- yield strength,
- break elongation and breaking load.

In the dynamic-mechanical evaluation, on the contrary, sinusoidal stresses or strains are applied in order to obtain the elastic dynamic modulus and mechanical dissipative factor (also called *internal friction*).

Polymers are, in fact, viscoelastic materials, provided intrinsically with an elastic component whose energy can be recovered and a nonrecoverable dissipative component. One component can prevail over the other according to the temperature and frequency range under consideration.

Finally, mechanical tests of *creep* (at constant stress) or *stress relaxation* (at constant strain) provide information on the chemical, physical, or geometrical stability of the system with time.

2.3. Polymers in Medicine

Biocompatible polymers that are designed (and increasingly employed) for medical purposes present very delicate aspects from the viewpoint of the interaction between biological systems and synthetic materials. Besides polymers for prosthetic insertions (hip, knees, ocular, cardiovascular, etc.) and for extracorporeal purification treatments (hemodyalysis, hemofiltration, plasmapheresis), employed at the present time by millions of patients, also biodegradable and "bioerodible" polymers play an important role in important therapeutical applications, such as the slow release of drugs or their targeting to specific organs.

Systems employing enzymes immobilized in both natural and synthetic polymers can find clinical application both for endocorporeal use and as components of extracorporeal circuits for specific blood detoxifications, a potentially important field of application.

The chemical, physical, and technological properties of biomedical polymers can be very different: from water-soluble or biodegradable ones, like poly(ethyleneglycol) or poly(lactic acid), to rigid polymers, hydrophobic and designed to resist for many years mechanical stress and the hydrolytic action carried out in the human body by chemical or enzymatic agents. Examples of this latter class are the aromatic polyesters, the poly(alkylsiloxanes), fluorinated polymers, and polyurethanes, which are preferably employed for permanent endocorporeal prostheses.

2.3.1. Synthetic Polymers

Synthetic polymers can be employed in various fields of application, as shown in Table 2.1. Polymers which, due to their fairly good intrinsic hemocompatibility properties, have been largely employed in endocorporeal permanent applications of prosthetic type include polyurethanes, silicone rubbers, hydrogels, teflon, and some vinyl polymers or copolymers.

Table 2.1. Application Fields of Synthetic Polymers

Type of polymer	Application fields
Vinyl polymers (Polyethylene LDPE, HDPE, UHMWPE; Polypropylene)	Sutures, ligament protheses, reconstructive surgery, orthopedics
Poly-vinyl-chloride	Tubing in biomedical applications
Vinyl copolymers	Hemodialysis filters
Fluorinated polymers (Teflon)	General surgery, cardiovascular, sutures
Polyamides (Nylon)	Sutures
Polyesters (Polyethylene-terephthalate)	Sutures, cardiovascular
Silicone rubber	Plastic surgery, orthopedics
Hydrogels (Polymethyl-methacrylate, Polyhydroxyethyl-methacrylate, Poly-*N*-vinyl pyrrolidone)	Ophthalmics
Polyurethanes	Blood-contact devices
Polymethyl-methacrylate	Orthopedics, dentistry

Segmented polyurethanes form a class of widely employed materials in the biomedical field to obtain catheters, blood oxygenators, filters, cardiac valves, and internal lining of artificial hearts. Their special molecular structure provides them with good properties like elasticity, abrasion resistance, durability, chemical stability, and easy processability, in a broad range of compositions easy to synthetize. They possess a "biphasic" structure, consisting of alternating "hard" and "soft" segments, possessing very different chemical structure; while the "hard" segments are responsible for the high mechanical resistance, due to their glassy or semicrystalline structure, the elastomeric behavior is due to the "soft" segments. This phase segregation influences markedly their behavior when surfaces of segmented polyurethane contact a biological system, and several studies (Takahara *et al.*, 1991; Silver *et al.*, 1993) have evaluated the effect on hemocompatibility of parameters like hydrophilicity, length, and chemical composition of the soft segment, as well as the surface composition expressed as a ratio between soft and hard portions (i.e., as free surface energy).

Due to its chemical inertia and hydrophobicity (even higher than that of silicones), poly(tetrafluoroethylene) is used for the construction of vascular grafts, consisting of expanded materials having a microporous structure, whose hemocompatibility would seem to originate from the fact that the filling of micropores by water would favor rapid endothelialization of the prosthesis, i.e., coating of the grafts by a layer of endothelial cells from the anastomosis points.

Organosilicon-based polymers have been employed successfully for more than thirty years in biomedical applications due to their outstanding *in vivo* stability, to the ease of producing them in an extremely pure form, to high oxygen permeability, and to the possibility of introducing different physicochemical properties by simple modification of the basic polymer composition (Lumsden *et al.*, 1996).

Also, the so-called "multiphase" polymers have proved to possess an improved hemocompatibility; this technique consists of realizing polymer blends both by simple physical mixing and by coating, or by "block-copolymerization." The following compositions have exhibited good thromboresistance:

- poly(ethyleneterephthalate) (Dacron®) coated with Urethane L325 (DuPont Adiprene®);
- Avocothane 51®, which is an elastomeric copolymer containing 90% poly(etherurethane) and 10% poly(dimethylsiloxane). It combines the good properties of both polymers and is provided with a very good flex life. For this reason it is largely employed in the construction of intra-aortic balloon pumps.

An ethylene–vinyl alcohol copolymer (EVAL), obtainable at different monomer ratios, is used in the commercial production of filters for dialysis. In these copolymers the olefinic backbone provides good mechanical properties while the hydroxy groups, besides increasing the hydrophilicity, can provide sites for the bonding of biologically active molecules (Marconi *et al.*, 1997).

Other applications of polymeric materials in endocorporeal permanent prostheses include: suture filaments (polypropylene of different diameters is now widely used); contact lenses, both hard (polymethyl-methacrylate) and soft (polyhydroxy-ethyl methacrylate); diaphragms by teflon (both inter-atrial and interventricular); components of pacemakers; acrylic cements, employed in dentistry or in orthopedic surgery (for example, in the fixation of hip prostheses into the femoral bone) (Lewis, 1997).

Polyethylene seems to be a promising material for the fabrication of artificial tendons due to its high strength, flexibility, and elastic recovery. This prosthetic application is particularly critical since, in order to achieve long-term successful clinical results, it is necessary to minimize the tissue reaction while simultaneously obtaining sufficient strength through tissue ingrowth. For this reason, sophisticated fabrication techniques of the tendons have been developed (double loop, porous tape fabric mash, porous woven tape). Nylons and aromatic polyesters have also been evaluated for this application (Shieh *et al.*, 1990).

Another important class of synthetic polymers used in medicine are hydrogels, i.e., hydrophilic macromolecular systems able to adsorb high amounts of water and consequently to swell, without dissolving. They are generally obtained by free radical polymerization of monomers of vinyl type, like acrylamide derivatives, *N*-vinyl 2-pyrrolidone, hydroxyalkyl methacrylates, etc. Water insolubility is obtained by cross-linking the polymer with small amounts of a bifunctional monomer (methylene bis-acrylamide, ethylene glycol dimethacrylate derivatives, etc.) added during the polymerization. The peculiar soft and rubbery structure of hydrogels guarantees some advantages, such as minimization of mechanical irritation to surrounding tissues and of interfacial tension with surrounding biological fluids, with consequent decrease in protein adsorption and blood cell adhesion and aggregation. Furthermore, the particular structure of the polymeric network of hydrogels, somehow mimicking that of living tissues, provides them with permeability to low (or even middle) molecular weight metabolites and salts.

Although preparation methodologies, properties, and applications of hydrogels will be treated in detail in another chapter of this book, it is important to specify that, owing to the generally poor mechanical properties of hydrogels, they have usually been regarded in biomedical applications as grafting to mechanically stronger, generally hydrophobic, polymers. An important advantage of this technique is that this hydrogel coating can be easily distributed even onto hard matrices having complex contours.

Although many biomedical applications of hydrogels have been described, few have found widespread clinical use. Ophthalmic hydrogels, largely employed for contact lenses of the "soft" type, are the most important materials of this class utilized in clinical applications. They consist of hydroxyethyl-methacrylate cross-linked by copolymerization with a few percent of bis-methacrylate of a glycol. Different degrees of crosslinking bring about different values of water adsorption at equilibrium (i.e., different degrees of swelling). These hydrogels are fragile and glassy when dry but, after swelling, become soft and flexible, permeable to oxygen and ions and, most important, optically transparent.

2.3.2. Biodegradable and Bioresorbable Polymers

Both natural and synthetic polymers are employed in medicine as biodegradable materials. For example, referring to natural polymers, polyaminoacids are used for drug control release and collagen or gelatin for soft tissue reconstruction.

Among the synthetic polymers, aliphatic polyesters were also employed for controlled release (Cohen *et al.*, 1995), but their most important utilization is as substitutes of metallic parts in the therapy of bone fractures (Yamamuro *et al.*, 1994), since the polymers possess adequate mechanical properties, and their flexibility makes possible bone healing via formation of a callus. Moreover, they are bioresorbable, and this property makes possible, by the newly forming bone, the replacement of degraded polymer particles with progressive transfer of mechanical stress to the bone. By this procedure, there is no requirement for a second surgical procedure that is, however, necessary when temporary implants of metallic type must be removed.

To date, the most suitable polymers are polyesters of aliphatic hydroxy acids, in particular α-hydroxy acids (like lactic or glycolic), but also the high molecular weight poly(β-hydroxy butyric acid), of microbial production (Sang, 1996); to a lesser extent, poly(caprolacton) can be employed. Their degradation rates are very different, ranging from a few weeks for the lactic–glycolic copolymer, to about 6 months for poly(glycolic) acid or for the highly crystalline poly(L-lactic acid). Poly(L-lactic acid) was also utilized as coating of carbon fibers employed as artificial tendons and ligaments; the polymer coating reduces drastically the flammatory reaction that would take place in case of migration of the carbon fibers in the surrounding tissues (Aragona *et al.*, 1981).

Besides intrinsic polymer properties like molecular weight, steric configuration, and crystallinity, other factors can influence the mechanical and biological behavior of poly(hydroxy acids), such as the presence of oligomers or monomer residues, and modifications introduced during the manufacture of prosthetic devices, thermal post-treatments, and sterilization. In particular, these latter treatments may be responsible for formation of oligomers due to degradation induced by heat or radiation.

An increasingly important application of biodegradable polymers is the controlled release of therapeutic agents like drugs or enzymes, i.e., the employment of these polymers in the fabrication of devices contacting various parts of the human body, and able to guarantee the release of the therapeutically active agent for a long period of time and at constant rate. For any drug entrapped in a polymeric matrix, it is fundamental to consider its partition coefficient between the matrix and the biological environment in which it must diffuse. The slow release of drugs can find interesting application both for intensive short-term therapy (as in the case of an intensive antibiotic therapy of infected wounds), and for long-term therapy. This latter is probably the most interesting field of application, and favorable results were obtained particularly in two clinical situations: (a) when it is necessary (as in the case of cytostatic agents) to obtain a high local concentration of a highly toxic drug; (b) when it is necessary to maintain for a long period of time a constant systemic concentration of a hormone (insulin, contraceptives, thyroid or growth hormone).

Polymers employed for this type of application belong mainly to three classes:

1. Water-soluble polymers, which are transformed into low molecular weight products through cleavage of chemical bonds in the main chain.
2. Water-soluble polymers made insoluble by cross-links that are, however, hydrolytically instable, and so undergo, under physiological conditions, more or less slow hydrolysis.
3. Hydrogels. These polymers, due to their capability of swelling to a high degree in water, are highly permeable to water-soluble drugs.

The administration forms of these drug–polymer conjugates are very different, and include implantable small cylinders or spheres, powder formulations, injectable microcapsules or multilayer films or capsules contacting skin or mucosa.

2.3.3. Polymers for Extracorporeal Enzymatic Detoxification

The use of immobilized enzymes or specific organ cells in extracorporeal circulation circuits is a novel and increasingly important tool for the elimination from blood of toxic or potentially dangerous metabolites

(Pozniak *et al.*, 1995; Ohshima *et al.*, 1997). Enzymes have unique selectivity and generally elevated catalytic activity, but usually cannot be administered orally without undergoing denaturation by the hydrochloric acid of stomach (followed by proteolitic digestion). If a protective coating is used (such as a polymeric capsule), then they are unable to pass through the intestinal barrier. Moreover, enzymes of human origin are often difficult to obtain and more expensive than the corresponding microbiological enzymes; these latter ones, however, when in contact with blood (as is necessary for their biomedical application), can activate the host immune system, with production of antibodies that deactivate them, and with generation of other reactions, even ominous as anaphylactic shock.

These drawbacks can be avoided by immobilizing the enzymes outside the human organism, as components of an extracorporeal circuit. Blood contacting immobilized enzymes cannot initiate immunoreactions, since macrophages cannot in this case incorporate the foreign protein by phagocytosis. Furthermore, modern immobilization techniques make it possible to obtain stable enzymatic preparations provided with good catalytic activity.

This technique, however, can be applied only to substrates dissolved in extracellular body fluids, mainly blood, and cannot replace the function of intracellular enzymes nor be used to transform intracellular substrates. In order to minimize (or hopefully avoid) the administration of anticlotting drugs, it is also necessary that the surfaces contacting the blood pumped into the extracorporeal circuit be provided with sufficiently good hemocompatibility.

The enzyme immobilization can be carried out by different systems:

- physical entrapment into gels, hollow fibers, or hollow microspheres of polymeric permeable materials (so-called artificial cells);
- chemical bonds between the enzyme and a polymer matrix.

This latter procedure is generally preferred, due to the higher stability of covalent bonds and consequent lower probability of enzyme leakage. All these enzymatic preparations (fibers, films, spheres, etc.) are then packed in a reactor, in a way able to guarantee, for a long utilization time, good flow conditions and elevated surface area.

Many polymers, both natural and synthetic, can be employed as matrices for enzyme immobilization. Synthetic polymers like poly(urethanes), poly(amides), and poly(esters) are generally preferred, due to their good mechanical properties and chemical stability under working conditions, and to the ease of obtaining from them the above-mentioned physical forms (films, fibers, etc.).

When polyamides or polyesters are used, they must previously be submitted to hydrolysis in order to generate in the macromolecule the functional groups (generally carboxy or amino) necessary for binding the

Table 2.2. Extracorporeal Enzymatic Reactors

Type of enzyme	Immobilization technique	Catalyzed reaction	Therapeutical application
Urease	Chemical bond to collagen membranes	Urea decomposition to NH_3 and CO_2	Renal failure
Asparaginase	Chemical bond to polymethacrylates and to cellulosic hollow fibers	Decomposition of asparagine to aspartic acid and NH_3	Malignant tumors
Phenylalanine ammonia liase	Hollow fibers	Deamination of phenylalanine and tyrosine to cynnamic or coumaric acid, respectively	Phenylketonuria Liver coma Malignant tumors
Carbonic anhydrase	Chemical bond to "silastic" membranes	Decomposition of HCO_3^- to CO_2 and H_2O	Membrane oxygenators
Heparinase	Covalent bond to sepharose	Heparin degradation to inert polysaccharides	Extracorporeal circuits requiring anticoagulant treatment
Bilirubin oxidase	Chemical bond to agarose or sepharose	Oxidation of bilirubin to biliverdin	Treatment of newborn jaundice
Enzymes from liver microsomes	Chemical bond to agarose or sepharose microspheres	Toxin elimination	Liver failure

enzyme by suitable bifunctional reagents. Table 2.2 lists the most important therapeutical applications of extracorporeal enzyme reactors for different types of disease or genetic failure. Enzymes were immobilized within or onto the polymer matrix, either through chemical bonds or by physical entrapment.

2.4. Requirements and Evaluation of Polymeric Materials

2.4.1. Bulk and Surface Properties

The possibility of clinical utilization of a polymeric material destined to be in intimate and continuous contact with organism tissues, or to vicariate delicate functions of the human body, depends on particular requisites, in particular biocompatibility, chemical and thermal stability, and suitable mechanical properties, which determine not only the functional properties of the device, but also the technologies that can be employed for its fabrication. Generally, the intimate structure of the material influences its bulk and surface physicochemical properties, affecting, in their turn, the interaction between the material and biological system.

Sometimes, we require polymeric materials to provide the structural support function usually exerted by bone tissue and collagen, while for different applications (such as for artificial skin or for slow release of hormones or drugs) strongly hydrophilic materials able to retain large amounts of water need to be available. Moreover, while for some applications the polymer will have to be absolutely stable versus degradation, for others easy biodegradation will be required, in order to make it possible that, after having performed its duties, it be adsorbed or eliminated by a metabolic pathway.

The special properties of polymeric materials are due to their macromolecular nature, i.e., to the fact that their main chain consists of a great number of monomer units bonded to each other by covalent bonds, and that intermolecular bonds occur between polymer chains. These latter ones can be of different types: covalent bonds (and in this case, as we discuss later, the polymer can become completely insoluble and infusible), or polar, generally weak bonds, but sometimes strong, such as when strong ionic bonds are involved. This anisotropy of properties at a molecular level often brings about anisotropy of physical and mechanical properties of the manufactured article.

Any chemical reaction or physical treatment involving a modification of the molecular weight or of the chemical structure of the polymer can irreversibly modify its properties, and even make it no longer suitable for its original application.

In order to avoid possible undesirable structural modifications due to severe processing conditions, aging, or sterilization procedures, stabilizers able to inhibit or slacken the degradation process, as well as processing aids are added. These low molecular weight products, however, can later migrate from the polymer bulk to its surface, and affect by their presence the interaction of the biomaterial with the biological system.

It is also important to know the molecular weight of a polymer, because an increase in the molecular weight as well as a narrow distribution of molecular masses bring about an improvement in some properties of the material, like stiffness and resistance to strain, to abrasion, to chemical agents, and to thermal degradation, and a decrease in solubility and adhesion properties.

For example, one of the most important orthopedic applications of polymers is the hip prosthesis, where it is mandatory to minimize wear between the contacting surfaces of the femoral head and acetabulum cap. It is also necessary to guarantee satisfactory mechanical resistance to the whole system, subjected to high flexural and torsional stresses. This can now be obtained by employing ultrahigh molecular weight poly(ethylene) (UHMWPE) (Wang *et al.*, 1995).

For these reasons, the determination of both molecular weight and its distribution curve is considered important for the characterization of a polymeric biomaterial, since it is also possible to obtain by these methodologies information about the possible presence of low molecular weight polymer chains (oligomers) that can influence negatively the mechanical properties or the interaction between the polymer surface and biological system. These oligomers can form directly in the polymerization step or by thermal or photooxidative degradation occurring in the processing step.

Generally, inter- and intramolecular forces due to the presence in the polymer chain of particular atoms or functional groups can influence the structure of the material and consequently its properties, such as stiffness, which increases if electrostatic, ionic, or dipolar interactions can take place. For instance, the tenacity of polyamides (nylons) employed for the production of suture monofilaments is due to the formation of electrostatic interactions (hydrogen bonds) between hydrogen atoms and oxygen atoms belonging to carboxy groups of the polyamide chains.

Another example is given by the extensive and diversified biomedical use of segmented polyurethanes, due to the particular physicomechanical properties related to their molecular structure. They can be classified as thermoplastic elastomers, i.e., as materials able to undergo remarkable deformation under relatively small stress, and quickly recover the original shape and dimensions when the stress is removed. Moreover, they are characterized by a biphasic structure consisting of a sequence of segments, defined as "soft" and "hard," whose chemical nature differs much (Figure 2.8). The interactions that can take place between these two phases provide these materials with mechanical resistance, flexibility, and elasticity, which are extremely important requisites conditioning their choice for specific biomedical application. In the realization of vascular prostheses, for instance, optimal resistance to various pressure regimens, elasticity sufficient to permit normal circulation dynamics, and the flexibility required by anatomic situations must be guaranteed.

In fact, detailed knowledge of the forces involved and of the mechanical behavior of the material employed is necessary for designing and fabricating prosthetic devices.

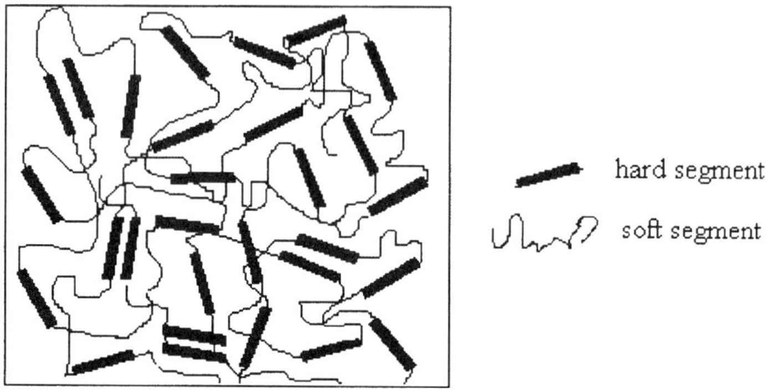

Figure 2.8. Biphasic structure of segmented polyurethanes consisting of a sequence of "soft" and "hard" segments.

As we have seen, it is necessary to evaluate, for any specific application of biomaterials, their response to mechanical stress. It is also necessary, however, to foresee the possible modifications induced over a long period of time by an "aggressive" environment such as the human body. The experimental evaluation of the mechanical behavior of an artificial device (or also of a natural tissue) takes place through a series of mechanical tests of static and dynamic type. The principles involved and the main techniques employed will be described in detail in another chapter of this book.

Since biomedical polymers must be used in the biological environment, mainly consisting of water, both the wettability of the surface and water adsorption by the polymer bulk are very important in order to determine whether a polymer can be employed for a specific application. Water adsorption, indeed, can influence the dimensional stability and mechanical properties of the prosthetic element and, moreover, water by itself can be a powerful degrading agent. So, for example, "soft" polymers like silicones and polyurethanes, containing hydrophobic groups which adsorb low amounts of water, are used for the production of catheters, implants, pipes, etc., while hydrophilic materials like poly(hydroxyethylmethacrylate) (p-HEMA), which adsorb high amounts of water, are largely employed for the fabrication of (soft) contact lenses (LaPorte,1997).

It is evident that a careful characterization of the bulk properties is fundamental for determining the structure–properties correlation. Moreover, since the *in vivo* biological response depends on the interactions taking place at the tissue–material interface, their surface characterization is also very important (particularly for blood in contact with materials).

Some authors (Andrade, 1973) suggested that, referring to biological interactions, the interfacial region can be classified at four levels: (a) the molecular level, extending from 3 to 15 Å from the surface, in which the structure of water, of ions, and of dissolved small molecules play an important role; (b) the macromolecular level, between ten and some hundreds Å from the surface, where interactions with biological macromolecules like proteins and polysaccharides occur; (c) the cellular level, 2–20 μm from the surface, where the reaction of platelets, and even of larger cells, can be observed; (d) events taking place more than 0.1 mm from the surface.

It was hypothesized that the polymer surface probably does not interact directly at all the above-mentioned levels, but it is apparent that some complex and sequential phenomena, like thrombosis, can originate from the polymer surface. In a polymer, the ratio between the relative amount of the crystalline and amorphous region influences the migration and consequent surface distribution of polymer chemical groups or segments.

Furthermore, in order to minimize the free energy at the interface, the polymer surface will orient or rearrange its chemical groups according to the nature of the surrounding microenvironment. In some cases, the free energy of a polymer–water interface is a driving force sufficient to orient dipolar groups toward the water phase, while in systems containing both hydrophilic and hydrophobic groups (such as some block copolymers), the hydrophilic phase will prevail at the interface with water while the hydrophobic one will extend prevailingly toward the polymer bulk or, for very thin films, at the air–polymer interface.

Increasing evidence that the nature of the response of a biological system is conditioned by the surface characteristics stimulated its investigation by many different techniques, due to the necessity of correlating their physicochemical properties with some biological ones like protein adsorption, adhesion of platelets and blood cells, and onset of thrombosis.

The techniques of surface analysis, which will be discussed in detail in another part of this book, can be classified on the basis of the information they provide:

- *Information on chemical composition*

The following spectroscopic techniques, utilizing the interaction between a surface and different radiations or high-energy particles, are employed:

1. Infrared spectroscopy using reflection and refraction of IR beams at the interface of two materials (Fourier Transformed Infrared Spectroscopy-Attenuated Total Reflection, FTIR-ATR), having different refraction index. By this technique information on molecular

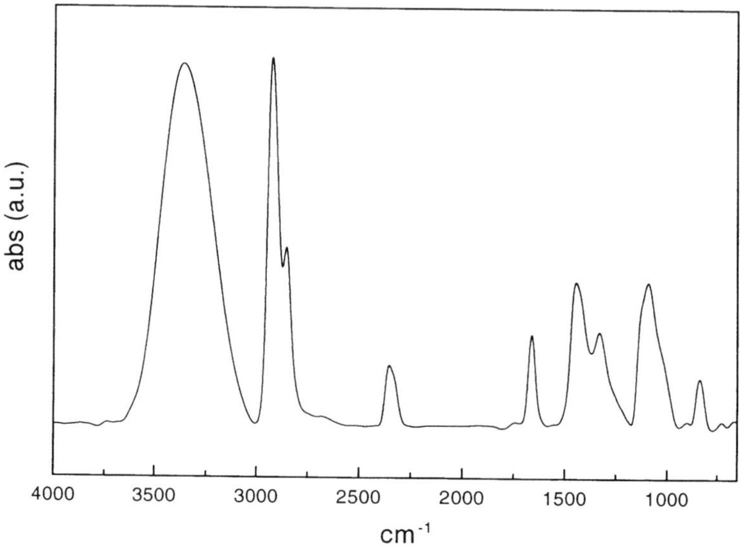

Figure 2.9. FTIR-ATR spectrum of an ethylene–vinyl alcohol copolymer (EVAL 40/60 molar ratio).

structure, crystallinity, and intramolecular interactions can be obtained (Figure 2.9).

2. SEM (Scanning Electron Microscopy). This well-known application of electron microscopy, coupled with energy dispersion spectroscopy (EDS), enables information on the atomic composition of the surface to be obtained.
3. XPS (X-ray Photoelectron Spectroscopy or Electron Spectroscopy for Chemical Analysis, ESCA). This technique, based on kinetic energy measurements of electrons emitted by surfaces irradiated with X-rays, gives information on the surface chemical composition.
4. SIMS (Secondary Ion Mass Spectroscopy). Similar information can be obtained by bombarding a surface with a beam of accelerated ions and analyzing the ionized fragments leaving the surface by a mass spectrometer.

- *Information on surface free energy*

Because of the energy difference between bulk and surface, due to the conformation of the macromolecules induced by the surrounding environment, it is important to determine (by measurements of the contact angle with static and dynamic techniques) the surface free energy and wettability of the material (Marconi *et al.*, 1999) (Figure 2.10).

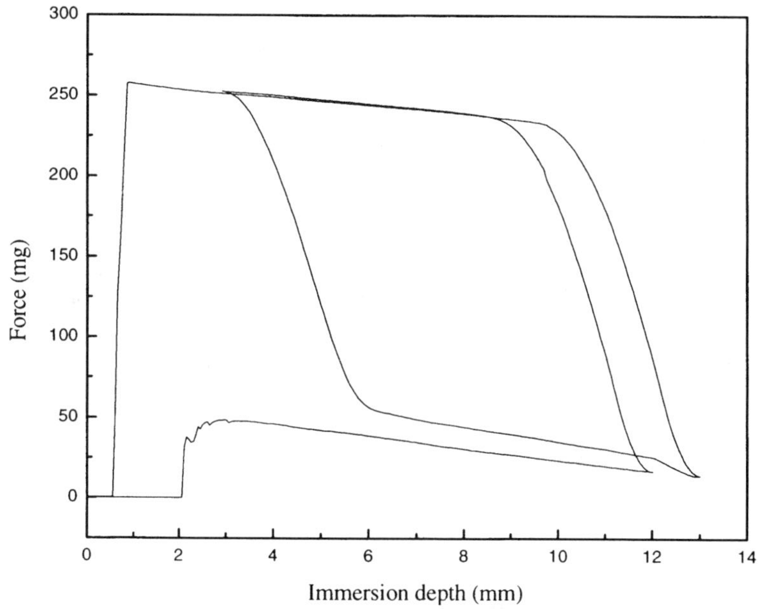

Figure 2.10. Force vs immersion depth (2 cycles) for EVAL employing water as liquid (Marconi, W. *et al.*, 1999. Synthesis and physicochemical evaluation of ethylene–vinyl alcohol–vinyl stearate polymers, *Macromol. Chem. Phys.* **200**, 1191).

• *Information on surface electric potential*

When polymers are used in biomedical applications, it was observed that the electric properties of their interface strongly influence the initial adsorption of the protein layer and of platelets. It was also noted that surfaces possessing an overall negative charge proved to be more thrombo-resistant. Their study is carried out by measuring the electrokinetic potential ("zeta potential") using different techniques (streaming potential, streaming current, electroosmosis, electrophoresis) to provide information on the presence of charges, their distribution, and the influence exerted on them by the pH, ionic force, and previous treatment processes of the material.

• *Information on surface area and porosity*

The hemocompatibility of artificial devices in direct contact with blood, like membranes and vascular or cardiac valvular prostheses, does not depend only on their chemical composition or physical properties, but also on the surface morphology. Indeed, deposition of platelets and of plasma proteins was observed on rough, much more than on smooth, surfaces. The structure of the surface as well as its roughness and porosity can be investigated by electron microscopy techniques (SEM).

It is clear that the development of an optimized biomedical device for long-term blood-contacting application requires the combination of appropriate mechanical properties (like mechanical compliance, shape invariance, flex life, and so on) and a thromboresistant surface. It is for this reason that in many cases modifications aimed at improving hemocompatibility are relevant only to the surface, as in the case of hydrogels, which cannot be used on their own as structural biomaterials because of their poor mechanical properties. However, they can be created, as a thin film, at the surface of sufficiently strong materials, by chemical treatment or graft-polymerization of hydrophilic monomers. Another important hemocompatibility-inducing treatment, discussed in detail later, is the surface bonding of biologically active molecules, able to interfere with some thrombogenesis mechanisms but leaving unmodified the polymer bulk structure and properties.

2.4.2. Chemical Modifications

The need to combine in the same material suitable bulk properties and specific surface requirements has promoted the development of several surface modification techniques, able to alter the biological response of the biomaterial to blood or tissue fluids. One way is chemical modification by surface copolymerization initiated by high-energy radiation, UV rays, chemical promoters, or plasma polymerization. This approach has mainly two different aims:

- to minimize the adsorption of plasma proteins on the material;
- to form a protein layer able to inhibit the platelet adhesion.

Hydrogels can be regarded in this category as an interesting example. Their insufficient mechanical properties, as mentioned above, require, however, that they be covalently grafted onto adequate matrices, such as polyurethanes.

The same category includes polymer surfaces grafted with poly(ethylene-oxide) molecules of different molecular weight (so-called "molecular cilia") designed to freely orient into the aqueous environment (Han *et al.*, 1991). The mobility and flexibility of this kind of hydrophilic chain is reported to be responsible for low protein adsorption and platelet adhesion.

Conversely, much research was oriented toward increasing the surface hydrophobicity by grafting fluorinated or long alkyl chains, which have proved to have high affinity toward albumin whose activity, in terms of inhibition of platelet activity, is well known. In this connection, Munro and co-workers and then Platè (Eberhart *et al.*, 1987; Platè and Matrosovich, 1976) observed that the introduction of alkyl groups onto polymer surfaces involved an increase in their albumin adsorption, and in particular a selective adsorption from blood of albumin, with respect to other proteins. Munro's hypothesis, that an increased concentration of albumin would have brought about a reduction in adhesion and aggregation of platelets, was confirmed by *in vivo* experiments. Also, reduced clot formation and decreased fibrinogen adhesion was noted. Since albumin binds to molecules provided with hydrocarbon chains (generally in the C_6–C_{18} range) due to the existence in its molecule of an apolar region, it was ingeniously envisaged that, by a similar mechanism, long-chain alkyl groups present on modified polymer surfaces would be able to interact with albumin. This bond strength shows a maximum for a C_{18} hydrocarbon chain. Furthermore, in the case of alkyl-functionalized polyurethanes, some influence of the length of the alkyl chain on the initial adsorption rate of albumin was confirmed.

2.4.2.1. Polymer Surfaces Modified by Biospecific Anticoagulants

Better knowledge of thrombogenic mechanisms made it possible to identify key components of biological type involved in its regulation and inhibition, and also to understand how foreign substances can interfere.

These substances presently appear to be of much interest for the realization of active surfaces able, due to their presence, to inhibit clot formation when blood contacts the surface. According to the modality of their action on hemostasis, the biospecific agents employed can be classified as follows:

- inhibitors of the coagulative cascade,
- antiplatelet agents,
- activators of the fibrinolysis,
- inactivators of the complement system.

The same class can also include so-called "biomimetic" surfaces, consisting of polymer materials coated with a lipid double layer able to mimic the membrane properties of endothelial cells; surfaces coated with proteins (like gelatin or collagen) cross-linked by glutaraldehyde; and "endothelialized" surfaces, where a cellular growth aimed at the complete coating of porous or fibrous matrices is induced, to obtain a physiologically hemocompatible interface.

Among substances participating in the fibrin-forming processes, heparin is the most extensively employed and has provided the best results in the

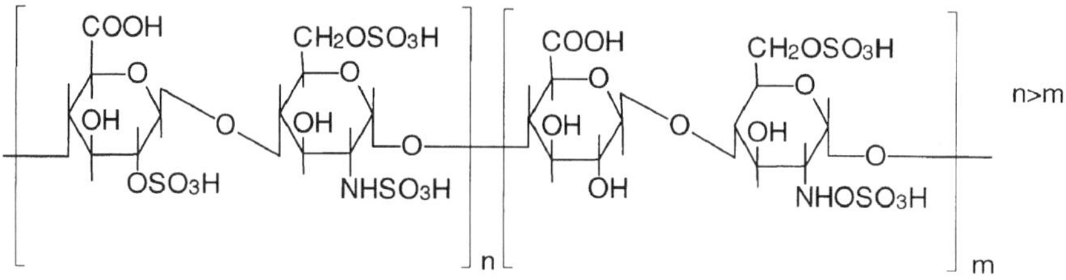

Figure 2.11. Formula of heparin.

realization of nonthrombogenic surfaces. The term *heparin* refers to a heterogeneous mixture of polysaccharides of different molecular weight. It belongs to the class of glycosamino-glycans and is preferentially obtained by extraction of pig intestinal mucous membrane (Figure 2.11).

It can be described as a copolymer alternating 2-amino-2-deoxy-D-glucose and L-iduronic acid units, bonded by an α (1,4) glycosidic bond. Every disaccharide unit contains mainly sulfate and also sulfamic and carboxy groups (besides the unsubstituted hydroxy groups). Heparin is not a pure polysaccharide, since it also contains a protein residue bonded to the polysaccharidic moiety through a serine molecule.

Due to its particular structure, heparin is able to inactivate, by complexing, several proteins of the hemostatic system, like the activated factors IX, X, XI, XII, plasmin and thrombin. The inactivation of thrombin (i.e., the main inhibition step involving the coagulative cascade) is greatly enhanced by the presence of the protein antithrombin III (ATIII), which is a powerful thrombin inhibitor. Two different hypotheses on the action mechanism of heparin stress respectively the previous formation of either of the Hep–ATIII or the Hep–Thrombin complex. In both cases, however, the role of heparin would be to induce a conformational change in the bonded protein (ATIII or thrombin), increasing the affinity toward the other protein, with final formation in both cases of a ternary Hep–ATIII–Thrombin complex. This latter complex would finally decompose, releasing the inactive binary ATIII–Thrombin complex and free Hep, able to exert again its catalytic action of thrombin inactivation.

Particular advantages in the employment of heparin were observed when heparinized prostheses are used in low blood-flow regions where, because of the slow circulation, the fibrin clots could be removed with difficulty. Heparinized surfaces can be classified on the basis of the type of heparin immobilization, which can involve either ionic or covalent bonds, with consequent substantial differences in the duration and mechanism of its activity.

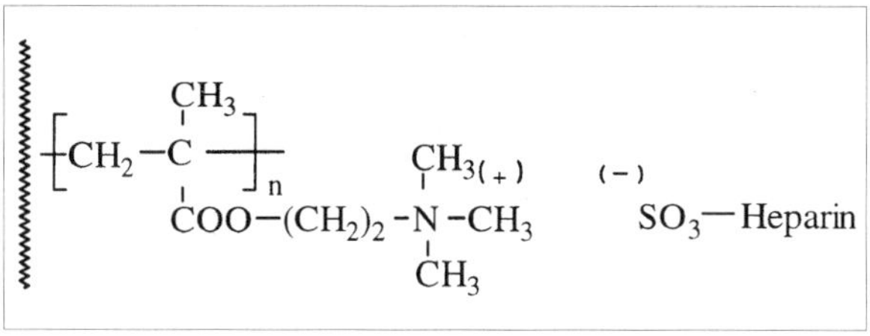

Figure 2.12. Surface grafting of quaternized dimethylaminoethyl methacrylate for the ionic adsorption of heparin.

(*a*) *Ionic Immobilization of Heparin.* Ionically heparinized polymer surfaces release heparin at a rate that depends both on the force of the heparin–matrix bond and on the physicochemical nature of the latter, which influences the phenomena of surface diffusion.

First, polymer matrices containing on their surface covalently bonded groups possessing quaternary ammonium groups have been realized. These groups, such as *N,N*-dimethylaminoethyl or *N,N*-diethylaminoethyl, were introduced by copolymerization with acrylic monomers containing them, or by subsequent chemical modification. The quaternization was further obtained by reaction with alkyl or alkyl-aryl halides (Falb *et al.*, 1975).

Surface polymerization by radiation or photosensitive initiators was also employed for obtaining surfaces able to adsorb ionically heparin, for example by grafting monomers like vinyl-pyridine or dimethylamino-ethyl-methacrylate, followed by quaternization with methyl iodide (Figure 2.12) (Tanzawa *et al.*, 1973).

An ingenious system for the ionic bond of heparin onto suitably quaternized tertiary ammonium groups was realized by the synthesis of poly(amidoamines), obtained from *N,N'*-methyl-diamines (of different molecular weight) and 1,4-bis-acryloyl-piperazine (Figure 2.13) (Ferruti and Provenzale, 1976).

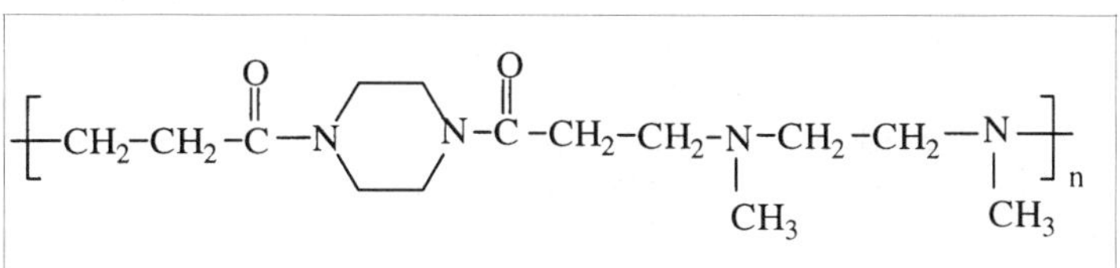

Figure 2.13. Formula of poly(amidoamine).

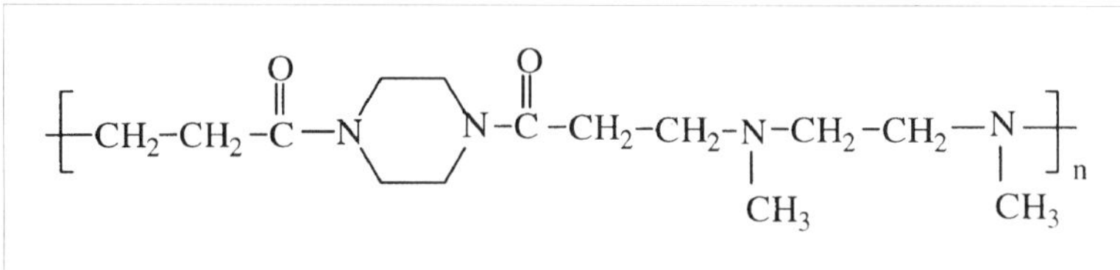

Figure 2.14. Functionalized glycols employed for the synthesis of segmented polyurethanes.

Poly(amidoamines) containing terminal vinyl groups have been used to synthesize block copolymers with styrene or vinyl chloride, while the terminal amino group of poly(amidoamines) was used in the block copolymerization with prepolymers of segmented polyurethane type (Barbucci *et al.*, 1989).

In order to introduce strongly basic amino groups in the main or in the side chain of segmented polyurethanes, functionalized glycols of the type shown in Figure 2.14 (Shibuta *et al.*, 1986; Ito *et al.*, 1986; Marconi *et al.*, 1992) have been employed as chain extenders in the polycondensation reaction. Ionic immobilization is presently the most common method for the preparation of heparinized surfaces, due to its simplicity and possibility of application to diversified polymer classes. A serious limitation to their long-term employment *in vivo*, however, derives from the fact that, by contact with physiological fluids, they leach their surface heparin rather rapidly.

(*b*) *Covalent Immobilization of Heparin.* When heparin is bonded to the polymer matrix by a much more stable type of bond, such as the covalent one, its leaching from the surface under the action of the body fluids is extremely slow and cannot generally be detected by the usual analytical techniques. It was also demonstrated that the thromboresistance of surfaces containing covalently bonded heparin is an intrinsic property of the solid phase, since the amount of released heparin is generally too small to contribute significantly to stop hemostasis.

The bifunctional reagents employed generally utilize either the nucleophilicity of the saccharidic hydroxy groups and of the amino groups of the serine residues bonded to heparin, or the moderate electrophilicity of the carboxy groups of the uronic residues. For example, cyanogen bromide can activate the hydroxy groups of some polymers and create a carbamic bond with the amino groups of heparin. This latter type of bond, however, is not sufficiently stable, and this type of immobilization does not hinder heparin release.

Hydrosoluble carbodiimides and Woodward's reagent are often and more efficiently employed to activate carboxy groups belonging both to heparin and to the matrix, while bifunctional reagents like glutaraldehyde or acyl chlorides of dicarboxylic acids possess the further advantage of acting as "spacing agents" of the heparin from the solid surface, so guaranteeing the anticoagulant molecule higher mobility and conformational freedom (Marconi *et al.*, 1993).

Different types of limitations and problems are involved in the covalent immobilization of heparin. Some are of a technical and practical nature, like the possibility of degradation during the immobilization procedure, while some difficulties are due to the fact that heparin dissolves only in water and, at a lower degree, in formamide. Other difficulties involve functional aspects, like the drastic activity decrease of bonded heparin with respect to the native one, due to its consequent lower mobility in the aqueous medium and to its reduced accessibility from the large molecules (thrombin and ATIII) with which it must interact.

In order to minimize this latter drawback, heparin was bonded to hydrophilic matrices able to swell in water, like sepharose, poly(vinylalcohol), or poly(hydroxyethyl-methacrylate) (Miura *et al.*, 1980). Since, however, these types of polymers usually possess poor mechanical properties, they are deposited by casting onto a sufficiently strong material, such as poly(urethane), and then (before reaction with heparin) crosslinked, to make them water-insoluble. A widely utilized methodology for increasing mobility and accessibility of heparin employs its bonding to suitable "spacers," i.e., to high molecular weight hydrophilic molecules, which enables it to get out of the polymer surface and lean forward into the aqueous phase. In particular, poly(ethyleneoxide) (PEO) of different molecular weight was used for this purpose, for example onto poly(urethane) matrices (Han *et al.*, 1989).

2.4.2.2. Surface Modifications by Different Hemocompatibility Enhancers

It has been noted that, also in the absence of heparinization treatment, segmented poly(urethane) surfaces containing PEO show a much lower platelet adhesion and a decreased adsorption of blood proteins like albumin and fibrinogen. Therefore, this procedure was extended to other polymers (e.g., of acrylic type) and the aforesaid good achievements were confirmed. This behavior was attributed to an improved molecular motion of the long hydrated chains of PEO, and to the thermodynamic repulsive forces deriving from the consequent excluded volume.

As a result of the great success obtained by pyrolytic carbon in the fabrication of components of cardiac valves, this technology was extended to the coating of prosthetic elements of different type (in particular, vascular prostheses) with a carbon structurally analogous to pyrolite. By techniques of ionic implantation under vacuum, it was possible to coat, at temperatures not exceeding 150 °C, different types of polymeric prostheses (Teflon®, Dacron®, polyolefins, etc.), which proved to maintain good long-term patency in human clinical applications.

The investigation of the heparin structure–properties correlation, and in particular of the role of its sulfate and sulfamic groups, has suggested synthesizing heparin-analogous polymers (in particular, of vinyl or urethane type) provided with sulfate and sulfonic groups (Van Der Does *et al.*, 1979; Han *et al.*, 1996). These "heparin-like" polymers, however, if compared to heparin, possess a remarkably lower capability of interaction with thrombin. The latter could be partially improved by increasing the surface density of the sulfate or sulfamic groups.

The grafting of platelet antiaggregants (such as dipyridamole) was also carried out on cellulosic polymers, or onto nylon or polyesters previously hydrolyzed in order to introduce onto their surfaces the functional groups necessary for the coupling with the drug (Marconi, 1981). Surfaces treated in this way showed in *in vitro* and *in vivo* animal tests superior antiaggregating properties.

Prostacyclin (PGI_2), whose role in the inhibition of platelet adhesion and activation is well known, has also been bonded both ionically and covalently to different polymer matrices. Unfortunately, due to its short stability and durability under *in vivo* operating conditions, these preparations cannot be employed to date for significant duration times (Ebert *et al.*, 1982).

Components of the fibrinolytic system, like plasminogen or its activators (urokinase and streptokinase), were also immobilized on polymer matrices, and promising results were obtained from their preliminary *in vitro* evaluation (Marconi *et al.*, 1996).

2.4.3. Production of Polymeric Materials

2.4.3.1. Introduction

Polymers employed in this field of application are generally commercial products, often synthetic and sometimes (as in the case of the production of cellulose membranes) transformation products of natural polymers. Consequently, the polymerization techniques are of traditional type, like polyaddition (for polyolefins, chlorinated or fluorinated polyolefines, silicones) and polycondensation (polyesters, polyurethanes, etc.). On the other hand, what is peculiar for "medical grade" polymers are the characteristics of purity, in particular the absence of oligomers, i.e., of polymers of lower molecular weight, which are generally provided with a higher reactivity when compared to high polymers and influence negatively the mechanical properties of manufactured articles, and sometimes exhibit (as in the case of polyesters) cytotoxicity. In addition, the presence of additives as plastifiers, antioxidants, stabilizers, etc., must be carefully controlled and often avoided due to their potential toxicity.

Essential requisites in the production of polymers for biomedical application are quality constancy, guarantee of a constant performance under the given conditions of employment, and a choice of fabrication techniques involving no polymer degradation or cross-linking.

Often, particular characteristics are required for the raw polymer [such as the extremely high molecular weight of poly(ethylene) employed for the acetabulum cup in hip prosthesis], or for the final manufactured article as in the case of the "controlled cut-off membranes" employed for blood detoxification, or for the textile components (fibers or microporous fabrics) used for producing vascular prostheses. Another general problem is the necessity of sterilizing all components of circuits, sutures, catheters, extracorporeal circuits, containers, etc., before their therapeutic employment. Since the thermal and chemical stability of polymers is often rather low, dry heat sterilization carried out in the range of 160°–190 °C cannot be employed for large classes of polymers, such as polyolefins, acrylic polymers, and polyamides. Also, steam sterilization in an autoclave, for which lower temperatures are necessary (125°–130 °C), cannot be used for polymers that can be damaged by high-pressure steam, like PVC, polyacetals, polyamides, and LDPE. In addition, γ-irradiation sterilization (using the ^{60}Co isotope) can seriously affect the quality and properties of polymeric materials, due to chain scission, cross-linking, oxidation, and other adverse reactions brought about by high-energy radiation. Chemical agents such as oxidizing water solutions of hypochloride, and particularly gaseous ethylene oxide, are now widely employed due to their ability to sterilize effectively at room temperature and for short times (10–12 h).

Another peculiarity of polymers used in medicine is that they must enable the fabrication of devices provided with different and sophisticated characteristics, like membranes employed for extracorporeal blood purification or oxygenation, and woven or knitted fabrics for cardiovascular prostheses.

Membranes for hemodialysis or hemofiltration, for example, must bring together mechanical strength and blood compatibility with very critical permeability properties (i.e., permeability to water and to solutes and impermeability to blood proteins and to microorganisms).

2.4.3.2. Polymer Classes

Polyurethanes, due to their versatility, are preferably employed in many biomedical applications, such as hemodialysis sets, blood bags, oxygenation circuits, parts of intraventricular assist devices and artificial hearts, etc. Besides their intrinsic favorable properties, their success is largely due to intensive research efforts in improving fabrication techniques and anticlotting properties. Furthermore, their flexibility and good elastomeric properties have made possible their use for surgical patches and other prostheses like artificial blood vessels (Anderheiden *et al.*, 1992).

The basic polycondensation for their synthesis consists of a first reaction between a diisocyanate and a polyether (like PEO, PPO, poly-1,4-butanediol, etc.) to give a prepolymer, which is then reacted with a linear diol like 1,4-butanediol, 1,6-hexanediol, etc., to give the final product of the general formula shown in Figure 2.15.

The soft segment and the region consisting of the monomeric diol and of the rigid aromatic diisocyanate residues form the hard one. Polyurethane can give either thermoplastic or thermosetting elastomeric materials. Even the thermoplastic elastomers are provided with high tensile strength and abrasion resistance, besides a high break elongation. These excellent properties made them able to substitute PVC, silicones, and acrylic polymers in the biomedical field where their present consumption exceeds 20,000 tons/year.

Some elastomeric PU, like Tecoflex®, have the further advantage that they can be formed by casting techniques. Acrylic cements find wide use in dentistry, and for fixing the femoral head (by metallic or ceramic composite material) into the bone in hip prosthesis surgery (Pascual *et al.*, 1996). In this case, curing of the cement takes place at room temperature. The cement is obtained by mixing a powder of completely polymerized poly(methyl-methacrylate, PMMA) to methyl methacrylate monomer and adding a polymerization catalyst. The polymerization occurs around the polymer particles that have been swollen by the monomer with a radical-initiation mechanism, and the formation of a hard polymer cement occurs rapidly. It

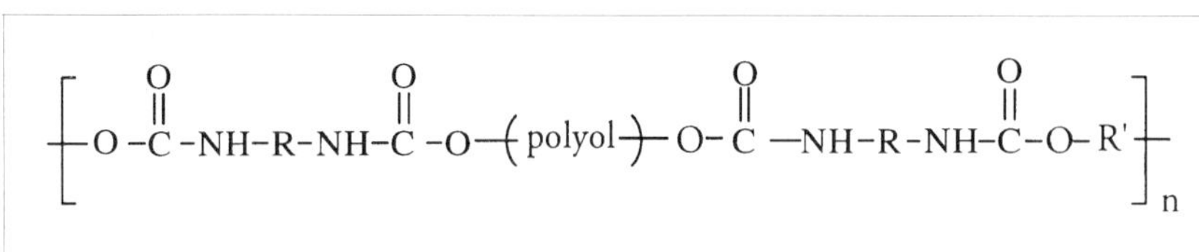

Figure 2.15. Formula of segmented polyurethane.

is possible to control the quality of the reaction product by varying the PMMA particle size, the catalyst amount, and also by adding to MMA other monomers such as styrene or butyl-methacrylate, able to provide the cement with some degree of elasticity. Prostheses of this type can also be made radio-opaque by the addition of barium sulfate.

An important class of acrylic polymers to be ascribed to the hydrogels, which will be described further, is represented by poly(hydroxyethyl-methacrylates), cross-linked with the bis-methacrylate of a glycol, largely employed for the production of contact lenses of the "soft" type (Refojo, 1979). The industrial polymerization process takes place in the absence of a solvent (mass polymerization), starting from a prepolymer dissolved-swollen in the monomer, by a free radical initiation mechanism. The obtained polymers are melted to obtain cylinders, from which the lenses are directly obtained by employing machine tools.

Water-swellable polymers, like hydrogels, have shown good hemocompatibility in evaluations including also *ex vivo* or *in vivo* tests. Due to their poor mechanical properties, however, they can be employed only as coatings of tough polymeric substrata, such as for vascular prostheses. This treatment might be done, in principle, by spreading solutions of the hydrophilic polymer on the surface to be coated, but in this case the adhesion of the hydrogel, even if the surface has been activated in a suitable way, is too poor to guarantee an acceptable long-term performance; for this reason, alternative techniques have been used. One of these is the formation of interpenetrating polymeric networks (IPN), obtained by polymerizing a hydrophilic monomer *in situ* in the rigid polymer substratum, the monomer being introduced both as vapor or dissolved in a solvent able to penetrate into the polymer matrix. IPN can also be obtained by hot-pressing a thin film of the hydrophilic polymer onto the surface of the plastic or elastomeric polymer.

Hydrogel coatings can also be realized by polymerizing the hydrophilic monomer (as water solution or as vapor) onto a polymer surface activated (in order to generate free radicals able to initiate the polymerization) by oxidizing agents like ozone, or cerium salts, or radiation. The employment of monomer vapors is particularly interesting, since it enables one to obtain a high purity monomer and to realize very uniform layers even onto polymeric devices of complex shape (Peppas and Mikos, 1986).

Aliphatic polyesters, whose applications as biodegradable and bioresorbable polymers were reported in brief earlier, are obtained by condensation from the corresponding α-hydroxy acids; they possess low molecular weight and poor mechanical and structural properties. Much more satisfactory polymers can, on the contrary, be obtained by ring-opening polymerization of the corresponding cyclic lactons, such as glycolide and lactide

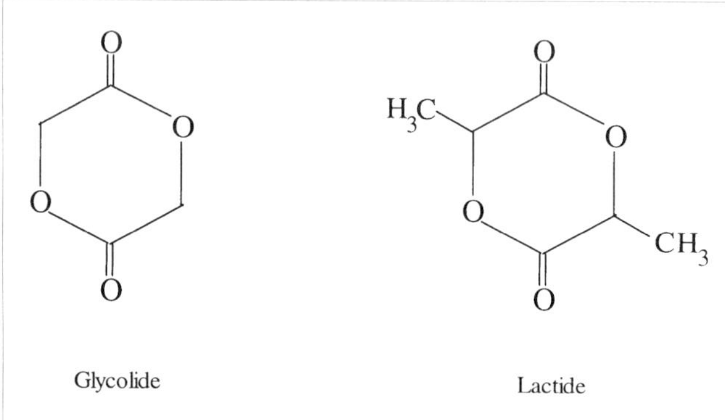

Figure 2.16. Cyclic lactons employed for the synthesis of biodegradable and bioresorbable polymers.

(Hu, 1983), as shown in Figure 2.16. The polymerization catalysts (for example, of cationic type such as SbF_3) respect the steric configuration of the starting hydroxy acid of the lactide by inserting the monomer units two by two (corresponding to the cyclic lactide) to give "polydimer." The polymerization rate of the racemic lactide is much higher than that of the L-lactide.

Many polymeric materials have been evaluated clinically for the fabrication of membranes in biomedical application, but only few (cellulose and cellulose derivatives, polyether polyurethanes, polysulfone, polyacrylonitrile, and ethylene-vinyl alcohol copolymers) are now used more or less extensively.

Regenerated cellulose membranes were the first to be largely employed in hemodialysis and still retain a dominant market position. The presence of β-glucosidic linkages and the high density of hydrogen bonds existing in its molecule provide its good mechanical performance; however, for this reason, it is also insoluble in almost all solvents. Furthermore, it cannot be melted without undergoing decomposition.

For this reason it is necessary to transform chemically cellulose (by functionalization of the hydroxy groups or complex formation), then to form a membrane by coating or wet spinning these solutions, and finally to regenerate the cellulose by treatment (with acids or alkali) of the cellulose derivative. The solubilization of cellulose can be carried out via formation of an acetate, or by formation of a copper-containing cellulose complex obtained by treatment with a cupro-ammonium solution. Since regenerated cellulose membranes are generally brittle in the dry state, a plasticizer (glycerol) is generally added.

In particular, when synthetic polymers are used for the membrane, this latter often consists of a tubular container filled with a huge number of hollow fibers, which have the advantage of an enormous surface-to-volume ratio. The production technology is the same as that employed for hollow textile fibers: extruding a melted polymer (melt spinning) or a polymer solution through the annular holes of a spinneret. The solid fiber is then obtained by coagulation in a nonsolvent (wet spinning) or by evaporating the organic solvent in a countercurrent with air (dry spinning).

Synthetic fibers play a very important role as basic materials for the preparation not only of sutures, but also of sophisticated biomedical devices, such as cardiovascular prostheses. Poly(ethylene terephthalate) fibers are at present largely employed for this purpose, in particular for medium or large diameter vascular substitution and for sewing rings of cardiac artificial valves. This is due both to the fairly good biocompatibility of the polymer, and to the commercial availability of many types (even complex) of filaments of different diameters, shapes, and manufacture characteristics. These "general purpose" materials are also provided with good mechanical and technical properties, resistance to sterilization procedures, and chemical inertia, and can be employed, after careful selection and upgrading treatment, in the biomedical field (King *et al.*, 1981). The polymer has the formula given in Figure 2.17) and is obtained by heating under vacuum at 270°–300 °C the ethylene glycol ester of terephthalic acid or a 1:1 mixture of ethylene glycol and dimethyl-terephthalate in the presence of a suitable catalyst (calcium or antimony or manganese salts). The number-average molecular weight of the polymer is in the range 15,000–20,000 and low molecular weight fractions (oligomers) should not be present, due to their chemical reactivity and suspected cytotoxicity.

The fibers are then formed by melt-spinning of the polymer (added with suitable stabilizers and antioxidants) under an inert atmosphere. After spinning the continuous filaments are stretched at high temperature, in order to increase the orientation (and consequently the crystallinity, originally rather poor) of the polymer matrix. This treatment, besides increasing the length of the monofilaments of almost one order of magnitude, markedly improves their dynamomechanical properties.

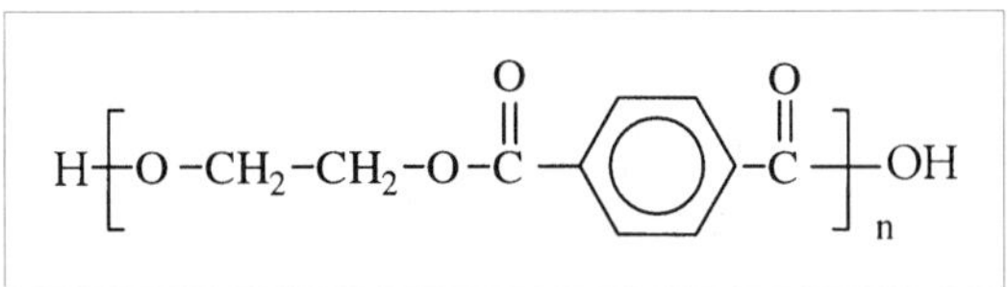

Figure 2.17. Formula of poly(ethylene terephthalate).

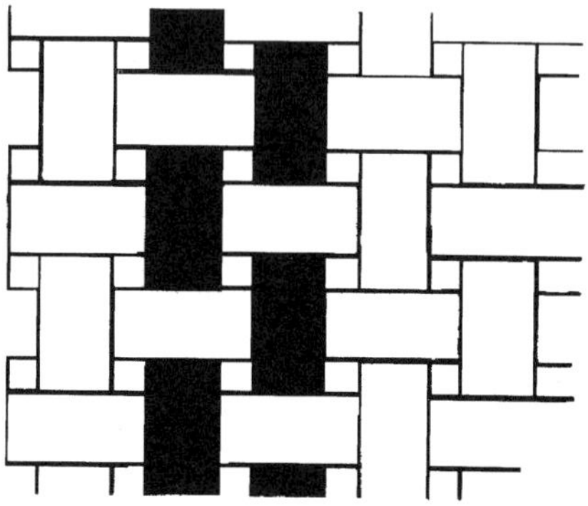

Figure 2.18. Woven fabric of polyester filaments used in vascular prostheses.

Vascular prostheses made with polyester filaments consist of seamless cylinders, where the configuration of the fabric is of the "woven" or "knitted" type. Woven fabrics consist of two sets of yarns interlaced orthogonally to each other in the a usual way (Figure 2.18). Knitted fabrics, on the other hand, consist of sets of yarns that, instead of being interlaced, are interloped around each other, an example of which is shown in Figure 2.19 (Mathisen *et al.*, 1987).

In spite of their good properties of mechanical resistance and shape stability, woven prostheses have proved to possess some negative properties like low water permeability, poor elongation, and particularly limited compliance with neointima. Knitted fabrics possess a more porous stucture and when used for grafts, have the advantage that the prostheses, before

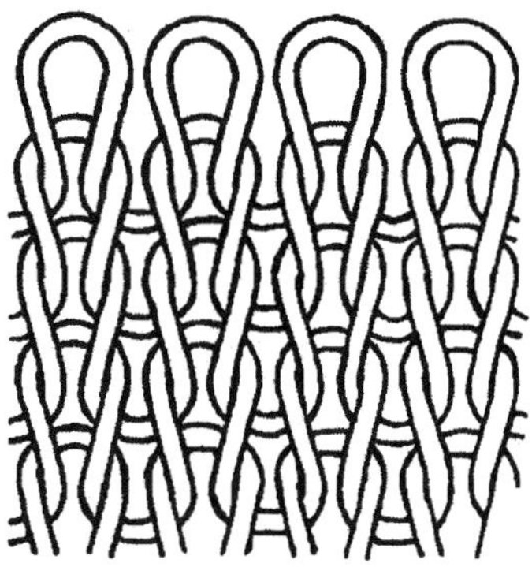

Figure 2.19. Knitted fabric of polyester filaments used in vascular prostheses.

implantation, can be submitted to preclotting. By this treatment, the pores are fitted with fibrin and it was observed that this is able to improve the hemocompatibility of the vascular prosthesis.

Also so-called "velour" fabrics, characterized by higher thickness and a smooth surface, belong to the class of knitted fabrics and have proved to exhibit good mechanical properties and yield improved hemocompatibility (Mathisen *et al.*, 1987).

2.4.4. Biological Interaction of Polymer Materials

The implantation site of a prosthesis is generally responsible for specific (and more or less rapid) interactions between the prosthesis and host tissues. To date it is generally recognized that a prosthesis must be considered as a foreign body, so an inflammatory reaction by the recipient organ or organism must be foreseen (Hanson and Harker, 1987).

The degree of this inflammation is first determined by surgical trauma and by the individual reactivity of the organism, but it also depends on the biological characteristics of tissues surrounding the prosthetic implant and on the reactions occurring at the prosthesis–biological system interface. For example, the material, or its impurities or decomposition products, can behave as an antigen or a hapten, stimulating immunoreactions.

By summarizing the present opinion on phenomena occurring successively on the material surface, it is generally believed that the first event is the adsorption of proteins from the body fluids, and that the type and degree of this adsorption are able to influence both the typology and activity of the cells which will subsequently coat the surface. Both the chemical composition and morphology of the surface are responsible for its behavior. Referring to the serum proteins, albumin thus inhibits the cell adhesiveness, which on the other hand is favored by fibrinogen, fibrinonectin, and probably globulins.

The cells that adhere to the surface produce chemical transmitters able to call other types of cells involved in the inflammatory process, and in particular macrophages, provided with important functions like phagocytosis and intracellular digestion. The evolution of the inflammatory process will then depend on the efficiency of the lymphocytes of different type in suppressing it. The by far most dreadful and difficult to control interaction is connected with coagulative phenomena occurring when blood contacts materials of nonbiological type. Blood is an aqueous solution of proteins and electrolytes, called plasma, where cellular components consisting of erythrocytes, leukocytes, and platelets are suspended. These latter are particularly involved in hemostasis, while the other two components, due to their entrapment into the thrombus, cause its increase.

In a healthy organism, blood flows freely through the vascular system in the absence of coagulation phenomena due to a delicate equilibrium among finely regulated mechanisms, involving many blood components, of both cellular and proteinic type. This equilibrium can be modified either by the effect of a vascular lesion or by contact of blood with a surface different from the endothelium internally coating blood vessels, such as a synthetic material or a foreign biological tissue. This brings about the activation of several concomitant and interconnected mechanisms aimed at stopping the bleeding phenomenon through the formation of a clot. However, a comprehensive knowledge of these mechanisms, necessary for the realization of hemocompatible surfaces, has not yet been achieved.

It was previously noted in brief that hemostasis takes place through two distinct pathways which, however, interconnect at various levels: the "platelet aggregation" process involving one of the blood cellular components and, as the final step of the "coagulation cascade," the formation of the fibrin clot. This latter pathway involves some proteinic components of blood. The final result is the formation of a strong and impenetrable agglomerate where platelets, and often other blood cells, are entrapped in the cross-linked fibrin network (Williams, 1987).

The adhesion of platelets involves their morphological modification and the release through their membrane of substances stimulating the aggregation. This release is caused by some substances like collagen, thrombin, thromboxane, and particularly adenosine diphosphate (ADP), coming both from the damaged tissues and by the platelet secretion itself, with a phenomenon of "autogeneration." The action of the release stimulators takes place through interaction with particular receptors of the platelet membrane, involving the activation of a complex intracellular mechanism mediated by prostaglandins, calcium, and cyclic AMP (adenosyl monophosphate). A last phase, called "secondary aggregation" and induced by ADP, follows with eventual formation of a platelet multilayer. It is called "secondary" since it is subsequent to adhesion and differs from the "primary" aggregation, which takes place under the action of the release stimulating agents in the absence of previous adhesion phenomena.

As for the coagulative cascade, it is formed by a series of pro-enzymes of proteolytic type in which the activated form of the preceding one activates the following pro-enzyme to its active form. These enzymes are called *coagulative factors* and some of them are serine-proteases (i.e., a serine residue is present in their active site).

Two biomedical pathways are present in the coagulative cascade. The first, called "extrinsic," is activated by a surface glycoprotein, called *tissue factor*, which is released in consequence of a trauma and, by interaction with the factor VII, is able to activate factor X. Conversely, the "intrinsic" way is

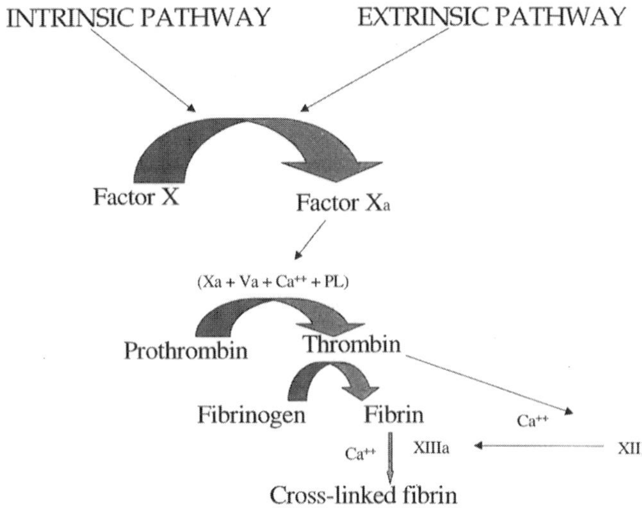

Figure 2.20. Intrinsic and extrinsic coagulation pathways.

started by contact with foreign surfaces, and for this reason is more related to the study of interaction of blood with hemocompatible materials. Both intrinsic and extrinsic pathways (see Figure 2.20) converge in the step of factor X activation, starting the so-called "common pathway" and leading, together with calcium ions, phospholipids, and activated factor V, to the formation of the prothrombinasic complex. This latter has the function of activating the prothrombin to thrombin, which is the key point of the whole thrombogenesis process. It is a proteolytic enzyme whose fundamental function is the transformation of fibrinogen into fibrin. Fibrinogen is a protein formed by three globular domains connected to each other by rod-like regions, and its activation brings about the detachment of oligopeptides (called *fibrinopeptides*) from the central region. The so-formed fibrin monomers associate spontaneously under the action of electrostatic interactions in ordered fibrous structures called *fibrin*.

Next, the fibrin clot is further stabilized by formation of covalent cross-links among different polymeric chains, by a reaction of *trans*-amidation taking place between residues of glutamine and lysine, catalyzed by an enzyme (called *factor XIII*) activated by thrombin.

The whole coagulation process is dependent on control and regulation systems which make possible clot formation not only very rapidly, but also localized to the injured region, and subsequently, after tissue repair, rapid clot dissolution.

The control is guaranteed by the short half-life of the coagulation factors, which are removed from the blood flow and degraded. Conversely, the regulation is affected by specific inhibitors like antithrombin III (as mentioned in the section relevant to the surface heparinization of polymers) whose action, enhanced by the association with heparin, has as an object the neutralization of thrombin and of other serine proteases.

Finally, the clot elimination is carried out by plasmin, which is a protein forming from an inactive precursor (plasminogen) under the action of some substances, mainly the urokinase. Since the fibrin network contains plasminogen and its activators, activated plasmin is able to hydrolyze the polymeric fibrin due to the porosity of the coagulum. This hydrolysis occurs at the level of the connecting rod-like regions.

In conclusion, it appears that the coagulation system is integrated and closely linked with the platelet aggregation mechanisms. For instance, the thrombin formed in the coagulative cascade can cause, by itself, the platelet primary aggregation phenomenon. Moreover, the strong propensity of fibrin to adsorb on the platelet surface is responsible for the fact that the deposition of the first one forms the deposition of the second, and vice versa. Several other factors are also adsorbed on the platelets, and for this reason a platelet clot can be a preferential site for the formation of the fibrin network.

References

Anderheiden, D., Klee, D., Hocker, H. 1992. Surface modification of a biocompatible polymer based on polyurethane for artificial blood vessels, *J. Biomed. Mater. Res.* **3**, 1.

Andrade, J.D. 1973. Interfacial phenomena and biomaterials, *Med. Instrum.* **7**, 110.

Aragona, J., Parson, J.R., Alexander, H., Weiss, A.B. 1981. Soft tissue attachment of a filamentous carbon-absorbable polymer tendon and ligament replacement, *Clin. Orthop.* **160**, 268.

Barbucci, R., Benvenuti, M., Dal Maso, G., Nocentini, M., Tempesti, F. 1989. Synthesis and physico-chemical characterization of a new material (PUPA) based on polyurethane and poly(amido-amine) components capable of strongly adsorbing quantities of heparin, *Biomaterials* **10**, 299.

Cohen, S., Chen, L., Apte, R.N. 1995. Controlled release of peptides and proteins from biodegradable polyester microspheres: An approach for treating infectious diseases and malignancies, *React. Polym.* **25**, 177.

Eberhart, R.C., Munro, M.S., Williams, G.B. 1987. Albumin adsorption and retention on C18 alkyl derivatized polyurethane vascular grafts, *Artif. Organs* **11**, 375.

Ebert, C.D., Lee, E.S., Kim, S.W. 1982. The antiplatelet activity of immobilized prostacyclin, *J. Biomed. Mater. Res.* **16**, 629.

Falb, R.D., Leininger, R.I., Grode, J., Crowley, J. 1975. Surface-bonded heparin, *Adv. Exp. Med. Biol.* **52**, 365.

Ferruti, P., Provenzale, L. 1976. A new thrombogenic polymeric material, *Transplant. Proc.* **7**, 103.

Han, D.K., Park, K.D., Ahn, K.D., Jeong, S.Y., Kim, Y.H. 1989. Preparation and surface characterization of PEO-grafted and heparin-immobilized polyurethanes, *J. Biomed. Mater. Res.* **23**, 87.

Han, D.K., Jeon, S.Y., Kim, Y.H., Min, B.G., Cho, H.I. 1991. Negative cilia concept for thromboresistance: Synergistic effect of PEO and sulfonate groups grafted onto polyurethanes, *J. Biomed. Mater. Res.* **25**, 561.

Han, D.K., Park, K.D., Ryu, G.H., Kim, U.Y., Min, B.G., Kim, Y.H. 1996. Plasma protein adsorption to sulfonated poly(ethylene oxide)-grafted polyurethane surface, *J. Biomed. Mater. Res.* **30**, 23.

Hanson, S.R., Harker, L.A. 1987. Evaluation of blood-material interactions, in: *Blood Compatibility, Vol. 1* (D.F. Williams, ed.), CRC Press, Boca Raton.

Hu, C.C. 1983. Survey of clinically important wound closure biomaterials, in: *Biocompatible Polymers, Metals and Composites* (M. Szycher, ed.), p. 477, Technomic Publishing Co., Lancaster, PA.

Ito, Y., Sisido, M., Imanishi, Y., 1986. Synthesis and antithrombogenicity of polyethereurethaneurea containing quaternary ammonium groups in the side chains and of the polymer/heparin complex, *J. Biomed. Mater. Res.* **20**, 1017.

King, M., Blais, P., Guidoin, R., Prowse, E., Marois, M., Grosselin, C., Norl, H.P. 1981. Polyethylene terephthate (Dacron®) vascular prostheses-material and fabric construction aspects, in: *Biocompatibility of Clinical Implant Materials, Vol 2*, p. 177 (D.F. Williams, ed), CRC Press, Boca Raton.

LaPorte, R.J. 1997. *Hydrophilic Polymer Coatings for Medical Devices*, p. 157, Technomic Publishing Co., Lancaster, PA.

Lewis, G. 1997. Properties of acrylic bone cement: State of the art review, *J. Biomed. Mater. Res.* **38**, 155.

Lumsden, A.B., Chen, C., Hanson, S.R. 1996. Nonporous silicone polymer coating of expandeal polytetrafluoro-ethylene grafts reduces graft neointimal hyperplasia in dog and baboon models, *J. Vasc. Surg.* **24**, 825.

Marconi, W. 1981. New non-thrombogenic polymer compositions, *Makromol. Chem. Suppl.* **5**, 15.

Marconi, W., Magnone, G., Martinelli, A., Piozzi, A. 1992. New polyurethanes able to bind high amounts of heparin, suitable as biomedical compositions, *Polym. Adv. Technol.* **4**, 319.

Marconi, W., Barontini, P., Martinelli, A., Piozzi, A. 1993. New polyurethane compositions containing high amounts of covalently bonded heparin, *Makromol. Chem.* **194**, 1347.

Marconi, W., Piozzi, A., Romoli, D. 1996. Preparation and evaluation of polyurethane surfaces containing immobilized plasminogen, *J. Biomater. Sci., Polym. Ed.* **8**, 237.

Marconi, W., Benvenuti, F., Piozzi, A. 1997. Covalent bonding of heparin to a vinyl copolymer for biomedical applications, *Biomaterials* **18**, 885.

Marconi, W., Cordelli, S., Napoli, A., Piozzi, A. 1999. Synthesis and physico-chemical evaluation of ethylene-vinyl alcohol-vinyl stearate polymers, *Macromol. Chem. Phys.* **200**, 1191.

Mathisen, S.R., Coan, D.E., Sauvage, L.R., Wu, H.D., Wechezak, A.R., Goff, S.G. 1987. A rapid in vitro test of the in vivo healing potential of vascular prostheses, *J. Biomed. Mater. Res.* **21**, 1081.

Miura, Y., Aoyagi, S., Kusada, Y., Miyamoto, K. 1980. The characteristics of anticoagulation by covalently immobilized heparin, *J. Biomed. Mater. Res.* **14**, 619.

Ohshima, N., Yanagi, K., Miyoshi, H. 1997. Packed-bed type reactor to obtain high density culture of hepatocytes for use as an artificial liver, *Artif. Organ* **21**, 1169.

Pascual, B., Vazques, B., San Roman, J. 1996. New aspects of the effect of size and size distribution on the setting parameters and mechanical properties of acrylic bone cements, *Biomaterials* **17**, 509.

Peppas, N.A., Mikos, A.G. 1986. Preparation methods and structure of hydrogels, in: *Hydrogels in Medicine and Pharmacy: Vol. 1 — Fundamentals* (N.A. Peppas, ed.), CRC Press, Boca Raton.

Platè, N.A., Matrosovich, M.M. 1976. Affinity chromatography of serum albumin for adsorption on synthetic polymers, *Akad. Nauk (URSS)* **220**, 496.

Pozniak, G., Krajeuska, B., Trochimczuk, W. 1995. Urease immobilized on modified polysulphone membrane: Preparation and properties, *Biomaterials* **16**, 129.

Refojo, M.F. 1979. Contact lenses in: *Kirk-Othmer: Encyclopedia of Chemical Technology*, 3rd edn., Vol. 6, p. 720, Wiley, New York.

Sang, Y.L. 1996. Bacterial polyhydroxyalkanoates, *Biotechnol. Bioeng.* **49**, 1.

Shibuta, R., Tanaka, M., Sisido, M., Imanishi, Y. 1986. Synthesis of novel polyaminoethereurethaneureas and development of antithrombogenic material by their chemical modifications, *J. Biomed. Mater. Res.* **20**, 971.

Shieh, S.J., Zimmerman, M.C., Parson, J.R. 1990. Prelimimary characterization of bioresorbable and non-resorbable synthetic fibers for the repair of soft tissue injuries, *J. Biomed. Mater. Res.* **24**, 789.

Silver, J.H., Marchant, J.W., Cooper, S.L. 1993. Effect of polyol type on the physical properties and thrombogenicity of sulfonate-containing polyurethanes, *J. Biomed. Mater. Res.* **27**, 1443.

Takahara, A., Okkema, A.Z., Wabers, H., Cooper, S.L. 1991. Effect of hydrophilic soft segment side chains on the surface properties and blood compatibility of segmented poly(urethaneureas), *J. Biomed. Mater. Res.* **25**, 1095.

Tanzawa, H., Mori, Y., Harumiya, N., Miyama, H., Hori, M., Ohshima, N., Idezuki, Y. 1973. Preparation and evaluation of new antithrombogenic heparinized hydrophilic polymer for use in cardiovascular system, *Trans. Am. Soc. Artif. Int. Organs* **19**, 188.

Van Der Does, L., Beugeling, T., Froehling, P.E., Bantjes, A. 1979. Synthetic polymer with anticoagulant activity, *J. Polym. Sci., Polym. Symp.* **66**, 337.

Wang, A., Stark, C., Dumbleton, J.H. 1995. Role of cyclic plastic deformation in the wear of UHMWPE acetabular cups, *J. Biomed. Mater. Res.* **29**, 619.

Williams, D.F. 1987. Blood physiology and biochemistry: Haemostasis and thrombosis, in: *Blood Compatibility, Vol 1*, p. 5 (D.F. Williams, ed.), CRC Press, Boca Raton.

Yamamuro, T., Matsusue, Y., Uchida, A., Shimada, K., Shimozaki, E., Kitaoka, K. 1994. Bioabsorbable osteosynthetic implants of ultra high strength poly-L-lactide. A clinical study, *Int. Orthop.* **18**, 332.

3

Fundamentals of Polymeric Composite Materials

Claudio Migliaresi and Alessandro Pegoretti

3.1. Introduction

Most engineering progress through the centuries was dependent on the discovery and availability of new structural materials. In fact many of our modern technologies require materials with unusual combinations of mechanical properties, lightness, and ease of processing that cannot be met by the conventional metal alloys, ceramics, and polymeric materials. For example, engineers working in research and development of aerospace, underwater, transportation, civil, and biomedical applications are increasingly searching for structural materials that have low densities, are strong, stiff, abrasion and impact resistant, and are not easily corroded. This is a rather unusual combination of characteristics, since strong materials are relatively dense and increasing strength or stiffness generally results in a decrease of impact strength. A possible way to extend material property combinations and ranges relies on the development of *composite materials*. Very simply, a composite is a material that is composed of two or more distinct constituent materials or phases, separated by definite interfaces. To a certain extent this definition depends upon the level of analysis, as all materials may be considered heterogeneous if the scale of interest is sufficiently small. It is only when the constituents have significantly different physical properties, and thus the composite properties are noticeably different from the constituent properties, that we have come to recognize these materials as composites (Agarwal and Broutman, 1990). Major con-

---

Claudio Migliaresi and Alessandro Pegoretti • Department of Materials Engineering, University of Trento, via Mesiano 77, 38050 Trento, Italy.

Integrated Biomaterials Science, edited by R. Barbucci. Kluwer Academic/Plenum Publishers, New York, 2002.

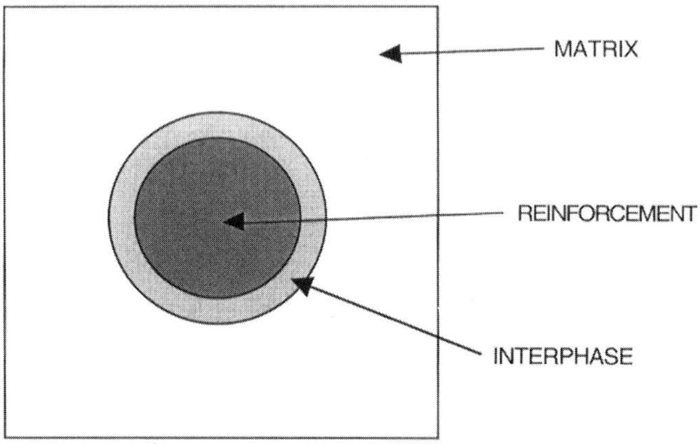

Figure 3.1. Schematic representation of the principal composite constituents.

stituents in a composite material are the *reinforcing agents* and a *matrix*, which act as a binder, and in most cases a distinct region (interphase) between reinforcement and matrix may also be found, as depicted in Figure 3.1.

Of course, mechanical properties represent only one of the targets that can be achieved using composite materials, it being possible, to some extent and based on the choice of components, to tailor other physical properties, such as electrical conductivity, mass transport properties, heat conduction, and so on.

Most composite materials fabricated so far, however, have been developed in order to improve mechanical performances such as elastic properties (modulus of elasticity) and ultimate properties (strength, toughness). It is consequently natural to group composite materials on the basis of the strengthening mechanism, which depends strongly on the geometry of the reinforcement. Therefore, it is convenient to classify composite materials on the basis of the geometry of the reinforcing representative unit, following the scheme proposed in Figure 3.2.

With reference to this classification, the characteristic feature of a particle is that it has approximately the same dimension in all directions (usually equiaxial, with the exception of platelets). It can have a variety of geometries like spherical, cubic, tetragonal, a platelet, or some other regular or irregular shape. There are many good reasons for using particles (talc and mica overall) in plastics, in addition to the obvious usual reduction in cost of the final product. In the case of plastics, the addition of particles provides a reduction of shrinkage during the cure of thermoset polymer or the

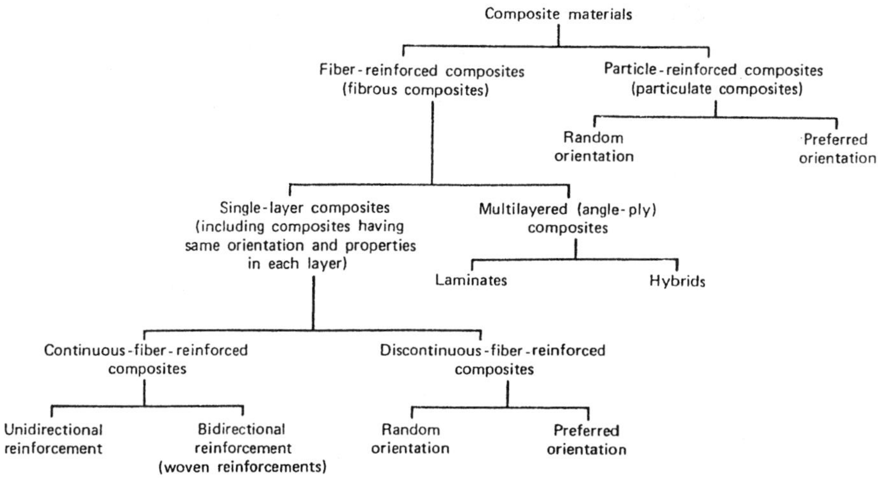

Figure 3.2. Classification of composite materials.Taken from Agarwal and Broutman (1990), p. 4, with kind permission of John Wiley & Sons, Inc.

injection molding of a thermoplastic resin. The addition of particles generally improves the elastic properties of a matrix, but produces contrasting effects on its ultimate properties, also depending on the mode of loading (i.e., tension rather than compression). Therefore, the particle-reinforced polymer has a much greater thermal conductivity and some higher mechanical properties. A much more efficient strengthening process can be achieved through the usage of fiber reinforcement, since the load transfer process from the matrix is greatly improved. A fibrous reinforcing element is characterized by the fact that its length is much greater than its cross-sectional dimensions.

3.2. Fiber Reinforcements

Fibers are inherently stronger than the bulk form of a material (as evidenced in Table 3.1) for a number of reasons, the two major ones being: (i) the fiber's small diameter, which strongly reduces the probability of the presence of critical defects; (ii) the alignment or preferential orientation of molecular crystal structures. In many cases, this latter is also the cause of the higher stiffness of the fibrous with respect to the bulk material.

Reinforcing fibers used in modern composites can be broadly classified into three main categories (Mallick, 1993): (i) inorganic fibers; (ii) carbon

Table 3.1. Comparison of the Mechanical Properties of Monolithic Materials and Their Fibrous Counterparts[a]

	Young's modulus (GPa)	Strength (MPa)
Glass		
monolithic	72	100
fiber (E)	72	3400
Alumina		
monolithic	380	330
fiber (Fiber FP)	350–380	1700
Silicon carbide		
monolithic	410	500
fiber (MF)	400	3400
Carbon		
monolithic	10	20
fiber (T-300)	235	3200
Polyethylene		
monolithic	0.4	26
fiber (S 1000)	170	3000

[a] Flexural and tensile strength for the fiber and monolithic materials, respectively, are reported.

fibers; (iii) polymeric fibers. They can be used in continuous (long fibers) as well as in discontinuous (short fibers) form. Some characteristics of the most common reinforcing fibers are reported in Table 3.2. It is noteworthy that, unlike carbon and polymeric fibers, inorganic fibers are mostly isotropic.

3.2.1. Inorganic Fibers

Examples of inorganic fibers are glass, boron, silicon carbide, alumina (Al_2O_3), and alumina borosilicate (Nextel). Glass fibers are the most common of all reinforcing fibers for polymeric matrix composites, mainly because they offer several advantages like low cost, high tensile strength, elevated chemical resistance, and excellent insulating characteristics. On the other hand, their main disadvantages are low tensile modulus, relatively high density, sensitivity to abrasion with handling, relatively low fatigue resistance, and poor adhesion to matrix resins, particularly in the presence of moisture. Manufacturing, structure, properties, and applications of glass fibers are reported in a number of texts (Loevenstein, 1983; Dockum, 1987; Vaughan, 1998). The glass fiber microstructure consists of a three-dimensional network of silicon, oxygen, and other atoms randomly arranged, which accounts for the amorphous state and isotropic properties. For structural composites the two commonly used types of glass fibers are

E-glass and S-glass, whose properties and typical compositions are reported in Tables 3.2 and 3.3, respectively.

The main reason for the widespread use of E-glass fibers in the composite industry is its lowest cost among all commercially available reinforcing fibers. S-glass reaches the highest tensile strength among all available fibers, but the compositional differences and higher processing cost make it more expensive than E-glass. S-2-glass, a lower-cost version of S-glass, was recently developed with tensile strength and modulus similar to those of S-glass. Another type, known as C-glass, is used in chemical applications requiring improved corrosion resistance to acids.

Boron fibers are currently produced with diameters of 100, 140, and 200 μm by chemical vapor deposition (CVD) on a resistively heated (up to 1260 °C) tungsten filament from the reduction of boron trichloride (BCl_3) with hydrogen (Tsirlin, 1985; Suplinskas and Marzik, 1987). Over the years, the ultimate properties of boron fibers have improved steadily from an average tensile strength of under 2.8 MPa to over 3.4 GPa.

The technological need for high-temperature reinforcing fibers has led to the development of inorganic ceramic fibers, like alumina (Birchall *et al.*, 1985) and silicon carbide (Yajima, 1985), which combine high strength and rigidity with elevated temperature and environmental attack stability. Alumina fibers were first developed and marketed by Du Pont de Nemours & Co. with the trade name "Fiber FP," as continuous yarns of α-alumina produced by wet spinning from an aqueous slurry and subsequent firing. FP fiber retains its strength up to about 1370 °C. Silicon carbide (SiC) fibers can be obtained by two main processes: (i) chemical vapor deposition (AVCO Specialty Materials Co.) and (ii) controlled pyrolysis of a polymeric precursor (Nippon Carbon Co. – Nicalon fibers). SiC fiber retains tensile strength well above 650 °C. Properties of alumina and silicon carbide fibers are summarized in Table 3.2.

3.2.2. Carbon (Graphite) Fibers

For the fabrication of high-performance polymeric composites, carbon fibers are by far the predominant high-strength, high-modulus reinforcing agents currently used (Donnet and Bansal, 1990; Peebles, 1995; Lafdi and Wright, 1998). As reported in Table 3.2, carbon fibers are commercially available for a wide range of mechanical properties, with tensile moduli from 160 to about 800 GPa, and tensile strengths from 1.4 up to about 7 GPa, depending on the degree of microstructural orientation. In fact, carbon fibers contain a mixture of amorphous and graphitic carbon. Their elevated tensile modulus and strength are related to the graphitic form, in which carbon atoms are arranged in crystallographic parallel planes of regular

Table 3.2. Properties of Some Common Reinforcing Fibers[a]

Fiber	Density (g/cm^2)	Tensile modulus (GPa)	Torsional modulus (GPa)	Tensile strength (GPa)	Compressive strength (GPa)	Strain to failure (%)	Coefficient of thermal expansion ($10^{-6} K^{-1}$)	Thermal conductivity (W/mK)
Inorganic fibers								
E-glass	2.58	72	28	3.4	>0.8	4.7	4.9	1.04
S-glass	2.46	87		4.3	>1.1	5.0	2.5	
Boron	2.5–2.6	415	139	3.5	5.9	0.8	4–8	
Nicalon	2.8	200		2.8	3.1	1.4	3.1	
Al_2O_3 (fiber FP)	3.7	350–380	122	1.7	6.9	0.4	6.8	
SiC (CVD)	3.3	400		3.4		0.9	5.7	
SiC (Nicalon)	2.6	180		2.0		1.1		
Asbestos (chrysolite)	3.1	169			2.5			
Pitch-based carbon fibers								
Amoco P-25	1.9	160		1.4	1.15	0.9		22
Amoco P-100	2.15	725	4.7	2.2	0.48	0.30	−1.5 (9.4)	500
Nippon NT-20		200		2.8				
Nippon NT-20		595		3.0				
PAN-based carbon fibers								
T-300	1.76	235	15	3.2	2.88	1.4	−0.5 (12)	15
T-1000	1.82	295		7.1	2.76	2.4		
GY-70	1.96	520		1.8	1.06	0.4	−1.1	
AS4	1.80	235	17	3.6	2.69	1.6		
M60J	1.94	585		3.8	1.67	0.7	−0.9	75

Polymeric fibers								
Kevlar 29	1.44	65	1.9	2.8	0.4	4.0		
Kevlar 49	1.44	125	1.4	3.5	0.4	2.3	−4.0 (59)	0.04
Kevlar 149	1.47	185	1.1	3.4	0.4		−1.5	
Nomex	1.38	10		0.5		22.0		
Vectran HS	1.41	65	0.6	2.8		3.3		
Vectran M	1.4	53		1.1		2.0		
Spectra 900	0.97	117		2.6		3.5	−9	
Spectra 1000	0.97	170	0.8	3.0	0.17	2.7	−10	
PBO	1.58	200–360	1.0	3.5–5.7	0.2	1–2	−7 to −10	
Textile fibers								
Polyester (PET)	1.39	3–10		0.4–0.8			−1000	0.25
Nylon	1.14	1–5		0.3–0.8			−300	0.14
Metal wires								
Stainless steel (18/8) (diameter 50–250 μm)	8.0	198	77	1.0–1.4			18	
Tungsten (diameter <25 μm)	19.3	360	140	5.5			4.5	

[a]Thermal expansion values are for longitudinal direction. Values in parentheses are for the transverse direction.

Table 3.3. Typical Compositions of E-Glass and S-Glass Fibers

Glass fiber type	SiO_2	Al_2O_3	CaO	MgO	B_2O_3	Na_2O
E-glass	54.5	14.5	17	4.5	8.5	0.5
S-glass	64	26	—	10	—	—

hexagons. The covalent bond between carbon atoms in the graphite basal planes leads to extremely high rigidity and strength, while the weak van der Waals bond between neighboring planes results in a lower modulus in that direction. This accounts for the highly anisotropic physical and mechanical properties of the carbon fibers. Advantages of carbon fibers are their extraordinary specific (i.e., properties divided by material specific weight) modulus and strength, very low (in most cases, negative) coefficient of linear thermal expansion, and high fatigue resistance. The disadvantages are their high electrical conductivity, which can be dangerous for some electrical equipment, and low impact resistance of the corresponding fiber-reinforced composites. Moreover, the relatively high cost has so far limited the widespread use of commercial applications, their main utilization being in the aerospace industry, where weight saving is usually more important than cost.

Currently available carbon fibers are produced using one of the following three precursor materials: polyacrylonitrile (PAN), mesophase pitch, and cellulose (in decreasing order of usage). The organic precursor materials are converted in carbon fibers through a quite complex pyrolysis process involving thermal treatment and stretching at elevated temperatures (up to 2000 °C), as reported schematically in the flow diagram of Figure 3.3. Resulting fibers have diameters in the range from 5 to 10 μm. For more information the reader is referred to Donnet and Bansal (1990) and Peebles (1995).

3.2.3. Polymeric Fibers

High-performance polymeric (organic) fibers can be broadly classified into the following three main categories (Kumar and Wang, 1997; Clements, 1998): (i) fibers from lyotropic liquid crystalline polymers, such as the aramid fibers (Kevlar); (ii) fibers from thermotropic liquid crystalline polymers, such as a copolymer of benzoic and naphthoic acids (Vectran); (iii) fibers from extended-chain flexible polymers, such as ultrahigh molecular weight polyethylene (Spectra, Dyneema).

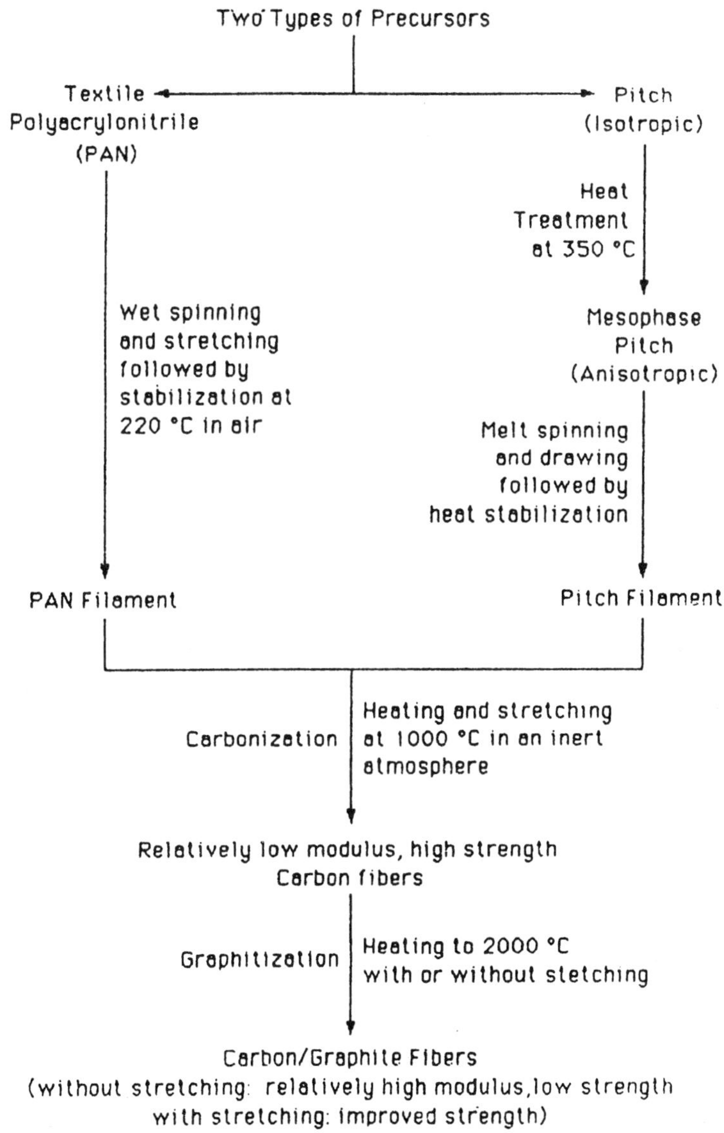

Figure 3.3. Flow diagram for carbon fiber fabrication. Taken from Mallick (1993), p. 31, with kind permission of John Wiley & Sons, Inc.

High-performance aramid fibers (Dobb, 1985) were first introduced in 1971 when the problem of spinning the poly(*p*-phenylene terephthalamide) (PPTA) was solved due to the discovery that the polymer would dissolve in strong acids to form a liquid crystalline solution. The polymer solution is extruded at elevated temperature through an air layer into a coagulating water bath. Commercially available aramid fibers include Kevlar (DuPont), Twaron (Akzo), and Technora (Teijin). Aramid fibers possess very good tensile properties, as reported in Table 3.1, but poor characteristics in compression, with compressive strength being one-eighth of the tensile value. Due to the anisotropy of their microstructure, aramid fibers have very anisotropic mechanical, thermal, and physical properties. Aramid fibers were mostly used in combination with other fibers (like carbon or glass) to obtain hybrid composites with improved impact resistance.

Fibers from thermotropic copolyesters (Jaffe, 1987) have been commercially available since 1985 by Celanese under the trade name of Vectran. These fibers are produced by a melt-spinning technique at a spinning temperature between the melting point of the crystalline phase and the liquid crystalline to amorphous transition temperature. Advantages offered by Vectran fibers are relatively good mechanical properties (see Table 3.2), excellent chemical resistance, low moisture pick-up, and reduced creep.

Ultrahigh molecular weight ($M_w > 10^6$) and low-polydispersity high-density polyethylene (UHMWPE) can be used to produce high-performance polyethylene fibers such as Spectra (Allied Signal) or Dyneema (DSM). UHMWPE fibers are produced by a gel-spinning technique in which the polymer is dissolved in a common solvent (such as decalin), at a concentration of about 2–8 weight percent with stirring at elevated temperatures. The solution is spun at 130–140 °C into a room temperature bath and the residual solvent is then removed during the hot drawing process. Drawing at very high draw ratios (from 30 to 100) leads to fibers with the highest specific strength of all commercial fibers available to date. Main disadvantages are the low melting point (about 147 °C), which is limiting their usage at temperatures lower than 80–90 °C, the high creep rate, and poor adhesion with all polymeric matrices.

3.3. Matrix Resins

In a fiber-reinforced composite, the role of the matrix is (i) to bind the fibers together, (ii) to transfer stresses between fibers, (iii) to protect them against environmental attack and damage due to mechanical abrasion. Moreover, the matrix controls processability, maximum service temperature, flammability, and corrosion resistance.

Polymers that can be used as matrices to make structural composites can be divided into two main classes: thermoplastics (individual molecules are linear in structure with no chemical linking between them) and thermosets (the molecules are chemically joined together by crosslinks, thus forming a three-dimensional rigid structure).

3.3.1. Thermoset Matrices

Polyester and epoxy resins are the most common thermoset matrices used for the preparation of high-performance fiber-reinforced composites.

3.3.1.1. Polyester and Vinyl Ester Resins

Unsatured polyesters (UP) are by far the most widely used resins in the composite industry. UP resins are used in the highest volume due to their relatively low cost and good combination of thermomechanical properties and environmental durability. Typical properties of a cast UP resin are reported in Table 3.4.

A UP resin is usually obtained from an unsaturated polyester dissolved in a reactive monomer. Unsaturated polyesters are linear polymers containing a number of carbon double bonds obtained by a condensation reaction between three chemical species: saturated aromatic acids (orthophthalic acid, isophthalic acid), unsaturated acids (maleic anhydride, fumaric acid), and glycols (ethylene, propylene, diethylene glycol). UP resins are classified as orthophthalic or isophthalic, depending on the type of saturated acid in the oligomer. The resulting polymeric liquid is dissolved in a reactive diluent containing carbon–carbon double bonds, such as styrene, which reduces its viscosity, making it easier to process, and acts as

Table 3.4. Typical Properties of Unsaturated Polyester and Vinyl Ester Resins

	Unsaturated polyester	Vinyl ester
Density (g/cm^3)	1.10–1.40	1.12–1.32
Tensile modulus (GPa)	2.10–3.45	3.0–3.5
Tensile strength (MPa)	34.5–103.5	73.0–81.0
Strain at break (%)	1–5	3.5–5.5
Coefficient of linear thermal expansion ($10^{-6}\,C^{-1}$)	55–100	—
Heat distortion temperature (°C)	60–205	93–135
Cure shrinkage (%)	5–12	5.4–10.3
Water sorption in 24 h (%)	0.15–0.6	0.01–0.2

a cross-linking agent by reacting with unsaturation points of polyester molecules. The curing reaction is initiated by adding small quantities of a catalyst that decomposes into free radicals as the temperature increases. The curing time for UP resins depends on the decomposition rate of the organic peroxide or aliphatic azo compounds used as catalysts.

Vinyl ester resins are obtained by using unsaturated vinyl ester resins produced from the reaction between an unsaturated carboxylic acid (e.g., methacrylic or acrylic acid) and an epoxy resin. A vinyl ester molecule contains carbon–carbon double bonds only at the ends and they are suitable to be dissolved in a reactive monomer (styrene) like UP resins. Styrene coreacts with the vinyl ester resin to form cross-links at the unsaturation points. Major advantages of vinyl ester resins with respect to UP resin is the lower susceptibility to chemical attacks and then lower cross-link density, which account for the higher strain at break. However, the volumetric shrinkage of vinyl ester resins is very high, being in the range 5–10%.

For more details about unsaturated polyester and vinyl ester resins, the reader is referred to Launikitis (1982), Updegraff (1982) and Cassis and Talbot (1998).

3.3.1.2. Epoxy Resins

For several reasons epoxy resins (Penn and Chiao, 1982; Juska and Puckett, 1997; Penn and Wang, 1998) are among the best matrices for continuous filament composites used in the most demanding structural application. The main reasons are (i) the broad range of properties achievable through a proper combination of epoxy resin and curing agent, (ii) good adhesion to most high-performance fibers, (iii) low shrinkage after curing, and (iv) elevated resistance to chemicals and good insulating properties. Starting materials for epoxy resin production are low molecular weight organic liquids containing a number of epoxide groups, which are three-atom rings of one oxygen and two carbons, also called oxirane rings or glycidyl groups:

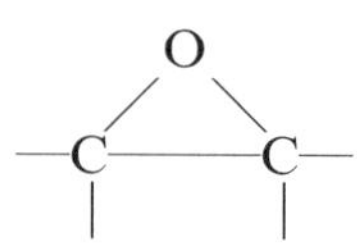

The most common epoxy resins are obtained by using diglycidyl ether of bisphenol A (DGBEA), which contains two epoxide groups at the ends of the molecule. The epoxy liquid is usually mixed with diluents to reduce the

Table 3.5. Typical Properties of an Epoxy Resin

Density (g/cm^3)	1.2–1.3
Tensile moduls (GPa)	2.75–4.10
Tensile strength (MPa)	55–130
Strain at break (%)	1–8
Coefficient of linear thermal expansion ($10^{-6}\,C^{-1}$)	50–80
Heat distortion temperature (°C)	70–170
Cure shrinkage (%)	1–5
Water sorption in 24 h (%)	0.08–0.15

viscosity and flexibilizers to increase the impact performances of the final epoxy resin. Epoxide molecules in the pure state normally do not react with each other at room temperature. The polymerization (curing) reactions involved in network formation fall into two categories: curing agents and catalysts. A curing agent is added in significant amounts into the liquid epoxy to form a solid network cross-linked polymer and it becomes a part of the final resin. Commercial curing agents are aromatic amines, aliphatic amines, or anhydrides. On the other hand, catalysts are added in extremely reduced quantities to cause the epoxide ring to open and react directly with each other, or, in other words, to homopolymerize. Typical catalysts are certain Lewis acids or Lewis bases that can induce a self-perpetuating cationic or anionic homopolymerization, respectively. Characteristic properties of a typical fully cured epoxy resin are reported in Table 3.5.

Other thermosetting resins used as matrices for structural composites are phenolics (Agarwal and Broutman, 1990), aromatic polyimides (Gibbs, 1998), and other special high-temperature resins like bismaleimides and cyanate esters (Shimp, 1998). Typical properties of some of the above-cited resins are reported in Table 3.6.

3.3.2. Thermoplastic Matrices

Thermoplastic polymers have very few or no chemical cross-links and can consequently be processed by increasing the temperature until the solid polymer becomes a high-viscosity liquid. When in this state, reinforcements can be added and the material can undergo injection, extrusion, and several other forming processes. Since no irreversible chemical reactions occur during the molding process, the thermoplastic can, in principle, be remolded many times. From the practical point of view, a certain thermal degradation during processing prevents the material from restoring the same physical properties when re-processed.

Table 3.6. Typical Properties of Phenolics, Polyimide, Bismaleimide, and Cyanate Ester Resins

	Phenolics	Polyimide (PMR-15)	Bismaleimide matrimid (5292)	Cyanate ester (AroCy B)
Density (g/cm^3)	1.30	1.31	1.23	1.20
Tensile modulus (GPa)	3.5	3.2	4.3	3.2
Tensile strength (MPa)	50–55	55	82	88
Strain at break (%)	1.7	1.5	2.3	3.2
Coefficient of linear thermal expansion ($10^{-6}\,C^{-1}$)	45–110	16	63	64
Glass transition temperature (°C)	—	335	295	289

Due to processing difficulties related to the very high viscosity of polymer melts, thermoplastic matrices are predominantly used to obtain short-fiber-reinforced composites. Molding compounds, typically reinforced with 20 to 40% by weight of short E-glass or carbon fibers, are transformed into the final product by injection molding processes directly adapted from the plastic technology. The most common matrices employed for the production of short-fiber-reinforced composites are polypropylene (PP), nylons (PA), polybutyleneterephthalate (PBT), polyethyleneterephthalate (PET), polycarbonate (PC), and polyphenylene sulfide (PPS), whose typical properties are reported in Table 3.7.

Recently, a number of commercial long-fiber composites based on thermoplastic matrices have emerged for high-temperature structural applications. In these newer high-performance thermoplastic matrices, mechanical properties, temperature stability, and solvent resistance have been greatly improved by the introduction of rigid aromatic rings instead of aliphatic chains in order to attain performances often equivalent to or even better than the best thermosets. The polymer chain is flexibilized by the introduction of groups such as carbonyl, ether, ester, amide, etc., between the aromatic rings, thus permitting the processability. Examples of such high-performance thermoplastic matrices are polyarylenesulfide (PAS), polyetheretherketone (PEEK), polysulfone (PSU), polyethersulfone (PES), polyamideimide (PAI), polyetherimide (PEI), and thermoplastic polyimide (TPI), whose characteristic properties are reported in Table 3.7. More information about thermoplastic matrices for composite materials are reported by Béland (1990) and Berglund (1998).

Table 3.7. Characteristic Properties of Some Typical Thermoplastic Matrices

Material	Tensile modulus (GPa)	Tensile strength (MPa)	Glass transition temperature, T_g (°C)	Melting temperature, T_m (°C)	Processing temperature (°C)
Polypropylene	1.1–1.6	30–40	−10	165	200–240
Nylon-6	3.0 (dry) 1.5 (wet)	80–90 (dry) 50 (wet)	47–57	225	238–270
Nylon-66	3.3 (dry) 1.7 (wet)	90 (dry) 60 (wet)	48	265	270–320
Polybutyleneterephthalate	2.6	50	50	230	260–290
Polyethyleneterephthalate	2.7–4.0	50–70	70	265	280–310
Polycarbonate	2.3–3.0	60–70	150	amorphous	280–330
Polyphenylene sulfide (Ryton, Phillips)	3.5	80	90	280	300–340
Polyarylenesulfide (PAS-2, Phillips)	3.2	100	215	amorphous	330
Polyetheretherketone (Victrex PEEK, ICI)	3.1–3.8	90–100	143	343	380–400
Polysulfone (Udel P1700, Amoco)	2.5	70	190	amorphous	300–350
Polyethersulfone (Victrex, ICI)	2.6	80	220	amorphous	300–320
Polyamideimide (Torlon, Amoco)	2.8–4.4	90–190	275	amorphous	50–400
Polyetherimide (Ultem, GE)	3.0	105	217	amorphous	335–420
Thermoplastic polyimide (Avimid, Du Pont)	3.5	100	250	amorphous	340–360

3.4. Fiber/Matrix Adhesion

The level of adhesion between fibers and matrix plays a major role in determining the mechanical performances and environmental stability of most types of advanced composite materials. In fact, many ultimate properties like interlaminar and in-plane shear strength (Mahdukar and Drzal, 1991a), longitudinal and transverse tensile and flexural strength (Mahdukar and Drzal, 1991b), longitudinal compressive strength (Mahdukar and Drzal, 1992a), and mode I and mode II fracture toughness (Mahdukar and Drzal, 1992b) increase with adhesion level. On the other hand, elastic properties at low strain levels were found to be relatively independent of the fiber/matrix interfacial strength.

A great deal of earlier work concerning fiber/matrix interfacial strength measurements has focused on the development of reliable experimental test procedures (Herrera-Franco and Drzal, 1992; Kim and Mai, 1998). The most common methods involve the use of single-fiber composites in order to perform micromechanical tests, such as the fragmentation test (Kelly and Tyson, 1965; Fraser *et al.*, 1975) and a variety of single-fiber pull-out (Broutman, 1969), microdebond (Miller *et al.*, 1987), and microindentation (Mandell *et al.*, 1980) tests. A schematic presentation of the above-mentioned tests is reported in Figure 3.4.

One of the most widely studied is the "embedded single fiber" or fragmentation test in which a single fiber is embedded in the centerline of a matrix tensile specimen. Upon application of a tensile force the embedded fiber breaks repeatedly at points where the fiber strength has been reached. Continued application of strain to the specimen results in fiber fragments so short that the shear stress transfer along their lengths can no longer build up enough tensile stress to cause further failures and a limiting fragment size, defining a critical length L_c, is reached ("saturation"). From the value of L_c and the extrapolated fiber mean strength at the critical length $\sigma_{f-b}(L_c)$, a mechanical parameter called "interfacial shear strength" (ISS) can be obtained on the basis of a simplistic force equilibrium, based on the hypothesis of a constant interfacial shear stress along the fiber, first proposed by Kelly and Tyson (1965):

$$\text{ISS} = \frac{r\sigma_{f-b}(L_c)}{L_c} \tag{3.4.1}$$

where r is the fiber radius. The Kelly and Tyson model is described later in Section 3.7.1.

In the pull-out and microdebonding tests, the force, F_P, needed to extract a single fiber from a certain embedding neat resin of length L_m is

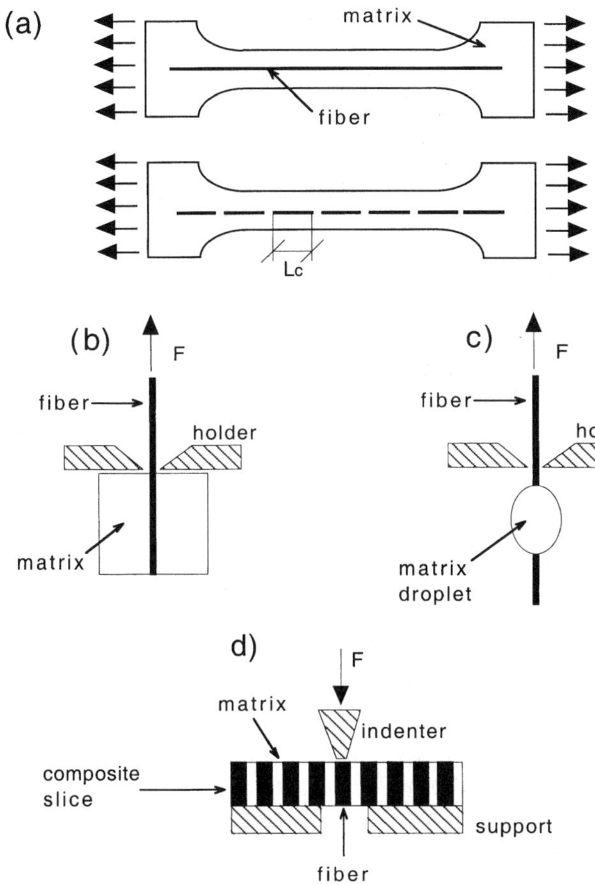

Figure 3.4. Schematic representation of the principal direct tests for evaluating the fiber/matrix interfacial shear strength: (a) fragmentation, (b) pull-out, (c) microdebonding, (d) microindentation.

measured in order to evaluate an interfacial shear strength value using the following expression:

$$\mathrm{ISS} = \frac{F_{\mathrm{p}}}{2\pi r L_{\mathrm{m}}}$$

Single-fiber methods are also called *direct tests* because they provide detailed information about the fiber/matrix interaction. For the purpose of quality control, or when the effects of environmental conditions on adhesion need to be determined, more rapid *indirect tests* are frequently used in which an interface-sensitive macroscopic property is evaluated. For example, several methods have been developed to measure the shear strength of composite laminates, like the $(\pm 45)_s$ tensile test (ASTM D 3518M, 1995), the Iosipescu shear test (Carlsson and Pipes, 1997), and the short-beam shear test (ASTM D 2344, 1995). It must be pointed out that indirect tests cannot be used to exactly quantify the fiber/matrix interfacial adhesion, but they can determine whether or not the adhesion level is acceptable.

The level of adhesion at the fiber/matrix interface depends strongly on the interactions between the composite constituents, which can be of mechanical and chemical type. Mechanical bonding depends strongly on the surface topography or morphology of fibers, as it is well known that surfaces of many fibers are neither smooth nor regular.

Chemical bonding is usually promoted by a number of fiber surface treatments or fiber coatings (sizings), depending on the nature of the fiber and matrix type. For example, immediately after the filaments are pulled from the melt, glass fibers are usually coated by a silane agent in aqueous solution which is intended to form a protective coating for the fiber surface and act as a coupling agent to improve the adhesion with various polymeric matrices (Plueddemann, 1991). When an organosilane is added to water, it hydrolyzes to form the corresponding silanol $R{-}Si{-}(OH)_3$:

$$R{-}Si{-}(OR')_3 + 3H_2O \rightarrow R{-}Si{-}(OH)_3 + 3HOR'$$

Hydroxyl groups of silanol are capable of forming hydrogen bonding with the hydroxyl groups of the glass surface, while the organofunctional R-group reacts with polymer matrix, thus promoting adhesion according to the following scheme:

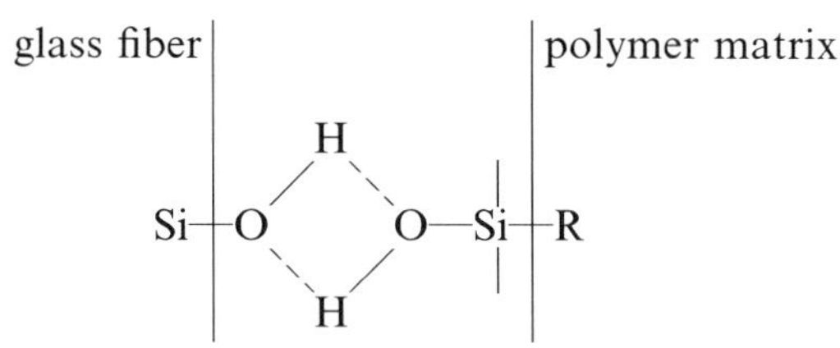

The organic end is resin-specific in order to optimize the adhesion with various polymeric matrices: the major contribution of silane coupling agents is to maintain the mechanical integrity of the interface in the presence of moisture.

Carbon fibers are also coated with a sizing agent whose main purpose is to protect them from damage, while the adhesion is usually improved through appropriate surface treatments (Hughes, 1991), which can be classified into oxidative (dry oxidation in the presence of gas, plasma etching, and wet oxidation) and nonoxidative treatments (whiskerization and plasma deposition of organic coatings).

3.5. Volume and Weight Fractions

Properties of composite materials are mainly determined by the relative proportions of matrix and reinforcing phases, which can be expressed as *weight* or *volume fractions*. Theoretical predictions of the composite properties are based exclusively on the volume fractions of the constituents, while during processing operations weight fractions are usually easier to control. In the case of a composite of volume v_c consisting of a volume v_f of filler (fibers or particles) and a volume v_m of matrix so that $v_c = v_f + v_m$, filler volume fraction, V_f, and matrix volume fraction, V_m, are defined as follows:

$$V_f = \frac{v_f}{v_c}; \qquad V_m = \frac{v_m}{v_c}$$

In the same way, filler and matrix weight fractions can be defined as

$$W_f = \frac{w_f}{w_c}; \qquad W_m = \frac{w_m}{w_c}; \qquad W_c = W_f + W_m$$

where w_c, w_f, and w_m are the corresponding weights of composite, filler, and matrix, respectively.

Conversion relations between volume and weight fractions can be established through knowledge of the composite density, ρ_c, which depends on the densities of the filler, ρ_f, and matrix, ρ_m, by the following relationship:

$$\rho_c = \rho_c V_f + \rho_m V_m$$

Now we can deduce that

$$W_f = \frac{w_f}{w_c} = \frac{\rho_f v_f}{\rho_c v_c} = \frac{\rho_f}{\rho_c} V_f$$

and in an analogous manner,

$$W_m = \frac{\rho_m}{\rho_c} V_m$$

3.6. Mechanics of Continuous-Fiber-Reinforced Composites

The most efficient and common way to build structures with continuous-fiber-reinforced composites is based on the use of so-called *laminates*. A laminate is obtained by stacking a number of *laminae* bonded together to act as an integral structural element whose behavior depends on the properties and orientation of its constituent laminae. Thus in order to analyze or design a laminate, knowledge of the behavior of single laminae is required. Models for predictions of the mechanical behavior of single laminae and multilayer laminates will be presented briefly. For a more detailed discussion the interested reader is referred to Agarwal and Broutman (1990), Mallick (1993), Gibson (1994), Barbero (1998), and Herakovich (1998).

3.6.1. Elastic Properties of a Unidirectional Lamina

As depicted in Figure 3.5a, a unidirectional lamina can be represented as a single composite layer with continuous fibers (of uniform properties and diameter) perfectly aligned along the longitudinal (L) direction. No slippage is considered to occur at the fiber/matrix interface. The L–T–Z coordinate axes in Figure 3.5a are referred to as the *principal material coordinates*, since they are associated with the reinforcement directions. An arbitrary set of reference axes X–Y–Z exists, where X and Y represent the *loading directions*. The angle θ between the positive x-axis and the L-axis is called the *fiber orientation angle*. A lamina referred to the principal material coordinates is called a *specially orthotropic lamina*, while a lamina referred to arbitrary axes is called a *generally orthotropic lamina*. At a first approximation the lamina thickness is considered very small in comparison with planar dimensions, so that a plane stress state can be reasonably assumed.

It can be proven that, for a two-dimensional case, the elastic behavior of an orthotropic lamina is fully defined by five *engineering constants* (Agarwal and Broutman, 1990), i.e., the longitudinal elastic modulus E_L, the transverse elastic modulus E_T, the in-plane shear modulus G_{LT}, the major Poisson ratio ν_{LT}, which gives the transverse strain caused by a longitudinal stress, and the minor Poisson ratio ν_{TL}, giving longitudinal strain caused by a transverse stress. It is noteworthy that even if five engineering constants have been mentioned, only four of them are independent since the following relationship exists:

$$\nu_{LT}E_T = \nu_{TL}E_L$$

The engineering constants can be derived from the constituent properties and respective volume fractions on the basis of widely diffused

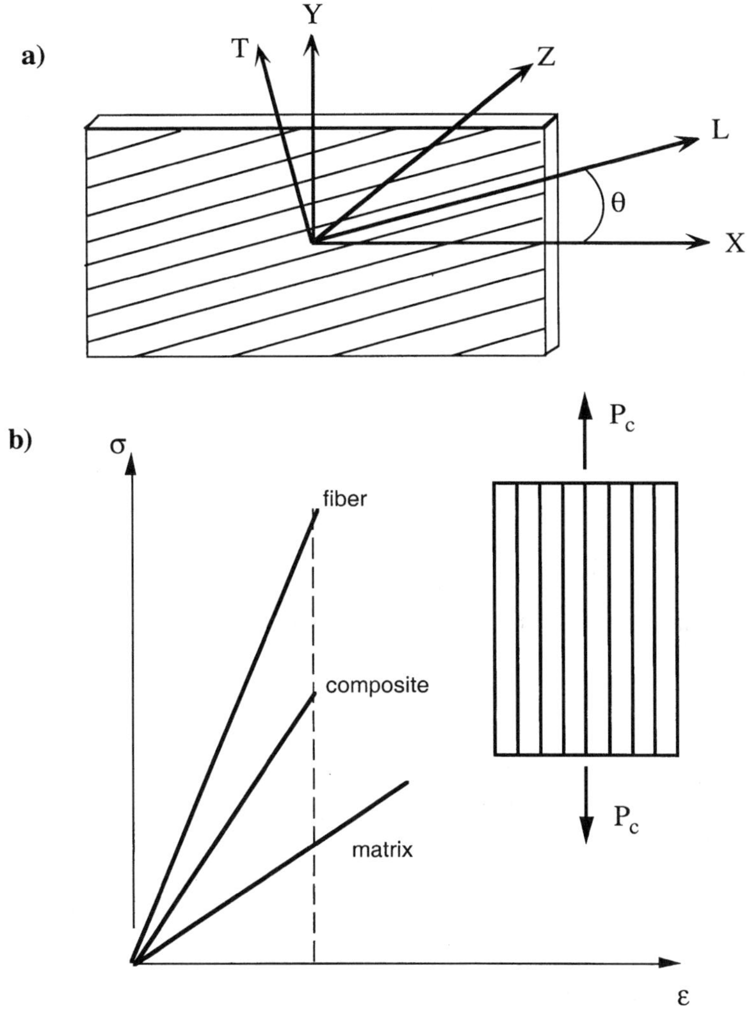

Figure 3.5. (a) Orthotropic composite lamina with principal (LTZ) and general (XYZ) coordinate systems; (b) stress–strain relationships for a continuous unidirectional lamina.

analytical and semiempirical models, which will be described briefly in the following.

Let us consider a specially orthotropic lamina with a load F_L applied along the L-direction (see Figure 3.5b). Since a perfect bonding is assumed to exist between the fibers and the matrix, the strains of the composite and its constituents must be the same, i.e.,

$$\varepsilon_L = \varepsilon_{\rm f} = \varepsilon_{\rm m} \tag{3.6.1}$$

while the load applied to the composite is shared between the fibers, $F_{\rm f}$, and the matrix, $F_{\rm m}$:

$$F_L = F_{\rm f} + F_{\rm m} \tag{3.6.2}$$

In term of stresses, equation (3.6.2) can be rewritten as

$$F_L = \sigma_L A_L = \sigma_{\rm f} A_{\rm f} + \sigma_{\rm m} A_{\rm m} \qquad \text{or} \qquad \sigma_L = \sigma_{\rm f}\frac{A_{\rm f}}{A_L} + \sigma_{\rm m}\frac{A_{\rm m}}{A_L}$$

where A_L, $A_{\rm f}$, and A_m are the composite, fiber, and matrix cross-sectional areas, respectively. By taking into account that area fractions are equal to volume fractions for composites with parallel fibers, it follows that

$$\sigma_L = \sigma_{\rm f} V_{\rm f} + \sigma_{\rm m} V_{\rm m} \tag{3.6.3}$$

Dividing the terms of equation (3.6.3) by the composite strain, it follows that

$$\frac{\sigma_L}{\varepsilon_L} = \frac{\sigma_{\rm f}}{\varepsilon_L} V_{\rm f} + \frac{\sigma_{\rm m}}{\varepsilon_L} V_{\rm m} = \frac{\sigma_{\rm f}}{\varepsilon_{\rm f}} V_{\rm f} + \frac{\sigma_{\rm m}}{\varepsilon_{\rm m}} V_{\rm m} \tag{3.6.4}$$

The composite, fiber, and matrix stress-to-strain ratios of equation (3.6.4) can be now replaced by the corresponding elastic moduli, thus giving

$$E_L = E_{\rm f} V_{\rm f} + E_{\rm m} V_{\rm m} \tag{3.6.5}$$

The above equation is called the *rule of mixtures.*

Figure 3.5b shows schematically that the composite stress–strain curve would lie between the stress–strain curves of the fiber and the matrix, with a slope depending on $V_{\rm f}$.

Prediction of the transverse and in-plane shear elastic moduli is more difficult than the longitudinal case, and an exact solution can be obtained only through quite complex micromechanics analyses. A detailed discussion of such models is reported in the review article of Chamis and Sendeckyj (1968). Nevertheless, for design purposes, satisfactory predictions can be obtained by the Halpin–Tsai equations (Halpin and Tsai, 1969; Halpin and Kardos, 1976), which represent an approximation of the generalized self-consistent micromechanics solutions developed by Hill (Hill, 1965). In general form, the Halpin–Tsai equations for oriented fibrous reinforcements can be expressed as follows:

$$\frac{P}{P_{\mathrm{m}}} = \frac{1 + \zeta \eta V_{\mathrm{f}}}{1 - \eta V_{\mathrm{f}}} \tag{3.6.6}$$

with

$$\eta = \frac{(P_{\mathrm{f}}/P_{\mathrm{m}}) - 1}{(P_{\mathrm{f}}/P_{\mathrm{m}}) + \zeta} \tag{3.6.7}$$

where P is a composite property; P_{f} the corresponding fiber property; P_{m} the corresponding matrix property; ζ is a constant depending on the reinforcement geometry, packing geometry, and loading condition; and V_{f} is the fiber volume fraction.

Engineering constants E_T and G_{LT} can be predicted by using equations (3.6.6) and (3.6.7) and appropriate values for the constant ζ. In particular, if E_T is the composite property of interest, then $P = E_L$; $\eta = 2$; $P_{\mathrm{f}} = E_{\mathrm{f}}$; $P_{\mathrm{m}} = E_{\mathrm{m}}$. In the case of G_{LT} it follows that $P = G_{LT}$; $\eta = 1$; $P_{\mathrm{f}} = G_{\mathrm{f}}$; $P_{\mathrm{m}} = G_{\mathrm{m}}$.

The major Poisson ratio ν_{LT} can be predicted satisfactorily by using a rule of mixture relation (Agarwal and Broutman, 1990):

$$\nu_{LT} = \nu_{\mathrm{f}} V_{\mathrm{f}} + \nu_{\mathrm{f}} V_{\mathrm{f}} \tag{3.6.8}$$

Characteristic values of the engineering constants and strengths for some unidirectional and cross-ply fabric reinforced laminae are reported in Table 3.8.

The stress–strain relation for a specially orthotropic lamina under plane-stress conditions can be then stated as follows:

$$\begin{Bmatrix} \sigma_L \\ \sigma_T \\ \tau_{LT} \end{Bmatrix} = \begin{bmatrix} Q_{11} & Q_{12} & 0 \\ Q_{12} & Q_{22} & 0 \\ 0 & 0 & 2Q_{66} \end{bmatrix} \begin{Bmatrix} \varepsilon_L \\ \varepsilon_T \\ \frac{1}{2}\gamma_{LT} \end{Bmatrix} \tag{3.6.9}$$

where the four independent *elastic constants* Q_{ij} are related to the engineering constants by the following simple relationships:

$$Q_{11} = \frac{E_L}{1 - \nu_{LT}\nu_{TL}}, \qquad Q_{22} = \frac{E_T}{1 - \nu_{LT}\nu_{TL}},$$

$$Q_{12} = \frac{\nu_{LT} E_T}{1 - \nu_{LT}\nu_{TL}} = \frac{\nu_{TL} E_L}{1 - \nu_{LT}\nu_{TL}}, \qquad Q_{66} = G_{LT}$$

Table 3.8. Properties of Some Commercial Fiber Composites (Adapted from Agarwal and Broutman, 1990)

			Elastic constants				Strengths				
Material	Fiber volume fraction V_f	Density (g/cm^3)	E_L (GPa)	E_T (GPa)	G_{LT} (GPa)	ν_{LT}	σ_{LU} (MPa)	σ'_{LU} (MPa)	σ_{TU} (MPa)	σ'_{TU} (MPa)	τ_{LTU} (MPa)
Glass-epoxy E-glass/epoxy	0.45	1.80	38.6	8.27	4.14	0.26	1062	610	31	118	72
Carbon-epoxy AS/H3501	0.66	1.60	138.0	8.96	7.10	0.30	1447	1447	51.7	206	93
Carbon-epoxy T300/N5208	0.70	1.60	181.0	10.30	7.17	0.28	1500	1500	40	246	68
Carbon-epoxy IM6/epoxy	0.66	1.60	203.0	11.20	8.40	0.32	3500	1540	56	150	98
Aramid-epoxy Kevlar 49/epoxy	0.60	1.46	76.0	5.50	2.30	0.34	1400	235	12	53	34
Boron-epoxy B-4/N5505	0.50	2.00	204.0	18.50	5.59	0.23	1260	2500	61	202	67
Carbon-PEEK AS4/APC2	0.66	1.60	134.0	8.90	5.10	0.28	2130	1100	80	200	160
Carbon-epoxy T300/Fiberite 934 (fabric 0.18 mm)	0.60	1.50	74.0	74.0	4.55	0.05	499	352	458	352	46

Stress and strain components for a lamina referred to arbitrary axes oriented at an angle θ with respect to the reference coordinate axes can be obtained as follows:

$$\begin{Bmatrix} \sigma_L \\ \sigma_T \\ \tau_{LT} \end{Bmatrix} = [T] \begin{Bmatrix} \sigma_x \\ \sigma_y \\ \tau_{xy} \end{Bmatrix} \quad \text{and} \quad \begin{Bmatrix} \varepsilon_L \\ \varepsilon_T \\ \frac{1}{2}\gamma_{LT} \end{Bmatrix} = [T] \begin{Bmatrix} \varepsilon_x \\ \varepsilon_y \\ \frac{1}{2}\gamma_{xy} \end{Bmatrix}$$

where the transformation matrix $[T]$ is related to θ in the following way:

$$[T] = \begin{bmatrix} \cos^2\theta & \sin^2\theta & 2\sin\theta\cos\theta \\ \sin^2\theta & \cos^2\theta & -2\sin\theta\cos\theta \\ -\sin\theta\cos\theta & \sin\theta\cos\theta & \cos^2\theta - \sin^2\theta \end{bmatrix}$$

The stress–strain relation for a generally orthotropic lamina is hence given by

$$\begin{Bmatrix} \sigma_x \\ \sigma_y \\ \tau_{xy} \end{Bmatrix} = [T]^{-1} \begin{bmatrix} Q_{11} & Q_{12} & 0 \\ Q_{12} & Q_{22} & 0 \\ 0 & 0 & 2Q_{66} \end{bmatrix} [T] \begin{Bmatrix} \varepsilon_x \\ \varepsilon_y \\ \frac{1}{2}\gamma_{xy} \end{Bmatrix} \tag{3.6.10}$$

where

$$[T]^{-1} = \begin{bmatrix} \cos^2\theta & \sin^2\theta & -2\sin\theta\cos\theta \\ \sin^2\theta & \cos^2\theta & 2\sin\theta\cos\theta \\ \sin\theta\cos\theta & -\sin\theta\cos\theta & \cos^2\theta - \sin^2\theta \end{bmatrix}$$

Equation (3.6.10) can be expressed in a more compact and useful form by introducing a $[\bar{Q}]$ matrix, which relates engineering strains to stresses, referred to arbitrary axes $X-Y$:

$$\begin{Bmatrix} \sigma_x \\ \sigma_y \\ \tau_{xy} \end{Bmatrix} = \begin{bmatrix} \bar{Q}_{11} & \bar{Q}_{12} & \bar{Q}_{16} \\ \bar{Q}_{12} & \bar{Q}_{22} & \bar{Q}_{26} \\ \bar{Q}_{16} & \bar{Q}_{26} & \bar{Q}_{66} \end{bmatrix} \begin{Bmatrix} \varepsilon_x \\ \varepsilon_y \\ \gamma_{xy} \end{Bmatrix}$$

where the following relations exist between elements of $[\bar{Q}]$ and $[Q]$ matrices:

$$\bar{Q}_{11} = Q_{11}\cos^4\theta + Q_{22}\sin^4\theta + 2(Q_{12} + 2Q_{66})\sin^2\theta\cos^2\theta$$

$$\bar{Q}_{22} = Q_{11}\sin^4\theta + Q_{22}\cos^4\theta + 2(Q_{12} + 2Q_{66})\sin^2\theta\cos^2\theta$$

$$\bar{Q}_{12} = (Q_{11} + Q_{22} - 4Q_{66})\sin^2\theta\cos^2\theta + Q_{12}(\cos^4\theta + \sin^4\theta)$$

$$\bar{Q}_{66} = (Q_{11} + Q_{12} - 2Q_{12} - 2Q_{66})\sin^2\theta\cos^2\theta + Q_{66}(\cos^4\theta + \sin^4\theta)$$

$$\bar{Q}_{16} = (Q_{11} - Q_{12} - 2Q_{66})\cos^3\theta\sin\theta - (Q_{22} - Q_{12} - 2Q_{66})\cos\theta\sin^3\theta$$

$$\bar{Q}_{26} = (Q_{11} - Q_{12} - 2Q_{66})\cos\theta\sin^3\theta - (Q_{22} - Q_{12} - 2Q_{66})\cos^3\theta\sin\theta$$

3.6.2. Elastic Properties of a Laminate

A laminate is obtained by stacking various laminae oriented to produce a structural element in which the bond between laminae is assumed to be perfect, so they cannot slip over each other. When loads are applied, the laminate stresses vary from layer to layer. For analysis purpose, it is convenient to define an equivalent system of forces and moments acting on the laminate midplane. With reference to the laminate depicted in Figure 3.6, whose thickness is h and which consists of n orthotropic laminae, the resultant forces per unit laminate width can be obtained by integrating the laminate stresses over the laminate thickness:

$$N_x = \int_{-h/2}^{h/2} \sigma_x \, dz, \qquad N_y = \int_{-h/2}^{h/2} \sigma_y \, dz, \qquad N_{xy} = \int_{-h/2}^{h/2} \tau_{xy} \, dz$$

In a similar manner, the resultant moments per unit width can be obtained as follows:

$$M_x = \int_{-h/2}^{h/2} \sigma_x z \, dz, \qquad M_y = \int_{-h/2}^{h/2} \sigma_y z \, dz, \qquad M_{xy} = \int_{-h/2}^{h/2} \tau_{xy} z \, dz$$

At this point the resultant forces and moments can be related to the midplane strain, ε^0, and curvature, k, through the following relationships:

$$\begin{Bmatrix} N_x \\ N_y \\ N_{xy} \end{Bmatrix} = \begin{bmatrix} A_{11} & A_{12} & A_{16} \\ A_{12} & A_{22} & A_{26} \\ A_{16} & A_{26} & A_{66} \end{bmatrix} \begin{Bmatrix} \varepsilon_x^0 \\ \varepsilon_y^0 \\ \gamma_{xy}^0 \end{Bmatrix} + \begin{bmatrix} B_{11} & B_{12} & B_{16} \\ B_{12} & B_{22} & B_{26} \\ B_{16} & B_{26} & B_{66} \end{bmatrix} \begin{Bmatrix} k_x \\ k_y \\ k_{xy} \end{Bmatrix} \qquad (3.6.11)$$

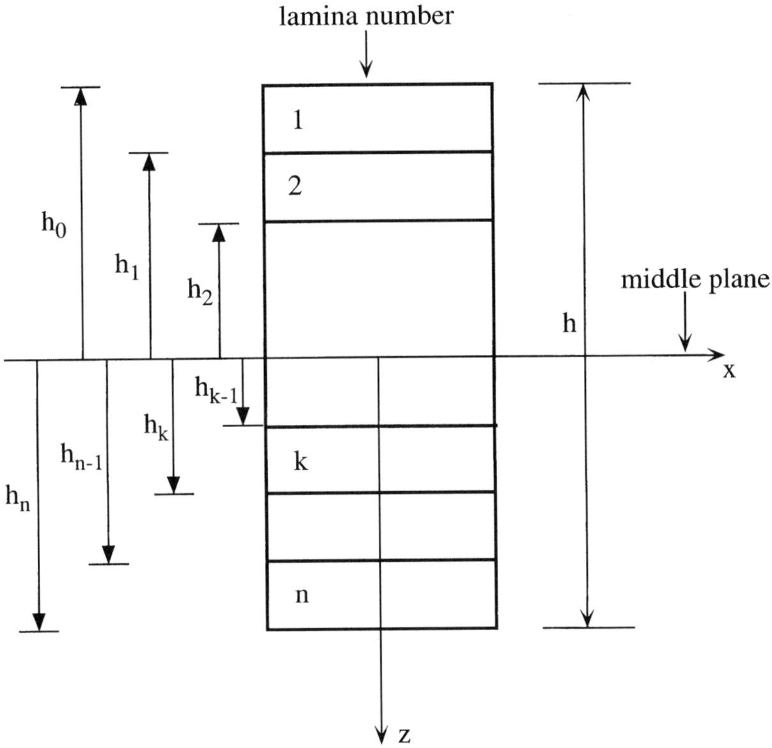

Figure 3.6. Cross-sectional geometry of a composite laminate. Adapted from Agarwal and Broutman (1990), p. 192, with kind permission of John Wiley & Sons, Inc.

and

$$\begin{Bmatrix} M_x \\ M_y \\ M_{xy} \end{Bmatrix} = \begin{bmatrix} B_{11} & B_{12} & B_{16} \\ B_{12} & B_{22} & B_{26} \\ B_{16} & B_{26} & B_{66} \end{bmatrix} \begin{Bmatrix} \varepsilon_x^0 \\ \varepsilon_y^0 \\ \gamma_{xy}^0 \end{Bmatrix} + \begin{bmatrix} D_{11} & D_{12} & D_{16} \\ D_{12} & D_{22} & D_{26} \\ D_{16} & D_{26} & D_{66} \end{bmatrix} \begin{Bmatrix} k_x \\ k_y \\ k_{xy} \end{Bmatrix} \tag{3.6.12}$$

where

$$A_{ij} = \sum_{k=1}^{n} (\bar{Q}_{ij})_k (h_k - h_{k-1}), \qquad B_{ij} = \frac{1}{2} \sum_{k=1}^{n} (\bar{Q}_{ij})_k (h_k^2 - h_{k-1}^2),$$

$$D_{ij} = \frac{1}{3} \sum_{k=1}^{n} (\bar{Q}_{ij})_k (h_k^3 - h_{k-1}^3)$$

Equations (3.6.11) and (3.6.12) can be combined to obtain the *laminate constitutive equation*, written as follows:

$$\left\{\frac{N}{M}\right\} = \left[\frac{A\ B}{B\ D}\right]\left\{\frac{\varepsilon^0}{k}\right\} \tag{3.6.13}$$

Matrix $[A]$ is called the *extensional stiffness matrix*, because it relates the resultant forces to the midplane strains, while matrix $[D]$ is called the *bending stiffness matrix* because it relates the resultant moments to the laminate curvature. The so-called *coupling stiffness matrix*, $[B]$, accounts for coupling between bending and extension, which means that normal and shear forces acting at the laminate midplane are causing laminate curvature, or that bending and twisting moments are accompanied by midplane strain.

It is noteworthy that if the laminate is balanced (i.e., it possesses the same number of laminae having fibers oriented at θ and $-\theta$), the coefficients A_{16} and A_{26} of the matrix A_{ij} are zero; moreover, if the laminate contains laminae with the same orientation at the same distance above and below the laminate geometric midplane (i.e., it is symmetric), all the coefficient of the matrix B_{ij} are equal to zero.

Equations (3.6.11) and (3.6.12) imply that forces applied in the x- or y-direction to a symmetric and balanced laminate do not provoke shear deformation (because the laminate is balanced) or bending (because the laminate is symmetric).

When midplane strain and curvature are obtained through equation (3.6.13), the strain at any point in the laminate can be easily obtained by taking into account that:

$$\begin{Bmatrix} \varepsilon_x \\ \varepsilon_y \\ \gamma_{xy} \end{Bmatrix} = \begin{Bmatrix} \varepsilon_x^0 \\ \varepsilon_y^0 \\ \gamma_{xy}^0 \end{Bmatrix} + z \begin{Bmatrix} k_x \\ k_y \\ k_{xy} \end{Bmatrix}$$

For symmetric and balanced laminates, a set of equivalent elastic moduli (E_x, E_y, G_{xy}, v_{xy}) can be easily evaluated from the A_{ij} coefficients (Barbero, 1998):

$$E_x = \frac{1}{h}\frac{A_{11}A_{22} - A_{12}^2}{A_{22}}, \qquad E_y = \frac{1}{h}\frac{A_{11}A_{22} - A_{12}^2}{A_{11}},$$

$$v_{xy} = \frac{A_{12}}{A_{22}}, \qquad G_{xy} = \frac{1}{h}A_{66}$$

3.6.3. Failure of a Unidirectional Lamina

From the stress analysis procedure presented in the above section, the actual stress components in each lamina of a loaded composite laminate can be determined and compared with the material strength (see Table 3.8) in order to asses the load-carrying capacity of the composite structure. A *failure criterion* must be applied in order to predict lamina strength under a biaxial stress state using strength data measured from uniaxial tests, which usually provide values along principal directions for both stress and strain at break.

Among available multiaxial composite failure criteria (Chamis, 1969; Hashin, 1980), the most widely known are based on maximum stress, maximum strain, and maximum work.

3.6.3.1. Maximum Stress Criterion

According to this criterion, in order to avoid failure the following set of inequalities must be satisfied:

$$\sigma_L < \sigma_{LU} \qquad (\sigma_L < \sigma'_{LU} \text{ in case of compressive stresses}),$$
$$\sigma_T < \sigma_{TU} \qquad (\sigma_T < \sigma'_{TU} \text{ in case of compressive stresses}),$$
$$|\tau_{LT}| < \tau_{LTU}$$

where σ_{LU} is the longitudinal tensile strength, σ_{TU} is the transverse tensile strength, σ'_{LU} is the compressive longitudinal strength, σ'_{TU} is the transverse compressive strength, and τ_{LTU} is the in-plane shear strength.

This criterion does not account for any possible interaction between the stress components, being the predicted limiting value of a certain stress component independently of the presence of other stress components. As shown in Figure 3.7, for this criterion the failure surface in the σ_L–σ_T space is a rectangle.

3.6.3.2. Maximum Strain Criterion

This criterion predicts failure when strain components along principal directions exceed the corresponding strain at break values. In other words, to avoid failure the following set of inequalities must be satisfied:

$$\varepsilon_L < \varepsilon_{LU} \qquad (\varepsilon_L < \varepsilon'_{LU} \text{ in case of compressive strains}),$$
$$\varepsilon_T < \varepsilon_{TU} \qquad (\varepsilon_T < \varepsilon'_{TU} \text{ in case of compressive strains}),$$
$$|\gamma_{LT}| < \gamma_{LTU}$$

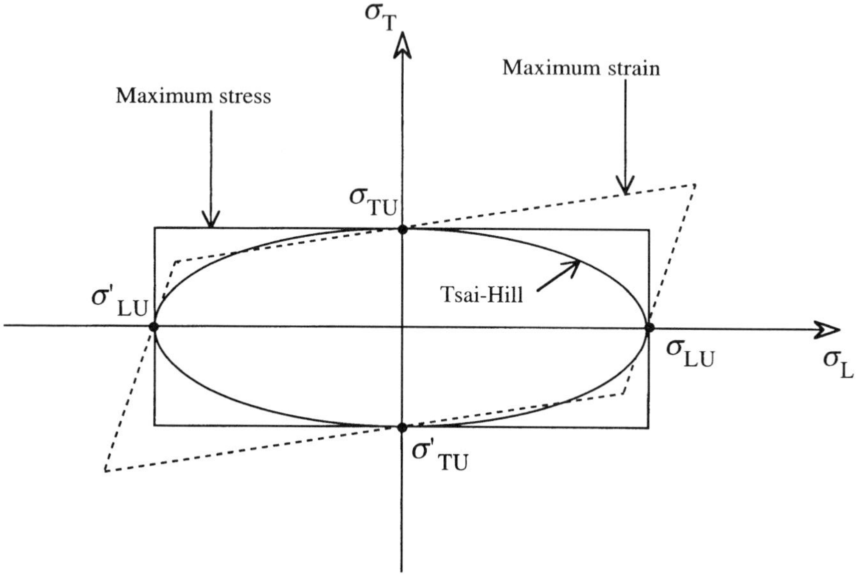

Figure 3.7. Failure surfaces in σ_L–σ_T space for the maximum stress, maximum strain, and Tsai–Hill criteria. Taken from Gibson (1994), p. 104, with kind permission of McGraw-Hill Companies.

where ε_{LU} is the longitudinal tensile strain at break, ε_{TU} is the transverse tensile strain at break, ε'_{LU} is the compressive longitudinal strain at break, ε'_{TU} is the transverse compressive strain at break, and ε_{LTU} is the in-plane shear strain at break.

In the σ_L–σ_T space, the failure surface for this criterion is a skewed parallelogram like that depicted in Figure 3.7, whose shape can be deduced from the lamina stress–strain relationships. In analogy to the maximum stress criterion, the maximum strain criterion does not account for possible interaction between strain components.

3.6.3.3. The Tsai–Hill (Maximum Work) Criterion

This energetic criterion predicts that failure occurs when the following inequality is violated:

$$\left(\frac{\sigma_L}{\sigma_{LU}}\right)^2 - \left(\frac{\sigma_L}{\sigma_{LU}}\right)\left(\frac{\sigma_T}{\sigma_{LU}}\right) + \left(\frac{\sigma_T}{\sigma_{TU}}\right)^2 + \left(\frac{\tau_{LT}}{\tau_{LTU}}\right)^2 < 1$$

The failure envelope in the σ_L–σ_T space is an ellipse, as shown in Figure 3.7. In the case of equal tensile and compressive strength values, the ellipse is symmetric about the origin; if the tensile and compressive strengths are different the failure surface will no longer be symmetric about the origin. The wide extent of this criterion is due to the fact that the equation defines one single function to predict strength, and that this approach does consider interaction between strength components, which is not the case for the maximum stress and maximum strain criteria.

3.7. Mechanics of Discontinuous-Fiber-Reinforced Composites

Composite materials containing short fibers as reinforcing agent are called *discontinuous-fiber-reinforced composites* or *short fiber composites.* The mechanical properties of these composites depend on various parameters like (i) constituents properties, (ii) fiber volume fraction, (iii) fiber orientation, (iv) efficiency of stress transfer at the fiber/matrix interface. Short fiber composites with a random fiber distribution are practically isotropic, while unidirectionally oriented short fiber composites are markedly anisotropic.

3.7.1. Fiber/Matrix Stress Transfer

Some aspects of the stress distribution in a discontinuous fiber embedded in a polymer matrix can be analyzed by considering the simple model presented in Figure 3.8a.

For static equilibrium of forces along x-direction the following expression can be written

$$(\sigma_f + d\sigma_f)\pi r^2 - \sigma_f \pi r^2 - \tau(2\pi r)\,dx = 0 \tag{3.7.1}$$

where σ_f is the axial fiber stress at distance x from the fiber end, τ the fiber/matrix interfacial shear stress at distance x from the fiber end, r the fiber radius, dx represents the length of a differential element of fiber, and $d\sigma_f$ is the differential element of stress. On simplifying and rearranging equation (3.7.1) the following differential equation can be easily obtained:

$$\frac{d\sigma_f}{dx} = \frac{2\tau}{r} \tag{3.7.2}$$

which can be integrated to give

$$\sigma_f = \frac{2}{r}\int_0^x \tau\,dx \tag{3.7.3}$$

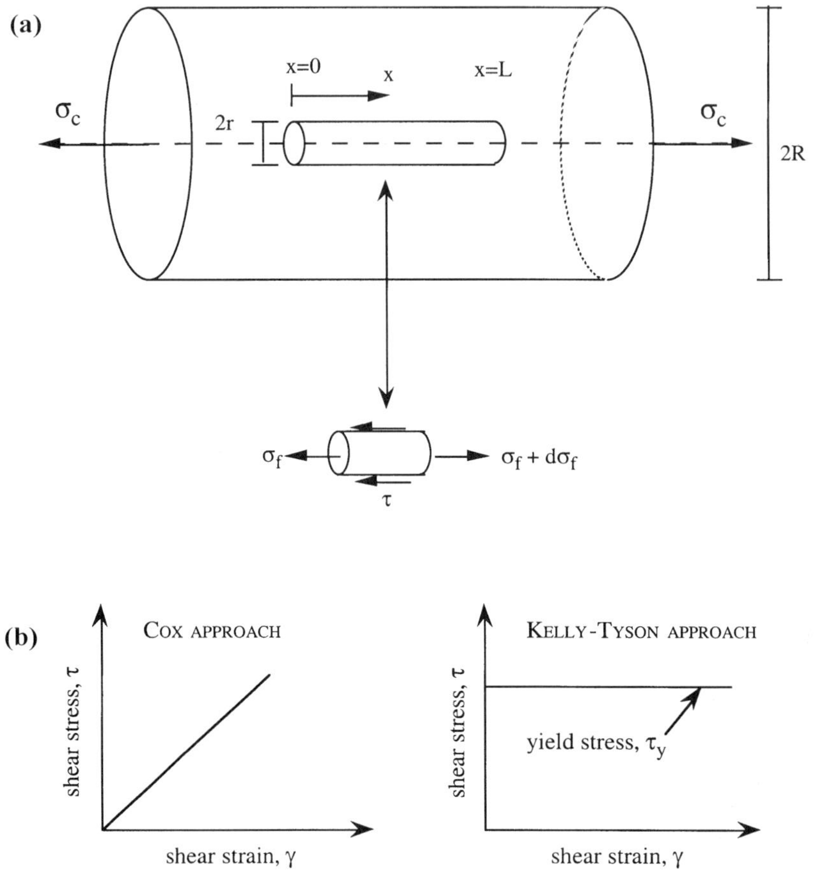

Figure 3.8. (a) Equilibrium on a differential element of a discontinuous fiber in the case of longitudinal tensile loading; (b) matrix behavior for Cox and Kelly–Tyson approaches.

It emerges from the latter equation that in order to determine the fiber axial stress, it is necessary to know the interfacial shear stress as a function of the distance x along the fiber. In the scientific literature two basic approaches have been proposed, based on different assumptions regarding the matrix behavior. Gibson (1994) summarizes the results of these analyses. In particular, Cox (1952) assumed that the matrix is linear-elastic, while Kelly and Tyson (1965) assumed a rigid perfectly-plastic matrix behavior (see Figure 3.8b). In both models the fiber is considered to behave in a linear-elastic manner up to fracture. For illustrative purposes, some results based on the Kelly–Tyson approach will be presented. This model implies that, along the entire fiber length, τ is a constant equal to the matrix shear strength, τ_y. Under this hypothesis it follows from equation (3.7.3) that

$$\sigma_f = \frac{2}{r}\tau_y x \tag{3.7.4}$$

This equation asserts that the axial fiber stress increases linearly from the fiber end ($x = 0$), where its value is zero. From the geometry of deformation we know that the axial fiber stress distribution must be symmetric with respect to the middle of the fiber, with $\sigma_f = 0$ for $x = L$. Consequently, the maximum fiber stress, σ_{f-max}, occurs at $x = L/2$ and thus

$$\sigma_{f-max} = \frac{\tau_y L}{r} \tag{3.7.5}$$

From equation (3.7.5) it is seen that, under a given composite stress, σ_c, the maximum fiber stress increases with fiber length. Of course, there is a limiting value for σ_{f-max}, which is given by the axial fiber stress in a continuous fiber composite, corresponding to $\sigma_c E_f / E_L$ (see Section 3.6.1). The minimum length required for the fiber stress to build up to the maximum value is called the *load transfer length*, L_t:

$$L_t = \frac{r E_f \sigma_c}{\tau_y E_L} \tag{3.7.6}$$

According to the Kelly–Tyson model, axial and shear stress are thus varying along the fiber length according to the scheme presented in Figure 3.9.

Another limiting value for σ_{f-max} is the fiber strength, σ_{f-b}. The minimum load transfer length required to have $\sigma_{f-max} = \sigma_{f-b}$ is called the *critical fiber length*, L_c, which is given by

$$L_c = \frac{r\sigma_{f-b}}{\tau_y} \tag{3.7.7}$$

Alternatively, this equation can be rearranged to give the interfacial shear strength expression reported in equation (3.4.1).

3.7.2. Elastic Properties of Discontinuous-Fiber Composites

Mechanical behavior of short fiber composites is quite a complex subject due to the fact that, as shown in Figure 3.10a, fibers are usually

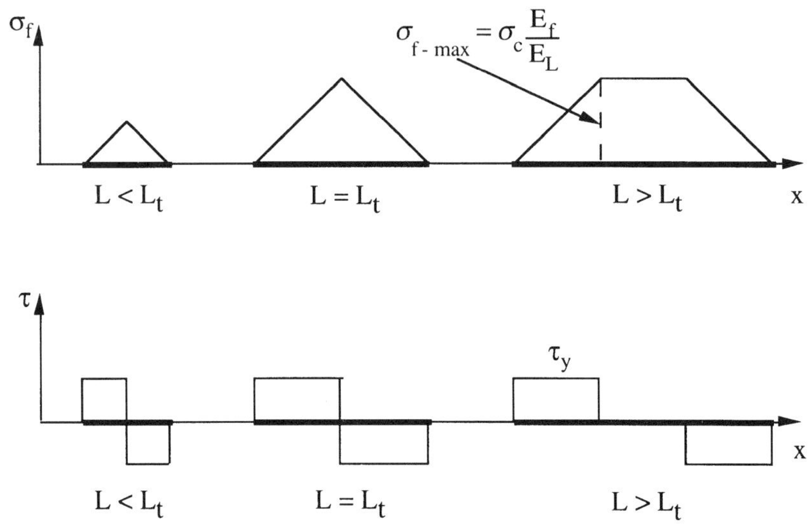

Figure 3.9. Axial and shear fiber stress distribution for various fiber lengths according to the Kelly–Tyson model.

randomly distributed inside the polymer matrix (or oriented to a certain degree), and because the load transfer efficiency depends strongly on fiber length (which, in general, is not a constant inside the composite) and on the fiber/matrix adhesion.

For discontinuous-fiber composites in which the fibers are aligned perfectly along the L-direction (depicted schematically in Figure 3.10b), the Halpin–Tsai equation can be profitably used to predict longitudinal, E_L, and transverse, E_T, moduli. In particular,

$$\frac{E_L}{E_m} = \frac{1 + (2L/d)\eta_L V_f}{1 - \eta_L V_f} \tag{3.7.8}$$

and

$$\frac{E_T}{E_m} = \frac{1 + 2\eta_T V_f}{1 - \eta_T V_f} \tag{3.7.9}$$

where

$$\eta_L = \frac{(E_f/E_m) - 1}{(E_f/E_m) + (2L/d)}, \qquad \eta_T = \frac{(E_f/E_m) - 1}{(E_f/E_m) + 2}$$

L is the fiber length and d the fiber diameter.

(a)

(b)

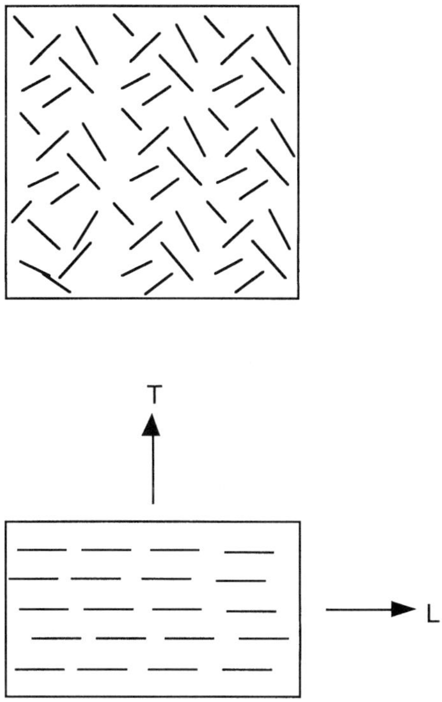

Figure 3.10. Schematic representation of (a) a random short fiber composite; (b) a perfectly aligned short fiber composite.

It is important to point out that for aligned discontinuous-fiber-reinforced composites, at a given fiber-to-matrix moduli ratio, the longitudinal elastic modulus increases as the fiber volume fraction and fiber aspect ratio (L/d) increase, as shown in the example ($E_f/E_m = 45$) reported in Figure 3.11a. On the other hand, the transverse modulus is not influenced by the fiber aspect ratio and depends only on the fiber volume fraction and on the fiber-to-matrix moduli ratio (see Figure 3.11b).

For a randomly oriented short-fiber composite (see Figure 3.10a), the elastic modulus, E_R, and shear modulus, G_R, can be predicted by knowing the longitudinal and transverse moduli, E_L and E_T, of an aligned discontinuous-fiber composite with the same fiber volume fraction, fiber aspect ratio, and fiber-to-matrix moduli ratio. In particular, for a two-dimensional isotropic case Tsai and Pagano (1968) proposed the following expressions:

$$E_R = \tfrac{3}{8}E_L + \tfrac{5}{8}E_T, \qquad G_R = \tfrac{1}{8}E_L + \tfrac{1}{4}E_T$$

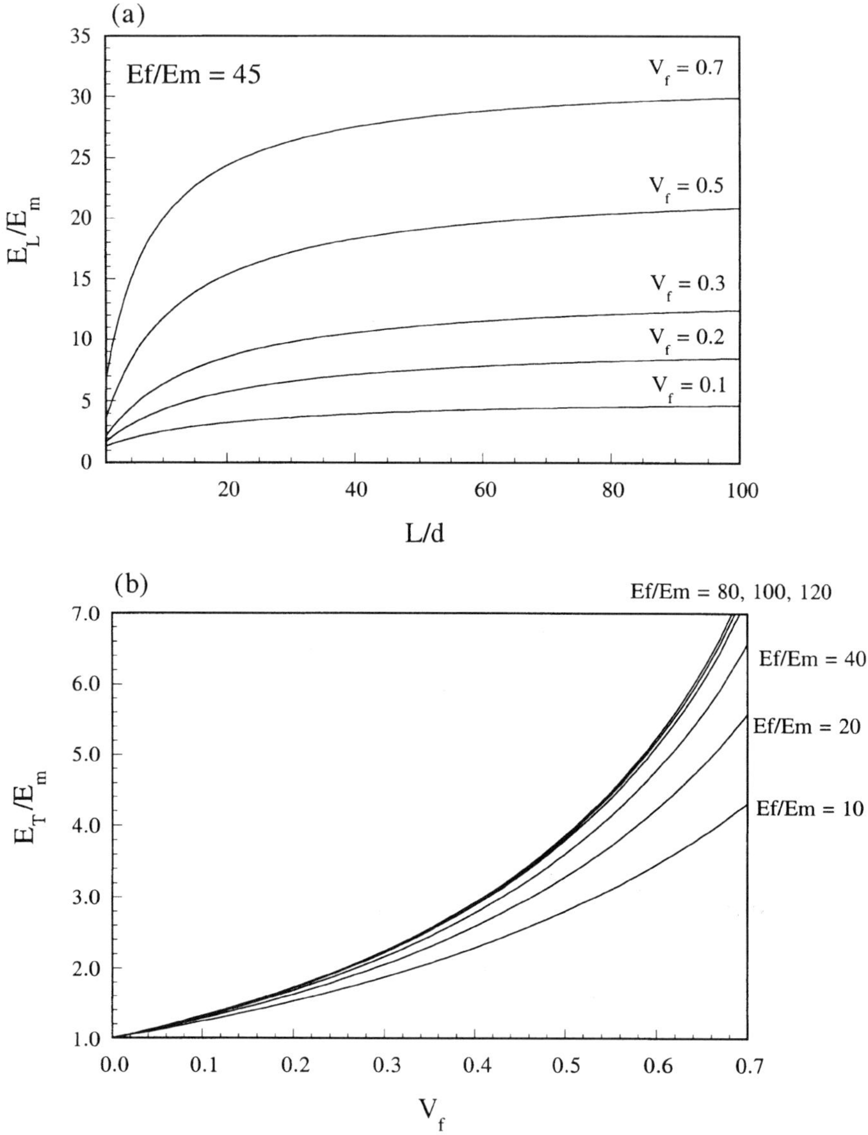

Figure 3.11. (a) Longitudinal modulus of a perfectly aligned short fiber composites (E_f/E_m = 45) as a function of fiber aspect ratio (L/d) for various fiber volume fractions; (b) transversal modulus of a perfectly aligned short-fiber composite as a function of fiber at various E_f/E_m ratios.

3.7.3. Ultimate Properties of Discontinuous-Fiber Composites

The load-carrying capacity of a short fiber can be analyzed on the basis of the fiber/matrix stress transfer mechanism. In particular, the average fiber stress, $\bar{\sigma}_f$ is given by

$$\bar{\sigma}_f = \frac{1}{L}\int_0^L \sigma_f \, dz$$

With reference to the Kelly–Tyson model described in Section 3.7.1, namely, the average fiber stress represented by the area under the curve of fiber axial stress plotted as a function of the fiber length L (see Figure 3.6), it can be found that

$$\text{if } L \leqslant L_t \quad \text{then } \bar{\sigma}_f = \tfrac{1}{2}\sigma_{f-\max} = \frac{\tau_y L}{2r}$$

while

$$\text{if } L > L_t \quad \text{then } \bar{\sigma}_f = \sigma_{f-\max}\left(1 - \frac{L_t}{2L}\right)$$

Considering that, on the basis of the rule of mixtures, the average longitudinal stress, $\bar{\sigma}_L$, in an aligned discontinuous-fiber composite can be evaluated as

$$\bar{\sigma}_L = \bar{\sigma}_f V_f + \sigma_m V_m$$

it follows that

$$\text{if } L \leqslant L_t \quad \text{then } \bar{\sigma}_L = \tfrac{1}{2}\sigma_{f-\max} V_f + \sigma_m V_m \tag{3.7.10}$$

while

$$\text{if } L > L_t \quad \text{then } \bar{\sigma}_f = \sigma_{f-\max}\left(1 - \frac{L_t}{2L}\right) V_f + \sigma_m V_m \tag{3.7.11}$$

Equations (3.7.10) and (3.7.11) can now be used to predict the composite longitudinal strength, σ_{LU}, of a perfectly aligned short-fiber composite which, depending on the fiber length, is given by

$$\sigma_{LU} = \tfrac{1}{2}\sigma_{f-max} V_f + \sigma_m V_m = \frac{\tau_y L}{2r} V_f + \sigma_{mu} V_m \quad \text{if } L \leqslant L_c \tag{3.7.12}$$

or

$$\sigma_{LU} = \sigma_{f-b}\left(1 - \frac{L_c}{2L}\right) V_f + \sigma_{m\varepsilon_{f-b}} V_m \quad \text{if } L > L_c \tag{3.7.13}$$

where σ_{mu} is the matrix strength and $\sigma_{m\varepsilon_{f-b}}$ is the matrix stress corresponding to the fiber strain at break, ε_{f-b}.

It is worth noting that when $L \gg L_c$, equation (3.7.13) reduces to the following expression:

$$\sigma_{LU} = \sigma_{f-b} V_f + \sigma_{m\varepsilon_{f-b}} V_m \quad \text{if } L \gg L_c \tag{3.7.14}$$

which can even be used to estimate the tensile longitudinal strength of a continuous unidirectional lamina.

Fibers increase the strength of the matrix, but only if their volume fraction is higher than a defined critical value V_{crit}. Below V_{crit}, the addition of fibers reduces the strength of the material. The higher the stiffness of the matrix and the lower the strength of the fibers, the higher V_{crit}, so that V_{crit} is very small (in most cases, less than 1%) for conventional polymeric composites, but it can become much higher for metal- or ceramic-based composites.

3.8. Mechanics of Particulate Composites

As already stated, the addition of rigid particles generally increases the elastic properties of a composite (but to a lower extent than fibers), while producing a contrasting effect on its ultimate properties. Of course, elastic properties decrease if particles less rigid than the matrix are used, and this could be the target for some specific applications (refer, for instance, to the use of rubber particles in glassy polymers in order to improve their toughness). In industrial applications, therefore, particles are added to a matrix in order to decrease its cost, or to improve specific properties like, for instance, electrical conductivity, thermal properties, or surface hardness.

From the standpoint of their application as biomaterials, particulate composites, however, assume a specific, important role being, for instance, already widely used in dentistry for teeth restoration, or being proposed as bone substitutes, often with the use of bioactive fillers coupled with biodegradable or not biodegradable matrices. In the former case particles are added to the acrylic matrix mainly to increase compressive mechanical properties and hardness, and to improve material dimensional stability. For bone substitutes, again the addition of particles can produce materials having compressive properties similar to the natural bone, with a moderate improvement of the tensile elastic properties.

Usually, particles used as fillers in polymeric composites are metallic or ceramic. Examples are calcium carbonate added to polyvinylchloride for the fabrication of pipes mainly in order to reduce the cost, the silica used, for instance, as reinforcing agent in silicon rubbers, or different metal powders (iron, nickel, aluminum, etc.) that are coupled to different polymeric matrices in order to produce electrically conductive devices.

The tensile elastic modulus of a particulate composite can be predicted by many equations, like the widely used Kerner equation (Ahmed and Jones, 1990):

$$E_c = E_m \frac{1 + ABV_f}{1 - \alpha_f BV_f}$$

with

$$B = \frac{(E_f/E_m) - 1}{(E_f/E_m) + A} \qquad \text{and} \qquad \alpha_f = 1 + \frac{1 - V_{max}}{V_{max}^2} V_f$$

where A is a parameter which depends on the particle shape and V_{max} represents the maximum packing fraction of the filler.

The addition of rigid particles reduces the deformation at break of the polymeric matrix, slightly increasing or not appreciably affecting its tensile strength, if particles adhere well to the matrix.

The adhesion again triggers the effect of the addition of particles on the material strength. In the case of poor adhesion the following equation, first developed by Nielsen (1967) and then modified by Nicolais and Narkis (1971), is in good agreement with experimental data for spherical inclusions:

$$\sigma_{cu} = \sigma_{mu}(1 - 1.21 V_f^{2/3})$$

where σ_{cu} and σ_{mu} are the tensile strengths of the composite and matrix, respectively, and V_f is the filler volumetric content.

3.9. Manufacture of Composites

The selection of a proper manufacturing or forming technique for a polymeric fiber-reinforced composite depends strongly on the type of matrix and fibers, on the required cost-effectiveness, and on the desired production rate. The manufacturing process is often the main point to consider in order to introduce a composite material for the fabrication of a given structural component (Richardson, 1987; Gutowski, 1997). The first fabrication method for fiber-reinforced polymer composites was the hand lay-up technique. Starting mostly from the mid-1970s, other methods for higher production rates like compression molding, resin transfer molding, pultrusion, and filament winding were developed, together with the extension of the traditional processing methods of the plastic industry (like extrusion and injection molding) to the fabrication of short-fiber thermoplastic composites.

3.9.1. Manufacture of Thermosetting Polymer Composites

3.9.1.1. Hand Lay-Up

By far, this is the most commonly used method for the fabrication of small and large fibrous reinforced composite structures (Agarwal and Broutman, 1990; Sidwell, 1998). Fibers and resin are placed manually on a open mold, made of wood, metal, or reinforced plastic, consisting of a flat surface, a cavity, or a convex shape. Reinforcements are usually glass-fiber mats, fabrics, or woven rovings, while resins are polyesters and epoxies. The mold usually requires some preliminary preparation with a releasing agent in order to facilitate removal of the composite part after the resin consolidation (cross-linking). When a good surface quality is desired, a specially formulated layer of resin (called the gel coat) is initially deposited on the open mold. The resin mixture is then applied to the reinforcement and compacted by using appropriate rollers in order to remove any entrapped air as carefully as possible. The procedure can be partially automated in a process (called spray-up) in which chopped fibers and resin are deposited simultaneously on the open mold by a special spray gun, as depicted schematically in Figure 3.12.

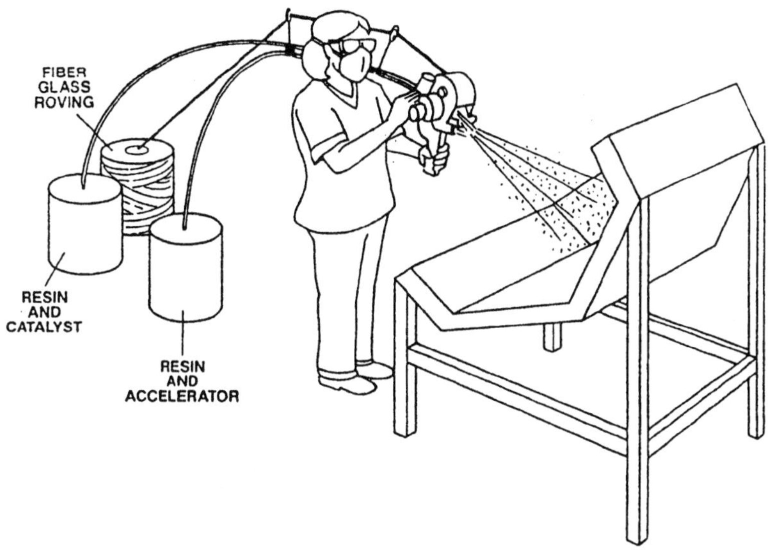

Figure 3.12. Schematic of a spray-up process. Taken from Agarwal and Broutman (1990), p. 34, with kind permission of John Wiley & Sons, Inc.

3.9.1.2. Bag Molding

This method is most important for the fabrication of high-quality composite components. The starting product for the bag molding is a *prepreg* (i.e., preimpregnate), which usually consists of a thin reinforcement layer (in the form of unidirectional fibers or woven cloth) impregnated with a partially cured resin (generally epoxy) to a typical fiber volume fraction of about 50%. A prepreg is generally stored at low temperature in order to prevent the resin reacting before the composite manufacture. Composite laminae are cut from the prepreg roll and positioned on each other according to the desired laminate sequence while ensuring that the fibers are aligned in the specified direction. The uncured laminate is then positioned between a bleeder, a breather, and various membranes and release materials, as shown schematically in Figure 3.13.

By means of an autoclave, the whole assembly is then subjected to a combination of external pressure, vacuum, and heat to consolidate and densify the various layers into a compact laminate. During this curing process part of the resin initially flows out of the prepreg, thus resulting in a typical fiber volume fraction of about 60%, which is an industrial standard for many structural applications. More details about this technique are

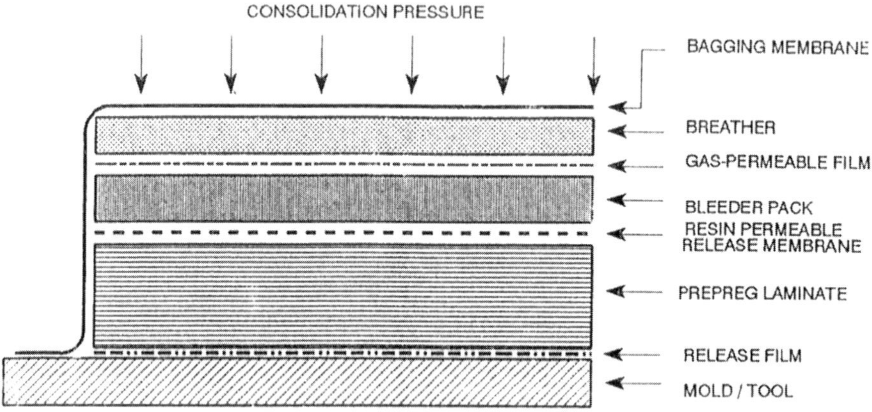

Figure 3.13. Typical setup for autoclave bag-molding of prepreg laminates. Taken from Bader and Lekakou (1997), p. 427, with kind permission of Marcel Dekker, Inc.

reported by Bader and Lekakou (1997), Dillon *et al.* (1997), and Sidwell (1998).

3.9.1.3. Filament Winding

Filament winding is a manufacturing process where continuous reinforcing fibers are wound on a mold, called the mandrel (Peters and Tarnopol'skii, 1997; Tarnopol'skii *et al.*, 1998). As depicted in Figure 3.14,

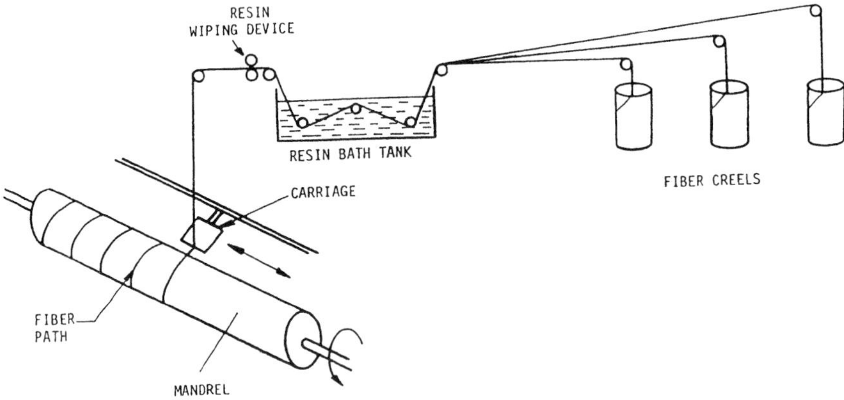

Figure 3.14. Schematic of a filament winding process. Taken from Mallick (1993), p. 345, with kind permission of Marcel Dekker, Inc.

fibers are passed through a resin bath before being placed on the mandrel, with a certain winding angle, by a carriage device.

The fabrication process is completed by the curing operation (which is usually performed in an oven) and the mandrel removal. The process can be used to manufacture objects with a surface of revolution, like tubes, pipes, pressure vessels, tanks, etc. In the case of cylindrical or conical open shapes the mandrel design is relatively simple, but when end closures have to be wound, the problem of mandrel removal arises. Available technological solutions are based on mandrels possessing segmented collapsible or inflatable parts, low-melting alloys, and frangible or soluble plasters.

3.9.1.4. Pultrusion

Figure 3.15 shows schematically how in the pultrusion process continuous fiber rovings and/or mats (generally of glass fibers) are pulled through a resin bath impregnator, then into a shape preformer, and finally across a heated die (Fanucci *et al.*, 1997; Sumerak, 1997; Wilson, 1998). During exposure to the elevated die temperature environment, the matrix resin undergoes rapid polymerization. The composite is then cooled by natural or forced air convection to a temperature level at which it can be gripped, pulled, and finally cut by a flying cut-off saw that enables the cutting without interrupting the continuous pull motion. The technique is a

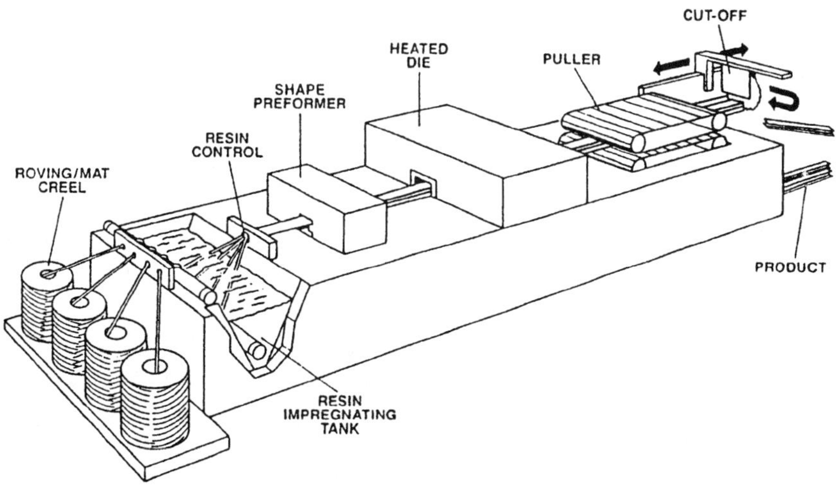

Figure 3.15. Schematic of a pultrusion process. Taken from Agarwal and Broutman (1990), p. 44, with kind permission of John Wiley & Sons, Inc.

highly automated process for the manufacture of composite materials into continuous, constant-cross-section profiles, like rods, tubes, and various structural shapes with a fiber content as high as 65–70% by volume.

3.9.1.5. Resin Transfer Molding (RTM)

Resin transfer molding is a process in which a fibrous preform is placed in the cavity of a closed mold (matched male and female parts) and a certain amount of premixed resin is transferred into the cavity by a pressure injection device (see Figure 3.16). Depending on the resin system and on the part thickness, an appropriate cure cycle is realized in the mold in order to attain sufficient green strength for the part removal. Final curing can be performed in an electric oven. The RTM process can be employed to produce complex structures and large near-net shapes at relatively low cost and with considerable time saving compared to conventional lay-up processes. More details on the RTM technique are reported by Fong and Advani (1998).

3.9.1.6. Compression Molding

As depicted schematically in Figure 3.17, compression molding is a manufacturing process wherein a molding compound (charge) is pressed in a matched metal mold and forced to fill the cavity. Heat and pressure are

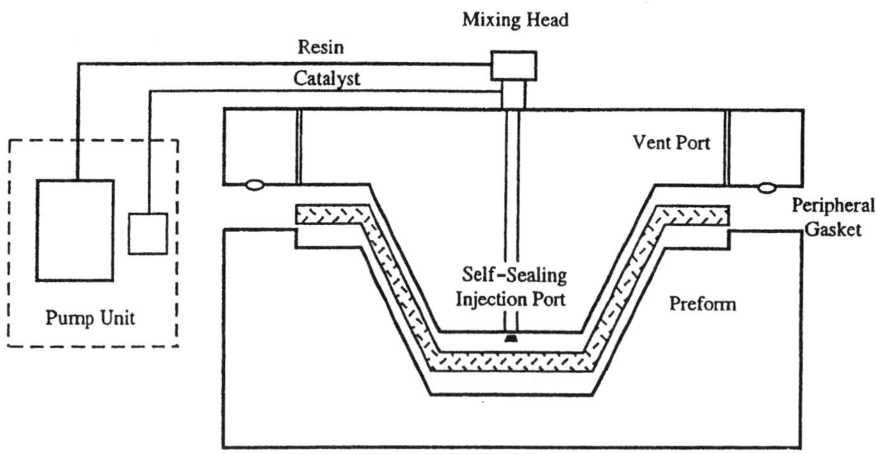

Figure 3.16. Schematic of a resin transfer molding process. Taken from Fong and Advani (1998), p. 433.

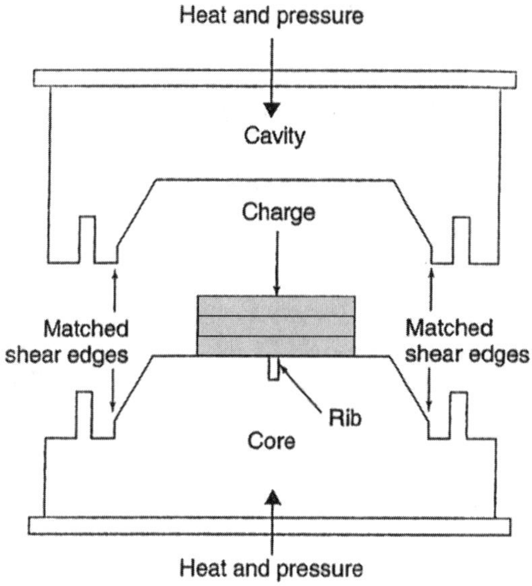

Figure 3.17. Schematic of a compression molding process. Taken from Haque and Leach (1998), p. 384.

then maintained until the composite charge solidifies. The charge can have two basic forms: (i) flat sheets, called sheet molding compound (SMC), invariably based on UP resin reinforced with chopped fibers mats; (ii) a doughlike mixture of short random fiber, resin, and filler, usually called bulk molding compound (BMC) or dough molding compound (DMC). These processes, presented in more detail by Castro and Griffith (1997) and by Haque and Leach (1998), enables large-scale production of wide surface area parts with tolerances acceptable for the quite restrictive automotive standards.

3.9.2. Manufacture of Thermoplastic Polymer Composites

The high viscosity of thermoplastic polymers in the molten state makes the fabrication of long (continuous) fiber-reinforced composites a quite difficult and complex task. For this reason thermoplastic matrices are predominantly used to obtain short-fiber composites, typically reinforced with 20–40% by weight of short E-glass or carbon fibers. Injection molding and extrusion are the principal techniques for the fabrication of short-fiber-reinforced thermoplastic composite parts. The fabrication machines are the same as for unfilled thermoplastics, but processing conditions are adapted for reinforced material. A detailed description of the above-mentioned processes is reported by Throne (1998).

During recent years a great deal of effort has been expended to assess innovative fabrication methods for continuous fiber-reinforced composites with thermoplastic matrices (Muzzy and Colton, 1998). Some high-performance thermoplastic matrices (like PEEK, PSU, PES, PEI) reinforced with carbon fibers are currently available as preimpregnated sheets (prepregs). Such composite layers are stacked to the desired sequence and spot-welded together along the outside edges in order to overcome the problem that they are not tacky (sticky) like the traditional thermosetting prepregs. The processing temperatures are much higher than the curing temperatures required for the thermosetting laminates, but the overall processing times are generally much lower. Other methods are based on the use of powder impregnated tapes, sheets and tows, or on commingled fiber tows or yarns (Okine, 1997).

References

Agarwal, B.G., Broutman, L.J. 1990. *Analysis and Performance of Fiber Composites*, 2nd edn., John Wiley & Sons, New York.

Ahmed, S., Jones, F.R. 1990. A review of particulate reinforcement theories for polymer composites, *J. Mat. Sci.* **25**, 4933–4942.

ASTM D 2344, 1995. Standard test method for apparent interlaminar shear strength of parallel fiber composites by short-beam method, in: *Annual Book of ASTM Standards*, Vol. 15.03, ASTM Philadelphia, PA.

ASTM D 3518M, 1995. Standard test method for in-plane shear response of polymer matrix composite materials by tensile test of a $\pm 45^\circ$ laminate, in: *Annual Book of ASTM Standards*, Vol. 15.03, ASTM Philadelphia, PA.

Bader, M.G., Lekakou, C. 1997. Processing for laminate structures, in: *Composites Engineering Handbook* (P.K. Mallick, ed.), pp. 371–479, Marcel Dekker Inc., New York.

Barbero, E.J. 1998. *Introduction to Composite Materials Design*, Taylor and Francis Inc., Philadelphia, PA.

Béland, S. 1990. *High Performance Thermoplastic Resins and Their Composites*, Noyes Data Corporation, Park Ridge, NJ.

Berglund, L.A., 1998. Thermoplastic resins, in: *Handbook of Composites*, 2nd edn. (S.T. Peters, ed.), pp. 115–130, Chapman & Hall, London.

Birchall, J.D., Brandbury, J.A.A., Dinwoodie, J. 1985. Alumina fibers: Preparation, properties and applications, in: *Strong Fibres* (W. Watt, B.V. Perov, eds.), pp. 115–154, Elsevier, Amsterdam.

Broutman, L.J. 1969. Measurement of the fiber-polymer matrix interfacial strength, in: *Interfaces in Composites*, ASTM STP 452, pp. 27–41, American Society for Testing and Materials.

Carlsson, L.A., Pipes, R.B. 1997. Experimental characterization of advanced composite materials, 2nd edn., Technomic Publishing Co., Lancaster, PA.

Cassis, F.A., Talbot, R.C. 1998. Polyester and inyl ester resins, in: *Handbook of Composites*, 2nd edn. (S.T. Peters, ed.), pp. 34–47, Chapman & Hall, London.

Castro, J.M., Griffith, R.M. 1997. Press molding processes, in: *Composites Engineering Handbook* (P.K. Mallick, ed.), pp. 481–513, Marcel Dekker Inc., New York.

Chamis, C.C. 1969. Failure criteria for filamentary composites, in *Composite Materials: Testing and Design*, pp. 336–351, ASTM STP 460, American Society for Testing and Materials.

Chamis, C.C., Sendeckyj, G.P. 1968. Critique on theories predicting thermoelastic properties of fibrous composites, *J. Compos. Mater.* **2**, 332–358.

Clements, L.L. 1998. Organic fibers, in: *Handbook of Composites*, 2nd edn. (S.T. Peters, ed.), pp. 202–241, Chapman & Hall, London.

Cox, H.L. 1952. The elasticity and strength of paper and other fibrous materials, *Br. J. Appl. Phys.* **3**, 72–79.

Dillon, G., Mallon, P., Monaghan, M. 1997. The autoclave processing of composites, in: *Advanced Composite Manufacturing* (T.G. Gutowski, ed.), pp. 207–258, John Wiley & Sons, New York.

Dobb, M.G. 1985. The production, properties and structure of high-performance poly(*p*-phenylene terephthalamide) fibres, in: *Strong Fibres* (W. Watt, B.V. Perov, eds.), pp. 673–704, Elsevier, Amsterdam.

Dockum, J.F. Jr. 1987. Fiberglass, in: *Handbook of Reinforcements for Plastics* (J.V. Milewski, H.S. Katz, eds.), pp. 233–286, Van Nostrand Reinhold Company, New York.

Donnet, J.B., Bansal, R.C. 1990. *Carbon Fibers*, 2nd edn., Elsevier/Marcel Dekker Inc., New York.

Fanucci, J.P., Nolet, S., McCarthy, S. 1997. Pultrusion of composites, in: *Advanced Composite Manufacturing* (T.G. Gutowski, ed.), pp. 259–295, John Wiley & Sons, New York.

Fong, L., Advani, S.G. 1998. Resin transfer molding, in: *Handbook of Composites*, 2nd edn. (S.T. Peters, ed.), pp. 433–455, Chapman & Hall, London.

Fraser, A.A., Ancker, F.H., DiBenedetto, A.T. 1975. A computer modelled single filament technique for measuring coupling and sizing agent effects in fibre reinforced composites, in: *Proceedings of the 30th Annual Tech. Conf. on Reinforced Plastics*, paper 22-A pp. 1–13, The Society of the Plastics Industry Inc., Washington D.C.

Gibbs, H.H. 1998. High temperature resins, in: *Handbook of Composites*, 2nd edn. (S.T. Peters, ed.), pp. 75–98, Chapman & Hall, London.

Gibson, R.F. 1994. *Principles of Composite Material Mechanics*, McGraw-Hill Inc., New York.

Gutowski, T.G. 1997. A brief introduction to composite materials and manufacturing processes, in: *Advanced Composite Manufacturing* (T.G. Gutowski, ed.), pp. 5–41, John Wiley & Sons, New York.

Halpin, J.C., Kardos, J.L. 1976. The Halpin–Tsai equations: a review, *Polym. Eng. Sci.* **16**, 344–352.

Halpin, J.C., Tsai, S.W. 1969. Effects of environmental factors on composite materials, AFML-TR-63-423.

Haque, E., Leach B.L. 1998. Matched metal compression molding of polymer composites, in: *Handbook of Composites*, 2nd edn. (S.T. Peters, ed.), pp. 378–396, Chapman & Hall, London.

Hashin, Z. 1980. Failure criteria for unidirectional fiber composites, *J. Appl. Mech.* **47**, 329–334.

Herakovich, C.T. 1998. *Mechanics of Fibrous Composites*, John Wiley & Sons, New York.

Herrera-Franco, P.J., Drzal, L.T. 1992. Comparison of methods for the measurements of fibre/matrix adhesion in composites, *Composites* **23**, 2–27.

Hill, R. 1965. Theory of mechanical properties of fibre-strengthened materials: III. Self-consistent model, *J. Mech. Phys. Solids* **13**, 189.

Hughes, J.D.H. 1991. The carbon fiber-epoxy interfaces — a review, *Compos. Sci. Technol.* **41**, 13–45.

Jaffe, M. 1987. High modulus polymers, in: *Encyclopedia of Polymer Science and Engineering*, Vol. 7, pp. 699–722, Wiley-Interscience, New York.

Juska, T.D., Puckett, P.M. 1997. Matrix resins and fiber/matrix adhesion, in: *Composites Engineering Handbook* (P.K. Mallick, ed.), pp. 101–165, Marcel Dekker Inc., New York.

Kelly, A., Tyson, W.R. 1965. Tensile properties of fiber-reinforced metals: copper/tungsten and copper/molybdenum, *J. Mech. Phys. Solids* **13**, 329–350.

Kim, J.K., Mai, Y.W. 1998. *Engineered Interfaces in Fiber Reinforced Composites*, Elsevier Science Ltd., Amsterdam.

Kumar, S., Wang, Y. 1997. Fibers, fabric, and fillers, in: *Composites Engineering Handbook* (P.K. Mallick, ed.), pp. 51–100, Marcel Dekker Inc., New York.

Lafdi, K., Wright, M.A. 1998. Carbon fibers, in: *Handbook of Composites*, 2nd edn. (S.T. Peters, ed.), pp. 169–201, Chapman & Hall, London.

Launikitis, M.B. 1982. Vinyl ester resins, in: *Handbook of Composites* (G. Lubin, ed.), pp. 38–49, Van Nostrand Reinhold Company Inc., New York.

Loevenstein, K.L. 1983. *The Manufacturing Technology of Continuous Glass Fibers,* 2nd edn., Elsevier, New York.

Mahdukar, M.S., Drzal, L.T. 1991a. Fiber-matrix adhesion and its effect on composite mechanical properties: I. Inplane and interlaminar shear behavior of graphite/epoxy composites, *J Compos. Mater.* **25**, 932–957.

Mahdukar, M.S., Drzal, L.T. 1991b. Fiber-matrix adhesion and its effect on composite mechanical properties: II. Longitudinal (0°) and transverse (90°) tensile and flexure behavior of graphite/epoxy composites, *J. Compos. Mater.* **25**, 958–991.

Mahdukar, M.S., Drzal, L.T. 1992a. Fiber-matrix adhesion and its effect on composite mechanical properties: III. Longitudinal (0°) compressive properties of graphite/epoxy composites, *J. Compos. Mater.* **26**, 310–333.

Mahdukar, M.S., Drzal, L.T. 1992b. Fiber-matrix adhesion and its effect on composite mechanical properties: IV. Mode I and mode II fracture toughness of graphite/epoxy composites, *J. Compos. Mater.* **26**, 936–969.

Mallick, P.K. 1993. *Fiber Reinforced Composites*, Marcel Dekker Inc., New York.

Mandell, J.F., Chen, J.H., McGarry, F.J. 1980. A microdebonding test for in situ fiber/matrix bond strength in composite materials, *Int. J. Adhes. Adhesiv.* **1**, 40–44.

Miller, B., Muri, P., Rebenfeld, L. 1987. A microbond method for determination of the shear strength of a fiber/resin interface, *Compos. Sci. Technol.* **28**, 17–32.

Muzzy, J.D., Colton, J.S. 1998. The processing science of thermoplastic composites, in: *Advanced Composite Manufacturing* (T.G. Gutowski, ed.), pp. 81–114, John Wiley & Sons, New York.

Nicolais, L., Narkis, M. 1971. Stress-strain behavior of styrene-acrylonitrile/glass bead composites in the glassy region, *Polym. Eng. Sci.* **11**, 194–199.

Nielsen, L.E. 1967. Mechanical properties of particulate-filled systems, *J. Compos. Mater.* **1**, 100–119.

Okine, R.K. 1997. Processing of thermoplastic matrix composites, in: *Composites Engineering Handbook* (P.K. Mallick, ed.), pp. 579–629, Marcel Dekker Inc., New York.

Peebles, L.H. 1995. *Carbon Fibers: Formation, Structure, and Properties*, CRC Press, Boca Raton.

Penn, L.S., Chiao, T.T. 1982. Epoxy resins, in: *Handbook of Composites* (G. Lubin, ed.), pp. 57–88, Van Nostrand Reinhold Company Inc., New York.

Penn, L.S., Wang, H. 1998. Epoxy resins, in: *Handbook of Composites*, 2nd edn. (S.T. Peters, ed.), pp. 48–74, Chapman & Hall, London.

Peters, S.T., Tarnopol'skii, Y.M. 1997. Filament winding, in: *Composites Engineering Handbook* (P.K. Mallick, ed.), pp. 515–548, Marcel Dekker Inc., New York.

Plueddemann, E.P. 1991. *Silane Coupling Agents*, 2nd edn., Plenum Press, New York.

Richardson, T. 1987. *Composites: A Design Guide*, Industrial Press Inc., New York.

Shimp, D.A. 1998. Speciality matrix resins, in: *Handbook of Composites*, 2nd edn. (S.T. Peters, ed.), pp. 99–114, Chapman & Hall, London.

Sidwell, D.R. 1998. Hand lay-up and bag molding, in: *Handbook of Composites*, 2nd edn. (S.T. Peters, ed.), pp. 352–377, Chapman & Hall, London.

Sumerak, J.E. 1997. The poltrusion process for continuous automated manufacture of engineered composite profiles, in: *Composites Engineering Handbook* (P.K. Mallick, ed.), pp. 549–577, Marcel Dekker Inc., New York.

Suplinskas, R.J., Marzik, J.V. 1987. Boron and silicon carbide filaments, in: *Handbook of Reinforcements for Plastics* (J.V. Milewski, H.S. Katz, eds.), pp. 340–363, Van Nostrand Reinhold Company, New York.

Tarnopol'skii, Y.M., Peters, S.T., Beil', A.I. 1998. Filament winding, in: *Handbook of Composites*, 2nd edn. (S.T. Peters, ed.), pp. 456–475, Chapman & Hall, London.

Throne, J.L. 1998. Processing thermoplastic composites, in: *Handbook of Composites*, 2nd edn. (S.T. Peters, ed.), pp. 525–555, Chapman & Hall, London.

Tsai, S.W., Pagano, N.J. 1968. Invariant properties of composite materials, in *Composite Materials Workshop* (S.W. Tsai, J.C. Halpin, N.J. Pagano, eds.), pp. 233–252, Technomic Publishing Co. Lancaster, PA.

Tsirlin, J. 1985. Boron filaments, in: *Strong Fibres* (W. Watt, B.V. Perov, eds.), pp. 155–199, Elsevier, Amsterdam.

Updegraff, I.H. 1982. Unsatured polyester resins, in: *Handbook of Composites* (G. Lubin, ed.), pp. 17–37, Van Nostrand Reinhold Company Inc., New York.

Vaughan, D.J. 1998. Fiberglass reinforcement, in: *Handbook of Composites*, 2nd edn. (S.T. Peters, ed.), pp. 131–155, Chapman & Hall, London.

Wilson, B.A. 1998. Pultrusion, in: *Handbook of Composites*, 2nd edn. (S.T. Peters, ed.), pp. 488–524, Chapman & Hall, London.

Yajima, S. 1985. Silicon carbide fibres, in: *Strong Fibres* (W. Watt, B.V. Perov, eds.), pp. 201–237, Elsevier, Amsterdam.

4

Biodegradable Polymers

Luca Fambri, Claudio Migliaresi, Kemal Kesenci, and Erhan Piskin

4.1. Introduction

At the end of World War II many classes of synthetic polymers, such as polystyrene (PS), polyvinylchloride (PVC), polymethylmethacrylate (PMMA), polyamides (PAs), polyester (PET), and polyethylene (PE), began to be produced and commercialized on a large scale. Due to their relative capability of being shaped, molded, or spun in the desired size by injection molding, extrusion, or other techniques, many products became available on the market for various applications in different fields. In the last 40 years, many other natural and synthetic polymers became available, both thermoplastic and thermosetting, either amorphous or semicrystalline, whose properties and formability depend on their chemical structure in terms of the number and type of chemical bonds.

Nowadays, several polymeric materials are widely used also in surgical and medical applications. The requirement of biocompatibility for all polymeric materials must also take into account the possible presence of plasticizers, fillers, catalyst residues, and various additives (heat stabilizers, antioxidants, external lubricants, colorants, etc.). In connection with biomedical polymers and depending on their behavior after an implant or when in contact with biological fluids, polymers can be classified as nondegradable or biodegradable. Typical nondegradable polymers are: polyethylene

---

Luca Fambri and Claudio Migliaresi • Department of Materials Engineering, University of Trento, via Mesiano 77, 38050 Trento, Italy. **Kemal Kesenci and Erhan Piskin** • Chemical Engineering Department and Bioengineering Division, Hacettepe University, Beytepe, 06530, Ankara, Turkey.

Integrated Biomaterials Science, edited by R. Barbucci. Kluwer Academic/Plenum Publishers, New York, 2002.

with ultrahigh molecular weight (UHMWPE), used in orthopedics (joints, total hip); polymethylmethacrylate (PMMA), polymerized *in situ* to form bone cements or used for contact lenses; polytetrafluoroethylene (PTFE), mainly known as Teflon™, with founding applications as vascular grafts; polyethyleneterephthalate (PET), known by the trademark name of Dacron, used for vascular grafts; polydimethylsiloxane (PDMS), an elastomeric silicone commercialized with the name of Silastic™, used, for instance, in soft tissue implants or in contact lenses.

Notwithstanding that the human body is a very aggressive environment, these materials are required to maintain their properties throughout their period of application. This objective can be achieved thanks to the specific stability of chemical bonds of the main backbone, which is constituted by carbon–carbon and silicon–oxygen bonds. On the other hand, various other polymers with one or more etheroatom in the main chain are susceptible of degradation, particularly by hydrolysis. Before the 1960s, hydrolyzable polymers were considered useless. However, Kulkarni *et al.* (1966) suggested using polylactic acid for degradable surgical implants, since the polymer hydrolysis would yield lactic acid, an intermediate in the Krebs cycle (Lehninger, 1977). Then, Schmitt and Polistina (1967) patented the synthetic absorbable suture application of polyglycolic acid, commercialized by Davis & Geck with the tradename of Dexon®.

The use of biodegradable polymers for the fabrication of biomedical implants offers at least two advantages: (i) the elimination of the need of a second surgery to remove the implanted prosthesis after the healing of the tissues, and (ii) the possibility of triggering and guiding the tissue regeneration via the degradation of the material.

Due to the above benefits, in the last 30 years the demand for biodegradable polymers has increased progressively, and several biodegradable polymer-based devices and prostheses have been proposed. Most of these systems are based on polyesters, such as polylactic or polyglycolic acids or their copolymers, that undergo hydrolytic degradation once implanted.

4.2. Definition

Williams (1981) considered *biodegradation* as degradation induced by the vital activity of an organism, and not simply the degradation of a material in a physiological environment. However, Feijen (1986) suggested broadening the concept of biodegradation to include all the degradation processes of a biomaterial, both *in vivo* and *in vitro*. Other terms such as bioresorption, bioabsorption, and bioerosion are also reported in the literature to describe the overall degradation phenomenon. In particular, a material is defined as bioresorbable if the degraded mass by-products enter into metabolic processes or are eliminated through natural pathways (Vert, 1989; Narayan, 1990). The term bioabsorption should refer to materials susceptible to be eliminated from their initial site with (Shalaby, 1988; Barrows, 1991) or without (Vert and Guerin, 1991) degradation of the polymer chain. Bioerosion implies the water dissolution of initially water-insoluble polymers at the surface and/or in the bulk (Park *et al.*, 1993).

Authors prefer to adopt the following definition proposed by Schacht (1990): *Biodegradable polymers are macromolecules that undergo chemical modifications when they enter into contact with a biological environment,... and the result is the formation of fragments of lower molar mass.*

4.3. Mechanisms

Degradation, according to Kronenthal (1975), proceeds schematically through four steps (water sorption, reduction of mechanical properties, reduction of molar mass, and finally weight loss), which in many cases occur with partial superposition or concomitantly, as shown in Figure 4.1. Initially, water and/or biological fluids diffuse into the material; then the mechanical properties change, i.e., usually the modulus and strength decrease, at the beginning due to the plasticizing effect of the fluids that reduce the polymer glass transition temperature and later on as an effect of the polymer molar mass reduction; shape modification and weight loss usually occur at later times. In particular, mechanical stress can induce material fragmentation, so producing particles with a larger surface/volume ratio. For instance, Figure 4.1 shows that after 2 weeks of degradation, water sorption reached about 10%, the residual strength and molar mass diminished by about 50% and 80%, respectively, while almost no variation of weight sample was registered. Only after 12 weeks was the residual weight about 80%, but the residual molar mass dropped to less than 50% and the specimen had no mechanical consistency (Fambri *et al.*, 2000).

Following Gilding (1981), biodegradation could occur through: (1) solubilization, (2) ionization followed by solubilization, (3) enzymatically catalyzed hydrolysis, (4) simple hydrolysis.

In the first two mechanisms, the degradation involves the dissolution of polymer chains directly or after ionization in aqueous medium while no break in the polymer backbone occurs.

Examples of polymers that undergo direct solubilization are many natural and synthetic polymers, such as dextran, polyvinyl alcohol,

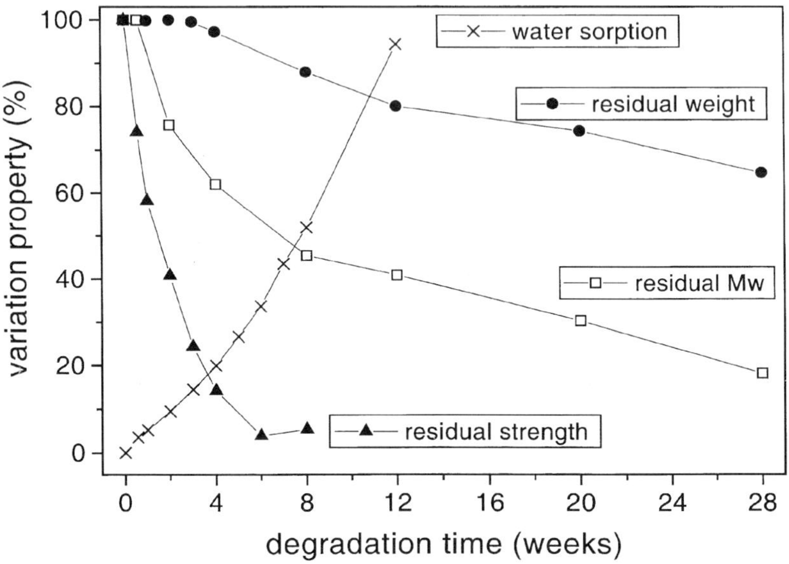

Figure 4.1. Typical variation of properties during degradation of biodegradable materials (dumbell specimens of PDLLA filled with degradable glass). Water sorption, residual tensile strength, molecular weight, and residual weight were considered.

polyethylene oxide, cellulose derivatives, and polyvinylpyrrolidone. The molecules of water first swell the polymer with disruption of its hydrogen bond, after which the polymer dissolves (MacGreger and Greenwood, 1980). The rate of this phenomenon depends on the type of polymer, the amount of available water and its flow, pH, the presence of salts, or other specific factors.

In this case of ionization, the polymer can form protonated or deprotonated species depending on pH; then it easily dissolves. For instance, derivative esters of cellulose, polyacrylic acid, or polyvinylacetate are used as enteric coating materials for pharmaceutical application (Chambliss, 1983; Murphy *et al.*, 1986). Another type of ionization involves the hydrolytic reaction of pendent groups, such as anhydride and ester. For instance, maleic anhydride copolymers become water soluble in a polyanion form (Heller *et al.*, 1990a); glutamic and aspartic acid derivatives resulted in being soluble depending on the grade of esterification and pH (Sidman *et al.*, 1980; Marck *et al.*, 1977).

On the other hand, the hydrolytic process causes fragmentation of the whole polymeric structure, either for enzyme catalysis or for simple water reaction. Hence, the physical or chemical process is responsible for the gradual modification of material properties during interaction with a physiological environment.

Polymers considered in this category are those susceptible to hydrolysis. In order to undergo hydrolysis, both linear and cross-linked polymers have to contain in the polymer backbone specific chemical functionalities, as reported in Table 4.1. Obviously in the case of biodegradable polymers, biocompatibility (Anderson, 1986; Williams, 1991) also depends on the newly-formed degradation products (organic acids, alcohols, amines).

Table 4.1 lists examples of degradable polymers in order of decreasing reaction rate. The more reactive the function, the higher the degradation rate. Polyureas, polyurethanes, and polyamides have been included, even if they are commonly considered to be stable polymers and if their degradation is really very slow. St. Pierre and Chiellini (1986) reported a comparative hydrolysis at room temperature as shown in Table 4.2.

Proteins and polysaccharides are natural polymers whose degradability in the body is well known, as a result of enzyme action. However, notwithstanding enzymes play a specific role in physiological reactions; enzymatic hydrolysis has been found to be effective also for many synthetic polymers especially with esterase activity, as reported in Table 4.3. It is well evident from the action of enzymes in polymers such as polyurethanes or polyamides, whose predicted simple hydrolysis would last many millennia. Enzyme-catalyzed degradation is also referred to in Chapter 7 of Park *et al.* (1993), where the type of body enzymes, and the specific action and effect that they have on modified proteins (albumin and gelatin) and polysaccharides (dextran, starch, amylose, and chitosan) is also reported.

Other degradation phenomena occur in a biological environment, such as oxidative biodegradation (Coury, 1996), which has been verified for

Table 4.1. Synthetic Polymers for Biomedical Applications

Nondegradable polymers	Biodegradable polymers
Polyethylene $[\text{—CH}_2\text{—CH}_2\text{—}]_n$	Polyanhydrides $[\text{—R—CO—O—CO}]_n$
Polymethylmethacrylate $[\text{—CH}_2\text{—CCH}_3(\text{COOCH}_3)\text{—}]_n$	Polyorthoesters $[\text{—O—CR(OR}')\text{—O—}]_n$
Polytetrafluoroethylene $[\text{—CF}_2\text{—CF}_2\text{—}]_n$	Polyphosphazenes $[\text{—N=PR}_2\text{—}]_n$
Polysilicones $[\text{—Si(CH}_3)_2\text{—O—}]_n$	Polyesters $[\text{—R—CO—O—}]_n$
	Polyureas $[\text{—R—NH—CO—NH—R}]_n$
	Polycarbonates $[\text{—R—O—CO—O—}]_n$
	Polyurethanes $[\text{—R—NH—CO—O—}]_n$
	Polyaminoacids $[\text{—NH—C*HR—CO—}]_n$
	Polyamides $[\text{—R—CO—NH—}]_n$

Table 4.2. Example of Polymer Hydrolysis (Decreasing Degradation Rate)

Polymers	Reaction	Hydrolysis time[a]
Polyanhydrides	(—R—CO—O—CO—R′) → R—COOH + R′COOH	5–10 minutes
Polyorthoesters	(—RO—CR′(OR″)—OR″) → ROH + R′—COOH + 2R″OH	4 hours
Polyacetals	(—R—O—CHR—O—R′) → R—OH + HRC═O + R′OH	9 months
Polyesters	(—R—CO—O—R′) → R—COOH + R′OH	3.3 years
Polyureas	(—R—NH—CO—NH—R′) → R—NH_2 + CO_2 + R′NH_2	33 years
Polycarbonates	(—R—OCO—O—R′) → R—OH + CO_2 + R′OH	42×10^3 years
Polyurethanes	(—R—NH—CO—O—R′) → R—NH_2 + CO_2 + R′OH	42×10^3 years
Polyamides	(—R—CO—NH—R′) → R—COOH + R′—NH_2	383×10^3 years

[a]Time required to reach 50% of hydrolysis at 25 °C and pH 7 (St. Pierre and Chiellini, 1986).

Table 4.3. Example of Enzymatic Hydrolysis (Decreasing Degradation Rate)

Polymers	Polymers	Enzymes	Reference
Polyesters	Polyglycolic acid	Bromelain, carboxypeptidase A, esterase, ficin, leucine aminopeptidase	Chu and Williams (1983)
	Polylactic acid	Bromelain, lipase, pronase, proteinase K	Williams (1981); Fukuzaki *et al.* (1989)
	Polycaprolactone	Esterase, lipase	Tokiwa and Suzuki (1977)
	Polydioxanone	Esterase	Williams *et al.* (1984)
	Polyhydroxybutyrate	Esterase	Kemnitzer *et al.* (1992)
	Polyhydroxybutyrate-co-hydroxyvalerate	Esterase	Parikh *et al.* (1992)
	Polyethylenterephthalate	Esterase, papain leucine, aminopeptidase	Smith *et al.* (1987a) Williams (1990b)
Polyureas	Polyesterurea	Elastase, substilisin	Britritto *et al.* (1979); Huang and Leong (1989)
Polyurethanes	Polyetherurethane	Cathepsin, esterase, trypsin, papain, urease	Smith *et al.* (1987b) Bouvier *et al.* (1991); Takahara *et al.* (1991b); Phua *et al.* (1987)
Polyamides	Polyamide 6,6	Chymotrypsin, papain, trypsin	Smith *et al.* (1987a)
	Polylysine	Chymotrypsin, elastase, ficin, papain, trypsin	Miller (1964)

various polymers, such as in the case of ultrahigh molecular weight polyethylene in joint prostheses or in antioxidant-free polypropylene. The polymer attack with the cleavage of a homoatomic bond derives from the phagocytic cells. In fact, polymorphonuclear leukocytes (neutrophils), macrophages, and giant cells produce a superoxide anion ($O_2^{-\cdot}$) that directly or through other derivative species—such as hydrogen peroxide, H_2O_2, and hypochlorous acid, HOCl (Test and Weiss, 1986)—attack organic polymers. Even urethane, urea, and amide bonds could be oxidized by HOCl. Moreover, traces of Fe^{2+} released in the implant site could catalyse the formation of the hydroxyl radical, which is a very aggressive oxidant (Klebanoff, 1982). Macrophages and giant cells can digest particles up to 50 micron or more in size.

It has been shown clinically that during inflammation processes, various implanted polymers exhibited a more rapid degradation, due to the so-called bacterial degradation (Williams, 1990a). However, the activation of mast cells that secrete chymase and tryptase, which behave as proteolytic enzymes with chymotrypsine-like and trypsine-like properties, must also be taken into account (Schwartz, 1990; Caghey, 1991).

Both aerobic and anaerobic bacteria displayed a large proliferation in the presence of polyesters, probably as a consequence of the metabolization of carbon derived from polymer hydrolysis. Finally, also a metal ion-induced oxidation has been reported for implanted polyurethanes for which, in the presence of metallic corrosion species, not only molecular degradation but also stress cracking phenomena occur, as a result of combined interaction between a metallic device, the biological environment, and the polymer. For this reason, the development of more biostable polyurethanes is recommended (Takahara *et al.*, 1991a).

4.4. Properties and Applications

The initial properties of the materials and the properties of a biodegradable polymer-made device determine its potential application. These properties depend on various factors, such as chemical structure, amorphous or crystalline structure, and glass transition temperature. In the literature, some papers review the physical-mechanical properties of various biodegradable polymers (Engelberg and Kohn, 1991), also of specific interest for orthopedic or surgical applications (Vainionpaa *et al.*, 1989; Daniels *et al.*, 1990).

Thermal and mechanical properties of selected biodegradable synthetic polymers are reported in Table 4.4. In principle, low glass transition temperature determines poor mechanical properties, especially for

Table 4.4. Thermal and Mechanical Properties of Selected Synthetic Biodegradable Polymers

Polymers	Tg (°C)	Tm (°C)	Modulus (GPa)	Strength (MPa)	Configuration	Reference
Polyglycolic acid (PGA)	35	225	6.5	57	tens	Christel *et al.* (1982)
fibers	—	233	13.4	750	tens	Authors' data
Polytrimethylenecarbonate (PTMC)	−15	*a*	0.003	0.5	tens	Engelberg and Kohn (1991)
Polyglycolide-co-trimethylenecarbonate fibers	—	222	3.17	606	tens	Benicewitz and Hopper (1991)
Polylactic acid (PDLLA)	55	*a*	2.0	42–49	tens	Authors' data
			3.5–3.6	84–85	flex	Authors' data
Polylactic acid (PLLA)	60	180	2.1	59–79	tens	Authors' data
			3.9–4.6	110–126	flex	Authors' data
fibers	57	184	8.5	700	tens	Hyon *et al.* (1984)
fibers	64	190	10.4	900	tens	Pegoretti *et al.* (1997)
Polycaprolactone (PCL)	−60	55	0.3	19	tens	Wehrenberg (1981)
			0.4	16	tens	Engelberg and Kohn (1991)
Polyhydroxybutyrate (PHB)	1	171	2.5	36	tens	Engelberg and Kohn (1991)
Polyhydroxybutyrate-co-hydroxyvalerate (7–22%)	−5/−1	137–160	0.6–1.4	16–20	tens	Engelberg and Kohn (1991)
Polydioxanone (PDS)	—	—	—	92	shear	Vainionpaa *et al.* (1989)
fibers	−16	110	1.7	549	tens	Benicewitz and Hopper (1991)
Polyimino carbonate	55/69	*a*	1.6–2.2	40–50	tens	Engelberg and Kohn (1991)
Polyorthoesters	55/95	*a*	0.8–1.2	20–27	tens	Engelberg and Kohn (1991)
Polyanhydride	—	46–49	0.04	4	tens	Engelberg and Kohn (1991)

[a] Amorphous.

Table 4.5. Mechanical Properties of Self-Reinforced or Oriented Biodegradable Polymers

Polymers	Modulus (GPa)	Strength (MPa)	Configuration	References
Polyglycolic acid	10–15	375	flex	Vainionpaa *et al.* (1989)
(PGA)		240	shear	Tormala *et al.* (1991)
Polylactic acid	—	180	flex	Vainionpaa *et al.* (1989)
(PLLA)		300–450	tens	Tormala *et al.* (1991)
		350–490	tens	Tunc (1995)
	13.7	215	flex	Ferguson *et al.* (1996)
	13	240	flex	Matsusue *et al.* (1992)

completely amorphous materials, and the lower the glass transition temperature, the higher the degradation rate. Crystalline materials and specifically fibers show higher mechanical properties, and in principle lower degradation rate. Table 4.5 reports the mechanical properties of PGA and/or PLA samples self-reinforced, i.e., combining fiber and matrix of the same composition, or having undergone a high-shear extrusion process.

Biodegradable polymers can be used in medicine (Gilding, 1981) as a temporary scaffold, a temporary barrier, and a drug delivery system. A temporary scaffold is utilized as an artificial implant temporary support able to promote tissue regeneration (Leung *et al.*, 1994; Hollinger, 1995; van der Elst, 2000). This category, maybe improperly, also includes suture materials that represented the first biodegradable polymer application (Chu, 1983; Benicewicz and Hopper, 1990, 1991; Goupil, 1996). Completely or partially biodegradable composite materials have also been properly developed for this type of application (Vainionpaa *et al.*, 1989; Daniels *et al.*, 1990).

Specific application of a biodegradable transient barrier is for the prevention of tissue adhesion, e.g., between the sliding surface of the tendon, or between the surface of the cardiac wall and the pericardic sac, or for prevention of soft tissue interference with osteogenesis during bone regeneration (Zellin *et al.*, 1995), or, furthermore, for burn dressing (Kane *et al.*, 1996; Sefton and Woodhouse, 1998).

Finally, biodegradable polymers can be used as drug delivery matrices, from which the drug, physically incorporated or covalently bound, is gradually released (Heller, 1983; Chasin and Langer, 1990; Park *et al.*, 1993; Ottenbrite *et al.*, 1996; Heller, 1996; Domb *et al.*, 1997).

Quite recently, biodegradable polymers were also used as scaffolds seeded by specific cells in order to promote the formation of specific tissues for later implantation (e.g., artificial skin). This field of application is in progressive evolution, and more frequently the literature reports tissue engineering methods able to reproduce bone, tendons, soft tissues, and so on (Patrick *et al.*, 1998). The reader will find both in Atala *et al.* (1997) and in Lanza *et al.*, (1997) a review of the synthesis and properties of biodegradable polymers utilized in tissue engineering, applications of these matrices to engineer a variety of tissue types, and relevant FDA and patent issues.

4.5. Natural Polymers

Natural polymers are formed in nature during the growth cycles of all organisms, hence they are also referred to as *biopolymers*. Their synthesis generally involves enzyme-catalyzed, chain growth polymerization reactions of activated monomers, which are formed typically within cells by complex metabolic processes. From the first appearance of natural polymers, (such as catgut, potato starch, and silk) more than 1000 years ago to their present use in products ranging from wound dressings to arterial and skin grafts, fibers and fabrics have been explored as potential materials for novel applications in medicine and surgery. In particular, biomaterial science demands materials which are compatible with human tissue and biological fluids and can meet demanding performance requirements over a long period. For such purposes a large variety of natural polymers are available with special properties and the advantage of enzymatic or hydrolytic degradability. There is an extensive list of these natural polymers including polysaccharides and proteins, while microbial polyesters are already being used in medicine as wound dressing (in membrane, sponge, and hydrogel form), drug delivery (in microsphere, sponge, and hydrogel matrix), surgical suture (in fiber form), and cell culture (in membrane, woven/nonwoven matrix) (Barrows, 1986; Peppas, 1987; Bogdansky, 1990; Hastings, 1992). This information suggests that the trend toward greater utilization of natural polymers will continue, depending on genetic engineering studies.

4.5.1. Polysaccharide-Based Polymers

Carbohydrates comprise one of the main groups of biochemical compounds present in the human body. In scientific terms they are described as polyhydroxy aldehydes/polyhydroxy ketones, or substances that yield such compounds upon hydrolysis, and they can exist either as single units (monosaccharides), or joined together in molecules ranging from two units (disaccharides) to hundreds of units (polysaccharides). The cyclic form can exist as one of two isomers, the α-isomer with an axial OH group on the ring or the β-isomer with an equatorial OH group. Glycosidic bonds link together monosaccharide units to form disaccharides. Linkages among disaccharides lead to large chains called polysaccharides (Kaplan *et al.*, 1994), which are among the three most important used in medicine as a biomaterial.

4.5.1.1. Starch

Starch is composed of the two polymers, amylose and amylopectin, as shown in Figure 4.2. Starch is obtained from potatoes, maize, wheat, and similar sources, from which it can easily be extracted in large quantities. The amylose molecule is essentially linear; a glucan chain and two glucosyl residues are linked in an α-glycosidic way. On the other hand amylopectin differs from amylose in being highly branched.

Starch can be properly modified in order to render its process easier, so forming membranes, fibers, microspheres, etc., for biomedical application. Moreover, starch can be used to prepare controlled-release matrix systems. Advantages are ease of tablet preparation, potential of a constant release rate (zero order) for an extended period of time, and the possibility to incorporate high percentages of drugs with different physicochemical properties (Wierik *et al.*, 1997). For drug delivery applications, starch and dextran microspheres were prepared using different techniques (Franssen *et al.*, 1999a and 1999b).

The hydrolysis of starch is induced by amylases. With the aid of an amylase (such as pancreatic amylase), water molecules access the linkages,

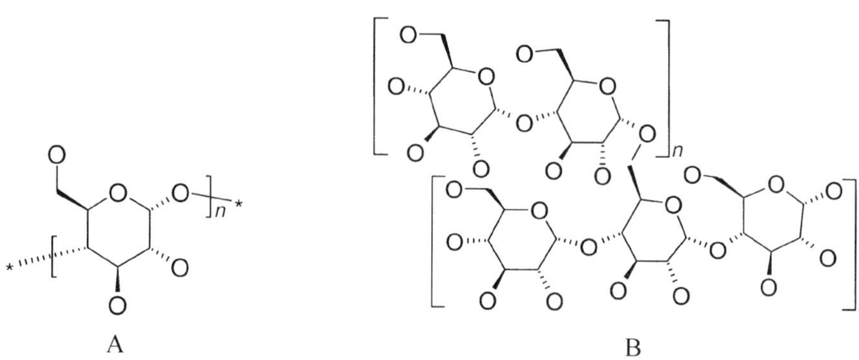

Figure 4.2. Chemical structure of starch (A) amylose and (B) amylopectin.

breaking the chains and eventually producing a mixture of glucose and maltose. Although these materials are sometimes claimed to be partially degradable, during a microbial amylase hydrolytic test the encapsulated starch can often not be reached by microorganisms producing the amylolytic enzymes and therefore the degradability is questionable (Brookfield *et al.*, 1997; Huijun *et al.*, 1998).

Hydroxyethyl starch is one of the most frequently used plasma substitutes. A variety of different hydroxyethyl starch solutions exist worldwide and differ greatly in their pharmacological properties (Treib *et al.*, 1999). Recently, degradable starch microspheres became available for use in patients with liver cancer. When degradable starch combined with a cytotoxic drug are infused through the hepatic artery, the steep drug concentration gradient to the tumor tissue results in a higher tissue drug concentration, which may elicit an increased antitumor response by blocking regional blood flow (Kumada *et al.*, 1999).

Films made from starch and its blends are of increasing scientific and commercial interest. These films are not only enzymatically degradable, they may also be recyclable as well as acceptable for pharmaceutical application. Amylose, hydroxypropylated starch, and dextrin films and hydrogels have also been formed as edible coatings on foods and pharmaceutics to provide an oxygen or lipid barrier, and to improve appearance, texture, and handling. (Heller *et al.*, 1990c; Lawton, 1996; Rindlav-Westling *et al.*, 1998; Ratto *et al.*, 1999).

The grafted starch solutions and the resulting hydrogels are both shown to be biodegraded by the enzyme α-amylase. These acidic hydrogels are potentially useful as enzymatically degradable protective coatings in self-regulated drug delivery system applications (Heller *et al.*, 1990c). A biodegradable starch hydrogel matrix releasing basic fibroblast growth factor on the basis of protein metal coordination with the protein drug, was studied by Tabata *et al.* (1998). The biodegradable hydrogel is prepared from amylopectin by its cross-linking with ethylene glycol diglycidyl ether, followed by introduction of diethylenetriaminepentaacetic acid residues for copper chelation. The degradation of dextran-HEMA hydrogels was studied by Franssen *et al.* (1999b). The hydrogels showed progressive swelling in time, followed by a dissolution phase. The total degradation time ranged from 25 to more than 80 days and depended on the initial water content of the gels.

4.5.1.2. Cellulose

Cellulose, shown in Figure 4.3, is a complex carbohydrate consisting of 3000 or more glucose units, where two glucosyl residues are linked with a β-glycosidic bond.

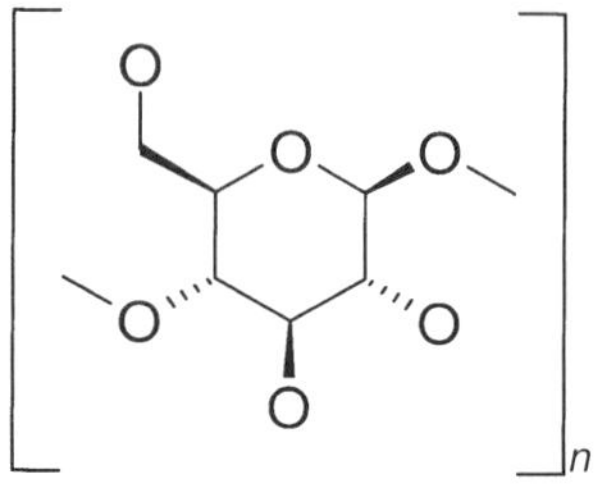

Figure 4.3. Chemical structure of cellulose.

Cellulose is the basic structural component of plant cell walls; 90% of cotton and 50% of wood is cellulose. It is the most abundant of all naturally occurring organic compounds, indigestible by humans, and is processed to produce membranes, sponges, and fibers. A wide variety of cellulose products are currently available in the medical field for use as dressing in treating surgical incisions, abrasions, and burns, and as an aid in the treatment of a variety of dermatological skin disorders. As liquid or antimicrobial agent loaded celluloses are useful as a wound dressing, surgical wipe, treatment pad, burn bandage, tissue/organ drope, and the like (David, 1986).

Today approximately 90% of artificial kidneys incorporate cellulose-based membranes for dialyzing (Nose, 1990). Due to many advantageous properties of cellulose membranes, such as balanced diffusive and convective transport of the toxic metabolic waste products and relatively low thrombogenicity, these membranes have made a fundamental contribution to the establishment of hemodialysis as a routine clinical therapy. Clinical investigation of the role of membrane structure on blood contact and solute transport characteristics of a cellulose membrane is studied by Hoenich and Stamp (2000).

A multifunctional drug delivery system based on hydroxypropyl methylcellulose placed within an impermeable polymeric cylinder (open at both ends) has been developed by Krogel and Bodmeier (1999). Depending on the configuration of the device, extended release, floating, or pulsatile drug delivery systems could be obtained.

Immobilization of enzymes or cells is of great importance to research and industry. That is why cellulose is another attractive matrix for the purification and immobilization of many of these proteins. For example, several affinity ligands such as protein A, human immunoglobulin G, iminodiacetate-copper, and cibacron blue F3GA were coupled to modified cellulose membrane matrices (Dongmei *et al.*, 1998). Another specific application, reported by Shi *et al.* (1999), is the growth of monoclonal antibodies in cellulose hollow fibers systems.

The usefulness of cellulose as a starting material for edible and biodegradable polymer can be extended by chemical modification to methyl cellulose, hydroxypropylmethyl cellulose, hydroxypropyl cellulose, and carboxymethyl cellulose. These celluloses, either films cast from aqueous or aqueous-ethanol solutions, have moderate strength, are resistant to oils and fats, and are flexible, transparent, odorless, tasteless, water-soluble, moreover acting as moderate barriers to moisture and oxygen for cell culture application (Hagenmaier and Shaw, 1990; Kester and Fennema, 1986; Nisperos-Carriedo, 1994). The enzymatic hydrolysis of bacterial cellulose was investigated by Samejima *et al.* (1997).

4.5.1.3. Chitin/Chitosan

Chitin is the second most abundant natural polymer in the world, only second to cellulose. It is also the most abundant naturally occurring polysaccharide that contains amino sugars. This abundance, combined with the specific chemistry of chitin and its derivative chitosan, make suitable materials with great potential for medical application (Zizokis, 1984; Muzzarelli *et al.*, 1986; Maeda *et al.*, 2000).

Chitin occurs as a component of crustacean shells, insect exoskeletons, fungal cell walls, microfauna, and plankton. It is found in association with proteins and minerals such as calcium carbonate. The different sources of chitin differ somewhat in their structure and percentage of chitin content. Chemically, chitin is a polymer formed primarily of repeating units of *N*-acetylglucosamine (Figure 4.4A).

Its structure resembles that of cellulose, except that the hydroxyl groups in position 2 have been replaced by acetylamino groups. Most commercial applications use the deacetylated derivative, chitosan, rather than chitin. Chitosan (Figure 4.4B) is a polysaccharide formed primarily of repeating units of D-glucosamine. Generally, about 80% of the units are

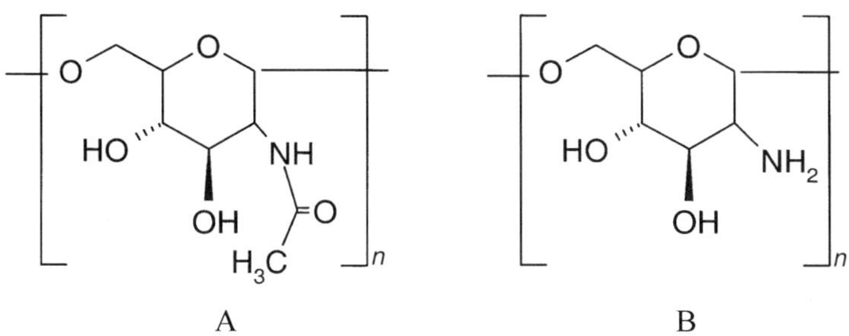

Figure 4.4. Chemical structure of chitin (A) and chitosan (B).

deacetylated, with the remaining 20% acetylated. These values can vary with chitin sources and with processing methods (Sandford, 1989). Chitin has been found to have an acceleratory effect on the wound healing process. Regenerated chitin fibers, nonwoven mats, sponges, and films show an increase in wound healing by over 30% (Hudson, 1994).

Chitin can also be used as a suture or a coating on biomedical materials (Benicewicz and Hopper, 1991). Standard silk and catgut sutures coated with regenerated chitin or chitosan show wound-healing activities only slightly lower than the all-chitin fibers. Surgical gauze coated with regenerated chitin demonstrates a substantially greater amount of activity than an uncoated control group (Chung *et al.*, 1994).

Chitosan is a very attractive candidate for burn treatment. This is true since chitosan can form tough, water-absorbent, biocompatible films. These films can be formed directly on the burn by application of an aqueous solution of chitosan acetate. The solution, although acidic, provides a cool and pleasant soothing effect when applied to the open wounds of burn patients. Another advantage of this type of chitosan treatment is that it allows excellent oxygen permeability (Sandford, 1989). This is important to prevent oxygen deprivation of injured tissues. Additionally, chitosan films have the ability to absorb water and are naturally degraded by body enzymes. This means that the chitosan need not be removed. In most injuries (and especially burns), removing the wound dressing can cause damage to the injury site. Deacetylated chitin, or chitosan, has been shown to bind aggressively to a variety of mammalian and microbial cells. Binding on cells and biodegradability of chitosan may lead to a variety of biomedical applications (Kuen *et al.*, 1995). In addition to the wound healing and burn treatment provided by chitosan, it has been shown to reduce serum cholesterol levels. To a certain degree, it has also been shown to stimulate the immune system (Muzzarelli, 1993).

The methods and structures described here provide a starting point for the design, fabrication, and degradation of a family of polysaccharide-based scaffold materials with potentially broad applicability. The degradation properties are still under investigation (Varum *et al.*, 1997; Kurita, 1998; Stankiewicz *et al.*, 1998).

4.5.1.4. Other Polysaccharides

Hyaluronan and related polysaccharides: Hyaluronan and related polysaccharides are called glycosaminoglycans. These substances are made up largely of repeating disaccharide units containing a derivative of an aminosugar (Figure 4.5).

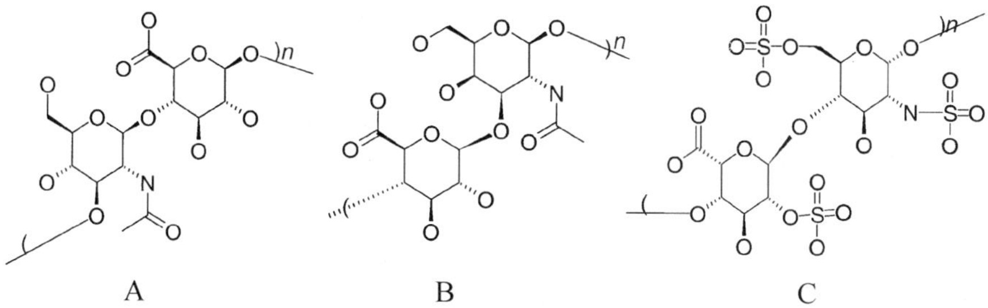

Figure 4.5. Chemical structure of hyaluronate (A), chondroitin (B), and heparin (C).

The most abundant glycosaminoglycans in the body are chondroitin sulfates; others are keratin sulfate, heparin and heparan sulfate, and dermatan sulfate. Applications of these compounds can include use in pharmaceutical preparations, cosmetics, medical and surgical devices (Laurent, 1970; Scott, 1989; Balazs, 1995). It is claimed that the compounds qualitatively possess the same or similar physical-chemical, pharmacological, and therapeutic properties as hyaluronic acid, but that they are considerably more stable, especially with regard to enzymatic degradation by hyaluronidase (Abatangelo *et al.*, 1997). There is evidence in the biomedical literature to suggest that hyaluronic acid is intrinsically involved in the progress of wound repair (Weigel *et al.*, 1986). Various formulations can be fabricated into gels, films, and woven materials (Rastelli *et al.*, 1990; Hoekstra, 1999).

Tissue adhesion after surgery occasionally causes serious complications. Materials that prevent tissue adhesion should be flexible and tough enough to provide for a tight cover over the traumatized soft tissues, and should be biodegradable after the injured tissue is completely regenerated. It was suggested that mucopolysaccharide gels may aid injured tissue repair in a bioactive manner (Chandra and Rustgi, 1998). Tomihata and Ikada (1997) prepared cross-linked hyaluronic acid films with a water content of 60 wt%; they exhibited practically no weight loss after 10 days of immersion in phosphate-buffered saline (pH 7.4) while undergoing *in vivo* degradation (30% weight loss after 7 days of subcutaneous implantation in rats). The inflammation reaction elicited around the implanted film was not found to be significant. Heparin is an another important hyluronan derivative. Although many techniques have been developed to immobilize heparin onto biomaterial surfaces, one of the most effective is based on the concept of "universal coating," in which the physiochemical properties of heparin are modified by incorporation of a specific binding agent onto the heparin molecules. The specific surface-modification requirements of a blood-contacting device depend on the length of time the product will be exposed to blood and on the criticality of the device or procedure. Platelet attachment rate and thrombus formation weight on canine jugular implants were studied by Anderson and Clapper (1998). They showed that platelet attachment and thrombus formation on heparin and heparin/coated implants is almost zero.

The resulting heparin coating material has a high affinity to a variety of synthetic surfaces and retains all biological properties of the unmodified heparin. Experiments have shown that the use of immobilized heparin provides greater benefits than does administration of systemic heparin. For example, the availability of heparin-coated bypass circuits has enabled surgeons performing open-heart surgery to decrease levels of systemic heparin, which has helped reduce patient blood loss and transfusion requirements while guarding against thrombus formation (Charles and Daniel, 1985; Gogly *et al.*, 1999; Pernerstorfer *et al.*, 1999).

Alginates: Alginates, commercially available as alginic acid, sodium salt, commonly called sodium alginate, are chain-forming heteropolysaccharides made up of blocks of mannuronic acid and guluronic acid (Figure 4.6).

Alginates, especially sodium alginate, are widely used in the textile industry because they form an excellent dressing material. Calcium alginate, which is insoluble in water, has been used in the manufacture of a medical dressing very suitable for burns and extensive wounds where a normal dressing would be extremely difficult to remove; the calcium alginate is extruded to make a fiber, which is then woven into a gauze-like product (Horncastle, 1995). Immobilization of cells in alginate is also a well-

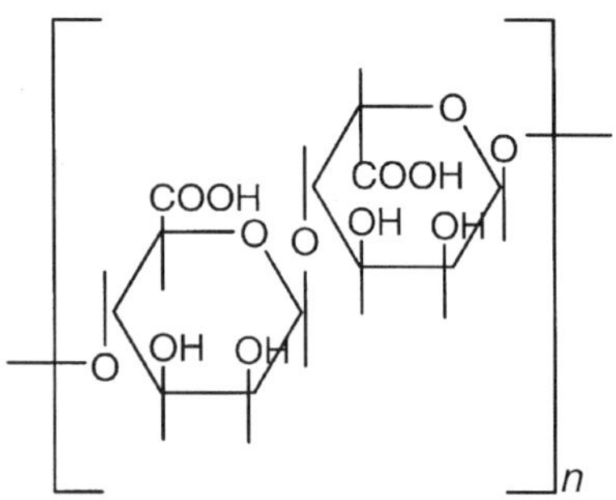

Figure 4.6. Chemical structure of alginate (mixed polymer of mannuronic and guluronic acid).

established technology in a broad range of biotechnology and biomedical fields. Due to a very gentle, simple, and rapid immobilization procedure, alginate entrapment is still the most promising method for islet encapsulating, and is in clinical evaluation for the treatment of diabetes (Smidsrod and Skjak-Braek, 1990). Chitosan-coated alginate microspheres (Ribeiro *et al.*, 1999) and microspheres containing human serum albumin (Edwards and Levy, 1999), can be prepared by evaporation of an aqueous alginate solution followed by ionic cross-linking with a calcium salt and the potential use as an oral controlled release system.

Other polysaccharides, such as inulin (Vervoort *et al.*, 1998), mannan (Ishihara *et al.*, 1998), and chondroitin (Sorell *et al.*, 1996), have also been recently investigated to prepare biodegradable matrices for different biomedical applications.

4.5.2. Protein-Based Polymers

Protein-based polymers are made up of chains of amino acids. Each amino acid has the same basic formula as shown in Figure 4.7. A central carbon, the α carbon, carries a carboxyl group, a hydrogen atom, and an amino group, and a variable R group and the 20 amino acids occurring in all living things (Lehninger, 1977).

The bond connecting amino acids is a peptide bond. It connects the amino end of one monomer to the carboxyl end of another. Longer chains of amino acids produce polypeptides (of less than 10 amino acids) and proteins (of 10 or more amino acids). Sometimes, the term polypeptide or peptide chain is used to describe even long chains of amino acids if they are only part of a complete active protein. The sequence of amino acids on the chain is the primary structure of the protein. The order of the amino acids determines all of the higher-order levels of structure of the protein.

Biomaterials created by protein-based polymers can revolutionize health care by providing a supply of soft (e.g., skin, cartilage, vessel, ligament) and hard (e.g., bone) connective tissues on demand. These polymers possess several interesting properties, such as elastomeric or thermoplastic

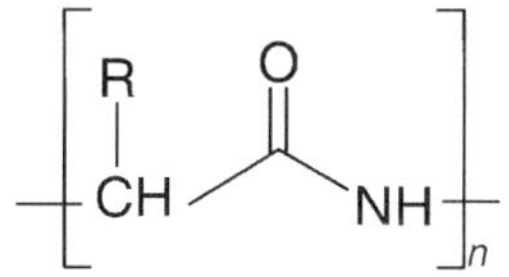

Figure 4.7. Structure of amino acid.

behavior (for example, collagen), oxygen permeabilities, and excellent biocompatibility. The potential uses include tissue restoration, biosensors, and drug delivery (Lee *et al.*, 1981).

4.5.2.1. Albumin

Albumin, a protein found in plasma, has been used for many years to treat burned patients, those with low levels of the protein, and to restore blood volume in other critically ill patients. They were first described by Kramer (1974). Blood compatibilities of blood-contacting biomaterials may be significantly improved by attaching albumin molecules on biomaterial surfaces. Because of its very high blood compatibility, it has been evaluated as a potential carrier matrix in intravascularly injectable drug delivery systems. The delivery of drugs from albumin microspheres was reviewed extensively by Davis *et al.* (1984).

Interaction of antiviral and antitumor photoactive drug hypocrellin A with human serum albumin was studied by Kocisova *et al.* (1999). The identification of the binding place for hypocrellin A as well as the model for the albumin–hypocrellin A complex were proposed. Biodegradable microspheres containing bovine serum albumin (BSA) were prepared by Bouillot *et al.* (1999) with high encapsulation efficiency (approximately 93%). This coating improves the performance of the release system compared with polylactide microspheres; the hydrophilic chains reduce the BSA adsorption onto the microspheres and increase the amount of BSA released in the supernatant.

The use of immobilized human serum albumin (HSA) as a stationary phase in affinity chromatography has been shown to be useful in resolving optical antipodes or investigating interactions between drugs and protein (Guillaume *et al.*, 1999).

Coating of extracorporeal systems with heparin does not prevent platelet activation and subsequent bleeding disorders. Borgdorff *et al.* (1999) investigated whether this could be due to elevated shear stress caused by a roller pump. Although a coating consisting of albumin and heparin is a suitable substrate for seeded endothelial cell, binding of endothelial cells to the substrate further improves when small amounts of fibronectin are present in the albumin-heparin coating. Therefore, albumin-heparin conjugate-coated surfaces form a suitable substrate for seeding of endothelial cells in low density (Bos *et al.*, 1999).

4.5.2.2. Collagen

The collagen molecule is a triple helix assembled from three individual protein chains. The collagen molecules, after being secreted by the cells,

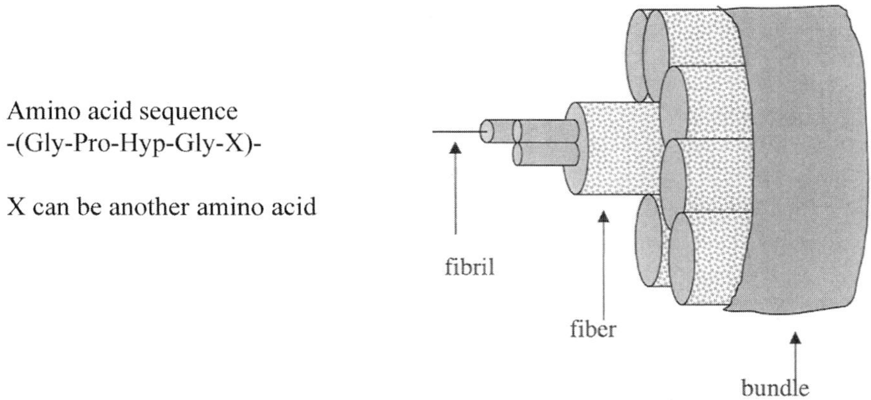

Figure 4.8. Schematic drawings of collagen structure.

assemble into characteristic fibers responsible for the functional integrity of tissues such as bone, cartilage, skin, and tendon. They contribute a structural framework to other tissues, such as blood vessels and most organs. A schematic representation of collagen bundle is given in Figure 4.8.

Six types of collagen have been isolated. Type I collagen forms striated fibers between 80 and 160 nm in diameter in blood vessel walls, tendon, bone, skin, and meat. It may be synthesized by fibroblasts, smooth muscle cells, and osteoblasts. Type II collagen fibers are less than 80 nm in diameter and occur in hyaline cartilage and in intervertebral discs. Type III collagen forms reticular fibers in tissues with some degree of elasticity, such as spleen, aorta, and muscle. Type IV collagen occurs in the basement membranes around many types of cells and may be produced by the cells themselves, rather than by fibroblasts. Although basement membranes were once regarded as amorphous (like glue), many of them are now thought to be composed of a network of irregular cords. Type V collagen is found prenatal in basement membranes and cultures of embryonic cells. Type V collagen has also been found in the basement membranes of muscle fibers, except at the point where muscle fibers are innervated. Type VI collagen is a tetramer of Type VI. It forms a filamentous network and has been identified in muscle and skin. The molecule consists of a short triple helix about 105 nm in length with a large globular domain at each end (Nimni, 1983; Veis, 1983; Arem, 1985).

Collagen, the principal protein component of skin, tendons, bone, and blood vessels, is not only one of the major structural proteins, but also plays an important role in many physiological processes. Collagen has found widespread use in the biomedical field where its applications in various forms abound (Ramshaw *et al.*, 2000). Medical applications in urology, dermatology, orthopedics, and vascular and general surgery utilize collagen in various forms, ranging from injectable solutions to sponge-like materials (Chvapil *et al.*, 1973; Pachence *et al.*, 1987; Silver *et al.*, 1995). In addition, collagens extracted from animal species, primarily bovine, are used in the preparation of a wide variety of commercial products including biological dressings, tissue culture applications, dermal injectables, food additives, and cosmetics (Ulrich *et al.*, 1992).

Wound care has become one of the first fields to see the benefit of a new technology: tissue engineering. Collagenous skin substitutes are produced by culturing keratinocytes on a matured dermal equivalent composed of fibroblasts included in a collagen gel and membranes (Rogalla, 1997; Auger *et al.*, 1998; Pandit *et al.*, 1999). Goissis *et al.* (1999) described the biocompatibility and biodegradation studies of anionic collagen membranes cast from collagen gels that were selectively hydrolyzed at the carboxyamide groups, as a function of the degree of cross-links induced by glutaraldehyde. Other clinical applications of collagen membranes for guided bone regeneration (Schlegel *et al.*, 1997) and for artificial skin (Sefton and Woodhouse, 1998) have been reported.

Basic knowledge about collagen biochemistry and the processing technology in combination with understanding of the physicochemical properties is necessary for an adequate application of collagen for controlled drug delivery systems, including a detailed description of the processing steps, i.e., extraction, purification, chemical cross-linking, and sterilization (Friess, 1998).

The most successful and stimulating applications are shields in ophthalmology, injectable dispersions for local tumor treatment, sponges carrying antibiotics, and minipellets loaded with protein drugs. Beside that, injectable collagen, i.e., a liquid made from the connective tissue of cows or pigs, is injected into and under the skin for cosmetic purposes (Coleman, 1996). The time between treatments varies, depending on the patient and the part of the face being treated. Generally, the effects of treatment last from a few months to about a year-and-a-half.

For clinical use, a recombinant human bone morphogenetic protein soaked onto an absorbable collagen sponge for bone regeneration has been studied by Friess *et al.* (1999). The results indicated that morphogenetic protein binds to the collagen system.

Collagen sutures are used extensively in general surgical procedures (Regan and Dunington, 1966; Brumback and McPherson, 1967; Bartone *et al.*, 1976; Benicewitz and Hopper, 1991). Multiple reports in the literature suggested that there was an increased frequency of postoperative adhesions, wound dehiscence, infection, and even intestinal obstruction along the line of suture material to which the patient had been sensitized during a previous surgery. Engler *et al.* (1986) reported a patient with a history of multiple abdominal surgical procedures. *In vitro* and *in vivo* degradation of collagen suture was investigated by Okada *et al.* (1992) with focusing on the change in the mechanical properties and weight. The *in vitro* hydrolysis assessed for catgut using collagenase (pH 7.4) and pepsin (pH 1.6), simulating the *in vivo* environments. The kinetic study on the weight loss of the fiber at the collagenase hydrolysis suggested that the degradation proceeded gradually from the surface of the fiber into the core. The enzymatic hydrolysis was different from the nonenzymatic acidic hydrolysis, which resulted in almost homogeneous degradation throughout the cross section of the fiber from the beginning of the hydrolysis reaction.

4.5.2.3. Gelatin

Gelatin is obtained by hydrolytic cleavage of collagen chains. It is an animal protein, consists of 19 amino acids joined by peptide linkages, and can be hydrolyzed by a variety of the proteolytic enzymes to yield its constituent amino acids or peptide components. Gelatin has been applied for biodegradable hydrogels and for various biomedical applications. It has been used to prepare film-based artificial skin that could adhere to an open wound and protect it against fluid loss and infection (Chandra and Rustgi, 1998). Also, edible coatings with gelatin reduce oxygen, moisture, and oil migration or can carry an antioxidant or antimicrobial agent. Gelatin can also encapsulate low-moisture or oil-phase food ingredients and pharmaceuticals. Encapsulation protects against oxygen and light and defines ingredient amounts or drug dosages (Reineccius, 1994). Cross-linked gelatin gels are used as biomaterials in living tissues, either as bioadhesives or as devices for sustained drug release. As these applications involve surgical insertion of gels, the effect of cross-linking on mechanical properties is relevant. The effect of cross-linking on the gel water uptake is also relevant for the kinetics of drug release (Lou and Chirila, 1999; Choi *et al.*, 1999). Tabata and Ikada (1999) investigated the biodegradation properties of glutaraldehyde cross-linked acidic gelatin. A mixture of gelatin and resorcinol polymerized by the addition of formaldehyde has been used as a glue for this purpose by Sung *et al.* (1999). Widespread acceptance of this glue, however, has been limited by reports of cytotoxicity, due to its release of formaldehyde upon degradation.

4.5.2.4. Silk Proteins

Silk proteins have found utility in textiles for thousands of years, and many new applications for these types of proteins are targeted. Besides collagen, silk fibroin from various species of silkworm and spiders has been proposed as biomaterials (Capello and McGrath, 1993; Heslot, 1998).

In ancient India and Egypt, and among ancient Greeks and Romans, wounds were sutured by using catgut and silk. For many surgeons, surgical silk represents the standard of performance by which newer synthetic materials are judged, especially due to its superior handling characteristics. Silk filaments can be twisted or braided, the latter providing the best handling qualities. To establish criteria for characterizing synthetic sutures, the handling characteristics of silk sutures were analyzed by Tomita *et al.* (1993). The characteristics that distinguish silk suture from other braided suture materials are its good knot security and relatively low tie-down resistance. Braided silk sutures often act as a non-immunologic foreign body and cause a granulomatous inflammatory reaction years after surgery. Kurosaki *et al.* (1999) reported a case of recurrent granulomas with remarkable infiltration of eosinophils that may have resulted from an IgE-mediated hypersensitivity reaction to silk fibroin, a component of the braided silk suture. Under normal circumstances exposure to fibroin is rather rare. One area of current research interest is the use of silk proteins in immobilization technology (Grasset *et al.*, 1977), based on glucose oxidase-immobilized silk fibroin membrane and oxygen electrode (Demura *et al.*, 1989; Liu *et al.*, 1997). Zhang *et al.* (1998) have developed an amperometric glucose sensor in flow-injection analysis. A simple and effective procedure was described for the immobilization of peroxidase in regenerated silk fibroin membrane prepared from waste silk (Qian *et al.*, 1996). A water-insoluble silk fibroin membrane was prepared by Minoura *et al.* (1990) by immersing a silk fibroin membrane as cast in 50 vol% aqueous methanol solution for different periods of time at 25 °C. The membranes of regenerated silk fibroin with or without peroxidase, before or after the ethanol treatment, were characterized by infrared spectra. To use the membrane as a biomaterial, oxygen and water vapor permeability, transparency, mechanical property, and enzymatic degradation behavior *in vitro* of the membrane in the wet state were investigated. Silk fibroins are also proposed as a burn wound dressing material (Minoura *et al.*, 1990; Santin *et al.*, 1999).

The growth of animal cells on silk fibroin-coated plates was examined by Inouhe *et al.* (1998). In this study the anchorage-dependent cells exhibited almost the same growth on both fibroin- and collagen-coated plates, and it was 30–50% higher than that on polystyrene plates coated with hydrophilic groups. Recently, Hara and Yamakawa (1995) investigated the antibacterial activity of the hemolymph from Bombyx Mori against Gram-negative bacteria.

Becker and Tuross (1993) found initial degradative changes in bombyx mori silk fibroin and the microbial degradation of silk was investigated by Seves *et al.* (1998). They found that initial biochemical degradative changes in bombyx mori silk fibroin are the appreciable loss of tyrosine and the loss of acidic and ionizable amino acids.

4.5.2.5. Other Proteins

Other proteins related to biomedical and pharmaceutical coating that have been studied included corn zein (Padgett *et al.*, 1998), wheat gluten (Kalimo and Vainio, 1980), soy protein isolate (Hawrylewicz *et al.*, 1995), and casein (Mitchell *et al.*, 1970). Besides collagen and gelatin, corn zein is the only other protein that has been promoted commercially as an edible film or coating. The barrier, vitamin adhesion, and antimicrobial carrier properties of zein film coatings have been used on a variety of foods. Zein is also used on pharmaceuticals for coating capsules for protection, controlling release, and masking flavors and aromas (Gennadios *et al.*, 1994).

4.5.3. Microbial Polyesters (Poly-β-hydroxyalkanoates)

Microbial polyesters are bacterial storage polymers produced by various microorganisms in response to nutrient limitation. When they are exposed to natural microorganisms in the ecosystem, degradation to carbon dioxide and water is achieved in about 1–6 months depending on composition. Chemical structures of poly(3-hydroxybutyrate) and poly (3-hydroxyvalerate) are given in Figure 4.9.

A random copolymer containing both hydroxyvalerate (HV) and hydroxybutyrate (HB) could be obtained by the manipulation of the growth

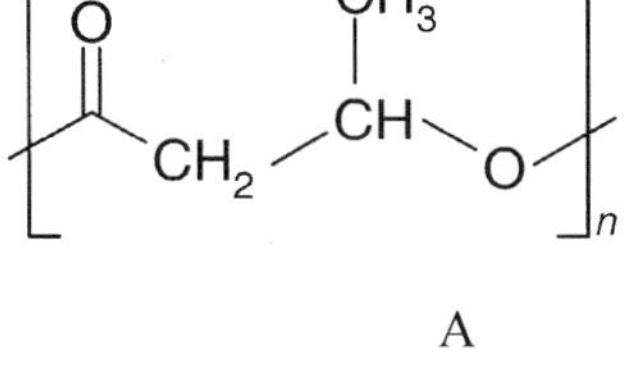

A

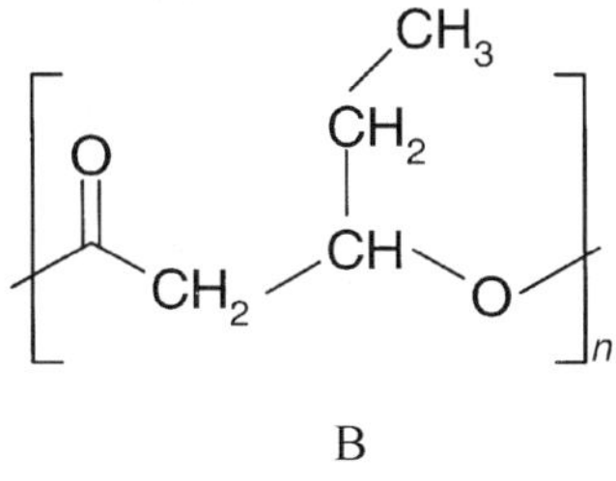

B

Figure 4.9. Chemical structure of poly(3-hydroxybutyrate (A) and poly(3-hydroxyvalerate) (B).

medium. The resulting copolymer poly(3-hydroxybutyrate)-co-(3-hydroxy-valerate) (PHB/V) is thermoplastic and fully biodegradable (Doi, 1990; Timmins *et al.*, 1993; Amass *et al.*, 1998). By changing the ratio of hydroxy-valerate to hydroxybutyrate, the resulting copolymer can be made to resemble either polypropylene or polyethylene, with regard to flexibility, tensile strength, and melting point (Engelberg and Kohn, 1991; Kemmish, 1993).

For the treatment of diseases, the design of a controlled release system seemed very appropriate for an effective, long-term result. Sendil *et al.* (1999) studied a novel, biodegradable microbial polyester, poly(3-hydroxybutyrate-co-3-hydroxyvalerate), PHBV, of various valerate contents containing a well-established antibiotic, tetracycline, known to be effective against many of the periodontal disease-related microorganisms, and was used in the construction of a controlled release system. Kassab *et al.* (1997) attempted to prepare microspheres from a microbial biodegradable polyester, i.e., polyhydroxybutyrate (PHB) as a potential chemoembolization agent. The drug-loaded PHB microspheres were prepared by a solvent evaporation technique, in which methylene chloride, distilled water, and polyvinyl alcohol were utilized as the solvent, dispersion medium, and emulsifier, respectively. Microspheres containing these ester prodrugs were prepared with poly(3-hydroxybutyrate) of different molecular weights. Poly(hydroxybutyrate) and poly(hydroxybutyrate-hydroxyvalerate) (PHBV) were also investigated by Gangrade and Price (1991) for use as sustained delivery carriers of a model drug, progesterone. Spherical microspheres containing the drug were prepared by an emulsion solvent-evaporation method with gelatin as an emulsifier. *In vitro* release of the drug was found slowest from microspheres made from copolymer containing 9% hydroxyvalerate. A less porous microsphere matrix was formed by this copolymer. Spherical bovin serum albumin loaded microporous matrix-type microspheres composed of P(HB-HV) blended with 20% polycaprolactone and fabricated using oil/water emulsification with solvent evaporation have been studied by Atkins and Peacock (1996). The greatest percentage weight loss was observed after incubation in newborn calf serum and decreased in the order:

newborn calf serum > pancreatin > synthetic gastric juice > Hanks' buffer

The effect of alkaline hydrolysis on several surface properties of poly(hydroxybutyrate-hydroxyvalerate) (92/8) (PHB/HV) and poly(ε-caprolactone) films and of poly(ethylene terephthalate) track-etched membranes has been characterized by Rouxhet *et al.* (1998), as well as the adsorption of three proteins normally encountered by mammalian cells *in vivo*, namely albumin, collagen, and fibronectin.

Polyhydroxyalkanoates were also good candidates for orthopedic applications. Boeree *et al.* (1993) evaluated the mechanical properties of a composite material comprising polyhydroxybutyrate with hydroxyapatite added in proportions varying from 0 to 50%. With the additional advantages of biocompatibility, biodegradability, and the potential for piezoelectric stimulation of new local bone formation, it was concluded that the injection-molded composite material has considerable potential for use in orthopedic surgery, both as a material to construct certain orthopedic implants and as an alternative to corticocancellous bone graft.

Kostopoulos and Karring (1994) explored the possibility of obtaining bone regeneration in jaw bone defects in rats after coverage of the defects with an occlusive polyhydroxybutyrate membrane. The defect on one side was covered with a polyhydroxybutyrate resorbable membrane, while the contralateral side received no membrane before closure of the wound. The histological analysis demonstrated increasing bone fill in the test specimens from 15–180 days, while only 35–40% of the defect area in the control sides was filled with bone after 3–6 months.

Clinically optimal situations for primary nerve repair are rarely observed. Crushed nerve ends result in either suboptimal repair or a need for nerve grafting. Functional results after nerve surgery are relatively poor, including major sensory deficits, which may be due to the death of primary sensory neurons that follows the nerve injury. Ljungberg *et al.* (1999) investigated the use of polyhydroxybutyrate (PHB), a resorbable nerve conduit, as an alternative to primary nerve repair in reducing loss of neurons.

4.6. Synthetic Polymers

Various aspects including degradation of aliphatic polyesters, polyesteramides, polyorthoesters, polyanhydrides, poly(alkyl 2-cyanoacrylates), polyiminocarbonates, and polyphosphazenes are reported in the following subsections, taking into consideration also synthesis, application, degradation effects, and relation with chemical structure. In the last three subsections, the degradation of polymers traditionally considered as stable materials, such as polyethyleneterephthlate, polyamides, and polyurethanes used for biomedical applications, are considered.

4.6.1. Aliphatic Polyesters

Aliphatic polyesters probably represent the most diffuse class of biomedical biodegradable polymers, in particular hydroxyacid-derived polymers encountered in major applications, as reported in some review chapters (Barrows, 1991; Shalaby and Johnson, 1994; Chu, 1995; Li and Vert, 1999).

In the following, some general concepts about synthesis are described (Sandler and Karo, 1974; Goodman, 1988). The most important reactions that can produce linear polyesters are those in which polymer backbone chain is grown up by a new ester bond at each step. Multistep water elimination from bifunctional compounds (containing hydroxy and carboxylic groups) in polycondensation reaction is the most diffuse method, not only for the multiplicity of available reagents, but also for the possibility to obtain copolymerized polyesters. Ring-opening polymerization (Johns *et al.*, 1984) of cyclic ester is always preferred whenever the potential precursor is available and sufficiently reactive, especially to synthesize higher molecular weight products. The two methods are intercorrelated according to the reaction scheme reported in Figure 4.10. The first step of the hydroxyacid (**I**) condensation can produce the dimeric hydroxyacid (**II**, $n = 2$) intermolecularly (a) or the cyclic ester (**III**) intramolecularly (b). Furthermore, the dimer hydroxyacid can react according to the different mechanisms (a,b) resulting in a trimer hydroxyacid or a dimer cycle, and so on, regarding all products derived from route (a). The higher the molecular weight, the lower the probability of a head–tail reaction for cyclization. Reverse reaction (c and d) represents the hydrolysis process. Favorable thermodynamics, i.e.,

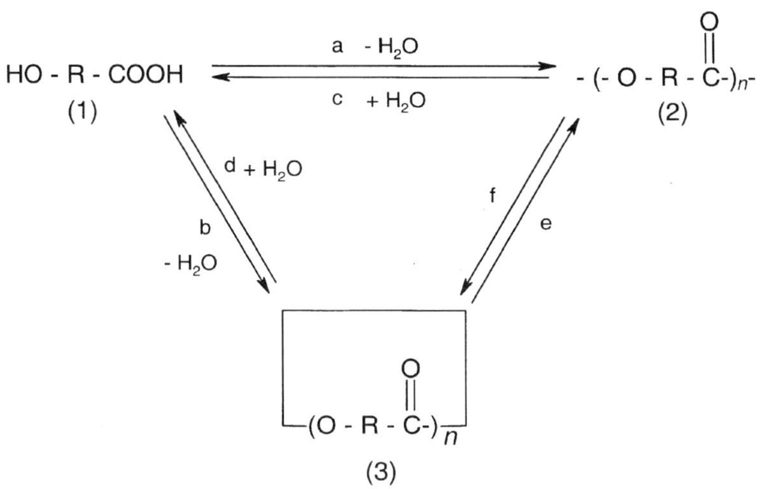

Figure 4.10. Scheme of polyhydroxyacids synthesis and degradation.

excess of water and relatively high temperature, does not necessarily mean favorable kinetics. Hydrolysis reactivity depends on structure and on ease of access to the reaction site. For instance, aliphatic polyesters will react faster than aromatic polyesters; an amorphous polymer will be more reactive than a crystalline polymer. Ring-opening polymerization is shown in route (e); its inverse reaction (f) represents depolymerization. No water is involved in either process. The structure of the reagents and products, the temperature and pressure conditions, and the presence of a catalyst affect the direction of reaction. In particular, the highest molecular weight polyesters can be synthesized according to this method at the lowest temperature in order to reduce the entropic factor. The higher the temperature, the higher the reaction entropy and the more favorable the depolymerization process. Starting from low molecular weight polymers, high temperature and low pressure are the usual conditions under which to obtain the cyclic ester of a 5–6 member ring.

After the first study on glycolide at the end of the century (Bischoff and Walden, 1893), Carothers *et al.* (1932) studied the polymerization of six-membered cyclic esters. Subsequently, ring-opening polymerization has been applied successfully for glycolide (Schmitt and Polistina, 1967; Chujo *et al.*, 1967; Frazza and Schmitt, 1971), lactide (Kulkarni *et al.*, 1966; Kulkarni *et al.*, 1971), dioxanone (Doddi *et al.*, 1977; Berry *et al.*, 1981; Ray *et al.*, 1981), caprolactone (Sinclair, 1977) and their copolymers (Gilding and Reed, 1979; Pitt *et al.*, 1981; Cohn and Younes, 1988; Leenslag *et al.*, 1988; Zhu *et al.*, 1990; Zhang *et al.*, 1993; Grijpma and Pennings, 1994; Karjalainen *et al.*, 1996) as shown schematically in Figure 4.11.

For instance, polylactic acid or polylactide (PLA) is polymerized from lactide, a condensed dimer of lactic acid, which is produced in mammalian muscles during glycogenolysis and correlated with the Krebs cycle through piruvic acid and acetyl CoA (Lehninger, 1977). Two different enantiomeric forms, D and L lactic acids, exist (but only the L configuration is in the body), so producing different corresponding enantiomeric polymers, consequent from the maintenance of the chiral center. While D,L polymers (both mesomeric and racemic D,L-lactide derivatives) are fully amorphous, as a result of the atacticity of methyl groups, poly-L-lactic acid (PLLA) can crystallize having an isotactic chain, and attaining a degree of crystallinity which depends on the molecular weight, annealing temperature, and time treatments. Figure 4.12 reports the Differential Scanning Calorimeter (DSC) curves of a PDLLA and an almost amorphous PLLA. Both samples have comparable molecular weights (around 100,000) and display similar glass transition (about 65 °C), but only PLLA exhibits a crystallization peak and the melting peak (around 185 °C).

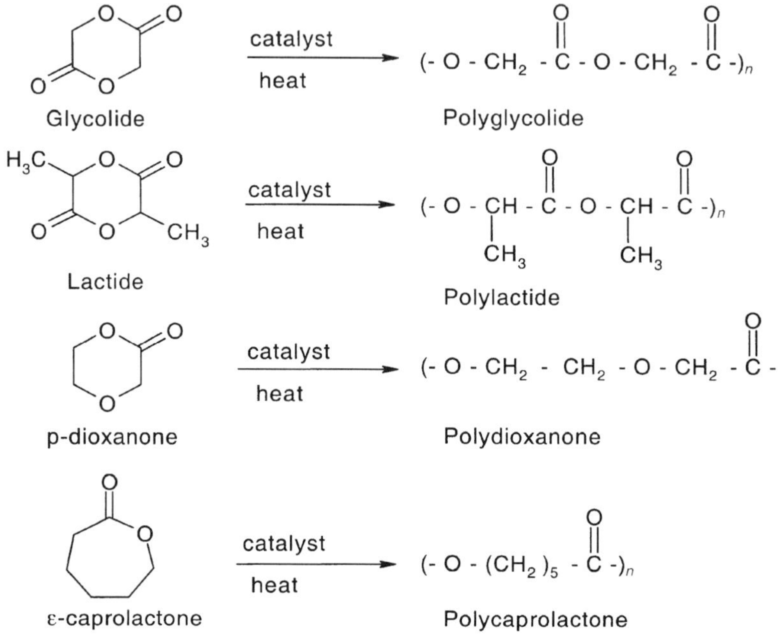

Figure 4.11. Synthesis of the most common aliphatic polyesters by ring-opening polymerization.

Depending on the polyester properties (Tg, molar mass, degree of crystallinity, processability, degradation rate), various applications have been proposed. Polymers and copolymers of polyglycolide/polylactide (Lewis, 1990) and polycaprolactone (Pitt, 1990) have been used as drug release carriers (Amass *et al.*, 1998; Li and Vert, 1999).

In the case of absorbable sutures, mofilaments/multifilaments are manufactured from semicrystalline polymers. Examples are polyglycolide as Dexon® by Davis&Geck (Schmitt and Polistina, 1967), polydioxanone as PDS™ by Ethicon (Doddi *et al.*, 1977; Trimbos *et al.*, 1991), and poly-L-lactide (Fambri *et al.*, 1997). Various copolymers were used to produce fibers having intermediate properties; for instance, a copolymer with 90% glycolide and 10% L-lactide (polyglactin 910, commercialized with the tradename of Vicryl™ by Ethicon), or a copolymer with about 65% glycolide and 35% trimethylencarbonate (commercialized with the tradename of Maxon™ by Davis&Geck), or a copolymer with 85% L-lactide and 15% caprolactone (Nakamura *et al.*, 1992). The degradation rate of commercial sutures, measured as a function of the residual strength percentage, increases

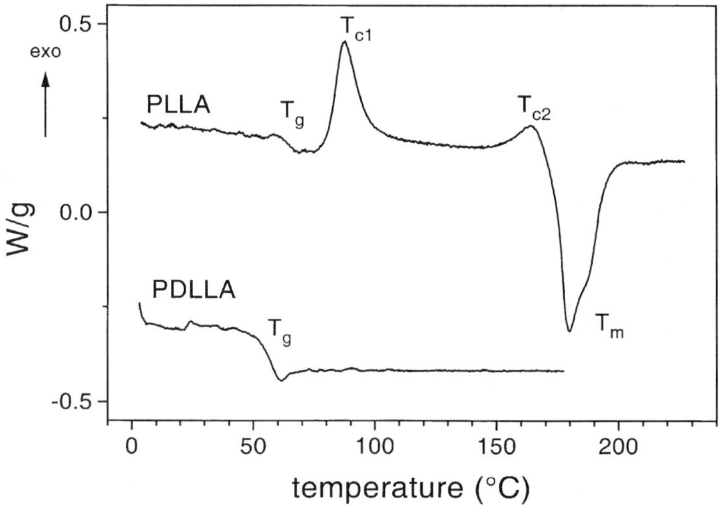

Figure 4.12. DSC thermograms of poly-L-lactide (PLLA) and poly-DL-lactide (PDLLA). Glass transition temperature (T_g), crystallization (T_{c1} and T_{c2}), and melting (T_m) peaks are indicated.

approximately in the following order (Saņz *et al.*, 1988; Greenwald *et al.*, 1994):

$$\text{PDS}^{\text{TM}} \leqslant \text{Maxon}^{\text{TM}} < \text{Vicryl}^{\text{TM}} < \text{Dexon}^{®}$$

The effect of superoxide ion on the *in vitro* degradation of absorbable sutures has been discussed by Chu and Lee (2000).

For many applications, when devices or prostheses have to bear loads, namely in orthopedics or maxillofacial surgery, the mechanical properties of polymers are not sufficient. Higher mechanical properties could be attained throughout specific treatments, such as by employing sintering starting from fibers to prepare self-reinforced rods (Tormala *et al.*, 1991), or the so-called orientrusion process (Matsusue *et al.*, 1992; Tunc, 1995; Ferguson *et al.*, 1996), or even by introducing inorganic fillers (Verheyen *et al.*, 1992) and fibers as reinforcing components. In this latter case, composite systems have been developed with fibers reinforcing the matrix, with a gain bounded from the moderate mechanical properties of the biodegradable polymers (Vainionpaa *et al.*, 1989; Daniels *et al.*, 1990).

On the other hand, a method to obtain biodegradable, less stiff polymers consists in the copolymerization of poly(ethylene oxide) (PEO) and polylactic acid (PLA) (Cohn and Younes, 1988, 1989). These poly(ether-esters) are characterized by hard semicrystalline PLLA domains and flexible, elastic, and hydrophilic PEO regions. Degradation kinetics suggested a biomedical application as replacement of soft tissue and drug delivery.

Poly(ester-urethane) and poly-L-lactide mixtures were intended to be used as biodegradable vascular prostheses and biodegradable nerve guides (Leenslag *et al.*, 1988). The two polymers are well known to degrade differently, and mechanical properties and degradation rate can be optimized as a function of composition and geometric factors.

A series of biodegradable aromatic polyester block copolymers, derived from polyethylene oxide and polybutylene terephthalate (PEO-PBT), have been recently produced with the tradename of Polyactive™ (HC Implants B.V.). Their elastomeric behavior and degradation kinetics varies with the block copolymer compositions (PEO-PBT ratio between 80/20 and 30/70) and several publications reported bone-bonding properties for these copolymers (van Blitterswijk *et al.*, 1992; Gaillard and van Blitterswijk, 1994; Radder *et al.*, 1994a). Polyactive copolymers have been extensively investigated for several applications, such as alloplastic tympanic membrane (Bakker *et al.*, 1990; Grote *et al.*, 1991), in orthopedic and dental surgery (Sakkers *et al.*, 1992; Radder *et al.*, 1994b; Meijer *et al.*, 1996; Bulstra *et al.*, 1996), and for cell culturing and artificial skin (Beumer *et al.*, 1994; van Dorp *et al.*, 1998, 1999).

Poly(phosphoester)s formally derived from phosphoric acid and hydroxyl terminated molecules represent a new interesting family of biodegradable polymers (Richards *et al.*, 1991) intended for drug delivering systems and tissue engineering scaffolds (Mao *et al.*, 1999). For instance, poly(phosphoester) urethanes (Dahiyat *et al.*, 1993) and poly(phosphoester) derived from poly(lactide-co-glycolide) oligomers have been considered.

Other classes of aliphatic polyesters, such as poly(ester-amides) and poly(orthoester)s, are presented in the following sections.

4.6.2. Poly(ester-amides)

The ester groups make the polymers easily hydrolyzable while the amide linkages provide mechanical stability.

This new class of copolymers was initially proposed by various authors (Katayama *et al.*, 1976; Shalaby and Jamiolkowski, 1980), and in 1983 Barrows *et al.* started to extensively study these materials for biomedical applications, in order to obtain polymers having mechanical

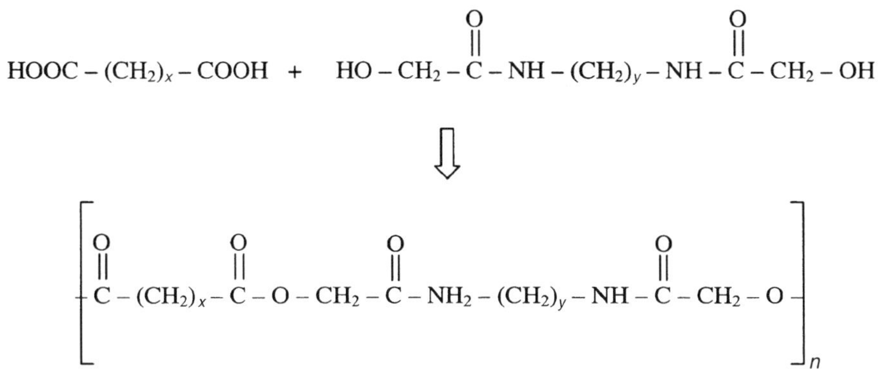

Figure 4.13. Synthesis of aliphatic polyamidoesters by condensation reaction.

properties nylon-like and degradability comparable to polyesters. Polymerization formally starts from a dicarboxylic acid (usually with succinic acid for $x = 2$) and an amidediol (or bishydroxyacetamide) produced from glycolic acid and a diamine, as shown in Figure 4.13. Aliphatic poly(ester-amides) with the name PEA-x,y have been distinguished from the number of methylenic groups in the diacid (x) and in the diamine (y), respectively.

Later, Barrows (1994) published a short review in which synthesis, properties, degradation, and toxicologic data were reported. These semicrystalline polymers have been found suitable for fiber, film, and molding processing. In particular, various experimental fibers were melt spun for applications as sutures; tensile moduli of 7.2 GPa and 3.8 GPa for PEA-2,6 and PEA-2,12 (derived from hexanediamine or dodecanediamine), respectively, and tensile strengths up to 630 MPa were measured.

The degradation properties depend on the amidediol and diacid compositions, and the hydrolysis of the ester bond was found to be the main mechanism. *In vitro* and *in vivo* experiment showed that PEA with the longer aliphatic chain ($x,y = 12$) exhibited the longer degradation time, and the PEA-x,2 polymers appeared to be more hydrolytically stable than the PEA-2,y ones. PEA-2,6 fibers required 8 months for bioabsorption, almost the same time as commercial PDS and Maxon monofilament, while the estimated time for PEA-2,12 is about 3 years.

Moreover, according to the reported standard assays, amidediol monomer, the major metabolite, appeared to be nontoxic, and neither were traces of ethylenediamine found nor was a carcinogenic effect found after 2 years of chronic study in rats.

4.6.3. Polyorthoesters

Polyorthoesters, extensively studied by Heller (1990), are hydrophobic, with hydrolytic linkages that are acid-sensitive. These polymers find their main application in drug delivery (Heller and Gurny, 1999); they degrade by surface erosion, and degradation rates can be controlled by incorporation of acidic or basic excipients (Heller *et al.*, 1990a).

Subcutaneous drug pellets based on nondegradable polymers have been used for continuous drug administration. However, these materials showed two main disadvantages: first, the need of a second surgical procedure to remove the drug-containing devices or the polymeric matrices after implantation, and second, their release profile was neither constant nor readily controlled in terms of precision of rate and duration of action. For these reasons, the development of biodegradable polymers as matrices able to incorporate drugs and to exhibit a well-defined kinetics release has been extensively investigated (Choi and Heller, 1978, 1979). In order to confine the erosion process at the polymer–water surface, the matrix should be reasonably hydrophobic to reduce the water penetration into the bulk and correspondingly highly reactive versus the hydrolytic process. In the 1970s, Alza Corp. first developed a poly(orthoester) matrix, designed with the tradename Chronomer (now Alzamer), obtained by a transesterification reaction between a diol and diethoxytetrahydrofuran. Its hydrolytic degradation, as reported in Figure 4.14A, involves a first step in which a diol and γ-butirrolactone are formed, and then by hydrolysis a γ-hydroxybutyric acid that accelerates the reactions with an autocatalytic effect. A second family, derived from the addition of polyols to diketene acetal 3,9-bis(ethylidene 2,4,8,10-tetraoxaspiro[5,5]undecane) without forming condensation by-products (Figure 4.14B), was developed by SRI International. The hydrolytic products are the diol and pentaerythritol dipropionate. The further hydrolysis of this latter compound produces propionic acid, but no autocatalytic reaction is observed because this hydrolysis results much more slowly than that of orthoester bonds. Another type of poly(orthoesters) are those derived from direct polymerization of a triol and an orthoester. Depending on the desired properties of the polymer, flexible or rigid triols such as 1,2,6-hexanetriol (Heller *et al.*, 1990b) or 1,1,4-cyclohexanetrimethanol (Heller *et al.*, 1992) can be used, as shown in Figures 4.14C and D, respectively. In both cases, the first hydrolysis step occurs at the orthoester bond with the formation of hydroxyester, whose hydrolytic cleavage is much slower, and hence the overall reaction is not autocatalytic. The final degradation products are the triol and acetic or propionic acid (Heller and Daniels, 1994). The surface analysis of biodegradable poly(orthoesters) was studied by Davies *et al.* (1991) with X-ray photo-

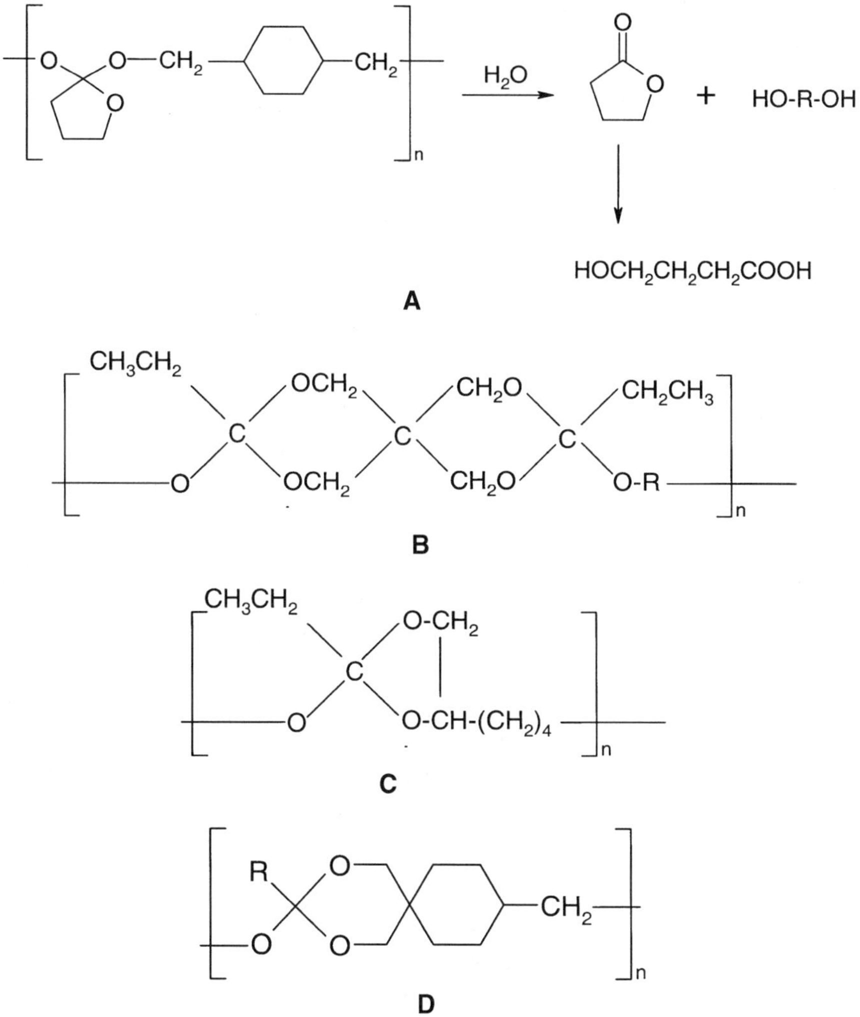

Figure 4.14. Chemical structure and hydrolysis (A) of some poly(orthoesters).

electron spectroscopy. They found very good agreement between the experimental and theoretical surface compositions, confirming the high surface purity of these polymers, and demonstrated the potential for the use of XPS in future studies of the solid state *in-situ* degradation of poly(orthoesters). Leadly *et al.* (1998) used SIMS, XPS, and AFM analyses to show that the kinetics of drug release from pH-sensitive poly(orthoesters) is predominantly controlled by the rate of polymer hydrolysis. Different biodegradable polymers, poly(orthoesters) included, were studied by Sinha and Khosla (1998) and were evaluated for controlled implantable drug delivery devices by using a variety of drugs. *In vitro* and *in vitro* degradation of poly(orthoesters) for internal tissue fixation devices has been recently reviewed by Andriano *et al.* (2000).

4.6.4. Polyanhydrides

Certainly polyanhydrides fall among the most hydrolytically unstable polymers, finding biomedical application as drug carriers (Chasin *et al.*, 1990; Domb *et al.*, 1994; Gopferich, 1999). The synthesis process formally requires the condensation of one or more diacids, usually with sebacic acid (SA). Two types of polyanhydrides, based on *p*-carboxyphenoxy propane (CPP) and fatty acid (FA), poly(CPP-SA) (Figure 4.15) and poly(FA-SA), have been mostly studied in various molar ratios. In particular, poly(CPP-SA) was approved by FDA for clinical trials and treatment of malignant brain tumor was studied (Chasin *et al.*, 1988). Engelberg and Kohn (1991) reported a physicochemical characterization of polyanhydrides derived from hexadecanedioic acid (HDA) and isophthalic acid (ISA), i.e., poly(CPP-SA-ISA) and poly(HDA-SA); due to their high hydrolytic rate and low mechanical strength, these polymers could be proposed for drug release applications only.

The hydrophobic character of anhydride polymers determines a very low water sorption, while the rate of hydrolytic degradation is much faster. Hence in this way the control of drug release can be easily optimized, resulting in a degradation process at the surface with concomitant zero-order drug release kinetics. In particular, Leong *et al.* (1985) first confirmed these data because they showed that the percentage of drug release is directly related to the percentage of the degradation (Figure 4.16). This surface mechanism erosion represents a potential advantage with respect to polyorthoesters, which usually require the incorporation of additives to

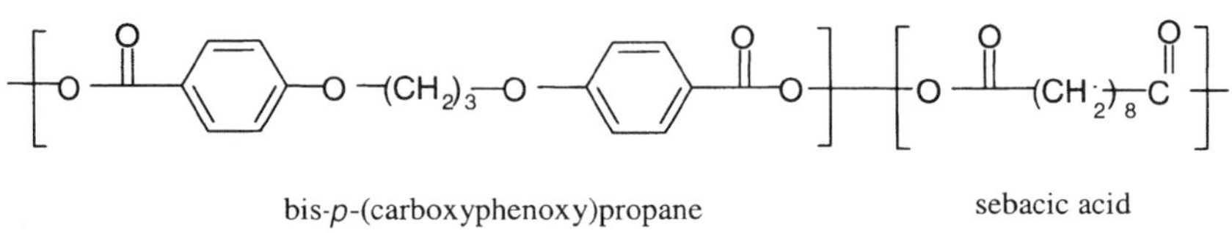

Figure 4.15. Chemical structure of poly(CPP-SA), polyanhydride derived from *p*-carboxyphenoxy propane (CPP) and sebacic acid (SA).

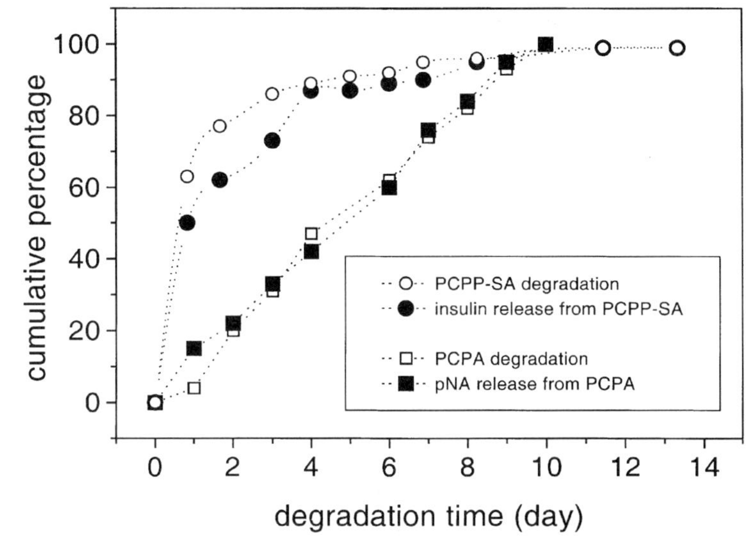

Figure 4.16. Release of insulin from microspheres of polycarboxyphenoxypropane–sebacic acid 50/50 (PCPP-SA) and release of *p*-nitroaniline (p-NA) from disks of polycarboxyphenoxyacetic acid (PCPA) compared to the polymer degradation *in vitro*. Adapted from Chasin *et al.* (1990), pp. 43–70, with kind permission of Marcel Dekker, Inc.

exhibit the same behavior. Depending on the diacids and their ratio, the degradation time of polyanhydrides can be properly ranged, for instance, between 1 day (poly-SA) and 3 years (polyCPP), as reported by Leong *et al.* (1985). Applications are for brain anticancer therapy, for the release of insulin, bovine somatotropin, angiogenesis inhibitors, immunosuppressive agents, for craniofacial growth, and for osteomyelitis treatment. Many tests to evaluate both biocompatibility and toxicity were performed as noted by Domb *et al.* (1994), including acute toxicity, irritation tests, and the potential of allergenic, carcinogenic, mutagenic, and teratogenic effects. In particular, both the safety of polyanhydride copolymer poly(CPP-SA) 20/80 (Brem, 1990) and the extended lifetime of a patient affected by brain cancer, with respect to conventional therapies after *in situ* treatment with a polymer wafer containing a chemotherapeutic agent, were demonstrated.

4.6.5. Poly(alkyl 2-cyanoacrylate)

This class of materials, derived from a polymerization reaction of cyanoacrylic monomers, was induced from traces of moisture directly *in situ*

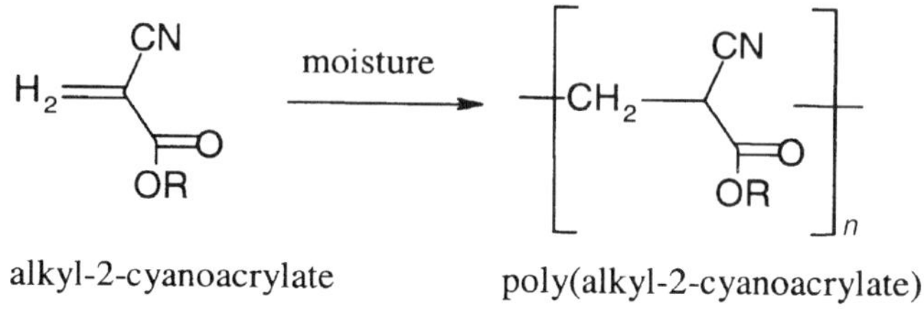

Figure 4.17. Polymerization reaction of cyanoacrylate.

according to a scheme reported in Figure 4.17. They find applications as tissue adhesives, and hemostatic, sealant, and embolization agent (Ronis *et al.*, 1984), and they undergo hydrolytic cleavage of the carbon–carbon bond due to the activated reactivity of methylenic hydrogens induced by two electron-withdrawing groups (—CN and —COOR). Depending on the substituent R, the rate of hydrolysis could be very fast (a few hours) especially at alkaline pH. Lower alkyl derivatives were found to degrade faster than higher homologs (Hegyeli, 1973), but they were more toxic. In particular, methyl cyanoacrylate, which was found to degrade consistently after 4–6 months of implantation (Kopecek and Ulbrich, 1983), has been progressively abandoned due to the toxicity, probably related to the formaldehyde release (Tseng *et al.*, 1990). Butyl (Ciapetti *et al.*, 1994; Amiel *et al.*, 1999), octyl (Wang *et al.*, 1999), and glycolate (where R is —CH_2CH_2COOR') (Jaffe *et al.*, 1986) derivatives are considered less toxic. Isobutyl cyanoacrylate was also proposed for drug delivery systems (Lenaerts *et al.*, 1984).

4.6.6. Polyimino Carbonates

Structure–property relationships for the design of polyiminocarbonates were well established. They are based on the investigation of thermal stability and processibility, morphology, tensile strength, hydrolytic degradation, and drug release profiles of different polyiminocarbonates (Kohn and Langer, 1986; Kohn, 1990; Pulapura *et al.*, 1990).

Some polyiminocarbonates were reported in the literature to be among the mechanically strongest, bioerodible polymers currently available (Engelberg and Kohn, 1991), very similar to PLLA. However, the iminocarbonate bond is highly unstable under physiological conditions, facilitating the design of rapidly degrading devices. The drug-release profiles of certain polyiminocarbonates exhibited lag periods, facilitating the design of pulsed-release or delayed-release devices. Possible limitations of the practical applicability of polyiminocarbonates as biomaterials are the low thermal

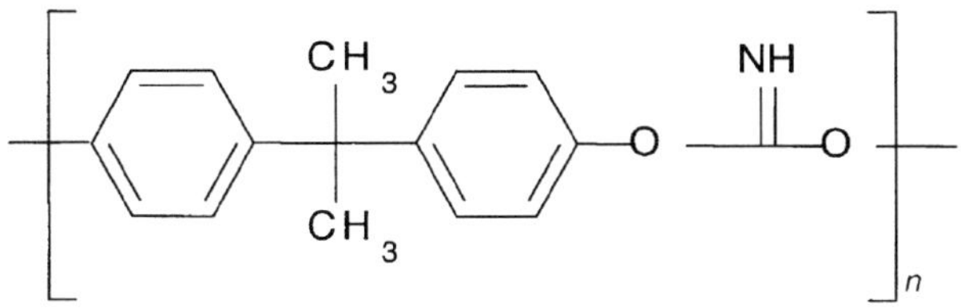

Figure 4.18. Structure of poly(Bisphenol A-iminocarbonate).

stability of the iminocarbonate linkage and the complicated, two-phase degradation mechanism that led to the formation of slowly degrading residues of low molecular weight. Degradation under basic conditions yielded bisphenol A, ammonia, and carbon dioxide, while under acidic conditions insoluble poly(Bisphenol A-carbonate) oligomers were also produced (Barrows, 1986).

Poly(Bisphenol A-iminocarbonate) (Figure 4.18) formed transparent films and strong fibers. It is a tough polymer with high tensile strength. Under physiological conditions, the complete erosion of a thin film of poly(Bisphenol A-iminocarbonate) required about 200 days (Kohn and Langer, 1986).

Compression-molded disks of two tyrosine-derived polymers derived from Bisphenol A [poly(Bisphenol A-iminocarbonate) and poly(Bisphenol A *N*-phenyliminocarbonate)] were studied by Silver *et al.* (1992). The two Bisphenol A-containing polymers elicited significantly more severe tissue responses. These results indicate that the use of derivatives of the natural amino acid L-tyrosine in the synthesis of degradable implant materials improved the tissue compatibility of these materials relative to chemically related polymers that contain Bisphenol A, an industrial diphenol.

4.6.7. Polyphosphazenes

Poly(organophosphazenes), POPs, represent a versatile class of inorganic–organic macromolecules (Allcock, 1972; De Jaeger and Gleria, 1998; Allcock, 1998) mostly prepared by ring-opening polymerization of hexachlorocyclophosphazene to polydichlorophosphazene and successive substitution reaction of the very reactive chlorines of this compound with a large variety of different nucleophiles. The properties of the obtained compounds derive from the combined characteristics of the inorganic —P=N— backbone of POPs and the features of the exploited phosphorus substituents.

In this context, biomedical applications of POPs could be derived both by the hydrolytic stability and by the hydrolytic instability of these

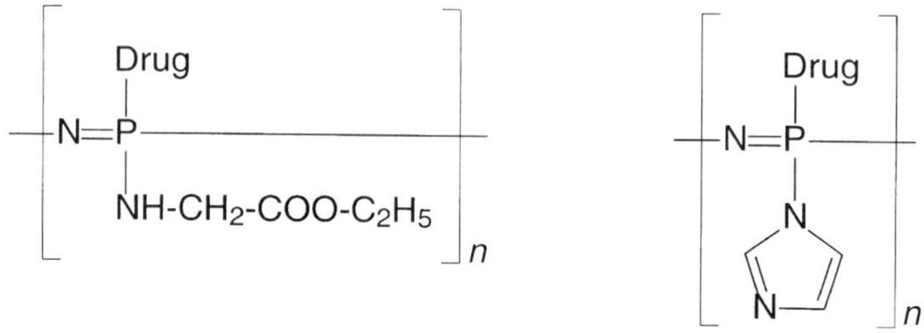

Figure 4.19A. Structure of biodegradable polyphosphazene macromolecules substituted with glycine or with imidazole for drug release.

materials (Allcock *et al.*, 1982; Allcock, 1990; Scopelianos, 1994). In the latter case, phosphazene macromolecules substituted with simple amino acid esters (glycine, alanine, etc.) (Allcock *et al.*, 1977; Schacht and Crommen, 1990; Crommen *et al.*, 1993) or with imidazole (Laurencin *et al.*, 1987) are characterized by a strong degradability under hydrolytic conditions to release the phosphorus-linked molecules of pharmacological interest (drugs) (Figure 4.19A). The ultimate degradation of the skeleton to ammonium salts and phosphates is reported in Figure 4.19B, where R_1, R_2, and R_3 are alkyl groups or other phosphazene substituents (Vandorpe *et al.*, 1997b).

Other phosphazene macromolecules functionalized with glycolic acid esters and lactic acid esters (Ibim *et al.*, 1997) or new types of phosphazene-based blends (Allcock *et al.*, 1994) were also explored as bioerodible materials for drug delivery systems and reported in the literature.

A very interesting phosphazene macromolecule recently synthesized by Allcock and Kwon (1989) is poly[bis(4-carboxylatephenoxy)phosphazene]. This polymer is insoluble in acid or neutral water, but is perfectly soluble under weakly alkaline conditions by the action of Na_2CO_3, and is easily ionically cross-linked under extremely mild experimental conditions by the action of di- (Ca^{2+}, Mg^{2+}, Zn^{2+}) or tri- (Al^{3+}) valent metal cations to produce very soft, highly swellable hydrogels able to encapsulate enzymes, living cells, antigens, proteins, etc. (Payne *et al.*, 1995a,b), as shown in Figure 4.19C. The successive coating of the produced microsphere with another polymer (e.g., poly-L-lysine) provides a semipermeable membrane through which the trapped species can be released by treatment with Na^+ ions in physiological solutions to reverse cross-linking and insolubilization of the phosphazene substrate. In addition to this first mechanism, a second process is available to attain the same goal and is based on the utilization of a phosphazene carboxylate phenoxy copolymer containing about 10% of glycine ester as a skeletal substituent. This substrate is able to hydrolytically

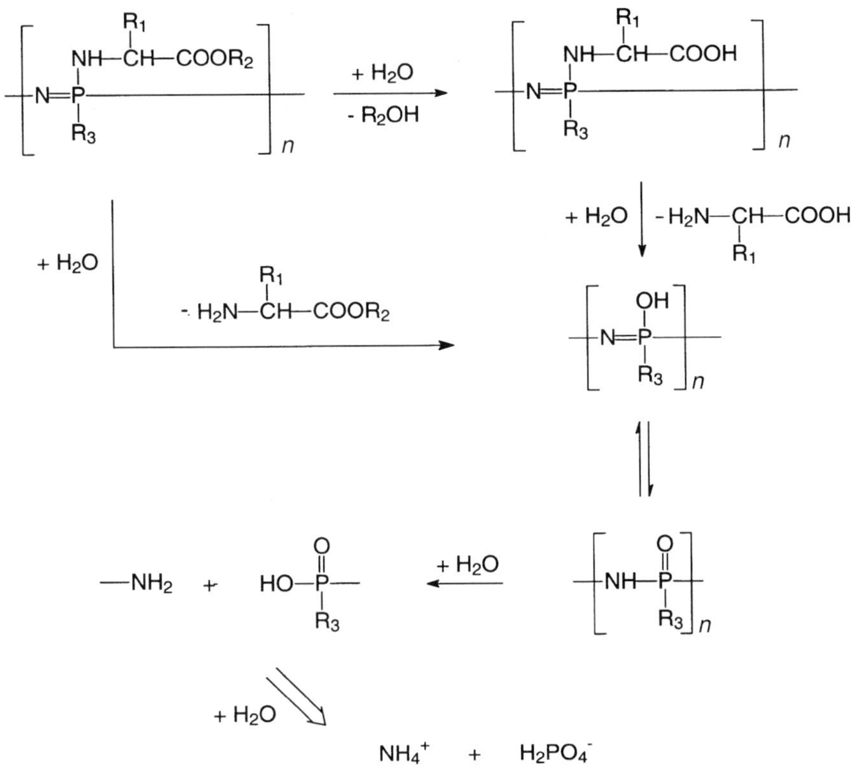

Figure 4.19B. Scheme of hydrolytic degradation of model polyphosphazene.

degrade in a few days under controlled conditions due to the presence of the amino acid residue.

The main clinical applications appear to be related to drug release, and a concerted research effort is being encouraged by Allcock (1990). *In vivo* experiments are in progress in order to evaluate, for instance, the biodistribution of degradation products (Vandorpe *et al.*, 1997a).

4.6.8. Polyethyleneterephthalate

Polyethyleneterephthalate (PET) is the most extensively used aromatic polyester in clinical applications. Synthesized from ethylene glycol and terephthalic acid and commercialized by DuPont with the tradename of Dacron®™, PET fibers have been manufactured for arterial prostheses,

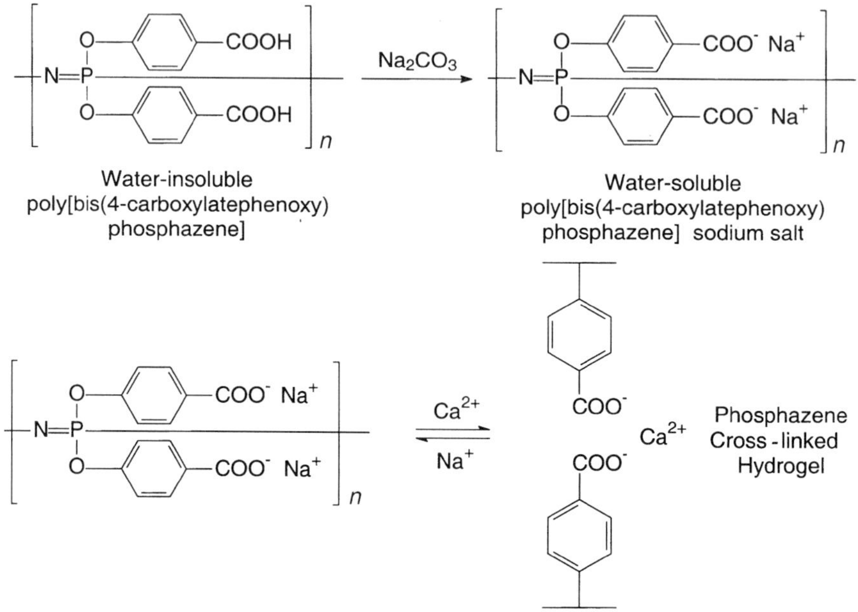

Figure 4.19C. Mechanism of solubilization and cross-linking of poly[bis(4-carboxylate-phenoxy)phosphazene].

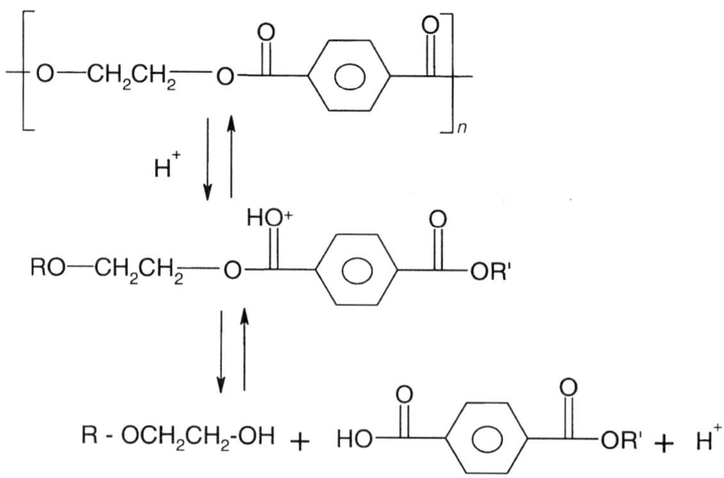

Figure 4.20. Mechanism of aromatic ester bond hydrolysis.

arterial patches, and valve sewing rings (Guidoin and Couture, 1991). After some decades, cases of long-term degeneration and failure of *in vivo* implanted prostheses were reported, and were attributed to various physicochemical factors such as hydrolytic degradation, structural defects, and processing/handling procedures (King *et al.*, 1985; Cardia and Regina, 1989). The hydrolytic cleavage of the aromatic ester bond is much slower than aliphatic groups (Table 4.2) and is represented schematically in Figure 4.20.

Rudakova *et al.* (1979) documented that during implantation in humans and subcutaneously in dog, the molecular weight of PET prostheses initially decreased, after which almost constant values were registered up to 8 years. However, expected times for the 50% reduction of filament strength and for the complete degradation of PET fibers of 10 ± 2 and 30 ± 7 years were reported, respectively. Further experiments (Gumargalieva *et al.*, 1982; Zaikov, 1985) in healthy and infected dogs exhibited in this latter case a much faster degradation due to the acid pH, and a 75% decrease in the average molecular weight after 1 year and the complete loss of properties after a few months were found. In particular, also a bulk fiber degradation was observed in SEM analysis. Other molecular weight analyses (Maarek *et al.*, 1984) confirmed the significant reduction of Mw and Mn of PET prostheses explanted after 6 months, mainly due to surface degradation which was frequently attributed to fiber damage that occurred during manufacture. In the first 15 years after implantation, this phenomenon appeared to be time-independent. The mechanical strength of commercial PET grafts after prosthesis failure was found to decrease by 2–75% of the virgin prostheses, and no apparent relation with the implantation time (ranging between 1 and 216 months) was exhibited (Vinard *et al.*, 1988). Moreover, other experimental evidence showed that infection, bacteria, and other microrganisms (Vinard *et al.*, 1991) were reported in 50 cases out of 212 of human explanted vascular grafts, and hence the graft failure could be associated to various effects in which simple hydrolysis, infection-induced degradation, fiber defects, and fatigue phenomena can also play synergistic roles. Finally, it is noteworthy that by studying the enzymatic degradation, Smith *et al.* (1987a) showed that ^{14}C-labeled poly(ethylene terephthalate) stability was affected *in vitro* by papain and esterase, while trypsine and chymotrypsine were ineffective.

4.6.9. Polyamides

Polyamide materials, or Nylons, are synthetic polymers which contain in the main backbone amide groups —NH—CO— similarly to natural polypeptides. Typical polymerization reactions are condensation from diacids and diamines or ring-opening polymerization of lactames, producing, for instance, PA-6,6 ($x = 6$, $y = 6$) and PA-11 ($z = 11$):

$$—[NH(CH)_x NH(CH)_y CO—]_n—$$
$$—[NH(CH)_z CO]_n—$$

These polymers are variously hygroscopic depending on the $CH_2/CONH$ ratio, attaining at 23 °C and at 100% RH an equilibrium water content of 15% for PA-4,6, about 9% for PA-6,6 and PA-6, and less than 2% for PA-11 and PA-12 (Williams *et al.*, 1995). The higher the water content, the more acceptable the hydrolysis. The reaction occurs under both acidic and basic conditions (Brown, 2000). After an initial effect of plasticization that reduces both modulus and strength, some hydrolytic reactions are in fact responsible for strength loosening after implantation *in vivo*. For instance, Kopecek and Ulbrich (1983) showed that the tensile strength of PA-6,6 was reduced by 75 and 17% after 89 and 726 days of implantation in dogs, respectively. Moreover, surface erosion phenomena are attributed to a proteolytic enzyme that could attack the amide group (Zaikov, 1985) with the formation of acid and amine by-products according to Figure 4.21, where an acid catalysis involves the protonation of the carbonylic bond. After *in vitro* degradation, radiolabeled PA-6 (Smith *et al.*, 1987a) was shown to be attacked by some enzymes such as trypsine, chymotrypsine, and papain, while esterase did not show any effect. The PA-6,6 suture represents a typical clinical use in which the maintenance of mechanical properties and the knot is the main requirement for the material. Another interesting application in which polyamide degradation is a desired effect is shown by the Biocompatible Osteoconductive Polymer, BOP, developed in the USSR. This material proposed for osteosynthesis, filling bone defects, neurosurgery, and stomatology comprises 50% of PA-6 fibers immersed in a matrix of vinylpyrrolidone and methylmethacrylate copolymer with 10% of calcium gluconate (Skondia *et al.*, 1987). Buron *et al.* (1994) documented that one year after implantation of a BOP rod in rabbit femur, only few fragments of PA-6 fibers were found.

On the other hand, aromatic polyamides such as Kevlar™ (*p*-phenylene terephthalate, by DuPont), which is commonly spun into high-strength fibers, are much less hydrolyzable due to the lower hydrophilicity and reactivity of the amide group conjugated with the aromatic ring.

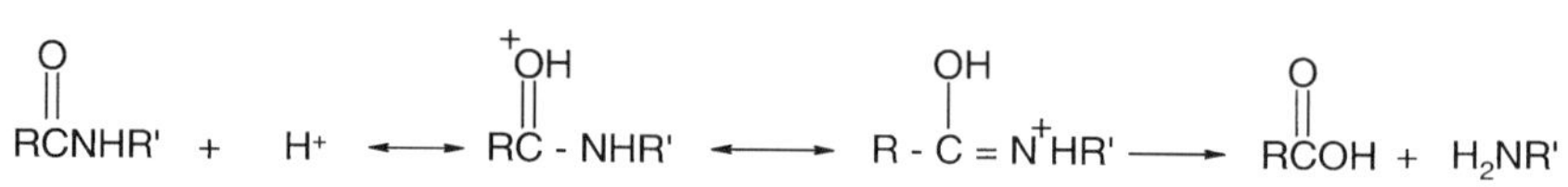

Figure 4.21. Mechanism of amide bond hydrolysis.

4.6.10. Polyurethanes

Polyurethanes are largely used for biomedical devices, such as small vessel prostheses, artificial heart, or tracheal prostheses. They represent another class in which biodegradation is an unlikely phenomenon, but which must be taken into account as a fraction of the composition (Lelah and Cooper, 1986; Szycher, 1991). Polyurethane materials are in fact segmented multiphase elastomers derived from a diisocyanate, a polyol, and a chain extender, with the formation of hard (urethane domains) and soft (polyol domains) segments. In particular, the hydrolytic stability decreases with the different type of polyol in the following order (Schollenberger and Stewart, 1973; Schollenberger, 1988):

$$\text{polyether} > \text{polycaprolactone} > \text{polyester}$$

Water sorption and hydrolysis can be increased with temperature and by changing the polyol used in making elastomer. For instance, polyester-diol polyurethanes were shown to be much more susceptible to *in vitro* degradation than polyurethanes derived from polyether diols both during an accelerated hydrolysis test at 70 °C (Ossefort and Testroet, 1966) and during a fungal degradation study. Clinical applications of polyester polyurethanes showed significant change in molecular structure and mechanical properties a few months after implantation (Mirkovitch *et al*., 1962). Moreover, while good hydrolytic stability was shown for polyester-urethanes based on poly(oxytetramethylene), poly(hexanediol-1,6-carbonate), polycaprolactone, and poly(butylene-1,4-adipate), higher degradation occurs for poly(ethylene adipate) and poly(diethylene glycol adipate) polyurethanes (Meckel *et al*., 1996). Similarly, polycaprolactone and polyether-based urethane elastomers were found to be more stable than polyadipate-urethanes during aging in water, dry air, and moist air (Magnus *et al*., 1966). Also, poly(alkylene tartrate) polyurethanes readily degraded both *in vitro* and *in vivo*. The autocatalytic effect of polyester-urethane during degradation was reported by several authors (Schollenberger and Stewart, 1973; Brown *et al*., 1980; Lelah and Cooper, 1986; Mormann and Wagner, 1988). Also, the different chain extender could affect hydrolytic stability (Masar *et al*., 1979). Under moderately acidic conditions, polyurethanes synthesized from aromatic diisocyanates should be less stable than those from aliphatic diisocyanates, and ureas were found to hydrolyze before urethanes (Chapman, 1989). Due to their higher stability, polyether-urethanes were preferred for biomedical applications.

Microbial and enzymatic degradation of some polyurethanes was reported in the literature, considering their degradation both in biological

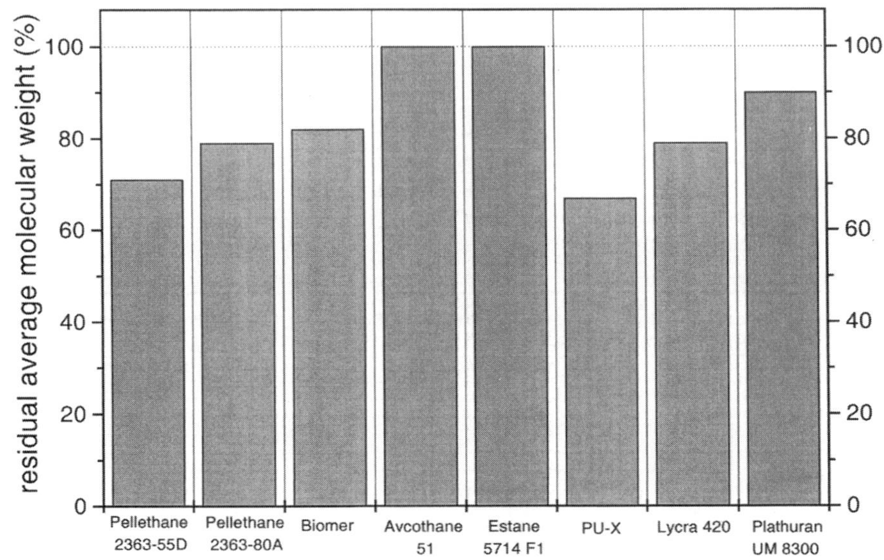

Figure 4.22. Residual molecular weight of various polyurethanes after 9 months of implantation in rats. Adapted from Lemm (1984), pp. 103–108, with kind permission of Elsevier.

environments for the long term (Lemm and Bucherl, 1983; Williams, 1984; Coury *et al.*, 1984; Santerre *et al.*, 1993; Smith *et al.*, 1987b; Zhao *et al.*, 1987; Ratner *et al.*, 1988; Phua *et al.*, 1987) and in accelerated tests at temperatures of 70–120 °C (Meijs *et al.*, 1993). Lemm (1984) reported that up to nine months of implantation in rats, several polyurethanes showed cracks and ruptures at the surface, and decreased molecular weight (Figure 4.22), but no direct influence on mechanical strength was found. Other experiments of *in vivo* strain tests on various biomedical polyurethanes reported by Lelah and Cooper (1986) showed that the resistance to surface crack propagation resulted in the following order:

Pellethane 2363-55D > Tecoflex EG-60D > Pellethane 2363-80A
> Cardiothane 51, Cardiomat 610
≫ Extruded Grade Biomer, Tecoflex EG-80A

The mechanism of degradation could be attributed to simple hydrolysis in the case of polyester-based polyurethanes, while effects of enzymatic, metal catalyst, and oxidative reactions can play synergistic roles in other materials.

In fact, polyether-based polyurethanes are much prone to undergo oxidative phenomena, as was also confirmed by the oxidation products found on the polymer surface after *in vivo* implantation.

4.7. Factors Affecting the Degradation of Polymeric Materials

Various factors influence the degradation of polymers (Kimura, 1993; Hasirci, 2000), as summarized in Table 4.6. They are: (i) the chemical and physical characteristics of polymer, (ii) the fabrication process, and (iii) the degradation conditions. Chemical structure influences both the hydrophobicity/hydrophilicity and the hydrolyzability of polymer bonds, as already described in earlier paragraphs. For instance, PCL is much more hydrophobic than PGA, due to the higher ratio of CH_2/COO methylenic/carboxylic groups. Moreover, the degree of crystallinity and the glass transition temperature play a relevant role, because at 37 °C the polymer could behave as a glass being below its T_g value (PDLLA, amorphous), or even above but with the amorphous chains blocked by the semicrystalline structure (PCL, PGA), or again as a glass but with less or more stiff/ductile behavior depending on the degree of crystallinity (PLLA). Experimental *in vitro* and *in vivo* degradation showed that degradation of polyglycolic acid occurs in 3–4 weeks (Chu, 1981; Chu and Williams, 1983), polylactic acid lasts much longer, even up to 3–4 years (Bergsma *et al.*, 1995), and crystalline polymers degrade slower than amorphous ones, e.g., PLLA and PDLLA, respectively (Migliaresi *et al.*, 1994; Zhang *et al.*, 1994).

Table 4.6. Factors Affecting the Degradation of Polymers

Characteristics of polymer	Chemical structure
	Molecular weight and distribution
	Crystallinity
	Enantiomeric purity
	Additives and impurities
Fabrication process	Type of process
	Thermal treatment
	Shape factor
	Superficial morphology
	Sterilization process
Degradation medium	Solution
	Site of implantation

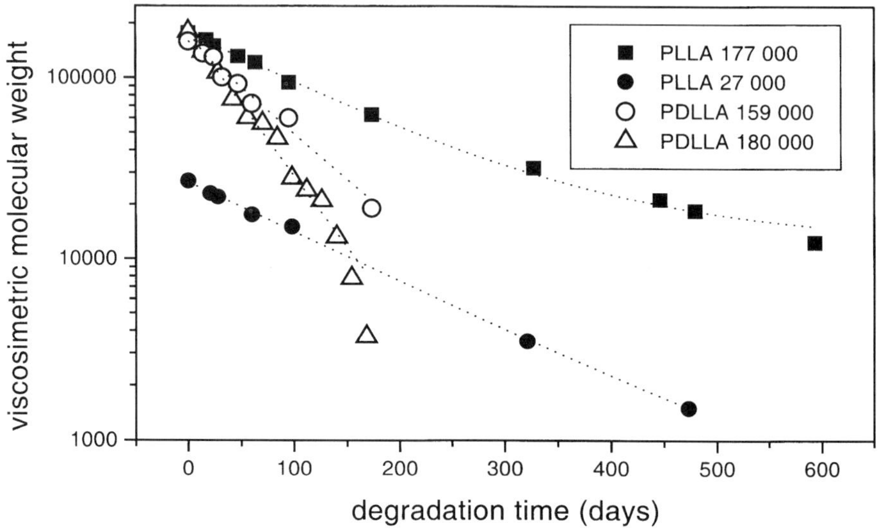

Figure 4.23. Viscometric molecular weight of poly-L-lactide (PLLA) and poly-DL-lactide (PDLLA) samples during *in vitro* degradation in Ringer solution at 37 °C. The numbers indicate the initial molecular weight.

Figure 4.23 depicts well the difference between polylactides with different enantiomeric purity (PDLLA and PLLA) during *in vitro* degradation. The linear dependence in a log scale diagram of the molar mass decrease is in good agreement with the kinetics mechanism of first order proposed by Pitt *et al.* (1979). In particular, both PLLAs with different initial viscometric molar mass showed a lower kinetics constant with respect to the PDLLAs. Mechanical properties showed a direct dependence on the molar mass decrease, and flexural strength was found to significantly decrease below 60,000 dalton for PDLLA and below 30,000 dalton for PLLA (Figure 4.24).

In amorphous copolymers, the degradation kinetics can be accelerated by increasing the amount of the lower T_g comonomer. As reported in Figure 4.25 for poly(DL-lactide-co-ε-caprolactone), the higher the percentage of caprolactone, the faster the reduction in the mechanical properties, as a consequence of the lower glass transition temperature and of the higher water sorption. Additives and impurities can modify either the hydrophilicity or the degradation mechanism. For instance, the presence of residual monomer was demonstrated to dramatically accelerate the degradation kinetics of poly-DL-lactide (Fambri *et al.*, 1995), due to the higher water sorption and to the autocatalytic effect of low molar mass by-products.

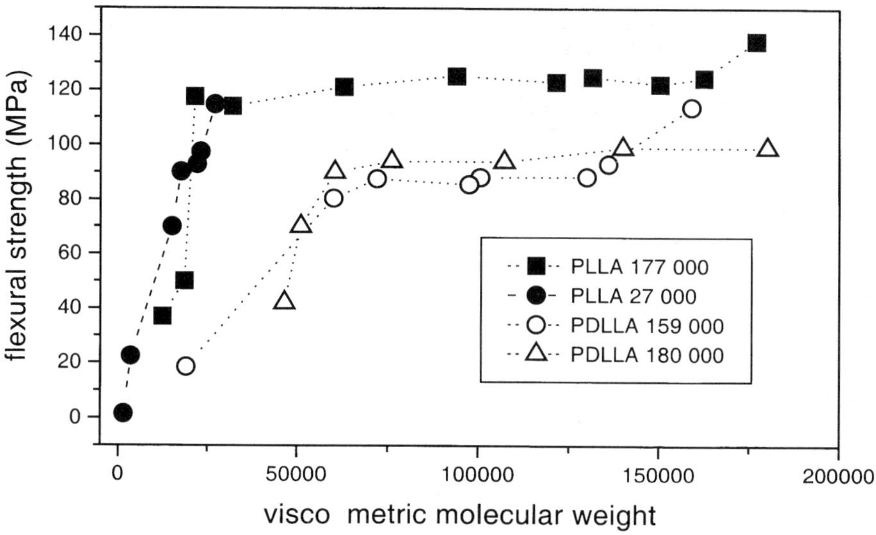

Figure 4.24. Flexural strength of poly-L-lactide (PLLA) and poly-DL-lactide (PDLLA) samples as a function of viscosimetric molecular weight during *in vitro* degradation in Ringer solution at 37 °C (see Figure 4.23).

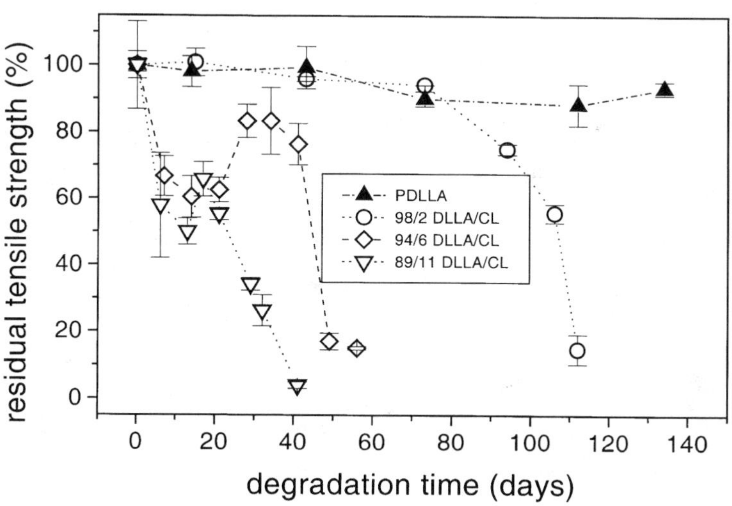

Figure 4.25. Residual tensile strength of poly-DL-lactide (PDLLA) and poly(DL-lactide-co-ε-caprolactone) copolymers (DLLA/CL) during *in vitro* degradation in Ringer solution at 37 °C. The numbers indicate the different DL-lactide/ε-caprolactone molar ratio.

Degradation can induce crystallization (Migliaresi *et al.*, 1994; Pegoretti *et al.*, 1997), as a consequence of the plasticizing effect of water and the higher mobility of the amorphous phase.

The processing condition of the biodegradable polymer can play a very important role on its final characteristics, some of them being sensitive to thermal degradation or resulting from the hydrolysis catalyzed by temperature, even if in the presence of very small amounts of water. For instance, sensible reduction in the molar mass of PLLA materials was found after compression molding (Migliaresi *et al.*, 1991a), thermal treatment (Migliaresi *et al.*, 1991b), or melt-spinning (Fambri *et al.*, 1997).

More specifically, von Oepen and Michaeli (1992) studied the injection molding of PLLA and the effect of various parameters on molar mass decrease during processing. In particular, the higher the percentage of moisture and the higher the processing temperature (see Figure 4.26) or the

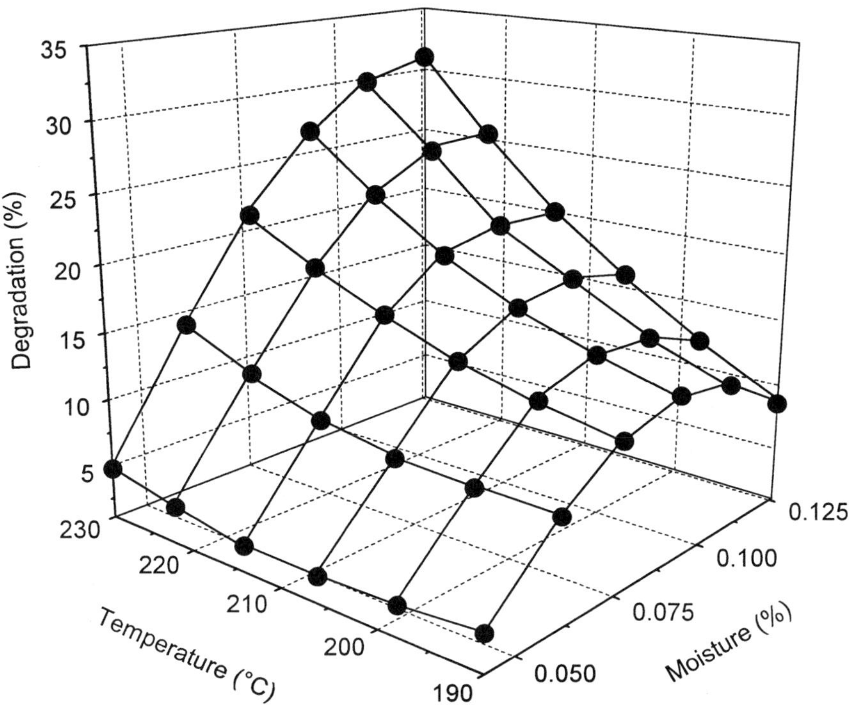

Figure 4.26. Percentage of PLLA molecular weight degradation during injection molding as a function of the residual moisture percentage and temperature processing. Adapted from von Oepen and Michaeli (1992), with kind permission of Elsevier.

Table 4.7. Viscosimetric Molecular Weight of Bulk PLLA and PDLLA Samples Before and After Sterilization with Beta-Rays, Ethylene Oxide, and Gamma-Rays

Polymer	Initial	After ETOX	After gamma-rays (2.5 MRad)
PLLA	240.000 (100%)	200.000 (83%)	138.000 (58%)
	165.000 (100%)	162.000 (98%)	86.000 (52%)
PDLLA	285.000 (100%)	—	151.000 (53%)
	209.000 (100%)	—	99.000 (47%)
	150.800 (100%)	148.000 (98%)	50.000 (33%)

higher the residence time (in the range 50–300 sec) and the higher the shear rate, the higher the percentage of degradation.

Furthermore, depending on the type and intensity of the sterilization procedure (ethylene oxide, beta-rays, gamma-rays), various degradation phenomena can occur and determine an anticipated/premature reduction of properties during application with respect to the expected values. Gamma radiation was found to be very critical for polyester-based material, as reported in the case of poly(lactide) (Goupta and Deshmukh, 1983) and for the enzymatic degradation of irradiated polyglycolide and polydioxanone sutures (Chu and Williams, 1983; Williams *et al.*, 1984). Table 4.7 shows that gamma-rays were more aggressive than ethylene oxide during sterilization of bulk polylactide samples, the residual molar mass being lower than 60% and higher than 80%, respectively. A parallel decrease in mechanical properties was also reported in the case of PLLA fiber before and after sterilization with beta-rays, ethylene oxide, and gamma-rays (Table 4.8). The hydrolytic degradation of commercial absorbable suture was also found to be affected by the gamma irradiation dose and the irradiation temperature (Chu *et al.*, 1995).

Finally, the degradation properties depend also on the site in which materials are implanted during *in vivo* applications and the effect of tissue

Table 4.8. Mechanical Properties of PLLA Fiber (diameter 115 ± 8 micron) Before and After Sterilization with Beta-Rays, Ethylene Oxide, and Gamma-Rays

Fiber samples	As produced	After beta-rays	After ETOX	After gamma-rays
Elastic modulus (GPa)	9.0(±0.7)	11(±0.6)	9.9(±0.2)	10.0(±0.1)
Yielding stress (MPa)	309(±27)	305(±43)	266(±14)	251(±14)
Stress at break (MPa)	780(±44)	651(±29)	630(±23)	483(±43)

vascularization or enzyme presence can play a specific role with respect to the simple hydrolytic reaction during *in vitro* experiments (phosphate buffer solution, Ringer solution, or enzymatic solution at 37 °C).

References

Abatangelo, G., Barbucci, R., Brun, P., Lamponi, S. 1997. Biocompatibility and enzymatic degradation studies on sulphated hyaluronic acid derivatives, *Biomaterials* **18**(21), 1411–1415.

Allcock, H.R. 1972. *Phosphorus–Nitrogen Compounds. Cyclic, Linear, and High Polymeric Systems*, Academic Press, New York.

Allcock, H.R. 1990, Polyphosphazenes as new biomedical and bioactive materials, in: *Biodegradable Polymers as Drug Delivery Systems* (M. Chasin, R. Langer, eds.), Ch. 5, pp. 163–193, Marcel Dekker, New York.

Allcock H.R. 1998, Functional polyphosphazenes, in: *Functional Polymers. Modern Synthetic Methods and Novel Structures* (A.O. Patil, D.N. Schulz, B.N. Novak, eds.), Vol. 704, Ch. 18, pp. 261–275, ACS Symposium Series, Washington.

Allcock, H.R., Kwon, S. 1989. An ionically cross-linkable polyphosphazene: Poly[bis(carboxylactophenoxy)phosphazene] and its hydrogels and membranes, *Macromolecules* **22**, 75–79.

Allcock, H.R., Fuller, T.J., Mack, D.P., Matsumura, K., Smeltz, K.M. 1977. Phosphazene compounds. Synthesis of poly[(amino acid alkylester)phosphazenes], *Macromolecules* **10**, 824–830.

Allcock, H.R., Fuller, T.J., Matsumura, K. 1982. Hydrolysis pathways for aminophosphazenes, *Inorg. Chem.* **21**, 515–521.

Allcock, H.R., Pucher, S.R., Scopelianos, A.G. 1994. Synthesis of poly(organophosphazenes) with glycolic acid ester and lactic acid ester side groups—Prototypes for new bioerodible polymers, *Macromolecules* **27**, 1–4.

Amass, W., Amass, A., Tighe, B. 1998. A review of biodegradable polymers: uses, current developments in the synthesis and characterization of biodegradable polyesters, blends of biodegradable polymers and recent advances in biodegradation studies, *Polym. Int.* **47**, 89–144.

Amiel, G.E., Sukhotnik. I., Kawar, B., Siplovich, L. 1999. Use of *N*-butyl-2-cyanoacrylate in elective surgical incisions—long-term outcomes, *J. Am. Coll. Surg.* **189**(1), 21–25.

Anderson, J.M. 1986. In vivo biocompatibility studies: perspectives on the evaluation of biomedical polymer biocompatibility, in: *Polymeric Biomaterials* (E. Piskin, A.S. Hoffman, eds.), pp. 29–39, Martin Nijhoff Publishers, Dordrecht.

Anderson, A.B., Clapper, D.L. 1998. Coatings for blood-contacting devices, *Med. Plast. Biomat.* **3**, 16–20.

Andriano, K., Daniels, A.U., Heller, J., 2000. In vitro and in vivo degradation studies of absorbable poly(orthoester) proposed for internal tissue fixation devices, in: *Biomaterials and Bioengineering Handbook* (D.L. Wise, ed.), Ch. 25, pp. 577–601, Marcel Dekker, New York.

Arem, A. 1985. Collagen modifications, *Clin. Plast. Surg.* **12**, 209–220.

Atala, A., Mooney, D.J., Vacanti, J.P., Langer, R. 1997. *Synthetic Biodegradable Polymer Scaffold: Tissue Engineering*, Birkhäuser, Boston.

Atkins, T.W., Peacock, S.J. 1996. In vitro biodegradation of poly(beta-hydroxybutyratehydroxyvalerate) microspheres exposed to Hanks' buffer, newborn calf serum, pancreatin and synthetic gastric juice, *J. Biomater. Sci. Polym.* **7**(12), 1075–1084.

Auger, F.A., Rouabhia, M., Goulet, F., Berthod, F., Moulin, V., Germain, L. 1998. Tissue-engineered human skin substitutes developed from collagen-populated hydrated gels: clinical and fundamental applications, *Med. Biol. Eng. Comput.* **36**(6), 801–812.

Bakker, D., van Blitterswijk, C.A., Hesseling, S.C., Koerten, H.K., Kuijpers, W., Grote, J.J. 1990. Biocompatibility of a polyether urethane, polypropylene oxide, and a polyether polyester copolymer. A qualitative and quantitative study of three alloplastic tympanic membrane materials in the rat middle ear, *J. Biomed. Mater. Res.* **24**(4), 489–515.

Balazs, E.A. 1995. Hyaluronan biomaterials: Medical applications, in: *Handbook of Biomaterials and Applications* (D.L. Wise, ed.), pp. 2719–2741, Marcel Dekker, New York.

Barrows, T.H. 1986. Degradable implant materials: a review of synthetic absorbable polymers and their application, *Clin. Mater.* **1**, 233-257.

Barrows, T.H. 1991. Synthetic bioabsorbable polymers, in: *High Performance Biomaterials* (M. Szycher, ed.), pp. 243–257, Technomic Publ., Lancaster, PA.

Barrows, T.H. 1994. Bioabsorbable poly(ester-amides), in: *Biomedical Polymers. Designed-to-Degrade Systems* (S.W. Shalaby, ed.), pp. 97–116, Hanser Publ., Munich.

Barrows, T.H., Grussing, D.M., Hegdahl, D.W. 1983. Poly(ester-amides): a new class of synthetic absorbable polymers, *Trans. Soc. Biomater.* **6**, 109.

Bartone, F.F., Shervey, P.D., Gardner, P.J. 1976. Long term tissue responses to catgut and collagen sutures, *Invest. Urol.* **13**(6), 390–394.

Becker, M.A., Tuross, N. 1993. Initial degradative changes found in bombyx mori silk fibroin, in: *Silk Polymers: Materials Science and Biotechnology* (D. Kaplan, W. Adams, B. Farmer, C. Viney, eds.), *ACS Symp. Ser.*, **544**, 254–268.

Benicewitz, B.C., Hopper, P.K. 1990, Polymers for absorbable surgical sutures — Part I, *J. Bioact. Biocomp. Polym.* **5** (October), 453–472.

Benicewitz, B.C., Hopper, P.K. 1991. Polymers for absorbable surgical sutures — Part II, *J. Bioact. Biocomp. Polym.* **6** (January), 64–94.

Bergsma, J.E., de Bruijn, W.C., Rozema, F.R., Bos, R.R.M., Boering, G. 1995. Late degradation tissue response to poly(L-lactide) bone plates and screws, *Biomaterials* **16**, 25–31.

Berry, A.R., Wilson, M.C., Thomson, J.W.W., McNair, T.J. 1981. Polydioxanone: a new synthetic absorbable suture, *J. R. Coll. Surg. Edinburgh* **26**, 170–172.

Beumer, G.J., van Blitterswijk, C.A., Ponec, M. 1994. Biocompatibility of a biodegradable matrix used as a skin substitute: an in vivo evaluation, *J. Biomed. Mater. Res.* **28**(5), 545–552.

Bischoff, C.A., Walden, P. 1893. Ueber das glycolid und seine homologen, *Berichte* **26**, 262–265.

Boeree, N.R., Dove, J., Cooper, J.J., Knowles, J., Hastings, G.W. 1993. Development of a degradable composite for orthopaedic use: mechanical evaluation of an hydroxyapatite–polyhydroxybutyrate composite material, *Biomaterials* **14**(10), 793–796.

Bogdansky, S. 1990. Natural polymers as drug delivery systems, in: *Biodegradable Polymers as Drug Delivery Systems* (M. Chasin, R. Langer eds.), pp. 231–259, Marcel Dekker Inc., New York.

Borgdorff, P., Van den Berg, R.H., Vis, M.A.., Van den Bos, G.C., Tangelder, G.J. 1999, Pump-induced platelet aggregation in albumin-coated extracorporeal systems, *J. Thorac. Cardiovasc. Surg.* **118**(5), 946–952.

Bos, G.W., Scharenborg, N.M., Poot, A.A., Engbers, G.H., Beugeling, T., Van Aken, W.G., Feijen, J. 1999. Blood compatibility of surfaces with immobilized albumin-heparin conjugate and effect of endothelial cell seeding on platelet adhesion, *J. Biomed. Mater. Res.* **47**(3), 279–291.

Bouillot, P., Ubrich, N., Sommer, F., Duc, T.M., Loeffler, J.P., Dellacherie, E. 1999. Protein encapsulation in biodegradable amphiphilic microspheres, *Int. J. Pharm.* **181**(2), 159–172.

Bouvier, M., Chawla, A.S., Hinberg, I. 1991. In vitro degradation of a poly(ether urethane) by trypsine, *J. Biomed. Mater. Res.* **25**, 773–789.

Brem, H. 1990. Polymers to treat brain tumours, *Biomaterials* **11**, 699–701.

Britritto, M.M., Bell, J.P., Brenckle, S., Huang, S.J., Knox, J.R. 1979. Synthesis and biodegradation of polymers derived from α-hydroxy acids, *J. Appl. Polym. Sci., Appl. Polym. Symp.*, **35**, 405–414.

Brookfield, P., Murphy, P., Harker, R., MacRae, E. 1997. Starch degradation and starch pattern indices; interpretation and relationship to maturity, *Post. Biol. Technol.* **11**(1), 23–30.

Brown, D.W., Lowry, R.E., Smith, L.E. 1980. Kinetics of hydrolytic aging of polyester urethane elastomers, *Macromolecules* **13**, 248–252.

Brown, R.S., 2000. Studies in amide hydrolysis: the acid, base and water reaction, in: *The Amide Linkage* (A. Greenberg, C.M. Breneman, J.F. Liebman, eds.), pp. 85–114, John Wiley & Sons, New York.

Brumback, G.F., McPherson, S.D., Jr. 1967. Reconstituted collagen sutures in corneal surgery. An experimental and clinical evaluation, *J. Ophthalmol.* **64**(2), 222–227.

Bulstra, S.K., Geesink, R.G., Bakker, D., Bulstra, T.H., Bouwmeester, S.J., van der Linden, A.J. 1996. Femoral canal occlusion in total hip replacement using a resorbable and flexible cement restrictor, *J. Bone Joint Surg. Br.* **78**(6), 892–898.

Buron, F., Bourgois, R., Burny, F., Chaboteaux C., d'Hericourt, J., El Banna, S., Pasteels, J.L., Sintzoff, S., Vienne, A. 1994. BOP: Biocompatible osteoconductive polymer: an experimental approach, *Clin. Mater.* **16**, 217–221.

Caghey, G.H. 1991. The structure and airway biology of mast cell proteinases, *Am. J. Resp. Cell. Mol. Biol.* **4**(5), 387–394.

Capello, J., McGrath, K.P. 1993. Spinning of protein polymer fibers, in: *Silk Polymers: Materials Science and Biotechnology* (D. Kaplan, W. Adams, B. Farmer, C. Viney, eds.), *ACS Symp. Ser.* **544**, 310–326.

Cardia, G., Regina, G. 1989. Degenerative Dacron graft changes: is there a biological component in this textile defect? A case report, *Vasc. Surg.* **23**(3), 245–247.

Carothers, W.H., Dorough, G.L., Van Natta, F.J. 1932. Studies of polymerization and ring formation. X. The reversible polymerization of six-membered cyclic esters, *J. Am. Chem. Soc.*, **54**, 761–772.

Chambliss, W.G. 1983. The forgotten dosage form: enteric-coated tablets, *Pharm. Technol.* September, 124–140.

Chandra, R., Rustgi, R. 1998. Biodegradable polymers, *Progr. Polym. Sci.* **23**, 1273–1335.

Chapman, T.M. 1989. Models for polyurethanes hydrolysis under moderately acidic conditions: a comparative study of hydrolysis rates of urethanes, ureas and amides, *J. Appl. Polym. Sci., Polym. Chem.* **27**, 1993–2005.

Charles, G.G., Daniel, M. 1985. The synthesis of some potentially blood compatible heparin-like polymeric materials, in: *Frontiers of Polymers and Advanced Materials, Advances in Biomedical Polymers Series* (G.G. Charles, ed.), pp. 277–284, Plenum Press, New York.

Chasin, M., Langer, R. 1990. *Biodegradable Polymers as Drug Delivery Systems*, Marcel Dekker, New York.

Chasin, M., Lewis, D., Langer, R. 1988. Polyanhydrides for controlled drug delivery, *Biopharm. Manuf.* **1**, 33–46.

Chasin, M., Domb., A., Ron, E., Mathiowitz, E., Langer, R., Leong, K., Laurencin, C., Brem, H., Grossman, S. 1990. Polyanhydrides as drug delivery systems, in: *Biodegradable Polymers as Drug Delivery Systems* (M. Chasin, R. Langer, eds.), pp. 43–70, Marcel Dekker, New York.

Choi, N.S., Heller, J. 1978. Drug delivery devices manufactured from poly(orthoesters) and poly(orthocarbonates), *US Patent*, 4 093 709, June 6.

Choi, N.S., Heller, J. 1979. Erodible agent releasing device comprising poly(orthoesters) and poly(orthocarbonates), *US Patent*, 4 138 344, Feb. 6.

Choi, Y.S., Hong, S.R, Lee, Y.M., Song, K.W., Park, M.H., Nam, Y.S. 1999. Studies on gelatin-containing artificial skin: II. Preparation and characterization of cross-linked gelatin-hyaluronate sponge, *J. Biomed. Mater. Res.* **48**(5), 631–639.

Christel, P., Chabot, F., Leray, J.L., Morin, C., Vert, M. 1982. Biodegradable composites for internal fixation, in: *Advances in Biomaterials. Biomaterials 1980*, Vol. 3 (D.G. Winter, D.F. Gibbons, J. Plench, Jr., eds.), pp. 271–280, John Wiley & Sons, New York.

Chu, C.C. 1981. Hydrolytic degradation of polyglycolic acid: Tensile strength and crystallinity study, *J. Appl. Polym. Sci.* **26**, 1727–1734.

Chu, C.C. 1983. Survey of clinically important wound closure biomaterials, in: *Biocompatible Polymers, Metals, and Composites* (M. Szycher, ed.), Ch. 22, pp. 477–523, Technomic Publ. Co., Lancaster, PA.

Chu, C.C. 1995. Biodegradable polymeric biomaterials: an overview, in: *The Biomedical Engineering Handbook* (J. D. Bronzino, ed.), pp. 611–626, CRC Press, Boca Raton.

Chu, C.C., Williams, D.F. 1983. The effect of gamma irradiation on the enzymatic degradation of polyglycolic acid absorbable sutures, *J. Biomed. Mater. Res.* **17**, 1029–1040.

Chu, C.C., Lee, K.H. 2000. The role of free radicals in degradation of biodegradable biomaterials, in: *Biomaterials and Bioengineering Handbook* (D.L. Wise, ed.), Ch. 5, pp. 157–177, Marcel Dekker, New York.

Chu, C.C., Zhang, L., Coyne, L.D. 1995. Effect of gamma irradiation and irradiation temperature on hydrolytic degradation of synthetic absorbable sutures, *J. Appl. Polym. Sci.*, **56**, 1275–1294.

Chujo, K., Kobayashi, H., Suzuki, J., Tokuhara, S., Tanabe, M. 1967. Ring-opening polymerization of glycolide, *Makromol. Chem.* **100**, 262–266.

Chung, L.Y., Shmidt, R.J., Hamlyn, P.F., Sagar, B.F., Andrews, A.M. 1994. Biocompatibility of potential wound management products: Fungal mycelia as a source of chitin/chitosan and their effect on the proliferation of human F1000 fibroblasts in culture, *J. Biomed. Mat. Res.* **28**, 463–469.

Chvapil, M., Kronenthal, R.L., van Winkle, W. 1973. Medical and surgical applications of collagen, *Int. Rev. Connect. Tissue Res.* **6**, 1–61.

Ciapetti, G., Stea, S., Cenni, E., Sudanese, A., Marraro, D., Toni, A., Pizzoferrato, A. 1994. Cytotoxicity testing of cyanoacrylates using direct contact assay on cell cultures, *Biomaterials* **15**(1), 63–67.

Cohn, D., Younes, H. 1988. Biodegradable PEO/PELA block copolymers, *J. Biomed. Mater. Res.* **22**, 993–1009.

Cohn, D., Younes, H. 1989. Compositional and structural analysis of PELA biodegradable block copolymers degrading under in vitro conditions, *Biomaterials* **10**, 466–474.

Coleman, W.P. 1996. Assessment of a new device for injecting bovine collagen—The ADG needle, *Dermatol. Surg.* **22**(2), 175–176.

Coury, A.J. 1996. Chemical and biochemical degradation of polymers, in: *Biomaterials Science: An Introduction to Materials in Medicine* (B.D. Ratner, A.S. Hoffman, F.J. Schoen, J.E. Lemons, eds.), pp. 243–260, Academic Press, San Diego.

Coury, A.J., Cahalan, P.T., Schultz, E.L., Stokes, K.B. 1984. In vitro aging of implantable polyurethanes in metal ion solutions, *Trans. Soc. Biomater.* **7**, 252.

Crommen, J., Vandorpe, J., Schacht, E. 1993. Degradable polyphosphazenes for biomedical applications, *J. Controlled Release* **24**, 167–180.

Dahiyat, B.I., Hostin, E., Posadas, E.M., Leong, K.W. 1993. Synthesis and characterization of putrescine-based poly(phosphoester-urethanes), *J. Biomater. Sci. Polym. Ed.* **4**(5), 529–536.

Daniels, A.U., Chang, M.K.O., Andriano, K.P., Heller, J. 1990. Mechanical properties of biodegradable polymers and composites proposed for internal fixation of bone, *J. Appl. Biomater.* **1**, 57–78.

David, F.R. 1986. Liquid loaded pad for medical applications, *US Patent*, 4 588 400.

Davies, M.C., Khan, M.A., Lynn, R.A., Heller, J., Watts, J.F. 1991. X-ray photoelectron spectroscopy analysis of the surface chemical structure of some biodegradable poly(orthoesters), *Biomaterials* **12**(3), 305–308.

Davis, S.S., Illum, L., McVie, J.G., Tomlinson, E. 1984. *Microspheres and Drug Therapy: Pharmaceutical, Immunological and Medical Aspects*, pp. 50–55, Elsevier, Amsterdam.

De Jaeger, R., Gleria, M. 1998. Poly(organophosphazene)s and related compounds: synthesis, properties and applications, *Progr. Poym. Sci.* **23**, 179–276.

Demura, M., Asakura, T., Kuroo, T. 1989. Immobilization of biocatalyst with bomboxy mori silk fibroin by several kinds of physical treatment and its application to glucose sensors, *Biosensors* **4**, 361–372.

Doddi, N., Versfelt, C.C., Wasserman, D. 1977. Synthetic absorbable surgical devices of poly-dioxanone, *US Patent*, 4052 988.

Doi, Y. 1990. *Microbial Polyesters*, Carl Hanser Verlag, New York.

Domb, A.J., Amselem, S., Langer, R., Maniar, M. 1994. Polyanhydrides as carriers of drugs, in: *Biomedical Polymers. Designed-to-Degrade Systems* (S.W. Shalaby, ed.), pp. 69–96, Hanser Publ., Munich.

Domb, A.J., Kost, J., Wiseman, D.M. 1997. *Handbook for Biodegradable Polymers*, Harwood Academic Publ., Singapore.

Dongmei, Z., Hanfa, Z., Jianyi, N., Li, Y., Lingyun, J., Yukui, Z. 1998. *Chin. J. Biotechnol.* **14**(4), 233–240.

Edwards-Levy, F., Levy, M.C. 1999. Serum albumin-alginate coated beads: mechanical properties and stability, *Biomaterials* **20**(21), 2069–2084.

Engelberg, I., Kohn, J. 1991. Physico-mechanical properties of degradable polymers used in medical applications: a comparative study, *Biomaterials* **12**, 292–304.

Engler, R.J., Weber, C.B., Turnicky, R. 1986. Hypersensitivity to chromated catgut sutures: a case report and review of the literature, *Ann. Allergy* **56**(4), 317–320.

Fambri, L., Guerriero, A., Grimaldi, M., Migliaresi C. 1995. Effect of polymer purity on the in vitro degradation of compression moulded poly-DL-lactic acid materials *12th European Conference on Biomaterials*, p. 38, Porto 10–13 September.

Fambri, L., Pegoretti, A., Fenner, R., Incardona, S.D., Migliaresi, C. 1997. Biodegradable fibres of poly(L-lactic acid) produced by melt spinning, *Polymer* **38**(1), 79–85.

Fambri, L., Pelz, M., Liedkte, H., Migliaresi, C. 2000. Production and characterisation of osteoinductive polylactide composites, *Proceedings of 6th World Biomaterials Conference*, p. 506, May 15–20, Kamuela, Hawaii.

Feijen, J. 1986. Biodegradable polymers for medical purpose, in: *Polymeric Biomaterials* (E. Piskin, A.S. Hoffman, eds.), pp. 62–77, Martinus Nijhoff Publishers, Dordrecht.

Ferguson, S., Wahl, D., Gogolewski, S. 1996. Enhancement of the mechanical properties of polylactides by solid-state extrusion. II. Poly(L-lactide), poly(L/D-lactide), and poly(L/DL-lactide, *J. Biomed. Mater. Res.* **30**(4), 543–551.

Franssen, O., Stenekes, R.J., Hennink, W.E. 1999a. Controlled release of a model protein from enzymatically degrading dextran microspheres, *J. Controlled Release* **59**(2), 219–228.

Franssen, O., Vandervennet, L., Roders, P., Hennink, W.E. 1999b. Degradable dextran hydrogels: controlled release of a model protein from cylinders and microspheres, *J. Controlled Release* **60**(2–3), 211–221.

Frazza, E.J., Schmitt, E.E. 1971. A new absorbable suture, *J. Biomed. Mater. Res. Symp.* **1**, 43–58.

Friess, W. 1998. Collagen-biomaterial for drug delivery, *Eur. J. Pharm. Biopharm.* **45**(2), 113–136.

Friess, W., Uludag, H., Foskett, S., Biron, R., Sargeant, C. 1999. Characterization of absorbable collagen sponges as rhBMP-2 carriers, *Int. J. Pharm.* **187**(1), 91–99.

Fukuzaki, H., Yoshida, M., Asano, M., Kumakura, M. 1989. Synthesis of copoly(D,L-lactic acid) with relatively low molecular weight and in vitro degradation, *Eur. Polym. J.* **25**, 1019–1026.

Gaillard, M.L., van Blitterswijk, C.A. 1994. Pre-operative addition of calcium ions or calcium phosphate to PEO/PBT copolymers (Polyactive™) stimulates bone mineralization in vitro, *J. Mater. Sci., Mater. Med.* **5**, 695–701.

Gangrade, N., Price, J.C. 1991. Poly(hydroxybutyrate-hydroxyvalerate) microspheres containing progesterone: preparation, morphology and release properties, *J. Microencapsul.* **8**(2), 185–202.

Gennadios, A., McHugh, T.H., Weller, C.L., Kroctha, J.M. 1994. Edible coatings and films based on proteins, in: *Edible Coating and Films to Improve Food Quality* (J.M. Kroctha, E.A. Baldwin, M.O. Nisperos-Carriedo, eds.), pp. 201–277, Technomic Publ. Co., Lancaster, PA.

Gilding, D.K. 1981. Biodegradable polymers, in: *Biocompatibility of Clinical Implant Materials*, Vol. 2 (D.F. Williams, ed.), pp. 209–232, CRC Press, Boca Raton.

Gilding, D.K., Reed, A.M. 1979. Biodegradable polymers for use in surgery—polyglycolic/polylactic acid homo- and copolymers: 1, *Polymer* **20**, 1459–1464.

Gogly, B., Dridi, M., Hornebeck W., Bonnefoix, M., Godeau, G., Pellat, B., 1999. Effect of heparin on the production of matrix metalloproteinases and tissue inhibitors of metalloproteinases by human dermal fibroblasts, *Cell. Biol. Int.* **23**(3), 203–209.

Goissis, G., Marcantonio, E. Jr., Marcantonio, R.A., Lia, R.C., Cancian, D.C., de Carvalho, W.M. 1999. Biocompatibility studies of anionic collagen membranes with different degree of glutaraldehyde cross-linking, *Biomaterials* **20**(1), 27–34.

Goodman, I. 1988. Polyesters, in: *Encyclopedia of Polymers Science and Engineering*, 2nd edn. (H.F. Mark, N.M. Bikales, C.G. Overberger, G. Menges, eds.), Vol. 12, pp. 1–75, John Wiley & Sons, New York.

Gopferich A. 1999. Biodegradable polymers: Polyanhydrides, in: *Encyclopedia of Controlled Drug Delivery* (E. Mathiowitz, ed.), Vol. 1, pp. 60–71, John Wiley & Sons, New York.

Gorham, S.D. 1991. Collagen, in: *Biomaterials, Novel Materials from Biological Sources* (D. Byron, ed.), Ch. 2, Stockton Press, New York.

Goupil, D. 1996. Sutures, in: *Biomaterials Science: An Introduction to Materials in Medicine* (B.D. Ratner, A.S. Hoffman, F.J. Schoen, J.E. Lemons, eds.), pp. 356–360, Academic Press, San Diego.

Goupta, M.C., Deshmukh, V.G. 1983. Radiation effects on poly(lactic acid), *Polymer*, **24**, 827–830.

Grasset, L., Cordier, D., Ville A. 1977. Woven silk as a carrier for the immobilization of enzymes, *Biotechnol. Bioeng.* **19**(4), 611–618.

Greenwald, D., Shumway, S., Albear, P., Gottlieb, L. 1994. Mechanical comparison of 10 suture materials before and after in vivo incubation, *J. Surg.Res.* **56**(4), 372–377.

Grijpma, D.W., Pennings, A.J. 1994. Copolymers of L-lactide. 2. Mechanical properties, *Macromol. Chem. Phys.* **195**, 1649–1663.

Grote, J.J., Bakker, D., Hesseling, S.C., van Blitterswijk, C.A. 1991. New alloplastic tympanic membrane material, *Am. J. Otol.* **12**(5), 329–335.

Guidoin, R., Couture, J. 1991. Polyesther prostheses: the outlook for the future, in: *Blood Compatible Materials and Devices. Perspectives Towards the 21st Century* (C.P. Sharma, M. Szycher, eds.), Ch. 13, pp. 221–236, Technomic Publ. Co., Lancaster, PA.

Guillaume, Y.C., Peyrin, E., Berthelot, A. 1999. Chromatographic study of magnesium and calcium binding to immobilized human serum albumin, *J. Chromatogr. B: Biomed. Sci. Appl.* **728**(2), 167–174.

Gumargalieva, K.Z., Moiseev, Y.V., Daurova, T.T., Voronkova, O.S. 1982. Effect of infections on the degradation of polyethylene terephthalate implants, *Biomaterials* **3**(3), 177–180.

Hagenmaier, R.D., Shaw, P.E. 1990. Moisture permeability of edible films made with fatty acid and hydroxypropyl methylcellulose, *J. Agric. Food Chem.* **38**, 1799–1803.

Hara, S., Yamakawa, M. 1995. Moricin, a novel type of antibacterial peptide isolated from the silkworm, Bombyx mori, *J. Biol. Chem.* **270**(50), 29923–29927.

Hasirci, V. 2000. Biodegradable biomedical polymers. Review of degradation of and in vivo responses to polylactides and polyhydroxyalkanoates, in: *Biomaterials and Bioengineering Handbook* (D.L. Wise, ed.), Ch. 4, pp. 141–155, Marcel Dekker, New York.

Hastings, G.W. 1992. *Cardiovascular Biomaterials*, pp. 10–25, Springer-Verlag, London.

Hawrylewicz, E.J., Zapata, J.J., Blair, W.H. 1995. Soy and experimental cancer: animal studies, *J. Nutr.* **125**(3 Suppl), 698S–708S.

Hegyeli, A. 1973. Use of organ cultures to evaluate biodegradation of polymer implant materials, *J. Biomed. Mater. Res.* **7**, 205–214.

Heller, J. 1983. Use of polymers in controlled drug release, in: *Biocompatible Polymers, Metals, and Composites* (M. Szycher, ed.), Ch. 24, pp. 551–584, Technomic Publ. Co., Lancaster, PA.

Heller, J. 1990. Development of poly(orthoesters), a historical overview, *Biomaterials* 11 (November), 659–665.

Heller, J. 1996. Drug delivery systems, in: *Biomaterials Science: An Introduction to Materials in Medicine* (B.D. Ratner, A.S. Hoffman, F.J. Schoen, J.E. Lemons, eds.), pp. 346–356, Academic Press, San Diego.

Heller, J., Daniels, A.U. 1994. Poly (ortho esters), in *Biomedical Polymers. Designed-to-Degrade Systems* (S.W. Shalaby, ed.), pp. 35–67, Hanser Publ., Munich.

Heller, J., Gurny, R. 1999. Polyorthoesters, in: *Encyclopedia of Controlled Drug Delivery* (E. Mathiowitz, ed.), Vol. 2, pp. 852–874, John Wiley & Sons, New York.

Heller, J., Sparer, R.V., Zentner, G.M. 1990a. Poly(ortho esters), in: *Biodegradable Polymers as Drug Delivery Systems* (M. Chasin, R. Langer, eds.), Ch. 4, pp. 121–161, Marcel Dekker, New York.

Heller, J., Ng, S.Y., Fritzinger, B.K., Roskov, K.V. 1990b. Controlled drug release from bioerodible hydrophobic ointments, *Biomaterials* **11** (May), 235–237.

Heller, J., Pangburn, S.H., Roskov, K.V. 1990c. Development of enzymatically degradable protective coatings use in triggered drug delivery systems. II. Derivatized starch hydrogels, *Biomaterials* **11** (July), 345–350.

Heller, J., Ng, S.Y., Fritzinger, B.K. 1992. Synthesis and characterization of a new family of poly(orthoester)s, *Macromolecules* **25**, 3362–3364.

Heslot, H. 1998. Artificial fibrous proteins: a review, *Biochimie* **80**(1), 19–31.

Hoekstra, D. 1999. Hyaluronan-modified surfaces for medical devices, *Med. Dev. Diagn. Ind. Mag.* **Feb**, 48–52.

Hoenich, N.A., Stamp, S. 2000. Clinical investigation of the role of membrane structure on blood contact and solute transport characteristics of a cellulose membrane, *Biomaterials* **21**(3), 317–324.

Hollinger, J.O. (ed.). 1995. *Biomedical Applications of Synthetic Biodegradable Polymers*, CRC Press, Boca Raton.

Horncastle, J. 1995. Wound dressings. Past, present, and future, *Med. Device Technol.* **6**(1), 30–36.

Huang, S.J., Leong, K.W. 1989. Biodegradable polymers. Polymers derived from gelatin and lysin esters, *Polym. Prepr.* **20**, 552–554.

Hudson, S.M. 1994. Review of chitin and chitosan as fiber and film formers, *J. Mater. Sci., Mater. Med.* **C34**(3), 375–437.

Huijun, L., Ramsden, L., Corke, H. 1998. Physical properties and enzymatic digestibility of acetylated and normal maize starch, *Carbohydr. Polym.* **34**(4), 283–289.

Hyon, S.-H., Jamshidi, K., Ikada, Y. 1984. Melt spinning of poly-L-lactide and hydrolysis of the fiber in vitro, in: *Polymers as Biomaterials* (S. Shalaby, A.S. Hoffmann, B.D. Ratner, T.A. Horbett, eds.), pp. 51–65, Plenum Press, New York.

Ibim, S.E.M., Ambrosio, A.M.A., Kwon, M.S., El-Amin, S.F., Allcock, H.R., Laurencin, C.T. 1997. Novel polyphosphazene/poly(lactide-co-glycolide) blends: miscibility and degradation studies, *Biomaterials* **18**, 1565–1569.

Inouhe, K., Kurokawa, M., Nishikawa, S., Tsukada, M. 1998. Use of Bombyx mori silk fibroin as a substratum for cultivation of animal cells, *J. Biochem. Biophys. Methods* **37**(3), 159–164.

Ishihara, C., Hiratai, R., Tsuji, M., Yagi, K., Nose, M., Azuma, I. 1998. Mannan decelerates the clearence of human red blood cells in SCID mouse, *Immunopharmacol.* **38**(3), 223–228.

Jaffe, R., Wade, C.W.R., Hegyeli, A.F., Rice, R., Hodge, J. 1986. Synthesis and bioevaluation of alkyl 2-cyanoacryloyl glycolates as potential soft tissue adhesives, *J. Biomed. Mater. Res.* **20**, 205–212.

Johns, D.B., Lenz, R.W., Leucke, A. 1984. Lactones, in: *Ring-opening Polymerization*, Vol. 1 (K.J. Ivin, T. Saegusa, eds.), pp. 461–521, Elsevier Applied Science Publishers Ltd., 1984.

Kalimo, K., Vainio, E. 1980. Wheat grain immunofluorescent antibodies as an indication of gluten sensitivity?, *Br. J. Dermatol.* **103**(6), 657–661.

Kane, J.B., Tompkins, R.G., Yarmush, M.L., Burke, J.F. 1996. Burn dressing, in: *Biomaterials Science: An Introduction to Materials in Medicine* (B.D. Ratner, A.S. Hoffman, F.J. Schoen, J.E. Lemons, eds.), pp. 360–370, Academic Press, San Diego.

Kaplan, D.L., Wiley, B.J., Mayer, J.M., Arcidiacono, S., Keith, J., Lombardi, S.J., Ball, D., Allen, A.L. 1994. Bioabsorbable poly(ester-amides), in: *Biomedical Polymers. Designed-to-Degrade Systems* (S.W. Shalaby ed.), pp. 189–212, Hanser Publ., Munich.

Karjalainen, T., Hiljanen, M., Malin, M., Seppala, J. 1996. Biodegradable lactone copolymers. III. Mechanical properties of ε-caprolactone and lactide copolymers after hydrolysis in vitro, *J. Appl. Polym. Sci.* **59**, 1299–1304.

Kassab, A.C., Xu, K., Denkbas, E.B., Dou, Y., Zhao, S., Piskin, E. 1997. Rifampicin carrying polyhydroxybutyrate microspheres as a potential chemoembolization agent, *J. Biomater. Sci., Polym. Ed.* **8**(12), 947–961.

Katayama, S., Murakami, T., Takahashi, Y., Serita, H., Obuchi, Y., Ito, T. 1976. Synthesis of alternating polyamide esters by melt and solution polycondensation of N,N′-di(6-hydroxycaproyl)diamines and N-6-hydroxycaproyl aminoalcohol with terephthalic and adipic dimethyl esters and dichlorides, *J. Appl. Polym. Sci.* **20**, 975–994.

Kemmish, D. 1993. The processing of poly(3-hydroxybutyrate-co-3-hydroxyvalerate)-PBHV, in: *Biodegradable Polymers and Packaging* (C. Ching, D. Kaplan, E. Thomas, eds.), pp. 225–232, Technomic Publ. Co., Lancaster, PA.

Kemnitzer, J.E., Gross, R.A., McCarthy, S.P. 1992. Stereochemical and morphoplogical effects on the degradation kinetics of poly(-hydroxybutyrate): a model study, *Proc. ACS Div., Polym. Mater. Sci. Eng.* **66**, 405–407.

Kester, J.J., Fennema, O. 1986. Edible films and coatings: a review, *J. Food Sci.* **40**, 47–59.

Kimura, Y. 1993. Biodegradable polymers, in: *Biomedical Application of Polymeric Materials* (T. Tsuruta, T. Hayashi, K. Kataoka, K. Ishihara, Y. Kimura, eds.), pp. 164–190, CRC Press, Boca Raton.

King, M.W., Guidoin, R., Blais, P., Garton, A., Gunasekera, R. 1985. Degradation of polyester arterial prostheses: a physical or chemical mechanism?, in: *Corrosion and Degradation of*

Implant Materials: Second Symposium (A.C. Fraker, C.D. Griffin, eds.), Vol. 859, pp. 294–307, ASTM STP.

Klebanoff, S. 1982. Iodination catalyzed by xanthine oxidase system: Role of hydroxyl radicals, *Biochemistry* **21**, 4110–4116.

Kocisova, E., Jancura, D., Sanchez-Cortes, S., Miskovsky, P., Chinsky, L., Garcia-Ramos, J.V. 1999. Interaction of antiviral and antitumor photoactive drug hypocrellin A with human serum albumin, *J. Biomol. Struct. Dyn.* **17**(1), 111–120.

Kohn, J. 1990. Pseudo poly(amino acids), in: *Biodegradable Polymers as Drug Delivery Systems* (M. Chasin, R. Langer, eds.), Ch. 6, pp. 195–229, Marcel Dekker, New York.

Kohn, J., Langer, R. 1986. Poly(iminocarbonates) as potential biomaterials, *Biomaterials* **7**(3) May, 176–183.

Kopecek, J., Ulbrich, K. 1983. Biodegradation of biomedical polymers, *Prog. Polym. Sci.*, **9**, 1–58.

Kostopoulos, L., Karring, T. 1994. Guided bone regeneration in mandibular defects in rats using a bioresorbable polymer, *Clin. Oral Implants Res.* **5**(2), 66–74.

Kramer, P.A. 1974. Albumin microspheres as vehicles for achieving specificity in drug delivery, *J. Pharm. Sci.* **63**, 1646–1647.

Krogel, I., Bodmeier, R. 1999. Development of a multifunctional matrix drug delivery system surrounded by an impermeable cylinder, *J. Controlled Release* **61**(1–2), 43–50.

Kronenthal, R.L. 1975. Biodegradable polymers in medicine and surgery, in: *Polymers in Medicine and Surgery* (R.L. Kronental, Z. Oser, E. Martin, eds.), pp. 119–137, Plenum Press, New York.

Kuen, Y.L., Wan, S.H., Won, H.P. 1995. Blood compatibility and biodegradability of partially N-acylated chitosan derivatives, *Biomaterials* **16**(16), 1211–1216.

Kulkarni R.K., Pani K.C., Neuman C., Leonard F. 1966. Polylactic acid for surgical implants, *Arch. Surg.* **93**, 839–843.

Kulkarni, R.K., Moore, E.G., Hegyeli, A.F., Leonard, F. 1971. Biodegradable poly(lactic acid) polymers, *J. Biomed. Mater. Res.* **5**, 169–181.

Kumada, T., Nakano, S., Sone, Y., Kiriyama, S., Hisanaga, Y., Rikitoku, T., Tamoto, A., Honda, T. 1999. Clinical effectiveness of degradable starch microspheres in patients with liver cancer, *Gan To Kagaku Ryoho* **26**(12), 1678–1683.

Kurita, K. 1998. Chemistry and application of chitin and chitosan, *Polym. Degrad. Stabil.* **59**(1–3), 117–120.

Kurosaki, S., Otsuka, H., Kunitomo, M., Koyama, M., Pawankar, R., Matumoto K. 1999. Fibroin allergy. IgE mediated hypersensitivity to silk suture materials, *Nippon Ika Daigaku Zasshi* **66**(1), 41–44.

Lanza, R.P., Langer, R., Chick, W.L. 1997. *Principles of Tissue Engineering*, Academic Press, San Diego.

Laurencin, C.T., Koh, H.J., Neenan, T.X., Allcock, H.R., Langer, R. 1987. Controlled release using a new bioerodible polyphosphazene matrix system, *J. Biomed. Mater. Res.* **21**, 1231–1246.

Laurent, T.C. 1970. Structure of hyaluronic acid, in: *Chemistry and Molecular Biology of the Intercellular Matrix* (E.A. Balazs, ed.), pp. 703–732, Academic Press, London.

Lawton, J.W. 1996. Effect of starch type on the properties of starch containing films, *Carbohydr. Polym.* **29**(3), 203–208.

Leadley, S.R., Shakesheff, K.M., Davies, M.C., Heller, J., Franson, N.M., Paul, A.J., Brown, A.M., Watts, J.F. 1998. The use of SIMS, XPS and in situ AFM to probe the acid catalysed hydrolysis of poly(orthoesters), *Biomaterials* Aug **19**(15), 1353–1360.

Lee, T.K., Sokoloski, T.D., Royer, G.P. 1981. Serum albumin beads: an injectable, biodegradable system for the sustained release of drugs, *Science* **213**, 230–235.

Leenslag, J.W., Kroes, M.T., Pennings, A.J., Van der Lei, B. 1988. A compliant, biodegradable vascular graft: Basic aspects of its construction and biological performance, *New Polym. Mater.* **1**(2), 111–126.

Lehninger, A.L. 1977. *Biochemistry*, 3rd edn., Worth Publishers Inc., New York.

Lelah, M.D., Cooper, S.L. 1986. *Polyurethanes in Medicine*, CRC Press, Boca Raton.

Lemm, W. 1984. Biodegradation of polyurethanes, in: *Polyurethanes in Biomedical Engineering* (H. Planck, G. Egbers, I. Sirè, eds.), pp. 103–108, Elsevier, Amsterdam.

Lemm, W., Bucherl, E.S. 1983. The degradation of some polyurethanes in vitro and in vivo, in: *Biomaterial and Biomechanics* (P. Ducheyne, G. Van der Perr, A.E. Aubert, eds.), pp. 319–324, Elsevier, Amsterdam.

Lenaerts, V., Couvreur, P., Christiansen-Leyh, D., Joiris, E., Roland, M., Rollman, B., Speiser, P. 1984. Degradation of poly(isobutyl cyanoacrylate) nanoparticles, *Biomaterials* **5**, 65–68.

Leong, K.W., Brott, B.C., Langer, R. 1985. Bioerodible polyanhydrides as drug carrier matrices I: characterization, degradation and release characteristics, *J. Biomed. Mater. Res.* **19**, 941–955.

Leung, K.S., Hung, L.K., Leung, P.C. 1994. *Biodegradable Implants in Fracture Fixation*, World Scientific Publ. Co., Singapore.

Lewis, D.H. 1990. Controlled release of bioactive agents from lactide/glycolide polymers, in: *Biodegradable Polymers as Drug Delivery Systems* (M. Chasin, R. Langer, eds.), pp. 1–41, Marcel Dekker, New York.

Li, S., Vert, M. 1999. Biodegradable polymers: Polyesters, in: *Encyclopedia of Controlled Drug Delivery* (E. Mathiowitz, ed.), Vol. 1, pp. 71–93, John Wiley & Sons, New York.

Liu, Y., Chen, X., Qian, J., Liu, H., Shao, Z., Deng, J., Yu, T. 1997. Immobilization of glucose oxidase with the blend of regenerated silk fibroin and poly(vinyl alcohol) and its application to a 1,1′-dimethylferrocene-mediating glucose sensor, *Appl. Biochem. Biotechnol.* **62**(2–3), 105–117.

Ljungberg, C., Johansson-Ruden, G., Bostrom, K.J., Novikov, L., Wiberg, M. 1999. Neuronal survival using a resorbable synthetic conduit as an alternative to primary nerve repair, *Microsurgery* **19**(6), 259–264.

Lou, X., Chirila, T.V. 1999. Swelling behavior and mechanical properties of chemically cross-linked gelatin gels for biomedical use, *J. Biomater. Appl.* **14**(2), 184–191.

Maarek, J.M., Guidoin, R., Aubin, M., Prud'homme, R.E. 1984. Molecular weight characterization of virgin and explained polyester arterial prostheses, *J. Biomed. Mater. Res.* **18**, 881–894.

MacGreger, E.A., Greenwood, C.T. 1980. *Polymers in Nature*, Chs. 3 and 6, John Wiley & Sons, New York.

Maeda, M., Inoue, Y., Kaneko, K., Sugamori, T., Iwase, H., Tsurutani, R. 2000. Chitin and its derivatives, in: *Biomaterials and Bioengineering Handbook* (D.L. Wise, ed.), Ch. 39, pp. 867–880, Marcel Dekker, New York.

Magnus, G., Dunleavy, R.A., Critchfield, F.E. 1966. Stability of urethane elastomers in water, dry air and moist air environments, *Rubber. Chem. Technol.* **39**, 1328.

Mao, H.Q., Kadiyala, I., Leong, K.W., Zhao, Z., Dang, W. 1999. Biodegradable polymers: Poly(phosphoester)s, in: *Encyclopedia of Controlled Drug Delivery* (E. Mathiowitz, ed.), Vol. 1, pp. 45–60, John Wiley & Sons, New York.

Marck, K.W., Wildevuur C.H., Sederel W.L., Bantjes, A., Fejen, J. 1977. Biodegradability and tissue reaction of random copolymers of L-leucine, L-aspartic acid and L-aspartic acid esters, *J. Biomed. Mater. Res.* **11**, 405–422.

Masar, B., Cefelin, P., Lipatova, T.E., Bakalo, L.A., Lugovskaya, G.G. 1979. Synthesis of polyurethanes and investigation of their hydrolytic stability, *J. Polym, Sci., Polym. Symp.* **66**, 259–268.

Matsusue, Y., Yamamuro, T., Oka, M., Shikinami, Y., Hyon, S.-H., Ikada, Y. 1992. In vitro and in vivo studies on bioabsorbable ultra-high-strength poly(L-lactide) rods, *J. Biomed. Mater. Res.* **26**, 1553–1567.

Meckel, W., Goyert, W., Wieder, W. 1996. Thermoplastic polyurethane elastomers, in: *Thermoplastic Elastomers*, 2nd edn. (G. Holden, N.R. Legge, R. Quirk, H.E. Schroeder, eds.), Ch. 2, pp. 16–45, Hanser Publishers, Munich.

Meijer, G.J., van Dooren, A., Gaillard, M.L., Dalmeijer, R., de Putter, C., Koole, R., van Blitterswijk, C.A. 1996. Polyactive as a bone-filler in a beagle dog model, *Int. J. Oral Maxillofac. Surg.* **25**(3), 210–216.

Meijs, G.F., McCarthy, S.J., Rizzardo, E., Chen, Y.C., Chatalier, R., Brandwood, A., Schindhelm, K. 1993. Degradation of medical grade polyurethane elastomers: the effect of hydrogen peroxide in vitro, *J. Biomed. Mater. Res.* **27**, 345–356.

Migliaresi, C., Cohn, D., De Lollis, A., Fambri, L. 1991a. Dynamic mechanical and calorimetric analysis of compression molded PLLA of different molecular weights: effect of the thermal treatments, *J. Appl. Polym. Sci.* **43**(1), 83–95.

Migliaresi, C., De Lollis, A., Fambri, L., Cohn, D. 1991b. The effect of the thermal treament on the crystallinity of different molecular weight PLLA biodegradable polymers, *Clin. Mater.* **8**, 111–118.

Migliaresi, C., Fambri, L., Cohn, D. 1994. A study on the in vitro degradation of poly(lactic acid), *J. Biomater. Sci. Polym. Ed.* **5**(6), 591–606.

Miller, A.G. 1964. Degradation of synthetic polypeptides. III. Degradation of poly-α-lysin by proteolytic enzymes in 0.20 M sodium chloride, *J. Am. Chem. Soc.* **86**, 3818–3822.

Minoura, N., Tsukada, M., Nagura, M. 1990. Physico-chemical properties of silk fibroin membrane as a biomaterial, *Biomaterials* **11**, 430–434.

Mirkovitch, V., Akutsu, T., Kolff, W.J. 1962. Polyurethane aortas in dogs. Three year results, *Trans. Am. Soc. Artif. Intern. Organs* **8**, 79.

Mitchell, J., Irons, L., Palmer, G.J. 1970. A study of the spread and adsorbed films of milk proteins, *Biochim. Biophys. Acta* **200**(1), 138–150.

Mormann, W., Wagner, J. 1988. Solvolytic degradation of aliphatic polyesteroligomers: poly(tetramethylene adipate) diol, *Angew. Makromol. Chem.* **160**, 1–15.

Murphy, K.S., Enders, N.A., Mahjour, M., Fawzi, M.B. 1986. A comparative evaluation of aqueous enteric polymers in capsule coating, *Pharm. Technol.* **October**, 36–45.

Muzzarelli, R.A. 1993. Biochemical significance of exogenous chitins and chitosans in animals and patients, *Carbohydr. Polym.* **20**, 7–15.

Muzzarelli, R.A., Jeuniaux, C., Gooday, G.W. 1986. Evaluation of chitosan as a new hemostatic agent: in vitro and in vivo experiments, in: *Chitin in Nature and Technology* (G. Fradet, S. Brister, D. Mulder, J. Lough, B.L. Averbach, eds.), pp. 78–85, Plenum Press, New York.

Nakamura, T., Shimizu, Y., Matsui, T., Okumura, N., Hyon, S.H., Nishiya, K. 1992. A novel bioabsorbable monofilament surgical suture made from (ε-caprolactone, L-lactide) copolymer, in: *Degradation Phenomena on Polymeric Biomaterials* (H. Planck, M. Dauner, M. Renardy, eds.), pp. 153–162, Springer-Verlag, Berlin–Heidelberg.

Narayan, R. 1990. Introduction, in: *Degradable Materials. Perspectives, Issues and Opportunities* (S.A. Barenberg, J.L. Brash, R. Narayan, A.E. Redpath, eds.), pp. 1–37, CRC Press, Boca Raton.

Nimni, M.E. 1983. Collagen: structure, function and metabolism in normal and fibrotic tissues, *Semin. Arthritis Rheum.* **XIII**(1), 1–86.

Nisperos-Carriedo, M.O. 1994. Edible coatings and films based on polysaccharides, in: *Edible Coatings and Films to Improve Food Quality* (J.M. Krochta, E.A. Baldwin, M.O. Nisperos-Carriedo, eds.), pp. 305–336, Technomic Publ. Co., Lancaster, PA.

Nose, Y. 1990. Artificial kidney, is it really not necessary?, *Artif. Organs* **14**, 245–251.

Okada, T., Hayashi, T., Ikada, Y. 1992. Degradation of collagen suture in vitro and in vivo, *Biomaterials* **13**(7), 448–454.

Ossefort, Z.T., Testroet, F.B. 1966. Hydrolytic stability of urethane elastomers, *Rubber. Chem. Technol.* **39**(6), 1308–1327.

Ottenbrite, R.M., Huang, S.J., Park, K. 1996. *Hydrogels and Biodegradable Polymers for Bioapplications*, ACS Symp. Ser. 627, Am. Chem. Soc., Washington DC.

Pachence, J.M., Berg, R.A., Silver, F.H. 1987. Collagen: Its place in the medical device industry, *Med. Device Diagn. Ind.* **9**, 49–55.

Padgett, T., Han, I.Y., Dawson, P.L. 1998. Incorporation of food-grade antimicrobial compounds into biodegradable packaging films, *J. Food Prot.* **61**(10), 1330–1335.

Pandit, A., Ashar, R., Feldman, D. 1999. The effect of TGF-beta delivered through a collagen scaffold on wound healing, *J. Invest. Surg.* **12**(2), 89–100.

Parikh, M., Gross, R.A., McCarthy, S.P. 1992. The effect of crystalline morphology on enzymatic degradation kinetics, *Proc. ACS Div., Polym. Mat. Sci. Eng.* **66**, 408–409.

Park, K., Shalaby, W.S.W., Park, H. 1993. *Biodegradable Hydrogels for Drug Delivery*, Technomic Publ. Co., Lancaster, PA.

Patrick, C.W., Mikos, A.G., McIntire, L.V. 1998. *Frontiers in Tissue Engineering*, Pergamon Press, New York.

Payne, L.G., Jenkins, S.A., Andrianov, A., Roberts, B.E. 1995a. Water-soluble phosphazene polymers for parenteral and mucosal vaccine delivery, in: *Vaccine Design: The Subunit and Adjuvant Approach* (M.F. Powell, M.J. Newman, eds.), Ch. 20, pp. 473–493, Plenum Press, New York.

Payne, L.G., Jenkins, S.A., Andrianov, A., Langer, R., Roberts, B.E. 1995b. Xenobiotic polymers as vaccine vehicles, *Adv. Exp. Med. Biol.* **371B**, 1475–1480.

Pegoretti, A., Fambri, L., Migliaresi, C. 1997. In vitro degradation of poly(L-lactic acid) fibers produced by melt spinning, *J. Appl. Polym. Sci.* **64**, 213–223.

Peppas, N.A. 1987. Hydrogels in medicine and pharmacy: properties and applications, in: *Hydrogels in Medicine and Pharmacy*, Vol. III, pp. 189–225, CRC Press Inc., Boca Raton.

Pernerstorfer, T., Jilma, B., Eichler, H.G., Aull, S., Handler, S., Speiser, W. 1999. Heparin lowers plasma levels of activated factor VII, *Br. J. Haematol.* **105**(4), 1127–1129.

Phua, S.K., Castillo, E., Anderson, J.M., Hiltner, A. 1987. Biodegradation of a polyurethane in vitro, *J. Biomed. Mater. Res.* **21**, 231–246.

Piskin, E. 1994. Biodegradable polymers as biomaterials, *J. Biomater. Sci. Polym. Ed.* **6**(9), 795–775.

Pitt, C. 1990. Poly-ε-caprolactone and its copolymers, in: *Biodegradable Polymers as Drug Delivery Systems* (M. Chasin, R. Langer, eds.), pp. 71–120, Marcel Dekker, New York.

Pitt, C.G., Jeffcoat, A.R., Zweidinger, R.A., Schindler, A. 1979. Sustained drug-delivery systems. I. The permeability of poly(ε-caprolactone), poly(DL-lactic acid), and their copolymers, *J. Biomed. Mater. Res.* **13**, 497–507.

Pitt, C.G., Gratzl, M.M., Kimmel, G.L., Surles, J., Schindler, A. 1981. Aliphatic polyesters. II. The degradation of poly(DL-lactide), poly(ε-caprolactone), and their copolymers in vivo, *Biomaterials* **2** (October), 215–220.

Pulapura, S., Li, C., Kohn, J. 1990. Structure-property relationships for the design of polyiminocarbonates, *Biomaterials* **11**(9) Nov., 666–678.

Qian, J., Liu, Y., Liu, H., Yu, T., Deng, J. 1996. An amperometric new methylene blue N-mediating sensor for hydrogen peroxide based on regenerated silk fibroin as an immobilization matrix for peroxidase, *Anal. Biochem.* **236**(2), 208–214.

Radder, A.M., Davies, J.E., Leenders, H., van Blitterswijk, C.A. 1994a. Interfacial behavior of PEO/PBT copolymers (Polyactive) in a calvarial system: an in vitro study, *J. Biomed. Mater. Res.* **28**(2), 269–277.

Radder, A.M., Leenders, H., van Blitterswijk, C.A. 1994b. Interface reactions to PEO/PBT copolymers (Polyactive) after implantation in cortical bone, *J. Biomed. Mater. Res.* **28**(2), 141–151.

Ramshaw, J.A.M., Glattauer, V., Werkmeister, J.A. 2000. Stabilization of collagen in medical devices, in: *Biomaterials and Bioengineering Handbook* (D.L. Wise, ed.), Ch. 32, pp. 717–738, Marcel Dekker, New York.

Rastelli, A., Beccaro, M., Biviano, F., Calderini, G., Pastorello, A. 1990. Hyaluronic acid esters, a new class of semisynthetic biopolymers: chemical and physico-chemical properties, in: *Clinical Implant Materials—Advances in Biomaterials*, Vol. 9 (G. Heimke, U. Soltesz, A.J.C. Lee, eds.), pp. 199–206, Elsevier, Amsterdam.

Ratner, B.D., Gladhill, K.W., Horbett, T.A. 1988. Analysis of in vitro enzymatic and oxidative degradation of polyurethanes, *J. Biomed. Mater. Res.* **22**, 509–527.

Ratto, J.A., Stenhouse, P.J., Auerbach, M., Mitchell, J., Farrell, R. 1999. Processing, performance and biodegrability of a thermoplastic aliphatic polyester/starch system, *Polymer* **40**(24), 6777–6788.

Ray, J.A., Doddi, N., Regula, D., Williams, J.A., Melveger, A. 1981. Polydioxanone (PDS); a novel monofilament synthetic absorbable suture, *Surg. Gynecol. Obstet.* **153**, 497–507.

Regan, E.F., Dunnington, J.H. 1966. Collagen sutures in cataract surgery: clinical and experimental observations, *Trans. Am. Ophthalmol. Soc.* **64**, 39–49.

Reineccius, G.A. 1994. Flavour encapsulation, in: *Edible Coatings and Films to Improve Food Quality* (J.M. Krochta, E.A. Baldwin, M.O. Nisperos-Carriedo, eds.), pp. 105–120, Technomic Publ. Co., Lancaster, PA.

Ribeiro, A.J., Neufeld, R.J., Arnaud, P., Chaumeil, J.C. 1999. Microencapsulation of lipophilic drugs in chitosan-coated alginate microspheres, *Int. J. Pharm.* **187**(1), 115–123.

Richards, M., Dahiyat, B.I., Arm, D.M., Brown, P.R., Leong, K.W. 1991. Evaluation of polyphosphates and polyphosphonates as degradable biomaterials, *J. Biomed. Mater. Res.* **25**, 1151–1167.

Rindlav-Westling, A., Stading, M., Hermansson, A.M., Gatenholm, P. 1998. Structure, barrier and mechanical properties of amylose and amylopectin films, *Carbohydr. Polym.* **36**, 217–224.

Rogalla, C.J. 1997. Autologous collagen: a new treatment for dermal defects, *Minim. Invasive Surg. Nurs.* **11**(2), 67–69.

Ronis, M.L., Harwick, J.D., Fung, R., Dellavecchia, M. 1984. Review of cyanocrylate tissue glues with emphasis on their otorhinolaryngological applications, *Laryngoscope* **94**, 210–213.

Rouxhet, L., Duhoux, F., Borecky, O., Legras, R., Schneider, Y.J. 1998. Adsorption of albumin, collagen, and fibronectin on the surface of poly(hydroxybutyrate-hydroxyvalerate) (PHB/HV) and of poly(epsilon-caprolactone) (PCL) films modified by an alkaline hydrolysis and of poly(ethylene terephthalate) (PET) track-etched membranes, *J. Biomater. Sci., Polym. Ed.* **9**(12), 1279–1304.

Rudakova, T.E., Zaikov, G.E., Voronkova, O.S., Daurova, T.T., Degtyareva, S.M. 1979. The kinetic specificity of polyethylene terephthalate degradation in the living body, *J. Polym. Sci., Polym. Symp.* **66**, 277–281.

Sakkers, R.J.B., de Wijn, J.R., van Blitterswijk, C.A. 1992. Relation between swelling pressure of PEO-PBT copolymers and bursting pressure of human femoral bones, in: *Biomaterial–Tissue Interfaces. Advances in Biomaterials*, Vol. 10 (P.J. Doherty, R.L. Williams, D.F. Williams, A.J.C. Lee, eds.), pp. 357–361, Elsevier, Amsterdam.

Samejima, M., Sugiyama, J., Igarashi, K., Eriksson, K.E.L. 1997. Enzymatic hydrolysis of bacterial cellulose, *Carbohydr. Res.* **305**(2), 281–288.

Sandford, P.A. 1989. Chitosan: commercial uses and potential applications, in: *Chitin and Chitosan: Sources, Chemistry, Biochemistry, Physical Properties and Applications* (T. Anthonsen, P. Sandford, eds.), pp. 51–69, Elsevier, New York.

Sandler, S.R., Karo, W. 1974. Polyesters, in: *Polymer Syntheses*, Vol. 1 (H.H. Wasseman ed.), pp. 55–72, Academic Press Inc., Orlando.

Santerre, J.P., Labow, R.S., Adams, G.A. 1993. Enzyme-biomaterial interactions: effect of biosystems on degradation of polyurethanes, *J. Biomed. Mater. Res.* **27**, 97–109.

Santin, M., Motta, A., Freddi, G., Cannas, M. 1999. In vitro evaluation of the inflammatory potential of the silk fibroin, *J. Biomed. Mater. Res.* **46**(3), 382–389.

Sanz, L.E., Patterson, J.A., Kamath, R., Willett, G., Ahmed, S.W., Butterfield, A.B. 1988. Comparison of Maxon suture with Vicryl, chromic catgut, and PDS sutures in fascial closure in rats, *Obstet. Gynecol.* **71**(3), 418–422.

Schacht, E.H. 1990. Using biodegradable polymers in advanced drug delivery systems, *Med. Dev. Technol.* **1**(1), 15–21.

Schacht, E., Crommen, J. 1990. Bioerodable sustained release implants, *US Patent*, 4 975 280.

Schlegel, A.K., Möhler, H., Busch, F., Mehl, A. 1997. Preclinical and clinical studies of a collagen membrane (Bio-Gide), *Biomaterials* **18**(7), 535-538.

Schmitt, E.E., Polistina, R.A. 1967. Surgical sutures, *US Patent* 3 297 033, Jan. 10.

Schollenberger, C.S. 1988. Thermoplastic polyurethane elastomers, in: *Handbook of Elastomers* (A.K. Bhowmock, H.L. Stephens, eds.), Ch. 11, pp. 375–409, Marcel Dekker Inc., New York.

Schollenberger, C.S., Stewart, F.D. 1973. Thermoplastic polyurethane hydrolysis stability, *Angew. Makromol. Chem.* **29/30**, 413–430.

Schwartz, L.B. 1990. Tryptase from human mast cells: biochemistry, biology and clinical utility, *Monogr. Allergy* **27**, 90–113.

Scopelianos, A.G. 1994. Polyphosphazenes as new biomaterials, in: *Biomedical Polymers. Designed-to-Degrade Systems* (S.W. Shalaby, ed.), pp. 153–172, Hanser Publ., Munich.

Scott, J.E. 1989. Secondary structures in hyaluronan solutions: chemical and biological implications, in: *The Biology of Hyaluronan*, Ciba Foundation Symposium Series No. 143, pp. 6–20, John Wiley & Sons, Chichester.

Sefton, M.V., Woodhouse, K.A. 1998. Tissue engineering, *J. Cutan. Med. Surg.*, Dec 3 (Suppl 1), 18–23.

Sendil, D., Gursel, I., Wise, D.L., Hasirci, V. 1999. Antibiotic release from biodegradable PHBV microparticles, *J. Controlled Release* **59**(2), 207–217.

Seves, A., Romano, M., Maifreni, T., Sora, S., Ciferri, O. 1998. The microbial degradation of silk: a laboratory investigation, *Int. Biodeterior. Biodegrad.* **42**(4), 203–211.

Shalaby, S.W. 1988. Bioabsorbable polymers, in: *Encyclopedia of Pharmaceutical Technology*, Vol. 1, (J. Swarbrick, J.C. Boylan, eds.), pp. 465–476, Marcel Dekker Inc., New York.

Shalaby, S.W., Jamiolkowski, D.D. 1980. Polyesteramides derived from bisoxamidodiols and dicarboxylic acids, *US Patent*, 4 209 607, June 24.

Shalaby, S.W., Johnson, R.A. 1994. Synthetic absorbable polyesters, in: *Biomedical Polymers. Designed-to-Degrade Systems* (S.W. Shalaby ed.), pp. 1–34, Hanser Publ., Munich.

Shi, Y., Ploof, J., Correia, A. 1999. Increasing antibody production with hollow-fiber bioreactors, *IVD Technology Magazine*, May, 37–40.

Sidman, K.R., Schwope, A.D., Steber, W.D., Rudolph, S.E., Poulin, S.B. 1980. Biodegradable, implantable sustained release systems based on glutamic acid copolymers, *J. Membrane Sci.* **7**, 277–291.

Silver, F.H., Marks, M., Kato, Y.P., Li, C., Pulapura, S., Kohn, J. 1992. Tissue compatibility of tyrosine-derived polycarbonates and polyiminocarbonates: an initial evaluation, *J. Long Term Eff. Med. Implants* **1**(4), 329–346.

Silver, F.H., Pins, G.D., Wang, M.C., Christiansen, D. 1995. Collagenous biomaterials as models for tissue inducing implants, in: *Encyclopaedic Handbook of Biomaterials and Bioengineering, Part A: Materials* (D.L. Wise, ed.), pp. 63–70, Marcel Dekker Inc., New York.

Sinclair, R.G. 1977. Copolymers of L-lactide and epsilon caprolactone, *US Patent*, 3 057 537, Nov. 8.

Sinha, V.R., Khosla, L. 1998. Bioabsorbable polymers for implantable therapeutic systems, *Drug Dev. Ind. Pharm.* **24**(12), 1129–1138.

Skondia, V., Davydov, A., Belykh, S., Heusghem, C. 1987. Chemical and physicochemical aspects of biocompatible orthopaedic polymer (BOP) in bone surgery, *J. Int. Med. Res.* **15**, 293–302.

Smidsrod, O., Skjak-Braek, G. 1990. Alginate as immobilization matrix for cells, *Trends Biotechnol.* **8**(3), 71–78.

Smith, R., Oliver, C., Williams, D.F. 1987a. The enzymatic degradation of polymers in vivo, *J. Biomed. Mater. Res.* **21**, 991-1003.

Smith, R., Williams, D.F., Oliver, C. 1987b. The biodegradation of poly(ether urethanes), *J. Biomed. Mater. Res.* **21**, 1149–1166.

Sorell, J.M., Carrino, D.A., Caplan, A.I. 1996. Regulated expression of chondroitin sulfates at sites of epithelial-mesenchymal interaction: spatio-temporal patterning identified with anti-chondroitin sulfate monoclonal antibodies, *Int. J. Dev. Neurosci.* **14**(3), 233–248.

Stankiewicz, B.A., Mastalerz, M., Hof, C.H.J., Bierstedt, A., Flannery, M.B., Briggs, D.E.G., Evershed, R.P. 1998. Biodegradation of the chitin-protein complex in crustacean cuticle, *Org. Geochem.* **28**(1–2), 67–76.

St. Pierre, T., Chiellini, E. 1986. Biodegradability of synthetic polymers used for medical and pharmaceutical applications: Part I — Principles of hydrolysis, *J. Bioact. Compatible Polym.* **1**, 467–497.

Sung, H.W., Huang, D.M., Chang, W.H., Huang, L.L., Tsai, C.C., Liang, I.L. 1999. Gelatin-derived bioadhesives for closing skin wounds: an in vivo study, *J. Biomater. Sci., Polym. Ed.* **10**(7), 751–771.

Szycher, M. 1991. Biostability of polyurethane elastomers: a critical review, in: *Blood Compatible Materials and Devices* (C.P. Sharma and M. Szycher, eds.), pp. 33–85, Technomic Publ., Lancaster, PA.

Szycher, M., Lee, S.J. 1992. Modern wound dressings: a systematic approach to wound healing, *J. Biomater. Appl.* **7**(2), 142–213.

Tabata, Y., Ikada, Y. 1999. Vascularization effect of basic fibroblast growth factor released from gelatin hydrogels with different biodegradabilities, *Biomaterials* **20**(22), 2169–2175.

Tabata, Y., Matsui, Y., Ikada, Y. 1998. Growth factor release from amylopectin hydrogel based on copper coordination, *J. Controlled Release* **56**(1–3), 135–148.

Takahara, A., Coury, A.J., Hergenrother, R.W., Cooper, S.L. 1991a. Effect of soft segment chemistry on the biostability of segmented polyurethanes. I. In vitro oxidation, *J. Biomed. Mater. Res.* **25**, 341–356.

Takahara, A., Hergenrother, R.W., Coury, A.J., Cooper, S.L. 1991b. Effect of soft segment chemistry on the biostability of segmented polyurethanes. II. In vitro hydrolytic degradation and lipid sorption, *J. Biomed. Mater. Res.* **26**, 801–818.

Test, S., Weiss, S. 1986. The generation of utilization of chlorinated oxidants by human neutrophils, *Adv. Free Radical Biol. Med.* **2**, 91–116.

Timmins, M.R., Gilmore, D.F., Fuller, R.C., Lenz, R.W. 1993. Bacterial polyesters and their biodegradation, in: *Biodegradable Polymers and Packaging* (C. Ching, D. Kaplan, E. Thomas, eds.), pp. 119–130, Technomic Publ. Co., Lancaster, PA.

Tokiwa, Y., Suzuki, T. 1977. Hydrolysis of polyesters by lipases, *Nature* **270**, 76–78.

Tomihata, K., Ikada, Y. 1997. Preparation of cross-linked hyaluronic acid films of low water content, *Biomaterials* **18**(3), 189–195.

Tomita, N., Tamai, S., Morihara, T., Ikeuchi, K., Ikada, Y. 1993. Handling characteristics of braided suture materials for tight tying, *J. Appl. Biomater.* **4**(1), 61–65.

Tormala, P., Vasenius, J., Vainionpaa, S., Laiho, J., Pohjonen, T., Rokkanen, P. 1991. Ultra-high-strength absorbable self-reinforced polyglycolide (SR-PGA) composite rods for internal fixation of bone fractures: in vitro and in vivo study, *J. Biomed. Mater. Res.* **25**, 1–22.

Treib, J., Baron, J.F., Grauer, M.T., Strauss, R.G. 1999. An international view of hydroxyethyl starches, *Intensive Care Med.* **25**(3), 258–268.

Trimbos, J.B., Booster, M., Peters, A.A. 1991. Mechanical knot performance of a new generation polydioxanon suture (PDS-2), *Acta Obstet. Gynecol. Scand.* **70**(2), 157–159.

Tseng, Y., Tabata, Y., Hyon, S., Ikada, Y. 1990. In vitro toxicity of 2-cyanoacrylate polymers by cell culture method, *J. Biomed. Mater. Res.* **24**, 1355–1367.

Tunc, D.C. 1995. Orientruded polylactide based body-absorbable osteosynthesis devices: a short review, *J. Biomater. Sci. Polym. Ed.* **7**(4), 375–380.

Ulrich, S., Kuntz, G., Anita, R. 1992. Haemostyptic preparations on the basis of collagen alone and as fixed combination with fibrin glue, *Clin. Mater.* **9**(3), 169–177.

Vainionpaa, S., Rokkanen, P., Tormala, P. 1989. Surgical applications of biodegradable polymers in human tissue, *Prog. Polym. Sci.* **14**, 679–716.

van Blitterswijk, C.A., Bakker, D., Leenders, H., Brink, J., Hesseling, S.C., Bovell, Y.P., Radder, A.M., Sakkers, R.J.B., Gaillard, M.L., Heinze, P.H., Beumer, G.J. 1992. Interfacial reactions leading to bone-bonding with PEO-PBT copolymers (Polyactive®), in: *Bone Bonding Materials* (P. Ducheyne, T. Kokubo, C.A. van Blitterswijk, eds.), pp. 13–30, Reed Healthcare Communications, Leiderdorp.

van der Elst, M., Klein, C.P.A.T., Patka, P., Haarman, H.J.T.M., 2000. Biodegradable fracture fixation devices, in: *Biomaterials and Bioengineering Handbook* (D.L. Wise, ed.), Ch. 22, pp. 509–524, Marcel Dekker, New York.

van Dorp, A.G., Verhoeven, M.C., Koerten, H.K., van der Nat van der Meij, T.H., van Blitterswijk, C.A., Ponec, M. 1998. Dermal regeneration in full-thickness wounds in Yucatan miniature pigs using a biodegradable copolymer, *Wound Repair Regen.* **6**(6), 556–568.

van Dorp, A.G., Verhoeven, M.C., Koerten, H.K., van Blitterswijk, C.A., Ponec, M. 1999. Bilayered biodegradable poly(ethylene glycol)/poly(butylene terephthalate) copolymer (Polyactive) as substrate for human fibroblasts and keratinocytes, *J. Biomed. Mater. Res.* **47**(3), 292–300.

Vandorpe, J., Schacht, E., Dunn, E., Hawley, A., Stolnik, S., Davis, S.S., Garnett, M.C., Davies, M.C., Illum, L. 1997a. Long circulating biodegradable poly(phosphazene) nanoparticle surface modified with poly(phosphazene)-poly(ethylene oxide) copolymer, *Biomaterials* **18**(17) 1147–1152.

Vandorpe, J., Schacht, E., Dejardin, S., Lemmouchi, Y. 1997b. Biodegradable polyphosphazenes for biomedical applications, in: *Handbook of Biodegradable Polymers* (A.J. Domb, J. Kost, D.M. Wiseman, eds.), Ch. 9, pp. 161–182, Harwood Academic Publisher, Singapore.

Varum, K.M., Myhr, M.M., Hjerde, R.J.N., Smidsrud, O. 1997. In vitro degradation rates of partially N-acetylated chitosans in human serum, *Carbohydr. Res.* **299**(1–2), 99–101.

Veis, A. 1983. Characterization of soluble collagens by physical techniques, in: *Methods in Enzymology* (L.W. Cunningham, D.F. Fredericksen, eds.), pp. 186–217, Academic Press, London.

Verheyen, C.C.P.M., de Wijn, J.R., van Blitterswijk, C.A., de Groot, K. 1992. Evaluation of hydroxylapatite/poly-(L-lactide) composites: Mechanical behaviour, *J. Biomed. Mater. Res.* **26**, 1277–1296.

Vert, M. 1989. Bioresorbable polymers for temporary therapeutic applications, *Angew. Makromol. Chem.* **166/167**, 155–168.

Vert, M., Guerin, P. 1991. Biodegradable aliphatic polyesters of the poly(hydroxy acid)-type for temporary therapeutic applications, in: *Biomaterial Degradation: Fundamental Aspects and Related Clinical Phenomena* (M.A. Barbosa, ed.), pp. 35–51, Elsevier, Amsterdam.

Vervoort, L., Rombaut, P., Van den Mooter, G., Augustijns, P., Kinget, R. 1998. Insulin hydrogels. II. In vitro degradation studies, *Int. J. Pharm.* **172**(1–2), 137–145.

Vinard, E., Eloy, R., Descotes, J., Brudon, J. R., Guidicelli, H., Magne, J. L., Patra, P., Berruet, R., Huc, A., Chauchard, J. 1988, Stability of performances of vascular prostheses retrospective study of 22 cases of human implanted prostheses, *J. Biomed. Mater. Res.* **22**, 633–648.

Vinard, E., Eloy, R., Descotes, J., Brudon, J.R., Guidicelli, H., Patra, P., Streichenberger, R., David, M. 1991. Human vascular graft failure and frequency of infection, *J. Biomed. Mater. Res* **25**, 499–513.

von Oepen, R., Michaeli, W. 1992. Injection moulding of biodegradable implants, *Clin. Mater.* **10**, 21–28.

Wang, M.Y., Levy, M.L., Mittler, M.A., Liu, C.Y., Johnston, S., McComb, J.G. 1999. A prospective analysis of the use of octyl acrylate tissue adhesive for wound closure in pediatric neurosurgery, *Pediatr. Neurosurg.* **30**(4), 186–188.

Wehrenberg, R.H. 1981. Polylactic acid polymers: strong, degradable thermoplastics, *Mater. Eng.* **94**(3), 63–66.

Weigel, P.H., Fuller, G.M., LeBoeuf, R.D. 1986. A model for the role of hyaluronic acid and fibrin in the early events during the inflammatory response and wound healing, *J. Theor. Biol.* **119**, 219–234.

Wierik, G.H., Eissens, A.C., Bergsma, J., Arends-Scholte, A.W., Bolhuis, G.K. 1997. A new generation starch product as excipient in pharmaceutical tablets. III. Parameters affecting controlled drug release from tablets based on high surface area retrograded pregelatinized potato starch, *Int. J. Pharm.* **157**(2), 181–187.

Williams, D.F. 1981. Enzymatic hydrolysis of polylactic acid, *Eng. Med.* **10**, 5–7.

Williams, D.F. 1984. The biodegradation of surgical polymers, in: *Polyurethanes in Biomedical Engineering* (H. Planck, G. Egbers, I. Sirè, eds.), pp. 93–102, Elsevier, Amsterdam.

Williams, D.F. 1990a. Biodegradation of medical polymers, in: *Concise Encyclopedia of Medical and Dental Materials* (D.F. Williams, ed.), pp. 69–74, Pergamon Press, Oxford.

Williams, D.F. 1990b. The role of active species within tissue in degradation processes, in: *Degradable Materials. Perspectives, Issues and Opportunities* (S.A. Barenberg, J.L. Brash, R. Narayan, A.E. Redpath, eds.), pp. 323–355, CRC Press, Boca Raton.

Williams, D.F. 1991. Objectivity in the evaluation of biological safety of medical devices and biomaterials, *Med. Dev. Technol,* **2**(1), 44–48.

Williams, D.F., Chu, C.C., Dwyer, J. 1984. Effects of enzymes and gamma irradiation on the tensile strength and morphology of poly(p-dioxanone), *J. Appl. Polym. Sci.* **29**, 1865–1877.

Williams, J.C.L., Watson, S.J., Boydell, S. 1995. Properties, in *Nylon Plastics Handbook* (M.I. Kohan, ed.), pp. 293–358, Hanser Publ., Munich.

Zaikov, G.E. 1985. Quantitative aspects of polymer degradation in the living body, *JMS-Rev. Macromol. Chem. Phys.* **C25**(4), 551–597.

Zellin G., Gritli-Linde, A., Linde, A. 1995. Healing of mandibular defects with different biodegradable and non-biodegradable membranes: an experimental study in rats, *Biomaterials* **16**, 601–609.

Zhang, X., Wyss, U.P., Pichora, D., Goosen, M.F.A. 1993. Biodegradable polymers for orthopedic applications: synthesis and processability of poly(L-lactide) and poly(lactide-co-ε-caprolactone), *Pure Appl. Chem.* **A30**, 933–947.

Zhang, X., Wyss, U.P., Pichora, D., Goosen, M.F.A. 1994. An investigation of poly(lactic acid) degradation, *J. Bioact. Compat. Mater.* **9**(1), 80–100.

Zhang, Y.O., Zhu, J., Gu, R.A. 1998. Improved biosensor for glucose based on glucose oxidase-immobilized silk fibroin membrane, *Appl. Biochem. Biotechnol.* **75**(2–3), 215–233.

Zhao, Q., Marchant, R.E., Anderson, J.M., Hiltner, A. 1987. Long term biodegradation in vitro of poly(ether urethane urea), a mechanical property study, *Polymer* **28**, 2040–2046.

Zhu, K.J., Xiangzhou, L., Shilin, Y. 1990. Preparation, characterization and properties of polylactide(PLA)-poly(ethylene glycol) (PEG) copolymers: a potential drug carrier, *J. Appl. Polym. Sci.* **39**, 1–9.

Zizokis, J.P. 1984. *Chitin, Chitosan and Related Enzymes*, pp. 75–85, Academic Press, Orlando.

5

Bioceramics and Biological Glasses

A. Krajewski and A. Ravaglioli

5.1. The Structure of Ceramics from Synthesis to Processing

The term *ceramic* is normally used in common speech when referring to a series for products for domestic use or connected with building construction. This brings to mind objects like artistic decorative kits, probably made by artisans (such as knickknacks, lampholders, ashtrays, fine boxes, etc.), kitchen pottery and food-containing sundries (pots, jars, jugs, dishes, bowls, etc.), or sanitary wares, bricks, and tiles (for roofs or for decorative and sanitary use on floors, walls, etc.). In this ambit of meaning, ceramic products are classified as earthenware, majolica, porcelain, etc.

Also, the term *glass* (generally transparent, but sometimes opaque or colored for decorative purposes) assumes in common speech a similar meaning connected with its use in making transparent slabs for windows, the lenses of spectacles, some Pyrex containers for liquids, various custom-jewelery parts, or many different decorative domestic sundries.

In reality, both are materials utilized for the manufacture of a wider range of products, in particular for technological and engineering applications, even biomedical applications, which is the field dealt with in this volume. Obviously, the semantics of these terms cannot be limited to narrow boundaries, even apart from any consideration as to whether they would be suitable materials or not. All ceramic typology originates from ancient times and is associated with traditional commercial terms accorded with use. It is therefore necessary not only to expand the meaning, but even

---

A. Krajewski and A. Ravaglioli • Research Institute for Ceramic Technology of the Italian National Research Council, Via Granarolo 64, 48018 Faenza (Ravenna), Italy.

Integrated Biomaterials Science, edited by R. Barbucci. Kluwer Academic/Plenum Publishers, New York, 2002.

to change the focus around which new definitions must be constructed for both materials.

5.1.1. Ceramics

Different definitions to be ascribed to the term "ceramic" were proposed at various times and, as a consequence, many are the criteria of the classification of the corresponding products. A first definition approaching the concept of material was: *ceramics are a class of inorganic products essentially nonmetallic, with prominent functional requisites.* This definition was based on criteria of functional classes, closely related to the specific uses. Moreover, it extended the concept of ceramics to cements and inorganic amorphous materials (or glass systems). Such a definition was useful for the commercial aims of all those industries that produced inorganic, nonmetallic materials. It is current practice to assume that a ceramic is endowed with functional requisites. However, it was not a correct definition of a material possessing specific physicochemical characteristics. If the term *ceramic* implies some more intimate specification concerning the characteristics and properties of the material, it must adopt and take into consideration all possible physical and physicochemical features via which inorganic hard substances arrange themselves in a similar way to conform to solid bodies we call *ceramic*. In particular, the reported definition says nothing about the structural and microstructural nature of such a material.

A second, more realistic and scientific approach followed this definition: *ceramics are polycrystalline consolidated materials based on compounds of the III and VI metalloid groups of Mendeleev's table with any metallic atomic species, made through technological treatments which allow the involvement of mass transfer, the latter resulting in the component bonding.* Although this definition involved chemical and physical information, it was too redundant and long. Today, the following definition is preferred and is as accurate as the previous one: *ceramic is any nonmetallic polycrystalline material consolidated through a sintering process.*

The sintering process takes place at high temperature and the technicians of the sector define it as *firing*. This process is not a special prerogative only of ceramics (metals, glass, and polymers can also be sintered), but it certainly involves a typical manufacturing process to obtain them. A hard body consolidated by sintering (ceramic or not) is obtained by starting with fine powders of the chemical compound(s) of which it is to be constituted. As opposed to casting of a melt (which is the main way to produce hard objects constituted from all other materials, such as metals, glass, and most polymers), recourse to the sintering process implies that the object is preformed before the warm consolidation. The preforming stage consists of a process of mixing powders with at least a binder (water, suitable high molecular weight hydrocarbons, fats, polymers) to obtain a plastic paste easily molded (by hand or machine) to impress on a required shape, which will be that of the object to be formed. The final body will be constituted with the starting compounds if no chemical reactions are involved, otherwise the final product will be constituted with different compounds and, in this case, we call the process reaction sintering. The temperature at which the sintering process is carried out depends mainly on the chemical nature of the starting powders, but also on the physical characteristics of the powders. It involves mass transfer mentioned in the previous definition, and links to each other the different crystalline grains, corresponding to the consolidation process. Through sintering the particle porosity is removed by dimensional shrinkage of the original volume of the preformed object.

The field of ceramics is divided into many subgroups, each delineated on the basis of a specific classification. There are many classifications in ceramic production: commercial, based on the properties, based on the functional use, etc. One simple classification, useful for the final outcome of this treatment, is to subdivide the ceramics into classical and special. The term *classical* involves all ceramics whose composition, production technology, and use have been known since ancient times (materials for pottery, jars, tiles, sanitary ware, etc.) or whose application is classical. However, the term *advanced* refers to all those compositions that have special characteristics (chemical and/or physical properties, strong mechanical performance, etc.) which warrant their use in advanced technology or in fields of application where ceramics were never before considered.

5.1.2. The Outstanding Properties of Ceramics

Great interest in the application of advanced ceramics stems from a combination of special properties that many of them possess. A series of advantages in technological applications is given below:

- Good mechanical resistance even at high temperatures; the compression strength is particularly high.
- High hardness.
- Good tribological properties with wear and erosion resistance.
- Low thermal expansion.
- High thermal refractoriness.
- High chemical refractoriness with particular reference to oxidation and corrosion resistance.

Many kinds of ceramics have particular physical, chemical, and biological properties. This enables devices with specific functions to be constructed where special care is devoted to the choice of raw materials, the starting compositions, and the processing.

5.1.3. The Drawbacks of Ceramics

The main drawbacks of ceramics are:

- High temperatures of sintering.
- Intrinsic brittleness (related to high hardness due mainly to the strong covalent nature of the chemical bonds which characterize substances possessing good performances that give rise to ceramics).
- Difficulty with good reproducibility of the same object in a series, due to the complex and difficult operations of processing, particularly when complicated shapes are involved.
- High cost of all mechanical processes, particularly those related to the finishing and polishing to conform to standard geometrical and dimensional tolerances.

The properties of ceramics change remarkably even with small operative differences during the processing. These changes are attributable in particular to:

- Chemical composition of the starting powders (with reference to the presence of impurities).
- The presence of different phases and the arrangement of their distribution (even if the chemical compound is unique).
- The chemical and physical nature and structure of the grain boundaries.
- Granulometric population, dimension, shape, and distribution inside the fired body.

All these drawbacks contribute to the properties assumed by a ceramic product and to its characteristic operative performance, particularly pertaining to parameters that are difficult to control. The compounds and phases present at grain boundaries generally represent the weak point across which a possible crack can propagate. However, the situation is not always as dramatic as reported. In the case of alumina (Al_2O_3) ceramic, the presence of small amounts of MgO represents a positive occurrence because it forms an intergranular material constituting spinel ($MgAl_2O_4$), which is even more resistant than alumina itself.

In spite of the most accurate controls, numerous defects are introduced at the various stages of the production process and also through the quality of the utilized raw materials. For instance, if they contain gasifiable substances, they free gaseous molecules during heating and produce porosity along their outlet paths from the firing body, so consequently a certain porosity is introduced in the final ceramic product.

It is really difficult, if not impossible, to produce ceramic products without defects. The more common typology of defects introduced in the production are:

- Porosity.
- Irregular or remarkable increase in crystalline grains.
- Microcracks.
- Inclusions.
- Closed cavities.
- Variation in densities.
- A nonhomogeneous random distribution of the different crystalline phases which are present.

The defects present at the interior of the ceramic body significantly influence its mechanical resistance in an unpredictable way. The major limitation of structural ceramics originates from their brittleness and, because the mechanical stress introduced by a load or a thermal action cannot be released through a plastic sliding (with deformation of the body), the concentration of stresses at a defect is the most probable reason for a breakage.

5.1.4. The Structural Properties of Ceramics and Their Possibilities

All mechanical, thermal, and functional properties (chemical, optical, electrical, magnetic, etc.) are, for ceramics, very structurally dependent. In fact they depend primarily on the microstructure: nature of the grains (type, shape, size, chemical quality, quantity), their distribution inside the volume of the ceramic body, grain boundaries (chemical and physical quality), porosity, nature of the defects (kind, quantity, and distribution). A secondary dependence is due to the atomic arrangement of the molecular structure of every type (or phase) of grain, particularly inside the crystallographic lattice. Many physical properties are closely connected with this structure, depending especially on the particular electronic distribution to which every type of arrangement gives rise. Electrical, magnetic, optical, and even mechanical elastic constants are strictly related to the electronic distribution. Some special characteristics (such as superconductivity, but also tensor mechanical constants) even depend on specific crystallographic planes. All types of crystallographic defects produce a weakening of all these properties. This illustrates the importance of the presence of various types of phases of every chemical compound: some phases can possess required properties to some degree, others not. However, one important noteworthy consideration is that the ceramic structure is not a homogeneous continuous system, but one with gaps represented by the grain boundaries. All crystallographic-dependent properties are valid only inside each grain going from one side of its boundary to the other. So, for example, it is easy to stimulate magnetic levitation on ceramic pieces at a high critical temperature of superconductivity because in this case electrons can run circularly around every grain, but it is difficult to obtain real electronic superconduction along the bar due to the presence of barriers represented by the grain boundaries.

However, it is possible to say that, in general, every different specific property is affected by:

- Properties of the starting compounds.
- Additive agents (of sintering, of control of the microstructure, to impart special physical functional character(s), to produce secondary phases, to prevent other spurious phases, etc.).
- Production technology.
- Methodology and parameters of sintering.
- Superficial characteristics.
- Structural and surface modifications owing to interaction with the environment.

5.1.4.1. Mechanical Performance

From the viewpoint of the mechanical properties, the size, placing, and distribution of defects may represent critical aspects for the fatigue performance of a ceramic product. It should be emphasized that there is a close relationship between the development capability of critical defects, their dimension and population, and the distribution of stresses on a ceramic body, the flux line of which passes through a stressed structure. The fracture mechanism supplies parameters to allow calculation of the critical defect dimension, which can be a few microns for a microcrack at the surface of a ceramic body or even some hundreds of microns for an internal inclusion. On the other hand, the critical dimension depends on the shape of the defect, in particular at its apex.

Among mechanical structural-dependent parameters is toughness, which is the ability of a material to oppose crack propagation or fracture resistance. Toughness depends in fact on the weakest chemical bond strength involved, Young's modulus, and crack size. Its parameter is K_{IC} (stress intensity factor of fracture toughness), which *represents the measure of the critical stress intensity beyond which a crack propagates catastrophically*. According to Griffith's theory, it can be obtained from the

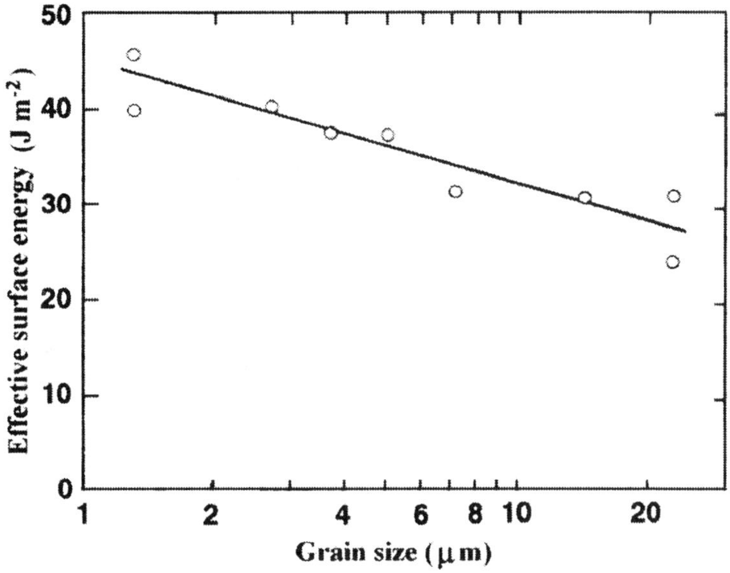

Figure 5.1. Variation of γ with grain size in alumina (Al_2O_3) ceramics.

following equation:

$$K_{IC} = \sigma L^{1/2}/\zeta \tag{1}$$

where σ is the applied stress, L the crack length, and ζ is a geometrical factor. The critical threshold stress factor σ_F is that value of applied stress σ beyond which a crack propagates. It is related to intrinsic parameters typical of every material, such as Young's modulus (E) and the superficial thermodynamic energy (of the particular crystallographic plane, if the material is crystalline), according to the equation:

$$\sigma_F = (2E\gamma/\zeta L)^{1/2} \tag{2}$$

where, in such a case, L is the initial length of the crack. In the crack geometry assumed by Griffith's theory, the geometric factor is $\zeta = \sqrt{\pi}$. Substituting σ_F for σ in equation (1), the K_{IC} value becomes equal to $(2E\gamma)^{1/2}$. The γ value is strongly dependent on grain size: the thinner the grains, the higher its value, as reported in Figure 5.1. Consequently, the σ_F value necessary to stimulate a critical crack to propagate increases as the grain size decreases.

5.1.4.2. Young's Modulus and Porosity

Young's modulus E is also influenced by the microstructure, in particular by the porosity and cavities. For these defects there is additionally a connection with their shape and distribution, governed by various equations. The most popular equation (and, statistically, that with the highest degree of success in the best-fit interpolation, because in practice it interpolates the experimental data directly) is the following:

$$E = E_0(1 - f_1 p + f_2 p^2) \tag{3}$$

where E_0 *is Young's modulus of the monolithic material*, p is the porosity measured as a fraction of overall volume, while f_1 and f_2 are two experimental coefficients. The value of E is also influenced by the presence of other substances dispersed randomly in the volume of the ceramic body, according to the different cases (shape, size, concentration, and E value of the dispersed particles and especially the mean degree of their aggregation or segregation, etc.).

5.1.4.3. Grains and Grain Boundaries in a Ceramic

Every ceramic body is formed from many crystalline micrograins. The reciprocal orientation of the crystallographic plains of these grains is random. As noted earlier, a ceramic is produced through a sintering process of powders in which the grains have no defined shape. The latter is, on the contrary, irregular because they originate from a milling process. Although irregular, the grains are, however, roundish, except in those cases for which a preferential growth prevails (possible, e.g., for compounds of the hexagonal crystallographic group). During sintering, the grains assume a more regular, polyhedral shape. A cross-section of a ceramic body exhibits a situation like that reported in Figure 5.2, where the numerals indicate the number of intergranular connections, better defined as the *intergranular coordination number*. These connections correspond to the grain boundaries through which all the various grains join closely together. In the case of Figure 5.2 the reported values refer only to the connections which are present in the plane (two-dimensional space) of the figure (for reasons of didactic immediateness) and not to all possible connections which can actually exist in three-dimensional space. On the other hand, the exhibited granulometric distribution is not good, these being present simultaneously big and small grains. This very variable situation must be avoided, because it lowers mechanical and tribological performance. The antiwear properties of ceramics are compromised in such cases because the big grains can easily

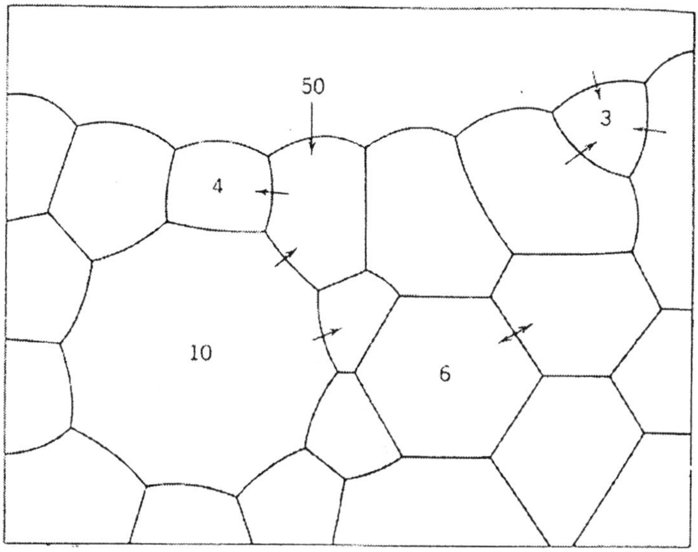

Figure 5.2. A sketch of the microstructure of a ceramic as seen on a cross section.

shell while running out their site and attaining the surface, where they can freely scrape off the sliding surfaces and form a cavity which can act as a crack initiator.

The attainable mean grain size during sintering can be controlled by the following factors:

- Sintering temperature.
- Duration of the steady temperature of sintering.
- Type and concentration of possible substances added to control grain growth.

These factors govern the microstructural evolution. The microstructure is related to grain size, its distribution, and the concentration of defects (cavities, inclusions, pores, cracks, etc.). The final density results from concurrence during the microstructural evolution. However, density and grain size are two independent factors. Instead, the ratio between density and the intergranular coordination number is not an independent factor in the comparison of density, as can be seen in Figure 5.3. This number ranges from 12.5 to 14.5 in dense structures, although a weak relationship with grain mean size exists in the case of high values.

The grain boundary is a region where the grains join together and in which there is the maximum concentration of defects (pores, impurities,

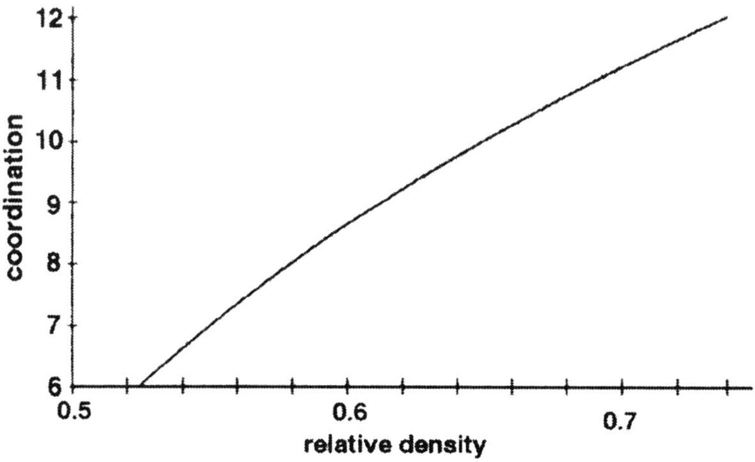

Figure 5.3. Relationship between relative density and mean coordination number calculated for irregular packing of monodimensional spheres.

secondary phases, etc.). Its characteristics influence all the properties of ceramics and they are the cause of all differences which arise between the monocrystal and ceramic body (when it is monophasic). Three types of deposits are formed at the grain boundary:

1. *Segregated deposits:* stratification of impurities from a few Å to some μm, which generally form a solid solution.
2. *Spread deposits:* present when the amount of impurities overcomes the saturation point and if the melting point of the precipitates is lower than the sintering temperature.
3. *Granular deposits:* present if the amount of impurities overcomes the saturation point and if the melting point of the precipitates is higher than the sintering temperature.

Some interesting properties of the grain boundary can be obtained by the addition of suitable substances.

The mean grain size Φ of a ceramic piece (a representative of some production) is measured by microphotography of a cross section taken through a (optical or scanning electronic) microscope equipped with a photocamera. This is Hilliard's method, which consists in drawing some circles of suitable diameter on the photo, as shown in Figure 5.4. The number of intersections N of every circle with the grains boundary traces is enumerated. If C indicates the length of the circumference and M the photographic magnitude, a mean grain size $D = C/NM$ is found from every

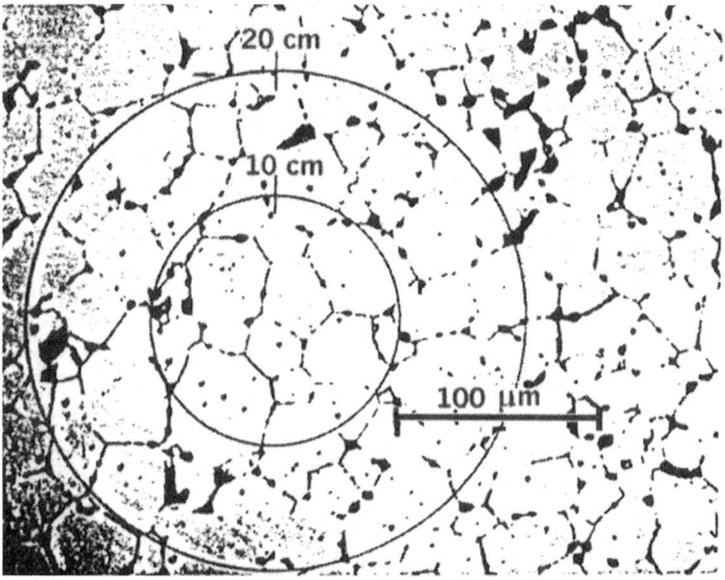

Figure 5.4. Example of Hilliard's method to calculate the mean grain size.

circle. The mean value Φ, and possibly its corresponding standard deviation, is obtained from all the *D* values originating from all the drawn circles. With this value one can calculate the number Γ_e, which represents the dimension of the grains following ASTM standards via the equation $\Gamma_e = -10000 + 6.64 \log(1/\Phi)$.

5.1.4.4. Tribological Performance

A good tribological characteristic for many ceramics under consideration in technological applications is their low wear, defined as the amount of removed material per unit surface while in contact with the applied load. This is a property closely related to the hardness of the material, its roughness, its husking, and its tribochemical sensitivity; the latter phenomenon is subject to the action of all the other indicated properties. What has been said could erroneously cause someone to think that wear is an intrinsic property of a material. Nothing is more unfounded than this. In reality *wear is the result of the interactive coupling through rubbing of two or more different materials.* This is the fundamental reason why it is difficult to introduce relevant standards.

5.1.5. Processing of Ceramics

The production process to obtain ceramic objects is connected to the requirements imposed by the sintering process. It follows a series of steps, consolidated during more than six millennia of human activity carried out by craftsmen engaged in improving pottery production. Obviously the introduction of technological ceramics has introduced some variations throughout the process, but no substantial strategic change has occurred. A flow chart of the series of production steps is sketched briefly in Figure 5.5. It represents the path from the raw materials to the finished product.

Every step should require a complex and articulated description. Furthermore, many of the powders used in the sintering process come from industrial production and not from controlled chemical syntheses in a laboratory. To understand ceramic processing it is absolutely necessary to examine the treatment of the powders, starting from an accurate control of their shape, dimension, and particle size distribution.

5.1.5.1. Powder Treatment

The powders are generally mixed with one or more additives (suitable organic binders) the nature and amount of which depend on the kind of shaping to be utilized in subsequent treatments and on the kind of powder material available. Complements of the binders are (if necessary) distilled water, some alcoholic substances, glycols, or glycerol. For certain types of forming processes one needs to add also deflocculants and sometimes plastifiers. All organic substances are suitable for restraining the single grains in the same position within the space allotted them during the shaping process. The material when mixed homogeneously and ready for shaping is called the *body*. To obtain a homogeneous body, the different substances employed are suitably and carefully mixed at room temperature by thermal action in jar mills or suitable mixers, depending on the type of body to be produced.

5.1.5.2. Shaping Methods

The shaping methods used to obtain a ceramic technological object are the following:

- *Pressing*, consisting in compressing a powder (sometime pretreated with the addition of a small amount of binder, generally stearic acid) through a piston within a disk.
- *Isostatic pressing*, consisting in applying very high pressure through a device comprising a compression camera filled with oil to a

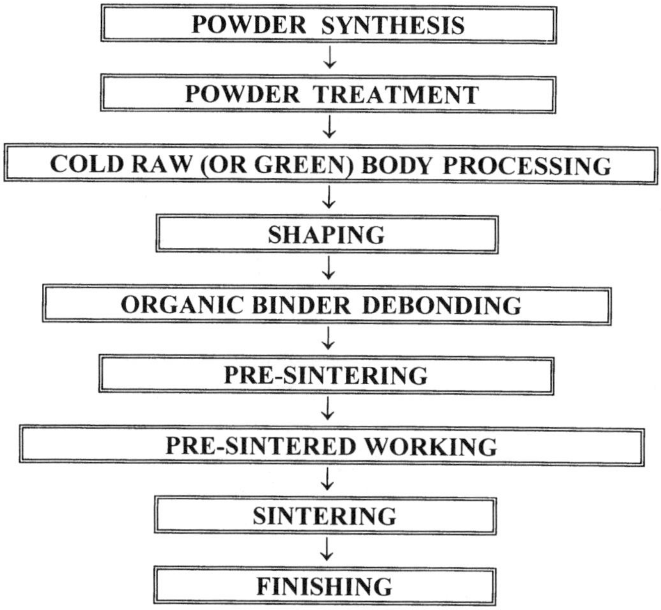

Figure 5.5. Steps of the production process to obtain a ceramic object.

preformed body, shaped while still in the form of powders (treated with the addition of a small amount of binder, generally stearic acid), and isolated from the environment by a thin impermeable latex rubber envelope (inside which a vacuum is created before any compression treatment) to preserve the body from contamination by oil.

- *Casting*, consisting in pouring a slip within an absorbent die (made, e.g., of gypsum).
- *Slip casting*, consisting in pouring a slip to check the thickness with a suitable barrier including adjustable knives upon a sliding tape suitably dried in it. (This technique is particularly useful in the production of flat and thin ceramic substrates.)
- *Extrusion*, consisting in driving (through a piston or a cochlea) a body across a mask which impresses a shape along the outlet direction to the exiting material. It is useful in the production of full bars with regular cross-section possessing symmetrical or at least simple geometry, or pipes of equivalent profile, or multiple honeycomb-like cells with triangular, square, or hexagonal cross-section profile.

- *Injection molding*, consisting in the introduction within suitable metallic dies (at a temperature of about 100–200 °C) of a slip driven through pressure constiting ceramic powder and polymers of suitable thermoplastic property (it must exhibit good plasticity, optimal viscosity and fluidity at the temperature under which the injecting device operates, and at the same time assume a solid consistency, without any sticking, at room temperature). The devices emloyed in the trade operate at low (about 10 atm) or high (about 100 atm) pressure, and the types of polymers, the microstructure of the powders, and the procedure used to prepare the slip vary greatly.

It is emphasized that for most techniques of shaping, it is necessary to proceed first to a prefiring process in order to obtain a body sufficiently sintered to be consistent as a solid, but not as hard as if it had been fired at the highest temperature. A prefired body allows mechanical refinements undertake dimensional and shape corrections using turning lathes and shaping grindstones, or even abrasive powders.

5.1.6. The Thermal Process

After shaping, much attention must be paid to the following operative steps, consisting in the drying and removal of all organic additives (binders, etc.) to avoid the formation of defects in the pieces up to 600 °C. Every obtained piece has a density ranging from about 40% to 70% with respect to its theoretical value (which is referred to the density of a monocrystal of the same substance in the same phase which will constitute the final consolidated ceramic body). In order to obtain as far as possible the highest final density, the first exigency is to obtain the greatest possible number of points of contact among grains and around each grain (the coordination number of the grains). This is facilitated by trying to produce some order in the grains through translation and rotation movements.

Prefiring. In the field of ceramics, this is an intermediate step of firing intended to refine the shape and dimensional tolerance. It is also called presintering. Recourse to this step is had especially when the green body is not sufficiently consistent to be worked cold. However, this step is often requested. Prefiring is carried out generally in the temperature range of 1000–1200 °C.

5.1.7. Sintering

Sintering is a physical process through which contiguous (crystalline or amorphous) grains join one another with a tendency to form bigger grains. When sintering takes place the following conditions are needed:

- A mechanism for the transport of material.
- An energetic source necessary to activate and support such transport.

The fundamental mechanisms which allow the transport are diffusion and viscous flow (sliding).

Heat is the primary source of energy which is suitable to activate transport processes in the solid state. Heat diffuses from external to inner parts of the firing piece and its permeation inside a body corresponds to an increase in molecular vibrations and electronic mobility. In crystalline materials this affects the crystallographic lattice vibrations. Energy gradients originate from contact among the particles and superficial tension associated with such a primary source of energy. When the temperature is sufficiently high, there is a sufficiently high number of molecular vibrations, the elongation of which allows migration of whole molecules or atoms leading to shifts of position. The molecular network of the surfaces of the grain boundaries and of the pores must attain a localized equilibrium of the forces in play. The local stresses are mainly connected to the shrinkage due to the progressive removal of porosity and to the increase in grain size, parameters that with time must take care of the angle of contact at which they join their surfaces. In conclusion, the fundamental interaction of the fusion of contiguous grains takes place thanks to the migration of atoms and/or molecules. Such migration is determined in many cases by their sliding along the surfaces (Figure 5.6). However, there are cases of migration through the local vapor phase. In this case, the physical process is promoted by elongations of the atoms or molecules at the surface wide enough to give rise to sufficient weakening of the involved chemical bonds to allow the interested particles to go away in a cloud whose state is in equilibrium with that of the surface. Obviously this kind of process can occur in the presence of sufficiently weak chemical bonds, light atoms or molecules, and typical modes and frequencies of vibrations. These physical characteristics depend on the type of compound in the state in which it lies at the sintering temperature.

The driving force leading to sintering originates from the difference ΔG_S between the free energy of the overall surface of the independent initial system of particles and that at the end, theoretically of a monolithic block (monocrystal if only one substance is involved). The rearrangement of the microstructure due to the action of the driving force leads to a sliding movement and/or rotation of the particles that constitute the geometry of the liquid meniscus. It ends when a strong packaged structure has formed. Long times are probably necessary to obtain the final theoretical state (e.g.,

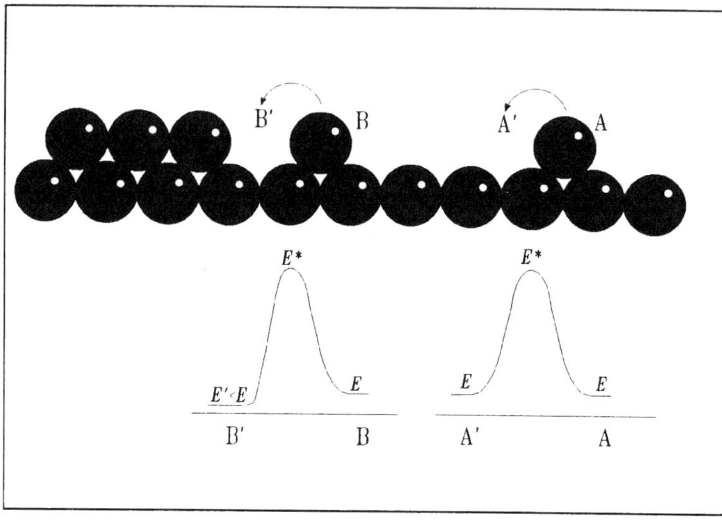

Figure 5.6. Example of atomic creep along the surface toward a zone at higher surface density. The creep from A to A′ leaves unchanged the involved energetic levels, in that from B to B′ a final greater energetic stabilization is expected because of the increase in the number of bonds.

the monocrystal) if one considers a process similar to that of the formation of crystalline rocks from volcanic lava (times measured in geological ages). The first steps in the formation of ceramics are sufficiently fast. When different aggregates of powders consolidate with time, a transfer of mass takes place so that the total volume of pores (and consequently of the whole piece) decreases. The driving force is governed by:

- Contact among the particles, due to an imbalance of the capillary pressures arising from the irregularity in their shape and dimensions.
- Density fluctuation.
- Distribution of a possible liquid film which behaves as an interparticle lubricant.

The sintering mechanism may take place according to different physicochemical events (Table 5.1).

Kinetics of grain growth. Under the action of the driving force, the mobility of the atoms which shift from less to more stable sites determines the establishment of a flux $J_A = dQ/dt = \rho dV/dt$, where Q is the quantity of moved atoms, t is the time, ρ is the density of the substance comprising the grains, and V is the transferred volume. If the grains are supposed to be

Table 5.1. A Summary of the Sintering Mechanisms and Their Characteristics

Sintering mechanism	Transport mechanism	Cause of the driving force	Notes
In vapor phase	Evaporation/ condensation	Difference in the vapor partial pressure which is a function of the surface bending	It does not produce shrinkage and densification
In liquid phase	Diffusion, viscous flux	Difference in the chemical potential of every atomic species which is at the base of a dissolution within the liquid phase due to capillary osmotic pressure or superficial tension	It does not give rise to shrinkage apart from the recovery of the bigger porosity
In solid state	Diffusion	Difference in the chemical potential of every atomic species which is at the base of a diffusion transport	The contribution coming from superficial diffusion does not give rise to shrinkage; that coming from volume diffusion does

spheroid, their volume is approximately $4\pi R^3/3$ and therefore $dV = 4\pi R^2 dR$, where R is their radius. If the flux is considered to be in a steady state, then J_A = constant = k and consequently $4\pi\rho R^2 dR = kdt$. Integration of this latter equation yields:

$$R^3 - R_0^3 = \lambda t \text{ or } D^3 - D_0^3 = 4\lambda t$$

where $D = 2R$ = the diameter of the grains.

If the assumed boundary conditions are not fitted to reality (e.g., a steady state is not reached, the atoms do not pack with the highest possible density ρ, lattice defects remain included, the mechanism of atomic transfer is closely related to the occurrence of other physical events which follow their own kinetic law, etc.), then the grain growth generally follows a kinetic law with exponent not equal to three. In general, the equation is the following:

$$D^n - D_0^n = 4\lambda t$$

where n is an integral number the value of which depends on the prevalent (or driving) kinetic law related to the grain growth. If the transfer process

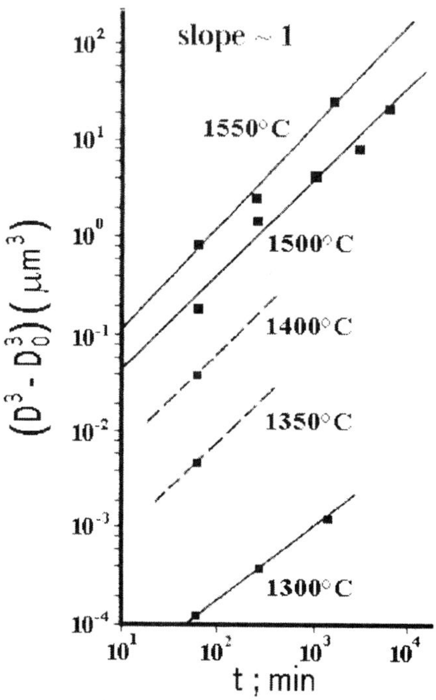

Figure 5.7. Example of the kinetic evaluation of grain growth (cubic in this specific example of alumina).

is related to more than one kinetic step in series, the slowest one determines the kind of kinetics followed.

The kinetics of grain growth can be determined experimentally. To obtain the value of the kinetic order, a large number of equal samples must be prepared. Different groups of samples must be sintered at various temperatures and times. The average dimension (radius or diameter) of the grains is then calculated for the resulting ceramic bodies by Hilliard's method. The values obtained from all the different groups of samples are then plotted on a bilogarithmic graph. An example of kinetic evaluation is reported in Figure 5.7. The plotted straight-line fitting isothermal points indicate a cubic trend (exponent $n = 3$) for grain growth of alumina.

The quantity λ is related to the transition free energy (ΔG^*) of the driving step by $\lambda = k_0 e^{-\Delta G^{*\prime} RT}$, where T is the absolute Kelvin's temperature of firing. If this expression is substituted into the equation in the previous paragraph and the result expressed in logarithmic form, the following equation is obtained:

$$\ln\{(D^n - D_0^n)/t\} = \ln(4k_0) - \Delta G^*/RT$$

By plotting $\ln\{(D^n - D_0^n)/t\}$ against $1/RT$ (the so-called *Arrhenius* plot) it is possible to obtain even ΔG^*. The resulting value is in general very indicative as it depends not only on the specific physical process involved, but even on the shape, roughness, porosity, and density of grain packing of the raw samples. In order to derive a reliable value, one must involve many different powders and select critically the more frequently occurring values.

5.2. Design and Duration of Ceramic Devices under Load

In all structural (including biomedical) applications the design assumes a particular importance particularly in the reproduction of devices made with other materials. Ceramics are endowed with great compression resistance, but meanwhile they do not react well to flexural and torque stresses. Consequently, all the various tensile and flexural load components need to be transformed into compressive ones. This is mostly possible through suitable technical projects. To develop such projects recourse can also be made to computer aiding design (CAD) which furnishes results originating from computerized simulation tests employing special mathematical procedures (such as finite element analysis).

Another difference in the behavior of ceramics with respect to metallic and polymeric materials more commonly utilized in technological applications is the rapidity with which any unforeseeable fracture occurs. A crack in a ceramic device happens unexpectedly without any warning sign of fatigue, even for a short time beforehand. This occurs because ceramics have a negligible or complete absence of a field of plasticity after the very short elastic one. Metallic and polymeric materials have, on the contrary, sufficiently wide fields of elastic and plastic (or yielding) behavior. Therefore, they undergo deformation when a threshold limit of mechanical fatigue is reached, producing seizure of moving parts which are the sign indicating that they need to be changed. The absence of any plastic behavior in ceramics prevents the formation of small plastic deformations, which are at the basis of fatigue signals and near-future yielding.

Therefore, in the design of a ceramic piece one needs to know how to choose the kind of ceramic material and to adopt operative criteria to obtain the best performance. A suitable microstructure, able to guarantee an optimal point of compromise between K_C and absolute resistance to the stresses, must be selected. In fact, during sintering some phenomena take place:

- Increase in the density.
- Increase in the volume of the grains.

Subcritical cracks form due to internal stresses via a detachment at the boundary between two grains, so the finer the grains the smaller the probability of forming cracks. In fact, since a ceramic consists of microscopic grains, the length of every microcrack formed will be proportional to the size of the relevant grains along that part of the grain boundary which is in tension and joined to another grain. Since $K_{IC} \propto \sigma L^{1/2}$ (where σ is the applied stress and L the length of the crack), the result is that the smaller the cracks the higher the sustained stress. Consequently, a ceramic will generally have high mechanical performance when it possesses high density and fine grains. Both conditions to some extent point in opposite directions because the densification process naturally involves an increase in grain size (on the other hand, the highest attainable densification originates uniquely from a monocrystal!). Therefore, a point of compromise should be reached by operating through sintering processes which guarantee high values of the *densification rate/rate of grain growth* ratio. Useful means to produce such conditions are:

- Application of pressure during densification.
- Optimization of the remaining sintering parameters: temperature, time, and chemical environment (in particular, the atmosphere of the kiln).
- Addition of suitable additives to the starting powder acting as inhibitors of grain increase.

These parameters are characteristic for every specific raw material or powder system and are closely related to the treatments that precede the sintering.

5.3. Ceramics for Surgical Implants

Many kinds of surgical intervention with the involvement of an internal device or prosthesis require that the objects to be implanted be made of ceramic materials. Ceramics are generally very well tolerated and integrated by living tissues and have no significant toxicity. The possibilities offered by ceramics are of three kinds: bioinert, bioactive, and bioresorbable. These are the classes of biological interactivity with living tissues.

5.3.1. Inert Bioceramics

Inert bioceramics are those which do not exert any influence on tissues and are not influenced by them. The most utilized are alumina, zirconia, hard porcelain, cordierite, sillimanite, etc. Their function is generally to sustain high mechanical loads. For this role they are in fact used to realize parts in which the applied compressive load is very high. However, they also offer very good tribological performance associated with high mechanical resistance, particularly to cyclic compressive loads. They are in fact particularly used to make parts in reciprocal movement which should run through sliding. Therefore, they are particularly employed to produce joint parts of prostheses (such as the head of a hip prosthesis or the plates of knee prostheses). The ceramics which are particularly suitable for this aim are alumina and stabilized zirconia. However, some carbides and nitrides are also useful as is porcelain for dental applications.

Alumina and zirconia exhibit good values of K_{IC} and their interaction with tissues appears to be least. The two sliding surfaces form a coupling; this can be homologous when the two surfaces are made from the same material (e.g., ceramic/ceramic of the same kind), or heterologous when one surface is made from one material and the other surface from a different material (e.g., ceramic/polymer). Obviously the size of the grains which comprise the ceramics must be particularly fine yet sufficiently homogeneous to avoid possible shelled grains. The more uniform the size of the grains, the less the probability of grain shelling. It needs to take into consideration that the grains of such ceramics are particularly hard and their abrading action is normally particularly catastrophic toward other, softer materials (such as metals and polymers). This is important particularly when a mixing coupling is chosen to reconstruct a joint. If large grains detach and move freely between the two sliding surfaces both made from these hard ceramics, they can produce disastrous rulings and roughening on parts of the sliding surfaces even if their nature is the same as that of the grains. On the other hand, a high amount of shelling grains produce debris which may deposit in the tissues that surround the implant. The debris is composed of ceramic grains and of the abraded particles originating from other materials (if any). This deposit generally produces phlogosis. It is hence clear that the safety of having at one's disposal a ceramic with low probability of shelling is a parameter of great importance.

The lubricating agent between the two surfaces in sliding is the synovia which is inserted between them. This is a viscous liquid produced by the human body, a fraction of the body's physiological fluids. In case of inflammation it contains a small percentage of proteins owing to draining of the catabolic products of the (human and bacterial) cell's death. These proteins can adhere to the surfaces, rendering them rough and making more difficult the functioning of the joint. Therefore, in the case of formation of wear particles, the inflammation of the tissues surrounding a joint may concur to promote blocking of the joint through a proteic deposit from synovia. To avoid such inconvenience, a ceramic/UHMWP (ultrahigh molecular weight polyethylene) coupling is normally adopted rather than a ceramic/ceramic one (such as a femoral head substituted by a ball made with alumina and acetabular side made with UHMWP, similar to, but more efficient than the corresponding metal/UHMWP coupling). The ceramic/UHMWP coupling (although it has a worse tribological performance at the beginning of its use than the ceramic/ceramic one) is that which has always been best in most applications.

5.3.1.2. Description of the Performance of the Main Inert Bioceramics

a. Alumina. Alumina (Al_2O_3) is one of the compounds most utilized to produce technological ceramic devices. It is also much used to produce biomedical products. It possesses one stable and many metastable phases. The stable phase (α-alumina) is a component of practically all ceramic products of this kind. It is also the structure of corundum. Only some applications require the presence (generally on the surface) of some other phases. The phase transformation is promoted particularly by grain size, disorder or degree of activity of the powders, environmental conditions (humidity, kiln atmosphere), impurities, and additives (which are added to promote or inhibit crystalline grain dimension). It should be noted that presence of some MgO favors the formation of η (particularly present at high temperatures) and γ phases. When a ceramic layer is deposited on a substrate by plasma spraying, the presence of some η phase is introduced. Table 5.2 lists all possible phases of alumina. Figure 5.4 reports the microstructure of an alumina ceramic with particular reference to grain boundary and grain growth.

b. Zirconia. The stable phase of zirconia (ZrO_2) at room temperature is the monoclinic phase. This phase is useless for technological application (except in some particular cases). However, similar to the austenitic/martensitic transformation of stainless steel, zirconia also undergoes phase transformation which can be rendered stable at room temperature thanks to the addition of suitable substances. The possible transformations that zirconia can undergo in relation to the cooling process once the preshaped object has been sintered are reported in Table 5.3.

Table 5.2. The Different Possible Phases of Alumina Ceramics

Phase	Transformation temperature (°C)	Crystallographic system	Molecules per unit cell (number)	Unit cell parameter(s) (Å)	Specific gravity (g/cm^3)
α		Rhombohedral	2	$a = 4.758$, $c = 12.991$	3.97
χ		Cubic	10	$a = 7.95$	3.00
η		Cubic	10	$a = 7.90$	2.5–3.6
γ	$\gamma \rightarrow \alpha \sim 1100\,°C$ (only on cooling)	Tetragonal		$a = 7.95$, $c = 7.79$	3.20
δ	$\delta \rightarrow \alpha$ at 705 °C	Tetragonal	32	$a = 7.967$, $c = 23.47$	3.20
ι		Orthorhombic	4	$a = 7.73$, $b = 7.78$, $c = 2.92$	3.72
θ	$\theta \rightarrow \gamma$ 850–900 °C	Monocline	4	$a = 5.53$, $b = 2.95$, $c = 11.86$ $\beta = 103.7°$	3.56
κ	$\kappa \rightarrow \alpha$ at 705 °C	Orthorhombic	32	$a = 8.49$, $b = 12.73$, $c = 13.39$	3.30
ε	$\varepsilon \rightarrow \alpha$ at 660 °C	Cubic		$a = 5.33$	

If a transformation from a tetragonal to a monoclinic phase were to occur during cooling, some tensile stresses may increase inside the ceramic body, generated by the modified contact relation between granules. The presence of these internal stresses can cause fracture, even delayed. The tetragonal to monoclinic transformation involves in fact a wide increase (5%) in molar volume. The grains which constitute the microstructure of the ceramic enlarge and change shape, and this generates local stresses tangentially to the formed axis. The transformation is not kinetically reversible and is denoted by the wide hysteresis which occurs from heating to cooling

Table 5.3. Some Crystallophysical Properties of Zirconia Phases

Phase	Transformation temperature (°C)	Space group	Unit cell parameter(s) (Å)	Specific gravity (g/cm^3)
Monoclinic	—	P2/c	$a = 5.156$, $b = 5.191$, $c = 5.304$, $\beta = 98.9°$	5.56
Tetragonal	1000–1200	P4/nmc	$a = 5.094$, $c = 5.171$	6.10 (calc.) 5.72 (exp.)
Cubic	2000–2400	Fm3m	$a = 5.124$	6.09

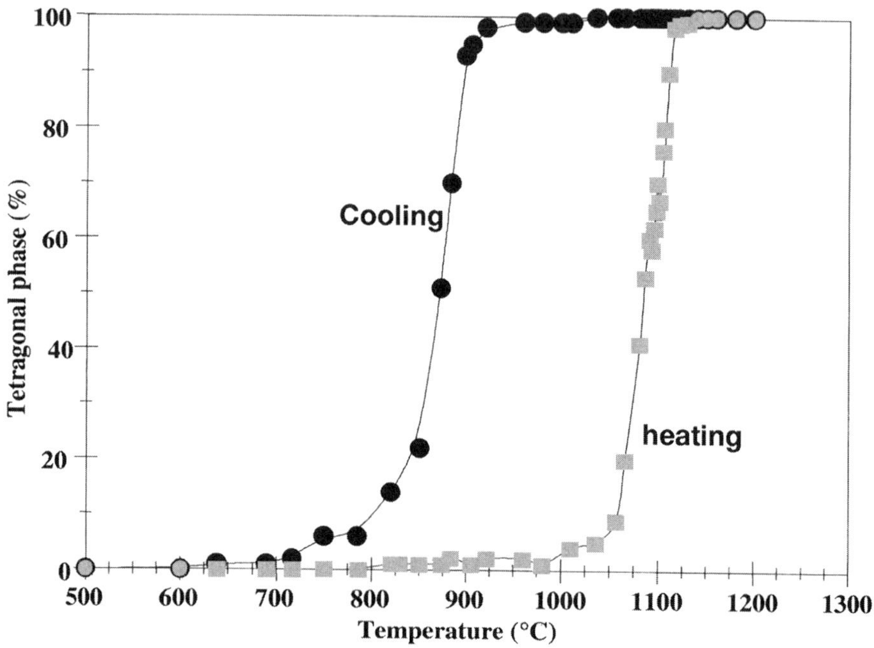

Figure 5.8. Percentage of tetragonal phase as detected by X-ray diffraction during heating and cooling of ZrO_2 in relation to the monoclinic–tetragonal transformation. Note the wide thermal hysteresis formed.

reported in Figure 5.8. Consequently it is not possible to utilize pure zirconia to produce ceramic pieces. On the other hand, natural zirconia contains HfO_2 as solid solution, and in some cases ThO_2, which renders more stable the monoclinic form and their chemical separation because of their very close affinity to zirconia. Medical grade zirconia does not contain any radionuclides and consequently no Th (and other radioactive contaminants such as Ra) is allowed. To improve the mechanical performances of zirconia it should be utilized in its allotropic forms: tetragonal and/or cubic phases. It is possible to stabilize these phases at room temperature by simply introducing in the crystallographic lattice a suitable amount of stabilizers. This is possible by chemical co-precipitation as dioxide from saturated solutions of both components (zirconium and stabilizer salts). These stabilizers are CaO, MgO, and Y_2O_3 which promote stabilization of the cubic phase, and CeO_2 which particularly promotes the tetragonal phase. For proper additions and treatments, zirconia can be also partially stabilized. In this case it may contain an appropriate quantity of the tetragonal phase as a precipitate of the cubic phase, thereby avoiding exaggerated fracturing.

c. Carbides and Nitrides. Carbides are considered for surgical grafting. These are substances with very high melting temperatures. An alloy comprising 80% of $TaC_{0.93}$ and 20% of $HfC_{0.93}$ has the highest melting point so far recorded, namely 4050 °C.

At high temperature they exist in three distinct forms, each of them nonstoichiometric. The α-phase has a metallic nature, rich in carbon (5–10%) and producing an eutectic with the β-phase when the carbon content exceeds the solubility limit. The β-phase belongs to the hexagonal crystallographic class and its average composition is M_2C, where M stands for the metallic cation partner. This phase is narrowly nonstoichiometric at low temperatures, though becoming more so at high temperatures. In this phase the nonstoichiometry is caused by carbon deficiency, not by an excess of metal. The γ-phase results either from an increase in the carbon content or from the peritectic decomposition of the β-phase at high temperature. This phase is largely nonstoichiometric and its composition, like the MC formula, has a rock-salt structure. Once again the nonstoichiometry is caused by carbon vacancies and not by an excess of metal. The γ-phase never appears to attain a 1:1 metal/carbon ratio, and each possible MC composition appears to be a mixture containing graphite. The MC composition is expected to be found in all sequences, but in practice it occurs only when the metal layer adopts a cubic stacking. Typical examples of this kind of carbide are TiC_x and TaC_x (with $x \leqslant 1$). Mechanical performances depend on the composition, since at room temperature the microhardness of the TiC_x and TaC_x phases may follow different behaviors. In the compositional range from $TaC_{0.82}$ to $TaC_{0.97}$ there is a linear decrease in microhardness from 2750 kg mm^{-2} to 1400 kg mm^{-2}, while from $TiC_{0.82}$ to $TiC_{0.97}$ there is a linear increase from 2000 kg mm^{-2} to 2750 kg mm^{-2}.

Similar considerations are possible for nitrides. Those involved in biomedical applications (TiN and TaN) have an α-phase MN. Nitrides exhibit a thermal expansion coefficient lower than that of carbides. Microhardness of TiN_x ranges from 1700 kg mm^{-2} to 1900 kg mm^{-2}.

The production of MC carbides requires very high temperatures (>1800 °C) with a synthesis through a voltaic arch in a suitable kiln with graphite electrodes. The equivalent nitrides are synthesized at much lower temperatures (about 1000 °C) in less expensive kilns. Nitrides are therefore more easily obtained and this is the reason for their preference in use with respect to carbides. All these compounds exhibit a very high tribological performance and are normally adopted to cover the sliding parts of the joints to avoid roughening. Nitride coverings of TiN are easily obtained by chemical vapor deposition on the metallic ball of a hip prosthesis made with titanium alloy.

d. Porcelain for Artificial Teeth. Artificial teeth are classified as "fritted porcelain" because they do not properly fit into the field of compositions and typical ceramic treatments classified classically as porcelain. A more appropriate definition should be feldspathic bodies, making reference to their typical composition. Different specialist books treating the matter classify these porcelains on the basis of their firing temperature. Three main levels of classification of these porcelains are commonly produced: the "high temperature" ones are fired over 1290 °C, the "average temperature" ones are fired between 1090 °C and 1260 °C, and finally the "low temperature" ones are fired between 870 °C and 1070 °C.

However, this is an arbitrary classification. The primary characteristic of these porcelain compositions must be their high durability and toughness, the absolute absence of porosity, and the remarkable brightness. The powders utilized for the production of these porcelains must be extremely pure and without substances which introduce chromatic effects, even if in traces. In particular, those chemical elements which can produce redox reactions must be absent due to the possible coloration they could introduce and/or the development of gaseous products which could give rise to the formation of undesired microbubbles. Consequently, with the exception of lanthanum, all transition elements must be absent ($\ll 0.02\%$; in particular iron and manganese) under whatever form and oxidation state. Particular care must be paid to the choice of the granulometry of these porcelain powders. It must be extremely uniform and fine, within a narrow range of grain size of $1.0 \pm 0.3\,\mu m$. Typical compositions of dental porcelain are reported in Table 5.4.

In mixtures of quartz and feldspar, the quartz must be dissolved in the viscous feldspar during the firing process, so obtaining a constant increase in the viscosity of the mixture with time while anticipating every possible distortion resulting from the different process used to prepare the synthetic teeth. Residual quartz must not remain, however, because its presence could cause mechanical weakness in the products. It was shown that an appropriate addition of ZnO produces a very complete dissolution of the quartz with consequent reduction in the thermal expansion coefficient, so improving the performance of the product in terms of thermal shock resistance. Small quantities of kaolin are introduced to mat the obtained body, which otherwise would be transparent. Because of its function, the purity and extreme finesse of the granulometry of kaolin are two very important attributes; generally only precalcined kaolin is used. During such precalcina-

Table 5.4. Typical Compositions of Dental Porcelains (wt%)

Component	German mixtures				American mixtures		
Feldspar	73	80	75	85	81	77	12
Quartz	25	20	24	13	15	18	60
Kaolin	—	—	1	2	4	—	—
Soda	—	—	—	—	—	—	8
Marble[a]	2	—	—	—	—	—	1
Bone powder[b]	—	—	—	—	—	5	—
Potash	—	—	—	—	—	—	8
Borax[c]	—	—	—	—	—	—	11

[a] Pure $CaCO_3$ (calcite).
[b] In practice, addition of $Ca_5(PO_4)_3OH$ (hydroxyapatite).
[c] B_2O_3.

tion a mullite phase develops, followed by a secondary one. To improve toughness and to avoid an excess of brightness, it is recommended that some alumina (Al_2O_3) and/or mullite be added, both very pure, very fine, and calcined. Calcium, sodium, and potassium oxides (in suitable proportions and prepared separately by roasting the respective carbonates, which decompose at sufficiently low temperatures) and borax (B_2O_3) can be introduced to an extent lower than 1% as fusibility correctors and opalescence and/or mat makers. Other possible opacity-makers, which can be introduced as ultrafine and pure powders up to a limit of 5%, are rutile (TiO_2), cassiterite (SnO_2), zirconia (ZrO_2), ceria (CeO_2), zircon ($ZrSiO_4$), and lantania (La_2O_3). Their function (apart from toughness) is to correct the white tone and adapt it to that of natural teeth.

5.3.1.2. Inert Ceramics as Bearing Materials

Inert ceramics based on alumina and zirconia exhibit their good adaptability in the production of small devices and prostheses in the various sectors listed in Table 5.5.

Generally, a fibrous layer forms all around the walls of an inert ceramic implanted in the bone. This layer is too soft, so it does not assure a good fixation (or anchorage) of the implanted object to the surrounding tissue. Sometimes, this result is even welcome to obtain the so-called "piston effect" (e.g., in the prostheses of the articulations of short bones some freedom in moving up and down inside the cavity of the phalanx bones, in which both their end-terminals are inserted, impart a general better behavior, either in allowing an easier re-intervention or from the functionality point of view). Later, it was found that the ingrowing bone tissue is

Table 5.5. Some Examples of Small Devices Produced with Ceramic Materials at IRTEC-CNR (Italy)

Surgical sector	Functions	Device	Material(s)
Generic	Fillers for bone cavities	Bioactive granulates, resorbable or not, porous or not, to fill cavities pre-existing or produced by surgical intervention to remodel bone shape, or after resection or removal of cysts, tumors, or to reproduce damaged volumes of bone (necrosis, infections, etc.)	Hydroxyapatite Other phosphates
	Cutting devices for surgery intervention	Bistoury, scissors, razor blades and tips of different shape and geometry.	Al_2O_3, ZrO_2
Articular extremities	Total or partial substitution of articulations	Metatarso-phalangeal of the foot	Al_2O_3
		Metacarpo-phalangeal	Hydroxyapatite
Orthopedics	Arthroplastics	Radial capitellum	Al_2O_3
	Bone and osteocartila-gineous synthesis	Screws and rods	Hydroxyapatite
	Corrective resolution of spine damages (discopathy).	Intervertebral spine spacer	Al_2O_3, ZrO_2
ENT	Microsurgical substitution in ear affected by otosclerosis or chronic otites	Total (TORP) or partial (PORP) ear ossicular chain substitution	Al_2O_3 Hydroxyapatite
		Mastoideal substitution	Hydroxyapatite
Dentistry	Guided bone regeneration	Semipermeable partially resorbable membranes	Polymer/ hydroxyapatite composites

surrounding the implanted device based on inert ceramic only in the zones subjected to a load. Dental roots made with alumina and having microstuds on their surface were experimented with some success. The microstuds contributed to induce a mechanical adhesion to the mandibular bone and give rise to points of compression to stimulate bone ingrowth. The quality of the success is, however, very similar to that attainable with titanium implants, less expensive, and less bulky.

5.3.2. Bioactive Ceramics

Differently from inert bioceramics, those which are defined as bioactive ceramics are able to exert some biological influence on tissues and are influenced by them. They are chemically composed with atomic species managed by the biological cycles, and generally they are calcium phosphates. The most utilized are hydroxyapatite, $Ca_5(PO_4)_3OH$, (HA), and in some cases tricalcium phosphate, $Ca_3(PO_4)_2$, (TCP). Their main application is in the bone, where there is a mineralized component whose chemical composition is similar to that of hydroxyapatite. Their function is generally to sustain repair or growth of bone. For this role they are in fact utilized to realize parts in which the bone is stimulated to grow.

Bioactivity is an interfacial response of the tissue toward material, which results at the end in a tissue bonding. On bone, the bioactivity of a material can be subdivided into osteoinduction (osteogenetic biostimulation of cellular and/or tissue activity to the repair or growth due to the ions freed in the biological environment) and osteoconduction (the process by which bone is directed so as to conform to the surface of the material). Bioactive materials can be subjected to bioresorption (the process of removal of material for biodegradation exercised by the biological environment) or can exhibit biostability (the capacity of a material to resist changes in a biological environment). For example, hydroxyapatite, being similar to the stable product present in the bone, is thermodynamically stable in that environment and so is biostable in bone while TCP is slowly bioresorbed (except for extensive volumes in which the surface became enveloped by a layer of hydroxyapatite which stops any further dissolution of the interior parts). Bioresorbable ceramics usually have high osteoinduction capability, while hydroxyapatite confers to the surface good bioattachment and bioadhesion (the state resulting between tissue and material from mechanical or chemical attachment, respectively). The use of hydroxyapatite is recommended not only for its total biotolerability, but also for its ability to influence the growth of neoformation bone and to become involved in it (*bioactivity*).

5.3.2.1. Calcium Phosphate Ceramics

Calcium phosphates, and in particular hydroxyapatite, were taken into consideration in early bioceramic studies for surgical application on bone (Osborn, 1985; De Groot, 1980; Bauer and Hohenberger, 1989; Jarcho, 1989). The production of hydroxyapatite for biomedical use became important about fifteen years ago thanks to its very high compatibility with bone tissue. Due to a not very high mechanical resistance, however, implant applications of objects based on ceramic calcium phosphates are—though numerous—limited to those sectors of skeleton implantology where considerably high loads are not involved. One such major application is the coating of metal prostheses with hydroxyapatite.

A calcium phosphate ceramic has a behavior which depends directly on its chemical nature and structure. A single compound may be liable to transformations by the action of the surrounding environment. Such transformations can take place in a wet environment, or with a solvent, or in a drying environment (particularly through heating). The compound in question may in fact undergo different transformations in each of the two environments. Because of their number and the number of relationships between themselves, phosphates build a complex class of chemical compounds.

Here, the calcium phosphate system is considered as a whole, paying due attention to the various kinds of inherent terminology. The contribution that a chemical interpretation can provide is its ability to foresee the different compounds which may form in relation to the different preparation procedures, making everybody aware of the transformations that take place and of their importance with a view, in particular, to avoiding the formation of specific compounds whose presence can weaken the mechanical strength (a physical parameter whose value has always been the weak spot of these ceramics in relation to their applicability in load conditions).

Once we have a clear perception of the basic concepts regarding the chemical and crystallochemical composition of calcium phosphates, as well as the concepts relative to phase mixtures and solid solutions in predetermined lattices, it will be possible to direct our efforts to devising ceramic materials which, thanks to the combination of their components (either pure or containing substituting ions in a known way) in the suitable crystal phases, can ensure the best results in terms of mechanical strength.

5.3.2.2. Calcium Phosphate Chemistry

Generally speaking, in a wet environment the compound will be influenced by the simultaneous acidic–basic equilibria relative to the phosphoric acid, while in a drying and heating environment the transformations will be mainly due to water loss as a result of molecular condensation, which leads to calcium pyrophosphate ($Ca_2P_2O_7$ or CPP) and even polyphosphates. But if the transformation (no matter if carried out by wet or dry means) starts from combinations of phosphates, it will not generally give rise to a combination of transformations as though each of the two components were independent, because the single components may interact with each other from the beginning and thereby lead to quite different and not previously forecasted products. Sometimes, there is even confusion between the chemical name of a compound and the mineralogical name of a specific crystallization phase of that compound. Table 5.6 provides the chemical and mineralogical names of the various calcium phosphate compounds of main interest for this work, while Table 5.7 presents the modified calcium phosphates that occur in the biological system of humans (LeGeros, 1991).

a. Transformations of Calcium Phosphates in Wet and Biological Environments. The chemical nature of a compound is the factor which is mainly responsible for the solubility product value. A role in influencing such a value may be played by the kind of crystallization and by the variously numerous molecules of crystallization water that could modify the crystallographic system of the crystallized compound.

In solution, when phosphates are present, the following multiple equilibria take place:

$$\begin{array}{llll} H_3PO_4 \rightleftarrows H_2PO_4^- & + H^+ & pKa_1 = & 2.1192 \\ H_2PO_4^- \rightleftarrows HPO_4^{2-} & + H^+ & pKa_2 = & 7.2076 \\ HPO_4^- \rightleftarrows PO_4^{3-} & + H^+ & pKa_3 = & 12.0000 \end{array}$$

In a very acidic solution $H_2PO_4^-$ will occur prevalently, in a moderately acidic solution HPO_4^{2-} will occur, and in a basic environment PO_4^{3-} will occur. Because of the solubility product (*SP*), the presence of Ca^{2+} in a slightly acid environment favors the precipitation of $CaHPO_4$ (DCP), while in a basic environment it favors the precipitation of hydroxyapatite instead of TCP, also with the help of the OH^- group which contributes to the formula of the solubility product. The more basic the environment, the more stable the hydroxyapatite. In fact, the two formulas of the solubility product:

(1) $SP_{TCP} = [Ca^{2+}]^2[PO_4^{3-}]^2$ for $Ca_3(PO_4)_2$

and

(2) $SP_{HA} = [Ca^{2+}]^5[PO_4^{3-}]^3[OH^-]$ for $Ca_5(PO_4)_3OH$

show that hydroxyapatite formation as precipitate is clearly favored, in particular in an alkaline environment. If, therefore, some TCP (e.g., crystallized in its β-phase, called witlockite) is placed in a basic environment, it will (however slowly) undergo the following transformation:

$$5Ca_3(PO_4)_2 + 3OH^- \rightarrow 3Ca_5(PO_4)_3OH + PO_4^{3-}$$

In such an environment the TCP, because of the phase transformation to hydroxyapatite, absorbs up to 7.6% water, and the resulting increase in

Table 5.6. Different Calcium Phosphate Substances that Can Be Involved in Ceramic Sintering

Compound name	Acronym	Chemical formula	Oxide notation	Ca/P ratio	Biological response
Calcium metaphosphate	CMP	$Ca(PO_3)_2$	$CaO \cdot P_2O_5$	0.5	Wide macrophagic activation
Calcium pyrophosphate	CPP	$Ca_2P_2O_7$	$2CaO \cdot P_2O_5$	1	Wide macrophagic activation
Di-calcium phosphate[a]	DCP	$CaHPO_4$	$2CaO \cdot P_2O_5 \cdot H_2O$	1	Low macrophagic activation
Tri-calcium phosphate[b]	TCP	$Ca_3(PO_4)_2$	$3CaO \cdot 2P_2O_5$	1.5	Resorbable
Tetra-calcium phosphate	TeCP	$Ca_4(PO_4)_2 \cdot$	$4CaO \cdot P_2O_5$	2	Without clinical relevance
Octa-calcium phosphate	OCP	$Ca_8H_2(PO_4)_6 \cdot 5H_2O$	$8CaO \cdot 3P_2O_5 \cdot 6H_2O$	1.333…	Resorbable
Hydroxyapatite[c]	HA	$Ca_5(PO_4)_3OH$	$10CaO \cdot 3P_2O_5 \cdot H_2O$	1.666…	Biologically active but stable

[a] The crystalline phase is named monetite; important is the hydrate crystalline phase brushite, the di-calcium phosphate di-hydrate (DCPD).
[b] Well known are the crystalline phases α- and β-TCP.
[c] This term commonly refers to the more accurate chemical definition of calcium hydroxyl apatite.

Table 5.7. Modified Calcium Phosphates in the Biological System of Humans (LeGeros, 1991)

Compound type	Chemical formula	Occurrences
HA	$(Ca, Z)_{10}(PO_4, Y)_6(OH, X)_2$	Enamel,[a] dentine,[a] bone,[a] dental calculi, stones, urinary calculi, soft tissue calcifications
OCP	$Ca_8H_2(PO_4)_6 \cdot 5H_2O$	Dental and urinary calculi
DCPD	$CaHPO_4 \cdot 2H_2O$	Dental calculi, chondrocalcinosis, crystalluria, decomposed bones
TCP	$(Ca, Mg)_9(PO_4)_6$	Dental and urinary calculi, salivary stones, dentinal caries, arthritic cartilage, soft tissue calcifications
ACP	$(Ca, Mg)_x(PO_4, Q)_x$	Soft tissue calcification
CPPD	$Ca_2P_2O_7 \cdot 2H_2O$	Pseudogout deposits in synovial fluids

[a] $Z = Na^+, Mg^{2+}, K^+, Sr^{2+}$, etc.; $Y = CO_3^{2-}, HPO_4^-$; $X = Cl^-, F^-$; $Q = P_2O_7^{2-}, CO_3^{2-}$.

volume brings about a disruption of the microstructure. In an acidic environment, owing to the simultaneous equilibria, TCP is transformed to $CaHPO_4$ (DCP) and $Ca(H_2PO_4)_2$ (MCP). Moreover, the TCP is not thermodynamically stable in H_2O, with the consequence that its phases suffer a pronounced loss of strength in aqueous solutions. A β-TCP bulk material may not undergo complete dissolution in a slightly alkaline environment because of the formation of a hydroxyapatite layer, which separates the β-TCP from the aqueous system.

On the other hand, the stability of hydroxyapatite in an acidic environment is not allowed because, as a result of the decrease in OH^- concentration and with the presence of H^+, the following transformation takes place:

$$Ca_5(PO_4)_3OH + 4H^+ \rightarrow 3CaHPO_4 + 2Ca^{2+} + H_2O$$

A series of equilibrium curves relative to isothermal solubility at 25 °C toward the pH and the Ca^{2+} concentration was produced (Brown and Chow, 1981). Hydroxyapatite is the most competitive product in the basic environment (its physiological pH is 7.2); in acid environment it is still very slowly soluble with a pH value of 4.3–4.8, below which the formation of $CaHPO_4 \cdot 2H_2O$ (DCPD) becomes very stable.

A ratio Ca/P = 1.5 allows one to obtain, in particular conditions, the formation of octacalcium phosphate (OCP) instead of $CaHPO_4$. LeGeros (1991) has pointed out that an OCP field exists in aqueous solution in terms of temperature and pH.

Table 5.8. Binding Capacity of Important Enzymes Relating to Ca^{2+} in Bones

Type of calcium-activating enzyme	Level of Ca^{2+} bound ($\mu g/\mu M$)
Phosphatase	28
Phosphorine	128
Calmoduline	8

The OCP is regarded not so much as a possible constituent to produce ceramic bodies, but rather as a precursor of biological hydroxyapatite, so that its presence may sometimes be an advantage.

The occurrence of particular substances such as Mg^{2+}, F^-, CO_3^{2+}, and of substances able to capture Ca^{2+} and PO_4^{3-} giving rise to *chelate** complexes in solution and to induce the formation of stable complexes, can considerably modify the stability of the crystallographic lattice of apatite and other calcium phosphates, favoring their formation and hence their presence in a precipitated stable phase. The mentioned *chelate* complexes exist in a living organism within specific proteins that function as transporters (Table 5.8) of Ca^{2+} and PO_4^{3-}. In particular, Mg^{2+} stabilizes the witlockite phase to the detriment of the apatite one, while the presence of F^- favors the existence of the apatite phase.

When foreign ions try to enter a chemical compound (such as hydroxyapatite) in an amount not sufficient to modify the lattice nature of the stable crystallized phase, the result is the creation of partially replaced compounds which show, however, a distribution of lattice defects. Such defects may be due to *steric* factors,† because the hosted ion settles in the sites that it finds more suitable for its chemical requirements. In this way the substituting ion becomes vicarious of the ion that really is present in its crystallographic site in the original pure compound.

Defects may also derive from the fact that the charge of the vicarious ion (no matter if it is of the same sign) does not correspond to the charge of the substituted one. So, in order to maintain the overall electroneutrality of the charge, there must be either a presence of other foreign suitable ions of opposite charge distributed in the complementary sites, or a suitable redistribution of vacancies in all kinds of sites.

* Terminology introduced in: Clifford, A. F. 1961. *Inorganic Chemistry of Qualitative Analysis*, p. 179, Prentice-Hall Inc., Englewood Cliffs, N.J.

† Chemical terminology, with the meaning of too wide a volume engaged by an assemblage of atoms which hampers possible chemical bonds and connections.

A stoichiometric representation of this complex arrangement in a defined constraining structure could be represented by a complicated formula whose display is practically impossible to write. This is because each new component introduced requires a new variable stoichiometric coefficient and all of these coefficients may participate also in the amount of the three different kinds of vacancies (in the following this concept will be better clarified).

According to the way in which the crystalline lattice has arranged itself there will be a remarkable change of chemical properties, and notably of thermal ones.

b. Thermal Transformations of Calcium Phosphates. The thermal behavior of phosphates is the subject of an intricate debate due to the fact that each phosphate can remarkably influence the overall process of the transformations which can occur at the different temperatures. Thermal transformations are awfully important, because a ceramic is obtained through a thermal treatment and consequently all eventual transformations that can occur at high temperatures must be expected as they form the base of the chemical quality of the original powders utilized for the production. We treat in a detailed way just this aspect of the overall problem due to its importance.

One of the main pollutants of the starting powders is $CaHPO_4$ (monetite) or its hydrated phase $CaHPO_4 \cdot 2H_2O$ (brushite), whose presence is generally noxious. The main condensation reaction is the following:

$$2CaHPO_4 \rightarrow Ca_2P_2O_7 + H_2O$$

with a transformation temperature lower than 600 °C.

Theoretically, in the presence of calcium oxide, the following reaction could occur:

$$6CaHPO_4 + 4CaO \rightarrow 2Ca_5(PO_4)_3OH + 2H_2O$$

from which hydroxyapatite could be obtained by pyrolysis.

The formation of pyrophosphate is revealed by a thermal peak at 1230 °C (CRC Handbook), corresponding to the temperature of the transformation indicated in the pure compound. To prevent the problem of the presence of $CaHPO_4$ in the starting powders, it is sufficient to wash the product many times by shaking at a temperature of 95 °C.

A pyrophosphate in a ceramic for implant use is noxious for two reasons: (1) its moderate toxicity, due to interference with ATP (adenosinetriphosphate) equilibria, and (2) its higher solubility compared to the calcium phosphates, which causes the implanted prosthesis to break up in time. The presence of CaO in the system during firing gives rise to the following reaction:

$$Ca_2P_2O_7 + CaO \rightarrow Ca_3(PO_4)_2$$

The canonical chain of transformation of CPDC reported in the literature is as follows:

$$CaHPO_4 \cdot 2H_2O \xrightarrow{200-260\,^{\circ}C} CaHPO_4 + 2H_2O$$

$$CaHPO_4 \xrightarrow{400-450\,^{\circ}C} \gamma\text{-}Ca_2P_2O_7 \xrightarrow{1200\,^{\circ}C} \beta\text{-}Ca_2P_2O_7 \xrightarrow{1250\,^{\circ}C} \alpha\text{-}Ca_2P_2O_7$$

c. Thermal Transformation of Tricalcium Phosphate. Tricalcium phosphate (TCP), $Ca_3(PO_4)_2$, may occur also at room temperature after its synthesis by the wet process [in polyhydrated form $Ca_3(PO_4)_2 \cdot nH_2O$]. In any case, the only phase existing above a temperature of 680–720 °C is the β-TCP, stable even at room temperature. The TCP canonical transformations are as follows:

$$\beta\text{-}Ca_3(PO_4)_2 \xrightarrow{1290\,^{\circ}C} \alpha\text{-}Ca_3(PO_4)_2 \xrightarrow{1540\,^{\circ}C} \alpha_S\text{-}Ca_3(PO_4)_2$$

The last phase (α_a) differs from the preceding one (α) because it acquires a molecular organization that gives rise to a superstructural lattice. The transformation of the β- into an α-phase does not necessarily appear at the canonical temperature of transformation. In the presence of other phosphates (such as hydroxyapatite) there may occur an allotropic phase α-TCP even at or above 650 °C as a secondary phase in small percentages. It is often assumed that the lower temperature limit at which the α-TCP may occur in a fair quantity is 1125 °C, but according to the current literature such a limit is 1200 °C (Torijama and Kawamura, 1986, 1987). The phase transformation involves a 7.3% decrement in volume of the elementary cell (Bauer and Hohenberger, 1989). The microstructure is therefore subjected to overstressing and cracking. As a parallel example one must remember that the enantiomorphic phase transformation of quartz from β to α at 573 °C is deleterious to the production of porcelains because of the formation of internal stresses with only just a 0.2% volume increase. Table 5.9 gives values of the thermal expansion coefficient of phosphates.

The formation of α-TCP is, of course, extremely deleterious for TCP as well as for hydroxyapatite products also from the point of view of thermal expansion.

Table 5.9. Thermal Expansion Coefficient of TCP and HA

Phosphatic phase	Thermal expansion coefficient
α-TCP	$60.0 \times 10^{-6}\ K^{-1}$
β-TCP	$13.1 \times 10^{-6}\ K^{-1}$
HA	$11.6 \times 10^{-6}\ K^{-1}$

In the presence of calcium oxide, the following reaction can occur:

$$Ca_3(PO_4)_2 + CaO \rightarrow Ca_4O(PO_4)_2$$

d. Thermal Transformation of Octacalcium Phosphate. Octacalcium phosphate (OCP), $Ca_8H_2(PO_4)_6 \cdot 5H_2O$, undergoes a thermal evolution represented by the following canonical chain of reactions:

$$Ca_2H_2(PO_4)_6 \cdot 5H_2O \xrightarrow{200\,^{\circ}C} Ca_8H_2(PO_4)_6 \cdot H_2O$$

$$\xrightarrow{400\,^{\circ}C} 2Ca_5(PO_4)_3OH + \gamma\text{-}Ca_2P_2O_7$$

However, as already explained, the production of pyrophosphate is a negative factor. Therefore the OCP is not a thermally stable compound and it is therefore an unsuitable constituent of a material destined for ceramic bodies.

When this substance occurs, either originally or through formation, it may react with calcium oxide or calcium carbonate (originating from the breaking up of other phosphates) to give rise to the reaction:

$$Ca_8H_2(PO_4)_6 \cdot 5H_2O + CaO \rightarrow 3Ca_3(PO_4)_2 + 6H_2O$$

or

$$Ca_8H_2(PO_4)_6 \cdot 5H_2O + 2CaO \rightarrow 2Ca_5(PO_4)_3OH + 5H_2O$$

e. Thermal Transformation of Hydroxyapatite. Each denomination (TCP, OCP, HA, etc.) refers to a chemical compound with a defined stoichiometric formula. Most of the compounds crystallize and have many crystallization phases. The crystallized phases generally have different names. Sometimes the name used is the chemical one, and a Greek letter is adopted to distinguish the different phases.

Hydroxyapatite is a well-defined chemical compound with formula $Ca_5(PO_4)_3OH$ (though the term apatite, in this case calcium hydroxyapatite, derives from a mineralogical definition). It belongs to a family of homologous compositions, crystallizing in the same spatial group, defined as apatites. The OH^- group can be replaced, for example, by F^- and Cl^-, so that fluorapatite and chlorapatite are obtained, respectively. Also, the cation can be replaced by other bivalent ions (such as Sr^{2+}, Ba^{2+}, Pb^{2+}) to give rise to strontium, barium, and lead hydroxyapatites. All these apatitic compounds crystallize with only one phase, with the specific lattice group $P6_3/m$.

Stoichiometric (calcium) hydroxyapatite is a very stable compound up to 1400 °C. At temperatures over 1200 °C the following reaction can occur:

$$2Ca_5(PO_4)_3OH \rightarrow 3Ca_3(PO_4)_2 + CaO + H_2O$$

particularly if associated with a CaO-consuming one. If calcium oxide is present, the following transformation can take place:

$$2Ca_5(PO_4)_3OH + 2CaO \rightarrow 3Ca_4O(PO_4)_2 + H_2O$$

By combining both equations, the following is obtained:

$$2Ca_5(PO_4)_3OH \rightarrow 2Ca_3(PO_4)_2 + Ca_4O(PO_4)_2 + H_2O$$

The main transformations under consideration are:

- Formation of oxyapatite $[Ca_{10}(PO_4)_6O]$—through condensation of hydroxyapatite, particularly above 1400 °C.
- Of great importance is the transformation that can take place in α-TCP and $Ca_4O(PO_4)_2$ at 1550 °C:

$$2Ca_5(PO_4)_3OH \rightarrow 2Ca_3(PO_4)_2 + Ca_4O(PO_4)_2 + H_2O$$

At 1550 °C, the last reaction is completely shifted to the right side.

There are also other cations and anions which, though unable to reach a complete substitution, may be available for playing a role in the formation of solid solutions confined within the apatitic crystal lattice. As regards the Mg^{2+}, it was ascertained to be a characteristic ion not favoring the apatitic structure (LeGeros, 1991). This ion can be incorporated into synthetic apatites in quantities lower than 0.4%. Similar ions are $P_2O_7^{4-}$, Sn^{2+}, and Al^{3+}, all of which tend to divert the formation of amorphous calcium phosphatic compounds (ACP).

Other ions, such as CO_3^{2-}, may be contained in the apatitic lattice in sufficiently large percentages on condition that Mg^{2+} is not present. A further ion that may occur in sufficiently large percentage proportions is HPO_4^{2-}.

In these cases we deal with the so-called nonstoichiometric hydroxyapatites which are, in reality, different solid solutions belonging to the same large family of isomorphous compounds, better defined by the general term of apatites. If the starting powders are not stoichiometric, the formation of other compounds, such as mainly CaO or amorphous phosphates, is expected.

f. The Apatitic Family and Its Importance in the Biomedical Field. The term hydroxyapatite commonly refers in the biomedical field to calcium hydroxyapatite, the chemical compound with stoichiometric formula $Ca_5(PO_4)_3OH$. The term comes from the mineralogical class of *apatites* to which the crystallized minerals of this compound belong (with the same name).

In many cases an imperfect understanding of the chemistry has produced confusion about the utilized terminology and, in particular, about the meaning of the term hydroxyapatite. This led, for example, to the erroneous concept that there are different calcium hydroxyapatites, as this term was intended to indicate a commercial name and not a chemical compound. Even a large number of experiments, once considered exhaustive, were carried out on numerous nonchemical aspects, but in some cases the results of these studies are improper because no distinction was made between the differences in chemical nature. It frequently happens that different laboratories have used powders of different origin (whether from the market or produced individually), with the result that there is an imperfect correspondence between the obtained data.

Considering all this, it would be more proper to speak of defective apatites, apatites containing substituting ions, or other apatites stable in their own right. In the past, many measurements used to be conducted on samples believed to be identical while in reality they were different in nature. This was due to the difficulty of dealing with a system made up of a myriad of equicomponent compounds existing in an equilibrium relationship to each other, not just individually but more than one at a time. Hence the difficulty of a deliberately systematic study, and also the ease with which they are spoken of in an improper way.

Various arrangement mechanisms are adopted by different ions that try to occupy sites which are more congenial to their requirements in terms of charge, volume, and molecular shape, or specific chemical properties. The greater the number and quantity of species substituting the original groups (bivalent cation, or site C; OH^- group, or site A; PO_4^{3-} group, or site B),

Table 5.10. Main Components that Can Fill the Three Sites of Hydroxyapatite[a]

Site of Ca^{2+} (C)	Site of PO_4^{3-} (B)	Site of OH^- (A)
Ca^{2+}	PO_4^{3-}	OH^-
Sr^{2+}	HPO_4^{2-}	CO_3^{2-}
Ba^{2+}	CO_3^{2-}	F^-
Cd^{2+}	(SiO_4^{2-})	Cl^-
Pb^{2+}	(HCO_3^-)	(S^{2-})
Eu^{2+}	$(P_2O_7^{4-})$	(O^{2-})
(M^+)[b]	(H_2O)	□
(D^{2+})[b]	□	
(T^{3+})[b]		
(Mg^{2+})		
□		

[a] Regular and vicarious ions without parentheses (those unusual and incompatible with the hydroxyapatite lattice in parentheses), □ = empty site or vacancy with no charge.
[b] M = Monovalent ions (Na^+, K^+); D = divalent ions (Fe^{2+}, Mn^{2+}); T = tervalent ions (Al^{3+}, Fe^{3+}, Mn^{3+}).

the more numerous are the possible combinations of solid apatitic solutions. Account must also be taken of sites that must remain empty in order to respect charge neutrality even at short distances. Such sites may involve each of the three original groups. Table 5.10 lists the most common, or regular, ions which can form specific apatitic molecules by filling the three sites. Some other ions are included in the list in parentheses, but they are not typical for the formation of apatitic compounds and can substitute regular ones in their own crystallographic site as vicarious. Classical vicarious substitutions are, e.g. HPO_4^{2-} and CO_3^{2-} for PO_4^{2-}. However, it must be emphasized that, for example, incorporation of CO_3^{2-} is extremely difficult in high-temperature syntheses, while at the same temperatures it is very much possible to incorporate $P_2O_7^{4-}$ groups (e.g., originating from the condensation of HPO_4^{2-}) into the apatitic groups.

5.3.2.3. The Role of Impurities Present in a Hydroxyapatite Powder

Impurities can play an important role during thermal transformation of hydroxyapatite. They can be divided into two categories:

(1) *Ionic impurities.* As previously noted in relation to hydroxyapatite substitutions, some ionic species may penetrate into the lattice and take the

place of each of the three groups: cation (Ca^{2+}), phosphate (PO_4^{3-}), and even hydroxyl (OH^-). Each kind of substitution modifies in a specific way the behavior of the resulting apatite in terms of its chemical and thermal stability. In the thermal evolution, in particular, these ionic impurities may (depending on their nature and quantity) lead to the existence of other phosphatic phases. Some possible cations which substitute Ca^{2+} in its site can be toxic (such as Ba^{2+}, Pb^{2+}), and this has induced authorities to introduce normative regulations and standards of production to prevent particular kinds of contaminants. Other impurities may be Sr^{2+}, Mg^{2+}, alkaline ions, etc., which may even influence—by their nature and quantity—the stability of the phosphates in question.

(2) *Foreign phases.* These may either occur in the starting powders or may develop as a result of thermal decomposition of the different phosphates. The latter aspect is particularly important in regard to thermal decomposition of defective hydroxyapatite. The foreign phases and more stoichiometric hydroxyapatite remain in physicochemical equilibrium between themselves at every temperature.

a. Ionic Impurities. X-ray analysis sometimes shows apatite peaks at a large band. This kind of compound appears to give rise to sudden transformations from 550 °C to 650 °C. Within this range there is a decrease in the crystallinity shown by X-ray, while at a higher temperature separate phases form such as, primarily, hydroxyapatite, TCP (in β- and α-phases), and OCP. In addition, the more different the compositions and physicochemical methods for obtaining the powders, the more variations will there be in the *thermal story* of hydroxyapatite following the disruption of the apatite lattice.

Regarding the behavior of elementary cells, there is seen in the original lattice a general tendency to high volumes, a circumstance which illustrates the difficulty of molecular rearrangement. An increase in thermal mobility brings about a collapse of the lattice, with a resulting decrease in crystallinity also due to the presence of crystallites. This event follows the destruction of the original lattice and prompts the formation of more stable lattices, which in the end leads to the existence of other foreign phases ascertainable by X-ray analysis from 700 °C upward.

Above this temperature, the volume of the elementary cell appears to decrease slowly up to about 1000 °C in relation to a loss of CO_2 and H_2O (if present). At around 1200 °C all the elementary-cell values coincide with and correspond to those considered canonical of stoichiometrically pure hydroxyapatite. The outcome is that a discharge of foreign ions allows the apatitic lattice to optimally rearrange the remaining fraction of atoms. While gaseous ions such as CO_2 and H_2O leave the system, there may still persist some equilibria between the various phases formed. The trend is in fact toward a combination of phases thermodynamically stable at that temperature. This also applies to the equilibria relative to the quantities of existing phases and the equilibria between the lattice defects of one phase and those of other phases.

A report on stoichiometric reactions is complicated, but experience indicates some guidelines:

- If OCP is present, at low temperatures there are reactions of the type:

$$\text{HA (highly defective and low crystalline)} + \text{OCP} \xrightarrow{700\,^\circ\text{C}} \text{HA (crystalline)} + \beta\text{-TCP} + \text{CaO}$$

With stoichiometric hydroxyapatite, a reaction like that leads to:

$$2Ca_5(PO_4)_3OH + Ca_8H_2(PO_4)_6 \cdot 5H_2O \rightarrow 6Ca_3(PO_4)_2 + 7H_2O$$

- At the highest temperatures there are phase equilibrium reactions that lead to a decrease in the lattice defects of hydroxyapatite (especially in the presence of CaO).

It must be stressed that if hydroxyapatite is stoichiometrically free from defects in terms of ionic impurities and free from the consequent defects due to vacancies, it would undergo no thermal transformation, apart from that of condensation to oxyapatite at a temperature of around 1400 °C.

All the transformations undergone by hydroxyapatite and leading to the formation of other compounds do not derive from stoichiometric hydroxyapatite, but from those apatitic/phosphatic compositions whose lattice hosts ions that, by their nature and for their complexity (in terms of distribution of charges, steric reasons, ionic/covalent ratio of the produced bond, etc.), differ from the canonical ones (Ca^{2+}, PO_4^{3-}, OH^-) that they proceed to substitute.

In general, the existence of impurities has some influence not only on thermal stability but also on biocompatibility and biological resorption in *in vivo* implants.

The deposition of a hydroxyapatite layer on the substrate answers two purposes:

1. To preserve the substrate and prevent its contact with physiological fluids.
2. To enable an anchoring to tissue as natural as possible (just like what happens with the introduction of hydroxyapatite in-bulk devices).

Care must be taken to evaluate the kind of porosity and the existing pinholes. These defects may in fact be harmful, because they allow the physiological liquids that are on the outside of the coated prosthesis to come into contact with the substrate. Such a contact can induce corrosion phenomena below the coating layer that are not easy to identify and are more dangerous than corrosion phenomena that might have developed directly on the uncoated substrate. The reason is that such substrate is not under the protection of corrosion or passivation treatments, whose effects were in any case cancelled by the cleaning procedures (etching and sand-blasting) applied to prepare the surface for plasma-spray coating.

b. Foreign Phases. Depending on the method adopted to synthesize the apatitic powder, the powder may or may not be accompanied by other separated phases such as $CaHPO_4$, $Ca_8(H_2PO_4)_6 \cdot 5H_2O$, and $Ca_2P_2O_7$. If present, these phases could be identified by X-ray diffractometry. The mentioned phases do not generally exceed just a few percent units in many commercial products, but are nonetheless noxious because they start a "story of reactions" with hydroxyapatite already at low temperatures (beyond 600 °C) and give rise to compounds in the ceramic body that are sufficiently soluble and consequently compromise in time the mechanical efficiency of an implanted device made with that ceramic.

It must be noted that a hydroxyapatite covering will bring the same biological benefits that would be brought by the introduction of an in-bulk hydroxyapatite ceramic. The use of hydroxyapatite as coating is evidently motivated by the fact that the substrate provides all the desired properties in terms of mechanical benefits. However, the minimum thickness of the deposited and properly evaluated layer should not be less than 70 μm. It was in fact observed that in animal and human implants there was in the phagocytic phase an average layer corrosion of around 40 μm. What was said above is valid provided that the deposited hydroxyapatite is crystalline, a condition ensuring greater physicochemical stability.

It may happen that a number of cells penetrate the porosity, affecting the walls of the ceramic pore. This event on the one hand vitalizes the covering hydroxyapatite layer but may, on the other hand, give rise to localized weakening that might in turn bring about a detachment from the substrate.

5.3.2.4. Transformations Induced at High Temperature by Plasma Spraying

Plasma spray application of hydroxyapatite on the substrate may give rise to a change (at least partial) in the nature of the latter.

The main transformations to be considered in producing a hydroxyapatite ceramic are:

- Presence or possibility of formation of CaO.
- Presence or possibility of formation of TCP whose β-phase undergoes a transformation of great importance in α-TCP at 1290 °C.

Powders must be precalcined to avoid any packing phenomenon. Grains must be rounded, possibly with a spherical shape, and carefully selected.

5.3.2.5. A Survey on Different Methods for Synthesizing Hydroxyapatite

The nature of a hydroxyapatite crystal lattice allows easy replacement of a number of chemical groups with others, endowing the resulting compound characteristics slightly dissimilar to those of the theoretical hydroxyapatite. In a synthesis, it is simpler to obtain partially substituted apatites than stoichiometrically theoretical ones. The required formulation could be achieved through small chemical or operative adjustments of the previously proposed methods.

The quality of the obtained hydroxyapatite is commonly represented by values assumed by the theoretical stoichiometric ratio Ca/P = 3/5 (or $1.\bar{6}$). Regarding the preparation of hydroxyapatite from an operative point of view, we shall discuss the following methods: (1) wet preparation; (2) sol-gel preparation; (3) mechanochemical preparation; (4) dry preparation; (5) preparation of hydroxyapatite as inorganic cement.

a. Wet Preparation. Several methods of hydroxyapatite synthesis from an aqueous solution have been proposed since 1961 (Mooney and Aia, 1961). One of the commonest is under ammoniac-alkaline conditions according to Asada *et al.* (1987):

$$5Ca(NO_3)_2 + 3NH_4H_2PO_4 + 7NH_4OH \rightarrow Ca_5(PO_4)_3OH + 10NH_4NO_3 + 6H_2O$$

This process, however, though very simple, requires not only a great amount of ammonia for the reaction, but also repeated washing with water on the filtered precipitate to try to eliminate any residual of it and of formed NH_4NO_3. An alternative method, the most widely adopted for small-scale productions, is that proposed by Akao *et al.* (1981):

$$5Ca(OH)_2 + 3H_3PO_4 \rightarrow Ca_5(PO_4)_3OH + 9H_2O$$

The above reaction occurs when H_3PO_4 is dropped in a $Ca(OH)_2$ aqueous suspension. Calcium hydroxide is in fact very weakly soluble in water, and consequently the reaction takes place between the PO_4^{3-} ions diffused from the drop plunged into the suspension and the surface of the colloidal particles. The alkaline pH of the aqueous environment, in which hydroxyapatite is stable, is maintained by the complete dissociation of the few dissolved molecules of $Ca(OH)_2$ which is a strong base. The hydroxyapatite-forming reaction is therefore linked to the rate of: (1) diffusion of the ionized phosphatic ionic groups (PO_4^{3-}, HPO_4^{2-}, $H_2PO_4^-$ and H_3PO_4 itself) connected to each other by well-known simultaneous equilibria; (2) dissolution of $Ca(OH)_2$ as well as that of diffusion of Ca^{2+} ions into the aqueous system; and (3) migration of the ionized phosphate groups within the colloidal grains of $Ca(OH)_2$. The success of the transformation depends on the value of the local pH, even if the overall solution may remain alkaline. There develops in fact, all around the plunged drop, an environment resulting from the diffusion of H_3PO_4 molecules and, according to the pH, the resulting ions are prevalently one of the above-cited allowed by the simultaneous equilibria. Therefore layers richer in PO_4^{3-}, or HPO_4^{2-}, or $H_2PO_4^-$, or H_3PO_4 will occur, starting from the periphery to the core of the drop. The hydroxyapatite-forming reaction is also linked to the concentration of OH^- ions, and through the formation of each molecule and the consequent trapping of an OH^- ion for each formed molecule the reaction contributes to a decrease in the local pH. In this way, unless the local pH is adequately checked, there is a risk that may give rise to a combination of residual $Ca(OH)_2$ in the core of the colloidal granules and to a certain quantity of phosphates of varying nature, such as dicalcium phosphate (DCP), tricalcium phosphate (TCP), and octacalcium phosphate (OCP).

Another factor to be considered is the presence of carbonate within the solution for all possible kinds of synthesis. It is in fact possible that CO_3^{2-} ions, even if not deliberately introduced as carbonate of some cation, are present in the solution at equilibrium with the CO_2 of the atmosphere. The dissolved fraction of carbonic acid may replace the anionic component of the calcium compounds and give rise to more stable $CaCO_3$ by operating in an alkaline environment. This is a further component which may be involved in the production of other kinds of phosphates, including the carbonate apatites.

Such a presence of CO_2 can be avoided by promoting a reaction inside a reactor and cause gas not contaminated by CO_2 to gurgle in the solution. All the foreign ions present in the synthesis solution may lead to the formation of molecules different from the hydroxyapatite molecule. These molecules may aggregate (and eventually crystallize in foreign phases), or may induce the formation of other phases and hinder the formation of hydroxyapatite, or may associate in the precipitation of hydroxyapatite crystals and, by co-precipitating, replace one or other of the component groups in their regular group. In this way, for example, HPO_4^{2-} and CO_3^{2-} may replace PO_4^{3-} in its site and CO_3^{2-} may also replace the OH^- group in its site.

If these replacements occur, defective hydroxyapatite is produced in which a number of empty sites are present inside the crystal lattice. Defective hydroxyapatites are always accompanied by lattice vacancies, which allow a rearrangement of the electroneutrality of the overall charge. The behavior during firing of these defective hydroxyapatite may cause alterations to the products, such as the formation by segregation of α- and β-TCP, free CaO, pyrophosphates, etc.

To favor the escape of foreign ions from the hydroxyapatite lattice and at the same time to increase the thickness and the rate of crystallization of synthesised hydroxyapatite, it is essential to allow a digestion of the solution once the synthesis has been completed, after the addition of the last drop which brings about the correct stoichiometric ratio between Ca^{2+} and PO_4^{3-} (in an atomic, or molar, ratio of 5/3).

The digestion consists in maintaining the solution at rest at a temperature of about 37 °C for at least 48 hours. It was ascertained that the highest degree of crystallinity was reached when the solution approached the boiling temperature (about 97 °C).

Another wet method for producing hydroxyapatite is to start from Ca^{2+} *chelate* complex [coming, e.g., from $Ca(NO_3)_2$ or calcium acetate] ions with EDTA (ethylene diamine tetra-acetic acid). This method is generally adopted either to impregnate spongy bodies or clothes with hydroxyapatite or to coat fibrous materials with a hydroxyapatite film.

It consists in placing the body to be impregnated in an aqueous solution based on $(NH_4)_2HPO_4$ with a pH brought to 7.5 thanks to a tris-buffer (trimethyl or triethyl amine). A solution of Ca^{2+} with EDTA is then added to the previous one and the whole is mixed carefully. The strength in forming the complex with Ca^{2+} exerted by EDTA is so great that it prevents the capture of Ca^{2+} from it by the phosphate groups. Therefore, it is impossible to link Ca^{2+} and PO_4^{3-} partners to give rise to a precipitate. When the solution is suitably homogeneous, H_2O_2 at 30 vol% is added. Oxygenated water oxidizes all the molecules of EDTA and thereby makes available the freed Ca^{2+} ions, which can now combine with the phosphate groups to form hydroxyapatite.

b. Sol-Gel Preparation. The sol-gel method, which has attracted attention as a new synthesis method for glass and ceramic materials (Sakka, 1983; Maki and Sakka, 1986), is expected to produce fine granules at high purity at the highest stoichiometric obedience. This method is also pursued to obtain either bulk objects or thin coating films of hydroxyapatite directly without a powdering step (Masuda *et al.*, 1990). Unlike what is commonly believed, the first paper concerning this method is very old, dating back to Ebelmen (1846), so belonging to history.

The procedure starts from molecular precursors dissolved in solutions that, unlike inorganic syntheses obtained by precipitation in aqueous solution, are organic solvents. The main conceptual difference comes just from the nature of such precursors. They are in fact organic molecules that include the inorganic atoms which will react afterward to give rise to the required chemical compound. This association of inorganic and organic parts is commonly called a metal-organic compound.

The name of the procedure originates from the constitution of a metal-organic component containing all the inorganic atoms in the correct stoichiometric proportion as required to obtain the required final inorganic compound, which is at first suspended as a sol solution in the suitable solvent utilized for the organic reaction. This metal-organic component is obtained by a series of organic reactions starting from the precursors, in their turn each containing one of the different inorganic atoms to be associated. With the introduction of a further solvent in which the previous one is soluble, but which does not allow the solvability of the present sol, a flocculation of roundish colloidal gel particles is obtained which precipitate under gravity.

Although apparently different, this particular procedure (taken as a whole) is not substantially different from the common techniques of chemical synthesis already in use in industry, such as precipitation, co-precipitation, thermohydrolysis, hydrothermy, etc. (Livage, 1994). Technologically speaking, the adoption of this method is not easy as the procedures involved are very sensitive to many variables (far more so than with other methods).

Anyway, all the reactions can be described via the same chemical models. The only question is to expand the classical chemical interpretation of acid–base ratios by Arrhenius into the scheme followed by Brönsted and Lowry. The procedure consists in creating required inorganic compounds by a coupling process involving metal-organic components. Such a coupling process is in the first place a polymerization, and subsequently a colloidal condensation of gel micellae.

The polymerization step generally involves condensation coupling. There can be many utilizable precursors: alkoxides, acetates, acethylacetonates, etc. Also, inorganic chemicals can be used provided they are soluble and/or captured by complexating agents in organic solvents. Mixtures of inorganic compounds as well as metal-organic precursors can be used too. All depends on the physicochemical operative conditions, on the ability to provide specific metal-organic precursors, and on the specificity of the required final compound.

The utilization of alkoxides is very popular owing to their easy availability in the market from many international companies. Generally speaking, their synthesis is carried out in various ways (Bradley *et al.*, 1978). The simplest method could be:

$$MCl_n + nROH \rightarrow M(OR)_n + nHCl \tag{1}$$

The chemical reactivity of alkoxides is connected to the impervious arrangement of the molecular structure of the metal-organic complex. This arrangement is conditioned by the inclination of the inorganic atom in a complex to assume a coordination with the largest number of molecules which produce *chelate* complexes, assuming its typical n-fold symmetry fashion. This depends on its external electronic configuration and on the consequent specific hybrid of coordination. However, the number of organic molecules coordinated in giving rise to the metal-organic complex depends not only on the maximum degree of coordination that is possible, but on the overall configuration arrangement induced by the steric situation which occurs in connection with the dimensions and the stereoisometry of the organic molecule that is able to produce *chelate* complexes. Therefore, different complexes having very different molecular structures can be found for the same inorganic atom possessing extremely variable reactivity.

Most alkoxides are extremely reactive compared to nucleophilic compounds:

$$M(OR)_x + yXOH \rightarrow M(OX)_y(OR)_{x-y} + xROH \tag{2}$$

The chemistry of alkoxides applied by the sol-gel method is founded on this equation. Therefore, with a reaction of chemical condensation such as this, new molecular precursors are synthesized and, in their turn, are involved as they are formed, so giving rise to more and more modified molecules having new structural arrangement, chemical complexity, and different steric factors. In this way, during the polymerization a continuous modification of reactivity and functionality of the whole system in reaction is involved. This process of polymerization is consequently modifiable, so allowing intervention to chemically control the structure and morphology of the required final product. Needle-like structures of the final powders come more easily, e.g., from polymerization in linear chains, while microcrystals with axial/basal ratio more prone to unity come more easily, e.g., from polymerization of clusters of multibranched polymers joined to each other.

A controller, or propagation stopper, of polymerization by polycondensation is acetylacetone (CH_3–CO–CH_2–CO–CH_3) which, by formation of a *chelate* complex with its own carbonyl groups the reacting sites of the head of propagation of the reacting polymeric molecules, stops the condensation process and so decreases the possibility of propagation of the polymerization process. The grain size of the powder of the required compound depends on when the condensation process is stopped.

As concerns the sol-gel preparation of hydroxyapatite, a method was recently proposed (Masuda *et al.*, 1990) which starts from calcium diethyloxide, $Ca(OC_2H_5)_2$, and triethylphosphite, $P(OC_2H_5)_3$. The procedure continues by dissolving calcium diethyloxide in ethylene glycol and the triethylphosphite in ethanol. These nonaqueous solvents are carefully dried for 24 hours by molecular sieves before use. This is to avoid the reaction of the metal-organic component with the more acidic molecules of water present inside the solvent before they have been reacted in the useful way. The starting materials are allowed to react with each other in a completely dried N_2 atmosphere (to reach a good result, N_2 must be dried by passing through a molecular sieve column). The ethylene glycol solution of $Ca(OC_2H_5)_2$ is mixed with the ethanol solution of $P(OC_2H_5)_3$ while stirring. When both solutions are well mixed to set the Ca/P molar ratio at 5/3, a mixture of water, ethanol, and acetic acid is in its turn added drop by drop (1 ml/min) always under stirring. The pH value will be maintained in a suitable range to favor gel flocculation and at the same time prevent possible reaction that may lead to a precipitate with a Ca/P ratio different from that theoretically required. In this manner the reagents undergo a number of reactions while the environmental solution changes its nature, favoring the formation of gel precipitates. The whole reactive process starts with the following dehydration of ethylene glycol by calcium diethyloxide:

$$C_2H_4(OH)_2 + Ca(OC_2H_5)_2 \rightarrow CH_3CHO + C_2H_5OH + Ca(C_2H_4O_2) \quad (3)$$

The formed aldehyde is a source of problems. In the first place, it causes an aldolic condensation if the solution is under alkaline conditions:

$$2CH_3CHO \rightarrow CH_3\text{—}\underset{}{\overset{\overset{\displaystyle OH}{|}}{C}H}\text{—}CH_2\text{—}CHO \rightarrow CH_3\text{—}CH{=}CH\text{—}CHO + H_2O \quad (4)$$

At the same time, the triethylphosphite reacts slowly with some of the added water to obtain

$$P(OC_2H_5)_3 + H_2O \rightarrow HPO\text{—}(OC_2H_5)_2 + C_2H_5OH \quad (5)$$

The phosphorylic ester so formed reacts with the aldehyde coming from reaction (3):

$$HPO\text{—}(OC_2H_5)_2 + CH_3CHO \rightarrow HPO(OC_2H_5)CH_2CHO + C_2H_5OH \quad (6)$$

But this reaction is slow, while if $Ca(OC_2H_5)_2$ is present the following faster reaction takes place:

$$HPO\text{—}(OC_2H_5)_2 + CH_3CHO + Ca(OC_2H_5)_2 \rightarrow [HPO(OC_2H_5)CHCHO]_2Ca^{2+}OH^- + C_2H_5OH \quad (7)$$

in which the calcium ion compound undergoes the dissociation

$$[HPO(OC_2H_5)CHCHO]_2Ca^{2+}OH^- \rightarrow HPO(C_2H_5)CH_2CHO + Ca(OH)_2 \quad (8)$$

The calcium ion derivative turns into calcium hydroxyde in the presence of a sufficient amount of water. Both hydroxyl calcium ion derivative $[HPO(OC_2H_5)CHCHO]_2Ca^{2+}OH^-$ and calcium hydrate are substantially all precipitated as gel colloids, while the phosphoric ester is sufficiently soluble. Consequently the required correct stoichiometric proportion is not guaranteed.

To avoid this problem it is necessary to stop the action of aldehyde. An addition of acetic acid yields

$$C_2H_5OH + CH_3COOH \rightarrow CH_3COOC_2H_5 \quad (9)$$

Ethyl acetate ester thus formed underwent an ester condensation in the presence of calcium diethyloxide as calcium source. An alternative insoluble and relatively stable calcium derivative ion is formed:

$$2CH_3COOC_2H_5 + Ca(OC_2H_5)_2 \rightarrow [CH_3COCHCOOC_2H_5]_2Ca^{2+}OH^- + C_2H_5COOH \quad (10)$$

This derivative ion is partially converted to calcium acetate, depending on the pH and the amount of introduced acetic acid:

$$[CH_3COCHCOOC_2H_5]_2Ca^{2+}OH^- + 2CH_3COOH \rightarrow CH_3COCH_2COOC_2H_5 + (CH_3COO)_2Ca \quad (11)$$

On the other hand, triethylphosphite would react with acetate to form phosphoric ester and ethyl acetate:

$$P(OC_2H_5)_3 + CH_3COOH \rightarrow HPO(OC_2H_5)_2 + CH_3COOC_2H_5 \quad (12)$$

A phosphoric-calcium-containing ion derivative is obtained at this point by condensation of the products from reactions (5), (11), and (12):

$$HPO(OC_2H_5)_2 + CH_3COCH_2COOC_2H_5 + Ca(OC_2H_5)_2 \rightarrow [HPO(OC_2H_5)CHCOCH_2COOC_2H_5]_2Ca^{2+}OH^- + C_2H_5OH \quad (13)$$

Since some amounts of phosphorus and calcium remain in the solution as soluble salts or organic compounds, a correct compromise to obtain a good Ca/P ratio of the gel precipitates to produce a high-purity hydroxyapatite is to balance all the existing reactions, both those with and without intervention of acetic acid. Such a compromise is reached when a relatively neutral environment (pH $\sim$ 7.5–8.5) is adopted, with a low concentration of acetic acid and no more than 20% ethanol.

The step that follows is to allow flocculation of the forming gel precipitate, possibly with the aid of a centrifugation process. The obtained gel mass is thus put in Pt crucibles and heated at 900 °C in a kiln, possibly in a flux of air. During firing all the organic part is pyrolyzed, producing CO_2 and H_2O, and the inorganic parts react together in giving rise to hydroxyapatite. Contamination of CO_3^{2-} for PO_4^{3-} can occur in the apatite lattice, depending on the amount of organic part and the rate of air flow. An enrichment of Ca^{2+} can derive from a pH > 8.5, which favors the lattice substitution of carbonate, while low values of the Ca/P ratio can derive from a pH < 6, which leads to formation of some calcium triphosphate.

c. Mechanochemical Preparation. The mechanochemical method consists in subjecting powder mixtures of suitable composition to pressure by the use of grinding media. The reaction to produce hydroxyapatite is (Toriyama *et al.*, 1995, 1996; Krajewski *et al.*, 1995, 1996)

$$3CaHPO_4 + 2CaCO_3 \rightarrow Ca_5(PO_4)_3OH + 2CO_2\uparrow + H_2O\uparrow$$

and can be activated by producing energy in the form of both heating and mechanical work. The reaction is generally promoted in large cylindrical jars filled with ZrO_2 balls of suitable dimensional distribution. Some have observed that Al_2O_3 balls cannot produce sufficient activation of the reaction. The reason for this, apart from any unreliable catalytic influence on the substance constituting the balls, is the higher density of ZrO_2 balls. Such a higher density determines a higher pressure on the powders, especially those lying between the balls and the internal wall of the jar. This means that the equilibrium of the reaction is shifted toward the right, owing to the variation in the pressure of the reaction system. The provision of the obtained product is guaranteed by the outflow of CO_2 and H_2O.

The best conditions were observed when use was made of a jar made from ZrO_2, and the efficiency appeared to increase with increase in the diameter of the jar. This also agrees with the thesis of pressure originating from both gravity and centrifugal forces of the column of balls incident on each point of the internal wall of the jar. On the basis of these observations, a threshold value of pressure will exist which is able to activate the reaction.

The operation consists in placing the powders to be reacted into the jar with a quantity of water ten times the overall weight of the powders. The overall weight of the balls must be at least five times as high as the amount of water. The best grinding conditions appeared to be at 24 hours and 280 rpm for the ZrO_2-based jar and at 48 hours, under the same reaction rate, for jars made from softer materials such as teflon. The hydroxyapatite synthesized in a jar with softer walls was more defective and gave rise in the sintering phase to a considerable TCP fraction which, however, was almost absent in the synthesis performed inside ZrO_2-based jars.

5.3.3. Ceramic and Polymeric Carbons

Polymeric carbons with either ceramic or fibrous structure are utilized in a variety of biomedical applications. The efforts of researchers have focused in particular on the production of two kinds of polymeric carbons: vitreous carbons and carbon-fibers reinforced carbons. Dental implants and heart valves based on vitreous carbons are manufactured. Obviously, their mechanical properties are correlated with the structures of the different varieties of polymeric carbons.

5.3.3.1. Vitreous Carbons

Vitreous carbon is prepared by controlled thermal degradation of some organic polymers, mainly from dehydration pyrolysis of phenol-formaldehyde resins. The properties of the material depend on the heat treatment to which it is subjected (Cowlard and Lewis, 1967). The applicable shaping techniques are those valid in the plastics industry. During firing, gases develop without any breakage of the mass; shrinkage is uniform and isotropic. The low permeability of vitreous carbons is surprising, due to its low density (if compared with other carbons) as well as to the remarkable gas volumes developed during the pyrolysis process which lead to polymerization in long chains of carbon atoms. Vitreous carbon is far more stable than a variety of other carbons or graphites. It should be pointed out that the maximum content of impurities observed in vitreous carbons is only just 200 ppm and these impurities can generally be removed from the starting material. Vitreous carbon is very inert, especially toward oxidation, and it is very stable also toward calcium fluorides, alkaline peroxides, and many acids. Properties of vitreous and pyrolytic carbons are reported in Table 5.11.

Specific performances of elementary carbons were investigated in the past (Benson *et al.*, 1973) for uses in orthopedic, percutaneous, internal, and dental applications. Surgeons have used vitreous carbon for skeletal fixation and in percutaneous interfaces (Mooney *et al.*, 1978). Reportedly, the degree of skeletal attachment is even higher than that of ceramics, though a number of problems may arise when the carbon is subjected to loading stress. Percutaneous electrodes made of vitreous carbon were used (Benson *et al.*, 1973) without any observed biodegeneration. It has, however, been noted (Mooney *et al.*, 1978) that certain current levels can alter the surface morphology of vitreous-carbon electrodes and may give rise to a number of transformations. In the dental field, vitreous carbons have been utilized for intrabone implantations.

Table 5.11. Properties of Vitreous and Pyrolytic Carbons

Properties	Vitreous carbon	Pyrolytic carbon
Density	1.47	1.5–2.2
Permeability (to He gas, cm/s)	$<2.5 \times 10^{-12}$	
Hardness (Knoop)	820	
Flexural strength (MPa)	150–250	50–80
Young's modulus (GPa)	20–28	$2.5–4 \times 10^{3}$
Compression strength (MPa)	690	
Electrical resistance (Ω cm^{1})	$1–5 \times 10^{-3}$	$2–5 \times 10^{-3}$
Thermal conductivity (cal/cm/s)	0.01–0.02	0.01
Thermal expansion coefficient (K^{-1}):		
from 0 °C to 100 °C	2.2×10^{-6}	$4–6 \times 10^{-6}$
from 100 °C to 1000 °C	3.2×10^{-6}	$4–6 \times 10^{6}$
Specific heat (cal/g/K)	0.3	
Max temperature of use (K)	<3270	

5.3.3.2. Carbon-Coated Implants

Experiments carried out on prostheses coated with LTI pyrolytic carbon have lead to tests on interesting new possibilities of application. In particular, some metal prostheses made with titanium alloy (Ti-6Al-4V) were provided with a porous surface (porosity has the advantage of enabling bone ingrowth on the surface in association with bone tissue expansion within the porosity of the substrate). A detectable difference in behavior between samples of only porous titanium alloy and samples of the same kind but coated with pyrolytic carbon was observed in relation to the shear strength at the interface with the ingrown bone tissue. The strength of the coated samples was 27 ± 3 MPa, while that of noncoated ones was 22 ± 3 MPa, a small but significant difference.

5.3.3.3. Pyrolytic Carbons

Thanks to their high resistance, pyrolytic carbons can be regarded as promising materials from a biological point of view. They were originally prepared by cracking-reforming decomposition of hydrocarbon gases and were originally produced for utilization at high temperatures in gas-cooled nuclear reactors. A pyrolytic carbon characterized by high compatibility toward blood and exhibiting a close and extremely adhesive interface with epithelium was also produced.

5.3.3.4. Graphite

Artificial graphite and carbons exhibit different values of absolute and apparent density. These values depend in fact on both the nature of the carbon (as well as, among other things, the degree of graphitization) and the porosity assumed by the manufactured piece, especially if this is obtained through ceramic procedures. Some indicative values are listed in Table 5.12. As far as its use as a biomaterial is concerned, graphite (or heparin-coated graphite) revealed the interesting surface property to be highly thromboresistant. In fact, the GBH (graphite-benzalkonium-heparin) has been applied to a wide number of materials, especially polymers, in order to increase their thromboresistance (FARB).

Properties of colloidal graphite were also investigated (Milligan *et al.*, 1970) in order to understand the surface properties of the material. Such materials have exhibited extremely low superficial load density and dielectric properties, resembling that of animal tissue. Colloidal graphite has uniform porosity and permeability.

Table 5.12. Indicative Values of Density (g cm^{-3})

Graphite (perfect monocrystal)	2.26
Agglomerated artificial graphite	1.5–1.9
Nongraphitized carbon	1.3–1.8
Pyrolytic carbon	2.0–2.25

5.3.3.5. Applications of the Carbons

Carbon-based materials have been regarded as particularly suitable because of their excellent biocompatibility and because they allow a wide range of modification of their physical properties. Carbon reinforced with carbon fibers was utilized to produce the stem of hip endoprostheses, exhibiting good adaptation of elastic properties in contact with bone. The orientation of the fibers and the degree of reinforcement have been evaluated and determined in such a way as to control elasticity all along the stem in order that the relative movement between the prosthetic stem itself and cortical bone may be minimal. Other devices produced with carbon based materials are screws.

However, the main application considered for these materials, dental implants, has not supplied too encouraging results. In fact, notwithstanding histological tests that have shown that implants with null mobility were firmly attached to the bone by direct contact, experiments with carbon implants implanted in mandible produced stresses in the crest area higher than those of alumina implants. Mechanical tests showed a load resistance five to ten times lower in the prostheses than in the natural teeth.

Good results are emerging from carbon fibers coated with pyrolytic graphite, employed to restore ligaments. No breakage was observed in the ligaments and, three months after implantation, there appears regeneration of tissue twice as mechanically resistant as that of natural ligament. The carbon fibers are tightly linked to the cords of the joints and, even after removal, it is very difficult to tear them off. The connection to the tissue appears warranted by the formation all around each single carbon fiber of two to four concentric layers of cells with the formation of a composite structure, called *composite ligament*. Most of these cells are fibroblasts surrounded by the formation of a reticulin matrix and mature collagen structures (Mendes *et al.*, 1987). A great number of patients today have been subjected to implantation of flexible carbon fibers aimed at strengthening the medial, lateral, collateral, and carpo-metacarpal ligaments as well as acromio-clavicular and clavicular joints. It suffices to say that after such interventions, some patients have been able to resume sports activities.

5.3.4. Biological Glasses

5.3.4.1. The Nature of Glass

In dealing with biological glasses, it is necessary to introduce some concepts in order to clarify what is meant by the term *glass*, at least in scientific language. The common definition of glass is based on chemical considerations: *a hard, amorphous, inorganic, usually transparent, brittle substance made by fusing silicates (sometimes borates and phosphates) of alkaline and alkaline-earth atoms and other bivalent* (Pb^{2+}, Zn^{2+}, Sn^{2+}) *or trivalent* (Al^{3+}, La^{3+}) *basic metal oxides, then rapidly cooling to prevent crystallization.* The typical anion is only oxygen. A glass is therefore typically based on silica (SiO_2) as main component and finds many of the usual applications due to its transparency and workability, known since ancient times. It is used to manufacture such common objects as drinking glasses, lenses for spectacles, window-glass sheets, and so on. The definition usually indicates an amorphous state of a siliceous body which, however, shares with crystalline bodies many important macroscopic physical properties, in particular mechanical.

The principal concept brought to mind by the term "glass" is a special state in which the matter is hard, as opposed to the concept of amorphous by which one commonly refers to other kinds of physical properties of substances (powdered, creamy, fatty, gummy, resinous, plastic, and so on). The term "amorphous" really pertains to a substance which is noncrystalline, having neither definite form nor structure, but generally intended to have the ability, in a more or less stable way, to maintain an impressed shape. In a nanometric scale of reference, rather than an ordered arrangement of the atoms (which is typical of a crystalline state), the amorphous state is characterized by the absolute absence of a particular spatial arrangement. In a crystal, the atoms are arranged in a way that responds to symmetrical units of grouped atoms (the so-called repetitive unit) which is repeated indefinitely in all directions (cyclic repetition); packing of the atoms into a crystal can be imagined as infinite reproduction of equal units (long-range symmetry) with formation of a "lattice." In an amorphous state, the atoms are all arranged randomly; there are only molecules joined chemically at specific points which can be imagined to form a "network." In a glass, however, although the long-range repetition is lost, a short-range symmetry remains (up to 2 or 3 shells of surrounding atoms per atom) with respect to the length and angle of chemical bonding between adjacent atoms.

The long-range symmetry can be lost due to small deviations around the correct values of bond lengths and angles associated with a specific compound; superposition of all deviations determines the removal of all possible symmetry at long range. A glass can therefore be regarded as an intermediate situation in the aggregation of matter between a crystalline solid and the liquid state.

The atomic components of a siliceous glass are divided into two main classes: the network formers and the network modifiers. The former give rise to the "skeleton" of the molecules which are able to produce fourfold coordination with formation of tetrahedral symmetry of oxygen atoms (with which they are bonded). The more network-former atoms, the harder the obtained glass. A sequence of tetrahedra produced by network formers is called a *chain*. Chains can be simple (pyroxene), double (when the vertex of every tetrahedron of a chain is in contact with a corresponding flanked chain), planar (or fillosilicatic, when the chains are arranged to form a plane of joined tetrahedra), or three-dimensional (when the chains are arranged so as to form a three-dimensional network of joined tetrahedra). The oxygen which is situated between two adjacent network-former atoms is said to be *bridging*; all other oxygen atoms are *nonbridging*. Network modifiers are those atoms whose presence breaks the length of adjacent tetrahedra chains or join two chains laterally.

The reference glass is amorphous silica, in which there is a three-dimensional network of tetrahedra possessing a Si^{4+} at the center. The substitution of tetrahedra by a trivalent ion like Al^{3+} implies that at least a univalent cation is present to compensate the loss of charge. A univalent cation (such as Na^{+}, K^{+}, etc.) acts as a chain terminator without connections between two chains. Therefore, univalent cations tend not only to shorten the chains but also to isolate them; consequently, the obtained glass will be less hard, very brittle, and low-melting. Bivalent cations (such as Ca^{2+}, Mg^{2+}, Pb^{2+}, etc.), on the other hand, assure a connection between chains, so hardening the glass. Trivalent cations can act as both former and modifier. With the exception of special cases (such as Pb^{2+}), in general almost all modifier atoms assume a sixfold coordination with, in particular, a bipyramidal octahedron coordination geometry. Depending on ionic size, polarizability, charge, bond strength, etc., and amount of each specific atom added into a composition, the physical and physicochemical properties of a glass will change. Each atom introduces its own individuality in imprinting properties to a glass. Linear (direct or inverse) relationships between specific properties (thermal expansion coefficient, hardness, Young's modulus, etc.) and the chemical composition of glasses were found at the end of the 19th century.

The term "glassy material" is equivalent to a particular amorphous state of that material, extended even outside the narrow inorganic field (such as Plexiglas, the tradename of a transparent plastic material made from methylmethacrylate). The related term "vitreous" is commonly used much more in connection with some optical performances of a body, such as translucency, transparency (or opacity), color (obtained generally with addition of oxides of transition elements), etc. Thanks to the random distribution of the molecules, a glassy material exhibits a pure isotropic behavior (e.g., for mechanical properties) not found in crystalline systems, even in the most isometric one (cubic).

However, the term "glassy state" mainly refers to an inorganic hard body in an "amorphous state," of a glass-like physical nature, but not necessarily siliceous. In any case, being amorphous the glassy state is thermodynamically unstable, because this stability is attained for solid bodies only with crystallization. However, generally a glass is far from appearing unstable. Thermodynamic explanations say that this is possible because the material is in effect at an energetic level higher than a stable crystalline state, but it resides in a sufficiently deep potential well; to produce a crystalline state it would need energy to overcome the energetic walls and fall into the field of the crystalline state. It is evident that the amount of energy (thermodynamically speaking) necessary to solve a glassy material is lower than that to solve the same material in its crystalline form. With respect to all possible existing amorphous material, their solidity and viscosity at room temperature increase in parallel to the complexity and weight of the molecules from which they are composed. Therefore, a glassy material is one in which the complex interrelationship among molecules does not allow the creep of the molecular chains either to give rise to their ordered rearrangement to produce a packing into a crystalline lattice, or to give rise to the complete release of free molecules typical of the liquids.

In the light of these considerations, another definition was introduced which considers a *glassy material as a liquid fluid very undercooled, the high viscosity* (η) *of which overcomes a threshold value* of about 10^7–10^8 poises (g/cm/s).

5.3.4.2. Glass in the Biomedical Field

A biological glass is a vitreous composition that, implanted in bone tissue, stimulates its ingrowth. The inducing properties of bone ingrowth from polyphosphates have been known for a long time (Kokubo, 1991). Such substances (in either crystalline or amorphous form) trend to solve rather rapidly when implanted in a tissue and consequently they are not utilizable in practice as biomaterials. Since the 1960s experiments were undertaken to trap phosphatic salts inside a foreign, but more stable, molecular network (Hench and Wilson, 1993; Hench, 1988, 1991). These salts were thus closed in a silicatic molecular trap, obtaining vitreous compositions which allowed a low release of the trapped salts. Some of these compositions exhibited interesting osteoconductive properties. With time, more and more suitable vitreous compositions were proposed.

As opposed to the action of hydroxyapatite ceramics which statically offer the bone tissue an opportunity to join them, biological glasses behave dynamically by reacting at any instant to the physicochemical state of the environment. While the surface of hydroxyapatite remains practically unchanged (in terms of both composition and physical state), biological glasses undergo a chemical transformation of their surface (Hench and Paschall, 1973; Kokubo, 1990a,b; Radin *et al.*, 1997). The transformation originates from a slow exchange of ions between the glass and the physiological liquids surrounding it: the glass releases some kinds of cations (the most mobile, like Ca^{2+}, Mg^{2+}, Na^{+}, K^{+}) while it capture hydrogen ions (H^{+}) from outside (Kim *et al.*, 1989). Glass also leaves to a lesser extent the same cations joined to proper anionic groups, such as phosphates and particularly silicates. The latter form in the neighborhood of the glass surfaces a cloud of colloidal micellae, which contribute in buffering the pH and in trapping proteins and phosphate ions. A complex mechanism is started, the steps of which are listed roughly in Table 5.13.

Obviously much depends on the chemical composition of the glass. All kinds of release must be allowed to the surrounding physiological liquid in a proper manner in due time. The concentration of released ions must not exceed some (above and below) threshold limits, while the values of these limits change with time. The fundamental components required to form these kinds of biological glasses are reported in Table 5.14.

Some other cations can be added to slow down the outlet flux of all different ions from biological glass in the presence of a physiological solution. Some of these are Al^{3+}, La^{3+}, and Ta^{5+}. Their role in the glass is to lock up the molecular network and consequently stiffen it, so further narrowing the existing small intermolecular channels. These channel allow the transit of small ions. The reader must imagine the possibility of transit not due to channels, like pipes, which have a diameter sufficiently larger than the diameter of the moving ions, but rather that (tetrahedral and octahedral) groups of relevant molecules rotate locally a bit (under the influence of charge induction of the advancing ion) just to allow the ion to proceed, restoring their original arrangement it has passed. It goes without saying that the amount of additional such network cations must not exceed some very low threshold limits, beyond which the stiffness of the glass is too high and consequently there is insufficient suitable rotation of molecular groups, so slowing down the possibility of a significant (for the biological interactions) amount of ionic flux until it is completely prevented. Since the bioactivity of these glasses depends strictly on a suitably balanced flux of the cells stimulating ions that flow from the glass surface, it is evident that

Table 5.13. Steps in the Interaction of a Biological Glass with Bone Tissue[a]

Step	Time	Action
1	Some hours	Diffusion toward the biological environment of the main components of the glass (Na^+, Ca^{2+}, silicates and phosphates ions), with exchange of cations of the glass with H^+ coming from the solution. Obviously this phenomenon is connected with the difference in concentration between the two systems in contact, and ionic motion occurs purely by diffusion. This process is probably initiated by the acidic activity of macrophages.
2	Some days	The above exchange causes the glass to undergo a modification for a thickness of up to 300–400 μm, called the degraded layer. This takes place in particular on the surface, where formation of silica gel occurs which results in the development of a 2- to 3-μm-thick layer rich in leached silica. Simultaneously the flow of suitable ions in a suitable amount contributes to stimulate osteoblastic cells to work in favorable conditions and to recognize the biological glass as an already existing suitable partner to be utilized during new bone reconstruction and growth.
3	One week	Release of complex molecules of alkaline silicates which give rise to a colloidal solution in the area surrounding the glass surface.
4	Some weeks	Increment in the degraded layer of the content of elements that do not diffuse (such as Al^{3+}, La^{3+}, Fe^{2+}, etc.). The presence of these ions contributes to impart specific physical properties, in particular the Z-potential, which plays an important role in the next steps (in particular, for the interaction with proteins which could compete with precipitation of salts).
5	Some weeks	Always by diffusion Ca^{2+} and PO_4^{3-} ions begin to shift from physiological liquids toward the interface with development of an initially electrostatic layer that progressively flocculates, like a gel, also aided by the presence of the silica gel particles (sized about 0.2 μm). Such ions diffuse into the degraded layer and their new values of concentration are high on the external side and low (or null) near the junction with the unmodified inner glass side. Phosphate groups comes from adenosintriphosphate of which physiological liquids are rich; Ca^{2+} comes through specific molecular drivers coming from erosion in neighboring parts of the bone (osteocyte erosion) or by systemic transport from blood.
6	Some weeks	The development of crystalline seeds by sedimentation of the interfacial colloid causes calcium phosphates to grow over the interface surface.
7	Two months	With time, when the conditions at the interface are changed (that is, they are no longer colloidal), a crystalline film of hydroxyapatite begins to form as a result of the action of the surrounding slightly alkaline environment.
8	Three months	The presence of large amounts of carbonates may interfere with the process of formation of calcium phosphates giving rise, at the end, to calcium hydroxyapatite.

[a] From L.L. Hench, on the occasion of the Founders Award, Society for Biomaterials 24th Annual meeting, San Diego, CA, April 22–26, 1998.

Table 5.14. Typical Ions for the Formation of Biological Glasses

Ion	Function	Biological role
Si^{4+}	Network former	Silica gel colloids which trap proteins and calcium phosphates
Ca^{2+}	Network modifier	Activator of cellular functions
Mg^{2+}	Network modifier	Activator of cellular functions, antagonistic to those of Ca^{2+}
Na^{+}	Low fluxing, network modifier	Activator of cellular functions
K^{+}	High fluxing, network modifier	Activator of cellular functions, antagonistic to those of Na^{+}
PO_4^{3-}	Low fluxing, network former	Stimulator of cellular functions (only in the first steps)
O^{2-}	Main anion, bridge bonding	
F^{-}	End chain anion	Stimulator of the reconstructive system of the bone

the action of network stiffening ions is depressive in terms of bioactivity until it is completely lost. Moreover, as opposed to La^{3+}, the Al^{3+} also exhibits small toxicity. Consequently, when selecting the type of ions to add in order to stiffen the glass, there is a preference toward La^{3+}, although Al^{3+} is a common classical amphoteric network former, cheaper than all other possible ions (with lower or null toxicity).

5.3.5. Coatings

When a barrier needs to separate a surface from an environment recourse is often made to ceramics. The barrier can serve to avoid chemical corrosion and formation of electrochemical reactions, and to change the physical or biological performance of a surface. There are many possible choices when coating substrates with ceramic materials, depending on the properties to be imparted to the surface. In the biomedical field ceramic coatings are considered for their biological inertia (Al_2O_3, ZrO_2, TiO_2) or for their capability to influence biological activity (hydroxyapatite and biological glasses) or to confer the highest tribological performance to the surface (some carbides and nitrides). Table 5.15 presents possible ceramics for biological coating.

The demand for coated components is increasing, in particular, to:

- face extreme physicochemical environmental situations;
- provide a defence to the support;
- produce a surface as biocompatible as possible, possibly even bioactive;

Table 5.15. Porosity, Grain Clustering, Separation and Bonds that Form between a Titanium Substrate and Various Ceramics Used as Coatings

Ceramic	Porosity	Grain agglomeration clustering	Adhesion to metal support	Sprayed component separation	Notes
ZrO_2	Low	Compact with irregular grains at variable size	Not optimal	White streaking	The separated elements from ZrO_2 act as phase stabilizers
Al_2O_3	Low	Streaked and parallel	Good		
Hydroxyapatite	Pitted microporosity	Amorphous grains with various dimensions and shape	Good	Some possible separation between Ca and P	Cathode luminescence image can indicate transformation in other calcium phosphates
Bioactive glasses					

Table 5.16. Comparison of Mean Indicative Values of Adhesive Shear Strength Obtained by Pushing-in Tests on Cylindrical Specimens Contained in the Sampling of Fresh Femoral Bone Volume Extracted from the Sacrificed Animal (Sheep) after 20 Weeks[a]

	Implanted material						
	Alumina ceramic	HA ceramic	A-W glass ceramics	45S5 Bioglass[b]	45S5F Bioglass[b]	Titanium alloys	AISI 316 L stainless steel
Mean value of the maximum strength of the biological bond with bone (MPa)	0.2	50	20	3.5	2.7	10	0.1
Standard deviation (MPa)	0.1	20	10	3.0	2.2	8	0.1

[a] In the case of hydroxyapatite ceramic, A-W glass ceramics and titanium alloys, some samples were partially porous, which partially reflects on the high standard-deviation value.

[b] The term Bioglass is a trademark of the University of Florida (Gainessville, Fl., USA); this term can be associated only with specific codes corresponding to the biological glasses studied and registered by the University of Florida and cannot be used with other different glass compositions. Therefore, to indicate a glass used in a biomedical field it is necessary to turn to a periphrasis like "biological glass" or "bioactive glass," if really bioactive. The term "Bioglaze®" is also registered for IRTEC-CNR by the authors of this chapter to mean a biological glass utilized to cover metallic or ceramic surfaces of devices for biomedical use; however, its use is free (but with a note which mentions the origin property) as well as that of "biological glass covering."

- provide technical defence;
- provide antiradiant defence;
- provide antifriction defence.

In fact, it must be emphasized that the possible physicochemical actions which can involve the surface of a component are friction, wear and erosion, thermal action, and biological action.

5.4. A Survey on the Adhesion of Ceramics to Bone Tissue

To end this presentation of ceramic material performance for biomedical application, information on the performance of adhesion with tissues is necessary. Various kinds of tests were conducted in many countries around the world using many devices and technologies. It is difficult to give precise values, however an indicative idea on what can be expected from each different material is useful to allow an engineering technician to correctly establish a project for some device. Table 5.16 compares adhesive shear strengths obtained by pushing-in tests carried out following common standards (though not officially accepted in all countries). From Table 5.16 it is possible to deduce that bioactive ceramics (hydroxyapatite and A-W glass ceramics) produce very high adhesion to bone. Also, titanium alloy exhibits quite a significantly high value. In the latter case, however, this is due to the formation on the surface of titanium alloy of a thin layer of rutile (TiO_2), a biologically very compatible compound. Rutile is one polymorph of the titanium oxide which could even be sintered to produce a ceramic, but the mechanical properties exhibited by the obtained ceramic product are poor.

References

Akao, M., Aoki, H., Kat, K., 1981. *J. Mater Sci.* **16**, 809.

Asada, M., Oukami, K., Nakamura, S., Takahashi, K., 1987. *Yogyo Kyokai Shi (The Ceramic Society of Japan)* **95**, 703.

Bauer, G., Hohenberger, G., 1989. Ursachen des unterschiedliches Verhaltens von bioactiven Calciumphosphatkeramiken im Organismus (Causes of behavioral variation of bioactive calcium phosphate ceramics in living organisms), *Ber. Dtsch. Keram. Ges.* **1-2**, 23–27.

Benson, J., Greener, E.H., Lautenschlager, E.P. 1973. *New Biomaterials: Advances in Biomedical Engineering*, pp. 156–159, Academic Press, New York/London/Oxford.

Bradley, D. C., Mehotra, R. C., Gaur, D. P., 1978. *Metal Alkoxides*, Academic Press, London.

Brown, W.E., Chow, L.C., 1981. Thermodynamics of apatite crystal growth and dissolution, *J. Cryst. Growth* **53**, 31–41.

Cowlard, F., Lewis J. 1967. *J. Mater Sci.* **2**, 507–512.

CRC Handbook of Chemistry and Physics, Calcium phosphate B-163.

De Groot, K., 1980. Bioceramic consisting of calcium phosphate salts, *Biomaterials* **1**, 47–50.
Ebelmen, A., 1846. *Compte Rendus de l'Academie des Sciences* **25**, 854.
Gibbons, D., Peckham, P., Martin, R. 1972. *J. Biomed. Mater Res., Symp.* **3**, 155–164.
Hench, L.L., 1988. Bioactive ceramics, in: *Bioceramics: Material Characteristics versus In Vivo Behavior* (P. Ducheyne, J.E. Lemons, eds.), p. 54, New York Academy of Sciences, New York.
Hench, L.L., 1991. Bioceramics: from concept to clinic, *J. Amer. Ceram. Soc.* **74**(7), 1487.
Hench, L.L., Paschall, H. A., 1973. Direct chemical bonding between bioactive glass-ceramic materials and bone, *J. Biomed. Mat. Res. Symp.* **4**, 25–42.
Hench, L.L., Wilson, J., 1993. *An Introduction to Bioceramics*, World Scientific Publ. Co., New York/London/Singapore.
Jarcho, M., 1989. The future of hydroxyapatite ceramics, in *Bioceramics 1*, Vol. 1, p. 57 (H. Oonishi, H. Aoki, K. Saway, eds.) Shiyaku-EuroAmerica Inc., Tokyo–Sant Louis.
Kim, C.Y., Clark, A.E., Hench, L.L., 1989. Early stages of calcium phosphate layer formation in bioglasses, *J. Non-Cryst. Solids* **113**, 195.
Kokubo, T., 1990a. Bonding mechanisms of bioactive glass-ceramic A-W to living bone, in: *Handbook of Bioactive Ceramics*, Vol. 1 (T. Yemerson, L.L. Hench, J. Wilson, eds.), p. 41–50, CRC Press, Boca Raton.
Kokubo, T., 1990b. Surface chemistry of bioactive glass-ceramics, *J. Non-Cryst. Solids* **120**, 138.
Kokubo, T., 1991. Bioactive glass ceramics: properties and applications, *Biomaterials* **12**, 155–163.
Krajewski, A., Ravaglioli, A., Celotti, G., Piancastelli, A., 1995. Characterization and annealing of wet prepared synthetic hydroxyapatite powders for high purity bioceramics, *Cryst. Res. Technol.* **30** (6), 843–852
Krajewski, A., Celotti, G., Ravaglioli, A., Toriyama, M., 1996. Spectrometric study of the thermal evolution of mechanochemically prepared hydroxyapatite-based powders, *Cryst. Res. Technol.* **31** (5), 637–646.
Lai, W., Ducheyne, P., Garino, J., 1999. Removal pathway of silicon released from bioactive glass granules in vivo, in: *Bioceramics*, Vol. 11 (R.Z. LeGeros, L. LeGeros, eds.), World Scientific Publishing Co., Singapore.
LeGeros, R.Z., 1991. Calcium phosphates in oral biology and medicine, in: *Monographs in Oral Science* (H.M. Myers, ed.), Karger Publ. A.G., Zürich.
Livage, J., 1994. *Mater. Tech.* (6–7) 23–27.
Maki, T., Sakka, S., 1986. *J. Mater Sci. Lett.* **5**, 28–30
Masuda, Y., Matubara, K., Sakka, S., 1990. *J. Ceram. Soc. Japan, Int. Ed.* **98**, 84–95.
Mendes, D.G., Roffman, M., Soundry, M.P. et al. 1987. Composite ligaments made of carbon fibre braid: biomaterials and clinical applications, in: *Biomaterials and Clinical Application: Advances in Biomaterials*, Vol. 7 (P.G. Marchetti, A. Ravaglioli, A.J.C. Lee, eds.), pp. 241–246, Elsevier Publishing B.V., Amsterdam.
Milligan, H., Davis, J., Edmark, K. 1970. *J. Biomed. Mater Res.* **4**, 121–138.
Mooney, R. W., Aia, M. A., 1961. *Chem. Rev.* **61**, 434.
Mooney, V., Hepenstall, M., Knapp, W., 1978. Direct skeletal attachment of an artificial limb, in: *Use of Ceramics in Surgical Implants* (S.F. Hulbert, F.A. Young, eds.), p. 115, Gordon and Breach Science Publ., London.
Osborn, J.F. 1985. *Implantatwerkstoff hydroxylapatitikeramik grundlagen*, Kliniske Anwendung Quintessenz, Springer-Verlag A.G., Berlin.
Radin, S., Ducheyne, P., Rothman, B., Conti, A., 1997. The effect of in vitro modelling conditions of the surface reactions on bioactive glass, *J. Biomed. Mat. Res.* **37**, 363.
Sakka, S., 1983. *Bull. Inst. Chem. Res., Kyoto Univ.* **61**, 376–396.
Torijama, M., Kawamura, S., 1986. *Yogyo-Kyokai-Shi (The Ceramic Society of Japan)* **94**, 1004–1008.

Torijama, M., Kawamura, S., 1987. Sinterable powder of mechanochemically synthetic β-tricalcium phosphate, *J. Ceram. Soc. Japan, Int. Ed.* **95**, 698–702.

Toriyama, M., Ravaglioli, A., Krajewski, A., Galassi, C., Roncari, E., Piancastelli, A., 1995. Slip casting of mechanochemically synthesized hydroxyapatite, *J. Mater Sci.* **30**, 3216–3221.

Toriyama, M., Ravaglioli, A., Krajewski, A., Celotti, G., Piancastelli, A., 1996. Synthesis of hydroxyapatite-based powders by mechanochemical method and their sintering, *J. Eur. Ceram. Soc.* **16**, 429–436.

6

Metallic Materials

Alberto Cigada, Roberto Chiesa, Maria Rosa Pinasco, and Kunihiro Hisatsune

6.1. The Crystalline Structure of Metallic Materials

Except for mercury, all other metals at room temperature are in a solid state. Under this condition atoms are arranged in space in a regular pattern forming in this way a three-dimensional structure, which is ordered and repeated, and is called a crystalline lattice.

In metallic materials the nuclei of atoms occupy the points of a crystalline lattice: the inner-shell electrons remain bonded to the nuclei while the electrons of the outer shell can easily move among the atoms of the crystalline lattice, forming the so-called electron cloud.

The bond between atoms (metallic bond) results from the electrostatic interaction of the nuclei with the electronic cloud. This type of bond determines the properties of this class of materials. On the one hand, the metallic bond is strong (e.g., stronger than the one that can bond different molecules together) and this determines the high mechanical properties of the metals. On the other hand, the ease of motion of the electrons among atoms of the crystalline lattice produces the electrical and thermal conductivity typical of the metals.

The metallic bond is produced by electrostatic attraction forces so it is adirectional (e.g., opposite to the covalent one). Therefore, the only factor that leads to the formation of a certain type of lattice rather than another type is the ability to fill the space. Consequently, metals will assume a

---

Alberto Cigada and Roberto Chiesa • Dipartimento di Chimica Fisica Applicata, Politecnico di Milano, via Mancinelli 7, 20131 Milano, Italy. **Maria Rosa Pinasco** • Dipartimento di Chimica e Chimica Industriale, Università degli Studi di Genova, via Dodecaneso 31, 16146 Genova, Italy. **Kunihiro Hisatsune** • Department of Dental Materials Science, Nagasaki University School of Dentistry, Nagasaki 852, Japan.

Integrated Biomaterials Science, edited by R. Barbucci. Kluwer Academic/Plenum Publishers, New York, 2002.

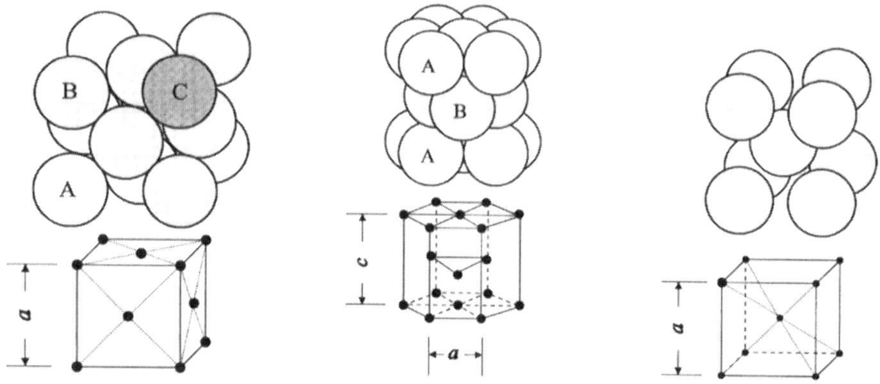

Figure 6.1. Crystal structures: (a) fcc, (b) hcp, (c) bcc.

compact crystalline structure, filling the available space with atoms as much as possible.

There are only 14 different ways to build a repeating lattice in the space, the so-called Bravais lattices. As a result of the special characteristics of the metallic bond, metallic materials may assume the structure corresponding to only 3 of the 14 possible Bravais lattices: the face-centered cubic (fcc) shown in Figure 6.1a, the hexagonal close-packed (hcp) shown in Figure 6.1b and the body-centered cubic (bcc) shown in Figure 6.1c.

Some metals may change their crystalline structure with temperature (allotropic transformations); for instance, iron at room temperature exhibits bcc structure which turns into fcc at 911 °C, bcc again at 1392 °C, before melting at 1536 °C. In the same way, titanium at room temperature has a hcp structure, turning into bcc at 882 °C before melting at 1670 °C.

6.2. Lattice Defects

The real structure of metals and alloys does not form a perfect monocrystal; defects of various type are present. They can be: localized in an extremely reduced zone of the crystal involving a very low number of atoms (in this case they are called point defects); of higher extension identified as line defects (called dislocations); planar defects (e.g., grain boundaries, stacking defects, twin boundaries, etc.). The main types of defects and their influence on the materials' properties will now be briefly examined.

6.2.1. Point Defects and Solid State Diffusion

Point defects consist of:

- Vacancies: reticular positions free from any atoms (Figure 6.2a).
- Self-interstitial atoms: atoms of the metal which do not occupy a normal lattice position (Figure 6.2b).

Solid state diffusion is the most important phenomenon of metallurgical interest in the context of point defects. It is connected to the fact that atoms in a crystal oscillate around their equilibrium position. These oscillations become so wide as to allow an atom to pass from a reticular position to another, so resulting in solid state diffusion.

The presence of point defects (vacancies in particular) makes diffusion processes easier, and in the absence of these defects those processes would never occur, at least at a low temperature.

6.2.2. Linear Defects and Plastic Deformation

When a crystalline structure, such as a metallic material, is subjected to a stress, it deforms. Deformation appears as a lattice distortion with a coordinate shift of the atoms when the stress is smaller than a certain value (called the elastic limit) and without any alteration of the crystalline structure. This deformation is of an elastic type. This means that when the stress is removed, the atoms retrieve their original position to eliminate the strain.

If the stress applied is higher than the elastic limit, a plastic deformation occurs on the material. When the stress is removed, only the elastic part of the strain remains; the material maintains an irrecoverable permanent deformation.

The presence of a permanent deformation is justified with relative slip of atoms in the crystal, or, more correctly, of a part of the crystal with

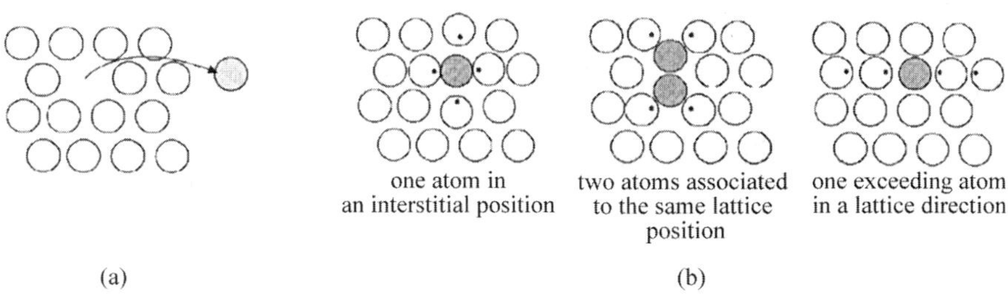

Figure 6.2. Point crystal imperfections: (a) lattice vacancies, (b) self-interstitial atoms.

respect to another (in the direction of well-determined crystalline planes). This deformation property is typical of metallic materials; it is, however, absent in ceramic ones, which also have a crystalline structure.

For metallic materials, the stress needed to obtain a plastic deformation is remarkably inferior than the calculated value according to the hypothesis of an ideal crystal, i.e., a defect-free one; a metallic crystal is more likely to be deformed than what one would expect.

It is now necessary to introduce the concept of dislocation, in order to understand why this happens. Dislocations are defined as defects present in crystals. They are composed of series of atoms placed at points not corresponding to their exact reticular positions. Two types of dislocations are known: edge dislocations (Figure 6.3a) and screw dislocations (Figure 6.3b). In real crystals, dislocations frequently show a mixed feature, i.e., they are partly edge and partly screw dislocations.

If dislocations did not exist, it would be necessary for a full atomic plane to slide on the adjacent one in order to deform a crystal. This would imply that at a certain instant a great number of bonds are simultaneously broken (to be formed again after the displacement of one or more reticular units), however calling for a much higher stress.

If, alternatively, dislocations are present in the crystal, strain will take place with a gradual slip of the dislocation inside the crystal (Figure 6.4). Strain slip involves the breaking of a reduced amount of atomic bonds (and their subsequent reformation in a different position), so calling for a much lower stress.

The effect of dislocations on the properties of metallic materials is strongly conditioned by two phenomena with opposed effects: work hardening and recrystallization.

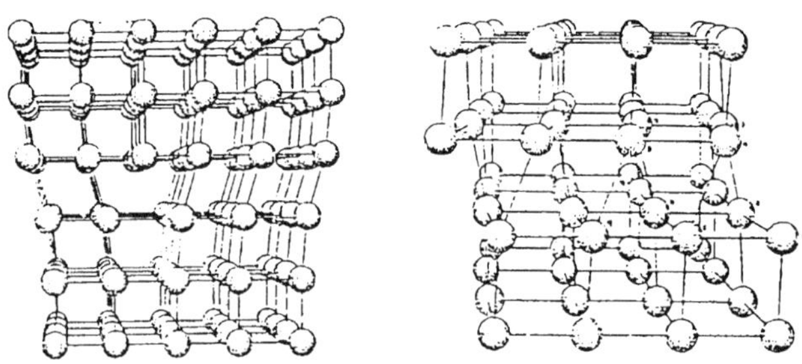

(a) edge dislocations (b) screw dislocations

Figure 6.3. (a) Edge and (b) screw dislocations.

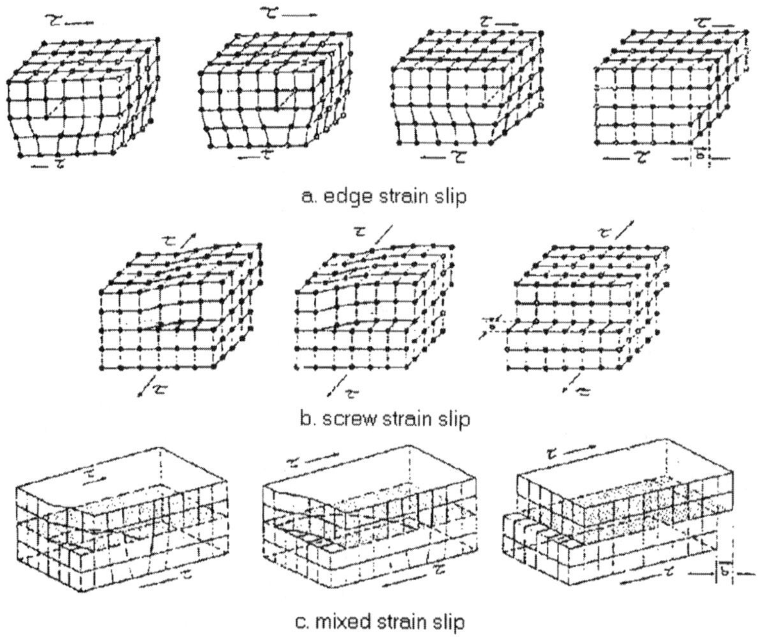

Figure 6.4. Slip between two lattice planes by the movement of a dislocation: (a) slip by the movement of an edge dislocation, (b) slip by the movement of screw dislocation, (c) slip by the movement of composite dislocations.

a. Work Hardening. In a crystalline lattice subjected to strain, the following phenomena occur:

- As the material gets more and more strained, the present dislocations grow correspondingly in number.
- During the sliding, the dislocations interact reciprocally, becoming less movable, and they tend to accumulate against obstacles inside the material (grain boundaries, inclusions).
- Both these phenomena (increase in the number of dislocations and their interaction) tend to make the dislocations less movable.
- Consequently, the stress necessary to determine a new strain increases, and therefore the mechanical properties of the material increases.
- This phenomenon is called work hardening.

b. Recrystallization. The condition of an imperfect crystalline lattice (owing to the presence of dislocations or grain boundaries) is characterized by a higher internal energy compared to a monocrystal, therefore it is thermodynamically unstable, and tends to evolve toward a condition of lower internal energy, i.e., with less defects. However, this evolution is possible only if the temperature is high enough to allow the movement of atoms which are necessary to diminish defectiveness.

Therefore, at a high temperature, the phenomenon of the rearrangement of the atomic position in the crystalline lattice occurs on metallic materials, defined as recrystallization. On the one hand, they reduce the number of dislocations and, on the other hand, as shown further, they determine a dimensional increase of some crystalline grains to the detriment of others.

c. Effect of the Plastic Deformation Temperature on Dislocations. If a metallic material is subjected to a high-temperature plastic strain (hot plastic deformation), there is a creation and movement of dislocations subject, however, to recrystallization, so in practice there is no hardening in the material. Consequently, hot plastic deformation is to be realized in a relatively simple way on metallic materials. In fact, on the one hand high temperature increases the deformability of the material while, on the other, work hardening does not occur. This would make the material less prone to further strain.

If, vice versa, plastic strain is realized at room temperature (cold plastic deformation), the dislocations that are being formed are permanent, so the material progressively work hardens. This increases its mechanical properties, but at the same time makes plastic strain more and more difficult.

6.2.3. Surface Defects and Grain Boundaries

A commercial metallic material is never composed of a single crystal but of many small crystals called grains, each one consisting of a crystal lattice with different orientation than the adjacent lattice.

One can intuitively understand why this could happen by hypothesizing that (Figure 6.5) during solidification of a molten metal, various randomly oriented solidification nuclei could begin to form more or less simultaneously. They then grow till complete solidification of the metal, hindering one another, and forming in this way grains with different crystallographic orientation.

Should bonds not exist among randomly oriented crystals, we could be in the presence of a material with low mechanical resistance (since the various bonds would tend to detach one another). However, the truth is that these bonds exist and are connected to surface defects called grain boundaries.

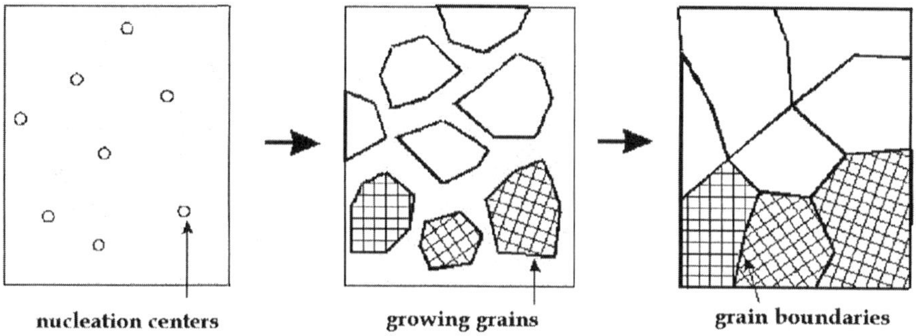

Figure 6.5. Formation of a polycrystalline structure.

At room (or not high) temperatures, grain boundaries are generally stronger than the core of the grain itself. Therefore, under high loads the material tends to fracture in the direction of surfaces which cross the grains and are not situated along the boundaries. This is called transcrystalline or transgranular fracture.

At high temperatures, the grain boundary is weaker than the core and the fracture spreads along the surfaces separating the grains. This is called intercrystalline or intergranular fracture.

As a consequence, it is possible to understand how, for example, one can improve the mechanical properties of a metallic object subjected to static charge, by reducing the mean dimension of the grain as much as possible if the object is to be operated at low temperatures. On the other hand, it would be advisable to increase the mean dimension of the grain if it works at high temperature.

A metallic structure is defined as fine, intermediate, and rough if the mean dimension of the grain is, respectively, about 0.4, 4, and 40 μm.

6.2.4. Effect of Plastic Deformation Temperature on Grain Size

Besides the creation and movement of the dislocations, plastic deformation on a metallic material also determines the breakage of crystal grains and consequently leads to a diminution of the grain size.

However, if deformation is realized at a high temperature (or if the material is maintained for a long time at a high temperature), recrystallization also takes place (as seen earlier) and determines the increase in the size of some grains to the detriment of others. Therefore, only cold plastic deformation (or a controlled temperature deformation) yields a diminution of the grain dimension.

6.3. Structure of Metallic Alloys

It has been seen how a pure metal could assume a structure formed by different grains in a single type of crystal lattice. The situation is more complex when in the presence of a metallic alloy formed by two or more metals (or also nonmetallic elements, such as carbon and hydrogen). We shall examine how two or more different metals coexist in a single crystal lattice, or vice versa form simultaneously two or more crystal lattices. This is possible thanks to the formation of interstitial and substitutional solid solutions or also intermetallic phases.

6.3.1. Interstitial Solid Solutions

The metal present in a higher quantity is defined as solvent, and as solute when it is present in a lesser quantity. Interstitial solid solutions are formed when solute atoms are small enough to occupy the empty space among the solvent atoms in their crystal lattice (Figure 6.6a).

The metallic structures are generally compact, so the dimension of the interstitial spaces are very small compared to the metal atom diameter. Therefore, only elements with quite small dimensions, such as carbon, hydrogen, and boron, give rise to interstitial solid solutions. Moreover, there exists a maximum number of solute atoms that place themselves in an interstitial position among the solvent atoms.

6.3.2. Substitutional Solid Solutions

In substitutional solid solutions, solute atoms replace the solvent ones inside its lattice, as shown schematically in Figure 6.6b, where an ordered (less frequent) and a disordered substitutional solid solution are shown.

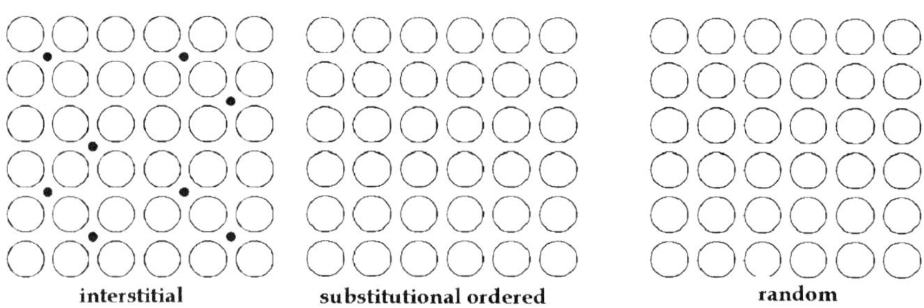

Figure 6.6. Solid solution: (a) (interstitial), (b) substitutional (ordered), substitutional (random).

Although the crystal structure remains unaltered, the dimension of a unit cell changes progressively with solute addition. However, these dimensional variations do not exceed a certain value.

Only few pairs of metals that are very similar to one another (as, for example, copper and nickel, or gold and silver) have complete solid solubility (i.e., all solvent atoms can be progressively substituted by solute atoms with no change in the crystal structure). In most cases the maximum solubility of solute in solvent (and vice versa) is limited.

6.3.3. Intermetallic Phases

Intermediate phases, also called intermetallic phases, are formed by crystal lattices different from those of the pure elements and characterized by particular ratios, but they are generally restricted to the two constituting elements. A typical example of an intermediate phase is iron carbide Fe_3C with complex orthorhombic crystalline lattice formed by a carbon atom every three iron atoms (weight ratio 6.67%).

6.3.4. Presence of More Phases

When a second alloying element is added to a pure metal in an amount higher than the maximum solubility in the solid state (substitutional or interstitial), and not exactly corresponding to an intermediate phase, the alloy in the solid state will not be constituted of a single type of crystal lattice (phase) but will be composed by at least two crystal lattices (two phases). A phase diagram is employed to study these phenomena.

6.4. Phase Diagrams

Phase diagrams are used for a graphic representation of equilibrium conditions. They allow one to know at any temperature which phases are present in a given metallic alloy.

6.4.1. Phase

A phase is a homogeneous portion of a heterogeneous physicochemical system. In practice, in a metallic alloy, the portions of the alloy (that can be a substitutional or interstitial solid solution, or intermediate phases) characterized by a well-defined crystal lattice are called phases.

6.4.2. Variance and Phase Rule

Specified independent variables which define unambiguously the state of the system are called the degrees of freedom.

The variance of a system is the maximum number of degrees of freedom, i.e., the number of variables that can be changed, independently of the others, without changing the number of phases present in the system.

The phase rule applied to a metallurgical system states that the number of degrees of freedom (F) is equal to the number of components (C) present in the system (2 in a binary metallic alloy, 3 in a ternary one, etc.), plus the number of the physical variables acting on the system (generally 2, temperature and pressure), minus the number of phases present (P), i.e.,

$$F = C + 2 - P$$

If we study only binary diagrams, $C = 2$. Metallurgical systems generally work at atmospheric pressure and therefore the pressure variable can be neglected (in practice, the degree of freedom neglected is to be used to impose a pressure equal to 1 atm). We can then express the phase rule for binary metallurgical diagrams as

$$F = 2 + 1 - P$$

6.4.3. Graphic Representation of Binary Phase Diagrams

The phase diagram of a binary alloy A-B is represented (neglecting the pressure) by a flat representation, where the vertical axis reports the temperature (the only acting physical variable) and the abscissa reports the chemical composition, the latter to be expressed as a weight percentage of B (the quantity value to be used later), the mole fraction of B or atomic percentage of B (obviously A% = 100 − B%).

If, for every chemical composition and every temperature value, a complete representation of the phases is made, a corresponding phase diagram will result. In practice, for every temperature and chemical composition of the alloys, it allows one to evaluate:

- the phases present (1, 2, or 3 in a transient situation),
- their chemical composition,
- the relevant quantity for each phase.

In the graphic representation of a given alloy under investigation, an empty

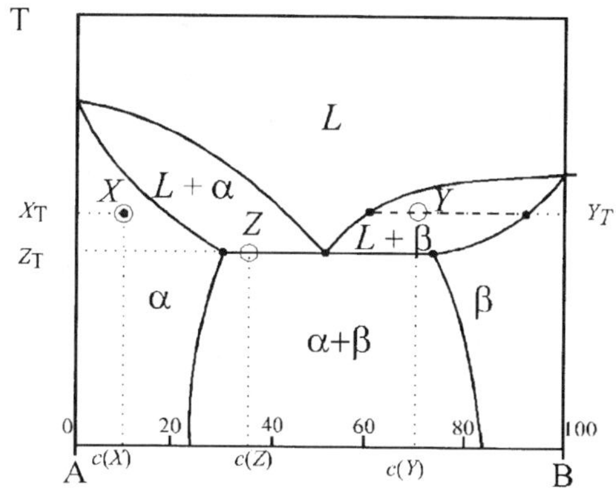

Figure 6.7. Phase diagram with the presence of an eutectic reaction.

circle will be used later to define the mean chemical composition of the alloy under investigation at a given temperature, and a filled dot to define the chemical composition of every phase present (the only ones with a real physicochemical meaning).

As an example, a phase diagram between two metals A and B, with limited solid solubility, is reported in Figure 6.7. It is possible to isolate the regions of existence of the liquid phase L, of the solid solutions α and β, and also the two-phase regions $L + \alpha$, $L + \beta$, and $\alpha + \beta$. The presence of one, two, or three phases is examined separately below.

6.4.4. Presence of One Phase

Let us consider, for instance, in Figure 6.7 an alloy with composition $c_{(x)} = 10\%B$ (i.e., 90%A–10%B at a temperature X_T represented by the empty circle X, falling in the region of the phase α.

The degrees of freedom are 2 ($F = 2 + 1 - P = 2 + 1 - 1 = 2$), so both the temperature and chemical composition of the alloy can be independently changed or chosen. In this case, the empty circle corresponding to the mean composition and the filled one corresponding to the real situation coincide.

The phase situation is as follows:

phase present:	α
composition of phase:	$C = c_{(x)} = 10\%B$
amount of phase:	100%

6.4.5. Presence of Two Phases and the Lever Rule

Let us consider in Figure 6.7 an alloy with composition $c_{(y)} = 70\%B$ (i.e., 70%A–30%B) at a temperature Y_T represented by the empty circle Y; the phase diagram indicates that we are in the two-phase region $L + \beta$.

If two phases are present, the degrees of freedom are

$$1\ (F = 2 + 1 - P = 2 + 1 - 2 = 1)$$

By fixing the temperature of the alloy (Y_T in this case), the chemical composition of the two phases present is imposed and does not coincide with the one we chose.

These compositions are found by tracing across Y a horizontal line until it meets the region of the phases L and β, and indicates the respective intersections with two filled circles representing the phases actually present. The related chemical compositions will be read on the abscissa axis (respectively the values 60%B and 90%B).

We can also calculate the amount of the two phases L and β with the lever rule. On the basis of this rule, the quantity of any phase at every temperature is inversely proportional to the segment connecting the filled circles (which represent the phases) with an empty one (denoting the mean chemical composition of the alloy). If we indicate by a the segment connecting the filled circle in the region of the phase L with the empty circle Y, and by b the line connecting the empty circle Y with the filled point placed on the region of phase β, the (weight) percentages of L and β can be calculated as follows:

$$\%L : \%\beta = b : a$$

This can also be written as

$$\%L : (\%L + \%\beta) = b : (b + a)$$

that is

$$\%L = [b/(a + b)] \cdot 100$$

In practice, %L is equal to the length of the opposite lever arm (b), divided by the full length of the lever ($a + b$), multiplied by 100.

The length of the lines a and b can be measured in any unit. To this end it is convenient to use the abscissa axis itself, it being a graduated scale. Therefore

$$\%L = [(90 - 70)/(90 - 60)] \cdot 100 = (20/30) \cdot 100 \approx 66.6\%$$

In the same way

$$\%\beta = [a/(a + b)] \cdot 100 \quad (\text{or} = 100 - \%\text{L})$$

that is

$$\%\beta = [(90 - 80)/(90 - 60)] \cdot 100 = (10/30) \cdot 100 \approx 33.3\%$$

The phase situation in the case just considered is therefore as follows:

phases present	L	β
composition of phases	C = 60%B	C = 90%B
amount of phases	$[b/(a+b)]\cdot 100$ (=66.6%)	$[a/(a+b)]\cdot 100$ (=33.3%)

6.4.6. Presence of Three Phases

Finally, let us consider in Figure 6.7 the case of an alloy with composition $C_{(Z)} = 35\%$B (that is, 65%A–35%B) at a temperature of 723 °C. This corresponds exactly to a horizontal line present in the phase diagram represented by the empty circle Z.

In this case, three phases are present at the same time, namely α, L, and β, whose composition is represented by the points at which the region touches the horizontal line described here with composition 30%B, 55%B, and 75%B.

If three phases are present, the degrees of freedom are

$$0 \ (F = 2 + 1 - P = 2 + 1 - 3 = 0)$$

Before the disappearance of one of the three phases it is not possible to modify a parameter, in particular the temperature. It is a transient situation, where it is meaningless to define the related percentage of the three phases as they are in evolution. The phase analysis is:

phases present:	α	L	β
composition of phases:	C = 30%B	C = 55%B	C = 75%B
amount of phases:	evolving	evolving	evolving

6.4.7. Iron–Carbon Phase Diagram

The application of iron alloys (steel and cast iron) is of great importance. Therefore, the study of the Fe–C phase diagram is of particular interest as it allows us to know the equilibrium structures for the various alloys as a function of carbon content and temperature.

Only the region of the diagram with carbon content lower than 6.67% (corresponding to the intermetallic phase iron carbide Fe_3C) will be described. Systems with a richer carbon content have no metallurgical meaning at all.

The Fe–C phase diagram is shown in Figure 6.8. The following phases are present:

- Liquid phase L.
- Fe-δ, Fe-γ, and Fe-α: they correspond to the allotropic forms of iron. Fe-δ and Fe-α have bcc structures, with very low interstitial solubility of carbon (maximum 0.1%), while Fe-γ has a fcc structure, characterized by high interstitial solubility of carbon (maximum 2.06%).
- Fe_3C phase (iron carbide); it is the intermediate phase formed by iron with a carbon content of 6.67%.

The most interesting part in the diagram is that with carbon content till 2.06%, corresponding to the steel region, while the part from 2.06% to 6.67% C corresponds to cast iron.

Consider a steel with carbon content of 0.4% at 900 °C. It is in a monophasic region corresponding to the only presence of Fe-γ with fcc

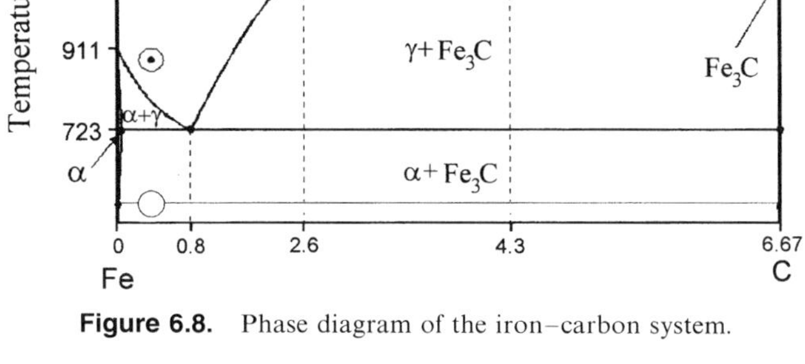

Figure 6.8. Phase diagram of the iron–carbon system.

structure (called also austenite). If this steel is slowly cooled till room temperature, it enters into a two-phase region constituted by Fe-α with bcc structure (ferrite) and iron carbide Fe_3C (cementite).

Consequently, at a high temperature, steel with carbon content 0.4% presents an austenitic structure that maintains inside all the carbon. After cooling it turns into ferrite (almost free of carbon) and cementite (carbon-rich).

6.4.8. Iron–Nickel and Iron–Chromium Diagrams

A study about the effect of nickel and chromium addition on allotropic transformations in iron (Fe-$\alpha \rightarrow$ Fe-γ and Fe-$\gamma \rightarrow$ Fe-δ) is very interesting. The iron–nickel phase diagram is shown in Figure 6.9a. Note that Ni tends to enlarge the region of Fe-γ.

In particular, it can be observed how for a certain Ni content (higher than 15–20%) the transformation Fe-$\alpha \rightarrow$ Fe-γ occurs at a temperature lower than room temperature, so it is possible that a steel containing nickel exhibits an austenitic structure (fcc) at room temperature.

The iron–chromium phase diagram is shown in Figure 6.9b. Chromium addition restrains the Fe-γ region, so beyond 13%Cr the Fe-$\alpha \rightarrow$ Fe-γ transformation no longer occurs, and the Fe-α region is joined with the Fe-δ one, so a steel containing chromium can exhibit a ferritic structure (bcc) from solidification to room temperature.

6.4.9. Titanium–Aluminum and Titanium–Vanadium Diagrams

Titanium–aluminum and titanium–vanadium phase diagrams are reported in Figure 6.10. Titanium presents an allotropic transformation

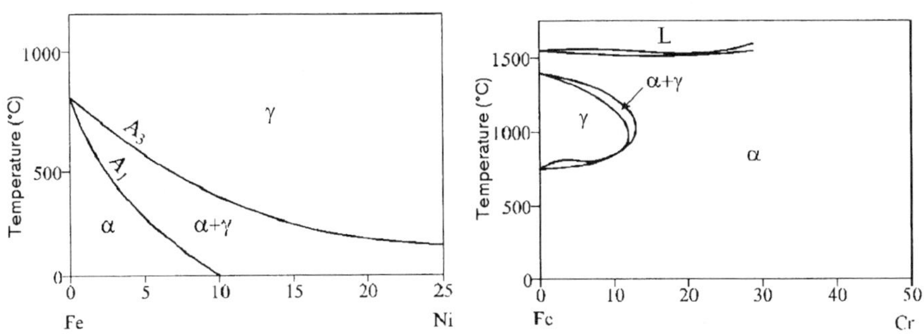

Figure 6.9. Phase diagrams of the iron–nickel system (a) and of the iron–chromium system (b).

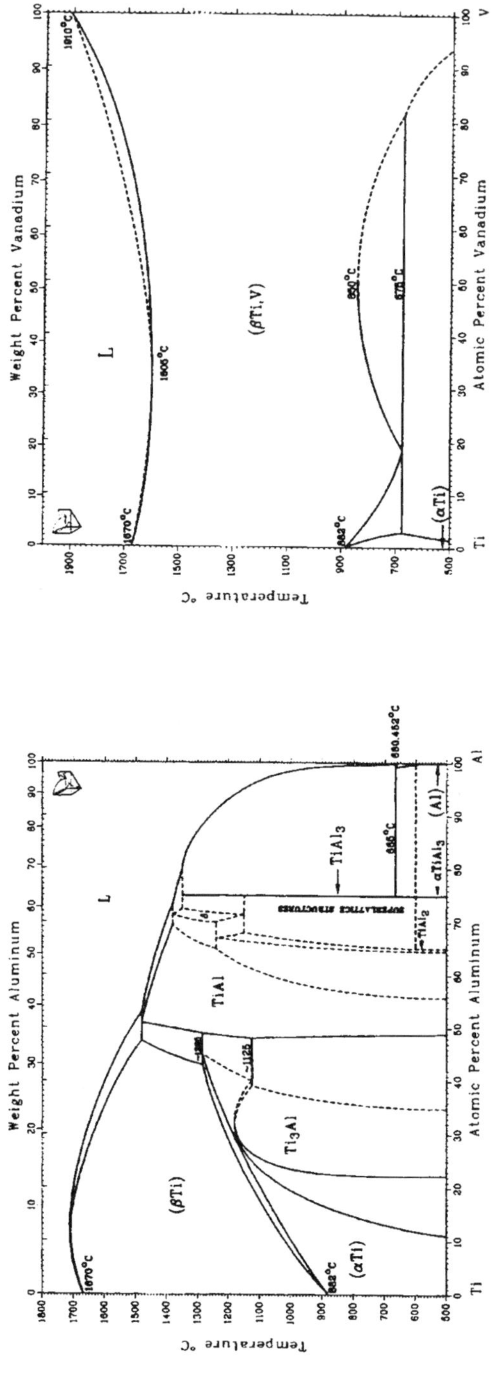

Figure 6.10. Phase diagrams of the titanium–aluminum system (a) and of the titanium–vanadium system (b).

from Ti-α (with a hcp structure) to Ti-β (with a bcc structure). Aluminum addition increases the temperature of transformation Ti-α°Ti-β, so stabilizing the Ti-α phase, while vanadium addition lowers the same temperature resulting in the stabilization of the Ti-β phase. The presence of the two elements in an alloy can lead to the presence of both phases Ti-α and Ti-β.

6.4.10. Other Phase Diagrams

It is well known that precious metal alloys are very useful as biomaterials, especially gold-base alloys which are used in dental applications. The essential components of commercial dental gold alloys are thought to be gold, copper, and silver. A knowledge of each equilibrium phase diagram is indispensable to understand them. According to the binary phase diagrams, three phase diagrams are relatively simple. The Ag–Cu has a typical eutectic system with a miscibility gap in the solid solution. Both Au–Cu and Au–Ag diagrams have typical isomorphous systems; in the lower temperature region, the former forms three kinds of superlattice; Au_3Cu, CuAu, and Cu_3Au. Thus, dental gold alloys are characterized by the formation of superlattice structures and phase separation. Generally, it takes time to obtain the equilibrium phase diagram in dental alloys. It is useful to represent the phase diagram by the coherent phase as defined by Allen and Cahn. In Au–Ag–Cu ternary alloy system, two types of calculated and experimental phase diagrams have been produced. Figure 6.11 shows an isothermal section at 573 K of a plausible Au–Cu–Ag ternary phase diagram which was constructed by superimposing the theoretical one calculated using the cluster variation method on experimental data. The shaded area in the figure indicates the composition region corresponding to commercial dental gold alloys. Figure 6.12 shows the coherent phase diagram of the $Au_x(Ag_{0.24}Cu_{0.76})_{1-x}$ section in the Au–Cu–Ag ternary system. The formation region of a long-period superstructure of CuAu II appears to coexist with a silver-rich disordered fcc a_2 phase. The Cu_3Au II long-period superstructure was also found in the $Cu_3Au + a_1 + a_2$ three-phase coexisting region.

In practice platinum and/or palladium is added to improve the properties in dental gold alloys. Therefore, a coherent phase diagram of more complex quaternary alloy systems was also determined as shown in Figures 6.13–6.15, respectively, each a pseudobinary phase diagram in Au–Cu–Pt ternary and Au–Cu–Ag–Pt quaternary systems. Various phase regions consisting of ordered phases (CuAu I, CuAu II, and Cu_3Au) and a disordered phase were detected in the coherent phase diagram. These coherent phase diagrams have various characteristic features which provide very useful information on the clinical application.

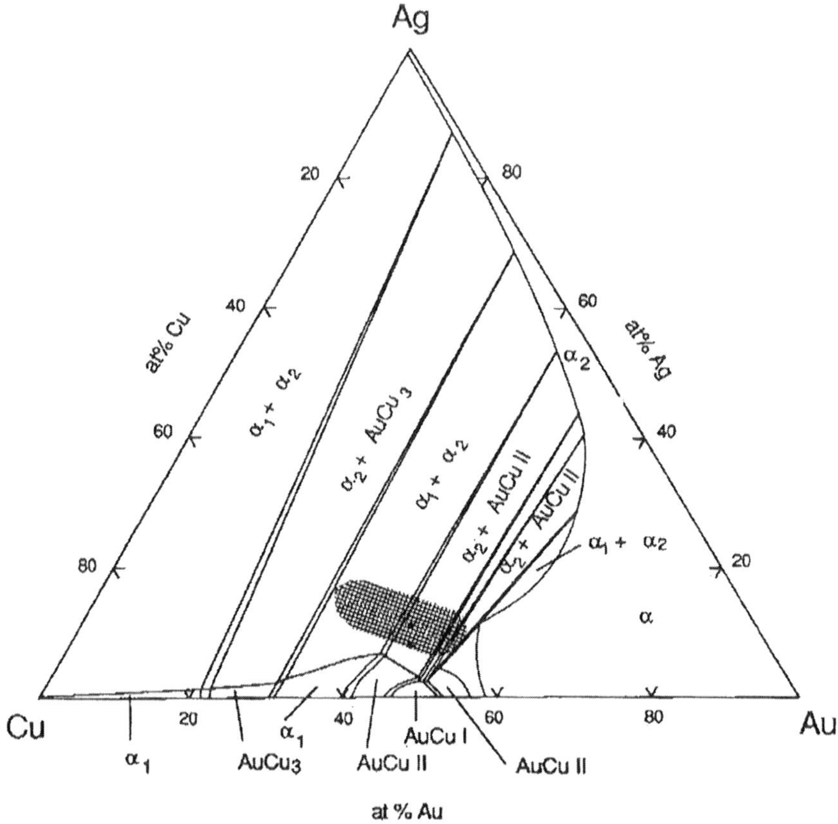

Figure 6.11. Isothermal section of a plausible phase diagram of Au-Cu-Ag ternary.

6.5. Thermal Treatments

Phase diagrams can describe transformations occurring in metal alloys after very slow equilibrium cooling. On the other hand, very often the cooling rate of metallic alloys is higher, leading to nonthermodynamical equilibrium structures. These operations of heating and subsequent fast cooling are called thermal treatments. They consist essentially of three operations:

- heating of the material;
- keeping it at a well-defined temperature;
- cooling at a suitable rate.

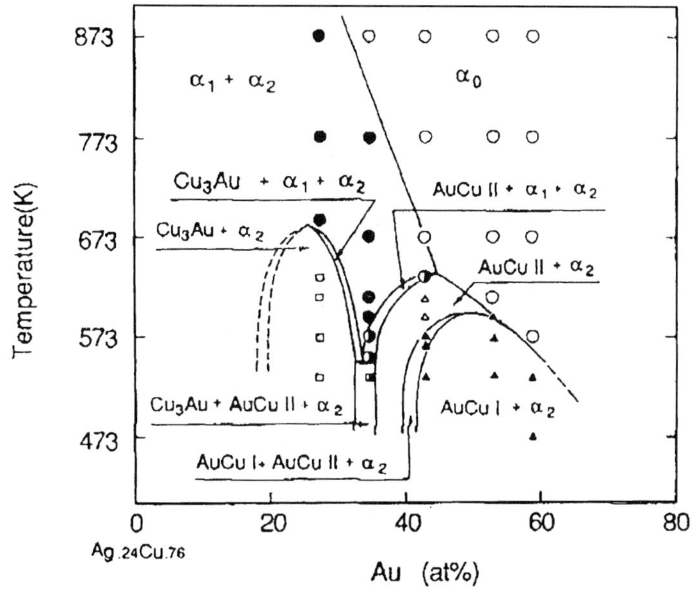

Figure 6.12. Experimental coherent phase diagram of the $Au_x(Ag_{0.24}Cu_{0.76})_{1-x}$ pseudobinary section in Au-Cu-Ag ternary system.

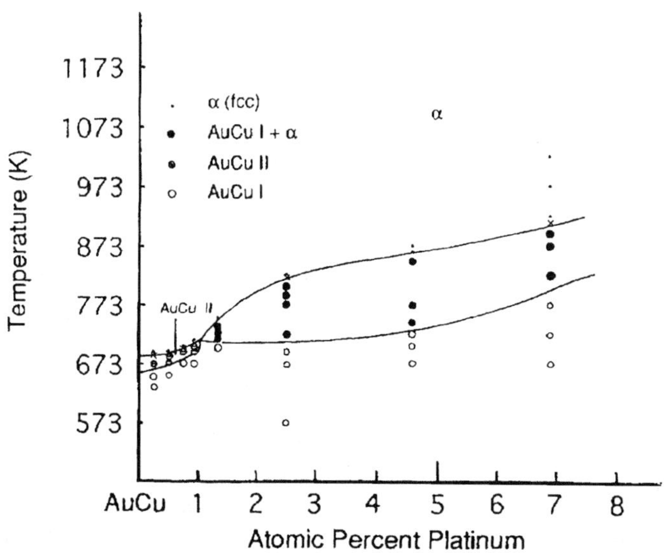

Figure 6.13. Experimental coherent phase diagram of the $(AuCu)_{1-x}Pt_x$ pseudobinary system.

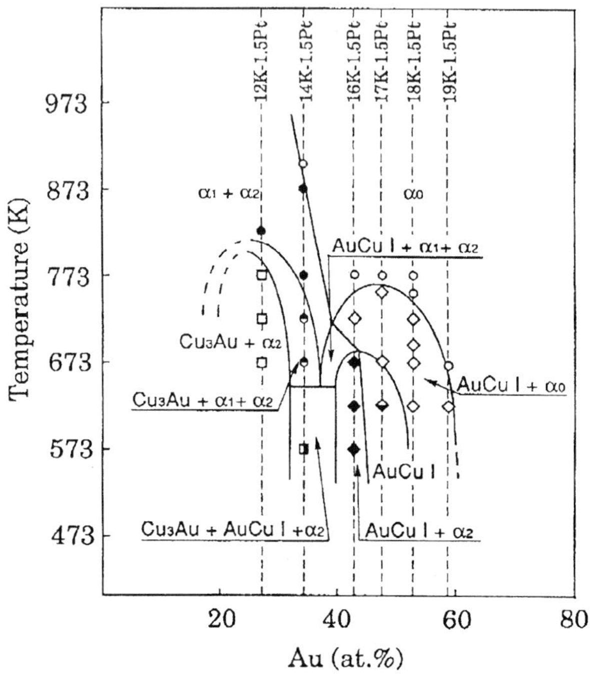

Figure 6.14. Experimental coherent phase diagram of the $[Au_x(Ag_{0.24}Cu_{0.76})_{1-x}]_{0.985}$ pseudobinary system.

The main thermal treatments on steel will be examined later. This is important both to understand these phenomena in the study of metallic materials and the undoubted applicative importance of steels. However, the same could be said for analogous classes of materials.

On the basis of the above considerations, we may predict the structures obtained after (in practice, very slow) equilibrium cooling.

In a steel containing only C (e.g., 0.4%) at high temperature, only Fe-γ (with fcc structure) is stable. During very slow cooling, it turns into Fe-α (bcc) plus iron carbide Fe_3C.

This transformation happens according to a nucleation and growing mechanism needing carbon diffusion, as shown in Figure 6.16. The first stage consists in the appearance of cementite Fe_3C nuclei on Fe-γ grain boundaries. Carbon concentration around these small cementite lamellae strongly diminishes until the value at which Fe-α nucleates, growing onto the Fe_3C surface. Since ferrite lamella contains practically no carbon, its growth

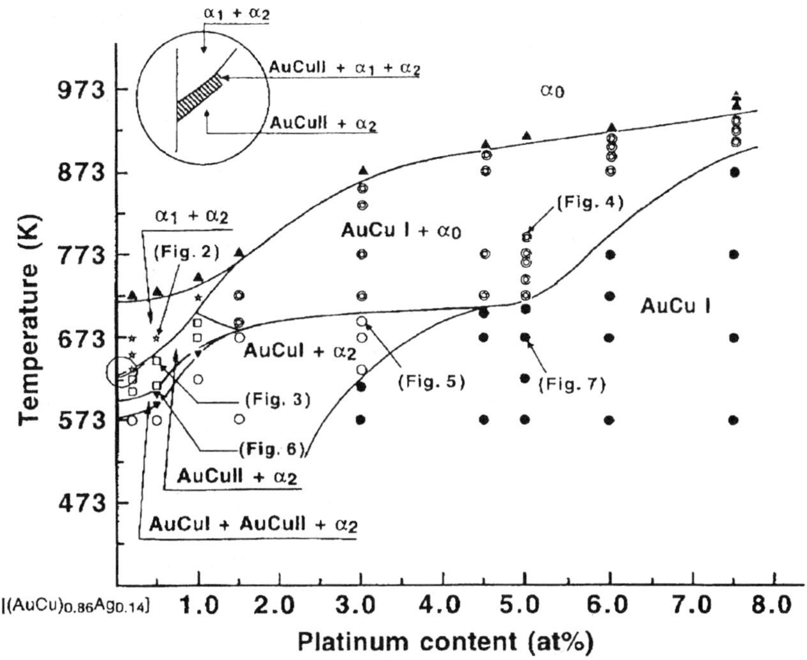

Figure 6.15. Experimental coherent phase diagram of the $[(AuCu)_{0.86}Ag_{0.14}]_{1-x}Pt_x$ pseudobinary system

results in carbon enrichment of the surrounding zones with subsequent nucleation of a new cementite lamella. This structure composed of small alternate cementite and ferrite lamellae is called pearlite.

On the other hand, by cooling at a high cooling rate, it is possible to obtain, at room temperature, a structure different than the equilibrium one,

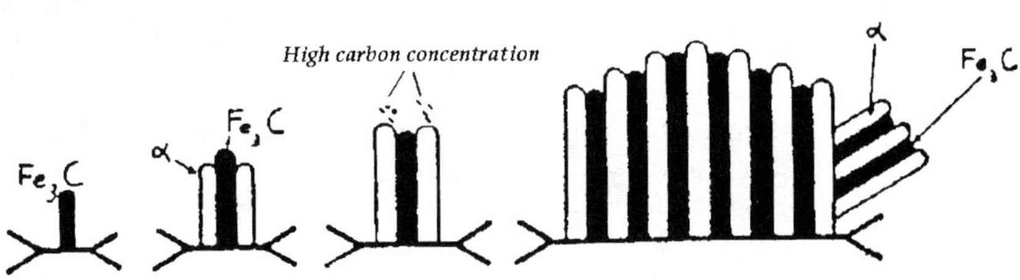

Figure 6.16. Pearlite nucleation and growing.

which in the case of steel takes the name martensite. The formation mechanism of martensite can be explained intuitively as follows.

When Fe-γ (fcc structure) is cooled, it should tend to transform into Fe-α (bcc), which can contain only little carbon, so calling for carbon to exit from the crystal lattice by diffusion to form Fe_3C.

When cooling is very fast, the lattice transformation from fcc to bcc tends to occur with no time for carbon to diffuse. A metastable phase is so obtained (metastable means that it tends to transform into a stable form) with a body-centered tetragonal lattice, obtained after distortion of the bcc lattice owing to the presence of interstitial carbon. This structure is called martensite.

Martensite is a nonequilibrium structure characterized by a strong reticular distortion, which makes it very hard and strong but at the same time too brittle to be used as it is. We shall show later that the toughness of a material can be improved by tempering.

After this introduction, it is now possible to examine the main thermal treatments on steel. Similar treatments based on phase transformation different from Fe-c to Fe-a + Fe_3C are possible for other metallic alloys too.

The basic principle is that fast cooling leads to nonthermodynamic equilibrium structures. These, when compared to equilibrium structures, are characterized by better mechanical properties.

6.5.1. Full Annealing

The term annealing indicates a thermal treatment characterized by:

- Progressive heating up to a temperature at which the steel structure turns into Fe-γ.
- Maintenance of this temperature for a sufficient time to complete austenitization (in the core of the piece).
- Slow cooling (switched off in the furnace), so that all transformations occur under conditions close to equilibrium for which the iron–carbon phase diagram is effective.

The aim of this treatment is to soften the material itself, to make it easier for machining, and to allow further cold deformation in case of work hardening by previous deformations. The aim of annealing is also to homogenize the composition of casting materials, so obtaining a homogeneous microstructure and, in the case of quenched steel, canceling the effect of quenching.

6.5.2. Normalization

This process involves heating steel at a temperature for which Fe-γ is stable, and maintaining it for a time sufficient for complete austenitization, after which it is extracted from the heating furnace and allowed to cool freely in air. The result of this treatment is a structure similar to that obtained after full annealing, but the process is simpler and cheaper.

6.5.3. Quenching

This consists in heating the steel in the region where Fe-γ is stable and maintaining it at this temperature for a sufficient time to attain complete austenitization. Subsequent fast cooling to room temperature leads to a martensitic structure, characterized by high hardness but high brittleness too.

The fast cooling necessary for steel quenching is obtained by immersing the piece in a quenching bath which can be in decreasing order of efficacy: water, oil, and in some cases also air.

6.5.4. Tempering

Martensite is hard and strong, but brittle too. Tempering is the process of heating martensite to obtain structures with the best result in terms of mechanical properties (referred to hardness) and toughness by diminishing the excessive brittleness of martensite to the partial detriment of hardness.

Tempering consists in heating a previously quenched steel at a temperature between 150° and 600 °C, maintaining it at that temperature for a suitable time, and then cooling it. The higher the treatment temperature, the higher the diminution of the hardness (and the increased toughness).

6.6. Strengthening of Metals

The intrinsic mechanical properties of pure metals are not so high, resulting essentially from intrinsic bond energy that determines crystalline structure. It is convenient for most industrial applications to increase the mechanical properties by exploiting various strengthening mechanisms.

We mention the following strengthening mechanisms:

- alloying,
- work hardening,
- addition of oligoelements,

- thermal treatments,
- order/disorder transformations.

Some strengthening mechanisms have already, yet briefly, been examined. At this stage, it is convenient to summarize their definitions and add some numerical examples in order to highlight the importance of the full exploitation of various strengthening mechanisms, even in a combined manner.

6.6.1. Strengthening by Alloying

The addition of an alloying element to a metal can give rise to solid solutions. A crystal lattice containing solute atoms (in substitutional or interstitial position) opposes more resistance to dislocation slip, making the material more resistant to deformations. A bigger force is necessary to deform it, which implies that the material has better mechanical properties. For instance, commercial refined copper (almost pure) has an ultimate tensile strength (UTS) of 235 MPa. Bronze is obtained by adding 10% tin. As a substitutional solid solution, it has the same crystal structure but with a UTS of 455 MPa.

6.6.2. Strengthening by Work Hardening

It was noted as a consequence of cold plastic deformation in a metallic material that there is a multiplication of the dislocations and of their mutual interaction, resulting in a hardening of the material. For instance, a strong cold deformation of pure copper determines an increase in its UTS from 235 MPa to about 400 MPa. Another example is the case of austenitic stainless steel, which has a UTS of about 200 MPa in the absence of hardening and can be work hardened to obtain a tensile yield strength (TYS) even higher than 1500 MPa.

6.6.3. Strengthening by Addition of Oligoelements

The addition of small amounts of other elements to a metallic material can determine the formation of small precipitates inside the crystal lattice of the solvent. The presence of these precipitates obstructs the deformation of the material, but reinforces it.

This is the case, for instance, of the alloy duraluminum (constituted by 96% of aluminum and 4% of copper). The addition of copper determines a stiffening by a solid solution with an increase in the UTS from 75 to 185 MPa. The treatment of solution quenching and aging, which lead to the formation of fine coherent precipitates, makes the UTS grow up to 485 MPa.

6.6.4. Strengthening by Thermal Treatments

Phase diagrams allow us to forecast the structures that metallic alloys should assume after very slow cooling under equilibrium conditions. If the cooling rate is increased (by so-called thermal treatments, quenching in particular), the crystal structure which is being formed can differ from the equilibrium one, forecast by the phase diagram.

For instance, steel containing iron and 0.4% carbon, after very slow cooling, forms a two-phase structure (ferrite and cementite); very fast cooling (quenching) of the same steel, on the other hand, leads to the formation of a structure (out of thermodynamic equilibrium) called martensite with a UTS of about 800 MPa, about twice the value compared to the equilibrium structure and about four times that of pure iron.

6.6.5. Strengthening by Order–Disorder Transformations

Ordered structures are produced in alloys and exhibit characteristic properties. In particular, hardening by the order–disorder transformation is of interest. We shall consider the order hardening in a Cu–Au alloy system, which is related to the dental gold alloys used as biomaterials. The binary Cu–Au system forms a continuous solid solution for all compositions at elevated temperatures. The equiatomic CuAu alloy, having an fcc structure above 410 °C becomes ordered below this temperature and forms two distinguishable superlattices. The first below 380 °C has a tetragonal structure with an axial ratio of 0.92, and is known as CuAu I. The second between 380 °C and 410 °C has an orthorhombic structure modified by CuAu I, and is known as CuAu II. Another type of ordered phase with an fcc structure forms near the stoichiometric compositions Cu_3Au and $CuAu_3$.

The former (CuAu) is accompanied by a change in symmetry, while the latter (Cu_3Au and $CuAu_3$) is not. The hardening depends on the type of superlattice structure; the former is more sensitive in hardening than the latter. Imperfect ordering can yield a remarkable hardening, followed by a softening in the development of the ordering. The hardness produced during the ordering of CuAu is twice as much as at 473 K with solution treatment. Figure 6.17 shows the hardening behavior by an ordering of CuAu. With increasing the annealing temperature, the ordering rate becomes fast, the hardness peak shifts to a longer aging time, and more hardening is obtained. Ordered plate-like CuAu I nuclei are formed which are coherent with and parallel to the $\{110\}$ planes of the disordered matrix. The increase in hardness is correlated to the coherency strains between ordered nuclei and disordered matrix and the decline in strength after further annealing to eliminate coherency strains by microtwinning.

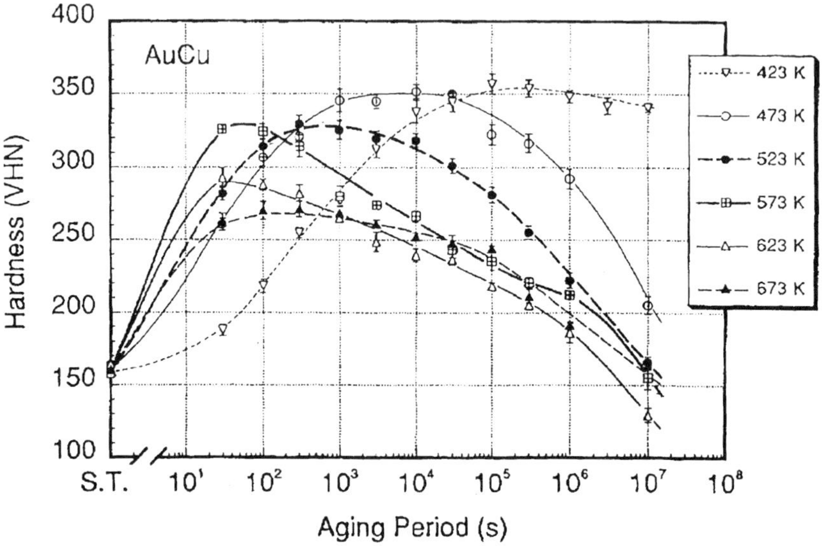

Figure 6.17. Hardening curves by the order-disorder transformation of equiatomic CuAl alloy.

In the case of no change in symmetry, such as the Cu_3Au ordered phase, considerable hardening is produced by the order–disorder transformation. The hardening in Cu_3Au-type alloys is due to an antiphase domain size effect.

Silver addition to the equiatomic CuAu alloy can achieve a combined strengthening of the atomic ordering based on CuAu I and the decomposition based on the Ag–Cu system. Figure 6.18 shows an example of age-hardening curves in CuAu–14% Ag alloy. Depending on the annealing temperature, various hardening characteristics are observed. Additional silver plays the role of retarding the ordering. The age-hardening was attributed to nucleation and growth processes of the CuAu I′ or CuAu II′ metastable ordered phase in the grain interior. Overaging followed by softening was induced by grain boundary precipitation of CuAu I and/or CuAu II ordered and silver-rich a_2 stable phases.

6.7. Working Technologies

The working technologies of metallic materials change much from one class of material to the other, also in relation to the object or component

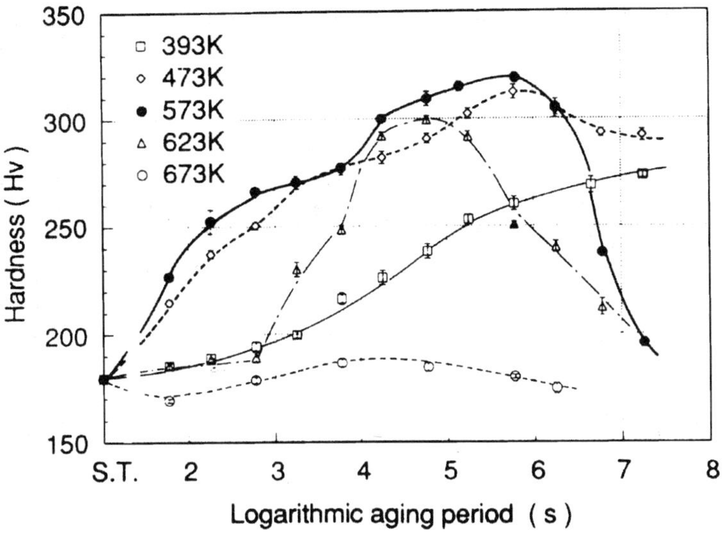

Figure 6.18. Age-hardening curves of CuAu-14%Ag alloy.

that one wishes to obtain. In particular, for metallic materials some common lines of working technologies can be identified schematically:

- Processes to obtain semimanufactured products with shape more or less close to the final component by means of hot or cold plastic deformation, molding, and powder metallurgy.
- Tool machining to obtain the desired final shape.
- Bonding operations between different pieces, warranting an adequate global mechanical strength.
- Surface finishing.

These technologies will be examined briefly with the aim of providing the most important and concise information.

6.7.1. Hot or Cold Plastic Deformation

In most cases the metallic materials produced by ingot molding must be transformed in semimanufactured products. Their shape must be as close as possible to that required for the final use. This is obtained by different techniques of plastic deformation that might be executed at a high or room temperature (respectively, hot and cold deformation).

- The material is more easily deformed at the high temperature, so the operations of hot plastic deformation allow the most important change in shape but do not cause any strain hardening in the material, as the recrystallization processes cancel the work hardening effects.
- The operations of cold plastic deformation performed at room temperature require more elevated power of the implants but allow less important variation in the shape of the material owing to the work hardening which occurs. However, the strain hardening allows the mechanical properties to increase. Furthermore, the surface finishing of cold rolled components can be regarded as final without any further treatment.

Among the several techniques of plastic deformation, mention should be made of rolling, forging, wire drawing, extrusion, deep drawing, and stretching.

a. Rolling. During rolling, the parts to be deformed are inserted in several series of two rollers at a suitable distance apart (Figure 6.19a). It is possible to use only one reversing rolling mill, where the part to be rolled is subjected to an alternate movement, or to use a succession of rolling mills through which the component moves in one direction only. Using shaped rolls and a proper punch it is possible to produce not only sheet, but also tubes (pipes) or rods (bars) of large diameter.

b. Forging. During forging the material is forced to assume a given shape by the action of a power hammer (determining a dynamic impact) or of a press (determining a progressive compression). In this way components of complex shape are obtained, with mechanical properties often far better than those of components of the same shape that were obtained by casting.

Two kinds of forging can be distinguished: open-die forging (Figure 6.19b), realized on components of big dimensions by dies that might be flat or have simple shapes (swage or vee dies); and closed-die forging (Figure 6.19c), performed on small pieces using two dies to reproduce the component shape or using a succession of dies that little by little approach the final shape.

c. Wire Drawing. In this technique metallic rods or wires are drawn through one or more drawing dies in very hard ceramic materials (e.g., tungsten carbide), as shown in Figure 6.19d. Dies with progressively smaller diameter are used until the desired rod or wire dimensions are obtained.

Products of small dimension can also be obtained and, in the case of cold drawing, these may be highly work-hardened (or hard-drawn).

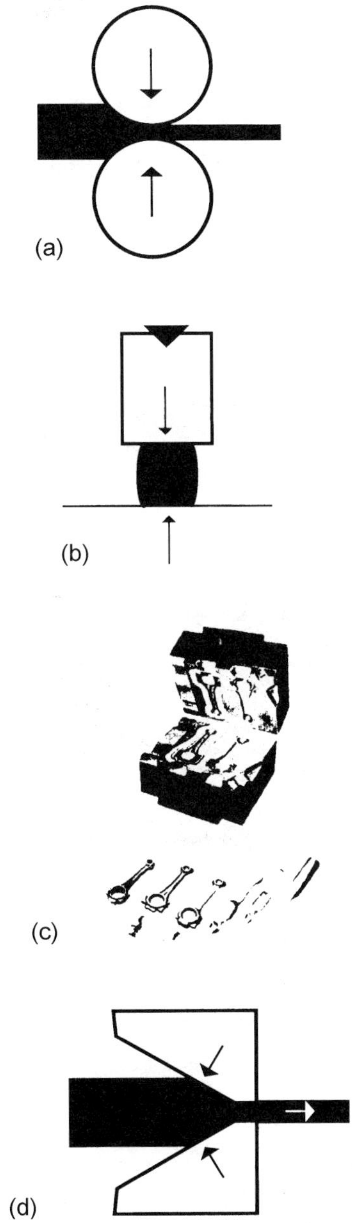

Figure 6.19. (a) Rolling. (b) Open-die forging. (c) Closed-die forging. (d) Wire drawing.

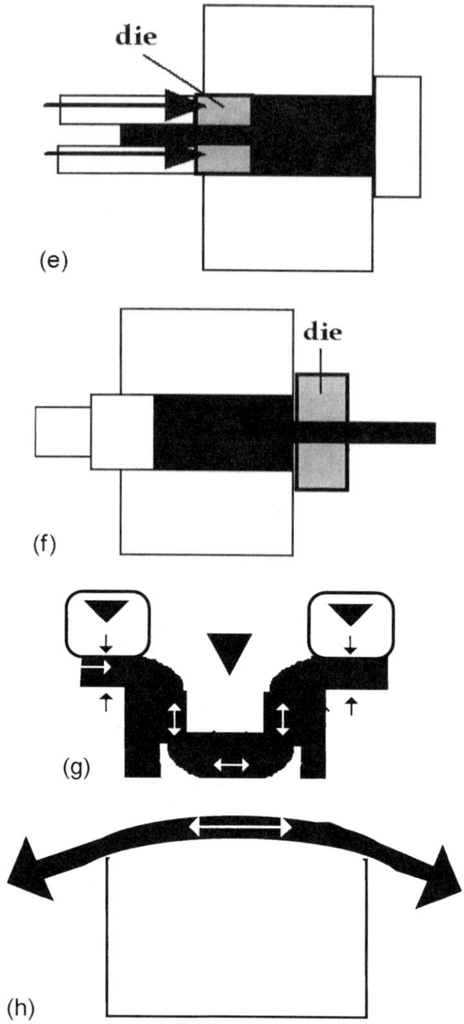

Figure 6.19. (e) Direct extrusion. (f) Indirect extrusion. (g) Deep drawing. (h) Stretching.

d. Extrusion. During extrusion, the material compressed by high pressure is forced to pass through a die of adequate shape. In this way rod and pipes can be obtained. With metals that can be easily deformed (such as aluminum), structural bars of complex section can be produced.

Direct extrusion (Figure 6.19e) consists of a piston that pushes the metal directly in the die, allowing one to apply strong pressures.

In the case of indirect extrusion, on the contrary, the piston supports the die (Figure 6.19f) while the head of the extruder is closed by a plate. In this way the extruded material exits from the die through the piston. This method allows for less friction; however, the use of a trunk piston allows one to exercise lower pressures than with direct extrusion.

e. Deep Drawing. With this technique, thin metallic sheets are deformed to realize a deep deformation that allows cup-shaped articles to be obtained. In this method, the metallic sheet is placed over a shaped die and then pressed into the die with a punch (Figure 6.19g). Usually, a hold-down device is used to allow the metal to be pressed smoothly into the die to prevent wrinkling of the metal.

f. Stretching. During the operation, the material is deformed by stretching on a suitable shape (Figure 6.19h) to obtain the desired deformation.

6.7.2. Molding

The aim of molding processes is to obtain directly components of complex geometry by a process of solidification. These components are also called castings. By this technique the tool machining, which will be necessary to obtain the same component starting from a semimanufactured item of standardized shape, is reduced to the required choice.

Once the chosen metal is melted, this is cast in molds with a shape very close to that of the desired final component.

Considerable care must be taken during the production of castings to eliminate, or at least reduce, the formation of internal defects (e.g., micro- and macrocavities, concentration of inclusions in particular zones, etc.) that can highly affect the mechanical properties of the casting up to to rendering it useless. In many cases it is necessary to perform nondestructive tests (e.g., X-ray radiographs, ultrasounds, etc.) to point out these defects and, when possible, to proceed with their elimination by removal and redeposition operations of material using welding-like techniques.

Depending on the kind of moulding and pouring techniques employed, it is possible to obtain sand castings, permanent-mold castings, and die castings, examined below. The castings then undergo a mechanical surface finishing, which can be more or less strong depending on the chosen kind of casting.

a. Sand Casting. This technique consists in pouring by gravity the melted metal inside an external wrapping made of foundry sand (i.e., a material with a very high melting point). Sand casting is mainly used for

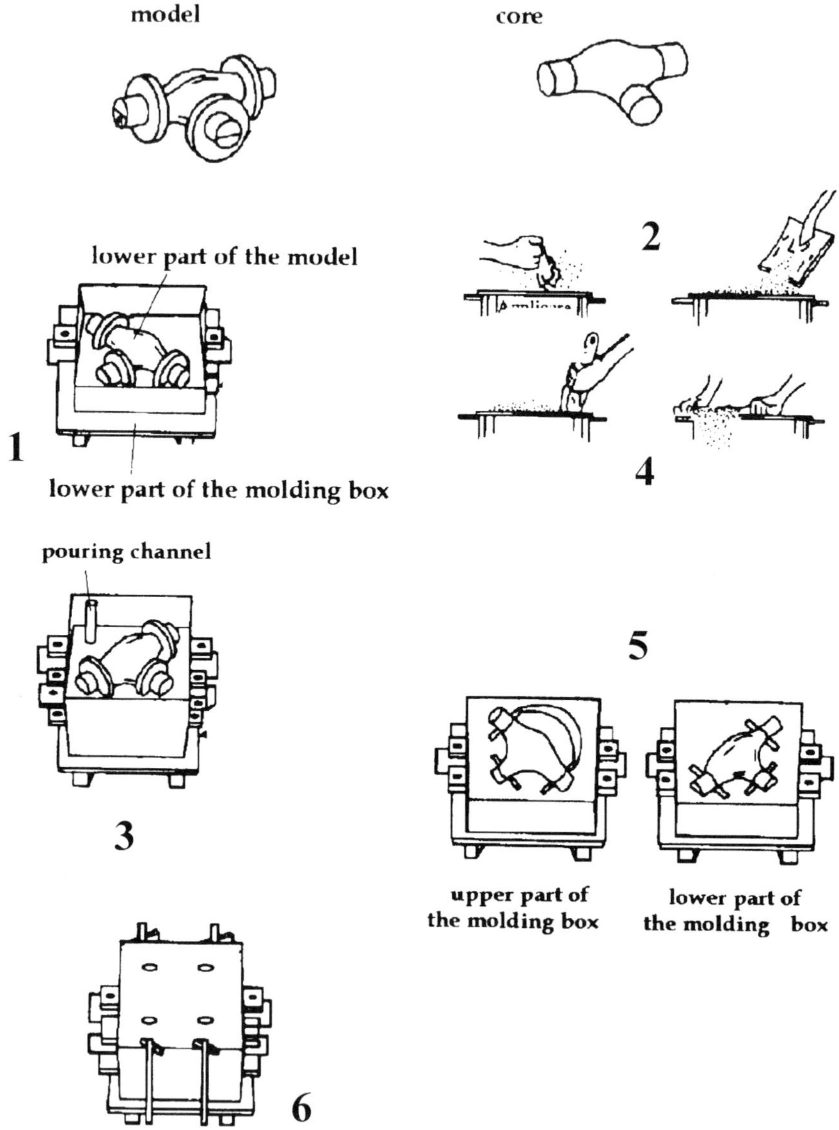

Figure 6.20. Production of castings by sand mold casting. Positioning the lower part of the model in the lower section of the molding box laying on the die shoe (1); setting up the lower part of the mould (2); positioning the upper part of the model and of the molding box upon the lower one (3); setting up the upper part of the mould (4); once the molding boxes separated, taking off the models, positioning the core and closing the molding boxes (5); molding boxes closed together ready to the pouring of the metal (6).

metals that possess a high melting point (such as steel, cast iron, and bronze) and for aluminum too.

The mold is realized by compacting the foundry sand all around the shapes and cores that must be removed before casting (Figure 6.20). The shape might also be made by wax or by expanded polymeric material, which is transformed in gaseous products before the casting of the melted metal (i.e., investment casting).

b. Permanent-Mold Casting. With this method the melted metal (that must have a low melting point, such as aluminum) is cast by gravity in metallic dies (Figure 6.21). The metals composing these dies have a melting point higher than the casting alloy. The separation of the casting from the mold is obtained by the use of adequate detaching agents that must be previously applied on the internal surface of the die. When compared with the previous technique, permanent-mold casting allows one to obtain better precision and surface finishing.

c. Die Castings. Using this casting method the melted metal is forced into a cavity under high pressures. The components produced by die castings are characterized by excellent surface finishing and, when compared with the previous casting methods, a lower concentration of microcavities and a possible smaller thickness of the walls of the casting. Nevertheless, only some alloys (primarily aluminum) can be used for this technique.

6.7.3. Powder Metallurgy

Powder metallurgy uses "metallic powders" produced by atomization of the melted metal and which solidify in small particles of controlled

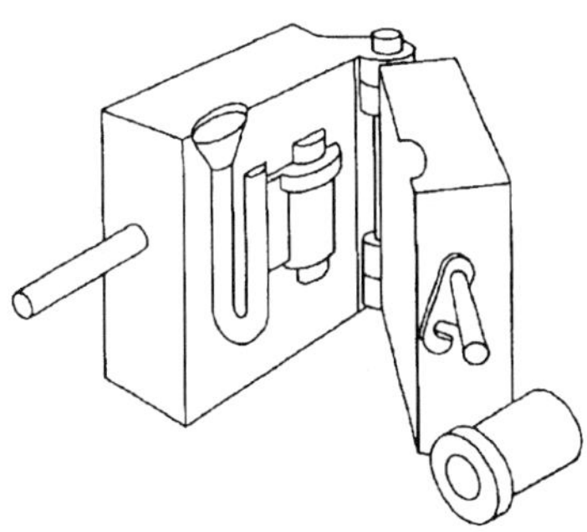

Figure 6.21. Permanent mold for shell molding.

dimensions. These powders are compacted in the required shape adding, if necessary, an adequate binder agent, after which they undergo a thermal process of sintering (i.e., heating at high temperature and high pressure). The sintered components can be tool-machined directly or after a previous thermal treatment that follows the sintering process.

Beside the advantages of the molding processes, powder metallurgy has the advantage of a low possibility of defect formation and a chance to use metals and alloys that are difficult to cast by traditional techniques. This technology will be developed in the future, even though at present it is limited by being more expensive than traditional techniques.

6.7.4. Tool Machining

Once semimanufactured items are produced (such as sheets, rods, bars, castings, etc.), it is often necessary to further machine them in order to obtain the final shape or to realize holes, millings, junctions, etc., or to more easily enhance the finishing of a piece, for example, by removing the surface layer of oxidized metal. These workings are normally realized by different tool machining procedures, the most important of which are turning, drilling, milling, broaching, boring, planing, shaping, sawing, shearing, abrading, grinding, and lapping.

Recently, new nontraditional machining techniques have been developed of which the following should be highlighted: electrical discharge machining, laser cutting, water-jet cutting, and plasma-jet cutting. For a more detailed description of these techniques, specialized publications should be consulted.

6.7.5. Bonding

A component cannot be produced in a single piece if it has a complex geometry or large dimensions. In this case it is necessary to link the different parts to one another while guaranteeing that the mechanical properties of the final component will be as close as possible to those of each single piece. It is altogether useless to perform operations that allow one to obtain single parts with high mechanical properties and then to produce a final component lacking the same resistance and toughness once the different pieces are linked together.

Common techniques performed in order to obtain fixed joints include welding, brazing, riveting, and structural adhesion.

6.7.6. Surface Finishing

Adequate preparation of surfaces must be conducted in order to realize the surface finishing of a component. The most used techniques include sandblasting, pickling, chemical etching, and degreasing.

It is possible to obtain the following surface coatings or finishings:

- Metal coatings obtained by dipping, plasma spray, or galvanic techniques.
- Ceramic coatings obtained by plasma spray.
- Painting or coating by polymeric materials.
- Physical vapor deposition (PVD) or chemical vapor deposition (CVD) in order to obtain coatings made by oxides, carbides, or nitrides.
- Ion implantation of the metallic surface by special ions (nitrogen, oxygen, etc.) in order to increase specific properties.
- Chemical or electrochemical passivation.

6.8. Main Metallic Materials Used as Biomaterials

A metallic material used in making orthopedic prostheses, osteosynthesis devices, or dental implants must possess the following properties:

- High mechanical properties, with yield strength often higher than 800 MPa.
- Corrosion resistance, both localized and generalized.
- Biocompatibility, i.e., ability of the organism to withstand the inevitable, though very restricted, metallic ions release without averse reaction that could in particular lead to allergic sensitization, local and systemic inflammation.

These conditions are so restrictive that practically only few classes of metallic materials can be used successfully, namely, austenitic stainless steels; cobalt alloys, both for casting and for plastic deformation; titanium and titanium alloys (with the best mechanical properties); precious metal alloys.

Other classes of materials, such as tantalum and nickel–titanium shape memory alloys, find applications limited to particular areas and functions.

It can be useful to underline the significant difference between the modulus of elasticity of stainless steels and cobalt alloys (E = 200–230 GPa, respectively) and titanium and its alloys (E = 110 GPa). A relatively low modulus of elasticity (as per titanium and its alloys) is useful when producing components (such as stems for a not cemented hip prosthesis) with relatively low stiffness, in order to prevent stress shielding. For other applications (such as stems for a cemented hip prosthesis, osteosynthesis devices) a higher stiffness should be requested, in which case the use of alloys with higher modulus, like stainless steels and cobalt alloys, is advisable.

The main metallic materials presently provided for by ISO Standards for biomedical applications and the most important metallic materials for dental applications are examined below.

6.8.1. Austenitic Stainless Steel

Most metallic components used in orthopedics are presently made with this material, in particular those for temporary use (osteosynthesis devices). The main advantages are:

- low cost,
- good mechanical properties in cold-worked conditions,
- easy working by plastic deformation,
- easy working by tool machining.

The main disadvantages are:

- presence of nickel, an element that can cause allergic reactions to many patients,
- sensitivity in the human body to localized corrosion, in particular crevice corrosion, mainly when steels with low molybdenum and nitrogen content are used.

Crevice corrosion appears in interstices like those forming between screw heads and their location in osteosynthesis plates, or in the contact zones between more endomedullary nails. It leads to a significant increase of metallic ions released in the tissues adjoining the implantation.

These ions can cause local irritations, systemic infections, and especially allergic sensitization phenomena, in particular for the presence of nickel. These phenomena occur in a not-negligible percentage of patients (mainly females). The insurgence of such phenomena implies the necessity to remove the metallic components in time. In the past various types of austenitic stainless steel were used; now, ISO Standards provide the use of three classes of steel: ISO 5832-1 Composition D, ISO 5832-1 Composition E, and ISO 5832-9.

The most traditional is ISO 5832-1 Composition D, corresponding practically to AISI 316L steel, containing chromium (17–19%), nickel

(13–15%), molybdenum (2.25–3.5%), and nitrogen (<0.1%). In comparison with AISI 316L, this steel is characterized by high purity (low sulfur, phosphorus, and inclusion contents). It is the cheapest metallic material provided by the Standards and is easily workable both by plastic deformation and by tool machining. Mechanical properties, not particularly high in the annealed state (UTS = 690 MPa, TYS = 190 MPa), can be increased by cold plastic deformation (UTS = 1100 MPa, TYS = 690 MPa). The steel is susceptible to crevice corrosion.

ISO 5832-1 Composition E steel contains chromium (17–19%), nickel (14–16%), molybdenum (2.35–4.2%), and nitrogen (0.1–0.2%). The higher molybdenum and nitrogen content, compared to traditional ISO 5832-1 Composition D steel, makes it more resistant to crevice corrosion, although it should not be considered unsusceptible to this type of corrosion. The mechanical properties are slightly higher than ISO 5832-1 Composition D steel.

ISO 5832-9 steel contains chromium (19.5–22%), nickel (9–11%), molybdenum (2–3%), manganese (2–4.25%), and nitrogen (0.25–0.5%). The high nitrogen content assures corrosion resistance to crevice corrosion (especially if the molybdenum content is near to 3%) and the best mechanical properties, both in the annealed condition (UTS = 740 MPa, TYS = 430 MPa) and in the cold worked condition (TYS up to 1800 MPa). It is, however, more expensive and more difficult to be worked by plastic deformation and tool machining.

6.8.2. Cobalt Alloys

Cobalt alloys may be divided into two categories: alloys for casting (cast) and alloys for plastic deformation (wrought).

a. Cast Alloys. Cobalt alloys have long been used as biomaterials because they are the only casting alloys with good mechanical properties (to which an adequate resistance to corrosion and biocompatibility are associated). Clearly the mechanical properties of these alloys, fatigue resistance in particular, depend strongly on the metallurgical quality of the castings. A remarkable diminution of these occurs when in the presence of defects like microcavities, cracks, metallurgical heterogeneity, and low control of the carbides present.

The main advantages of cast alloys are:

- high (for a casting) mechanical properties (for casts),
- good corrosion resistance, especially to fretting corrosion.

The main disadvantages are:

- high cost,
- low fatigue resistance, especially in the presence of metallurgical defects,
- impossibility of working by plastic deformation,
- difficulty of working by tool machining.

Casting alloys (ISO 5832-4) contain, besides cobalt (balance), chromium (26.5–30%) and molybdenum (4.5–7%). They have UTS = 655 MPa and TYS = 450 MPa.

b. Wrought Alloys. Cobalt alloys for plastic deformation (wrought alloys) were introduced more recently. They are (compared to titanium alloy, too) also characterized by the presence of nickel. The main advantages of wrought cobalt alloys are:

- good mechanical properties,
- good corrosion resistance.

The main disadvantages are:

- high cost,
- complex and expensive technology of production,
- presence of nickel.

The wrought Co–Cr–W–Ni alloys (ISO 5832-5) contains cobalt (balance), chromium (19–21%), tungsten (14–16%), and nickel (9–11%). They have UTS = 860 MPa and TYS = 310 MPa.

The wrought Co–Cr–Ni–Mo–Fe alloys (ISO 5832-7) contain cobalt (39–42%), chromium (18.5–21.5%), nickel (14–18%), molybdenum (6.5–8%), and iron (balance). They have very high mechanical properties with UTS exceeding 1650 MPa.

Finally, the wrought Co–Ni–Cr–Mo–W–Fe alloys (ISO 5832-8) contain cobalt (balance), nickel (15–25%), chromium (18–22%), molybdenum (3–4%), tungsten (3–4%), and iron (4–6%). They have high mechanical properties with UTS exceeding 1580 MPa.

6.8.3. Titanium and Titanium Alloys

Titanium is generally considered a metallic material with the best biocompatibility properties and, as a consequence, it finds more and more application as a biomaterial. However, pure titanium is characterized by relatively low mechanical properties, so in many applications it is replaced by titanium alloys, which are more expensive, less biocompatible, but with better mechanical properties.

Titanium and titanium alloys have very good resistance to crevice corrosion; however, they are extremely sensitive to fretting corrosion. This type of corrosion may occur only when a metallic surface is in contact with another surface (metallic or not), in the presence of a compression stress and slight reciprocal movements. This can happen, for example, in orthopedic applications, in the tape morse of joint prostheses (between the femoral head and stem), and under the heads of screws in ostheosynthesis devices. In these cases, the onset of fretting corrosion on titanium alloys has been confirmed by microscopic analyses at the damaged parts and by the presence of black titanium powder on the surrounding tissues, which seem to tolerate it. The sensitivity to fretting corrosion is the main limit of titanium and its alloys for orthopedic applications, especially because the fatigue or simply brittle fractures start very often at the corresponding sites of corrosion.

a. Pure Titanium. The main advantages of commercially pure titanium are:

- very good biocompatibility, especially as far as osseointegration capability is concerned,
- good workability by tool machining,
- possibility of hot plastic deformation.

The disadvantages are:

- low mechanical properties,
- sensitivity to fretting corrosion,
- difficulty of cold plastic deformation.

The Standard ISO 5832-2 provides 4 degrees of commercially pure titanium (degrees 1, 2, 3, and 4,), depending essentially on oxygen content (0.18–0.45%), whose increasing content determines an increase in the mechanical properties (with UTS varying from 240 MPa for degree 1, to 550 MPa for degree 4 annealed, to 680 MPa for degree 4 work hardened), however accompanied by a decrease in elongation and more difficult workability by tool machining.

b. Titanium Alloys. Titanium alloys can be subdivided into three categories according to their structure: one phase of type α (hcp), one phase of type β (bcc), two phases of type $(\alpha + \beta)$. Commercially pure titanium presents, at room temperature, a structure type α, while the more used titanium alloys present a two-phase structure $(\alpha + \beta)$. Materials presenting structure α are more ductile and weldable, but their mechanical properties cannot be increased by thermal treatments, in contrast with the $\alpha + \beta$ alloys. The β alloys are generally characterized by higher mechanical properties, but it is very difficult to work them by plastic deformation.

As far as $\alpha + \beta$ alloys are concerned, the main advantages are:

- high mechanical properties,
- good corrosion resistance (generalized and localized).

The main disadvantages are:

- sensitivity to fretting corrosion,
- biocompatibility less than pure titanium,
- no cold workability,
- difficulties of working by tool machining.

The more used titanium alloy is ISO 5832-2, with composition Ti6Al4V and UTS of 860 MPa, in the annealed state. This can be significantly increased with a thermal treatment of quenching and aging.

In practice, rapid cooling is performed from a temperature at which an $\alpha + \beta$ two-phase structure is stable. This treatment is followed by heating at lower temperature (aging). The rapid cooling rate avoids partial transformation of the β phase that occurs during a slow cooling rate (equilibrium state). The subsequent aging treatment causes the formation of very fine precipitates of α particles dispersed in β matrix. This improves the mechanical properties with respect to an annealed $\alpha + \beta$ structure. The fatigue resistance is the mechanical property that shows the highest improvement.

There is an attempt to substitute vanadium, as many doubts on its biocompatibility have been raised. The following alloys have been introduced: ISO 5832-10 alloys with composition $Ti_5Al_{2.5}Fe$ and ISO 5832-11 alloy with composition Ti_7Al_8Nb. These alloys have very similar characteristics to Ti_6Al_4V, in terms of corrosion resistance and mechanical properties. However, at present they are more expensive and less widespread.

6.8.4. Precious Metal Alloys

Precious metal alloys are very useful for biomedical applications, because they have excellent chemical stability in the oral environment and desirable mechanical properties. They are mainly classified as Au-base and Ag-base alloys in dental materials.

Dental gold alloys for crown and bridge are made by the addition of copper, silver, platinum group metals, and zinc. The role of each element is known as follows. Gold contributes to the color, corrosion resistance, and ductility. Copper contributes to the strength in combination with gold, and also platinum and palladium. Silver is added to the alloy to neutralize the red color afforded by copper. The platinum group metals added to dental gold alloys are platinum, palladium, iridium, and rhodium. Platinum and palladium contribute to an increase in strength. However, the amount of their addition is limited, because they raise the melting point and whiten the color. A small amount of iridium or rhodium plays a role as a grain refiner. Zinc acts as a deoxidizing element. According to International Standard ISO 1562, dental casting gold alloys are classified as Type I, II, III, or IV depending on their gold and platinum group metal contents and their mechanical properties. The composition has at least 65 wt% of gold and at least 75 wt% of gold and platinum group metals. Only Type IV group can be age-hardened.

Two types of alloys are used for a system in which porcelain is fused to metal. The alloys have a coefficient of thermal expansion matched to porcelain The first mainly consists of the noble metals such as gold, platinum, and palladium. Iron, tin, and indium are added to produce hardening and form an oxide layer that bonds with porcelain.

Palladium–silver alloys are the second type, which contain 50–60% palladium, 30–40% silver, and some base metals for hardening. Compared with high gold alloys, these alloys differ with regard to lower density and lower cost. The main problem is a discoloration by silver.

Dental silver alloys are made by palladium, copper, gold, iridium, and zinc. Palladium prevents the sulfide blackening in silver. Copper contributes to the strength in combination with palladium and silver. Gold contributes to the corrosion resistance. Iridium and zinc play a similar role in gold alloys.

The precious metal alloys are characterized not only by good biocompatibility, but also good castability and age-hardenability. Superlattice structures of CuAu I and CuPd are utilized in dental gold and silver alloys, respectively.

In dental gold alloys, corrosion resistance is thought to be controlled by the total amount of precious metals, namely nobility. A two-phase microstructure lowers the corrosion resistance compared with the single-phase alloys. The anodic potentiodynamic polarization curve of the two-phase microstructure can be explained by superimposing the curves of each phase using the principle of additivity. In fact, the potential at which the current density increased significantly corresponds to that of each phase, and the amount of current density is calculated as the summation of each phase in proportion to their volume fractions.

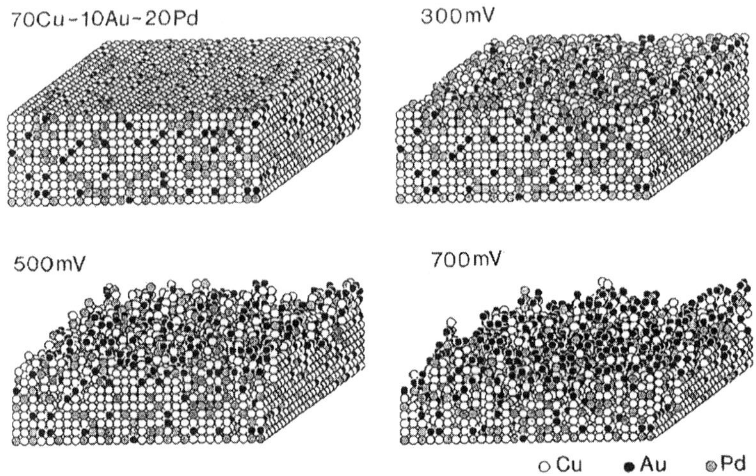

Figure 6.22. Computer simulated picture of anodic dissolution of the Cu-10at%Au-20at%Pd alloy.

In noble metal alloys, preferential or selective dissolution and surface enrichment with noble elements take place if the alloy has a lower potential than that of the anodic reaction of the noble elements. Figure 6.22 shows a result by computer simulation of the anodic dissolution process in a Cu–10 at% Au–20 at% Pd ternary alloy. It can be seen that remarkable dissolution occurs and the surface of the alloy becomes rougher with increasing polarization potential.

7

Degradation Processes on Metallic Surfaces

Emma Angelini, Angelo Caputo, and Fabrizio Zucchi

7.1. Introduction

Metallic materials in contact with physiological fluids are subjected to the aggressive action of organic and inorganic anions. The interaction may result in a tarnishing action with subsequent aesthetic modifications of the device; modification of the surface polishing degree; corrosive attack more or less localized and deep, that leads to a loss of performance or to a failure of a component (Fraker and Griffin, 1985). The specific environment in which these phenomena may occur must be taken into consideration. In certain environments, such as the oral cavity, extremely low limits of the corrosion products may be tolerated. Large amounts of corrosion products may lead to necrosis, cellular modifications, or poisoning.

Notwithstanding the specificity of the environment in which metallic materials are put, the behavior falls within the general phenomenon of metallic corrosion briefly described below.

7.2. The Biological Environment

The biological environment in which biomaterials operate, both the physiological fluids and the saliva, is a rather complex buffered aqueous

---

Emma Angelini • Dipartimento di Scienza dei Materiali ed Ingegneria Chimica, Politecnico di Torino, Corso Duca degli Abruzzi 24, 10129 Torino, Italy. **Angelo Caputo** • Advanced Prosthodontics, Biomimetics and Hospital Dentistry Department, UCLA School of Dentistry, Box 951668, B3-081 CHS, Los Angeles, California 90095-1668, United States. **Fabrizio Zucchi** • Centro Studi Corrosione A. Daccò, Università di Ferrara, Via Luigi Borsari 46, 44100 Ferrara, Italy.

Integrated Biomaterials Science, edited by R. Barbucci. Kluwer Academic/Plenum Publishers, New York, 2002.

medium containing various anions, in addition to chlorides that are prevalent, phosphate and bicarbonate ions, various cations mainly of sodium, potassium, calcium, and magnesium, variable amounts of organic compounds, from low molecular weight species to high molecular weight polymeric species, and finally dissolved oxygen. The pH in normal conditions, i.e., not in the presence of pathological alterations, is buffered in physiological fluids around values of 7.4 and in saliva around values of 6.7.

For *in vitro* tests an extensively utilized electrolyte, which simulates the physiological fluids, is the Ringer's solution, whose chemical composition is the following: 9.00 g NaCl, 0.24 g $CaCl_2$, 0.43 g KCl, 0.20 g $NaHCO_3$, distilled water up to 1 dm^3, while several similar receipts for artificial saliva may be found in the literature (Marek, 1983). A diffused one is the following: 0.25 g KH_2PO_4, 0.26 g Na_2HPO_4, 0.33 g KSCN, 0.70 g NaCl, 1.20 g KCl, 1.50 g $NaHCO_3$, 0,13 g NH_2CONH_2, distilled water up to 1 dm^3 buffered with diluted lactic acid at pH = 6.7.

One of the main obstacles to take into account in the *in vivo* and *in vitro* studies is the inconstancy of the biological environment. With time, with the location of the device, and with the health status of the body, the above-described characteristics may suffer variations in the oxygen level, in the variation of cellular activity with availability of increasing amounts of free radicals, and in the pH value, with the ultimate effect of a change of the aggressivity level versus the metallic devices.

7.3. Metallic Corrosion

The corrosion of metals is either an electrochemical process or a spontaneous chemical process. These processes take place between the metallic materials and the surrounding environment, with a subsequent technological degradation of the materials (Uhlig and Winston Revie, 1984; Bianchi and Mazza, 1989).

Referring to the basic corrosion principles, degradation phenomena may be divided into dry corrosion and wet corrosion.

7.3.1. Dry Corrosion

Dry corrosion occurs in the absence of condensed water at high temperature in the presence of oxygen, following this scheme:

$$2Me + O_2 \rightarrow 2MeO \quad (1)$$

This process depends on temperature, the type of metal or gas of interest, and on the characteristics of the layer of the corrosion products formed. Dry corrosion is not encountered in the usual applications of biomaterials.

7.3.2. Wet Corrosion

Wet corrosion, which takes place when a metal comes into contact with condensed water following different reaction schemes as a function of the pH of the solution, is the most pertinent kind of corrosion related to metallic biomaterials in the biological environment. The overall reactions (2) and (3) that may occur when a metallic surface comes into contact with an aqueous medium are two redox reactions. These reactions may be written as the sum of an anodic oxidation reaction, which yields metallic ions, and a cathodic reduction reaction, in which the electrons so generated are consumed.

In an acidic environment,

$$\begin{array}{ll} Me \rightarrow Me^{2+} + 2e & \text{anodic oxidation} \\ 2H^{+} + 2e \rightarrow H_2 & \text{cathodic reduction} \end{array}$$

$$Me + 2H^{+} \rightarrow Me^{2+} + H_2 \qquad (2)$$

In a neutral environment,

$$\begin{array}{ll} Me \rightarrow Me^{2+} + 2e & \text{anodic oxidation} \\ 1/2O_2 + H_2O + 2e \rightarrow 2OH^{-} & \text{cathodic reduction} \end{array}$$

$$Me + 1/2O_2 + H_2O \rightarrow Me(OH)_2 \qquad (3)$$

As shown, the precise cathodic reaction depends on the nature of the electrolyte, but two of the most important reactions are the reduction of hydrogen or of dissolved oxygen.

It is useful to remember a basic principle of electrochemically based metallic corrosion: in all corrosion processes, the rate of the anodic reaction must equal the rate of the cathodic one; this justifies the attention paid to the above-mentioned possible local variations of the biological environment which can affect dramatically either the anodic or cathodic reactions. The whole corrosion process can be arrested by preventing either of these reactions.

By examining from a thermodynamic point of view the anodic dissolution reaction of a metal in a solution containing its cations, the

Table 7.1. The Electrochemical Series

Metal	Standard electrode potential V (NHE)	Metal	Standard electrode potential V (NHE)
Gold	+1.50	Iron	−0.440
Platinum	+1.20	Gallium	−0.529
Palladium	+0.987	Chromium	−0.744
Mercury	+0.854	Zinc	−0.763
Silver	+0.799	Titanium	−1.63
Copper	+0.337	Aluminum	−1.66
Hydrogen	0.0000	Magnesium	−2.36
Lead	−0.126	Sodium	−2.71
Tin	−0.136	Calcium	−2.87
Nickel	−0.250	Sodium	−2.71
Cobalt	−0.277	Lithium	−3.04

following considerations may be applied. When the metal comes into contact with the solution, a net dissolution reaction occurs since the Gibbs free energy variation ΔG for the dissolution reaction is less than that for the replacement reaction. This leaves the metal with a net negative charge, thus making it harder for the subsequent dissolution reaction and increasing its ΔG. When the ΔG of the two reactions becomes equal, a dynamic equilibrium is reached and a potential difference is set up across the charged double layer surrounding the metal. The potential difference is characteristic of the metal or, in general, of the metallic material, and can be measured against a standard reference electrode. The standard electrode potential for a metal, E_0, is obtained when the measure is done in a solution 1 M of its cations, at 25 °C, against the normal hydrogen electrode (NHE).

The list of the standard electrode potentials, shown in Table 7.1, is called the electrochemical series and may be utilized as a general guide for the reactivity of metallic materials in aqueous solutions. At the top are the noble metals relatively unreactive, while those at the bottom are the more reactive ones. Mostly in the biological environment, characterized by a high complexity, the electrochemical series has to be considered only a first guide to corrosion resistance. For this reason other classifications of reactivity have been attempted, referred, for example, to blood plasma. Coming back to the electrochemical series, in conditions different from the standard ones, the electrode potential at equilibrium is shifted from the standard electrode potential and may be defined by the Nernst equation, in its general form:

$$E = E_0 + RT/nF \ln(a_{\text{anod}}/a_{\text{cathod}}) \tag{4}$$

where E_0 is the standard electrode potential, RT/F is a constant, n is the number of electrons transferred, and a is the activity of the anodic and cathodic reactants, approximable to the concentration (at low concentrations) situation in which a net dissolution of the metal takes place.

Consequently the redox potentials of the oxidation and reduction half reactions involved in the overall reactions (2) and (3) may be evaluated from the Nernst equation applied to the following equilibria at 25 °C:

$$Me^{2+} + 2e \leftrightarrow Me \qquad E_{Me^{2+}Me} = E_0 + 0.059/2 \log[Me^{2+}] \tag{5}$$

$$2H^+ + 2e \leftrightarrow H_2 \qquad E_{H^+/H_2} = E_0 + 0.059 \log[H^+] = -0.059\,pH \tag{6}$$

$$1/2O_2 + H_2O + 2e \leftrightarrow 2OH^- \qquad E_{O_2/OH^-} = E_0 - 0.059\,pH \tag{7}$$

The spontaneity condition of a corrosion process is $E_C > E_A$, where E_C is E_{H^+/H_2}, or E_{O_2/OH^-} and E_A is $E_{Me^{2+}/Me}$, so $\Delta E = E_C - E_A > 0$. Furthermore, remembering that $-\Delta G = nF\Delta E$, it may be observed that the process takes place with a decrease of Gibbs free energy (Bockris and Reddy, 1970).

It is possible to collect all the thermodynamic information about the equilibria that take place when a metal is immersed in an aqueous medium, like the biological environment, in a pH/potential diagram, the so-called Pourbaix diagram (Pourbaix, 1974). In Figure 7.1, lines a and b correspond to equilibria (6) and (7), consequently the area between the two lines is the field of stability of water. In the area under line a, water reduction by hydrogen evolution occurs, and up the line b, oxidation of water by oxygen evolution occurs.

The equilibrium potential of reaction (5), $E_{Me^{2+}/Me} = E_0 + 0.059/2 \log[Me^{2+}]$, will be represented by a line parallel to the abscissa and shifted more and more in the negative direction with respect to E_0 as a function of the decrease in the Me^{2+} concentration; when $[Me^{2+}] < 10^{-6}$ M the corrosion process stops. By increasing the pH value, the solubility product K_{ps} of the hydroxide may be reached:

$$Me^{2+} + 2OH^- \leftrightarrow Me(OH)_2 \qquad K_{ps} = [Me^{2+}]\cdot[OH^-]^2 \tag{8}$$

On the Pourbaix diagram this equilibrium is represented as a line perpendicular to the abscissa, and depends only on the pH value, not on the

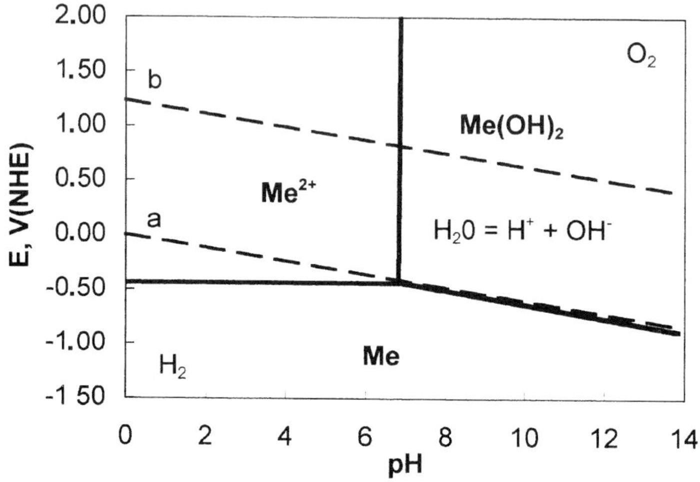

Figure 7.1. Pourbaix diagram of a metal showing the equilibrium hydrogen/water, line a, and water/oxygen, line b, at 25 °C.

potential value. At pH values higher than the equilibrium one, also the line representative of the equilibrium (5) shifts as a function of pH, because of the decrease in $[Me^{2+}]$ due to the shift of equilibrium (8) vs. the hydroxide formation.

Assuming a protective action of the solid corrosion products, the E/pH diagram of a metal may be divided into the following regions:

1. *Immunity region*, where only the reduced metal is thermodynamically stable, so the metal cannot undergo corrosion phenomena.
2. *Corrosion regions*, where the soluble forms (metallic ions, anions) are stable.
3. *Passivity zone*, where the thermodynamic conditions of corrosion exist, but the corrosion rate is extremely low for kinetic control of the corrosion products and may be considered negligible.

The Pourbaix diagrams furnish useful information on the behavior of metals in aqueous media, but they have to be considered with caution when choosing a metallic material for biomedical applications. While the immunity region may be detected with accuracy, the borders of the regions of corrosion and passivity may be changed by kinetic hindrances or by metastability conditions.

7.3.3. Kinetics

The rate of the corrosion process may be determined from knowledge of the kinetics of the cathodic and anodic processes. Consider hydrogen and oxygen reduction.

a. Hydrogen Reduction. In this case, the metal on which the H^+ reduction takes place has a noticeable influence on the kinetics. As a matter of fact, at the equilibrium potential of the reaction of equation (6), the reduction reaction rate equals the oxidation rate. By applying Faraday's laws and transforming the mass into current, it can be seen that $i_c = i_a = i_0$, where i_0 is the exchange current. The i_0 values for the equilibrium of equation (6) range from 10^{-12} A/cm^2 for mercury to 10^{-3} A/cm^2 for platinated platinum. Shifting the potential from E_0 in the positive or negative direction we can shift the equilibrium of equation (6) to oxidation or to reduction. The shift of the equilibrium potential is indicated as overpotential η, which is related to the current density through the Tafel law:

$$\eta = a + b \log i \tag{9}$$

Plotting in a semilogarithmic diagram, the current density i_c vs. the overpotential η lines with a slope of 0.1 V per decade may be obtained. The reduction of hydrogen ion is controlled by activation.

b. Oxygen Reduction. This process is controlled by diffusion processes; oxygen is a gas whose solubility in water or electrolytic solutions is 8–10 μg/l. Going far from the equilibrium potential, after a small range in which the Tafel law is followed because of the low oxygen concentration, all the oxygen that arrives on the metal is instantaneously reduced. The reduction rate, expressed as current density, is not a function of the overpotential, but of the oxygen diffusion rate in the electrolyte. The current density in these conditions is i_L, the limit diffusion current:

$$i_L = nFCD/\delta \tag{10}$$

where C is the oxygen concentration in the bulk solution, D is the oxygen diffusion coefficient, and δ is the limit diffusion layer, i.e., the liquid layer between the electrode surface with null oxygen concentration and the solution where the oxygen concentration is C.

From equation (10) it can be seen that i_L may increase by increasing the oxygen concentration, the diffusion coefficient, or by decreasing δ, changing the hydrodynamic conditions of the electrolyte. In a $E/\log i$ plot, the oxygen reduction reaction has the shape shown in Figure 7.2.

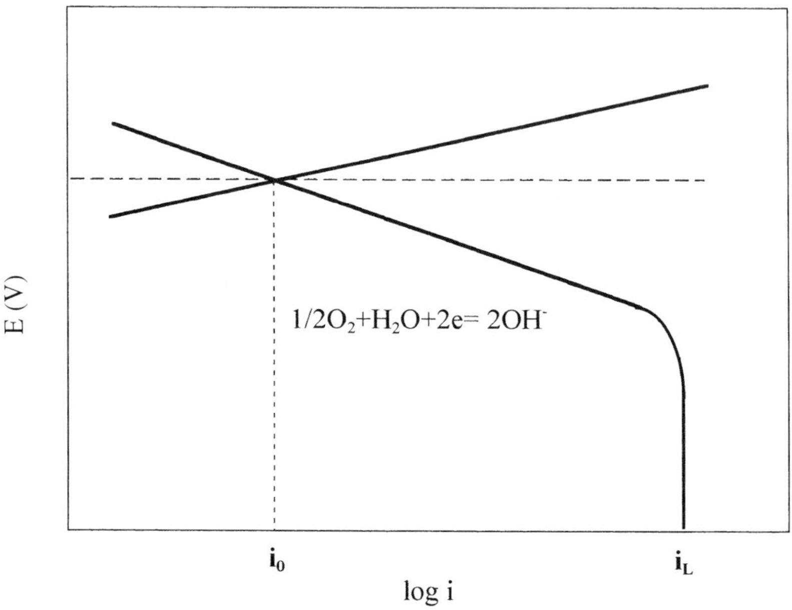

Figure 7.2. Oxygen reduction reaction on a metallic surface in neutral or alkaline solution.

c. Metal Oxidation Reaction. The shape of the oxidation reaction of all metals with low overpotential values is similar and follows the Tafel law. For some metals or alloys, by increasing the anodic current density (η_A) we reach a maximum value, the critical passivation current (i_{cr}), which then decreases abruptly and stabilizes at very low values. This value corresponds to the passivation current density i_p. The current density is independent of the overpotential, in a certain range, due to the formation of protective oxides which leads to the passivation of the metal. If the oxides possess insulating properties or low electronic conductivity, such as Al, Ti, Ta, and Zr oxides, the passive state is maintained until high potential values are reached. If the formed oxides possess electronic conductivity, or may be transformed into soluble oxides, the passive zone is followed by a transpassive one. Here, metal dissolution may take place in addition to water oxidation with oxygen evolution (Figure 7.3).

The current and potential values that characterize the anodic polarization curve of a material with an active–passive behavior are i_{cr}, i_p, E_{pp}, and E_{trans}. The wider the potential range between E_{pp} and E_{trans}, the more negative E_{pp} and the lower the i_{cr} value, the higher the passivation tendency of the metal.

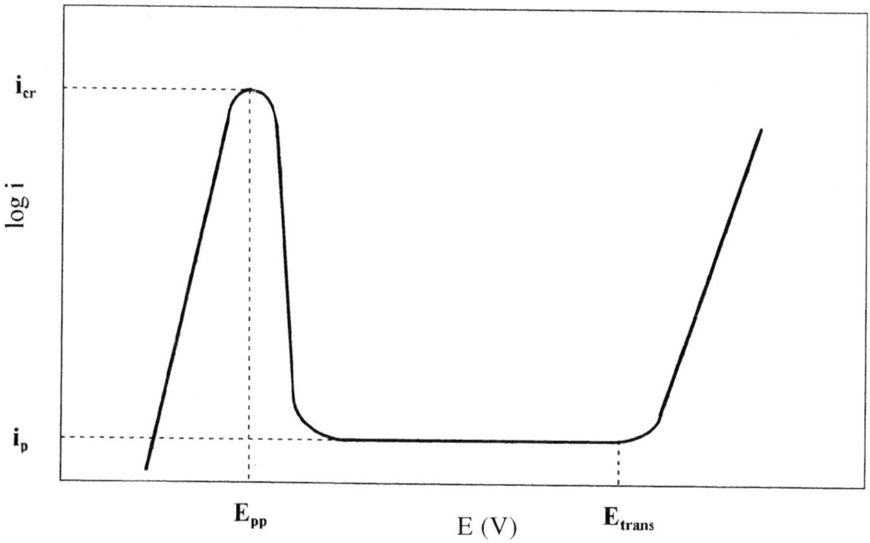

Figure 7.3. Potentiodynamic anodic polarization curve for a passivable metallic surface.

Let us examine again the overall corrosion process, taking into account a metal immersed in a HCl 1 N solution. The metal dissolves, $Me \rightarrow Me^{2+} + 2e$, and simultaneously gas bubbles detach from the metal surface, $2H^{+} + 2e \leftrightarrow H_2$.

A metal in a solution containing its ions has the following reversible potential:

$$E_{\text{rev A}} = E_0 + 0.059/2 \log [Me^{2+}] \tag{11}$$

On the metal the equilibrium (6) also may be established with the following potential: $E_{\text{rev C}} = E_0 + 0.059 \log[H^{+}]$. The metal is an electron conductor, consequently no accumulation or loss of electrons on the metal may occur, and the metal has a potential value intermediate between $E_{\text{rev A}}$ and $E_{\text{rev C}}$. The corrosion potential E_{corr} for satisfying the above-mentioned conditions should be the potential at which $i_A = i_C = i_{\text{corr}}$, as in Figure 7.4 it is clearly shown that only at E_{corr} does i_C equal i_A; all the electrons of the oxidation reaction are used in the reduction reaction. If in the solution the reduction reaction involves two species, E_{corr} will coincide with the point at which the sum of the cathodic currents equals the anodic current.

It is possible to hypothesize that useful information on the reaction rate cannot be obtained only from the thermodynamic conditions ($\Delta E = E_C - E_A > 0$).

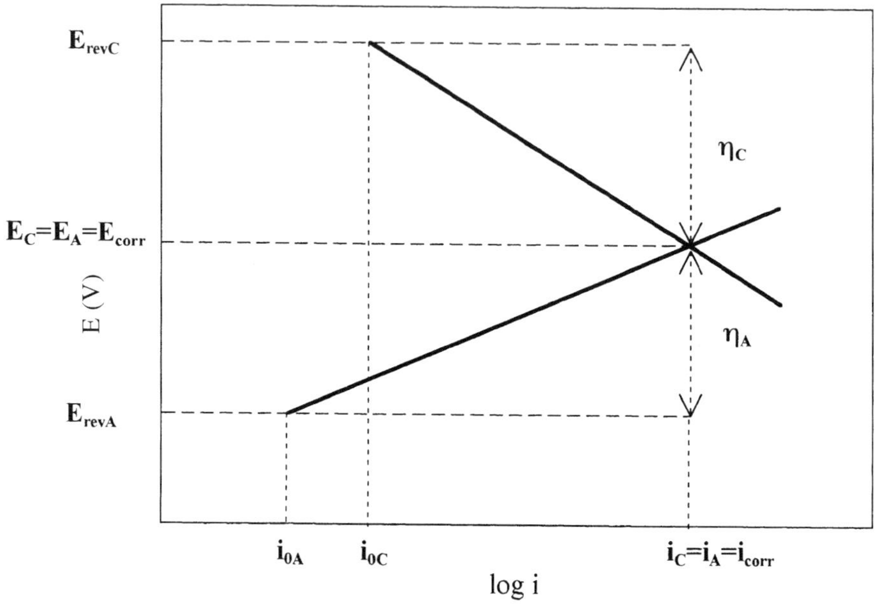

Figure 7.4. Polarization diagram illustrating the mixed potential theory.

As an example, Figure 7.5a shows a $E/\log i$ diagram for a zinc sheet immersed in HCl 1 N solution, with $[Zn^{2+}] = 1$ M. Figure 7.5b shows an analogous situation with an iron sheet immersed in HCl 1 N solution, with $[Fe^{2+}] = 1$ M. The corrosion rate, expressed as i_{corr}, is lower for zinc with respect to iron because of the difference of i_0 for H^+ reduction on the two metals, notwithstanding the fact that ΔE for Zn is 0.77 V(NHE) and for Fe it is 0.44 V(NHE).

The mixed potential theory illustrates the corrosion process: it is assumed that the whole surface behaves simultaneously as cathode and anode, making it impossible to distinguish between anodic and cathodic areas. However, cathodic and anodic regions may differentiate because of solution inhomogeneity, differences in flux rate, and metallurgical conditions. In these cases the corrosion process may be better illustrated with the theory of short circuit galvanic elements. In a short circuit galvanic element, all the free energy at our disposal is dissipated as heat, partially as cathodic and anodic overpotential and partially as ohmic decay:

$$\Delta E = (E_{\text{rev C}} - \eta_C) - (E_{\text{rev A}} - \eta_A) + iR \tag{12}$$

where η_A and η_C are the anodic and cathodic overpotentials, i is the current density, and R the solution resistance.

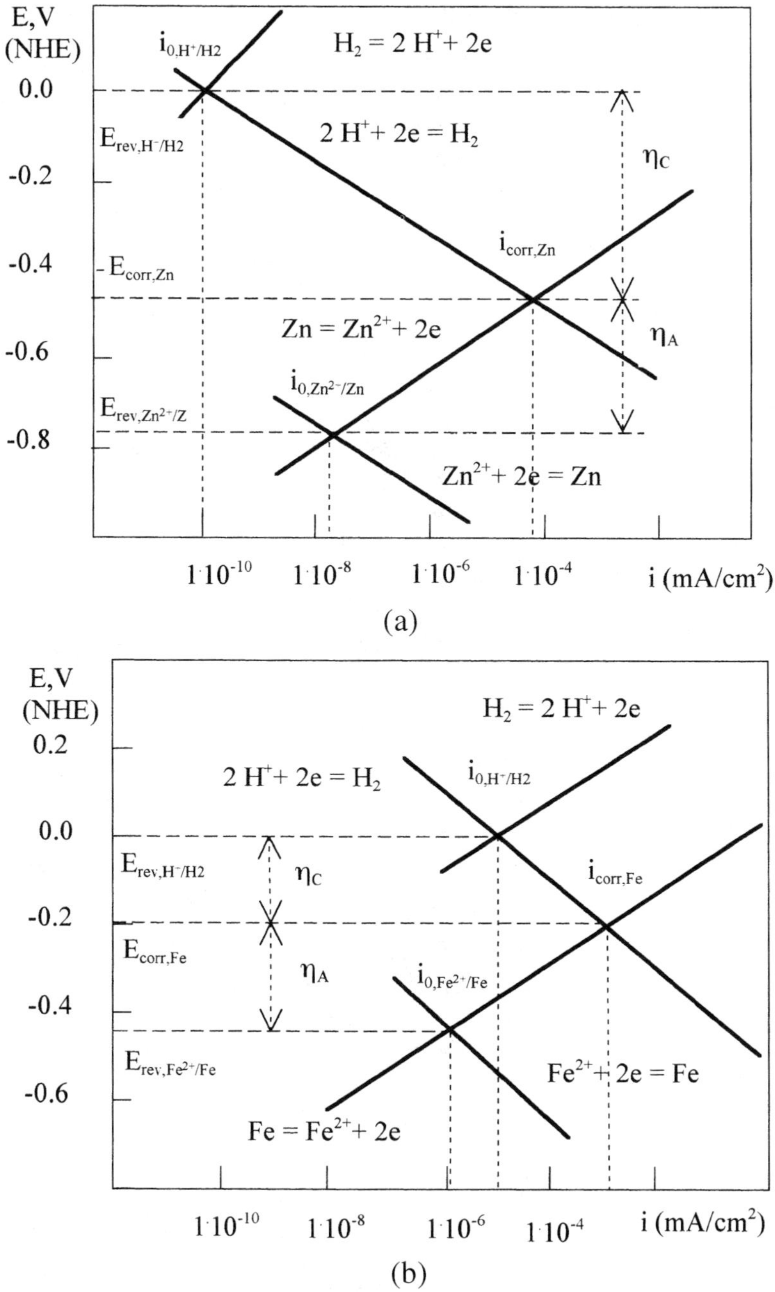

Figure 7.5. Corrosion process of zinc (a) and iron (b) in acid solution.

7.3.4. Influence of the Biological Environment

The prediction of the corrosion resistance of a metal in an aqueous medium may be done in theory from the standard electrode potential values listed in the electrochemical series. Also, if the nobility of some metals and the reactivity of others may be explained, unfortunately in practice information on the occurrence of corrosion of most metallic systems in the biological environment cannot be derived in this way.

As a matter of fact, the corrosion resistance of many metallic systems is determined by their tendency to passivation, i.e., to build up, when in contact with an electrolyte, an oxide layer which protects the underlying metal.

Reasonably, it may be assumed that in the biological environment the corrosion mechanisms discussed above are still valid, also if the presence of biological macromolecules may influence the rate of the corrosion processes by interfering with the anodic and/or cathodic reactions described. For example, proteins may bind to metal ions coming from the anodic dissolution of an implanted metallic device and transport them away from the surface, decreasing ΔG for the dissolution reaction.

The absorption of proteins onto the surface of metallic materials could limit the oxygen diffusion to certain areas of the device surface, thus causing preferential corrosion of the oxygen-deficient zones and leading to a breakdown of the passive layer.

Bacteria grown in the vicinity of an implant could utilize the hydrogen coming from the cathodic reaction, thus depressing the inhibiting action of the presence of hydrogen itself on the prosecution of active corrosion.

Although from an electrochemical point of view several studies have shown that parameters such as the electrode potential, the polarization behavior, the current density at fixed potentials, etc., of several metallic systems are not influenced noticeably by the presence of proteins in the electrolyte, the evaluation of the corrosion rate of metallic devices by means of weight loss measurements and analysis of the electrolyte has revealed significant differences in the presence of low protein concentration, from high increases to slight decreases as dependent on the operative conditions.

7.4. Corrosion Forms

Corrosion on a metallic surface in contact with an electrolyte may assume different forms as a function of the metallurgical and environmental conditions, all causing in some way the loss of structural integrity of the material, of volume, and function (Marcus and Oudar, 1995).

7.4.1. Generalized Corrosion

The attack develops on the overall metallic surface in a more or less uniform way. This attack is typical of metals in acid environments or of nonpassive metals in natural environments, such as atmosphere, soil, waters. Generalized corrosion is rarely encountered with biomaterials; it may be avoided thanks to the previous choice of the material in order to assure minimal corrosion, and because of the characteristics of the biological environment, an almost neutral buffered electrolyte.

7.4.2. Localized Corrosion

A much more insidious corrosion form in the biological environment is the localized corrosion, which may assume, as shown below, different shapes such as pits and intergranular or transgranular cracks (Sedriks, 1996). In this form of corrosion the surface of the anodic zones is smaller than the surface of the cathodic zones where the oxygen reduction generally takes place. These degradation processes are not necessarily continuous and the rate may either increase or decrease with time, depending largely on local and temporal variations in microstructure and environment, but metal ions are released anyway in the environment around the metallic device. This is particularly important with biomaterials, since the ultimate effect of these potentially toxic and irritant ions is the most important consequence of their employment in the human body.

7.4.2.1. Pitting Corrosion

This type of attack takes place on metals covered by passive layers in the presence of aggressive anions, like chlorides. This situation is rather frequent in the field of biomaterials because passivated metals are extensively used in the body instead of noble metals of high cost and relatively poor mechanical properties and the biological environment, as shown before, is rich in chlorides.

In particular these anions act deleteriously on the anodic polarization curve of passivable metals (Figure 7.3); the critical passivation current (i_{cr}) and passivation current density (i_p) are increasing, while the potential range of the passive zone is reducing, thereby decreasing the value of the transpassivity potential, E_{trans}. As an example Figure 7.6 shows the polarization curves of a stainless steel passivated by the chromium oxide that forms on the surface, in a deaerated environment, without chlorides (the lower curve) and with increasing chlorides contents. By increasing the chlorides concentration, E_{trans}, also called the pitting potential or breaking potential,

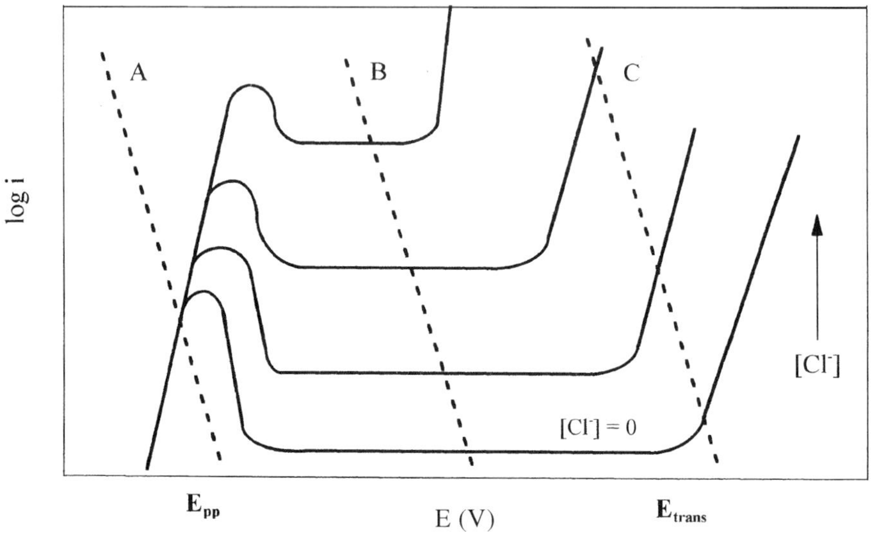

Figure 7.6. Typical polarization curves for a stainless steel in a sulfuric acid solution containing increasing amounts of chlorides; A, B, and C are three different cathodic processes.

decreases. Moreover, in addition to the presence of chlorides, in order for pitting corrosion to occur, it is necessary that there be the onset of a cathodic process that stabilizes the potential at values higher than E_{trans}. Among the three cathodic processes A, B, and C, only the last one will lead to the breakdown of the passive film and subsequently to pitting formation. This kind of corrosion is characterized by an onset period followed by a growing period. During the onset period, the chlorides damage the passive layer corresponding to grain boundaries, dislocations, inclusions, hardening zones, etc. The layer will not repassivate and these localized spots will actively corrode and pits will form on the surface of the material. The oxygen reduction, which can take place on the passive oxide layer, leads to an alkalinization that ameliorates the passive film. The solution inside the pit increases its concentration in metallic ions and induces an influx of chlorides. Similar to crevice corrosion, discussed below, the growing rate of pits is accelerated by hydrolysis of acid salts; the pH value of the solution inside a pit is 1–2, while the electrolyte has a pH value of 7–8. The pit growth mechanism is summarized in the scheme of Figure 7.7.

Figure 7.8 shows the cross section of a pit grown on the surface of a stainless steel implantable device after exposure to Ringer's solution.

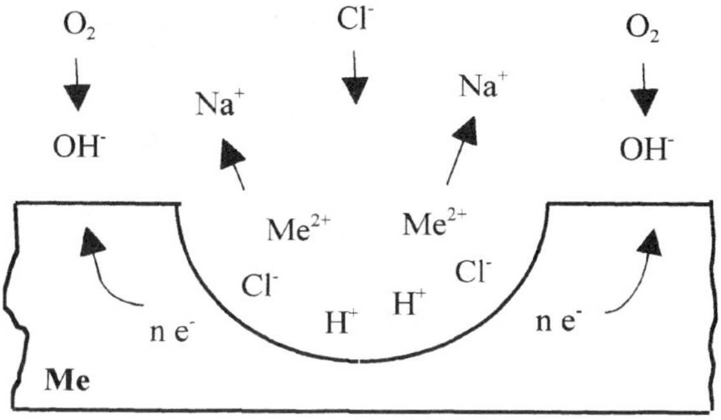

Figure 7.7. Schematic illustration of the pit growth mechanism.

7.4.2.2. Intergranular Corrosion

This corrosive attack occurs in a localized form on the grain boundaries of a sensitized alloy, such as stainless steels used extensively in the biomaterials field, as said before, in an electrolyte of medium aggressivity, as the biological environment itself. It is again a situation not so rarely observed

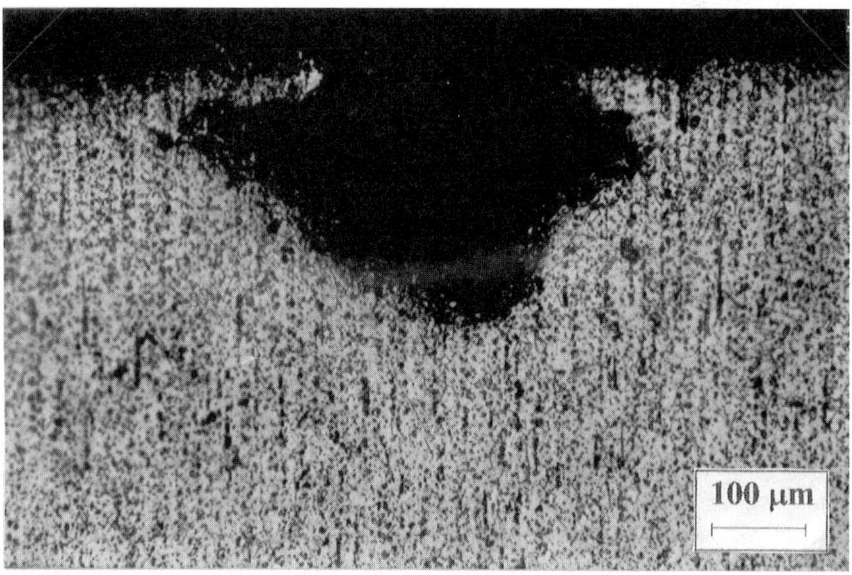

Figure 7.8. Cross section of a stainless steel implantable device showing a pit grown after exposure of the alloy to Ringer's solution at 37 °C.

on retrieved implants and may cause severe problems, since once initiated it will proceed rapidly and may cause the fracture of the implant and the release of large amounts of corrosion products in the surrounding tissues.

Sensitization is a heat treatment which causes precipitation of different phases on the grain boundaries and consequently induces a modification of the alloy composition near the precipitates. The grain center remains passive, while the grain boundary is in an active condition.

Austenitic stainless steels, when aged between 450 and 850 °C, for example in welding procedures, suffer intergranular corrosion, because of the precipitation on the grain boundaries of chromium carbides, $M_{23}C_6$. The diffusion coefficient of Cr is lower than that of C, causing the zones surrounding the carbides to become depleted in Cr. The passivity of the surface of stainless steels is guaranteed by a Cr content of at least 12%, while in the regions surrounding carbides the Cr content decreases to 5%. This zone has a thickness of a few microns. If a sensitized stainless steel is exposed to an aggressive environment, the zone depleted in Cr is active and easily corrodes, while the grain center is passive. The attack proceeds very quickly in the interior of the alloy, involving a little amount of the alloy itself.

Sensitization may be inhibited by reducing the C content under 0.03%, or by adding elements like Ti, Nb, or Ta which have greater affinity for C than for Cr.

Figure 7.9 shows an example of intergranular corrosion attacks on a partial denture framework after 30 days immersion in Ringer's solution (Angelini *et al.*, 1988).

7.4.2.3. Crevice Corrosion

Crevice corrosion occurs in zones where there is a limited recycling of the electrolyte, such as in crevices due to geometric conditions, at the contact between two surfaces, in the porosity of welds, or in crevices due to the deposition of corrosion products. Crevice corrosion takes place on passive metals immersed in electrolytic solutions, and is characterized by an onset period followed by a growing period.

In the biomaterials field, crevice corrosion may occur in diverse locations with implants: between screws and fixation plates, between metals and plastic devices, and between metallic devices and hard and soft tissues. It may occur also in the mouth. In the presence of the electrolyte saliva there are several possibilities for the onset of crevice corrosion phenomena: in contact areas between partial fixed or removable dental prostheses and the residual teeth at which the denture is fixed, or at the other systems of fixation.

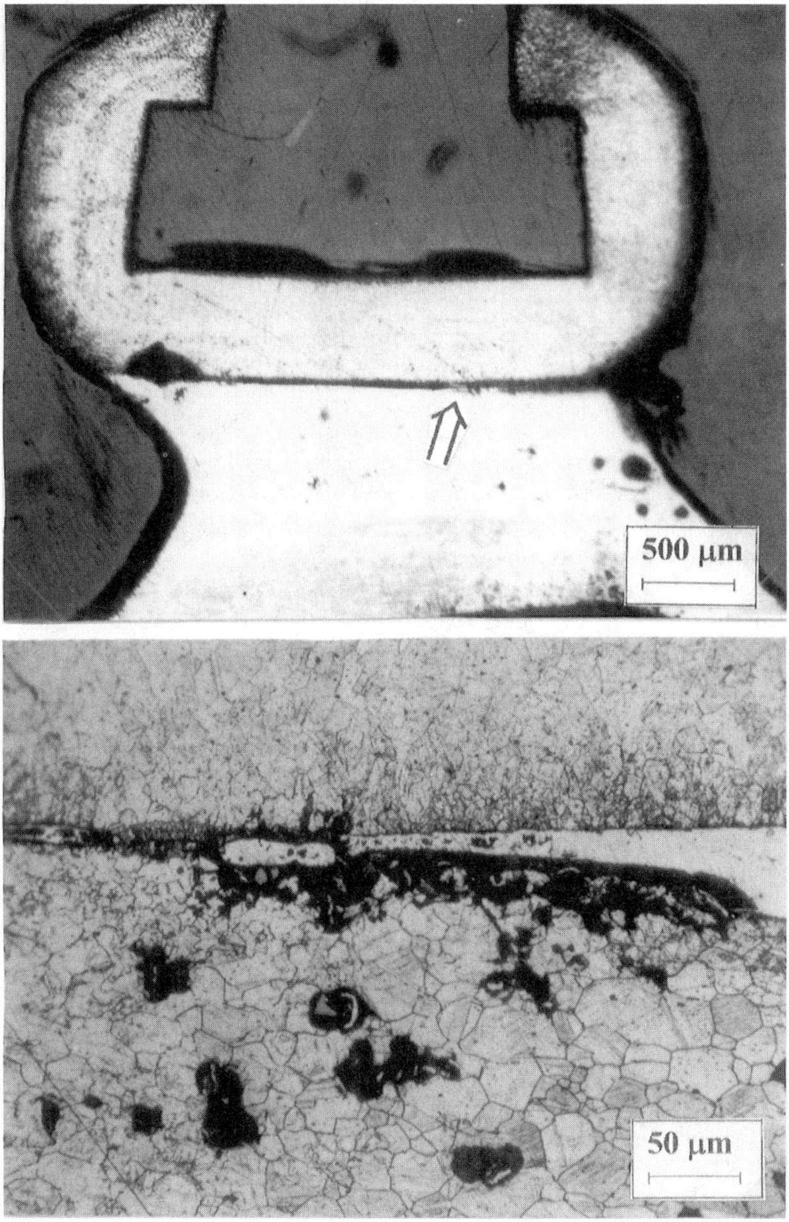

Figure 7.9. Intergranular corrosion attacks on a partial denture framework after 30 days immersion in Ringer's solution at 37 °C.

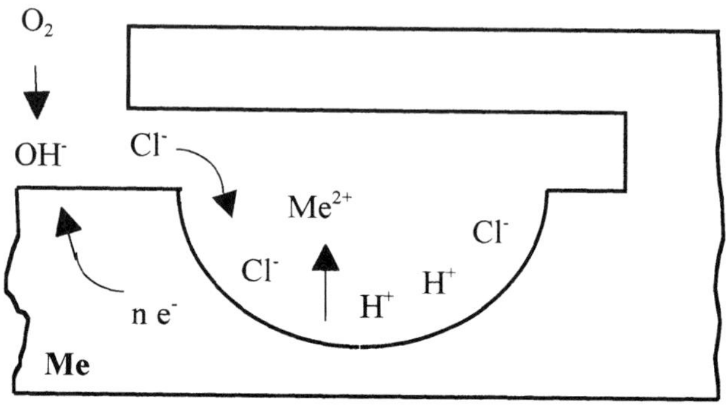

Figure 7.10. Schematic illustration of the crevice corrosion mechanism.

This kind of corrosion may be explained by looking at the working mechanism of a differential aeration cell. If a portion of a metal surface becomes depleted of oxygen, it becomes anodic, while the zone where the oxygen arrives freely becomes cathodic. Figure 7.10 shows a scheme of the crevice corrosion mechanism working in a NaCl aerated solution. Initially the anodic reaction of metal oxidation (2) and the cathodic reaction of oxygen reduction (3) occur uniformly over the surface, including the crevice. If the crevice is narrow enough, only a small quantity of the solution is inside and rather quickly becomes totally depleted of oxygen. Because solution recycling is hindered and because of oxygen diffusion, only the anodic reaction may occur on the metal surface in the interior of the crevice. On the external surface, where the oxygen arrives, the cathodic reaction causes an increase in pH of the solution which becomes alkaline, and consequently increases the stability of the passive film.

The metallic ions migrate from the interior of the crevice to the exterior and precipitate as hydroxides, thereby hindering a change of the solution. Moreover, the build-up of metal ions within the crevice causes the influx of chloride ions to balance the charge by forming metal chlorides. The crevice corrosion has overcome the onset period and is in the growing step. In the presence of water the chlorides of the transition metals (Fe, Cr, Ni) hydrolyze and produce an acidic solution. The decrease in pH and the high concentration of aggressive anions hinder the surface repassivation inside the crevice. This is a rapidly accelerating process.

The parameters affecting the crevice corrosion are the passive film stability, the conductivity of the solution, the hydrodynamic conditions, and the crevice dimensions.

Figure 7.11 shows a crevice grown on an orthopedic screw, in contact with a fracture fixation plate.

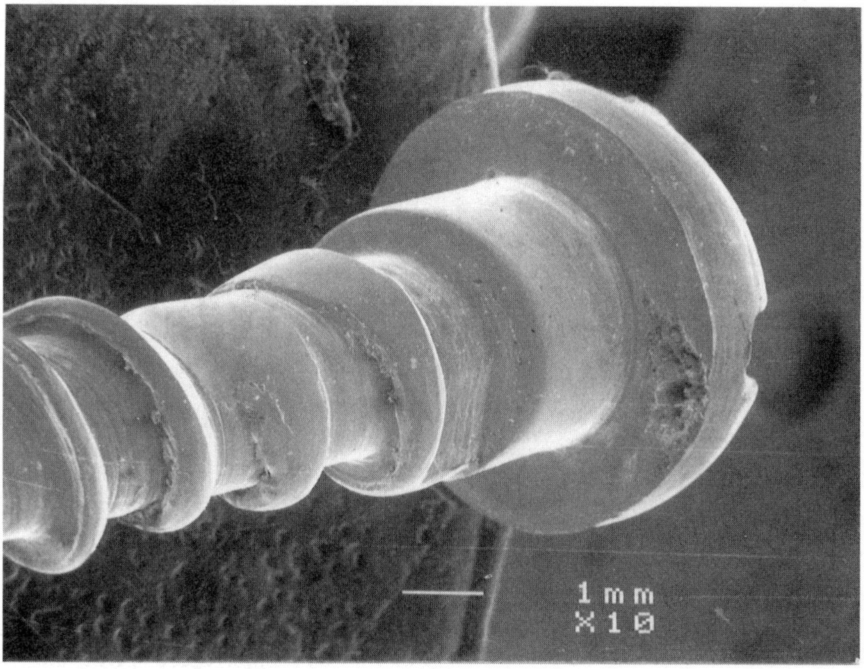

Figure 7.11. Example of crevice corrosion on an orthopedic screw in contact with a fracture fixation plate.

7.4.2.4. Stress Corrosion Cracking

An applied stress and a corrosive environment can work together to cause the complete failure of a component, when neither stress nor the environment alone would damage the material. Different alloys suffer stress corrosion cracking (SCC) in specific environments, for example, austenitic stainless steels in chlorides, ferritic stainless steels in the presence of hydrogen sulfide, carbon steels in nitrate solutions, and copper alloys in ammonia solutions.

In the field of biomaterials this form of corrosion is particularly insidious for stainless steel devices for orthopedic application that, implanted in the body, are subjected to mechanical stresses in the biological environment rich in chlorides.

Stress corrosion cracking cannot be explained by only one mechanism: two models have been developed. In accordance with the first model, the combined action of stress and environment leads to a breakdown of the passive film, giving rise to the onset of a crack. Under the action of the stress, the microscopic crack tip remains active, while the crack walls repassivate, because of the lack of stress. In the second model, the reaction between the crack tip and the solution leads to hydrogen evolution. Hydrogen is partially adsorbed by the surrounding metal which becomes brittle and breaks mechanically, layer by layer, until the complete failure of the device. Stress corrosion cracking may take place under the action of applied loads or because of residual internal stresses due to cold working. Generally the environments are of medium aggressivity, allowing most of the metallic surface and the crack wall to remain passive.

In stress corrosion cracking the onset period can be long, while the crack growth can be very rapid and lead to a catastrophic failure of the component, whose life depends on the onset time and on the toughness of the material. Figure 7.12 shows the result of SCC on a hip prosthesis of stainless steel.

7.4.2.5. Fatigue Corrosion

Another potential source for implanted devices may be fatigue corrosion, due to the combined action of an aggressive environment and of an applied cyclic stress that causes the onset of a series of cracks perpendicular to the applied stress. The cracks originate from surface defects: mechanical ones such as roughness and low polishing, or corrosive ones such as pits and fretting zones. On a fracture surface due to fatigue corrosion, a corroded zone appears. This zone is characterized by more or less evident strips, caused by intermittent growth of cracks. Further, this zone is a function of the applied load and by a zone of mechanical fracture, more or less wide depending upon the toughness of the metal. The influence of the environment is not so specific as in the previous case, because application of a variable load facilitates the mechanical breakdown of the passivated film. Fatigue resistance of the material is dramatically lowered in the presence of an aggressive medium; the corrosive action overlaps the mechanical action and is inversely proportional to the frequency of the applied load. Figure 7.13 a,b,c shows an example of fatigue corrosion on a stainless steel intra-femoral nail.

7.4.3. Galvanic Corrosion

Galvanic corrosion takes place when two different metals are in electric contact by means of an electrolyte. The corrosion potential of the metal, E_{corr}, is taken as reference potential, not the standard reduction potential, E_0, because several metals passivate in aqueous solution. In the passive state, E_{corr} is much more positive than E_0.

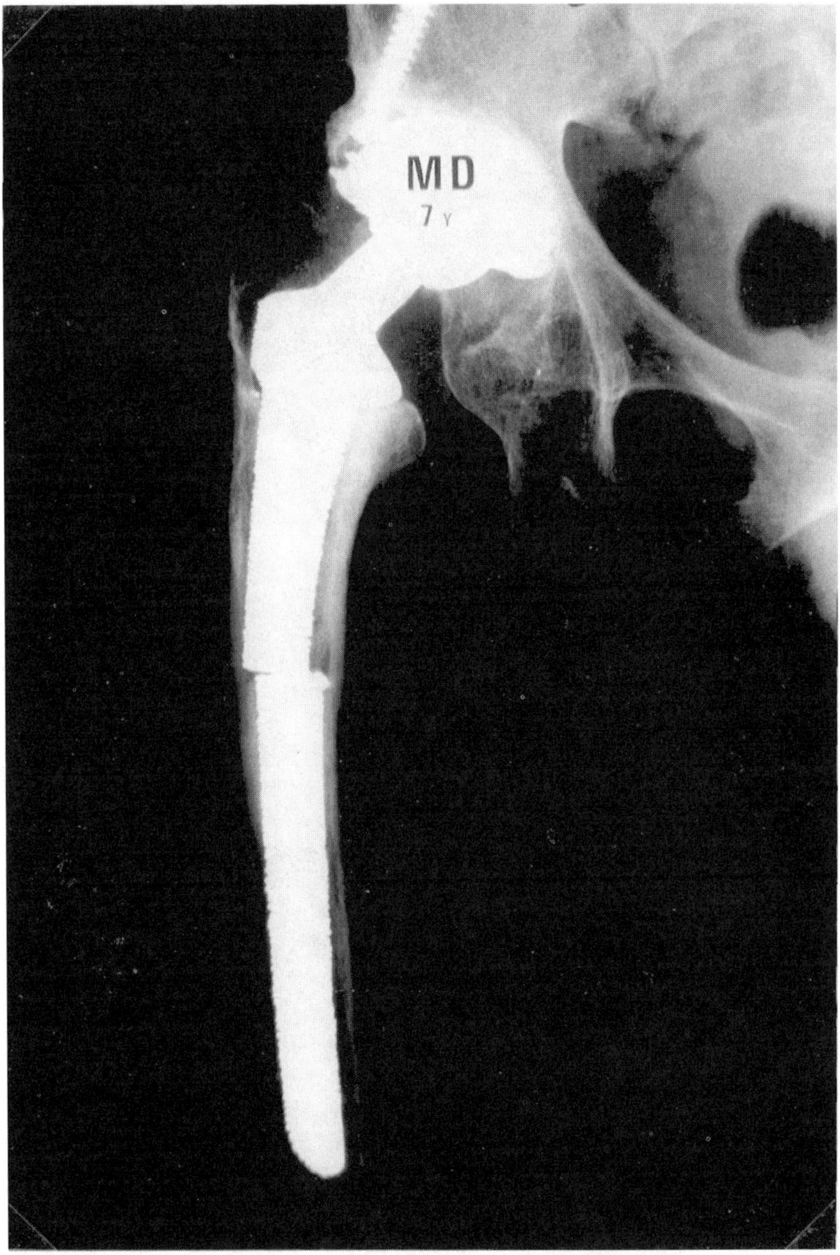

Figure 7.12. Stress corrosion cracking on a hip prosthesis of stainless steel.

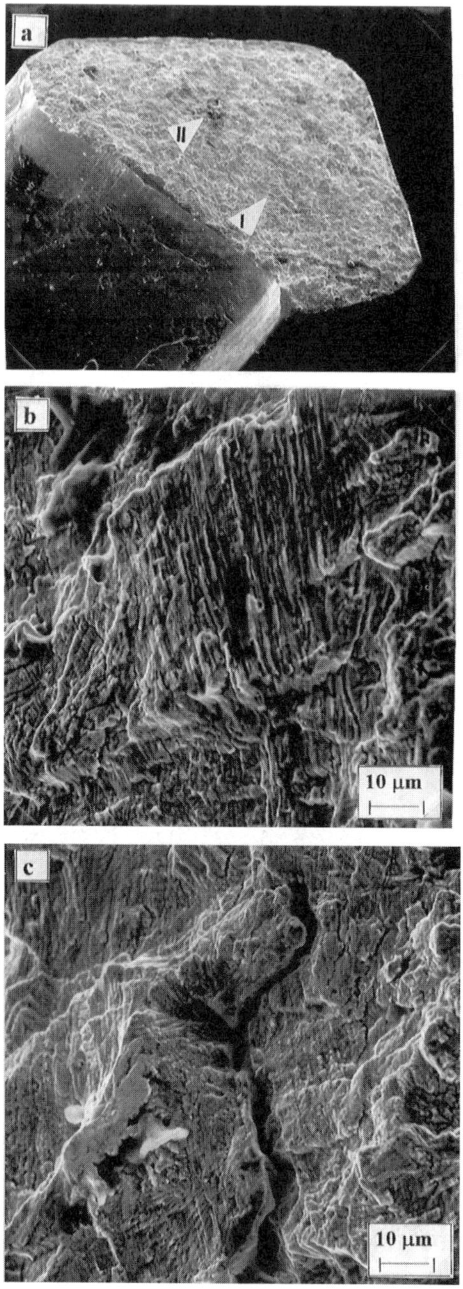

Figure 7.13. Fatigue corrosion on a stainless steel intrafemoral nail (a), SEM micrographs of areas I (b) and II (c).

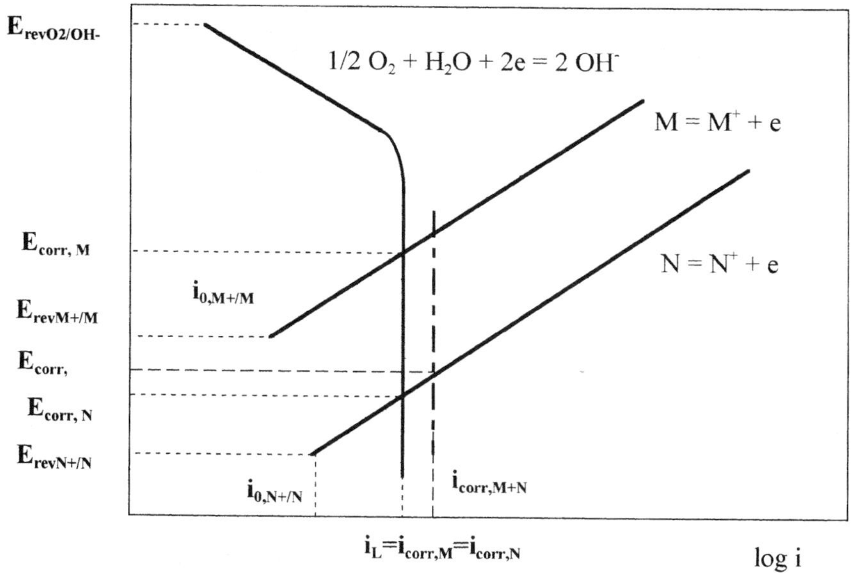

Figure 7.14. Short-circuited galvanic element in neutral solution with complete protection of the nobler metal.

For example, Cr and Ti show E_0 values more negative than Fe, but they easily passivate and the passivated layer is extremely resistant and protective. The reason lies in the fact that their E_{corr} are more positive than that for iron. Generally, E_{corr} of stainless steels in the active state are more negative than in the passive state.

The mixed potential theory allows one to explain the galvanic corrosion phenomena. Figure 7.14 shows an example of two metals M and N, with M nobler than N, in a neutral solution. The cathodic process is oxygen reduction under diffusion control. Conditions of total protection of the nobler metal occur. The reversible potential $E_{M^+/M}$ is more positive than the mixed potential, $E_{corr,M+N}$ so the oxidation reaction of M cannot take place. In these conditions M will act only as a cathodic area in the short-circuit element constituted by M + N and the electrolyte. On N both anodic and cathodic reactions will occur.

Other important parameters are the different areas of the short-circuited metals (the current density is higher on the lower area), the ΔE between the metals, and the conductivity of the solution (the higher the conductivity, the lower the ohmic decay).

This kind of corrosion may be observed in the human body if two different alloys are used in an implantable device when the more reactive may corrode freely; whenever stainless steel is coupled with another alloy it will suffer from galvanic corrosion. If both the alloys remain within their passive region when coupled in this way the additional corrosion may be minimal: some modular orthopedic systems are made of titanium alloys and cobalt base alloys, on the basis that both should remain passive.

Galvanic corrosion may also take place in the oral cavity where at various times different restoration materials (amalgams, gold bridges, non-precious alloy crowns, etc.) may be utilized and come into contact through the electrolyte saliva.

7.4.4. Selective Corrosion

Polyphasic alloys, with noticeable compositional differences among the various phases, may suffer corrosive attacks on the less noble phases, which is worsened by galvanic coupling with the more noble ones. For example, amalgam restorations exhibit this kind of corrosion in oral fluids. Figure 7.15 a,b shows a mercury dental amalgam after 30 days immersion in artificial saliva at 37 °C, together with the X-ray map for tin. A selective corrosion of the various phases present in the restorative material is observed (Zucchi and Angelini, 1982; Marek, 1983). The spheres of the quaternary Ag–Cu–Sn–In phase are partially covered by tin corrosion products reprecipitated.

7.4.5. Wear Corrosion

Wear corrosion occurs when two surfaces of the same material, or of different materials (metallic, polymeric, ceramic), in contact under load move with respect to each other in an aggressive medium. The passive layer is removed by the mechanical process and, moreover, if the process is continuous and cyclic, any reformed passive layer is continuously removed and the corrosion rate is high. In magnetically retained overdentures, the couple's magnet-keeper experiences biomechanical stresses during mastications (Angelini *et al.*, 1991). Figure 7.16a shows the surface of a stainless steel cap of the magnet Sm–Co, after 30 days of continuous wear in artificial saliva in the apparatus shown in Figure 7.16b.

7.5. Corrosion Prevention

Corrosion prevention may be achieved by modifications to the environment or to the metallic materials themselves. Modification of the environment by the addition of inhibitors is difficult to perform on biomaterials

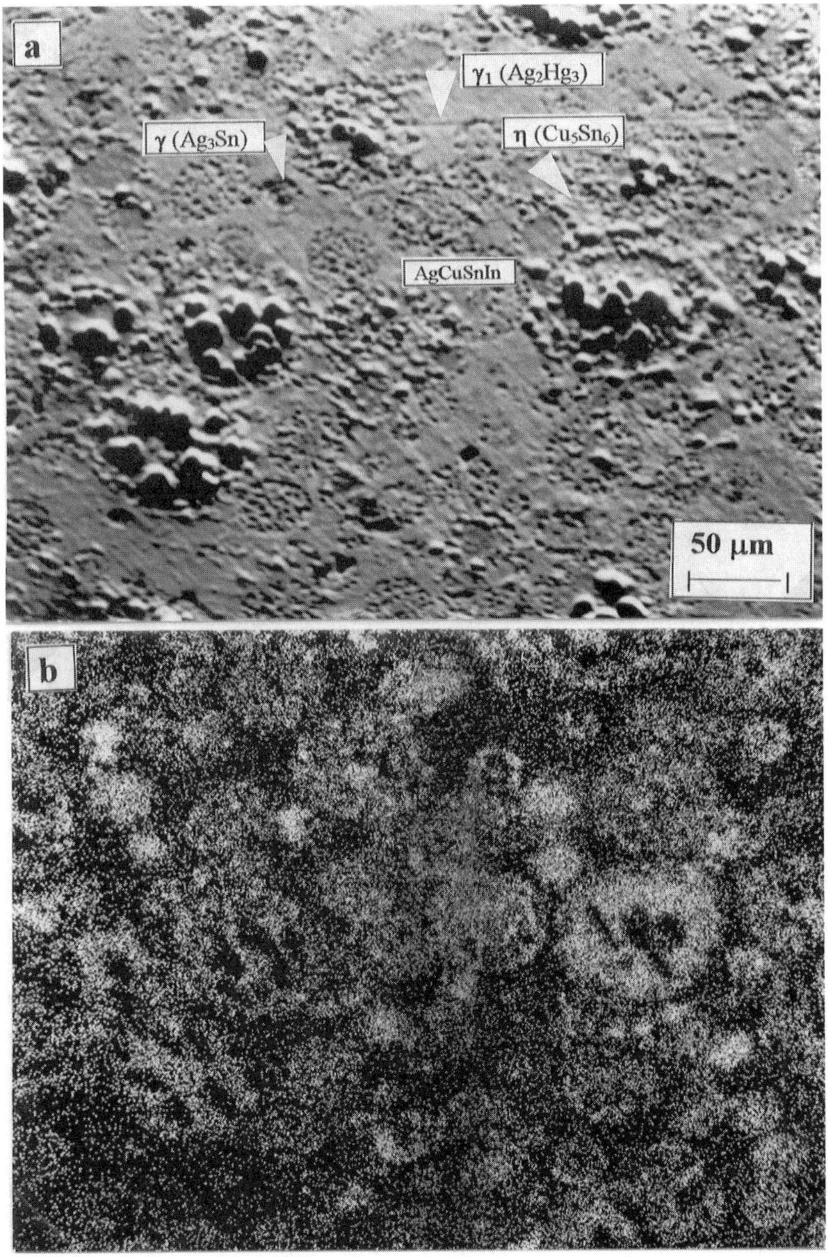

Figure 7.15. Backscattered electron micrograph (a) of a mercury dental amalgam after 30 days immersion in artificial saliva at 37 °C and X-ray map for tin (b).

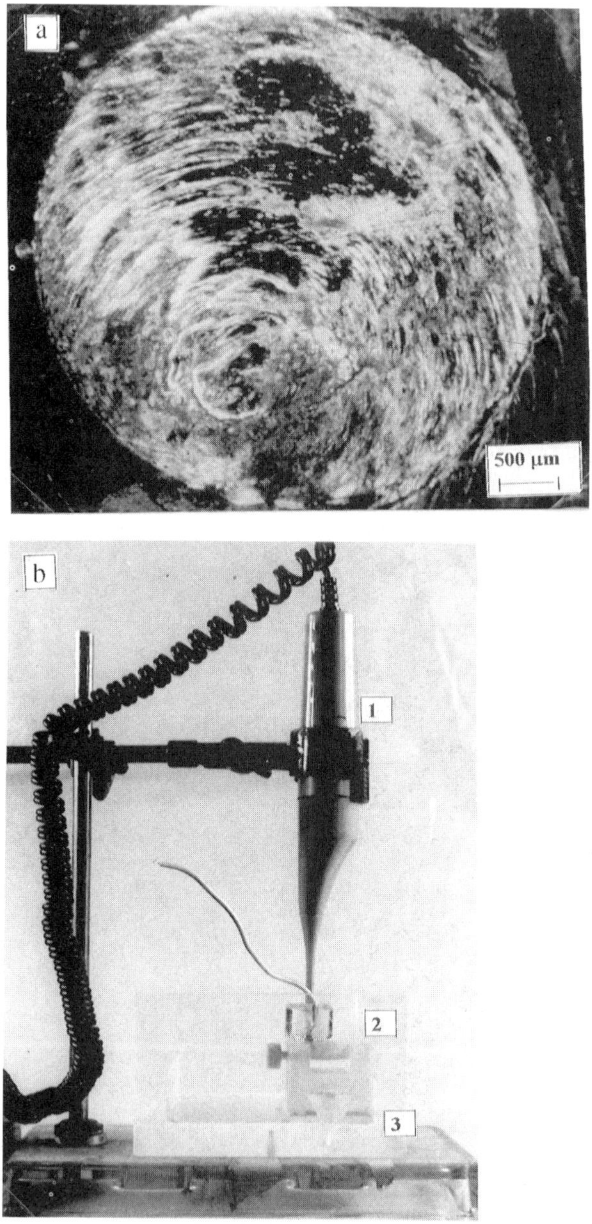

Figure 7.16 Surface of a stainless steel cap of a magnet employed for magnetic retention in dentistry (a) after continuous wear test in artificial saliva at 37 °C, in the apparatus (b) constituted by an electric toothbrush (1), the magnet (2), and a sample of Pd–Co ferromagnetic alloy (3).

in direct contact with physiological fluids. Only in the oral cavity is it possible to avoid the onset of dangerous conditions (such as plaque formation and the local increase of acidity due to the presence of food residuals) with a good oral hygiene.

Prevention on the metal may be obtained by direct modification of the metal surface with chemical or electrochemical methods, by applying a potential from the exterior in order to stabilize the material in the passive zone (anodic protection), or near the immunity potential (cathodic protection). With biomaterials only a direct modification of the metal surface may be performed; titanium nitridation is an example of this kind of action.

In the field of biomaterials the corrosion prevention is based mainly on the choice of materials, on the device design and execution, and on the care of surgical placement.

The choice of materials that may be used in biomaterials applications is not very extensive. In orthopedics, the choice is limited to stainless steels, Ti and Ti alloys, or Co–Cr–Ni alloys, materials that are easy to passivate and whose employment as biomaterials has a long history of success. The material has to be employed in conditions that allow the development of the best mechanical properties and of the best corrosion resistance properties. For example, the employment of a stainless steel involves starting with a cold worked material. The material should be of a high degree of purity in order to avoid the presence of inclusions. The surface should be highly polished and the design should avoid stress concentrating geometric discontinuities. Also, during surgical placement of the device, no excessive deformation or stress should be introduced, nor should the finishing degree be damaged.

References

Angelini, E., Bonino, P., Pezzoli, M. 1988. Corrosion resistance of solder joints for removable partial dentures, *Dent. Mater.* **4**, 255–260.

Angelini, E., Pezzoli, M., Zucchi, F. 1991. Corrosion under static and dynamic conditions of alloys used for magnetic retention in dentistry, *J. Prosthet. Dent.* **65**, 848–853.

Bianchi, G., Mazza, F. 1989. *Corrosione protezione dei materiali metallici*, Masson Ed., Milano.

Bockris, J.'O., Reddy, A.K.N. 1970. *Modern Electrochemistry*, Plenum Press, New York.

Fraker, A.C., Griffin, D. 1985. ASTM special technical publication: 859, *Corrosion and Degradation of Implant Materials* (A.C. Fraker and D. Griffin, eds.) , ASTM Publ. Code Number 04-859000-27.

Marcus, P., Oudar, J. 1995. *Corrosion Mechanism in Theory and Practice*, Marcel Dekker Inc., New York.

Marek, M. 1983. Corrosion: acqueous processes and passive films, in: *Treatise on Materials Science and Technology*, Vol. 23 (J.C. Scully, ed.), pp. 331–394, Academic Press, London.

Pourbaix, M. 1974. *Atlas of Electrochemical Equilibria in Aqueous Solution*, NACE, Houston, Texas.

Sedriks, J.A. 1996. *Corrosion of Stainless Steels*, 2nd edn., John Wiley & Sons Inc., New York.

Uhlig, H.H., Winston Revie, R. 1984. *Corrosion and Corrosion Control*, 3rd edn., John Wiley & Sons Inc., New York.

Zucchi, F., Angelini, E. 1982. In vitro corrosion of dental amalgams, *Surf. Technol.* **17**, 341–355.

8

Characterization of Biomaterials

Donald Lyman

8.1. Requirements of Biomaterial Characterization

Both the bulk and the surface properties of a biomaterial must be adequately characterized, since this provides baseline information upon which the performance of an implant material can be related. Several levels of testing need to be done (see Table 8.1). Initial tests are used to define the general properties of a potential biomaterial and can also be used for quality assurance on new batches of a material. These include determination of chemical composition and contaminants as well as tests of basic mechanical properties, such as tensile strength, elongation, elastic modulus (these should be measured under both dry and wet conditions for polymers), hardness, density, surface roughness (using light microscopy or SEM) and surface energy by contact angle measurements. For polymeric materials, an infrared transmission spectrum, molecular weight, and molecular weight distribution also provide important information for this initial baseline characterization. In many instances, solution viscosity measurement (inherent or intrinsic viscosity) can be used instead of a molecular weight measurement. The property values from most of these initial characterizations should be known and used in the preliminary selection of any biomaterial.

The second level of characterization defines the properties more closely related to the potential end-use applications of the biomaterial, and thus can help to differentiate between several possible candidate materials. These tests also provide for assurances of surface reproducibility. Tests should be done on materials which have been processed in a manner similar to that used in the fabrication of the final implant device (including

---

Donald J. Lyman • Department of Materials Science and Engineering and Department of Bioengineering, University of Utah, Salt Lake City, Utah 84112, United States.

Integrated Biomaterials Science, edited by R. Barbucci. Kluwer Academic/Plenum Publishers, New York, 2002.

Table 8.1. Characterization of Biomaterials

Initial tests (for baseline property values and quality assurance)
- Chemical composition
- Mechanical properties
  - Tensile strength, elongation, elastic modulus
- Hardness
- Density
- Surface texture (light and electron microscopy)
- Contact angle
- Infrared spectrum (for polymers)
- Molecular weight (for polymers)

Level II tests (for properties related to potential end-use)
- Bulk properties
  - Porosity, creep, stress relaxation, fatigue, and wear testing
  - X-ray diffraction
- Thermal properties
  - DSC (differential scanning calorimetry), DTA (differential thermal analysis), TGA (thermal gravimetric analysis), and DMTA (dynamic-mechanical-thermal analysis)
- Surface properties
  - Contact angle
  - SEM (scanning electron microscopy), TEM (transmission electron microscopy)
  - FT-IR ATR (Fourier transform infrared spectroscopy using attenuated total reflectance)
  - ESCA (electron spectroscopy for chemical analysis or XPS, X-ray photoelectron spectroscopy)
  - SIMS (secondary ion mass spectrometry)
  - ISS (ion scattering spectroscopy)
  - EDAX (energy dispersive X-ray analysis)
  - Protein adsorption
  - Solvent response

Level III tests (for specialized characterizations)
- Histological characterization of implanted samples
- Molecular biological analyses of implanted samples
- AFM (atomic force microscopy)
- STM (scanning tunneling microscopy)

sterilization) since these conditions could alter both the bulk and the surface properties of the biomaterial. These tests include, for example, bulk measurements of porosity, creep, stress relaxation, fatigue and wear testing, as well as surface measurements using techniques such as contact angle, ESCA, SIMS, ISS, FT-IR-ATR, and SEM. If the polymeric biomaterial is melt formed or is subjected to heat in any processing or sterilization steps, then thermal property measurements, such as DTA and DMTA, may also provide useful structural information since the morphology and the crystallinity of a polymer may be affected during these steps.

In addition, information on protein adsorption and the response of the biomaterial to solvents (water, saline, lipids, etc.), which may affect the material surface (and in some cases the material bulk structure), could be of importance in assessing the interaction of the biomaterial with the biological environment. Retrieved materials should also be retested after *in vitro* and *in vivo* exposure to the biological environment to determine what, if any, changes have occurred in the material which may adversely affect its long-term use.

The third level of testing involves measuring the histological response of blood and tissue to the presence of the implanted biomaterial using both standard histological test methods for particular applications (soft and hard tissue, blood, etc.) as well as newer molecular biological analyses for the presence of specific cell types and molecules such as matrix proteins, growth factors, etc. The results of these tests help in defining hypotheses of blood and tissue compatibility, assist in development of new biomaterials, and assist in the modification of implant design. Also, level III testing can involve newer techniques, such as AFM and STM. These surface characterizations, which allow three-dimensional imaging of surfaces from molecular to micron scales, may assist the biomaterials investigator to more accurately determine the surface of his biomaterial as well as defining possible molecular level interactions that might occur at the interface of the biomaterial with blood and tissue.

Since each of the above characterization methods examines the biomaterials structure in a different manner, one must be sure to use multiple techniques so as to obtain a meaningful understanding of the nature of the biomaterial surface and its interaction with the living system.

8.2. Structure of Materials

The bulk structure of materials has been well discussed in the individual chapters on Metals and Alloys (Chapter 6), Ceramics (Chapter 5), Polymers (Chapter 2), and Polymeric Composites (Chapter 3) and will not be amplified on here. However, although a solid material is defined as a portion of matter whose bulk is rigid and resists stress, it must be kept in mind that the fabrication of an implant as well as any post-fabrication processing (including sterilization) may alter the bulk structure of the biomaterial. This is particularly true for polymer materials. Thus, it is essential that both the original biomaterial as well as the biomaterial from the device being implanted be adequately characterized.

The surface structure of a biomaterial presents different types of problems for the investigator since the composition and spacial arrangement of the molecular segments on the surface may not be representative of the bulk structure. In addition, the surface is the interface where the biomaterial meets and interacts with the molecular constituents of the biological system (i.e., bone, soft tissue, blood). These reactions can alter the material as well as lead to macroscopic events in the biological media which ultimately determine whether or not the material will be successful in its performance in the body. Thus, the nature of a surface and its characterization will be discussed in somewhat more detail in this chapter.

8.3. The Nature of Surface Dynamics and Surface Analysis

Segments of the molecules of which a material is comprised extend up to the surface and are thus in an environment which is different than that seen by the same molecular segments in the bulk of the material. These surface molecules may be affected by this environment in several ways, ranging from oxidation of the surface molecules, the adsorption of contaminants, to changes in the spacial arrangement of the molecular segments on the surface.

8.3.1. Metal and Ceramic Surfaces

The surface structures of metals and ceramics are relatively stable in terms of molecular mobility. That is, the molecules present a rigid and immobile surface at equilibrium and the molecules do not re-orientate when coming in contact with water or the biological environment. However, the surface structures of pure metallic materials do oxidize readily in air (time frame for oxidation is approx. 1 s) and so the actual surface differs from the bulk in that it is primarily a metallic oxide surface. Exceptions to this are metals like gold and platinum. While these oxide surfaces are also immobile and do not show molecular movements due to contact with the aqueous biological medium, they can become altered. The presence of water, oxygen, and inorganic ions in the biological medium can result in the remodeling of a metallic surface by corrosive degradation, with different metals corroding at different rates. It is interesting to note that the presence of proteins and other organic molecules in the biological medium often appear to reduce the *in vivo* degradation rate of metals compared to that observed *in vitro* (Revie and Greene, 1969; Buchanan and Lemons, 1982).

The biological response to a metallic interface appears to be primarily due to conformational changes in proteins being adsorbed, then desorbed from the metallic surface. However, since metal surfaces are high energy surfaces, they tend to be easily contaminated by lower energy organic material. This contamination may occur, for example, during the polishing of the metallic parts or even during autoclave sterilization. Since this organic surface contamination would reduce the surface energy of the metallic biomaterial, it could alter the nature of the interaction with the biological environment. For example, titanium implants appear to show improved results when hydrocarbon contamination is high (Ratner 1990). However, since it is not known which surface properties are most relevant for an optimal biological response, there is a need for accurate characterization of metallic surfaces being implanted (Lausmaa *et al.*, 1988).

Since ceramics are composed of metallic and nonmetallic oxides, the surface compositions more closely resemble the bulk composition. The more ionic nature of the bonds in ceramic materials makes ceramic surfaces potentially more reactive than metals toward the water, ions, and molecules of the biological medium. As a result, only a few of the large number of available ceramic materials are suitable for use as permanent biomedical implants (Hench and Ethridge, 1982). The Al_2O_3 ceramics are considered to be bio-inert and appear to be more stable than metals under implant conditions. As with metals, surface changes can occur in ceramic biomaterials due to contamination of these high energy surfaces in a laboratory environment or during autoclave sterilization, and due to corrosion of the ceramic material when implanted. This also applies to the newer bioactive ceramic materials which are being explored, for example, as coatings on metals. Thus, as with metallic biomaterials, accurate surface characterization is needed for ceramic biomaterials.

8.3.2. Polymer Surfaces

In contrast to metals and ceramics, polymeric materials present more dynamic surfaces with the mobility of the surface molecules ranging from little mobility to an almost liquid-like mobility. Because of this mobility, the surface molecular segments of a polymeric material can reorient themselves to a variety of conformations depending on the nature of the environment that the polymer comes in contact with. This reorientation of the polymer surface can occur during the implant fabrication process due to contact with a mold or casting plate, or when the polymer comes in contact with water or the aqueous biological media. This is especially true for those polymeric materials with side chains. However, even the main polymer chain can undergo molecular motions when the barriers to single-bond rotations are low.

Contamination of the polymer surface can also occur. However, this is more often due to a migration to the polymer surface of additives (such as plasticizers and antioxidants) or impurities (from the polymerization process) that are present in the polymeric biomaterial. In addition, the surfaces of polymers formed by melt techniques can form an oxidized layer at the surface. For example, polyethylene, which is represented by the formula $(\text{—}CH_2CH_2\text{—})_n$, can have a variety of polar carbon–oxygen structures present on its surface due to oxidation. As a result, its surface reactions are different than what the pure hydrocarbon surface would show (Baszkin and Boissonnade, 1983).

The sensitivity of many polymer surfaces to their environment can also complicate the determination of their surface structure and thus characterization information from multiple techniques may be necessary. Therefore, the nature of polymeric biomaterial surfaces will be presented in some detail.

8.4. Organization of Polymer Surfaces

One would like to be able to describe the polymer surface in terms of the kinds of molecular groups and their spacial arrangement on the surface (i.e., their conformation). With this information one would know the types of bonding (that is, hydrogen bonds, polar bonds, ionic bonds, and dispersion force bonds) that are available on the surface for interacting with water and the other molecules of the biological medium (especially proteins), as well as the overall surface energy that would provide the driving force for these interactions.

The overall conformation of the surface molecular segments of a pure polymer is primarily dependent on the types of atoms and their arrangement in the polymer chains (i.e., their configuration) which make up the polymeric biomaterial. Thus, knowledge of the configuration of the polymeric biomaterial is necessary for interpretation of surface analysis data. The molecular segments on the surface tend to change their molecular conformation from that seen in the bulk phase so as to minimize the surface energy of the polymer. However, two factors affect the degree to which this lower energy surface conformational structure forms.

The first factor is that barriers to single-bond rotation in the polymer chain (i.e., chain flexibility) reduce the mobility of the surface segments, often preventing the lowest energy conformation from being formed. Thus, polymeric surfaces are usually in a thermodynamically metastable state. The glass transition temperature, T_g, of a polymer relates to the overall flexibility of the chains comprising the bulk material. As a polymeric material is warmed, the chain atoms vibrate around their equilibrium position. When the glass transition temperature is reached, there is sufficient free volume in the bulk so that longer chain segments (possibly up to 20 atoms in length) can begin to rotate, thus showing more liquid-like mobility. At this temperature the material goes through a transition from a glassy state to a rubbery state. More flexible chains have a lower T_g, stiffer chains have a higher T_g. While T_g is a property of the bulk material, it also gives an indication of the mobility of the chain segments on the surface of the polymer. Probably the most important factor in determining T_g is the hindrance to free rotation along the polymer chain resulting from the presence of bulky side groups. For example, polypropylene, $(\text{—CH}_2\text{—CHCH}_3\text{—})_n$, which has a T_g of $-20\,^\circ$C, has a more mobile surface than polystyrene, $(\text{—CH}_2\text{—CHC}_6\text{H}_5\text{—})_n$, which has a T_g of $100\,^\circ$C. Poly(oxydimethylsilylene), $(\text{—Si(CH}_3)_2\text{—O—})_n$, in which the barriers to single-bond rotation are very low due to both the Si—O bond length and bond angle, has a T_g of $-127\,^\circ$C. The surface chain segments on this siloxane polymer have an almost liquid-like mobility.

The second factor affecting the degree to which the lowest energy surface conformation is formed relates to how the polymeric biomaterial is fabricated into a test specimen or implant device. During fabrication into some end-use form, the surface composition and structure may be somewhat altered due to its contact with an external surface other than air. Thus, a film may have two distinct surface compositions and structures, the air side being one and the mold side being the other. This may result in each side of the polymer showing a different biological response.

8.4.1. Anisotropy of Polymer Surfaces

An early example of the affect of fabrication on the anisotropy of the surfaces of a polymeric biomaterial surface was shown by Avcothane® 51, a polyether-urethane/polydimethylsiloxane (90/10 by wt) material prepared by the reaction of a copolyether-urethane with a polydimethylsiloxane containing 3% acetoxy groups (Nyilas and Ward, 1975). When the copolymer solution was solvent cast on a metal substrate, then dried and cured, it was found that the two sides of the film responded differently to various *in vitro* blood tests. Preliminary surface analysis using IR-ATR indicated that the distribution of siloxane segments on the surfaces was anisotropic. The air side of the film had a higher concentration of siloxane segments compared to the substrate side. Later analyses using more sophisticated techniques confirmed that there were differences in composition between the two surfaces, but also showed some of the problems that investigators face in the determination of surface composition and conformation.

Analysis of an Avcothane® intraaortic balloon by FT-IR ATR using a KRS-5 ATR crystal, which allows a fairly deep depth of penetration (dp) of the IR beam (a calculated dp of 1.5 μm), gave data which appeared to be contrary to what had been found by Nyilas and Ward (1975). That is, the blood contacting side of the balloon appeared to have a lower siloxane content than did the substrate side. However, by reducing the dp of the IR beam to 0.8 μm using a barrier film on the ATR crystal, a higher siloxane content was measured on the more surface layer of the outer, blood-contacting side of the balloon (Sung *et al.*, 1978). Additional analyses using Auger Electron Spectroscopy (Sung and Hu, 1979a) and ESCA (Sung and Hu, 1979b) also supported the earlier data indicating that the outer, blood-contacting side of the intraaortic balloon had a higher concentration of siloxane segments on its surface.

However, a later study (Graham and Hercules, 1981) gave data which appears to be contrary to that reported by Sung and co-workers. These data, from an ESCA, ISS, and SIMS analysis of an Avcothane® intraaortic balloon pump, indicated that the higher siloxane concentration was on the inner side of the balloon. In addition, a fluorine-rich surface layer was found on this inner surface. The presence of the fluorine-rich surface layer on the inner side of the balloon could be from a mold release agent; in turn, this fluorine coating could have affected the composition and conformation of the surface molecules on the mold side of the balloon. An alternative explanation for these differences in data could be that after fabrication, the balloon was turned inside-out (a known practice in some balloon technology), thus reversing the surfaces. In this case the fluorine layer could be from a surface coating applied to the outside of the fabricated balloon, before it was turned inside-out, so that the siloxane-rich surface would not adhere to itself. Also, since the Avcothane® 51 was shown to give different results depending on how it was dried and cured (Nyilas and Ward, 1975), these differences may just reflect variations in the fabrication process.

Thus, in polymeric biomaterial characterizations, it is important to document the configuration of and potential additives or contaminants in the biomaterial being used, as well as all fabrication and post-fabrication steps that the material has undergone. Also, since the various surface characterization methods give different surface information (such as molecular versus elemental data) and different probe surface depths (see Table 8.2), it is advisable to use multiple techniques when relating the surface structure of a polymer to its biological response.

8.4.2. Microphase Heterogeneous Surfaces

One of the most widely used types of biomaterials (and probably the most complex to analyze) are the microphase-separated block copolymers (Allport and Janes, 1973). Of particular importance are the microphase-separated, linear, block copolyether-urethane-ureas. These were initially

Table 8.2. Depths of Penetration in Polymer Surfaces by Various Characterization Methods

Method[a]	Penetration depth (Å)
Contact angle	1–10
ISS	1–10
SIMS	1–10
ESCA	15–150
EDAX	1000
FT-IR-ATR	500–10,000[b]

[a] See Table 8.1 for definition of abbreviations.
[b] The depth of penetration is dependent on IR wavelength, refractive index of the ATR crystal, and the angle of incidence.

studied as implant materials because of their excellent mechanical properties (Boretos and Pierce, 1968; Lyman *et al.*, 1969). However, it was shown that this microphase-separated bulk structure resulted in a microheterogeneous surface, which appeared to play an important role in the improved blood and tissue compatibility shown by these polyurethane biomaterials (Lyman *et al.*, 1974, 1975).

A typical synthesis of a segmented copolyether-urethane-urea (shown in Figure 8.1) involves the reaction of an aromatic diisocyanate (I) with a dihydroxy oligomeric ether molecule (II) and a diamine (IV). This polymerization may be conducted by mixing all the ingredients together or by a stepwise reaction (as illustrated in Figure 8.1) in which the diisocyanate-capped oligomer (III) is first formed, then is chain extended by the diamine. In the two early studies, one copolyether-urethane-urea (Lycra®) was based on polytetramethylene oxide glycol (Boretos and Pierce, 1968), and the other copolyether-urethane-urea was based on polypropylene glycol (Lyman *et al.*, 1969, 1971). The Lycra® material was later replaced by Biomer®. Although Biomer® is still based on polytetramethylene oxide glycol, other aspects of its chemical structure have been changed over time. In addition, it appears to have a silicone contaminant (Lelah *et al.*, 1983).

The segments, or blocks of these linear copolymers are comprised of oligomeric ether blocks (or soft segments) and oligomeric urea blocks (or hard segments), with the urethane linkages interconnecting these blocks. The microphase separation into domains of hard segments imbedded in a matrix of soft segments results from the steric and chemical incompatibilities of the hard and soft segments. The size of the domains is in the range of 30 to 100 Å. The domains are separated in the matrix by about 100 to 200 Å. It is interesting to note that the sizes of the various proteins which are first to adsorb on a polymer surface range from tens to several hundred Å.

$$2\ OCNC_6H_4CH_2C_6H_4NCO \quad + \quad HO(CHCH_3CH_2O)_xCHCH_3CH_2OH \quad \rightarrow$$

I II

$$OCNC_6H_4CH_2C_6H_4NHCOO(CHCH_3CH_2O)_xCHCH_3CH_2OOCNHC_6H_4CH_2C_6H_4NCO$$

III

$$III \quad + \quad H_2NCH_2CH_2NH_2 \quad \rightarrow$$

IV

$$[-CONHC_6H_4CH_2C_6H_4NHCONHCH_2CH_2NHCONHC_6H_4CH_2C_6H_4NHCOO(CHCH_3CH_2O)_xCHCH_3CH_2O-]_n$$

V

(urethane link) ------------ urea "hard" segment ------------ (urethane link) ...... ether "soft" segment .....

Figure 8.1. Synthesis of a block copolyether-urethane-urea.

Preliminary surface characterization of these two copolyether-urethane-ureas using FT-IR ATR and ESCA (Knutson and Lyman, 1982; Lyman *et al.*, 1974, 1975; Sung *et al.*, 1978, Sung and Hu, 1979a, 1979b) have indicated that while these materials show much less anisotropy than that shown by Avcothane®, there is still more of the lower energy ether segments on the air side of a solvent cast film than there is on the mold side of the film. However, the surface is not overlaid with ether segments, but does have some urethane/urea segments on both surfaces.

Since these early implant studies, there have been many contradictory observations on the biological response to many implanted polyurethane materials. Some of these differences in biological response may be due to the use of commercially available polyurethane materials (either unmodified or modified by the investigator), since these materials often contain additives such as lubricants (bis-stearamides), silicones, and stabilizers which can migrate to the surface. The two copolyether-urethane-ureas used in the early studies were additive-free.

However, these differences in biological response are more likely related to changes in the microheterogeneous surface structure due to changes in the configuration of the block copolyurethane chains. For example, the chemical structure of the diisocyanate and the small difunctional molecule used to chain extend the prepolymer, the chemical structure and molecular weight of the oligomeric dihydroxy molecule, the molar ratio of these three reactants, and the polymerization conditions (Wang and Lyman, 1993) all contribute to the chain configuration of the resulting segmented copolyurethane. Any changes in chain configuration resulting from these variables will affect the steric and chemical compatibilities of the blocks and thus the phase separation of the segmented copolyurethane. This in turn will affect the mechanical, physical, and biological performance of the copolyurethane. For example, using an alicyclic diisocyanate will result in less phase separation than when an aromatic diisocyanate is used. If a diol is used in the chain extension (forming a copolyether-urethane) there will be less phase separation than when a diamine is used (forming the copolyether-urethane-urea). The molecular weight of the oligomeric ether segment and its chemical structure will also influence the amount and the mobility of the ether segments on the surface of the copolyurethane material. Even changes in the solvent used to solvent-cast films of the test material can influence phase separation. Thus, it must not be assumed that a surface has a microheterogeneous phase-separated surface and will be compatible with blood and tissue just because it is a polyurethane material.

Although the emphasis has been on only several types of polymeric biomaterials, these general principles have been found to apply to all polymeric surfaces being studied. Thus while a single characterization technique may suffice for a quality assurance determination, multiple characterization techniques must be used when determining the actual surface structure and its relationship to the biological response.

References

Allport, D.C., Janes, W.H. 1973. *Block Copolymers*, John Wiley, New York.

Baszkin, A., Boissonnade, M.M. 1983. Characterization and albumin adsorption on surface oxidized polyethylene films, in: *Polymers in Medicine I. Biomedical and Pharmacological Applications: Polymer Science and Technology* (E. Chiellini, P. Giusti, eds.), pp. 271–286, Plenum Press, New York.

Boretos, J.W., Pierce, W.S. 1968. Segmented polyurethane: A polyether polymer—an initial evaluation for biomedical applications, *J. Biomed. Mater. Res.* **2**, 121–130.

Buchanan, R.A., Lemons, J.E. 1982. In-vivo corrosion-polarization behavior of titanium and cobalt-base surgical alloys, *Trans. Soc. Biomat.* **5**, 110.

Graham, S.W., Hercules, D.M. 1981. Surface spectroscopic studies of Avcothane, *J. Biomed. Mater. Res.* **15**, 349–361.

Hench, L.L., Ethridge, E.C. 1982. *Biomaterials: An Interfacial Approach*, Academic Press, New York.

Knutson, K., Lyman, D.J. 1982. The effect of polyether segment molecular weight on the bulk and surface morphology of copolyether-urethane-ureas, in: *Biomaterials: Interfacial Phenomena and Applications* (S.L. Cooper, N.A. Peppas, eds.), pp. 109–132, Adv. Chem. Series 199, American Chemical Society, Washington, D.C.

Lausmaa, J., Kasemo, B., Rolander, U., Bjursten, L.M., Ericson, L.E., Rosander, L., Thomsen, P. 1988. Preparation, surface spectroscopic and electron microscopic characterization of titanium implant materials, in: *Surface Characterization of Biomaterials* (B.D. Ratner, ed.), pp. 161–174, Elsevier Science Publishers, Amsterdam.

Lelah, M.D., Lambrecht, L.K., Young, B.R., Cooper, S.L. 1983. Physiochemical characterization and in vivo blood tolerability of cast and extruded Biomer, *J. Biomed. Mater. Res.* **17**, 1–22.

Lyman, D.J., Brash, J.L., Klein, K.G. 1969. The effect of chemical structure and surface properties of synthetic polymers on the coagulation of blood, in: *Artificial Heart Program Conference Proceedings* (R.J. Hegylei, ed.), pp. 113–119, U.S. Dept. Health, Education and Welfare, NIH, Washington, D.C.

Lyman, D.J., Kwan-Gett, C., Zwart, H.H.J., Bland, A., Eastwood, N., Kawai, J., Kolff, W.J. 1971. The development and implantation of a polyurethane hemispherical artificial heart, *Trans. Am. Soc. Artif. Int. Organs* **17**, 456–463.

Lyman, D.J., Metcalf, L.C., Albo, Jr., D., Richards, K.F., Lamb, J. 1974. The effect of chemical structure and surface properties of synthetic polymers on the coagulation of blood: III. In vivo adsorption of proteins on polymer surfaces, *Trans. Am. Soc. Artif. Int. Organs* **20**, 474–478.

Lyman, E.J., Knutson, K., McNeill, B., Shibatani, K. 1975. The effects of chemical structure and surface properties of synthetic polymers on the coagulation of blood. IV. The relation between polymer morphology and protein adsorption, *Trans. Am. Soc. Artif. Int. Organs* **21**, 49–53.

Lyman, D.J., Albo, Jr., D., Jackson, R., Knutson, K. 1977. Development of small diameter vascular prostheses, *Trans. Am. Soc. Artif. Int. Organs* **23**, 253–260.

Nyilas, E., Ward, Jr., R.S. 1975. Development of blood compatible elastomers. V. Surface structure and blood compatibility of Avcothane® elastomers, *Polym. Prepr., Am. Chem. Soc., Div. Polym. Chem.* **16**, 681–686.

Ratner, B.D. 1990. Surface structure and properties, in: *Concise Encyclopedia of Medical & Dental Materials* (D. Williams, ed.), pp. 337–346, Pergamon Press, New York.

Revie, R.W., Greene, N.D. 1969. Comparison of in-vivo and in-vitro corrosion of 18-8 stainless steel and titanium, *J. Biomed. Mater. Res.* **3**, 453–465.

Sung, C.S.P., Hu, C.B., Merrill, E.W., Salzman, E.W. 1978. Surface chemical analysis of Avcothane and Biomer by Fourier transform IR internal reflection spectroscopy, *J. Biomed. Mater. Res.* **12**, 791–804.

Sung, C.S.P., Hu, C.B. 1979a. Application of auger electron spectroscopy for surface chemical analysis of Avcothane, *J. Biomed. Mater. Res.* **13**, 45–55.

Sung, C.S.P., Hu, C.B. 1979b. ESCA studies of surface chemical composition of segmented polyurethanes, *J. Biomed Mater. Res.* **13**, 161–171.

Wang, D.T.L., Lyman, D.J. 1993. Morphology of block copolyurethanes: IV. Effect of synthetic procedure on chain structure, *J. Poly. Sci., Polym. Chem. Ed.* **31**, 1983–1995.

9

Tissues

Luigi Ambrosio, Paolo A. Netti, and Peter A. Revell

9.1. Introduction

Tissues consist of a network of intertwining fibers with polysaccharide ground substance immersed in ionic fluid. Attached to the fibers are cells whose responsibility is nutrition of the fibers and ground substances that carry out the physical function (Park, 1979). The basic component of the tissues is the extracellular matrix, which is characterized by the following functions: mechanical support for cell anchorage, determination of cell orientation, control of cell growth, maintenance of cell differentiation, scaffolding for orderly tissue renewal, establishment of tissue microenvironment, and sequestration, storage, and presentation of soluble regulatory molecules. The extracellular matrix consists of large molecules linked together into an insoluble composite. It is composed of fibers (collagen and elastin) and a largely amorphous interfibrillary matrix (mainly proteoglycans, noncollagenous glycoproteins, solutes, and water). Two types of matrices can be defined: the interstitial matrix and the basal lamina, both mainly containing collagen, a cell-binding adhesive glycoprotein, and proteoglycans. The interstitial matrix is produced by mesenchymal cells and contains fibrillar collagens, fibronectin, hyaluronic acid, and fibril-associated proteoglycans. The basal laminae, produced by overlying parenchymal cells, contain a meshlike collagen framework, laminin, and a large heparan sulfate proteoglycan. Extracellular matrices are generally specialized for a particular function, such as strength (tendon, ligament), filtration (kidney

---

Luigi Ambrosio and Paolo A. Netti • Institute of Composite Materials Technology C.N.R. and C.R.I.B., University of Naples "Federico II," Piazzale Tecchio 80, 80125 Naples, Italy. **Peter A. Revell** • Department of Histopathology, Royal Free and University College Medical School, Royal Free Campus, Rowland Hill Street, London NW3 2PF, United Kingdom.

Integrated Biomaterials Science, edited by R. Barbucci. Kluwer Academic/Plenum Publishers, New York, 2002.

glomerulus), or adhesion (basement membranes). To produce additional mechanical strength, the extracellular matrix becomes calcified during the formation of bones and teeth.

The basic tissues play specific functional roles and have distinctive microscopic appearances. They include over one hundred distinctly different types of cells, which are separated into four groups: epithelium, connective tissue, muscle tissue, and nerve tissue. Epithelium covers the internal and external body surfaces, it provides a protective barrier (skin, epidermis) and an absorptive surface (gut lining), and generates internal and external secretions (endocrine and exocrine glands, respectively). Examples of exocrine secretion are the glandular elements associated with the gastrointestinal tract (for example, salivary glands, specialized epithelia in the stomach, small and large bowel, pancreas). Epithelium derives mostly from ectoderm and endoderm, but also from mesoderm. Connective tissues support the other tissues and organs of the body. It includes adipose tissue, blood cell-forming tissue, supports for blood vessels and nerves, cartilage, and bone. Muscle tissue is characterized by muscle cells containing the contractile proteins actin and myosin in varying amounts and configuration depending on cell function. There are smooth muscle, skeletal muscle, and cardiac muscle. Nerve tissue is highly specialized with respect to irritability and conduction. Nerve cells not only have cell membranes that generate electrical signals called action potentials, but also secrete neurotransmitters (Shoen, 1996).

The different tissue functions due to the specific roles make the tissue very distinctive at the microscopic and macroscopic level; a general distinction of the tissues can be made by considering their physical aspects: *soft tissue and hard tissue.*

9.2. Soft Tissues

As soft tissues we refer to a large family of tissue such as loose and dense connective tissues, muscles, heart, and nerve. Epithelia and endothelia require connective tissue scaffolds. The structure and the composition of soft tissues change significantly upon the site depending on the specific function. Soft tissues, such as tendons, ligaments, and cartilage, perform mainly a mechanical function while loose connective tissues provide mainly a natural scaffold for cell function. Although the functions may be very different, the basic constituents of all soft tissues are essentially the same. It is therefore the microstructural organization and nature and strength of interactions among the constituents that makes the difference in biological function of soft tissue. The underlying paradigm of organization of soft tissues is that structure is adapted to perform a specific function. To fulfil all the biomechanical and biological functions, soft tissues must have a set of unique mechanical and physiochemical properties which are modulated by the composition of the tissues, mainly collagen and proteoglycans, their assembly at ultramolecular level, and their interactions with the interstitial fluids.

The macroscopic properties of soft tissues are determined by the composition and the assembly of the fibrillar and ground substance components. All soft tissues have a hierarchical structure at various scale lengths: the molecular scale (nanoscale: 1–100 nm), the ultramolecular scale (microscale: 0.1–100 μm), and the tissue scale (0.1–10 mm) (Fung, 1993). At each hierarchical level, the structure has a significant role in determining the physical and physiological properties of the tissue (Ratcliffe and Mow, 1996).

In the following chapters the structure–properties relationship for tendons, ligaments, skin, and cartilage will be presented along with the specific functions of the tissue. It will be evident that, depending on how the fibers, cells, and ground substance are organized into a structure, the biofunction of the tissues vary. The simplest structure, in terms of organization of collagen, is presented by tendons, ligaments, and cornea, which are organized in an array of parallel fibers (Fung, 1993). The strict parallelism of collagen fibers in the lamina of the cornea guarantee the optical function of the tissue. Similar collagen organization is adopted in tendons whose main function is to transmit tension from a muscle to a bone. The fiber bundles are wavy in the relaxed state and become straighter under tension (Woo and Levine, 1998). A joint ligament has similar structure but is less regular, and different fibers in the ligament are stressed differently depending on the mode of function.

The two- and three-dimensional networks of the skin are more complex than in ligaments. These fibers are woven in a rhombic-like pattern, which allows considerable deformation without requiring elongation of the individual collagen fiber (Fung, 1993). A complex three-dimensional fiber organization is found also in cartilage. The collagen content and structure in cartilage varies from the surface to the deep zone (Mow *et al.*, 1992). In particular, collagen content is the highest in the surface zone and decreases approximately by 15% in the middle and deep zone. Conversely, the PG content is the lowest at the surface and increases by 15% in the middle and deep zone. At the surface, collagen fibers are aligned parallel to the articular surface; in the middle zone the fibers have a larger diameter and are arranged randomly; in the deep zone the fibers are woven in bundles and aligned perpendicular to the surface.

More complex is the organization of blood vessels (Fung, 1993). Blood vessels consist of three layers: the intima, media, and adventitia. The intima is the innermost layer, the media is the middle layer, and the adventitia is the outermost layer composed mainly of collagen and PGs. The structure of blood vessels varies along the arterial tree and there are several differences between the structure of veins and arteries. The structural organization of the fibers in the adventitia is rather complex with a circular organization around the direction of the blood stream. The most complex organization of tissues are those found in intestinal mucosa and female genital tracts.

This brief introduction shows that although the basic components of soft tissues are the same, their organization may vary in different structures which result in the different functions of the several kinds of tissues.

9.3. Hard Tissues

Hard tissue is often used as a synonym for bone when describing the structure and properties of bone or tooth. "Hard" is self-explanatory in comparison with all the other mammalian tissues, which are often referred to as soft tissue.

Bone is a composite constituted of 40% organic material, of which 90–96% is collagen (most is Type I) and the rest is mineral. The major subphase of a mineral consists of a submicroscopic crystal of an apatite of calcium and phosphate resembling hydroxyapatite in crystal structure [$Ca_{10}(PO_4)_6(OH)_2$]. There are other mineral ions, such as citrate ($C_6H_5O_7^{4-}$), carbonate (CO_3^{2-}), fluoride (F^-), and hydroxyl ions (OH^-), which may give some other differences in the microstructural features of bone (Park, 1979). The collagenous organic matrix and highly oriented calcium phosphate mineral are arranged in a highly organized hierarchical structure which has a strong effect on the mechanical properties of the bone. Thus it is important to describe the structure of the mammalian bone (Figure 9.1) (Lawson and Czernuska, 1998) in order to understand the related properties. The basic structural unit of collagen is the tropocollagen chain that is bundled in microfibrils. At the molecular level, the tropocollagen molecules are made up of three individual left-handed helical polypeptyde chains coiled into a right-handed triple helix.

The apatite crystallites, about $2 \times 50 \times 20$ nm in size, are associated with the tropocollagen, and have been found to be carbonate-substitute hydroxyapatite, which is generally thought to be nonstoichiometric.

At the ultrastructural level, the collagen and apatite crystallites are intimately associated and assembled into a microfibrillar composite. At the next level, the microstructural, these fibers are either randomly arranged (woven bone) or organized into concentric lamellar groups (osteons) or linear lamellar groups (plexiform bone). The highest level of organization differentiates between compact and cancellous bone.

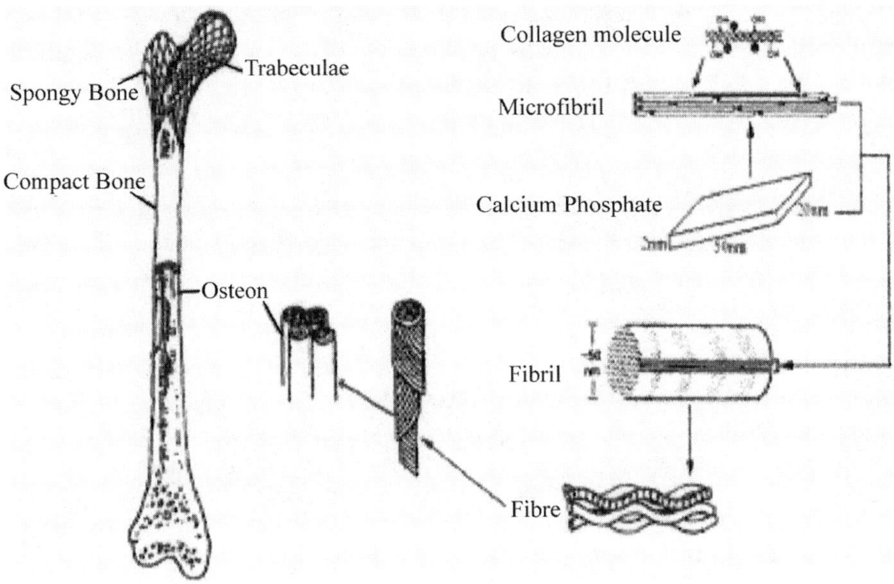

Figure 9.1. Hierarchical levels of structure in a human femur. Reproduced from Lawson and Czernuszka (1998), by permission of the Council of the Institution of Mechanical Engineers.

As a consequence of its structure, bone is an anisotropic, heterogeneous, inhomogeneous, nonlinear, thermorheologically complex viscoelastic material. It exhibits electromechanical effects, presumed to be due to streaming potentials, both *in vivo* and *in vitro* in wet conditions. In the dry state, bone exhibits piezoelectric properties (Katz, 1995).

The adult human skeleton consists of 206 distinct bones. Although the bones vary in size and shape, they are similar in structure and development, and may be classified into a few basic shapes: long bone (femur, tibia, radius), short bone (carpal, tarsal), flat bone (sternum, ribs, skull, ilium, scapula), irregular bone (ischium, pubis, vertebrae), and sesamoid (patella).

Long bones can be described based on their centers of ossification. The epiphyses develop from secondary ossification centers and are located at the end of long bones. The epiphyses articulate with other bones and are protected by a layer of articular cartilage. Between the two epiphyses is the shaft of the long bone, the diaphysis, which is a hollow structure surrounding the medullary cavity.

The medullar cavity is used as a fat storage site, it is lined by a thin, largely cellular connective tissue membrane, the endosteum: There is no medullary cavity in the flat bone. The portions of the flared ends of the long bones between the epiphyses and the diaphysis are called the metaphyses and are the growth zone during development. The bone is surrounded by a tough, vascular, fibrous tissue called the periosteum, whose fibers are intertwined with fibers of tendons, which provide attachment for muscles (Nigg and Grimston, 1994).

In the adult skeleton all bones have two main structural components: (a) Compact or cortical bone is the solid, dense material comprising the walls of diaphyses and external surfaces of bones. Compact bone is strong and resistant to mechanical stresses; its thickness varies between and within bones as a function of the mechanical requirements. (b) Cancellous or spongy bone is named after the thin bony spicules that form it, called trabeculae. These trabeculae have been observed to orient themselves in the direction of the forces applied to the bone. The spongy bone is located in the vertebral bodies, in the epiphyses of long bones, in short bones, and sandwiched between the two layers of compact bone that make up the flat bones. The flat bones are characterized by the presence of irregular interconnecting spaces (filled with bone marrow), between the trabeculae, reducing the weight of the bone.

Bone is a living tissue and this is made most evident by the blood circulation that transports materials to and from bone. The principal artery enters the bone through a distinct foramen. Within the medulla, the artery branches into ascending and descending medullary arteries. These subdivide into arterioles that penetrate the endosteal surface to supply the diaphyseal cortex. Epiphyseal arteries penetrate the articular cartilage from below; the orientations of vessels are different as their function varies at any specific location (Brookes, 1971).

Mechanical stresses modulate the change, growth, and resorption of bone, so that an understressed or overstressed bone can become weaker. There is a proper range of stresses that is optimal for the bone. That the evolution process has resulted in an optimum design of bone is borne out by the following: the general shaping of the structure to minimize stresses while transmitting prescribed forces acting at specific points, and the distribution of materials to achieve a minimum weight. For bone, Roux formulated the principal of functional adaptation, which means the “adaptation of an organ to its function by practising the latter,” and the principle of maximum–minimum design, which means that a maximum strength is to be achieved with a minimum of constructional material. Julius Wolff (1884) first advanced the idea that living bone changes according to the stress and strain involved. Changes in the external shape of bone are called external or surface remodeling, while changes in porosity, mineral content, X-ray opacity, and mass density of bone are called internal remodeling (Fung, 1993).

References

Brooks, M. 1971. *The Blood Supply of Bone. An Approach to Bone Biology*, Butterworths, London.

Fung Y.C. 1993. *Biomechanics, Mechanical Properties of Living Tissue*, 2nd edn., Chapter 12, Springer-Verlag, New York.

Katz, J.L. 1995. Mechanics of hard tissue, in: *The Biomedical Engineering Handbook* (J.D. Bronzino, ed.), CRC Press, Salem, MA.

Lawson, A.C., Czernuska, J.T. 1998. Collagen-calcium phosphate composites, *J. Eng. Med., Proc.*, Part H, **212**(6), 413–425.

Mow, V.C., Ratcliffe, A., Poole, R.A. 1992. Cartilage and diarthrodial joints as paradigms for hierarchial materials and structures. *Biomaterials* **13**, 67–97.

Nigg, B.M., Grimston, S.K. 1994. Bone, in: *Biomechanics of the Musculo-skeletal System*, Chapter 2.1 (B.M. Nigg and W. Herzog, eds.), John Wiley & Sons, Chichester.

Park, J.B. 1979. *Biomaterials: An Introduction*, Chapter 7, Plenum Press, New York.

Ratcliffe, A., Mow, V.C. 1996. Articular cartilage, in: *Extracellular Matrix* (W.D. Comper, ed.), pp. 234–302, OPA, Harwood Academic Publisher, Amsterdam.

Shoen, F.J. 1996. Tissue, in: *Biomaterials Science* (B.D. Ratner, A.S. Hoffmann, F.J. Shoen, eds.), Chapter 3.4, Academic Press, San Diego.

Woo, S. L-Y., Levine, R.E. 1998. Ligament, tendon and fascia, in: *Handbook of Biomaterials Properties* (J. Black, G. Hastings, eds.), Chapman and Hall, London.

10

Soft Tissue

Luigi Ambrosio, Paolo A. Netti, and Luigi Nicolais

10.1. Structure–Property Relationship of Soft Tissue

10.1.1. Introduction

The structural element of soft tissue is the extracellular matrix which is secreted by cells. The function of the extracellular matrix includes mechanical support for cell anchorage, determination of cell orientation, control of cell growth, maintenance of cell differentiation, scaffolding for orderly tissue renewal, establishment of tissue microenvironment, sequestration, storage and presentation of soluble regulatory molecules. Extracellular matrix consists of large molecules linked together in an insoluble composite (Shoen, 1996). The fibrillar components of the extracellular matrix include collagen and elastin. Collagen provides a major component of tissue strength, while the elastin fibers confer an elastic flexibility to tissues. The amorphous interfibrillary matrix (ground substances) is composed mainly of proteoglycans, noncollagenous glycoproteins, solutes, and water. Physically, a ground substance behaves as a glue, lubricant, and shock absorber in various tissues (Park, 1979).

The structure and hence the properties of a given soft tissue are dependent on the chemical and physical nature of the components present and their relative amounts. Moreover, depending on how the fibers, cells, and ground substance are organized into a structure, the mechanical properties of the tissues vary. The simplest structure, from the point of view of collagen fibers, consists of parallel fibers, as in tendon and ligament tissue, whose function is mainly to transmit tension. The fiber bundle appears

---

Luigi Ambrosio, Paolo A. Netti, and Luigi Nicolais • Institute of Composite Materials Technology C.N.R. and C.R.I.B., University of Naples "Federico II," Piazzale Tecchio 80, 80125 Naples, Italy.

Integrated Biomaterials Science, edited by R. Barbucci. Kluwer Academic/Plenum Publishers, New York, 2002.

somewhat wavy in relaxed conditions but becomes straighter under tension (Kastelic *et al.*, 1978).

A cruciate ligament has similar structure ligament, but less regular, with collagen fibers sometimes curved and laid out of the direction of load, and they are stressed differently in different modes of function of the ligament. Most ligaments are purely collagenous, but the ligamenta flava of the spine is mostly elastin, conferring higher elastic flexibility. The tissue that shows the most parallel-fibered structure of collagen is found in each lamina of the cornea, and in its adjacent laminae the fiber orientations vary.

The structure of collagen in the skin must be considered as a three-dimensional network, although the predominant direction of fibers is parallel to the surface; interwoven with the bundle of collagen is a network of elastin fibers (Fung, 1993b).

The type and orientation of collagen in the intervertebral disc have an important influence on how load is distributed. In the disc there is a gradation of collagen type and orientation from nucleus to annulus. The collagen fibers, contained in the concentric lamellae, are inclined with respect to the vertical axis of the spine in a lay-up structure. From the edge of the disc inward to the nucleus, the angle fiber orientation decreases from 62 to 45 degrees (Hiltner *et al.*, 1985).

In the cartilage, the orientation of collagen can generally be considered as a three-dimensional network. Indeed their organization depends on the zone: (1) In the superficial zone the crimped collagen is oriented mainly in the direction parallel to the joint movement; (2) in the transitional zone the collagen fibrils present larger diameter and appear less parallel to the join motion; (3) in the deep zone a large number of big collagen are oriented perpendicular to the plane of joint motion (Shrive and Frank, 1994).

In these latter tissues the distribution of interstitial water is very high. About 70% of the interstitial water is entrapped in the solution domain of proteoglycan molecules while the remainder is within the intrafibrillar compartment of collagen. The total amount of interstitial water depends mainly upon the number of hydrophilic groups present on the PG chains and their degree of hydrolysis, the ionic strength of the interstitial fluid, the organization and the mechanical strength of the collagen-PG network (Mow *et al.*, 1984).

High water content is present in the vitreous body in which an ordered network of fine collagen fibrils is immersed in a high hydrated hyaluronic acid and aggregate glycosaminoglycans. This structure makes the vitreous act as gel-like materials (Denlinger and Balaz, 1989; Mensitieri *et al.*, 1994).

10.1.2. Mechanical Properties

The constituents of soft tissue are organized into many different kinds of structures in order to perform in specific functions; as a result the mechanical properties are different. Collagen and elastin are organized so as to optimize mainly the strength and elasticity of the tissue while the ground substances (proteoglycans, water, hyaluronic acid, cells, etc.) are mostly responsible for the viscoelastic properties.

10.1.2.1. Stress–Strain Properties

All soft tissues present a peculiar behavior when they are tested in a uniaxial mode as a simple elongation at constant strain rate. The related diagrams of load versus elongation, for tensile rather than compressive test, show an upward concavity with an initial low modulus region (toe region) followed by a progressive increase in modulus up to a "linear" load–strain characteristic. The linear behavior held up to the failure of the tissue. The toe region is usually the physiological range in which the tissue normally functions, and generally depends on the composition of the ground substances and its interaction with collagen fibers and their orientation. For tendons and ligaments with parallel fiber, the toe region is less extended than the one obtained from a more random structure such as the skin. At the end of the toe region the collagen fibers begin to become straightened, resisting deformation and generating load up to failure (Viidik, 1980; Lanir, 1978).

This nonlinear behavior has been usually described with a fiber-recruitment model in which the progressive alignment of the collagen fibers along the direction of the load is modeled by several exponential constitutive equations (Kenedi *et al.*, 1964):

$$\sigma = K\varepsilon^d, \qquad \sigma = E(e^{\alpha\varepsilon} - 1)$$

or (Ridge and Wright, 1964):

$$\varepsilon = C + k\sigma^b, \qquad \varepsilon = x + y \log \sigma$$

The stress–strain behavior of intervertebral disc is best described by a cubic relationship (Skaggs *et al.*, 1994; Ebara *et al.*, 1996):

$$\sigma = A\varepsilon + B\varepsilon^3$$

The exponential law is suggested by the experimental data and leads to the result that the elastic modulus increases linearly with stress as more and more collagen fibers become stretched, according to the concept of fiber recruitment.

The uniaxial experiments may provide enough information for some tissues such as tendons, but not a full relationship between all stress and strain components for tissue such as skin. To obtain the tensorial relationship, it is necessary to perform biaxial and triaxial loading tests. Biaxial experiments on rabbit abdomen skin have been reported by Lanir and Fung (1974a, 1974b), from whose data Tong and Fung (1976), gleaned the pseudostrain–energy function for a loading process.

10.1.2.2. Viscoelastic Properties

The term *viscoelastic* refers to materials which exhibit elastic and at the same time viscous behavior. The elastic response is attributed to the instantaneous and reversible deformation under the external load, while slow relaxation due to configurational rearrangement of the material characterizes the viscous response. The ratio between deformation rate and the molecular configuration relaxation velocity determines the mechanical response of the material. When the deformation rate is well beyond the characteristic velocity of the relaxation phenomena, elastic behavior is attained, while at the other extreme (i.e., when the deformation is slower than relaxation) viscous behavior is registered. Viscoelastic response is attained when the two characteristic velocities are of the same order of magnitude. Virtually all materials are viscoelastic in nature, but this behavior is much more marked for macromolecular materials in which the poor molecular mobility renders the characteristic relaxation velocity of the same order of magnitude of the commonly used deformation rate (Christensen, 1971).

Features of viscoelasticity are relaxation, creep, and hysteresis. When a tissue is suddenly strained and then the strain is maintained constant afterward, the corresponding stresses induced in the tissue decrease with time. This phenomena is called *stress relaxation.*

If the tissue is suddenly stressed and the stress is maintained constant afterward, the tissue continues to deform, and the phenomena is called *creep.*

If the tissue is subjected to cycling loadings, the stress–strain relationship in the loading process is somewhat different from that in the unloading process; this phenomena is called *hysteresis.*

The viscoelastic behavior of materials is often discussed by using the mechanical models of Maxwell, Voigt, and Kelvin, all of which comprise a combination of linear spring and dashpot. The linear spring is supposed to produce instantaneously a deformation proportional to the load, while the dashpot is supposed to produce a velocity proportional to the load.

Different combinations of these models are analyzed in order to model the different viscoelastic behaviors of the soft tissues.

To analyze the viscoelastic properties of soft tissues, the QLV theory (Fung, 1993a, 1993b) has been successfully used (Kwan *et al.*, 1993). The QLV theory assumes that when the material is subject to a step increase of strain, ε_A, the subsequent stress relation is given by

$$\sigma(\varepsilon_A, t) = G(t)\sigma^e(\varepsilon_A) \tag{1}$$

where $\sigma(\varepsilon_A)$ is called the elastic response which, in general, is a nonlinear function of strain, and $G(t) = \sigma(t)/\sigma(0)$ is a time-dependent function called the reduced relaxation function, with $G(0) = 1$. Because of the implicit quasi-linear nature of equation (1), the stress response at time t can be obtained for a general applied strain history, $E(t)$, by using the Boltzmann superposition principle:

$$\sigma(t) = \int_0 G(t - \tau)\frac{\partial\sigma(\varepsilon)}{\partial\varepsilon}\frac{\partial\varepsilon}{\partial\tau}\,d\tau$$

By using the same approach and defining the reduced creep function, it is possible to write an equation for creep test (Fung, 1993a, 1993b).

Viscoelastic analysis can be carried out by imposing a sinusoidal excitation function and monitoring the resultant response. If a sinusoidal force is imposed on the sample, the deformation response of the material is composed of two components: the elastic (in-phase with excitation) and viscous (out-of-phase); the total response will lag behind the excitation by a phase angle ϕ. The phase lag results from the time necessary for molecular rearrangements and is associated with the relaxation phenomena. The stress σ and strain ε can be expressed as follows:

$$\sigma = \sigma_0 \sin(\omega t + \phi), \qquad \varepsilon = \varepsilon_0 \sin \omega t$$

where ω is the angular frequency. Applying simple trigonometric rules, we have

$$\sigma = \sigma_0 \sin \omega t \cos \phi + \sigma_0 \cos \omega t \sin \phi \tag{2}$$

where $\sigma_0 \cos \phi$ and $\sigma_0 \sin \phi$ are the in-phase and out-of-phase components, respectively. The in-phase modulus (elastic) and out-of-phase modulus (viscous) can be obtained on dividing the relation (2) by the strain:

$$E' = \sigma_0/\varepsilon_0 \cos \phi, \qquad E'' = \sigma_0/\varepsilon_0 \sin \phi$$

The vector composition of E' and E'' in the rotating vector plan leads to the complex modulus E_0^*. The elastic part of the complex modulus is also called the storage modulus, being correlated with the part of energy that is stored in the material. The viscous part E'' is also called loss modulus, being correlated with the dissipated energy.

The nonlinear flow properties of the biofluids, such as synovial fluids in a vitreous body, are evaluated through steady shear measurements to determine the viscosity η as a function of shear rate γ, while the small-amplitude oscillatory shear experiments allow measurement of the unsteady response of the samples and hence determination of their linear viscoelastic properties. Moreover, this technique is very useful for the determination of structure–mechanical property relationships.

In this dynamic experiment the material is subjected to a sinusoidal shear strain:

$$\gamma = \gamma_0 \sin(\omega t)$$

where γ_0 is the shear strain amplitude, ω the oscillation frequency, and t the time. The mechanical response expressed as shear stress τ of viscoelastic materials is intermediate between an ideal pure elastic solid (obeying Hooke's law) and an ideal pure viscous fluid (obeying Newton's law) and therefore is out of phase with respect to the imposed deformation as expressed by

$$\tau = G'(\omega)\gamma_0 \sin(\omega t) + G''(\omega)\gamma_0 \cos(\omega t)$$

where $G'(\omega)$ is the shear storage modulus and $G''(\omega)$ the shear loss modulus. Here, G' gives information about the elasticity or the energy stored in the material during deformation, while G'' describes the viscous character or the energy dissipated as heat.

Strain sweep tests at fixed oscillation frequency (consisting in monitoring the viscoelastic properties while logarithmically varying the strain amplitude γ_0) were previously performed on these materials to determine the strain amplitudes at which linear viscoelasticity is valid.

10.1.3. Transport Properties

As discussed before, soft tissues are generally composed of a fibrillar collagen network interpenetrated with a more hydrophilic macromolecular phase (hyaluronate and proteoglycan). Interspersed with this solid component is the free interstitial fluid, which moves relative to deformable solid material. This free interstitial fluid can serve for a number of biological purposes, including a convection path for molecules (e.g., nutrients, metabolites, drugs), tissue thermal regulation (heating and cooling), as well as to contribute to the mechanical function of the structure.

There are two continuum models commonly used to describe the mechanics of soft tissues, i.e., the poroelastic theory and the theory of mixtures. The former considers the soft tissue to be a fluid-saturated poroelastic solid (sponge-like material); the latter assimilates the soft tissue to an intimate mixture of solid and fluid phases (concentrated macromolecular solution). The poroelastic theory was originally formulated by Biot for the analysis of the consolidation of wet soil (Biot, 1941) and then applied to soft tissue mechanics. The theory of mixtures as developed by Truesdell and Toupin (Truesdell and Toupin, 1960; Bowen, 1980) and others was applied to soft tissue mechanics by Mow (Mow *et al.*, 1984) using a linear biphasic model. Although the derivation of the field equations is slightly different, when applied to biomechanical studies the two models are equivalent (Simon, 1992). These models have been used to successfully describe the mechanics of articular cartilage (Mow *et al.*, 1992; Spilker and Suh, 1990), intervertebral disc (Simon and Gaballa, 1988b), artery wall (Keynton, 1976; Simon and Gaballa, 1988a), and brain tissue (Basser, 1992; Nagashima *et al.*, 1987), as well as hydrogels (Barocas *et al.*, 1995; Grimshaw *et al.*, 1989).

Both concepts of a *mixture* or *pore in a solid matrix* are continuum approximations of the actual structure of soft tissue that includes proteins, fiber, and fluid. These allow a macroscopic view of the phenomena on a scale of several pore sizes ($\sim 100\,\mu$m), and the field variables are regarded as average quantities over this scale. All fluid movement is *passive*, i.e., driven by hydrostatic and osmotic pressure gradients and regulated by the structure and composition of the interstitial space and the vascular wall (Fung, 1990), and is particularly important for delivery of macromolecules or particles which transport and mainly rely on convection (Rippe and Haraldsson, 1994).

10.2. Skin

The human skin is a complex organ, distributed as a sheet covering in an adult human and exceeding two square meters. It functions as a physical barrier to loss of water and electrolytes from the body, playing a major role of thermoregulation with the assistance of sweat glands and vasculature, including the transduction of signals from the environment such as touch, pressure, and temperature (Clary, 1996). It must resist mechanical, chemical, physical, UV radiation, and microbial insults (Gilchrest, 1991). Its structure must permit adjustment to its range of movement, aging, and growth of the underlying organism (Montagna and Carlisle, 1979).

10.2.1. Composition and Structure

The skin is organized in four principal types of tissue: the epidermis, the dermis, the basement membrane, and the subcutis (Figure 10.1).

The epidermis is outside a 0.1-mm-thick continous sheet, containing about ten layers of keratinocytes. It is perforated only at the pores of sweat glands and by the hair follicles. The epidermis contains also melanocytes, dentritic cells, and Langerhan's cells (Odland, 1991; Lavker and Sun, 1983).

The dermis is a 2–5-mm-thick layer of vascularized and innervated connective tissue with few cells, mainly fibroblasts. It consists principally of a dense arrangement of extracellular matrix components, collagen, and elastic tissue embedded in a ground substance of proteoglycans and glycoproteins (Odland, 1991). The dermis is a massive tissue, accounting for 15–20% of total body weight.

At the interface between the epidermis and the dermis there has developed a basement membrane, an approximately 20-nm-thick multilayered membrane, which is responsible for adherence between the epidermis and the dermis and for the mechanical support of the epidermis. It comprises the basal cell membrane with a specialized attachment device, lamina lucida, lamina densa, and reticular layer containing fibrous components (Briggmann and Wheeler, 1975).

The subcutis underneath the dermis is 0.4–4 mm in thickness and comprises loose areolar connective tissue and fat.

The dermis is most responsible for the mechanical performance of the skin. As a consequence particular attention should be paid to its structure. The dermis is a moderately dense fibroblastic connective tissue composed of collagen (Type I and Type III) and elastin fibers embedded in a hydradet gel, called ground substance, which is rich in proteoglycans and glycoproteins (Odland, 1991; Fleischmajer *et al.*, 1972).

Collagen makes up over 75% of the dry fat weight of the skin and is held to account for its tensile strength. The principal cells are fibroblast, which are typically elongated cells with a thin branching cytoplasmic process. The reticular dermis which lies on the lower part of the dermis is relatively acellular, and is composed of densely interwoven, larger bundles of collagen, a meshwork of thicker elastin fibers, and a lesser content of interfibrillar ground substance components (Clary, 1996).

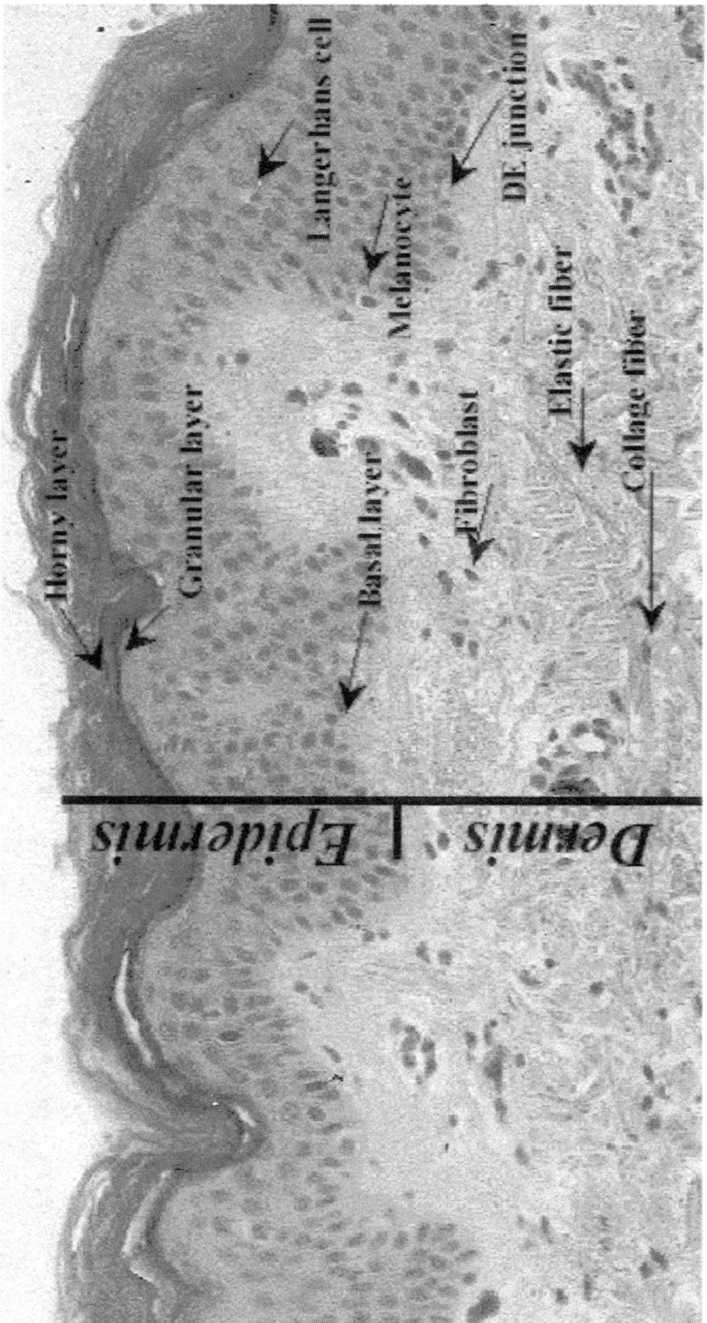

Figure 10.1. Structure of skin.

10.2.2. Mechanical Properties

The physical and mechanical properties of the skin are known to vary with the body region, age, and sex, but the analysis of how the various components of the skin affect these properties is still not completely understood. However, the mechanical properties of the skin are generally dependent on the relative composition of the extracellular matrix components and the organization of the collagen and elastin. The structure of collagen in the skin must be considered as a three-dimensional network, although the predominant direction of fibers is parallel to the surface. Interwoven with the bundle of collagen is a network of elastin fibers. This complex structure is responsible for the peculiar anisotropy mechanical properties of the skin; they vary according to the direction in which the load is applied.

Tensile properties of rabbit abdominal and human skin revealed that the application of either uniaxial or biaxial forces yielded a deformation pattern which is dependent upon test-piece orientation with respect to Langer's lines (Kenedi *et al.*, 1965; Ridge and Wright, 1966). The response is typical of soft tissue, which presents a toe region and a linear region due to the straightening and alignment of the fibrous component (Bader and Bowker, 1983; Lanir and Fung, 1974a, 1974b). The curve pertaining to the skin across the orientation with respect to Langer's line shows a wider toe region compared to that along the orientation. In the former case the deformation at break can reach a value of 40%, while a maximum of about 20% is obtained in the other direction (Bader and Bowker, 1983) (Figure 10.2).

Biaxial experiments on rabbit abdomen skin have been reported by Lanir and Fung (1974a, 1974b) from whose data Tong and Fung (1976) gleaned the pseudo-strain–energy function for a loading process. It was first observed that the mechanical property was orthotropic, and that in cyclic loading and unloading at constant strain rates the stress–strain relationship is essentially independent of the strain rate (Fung, 1993a, 1993b).

Among the *in vivo* testing methods, indentation has been the most implemented technique although it sums up the contribution of various tissue layers. The derived properties can be expected to vary depending on anatomical location, age, and environmental conditions.

Idendation behavior of human skin for the young male, young female, and aged female forearm was measured by Bader and Bowker (1983) by applying a constant pressure of 11.7 and 7 kPa for a two-minute period. The calculated moduli were calculated to be 1.51, 1.09, and 1.11 kPa, respectively. Lanir *et al.* (1990) measured the indentation behavior of human forehead skin with pressure up to 5 kPa; the calculated moduli were from 4 to 12 kPa (Mak and Zhang, 1998).

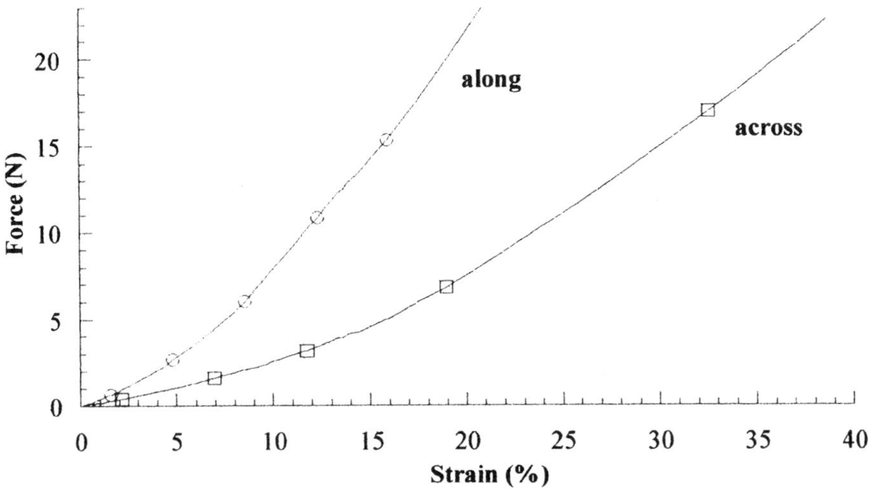

Figure 10.2. Tensile properties of skin with respect to Langer's lines.

The loading produced deformation–time curves which were typical of viscoelastic materials. After an almost linear response, a creep phase is followed in which deformation increased with time. On load removal, an instantaneous recovery is followed by long-term recovery, which is not usually fully complete during the testing time (Bader and Bowker, 1983).

10.3. Tendons and Ligaments

The main mechanical function of tendons and ligaments is to transmit loads between the elements that they connect. The tendons are fibrous composite cords that link together muscles and bones to ensure the mechanical continuity, transmitting tensile load from the muscle to the bone and therefore producing joint motion. The ligaments, from the Latin "ligare" which means to bind, connect together the articular extremities of the bones, reducing the degrees of freedom of the articulation by constraining non-physiological movements. In particular, the major function of ligaments is to guide joint movement, to maintain joint congruency, and to act as positional bend or strain sensor for the joint (Frank and Shrive, 1994).

Tendons and ligaments accomplish their various mechanical tasks thanks to synergistic cooperation among the constituents of their own structure (Figure 10.3).

Tendons and ligaments are dense connective tissues consisting of a protein phase (collagen and elastin) and a polysaccharide phase (proteo-

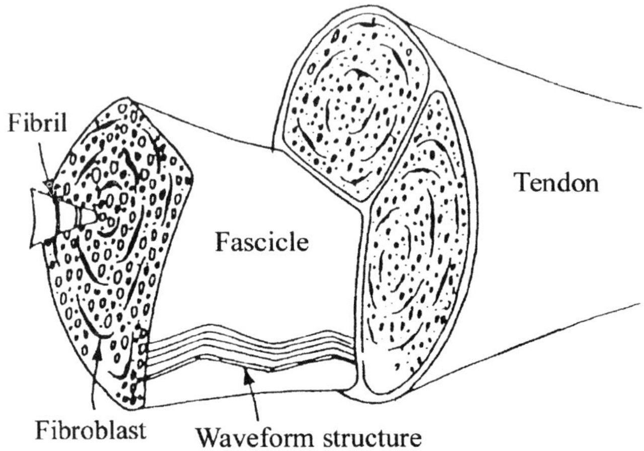

Figure 10.3. Structure of tendons (rearranged from Kastelic *et al.*, 1978).

glycans). The overall mechanical properties are determined, apart from the relative amounts of the two phases, by geometrical factors, conformation, and orientation of the single constituent (Hiltner *et al.*, 1985). The structural architecture of the tissue plays a very important role in the determination of the mechanical properties. In fact, tissues formed by the same elements show completely different behaviors.

10.3.1. Composition and Structure

The tendons and ligaments consist of fibroblasts and the more abundant extracellular matrix. The fibroblasts vary in size, shape, orientation, and number. They are ovoid and spindle-like and are generally oriented longitudinally along the length of the tendon and ligament body. The interactions between fibroblast and extracellular matrix, particularly in cell-to-cell adhesion, fibroblast-to-collagen attachment, and cell migration, are ensured by the Fibronectin, which is a large glycoprotein (Herzog and Loitz, 1994). The components of the extracellular matrix are proteoglycans, water, elastin, and collagen.

Collagen is the most abundant macromolecule and is presented mainly in Type I, while Type III is the second most common in ligaments. A small quantity of collagen Type V, VI, X, and XII is present in several ligaments (Herzog and Loitz, 1994).

In the tendons, the collagen fibers are arranged along the axial direction rendering anisotropy to the material, which will show higher stiffness in the fiber direction in order to resist axial tensile stress. It is characterized by having a hierarchical structure with six levels of organization. Beginning at the molecular level with the triple-helical tropocollagen macromolecule, a progressively larger and more complex structure is built up on the nano and microscopic scales. The macromolecules aggregate during biosynthesis to form nanoscale microfobrils, which in turn are packed into thicker discrete subfibrils; these subfibrils form fibrils. These basic building blocks form a tendon fascicle. At the fascicular level the collagen fibrils are in the crimp or wavy form. Two or three fascicles packaged together for a reticular membrane form a tendon (Kastelic *et al.*, 1978).

The microarchitecture of the cruciate ligaments has often been linked to the hierarchical arrangement described for a tendon in which collagen fibrils are grouped into fibers that, in turn, make up subfascicular units, which are bound together to form a fasciculus (Girgis *et al*, 1975; Amis and Dawkins, 1991) that in turn is enclosed in sheaths of loose connective tissue.

The ACL (anterior cruciate ligament) has a complex structure which can be separated into two major bundles: an anteromedial bundle and posterolateral bundle (Race and Amis, 1994). The bundles are oriented in different directions, causing the ACL to twist medially and to resist multiaxial stresses. In tendons, the collagen fibers have a strict waveform parallel arrangement to resist unidirectional tensile load.

The mechanical properties and configurations of collagen give the tendons and ligaments their characteristic strength, flexibility, and an ideal physical adaptation for tensile force transmission. The collagen content in tendons and ligaments is different: in tendons the collagen concentration is about 87%, while in ligaments it reaches about 80% (Amiel *et al.*, 1984; Crisp, 1972).

10.3.2. Mechanical Properties

The mechanical properties of tendons and ligaments depend not only on the properties and the arrangement of their constituent, but also on the proportion of various components. The elastin, scarcely present in tendons and extremity ligaments, probably enables the natural structures to recover the imposed deformations. The elastin, present in ligaments in only small amounts (about 5%), forms networks interdigitated among ligament collagen fibril fascicle contributing to the organization and function of the ligament matrix.

Water contributes about 60% or more of the wet weight of most ligaments and tendons, and in association with the proteoglycans provides the lubrication and spacing that are crucial to the gliding function at the fiber–matrix interface. Water and proteoglycans confer the viscoelastic properties to the tissue structure (Arnoczky *et al.*, 1993).

The mechanical properties of tendons and ligaments also depend on the presence of fibrocartilage and their insertions. Fibrocartilage might afford a gradual change in elastic moduli at insertion sites due to the variation in mineralization. The change of elastic modulus at an insertion site decreases the chance of failure, namely enhancing the ability of insertion to dissipate deformation energy (Arnoczky *et al.*, 1993).

10.3.2.1. Tensile Properties

Static load–strain curves of a fresh rabbit Achilles' tendon and an ACL are reported in Figure 10.4. These curves, according to many authors relative to collagenous tissues and reported in the literature (Herrick *et al.*, 1978; Woo, 1982), show an upward concavity with an initial low modulus region (toe region), followed by a progressive increase in modulus up to a "linear" load–strain characteristic. The linear behavior held up to the failure of the specimen, which occurred around 40 MPA for tendons and 30 MPA for ligaments.

Comparison of the two curves shows that ligament presents a wider toe region and consequently a lower initial elastic modulus. These behaviors can be easily explained in terms of differences in collagen fiber composition and configuration between tendon and ligament. Moreover, the latter contains a higher proportion of elastin and this results in higher elongation before fracture (Park, 1979). However, mechanical properties of ligaments

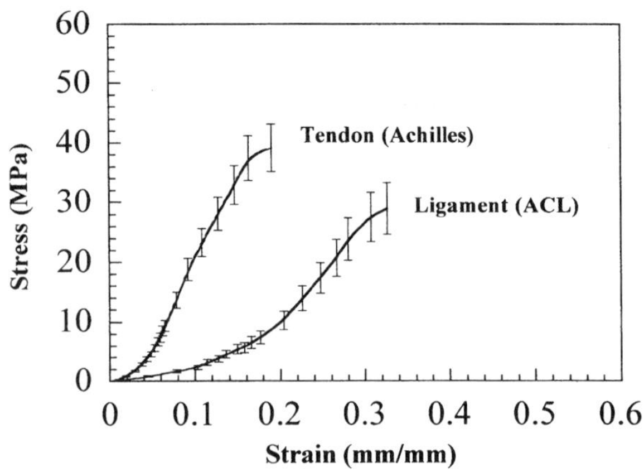

Figure 10.4. Tensile properties of ligaments and tendons.

Table 10.1. Tensile Properties of Tendons and Ligaments

Tissue	Modulus (MPa)	Stress at break (MPa)	Strain at break (%)
Tendons	300–2000	24–61	6–20
Ligaments	70–350	25–50	13–30

and tendons may vary in a wide range, depending on their location and the points where they attach to bone which influence the relative composition of these tissues. Tensile properties of tendons and ligaments are reported in Table 10.1.

10.3.2.2. Viscoelastic Properties

Natural tendons and ligaments, like most soft tissues, exhibit viscoelastic behavior such as stress relaxation and creep (Fung, 1993a, 1993b; Haut, 1993; Kwan *et al.*, 1993; Woo, 1982). This behavior shows the ability of the ligament and tendon to attenuate the stresses experienced when they are deformed and to limit rapid deformations when they are stressed, deformations which could damage them and/or other surrounding structures. The stress-relaxation characteristics help reduce the risk of injury to tendons and ligaments in the case of prolonged static deformation. Generally, the stress relaxation is rapid initially and becomes gradual over time. In the ACL AM bundle, the reduction in stress exceeded 50% of the peak value over two hours of experiments. Also, the reduced relaxation function was not a linear function of logarithmic time. Mathematical models were implemented, including a quasi-linear viscoelasticity theory for soft tissue (Fung, 1993a, 1993b; Kwan *et al.*, 1993).

Dynamic-mechanical tests have been performed in order to identify the elastic and viscous contribution or time-dependent contribution and correlate them to the structure (Netti *et al.*, 1996).

The dynamic behavior can be characterized by just two parameters, typically the storage and the loss moduli. These properties are functions only of frequency and temperature and must be determined experimentally.

However, the theory of linear viscoelasticity allows only a linear dependence of stress on strain. The stress–strain curves of natural ligaments and tendons are nonlinear. This fact represents the most obvious departure of natural ligament and tendon viscoelasticity.

Viscoelastic behavior of natural ligaments and tendons are easily inferred by the trend of the loss modulus with frequency and different static loads as reported in Figures 10.5 and 10.6. At low load, only a few collagen

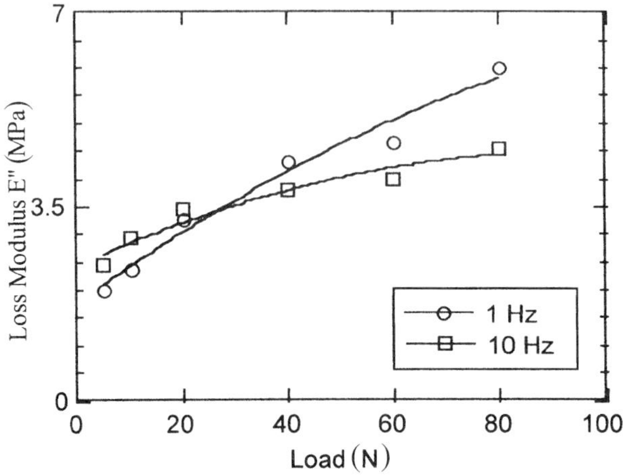

Figure 10.5. Loss modulus as a function of static load of ACL.

bundles are effectively loaded and the mechanical response of the specimen can be attributed mainly to the properties of the proteoglycans matrix. This is evident from the toe region of the static curve (low modulus region) and from the rubber-like behavior shown by the dynamic-mechanical analyses. The increase in the loss modulus with frequency, shown by the low static load, is typical of rubbery materials. Conversely, at high strain most of the collagen bundles are almost completely extended and the mechanical

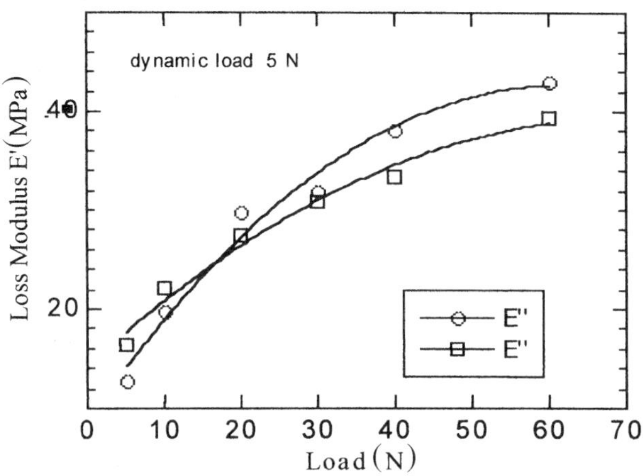

Figure 10.6. Loss modulus as a function of static load of Achilles' tendon.

response of the tissues is governed by the properties of the collagen fibers. The decrease in loss modulus with frequency, shown by the higher static load, is characteristic of glassy materials (Netti *et al.*, 1996). The dual behavior of the natural ligaments and tendons is evident by the crossing of the two curves. In the case of tendons, the crossing point occurs at a lower value of the load (16 N) than that of the ligament (28 N). This confirms the different tensile properties and structure of the two systems: the mechanical contribution of collagen fiber in tendon occurs earlier than in ligament. In fact, the collagen fibers in the tendon have a unidirectional waveform arrangement, while in the ligament they are waveform but oriented in different directions, and organized in two separated bundles, according to the structure of the natural systems.

References

Amiel, D., Frank, C., Harwood, F., Fronek, J., Akeson, W. 1984. Tendons and ligaments: morphological and biochemical comparison, *J Orthop. Res.* **1**, 257–265.

Amis, A.A., Dawkins, G.P.C. 1991. Functional anatomy of the anterior cruciate ligament, *J. Bone Jt. Surg.* **73-B**, 260–267.

Arnoczky, S.P., Matyas, J.R., Buckwalter, J.A., Amiel, D. 1993. Anatomy of the anterior breviate ligament, in: *The Anterior Cruciate Ligament: Current and Future Concepts* (D.W. Jackson *et al.*, eds.), Chap. 1, pp. 5–22, Raven Press Ltd., New York.

Bader, D.L., Bowker, P. 1983. Mechanical characteristics of skin and underlying tissue in vivo, *Biomaterials* **4**, 305–308.

Barocas, V.H., Knapp, D.M., Tranquillo, R.T. 1995. Biphasic mechanical theory of fibrillar gels, BED-29, pp. 309–310, ASME, Beaver Creek, Colorado.

Basser, P.J. 1992. Interstitial pressure, volume and flow during infusion into brain tissue, *Microvasc. Res.* **44**, 143–165.

Biot, M.A. 1941. General theory of three-dimensional consolidation *J. Appl. Phys.* **12**, 155–164.

Bowen, R.M. 1980. Incompressible porous media models by use of the theory of mixtures, *Int. J. Eng. Sci.* **18**, 1129–1148.

Briggmann, R.A., Wheeler, C.E. 1975. The epidermal-dermal junction, *J. Inest. Dermatol.* **65**, 71–74.

Christensen, R.M. 1971. *Theory of Viscoelasticity: An Introduction*, Academic Press, New York.

Clary, E.G. 1996. Skin, in: *Extracellular Matrix* (W.D. Camper, ed.), Vol. 1, Chap. 4, p. 109, Harwood Academic Publisher, Melbourne.

Crisp, J.D.C. 1972. Properties of tendon and skin, in: *Biomechanics: Its Foundations and Objectives* (Y.C. Fung, N. Perrone, M. Anliker, eds.), Chap. 6, pp. 141–179, Prentice Hall Inc., Englewood Cliffs, N.J.

Denlinger, J.L., Balaz, E.A. 1989. Viscoelastic materials, in: *Vision and Visual Health Care* (E.S. Rosen, ed.), vol. 2, Pergamon Press, Oxford.

Ebara, S., Iatradis, J.C., Setton, L.A., Foster R.J., Mow V.C, Weidenbaun, M. 1996. Tensile properties of non-degenerated human lumbar annulus fibrosus, *Spine* **19**(12), 1310–1319.

Fleischmajer, R.S., Perlish, J.S., Bashey, R.I. 1972. Human dermal glycosaminoglycans and aging, *Biochim. Biophys. Acta* **279**, 265–275.

Frank, C.B., Shrive, N.G. 1994. Ligament, in: *Biomechanics of the Musculo-skeletal System* (B.M. Nigg, W. Herzog, eds.), Chap. 2.3, pp. 106–132, John Wiley & Sons Ltd., Chichester.
Fung, Y.C. 1990. *Biomechanics: Motion, Flow, Stress and Growth*, Springer, New York.
Fung, Y. C. 1993a. *Biomechanics: Mechanical Properties of Living Tissues*, Springer-Verlag, New York.
Fung, Y.C 1993b, Bioviscoelastic solids, in: *Biomechanics, Mechanical Properties of Living Tissue*, second edition, Chap. 7, pp. 242–320, Springer-Verlag, New York.
Gilchrest, B.A. 1991. Physiology and pathophysiology of aging skin, in: *Physiology, Biochemistry and Molecular Biology of the Skin* (L.A. Goldestein, ed.), pp. 1425–1444, Oxford University Press, New York.
Girgis, F.G., Marshall, J.L., Al Monajem, A.R.S. 1975. The cruciate ligaments of the knee joint, *Clin. Orthop. Relat. Res.* **106**, 216–231.
Grimshaw, P.E., Grodzinsky, A.J., Yarmush, M.L., Yarmush, D.M. 1989. Dynamic membranes for protein transport: Chemical and electrical control, *Chem. Eng. Sci.* **44**, 827–840.
Haut, R.C. 1993. The mechanical and viscoelastic properties of the anterior cruciate ligament and ACL fascicles, in: *The Anterior Cruciate Ligament: Current and Future Concepts* (D.W. Jackson *et al.*, eds.), Chap. 5, pp. 63–73, Raven Press Ltd., New York.
Herrick, W.C., Kingsburry, H.B., Lou, D.Y.S. 1978. A study in the normal range of strain, strain rate, and stiffness of tendons, *J. Biomed. Mater. Res.* **12**, 877–894.
Herzog, W., Loitz, B. 1994. Tendon, in: *Biomechanics of the Musculo-skeletal System* (B.M. Nigg, W. Herzog, eds.), Chap. 2.4, pp. 133–153, John Wiley & Sons Ltd., Chichester.
Hiltner, A., Cassidy, J.J., Baer, E. 1985. Mechanical properties of biological polymers, *Ann. Rev. Mater. Sci.* **15**, 455–482.
Kastelic, J., Galesky, A., Baer, E. 1978. The multicomposite structure of tendon, *Connect. Tissue Res.* **6**, 11–15.
Kenedi R.M., Gibson, T., Daly, C.H. 1964. Bioengineering studies of the human skin; the effect of unidirectional tension, in: *Structure and Function of Connective and Skeletal Tissue* (S.F. Jackson, S. M. Harkness, G.M. Trismann, eds.), pp. 388–395, Scientific Committee, St. Andrews, Scotland.
Kenedi, R.M., Gibson, T., Daly, C.H. 1965. Bioengineering studies of the human skin, in: *Biomechanics and Related Bioengineering Topics* (R.M. Kenedi, ed.), pp. 147–158, Pergamon, Oxford.
Keynton, D.E. 1976. Transient filtration in a porous elastic cylinder, *Trans. ASME J. Appl. Mech.* **98**, 594–598.
Kwan, M.K., Lin, T.H-C, Woo, S.L-Y. 1993. On the viscoelastic properties of the anteromedial bundle of the anterior cruciate ligament, *J. Biomech.* **26**, 447–452.
Lanir, Y. 1978. Structure-strength relations in mammalian tendon, *Biophys. J.* **24**, 541–554.
Lanir, Y., Fung, Y.C. 1974a. Two-dimensional mechanical properties of rabbit skin. I. Experimental system, *J. Biomech.* **7**, 29–34.
Lanir, Y., Fung, Y.C. 1974b. Two-dimensional mechanical properties of rabbit skin. II. Experimental results, *J. Biomech.* **7**, 171–182.
Lanir, Y., Dikstein, S., Hartzshartark, A. 1990. In vivo indentation of human skin, *J. Biomech. Eng.* **112**, 63–69.
Lavker, R.M., Sun, T.T. (1983). Epidermal stem cell, *J. Inest. Dermatol.* **81** 121–127.
Mak, A.F.T., Zhang, M. 1998. Skin and Muscle, in: *Handbook of Biomaterials Properties* (J. Black, G. Hastings, eds.), pp. 66–69, Chapman & Hall, London.
Mensitieri, M., Lepore, D., Ambrosio, L., Balzano, L., Nicolais L. 1994. The rheological behaviour of vitreal substitutes and its comparison with vitreous of animal origin, *J. Mater. Sci. Materials in Medicine* **5**, 743–747.

Montagna, W., Carlisle, K. 1979. Structural changes in aging human skin, *J. Inest. Dermatol.* **73**, 47–53.

Mow, V.C., Holmes, M.H., Lai, W.M. 1984. Fluid transport and mechanical properties of articular cartilage, *J. Biomech.* **17**, 377–394.

Mow, V.C., Ratcliffe, A., Poole, A. R., 1992, Cartilage and diarthrodial joints as paradigms for hierarchical materials and structures, *Biomaterials* **13**(2), 67–97.

Nagashima, T., Tamaki, N., Matsumoto, S., Horwitz, B., Seguchi, Y. 1987. Biomechanics of hydrocephalus: a new mathematical model, *Neurosurgery* **21**, 898–904.

Netti, P.A., D'Amore, A., Ambrosio, L., Ronca, D., Nicolais, L. 1996. Structure–mechanical properties relationship of natural tendons and ligaments, *J. Mat. Sci. Materials in Medicine* **7**, 525.

Odland, F.F. 1991. Structure of the skin, in: *Physiology, Biochemistry and Molecular Biology of the Skin* (L.A. Goldestein, ed.), pp. 3–62, Oxford University Press, New York.

Park, J.B. 1979. *Biomaterials: An Introduction*, Chap. 7, pp. 97–130, Plenum Press, New York.

Race A., Amis, A.A. 1994. The mechanical properties of two bundle of the human posterior cruciate ligament, *J. Biomech.* **27**, 13–24.

Ridge, M.D., Wright, V. 1964. The description of skin stiffness, *Biorheology* **2**, 67–74.

Ridge, M.D., Wright, V. 1966. The directional effects of skin, *J. Inest. Dermatol.* **46**, 341–346.

Rippe, B., Haraldsson, B. 1994. Transport of macromolecules across microvascular walls: the two pore theory, *Phys. Rev.* **74**, 163–218.

Shoen, F.J. 1996. Tissue, in: *Tissue in Biomaterials Science* (B.D. Ratner, A.S. Hoffmann, F.J. Shoen, J.E. Lemons, eds.), pp. 147–164, Academic Press, San Diego.

Shrive, N.G., Frank, C.B. 1994. Articular cartilage, in: *Biomechanics of the Musculo-skeletal System* (B.M. Nigg, W. Herzog, eds.), Chap. 2.4, pp. 79–105, John Wiley & Sons Ltd., Chichester.

Simon, B.R. 1992. Multiphase poroelastic finite element models for soft tissue structure, *Appl. Mech. Rev.* **45**, 191–218.

Simon, B.R., Gaballa, M. 1988a. Finite strain poroelastic finite element models for large arterial cross sections, in: *Computational Methods in Bioengineering* (R.L. Spilker, B.R. Simon, eds.), pp. 325–331, ASME, New York.

Simon, B.R., Gaballa, M. 1988b. Poroelastic finite element models for the spinal motion segment including ionic swelling, in: *Computational Methods in Bioengineering* (R.L. Spilker, B.R. Simon, eds.), 93–99, ASME, New York.

Skaggs, D.L., Weidenbaum, M., Iatradis, J.C., Rartcliffe, A., Mow, V.C. 1994. Regional variation in tensile properties and bichemical composition of the lumbar annulus fibrosus, *Spine* **19**(12), 1310–1319.

Spilker, R.L., Suh, J.K. 1990. Formulation and evaluation of a finite element model for the biphasic model of hydrated soft tissue, *Comput. Struct.* **35**, 425–439.

Tong, P., Fung, Y.C. 1976. The stress-strain relationship for the skin, *J. Biomech.* **9**, 649–657.

Truesdell, C., Toupin, R.A. 1960. The classical field theories, in: *Handbuch der Physik III/I*, Springer, Berlin.

Viidik, A. 1980. Interdependence between structure and function in collagenous tissue, in: *Biology of Collagen* (A. Viidik, J. Vuust, eds.), pp. 257–280, Academic Press, London.

Woo, S. L-Y. 1982. Mechanical properties of tendons and ligaments, quasi-static and nonlinear viscoelastic properties, *Biorheology* **19**, 385–396.

11

The Eye

Domenico Lepore, Luigi Ambrosio, Roberto De Santis, Luigi Nicolais, and Luigi Scullica

11.1. Introduction

The eye of the vertebrates provides sensitivity to light, good visual acuity, and a wide field of vision through a camera-like arrangement. The delicate light-sensitive nervous tissue, the retina, is well protected beneath the surface, while a lens system focus images on it (Figure 11.1). Tissues in the light pathway must be transparent and formed into a curved surface, stable and strong enough to avoid distortion or disruption from external impacts. They must be able to repair injuries by active intervention of living cells or by constant renewal of the tissue. Furthermore, these properties must be constant over the years.

The eye can be viewed as a deformed sphere with a diameter of 23–24 mm, largely filled with water and tissues, such as the lens and iris. The wall of the sphere is a three-layered structure: the internal layer is posteriorly composed by the neuroretina, where light transduction take place; the intermediate layer is composed by uveal tissue, which provides nutrition for the other components (Fatt and Weissman, 1992). The outer sheath is a real shell for the eye globe. The anterior portion of this shell, the cornea, must be transparent to allow light passage; it represents 7% of the entire human eye surface and measure 0.5–0.7 mm in thickness. The sclera, which cover the rest, is 0.1–1.0 mm thick.

As in other parts of the body, collagen, a protein with high tensile strength and low extensibility, is the principal constructional material of the

---

Domenico Lepore and Luigi Scullica • Department of Ophthalmology, Catholic University of the Sacred Heart, Largo F. Vito 1, 00168 Rome, Italy. **Luigi Ambrosio, Roberto De Santis, and Luigi Nicolais** • Institute of Composite Materials Technology C.N.R. and C.R.I.B., University of Naples "Federico II," Piazzale Tecchio 80, 80125 Naples, Italy.

Integrated Biomaterials Science, edited by R. Barbucci. Kluwer Academic/Plenum Publishers, New York, 2002.

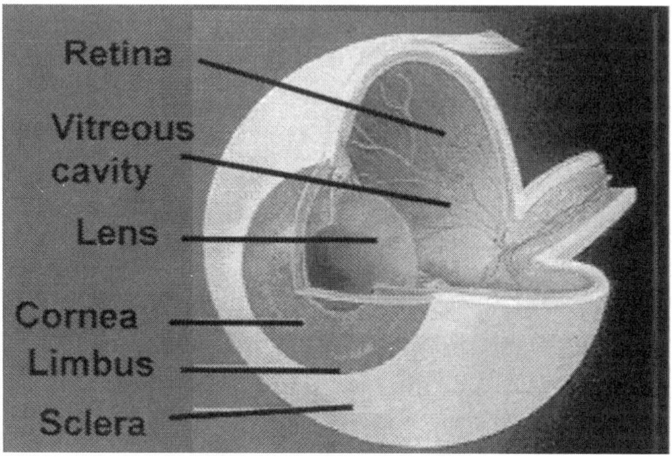

Figure 11.1. Structure of the eye.

eye globe. In particular, it constitutes the deformed spherical external eye shell. The collagen structure of this structure should not be condensed enough to block the growth of the eye. Moreover, it must be resistant to impact like a ping-pong ball, where the resilience to a blow is not in the elasticity of its contents but in the coat itself, which can equalize the strain over its entire surface (Maurice, 1988).

11.2. The Cornea

The cornea is the anterior part of the eye shell. Its geometry is essential for the eye refractive power: the radius of curvature of the external surface is 7.8 mm horizontally and 7.7 mm vertically (Figure 11.2). The cornea is a multilayered tissue, with a superficial layer of the epithelial cells, followed by Bowman's membrane, stroma, Descemet's membrane, and a monolayer endothelium (Figure 11.3).

Water content of the corneal stroma ranges from 65% to 75%; collagen (75% of the dry weight) provides the main structural component, while noncollagenous proteins (5%) and glycosaminoglycans (1%) represent a smaller fraction (Fatt and Weissman, 1992).

The geometry of the collagen fibers in the cornea is extremely regular (Figure 11.4). It is divided into very uniform fibrils, which reduce its light scattering and help make the tissue transparent (Gallagher and Maurice,

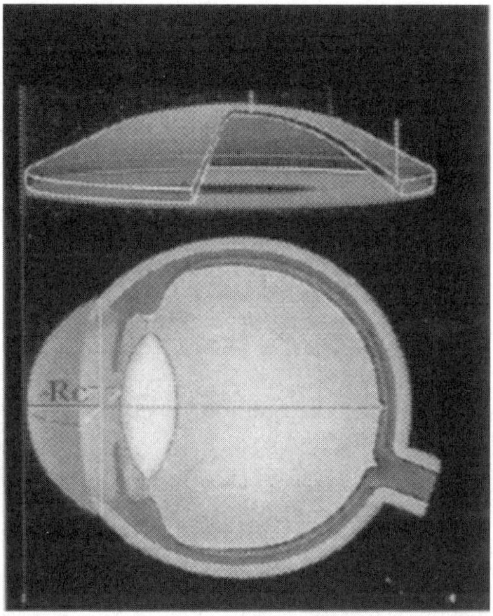

Figure 11.2. Geometry of the cornea: Rc is the radius of curvature.

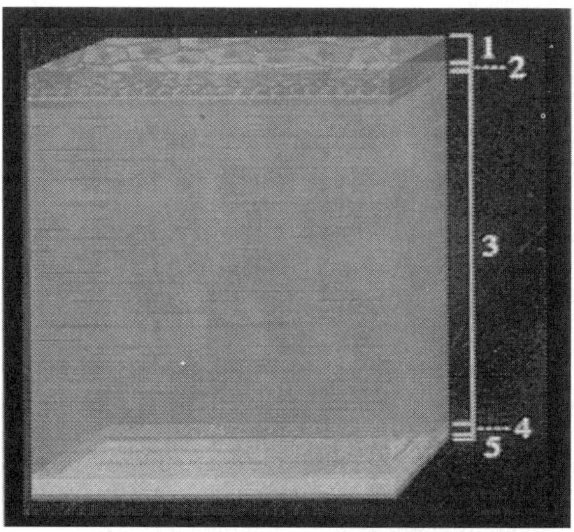

Figure 11.3. Structure of the corneal tissue: (1) epithelium; (2) Bowman's membrane; (3) stroma; (4) Descemet's membrane; (5) endothelium.

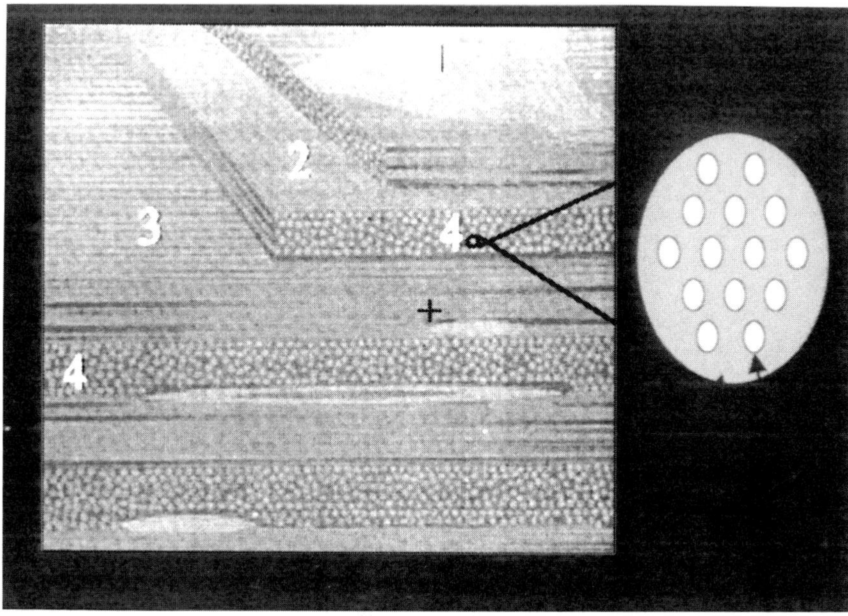

Figure 11.4. Collagen structure in the corneal stroma: (1) keratocyte; (2) perpendicular lamellae; (3) parallel lamellae; (4) collagen fiber; (5) ground substance; (6) collagen fibril.

1977). There are 200 lamellae or bundles parallel to the 2-μm-thick surface (Figure 11.4): fibers have a relatively constant center-to-center spacing (60 nm). The total length of the corneal collagen fibrils is about 15,000 km. Fibrils are braced apart from one another by packing of polysaccharides (Scott and Haigh, 1985). This structure further aids the transparency by spacing the fibrils apart in a regular manner and also provides the open structure required, allowing the diffusion of metabolites that can nourish the cells of the epithelium and the stroma. With fluid access to the stroma, it swells as a result of the expansive force of the polysaccharides (Scott and Haigh, 1985).

The complex structure of the corneal stroma (and of the sclera) can be simplified in the following model (Figure 11.4). Collagen fibrils are arranged in hexagonal arrays of cylinders within each lamella and, on a larger scale, the lamellae themselves form hexagonal arrays of parallel cylinders of 1 μm radius (there is some interweaving if the lamellae are in the sclera). Both the collagen fibrils within the lamellae and the lamellae themselves are surrounded by ground substance, an amorphous gel, consisting of the proteoglycan complexes: GAG-associated protein constitutes 1.5% of the total mass in the corneal stroma (Axelsson and Heinegard, 1978).

It is reasonable to suppose that the fibril disposition, running circumferentially at the limbus, can protect the cornea from rupture in case of high intraocular pressure (Figure 11.5). The orientation of the lamellae in the cornea (and in the sclera) therefore seems to be related to their mechanical functions (Maurice, 1988).

Measurements of the stress–strain relationship under shear clearly show that corneal lamellae must lie on one another without interweaving (Eliason and Maurice, 1981). Although this observation implies that tension in the stroma could not necessarily be uniform, it is possible to show experimentally that it is equal across the stromal thickness. The more interwoven structure of the sclera resists shear much more rigidly (Maurice, 1988).

The mechanical behavior of these tissues can be studied in an isolated strip by the use of a digitally controlled electromechanical testing system. This approach allows one to calculate a stress/strain curve that can document the time course of specimen deformation, load bearing, and wound rupture. It allows evaluating the biomechanical behavior of intact corneal tissue based on parameters such as the elastic modulus, the stress at break, and the strain at break (Bryant *et al.*, 1995).

Although the macrostructure of the collagen is really complex, with evidence of anisotropy, mechanical properties of the cornea are certainly related to the collagen fibril organization, in particular to their three-dimensional distribution.

The "J-shaped" stress–strain curve of rabbit corneal tissue is characterized by an initial toe region where the elongation does not produce any

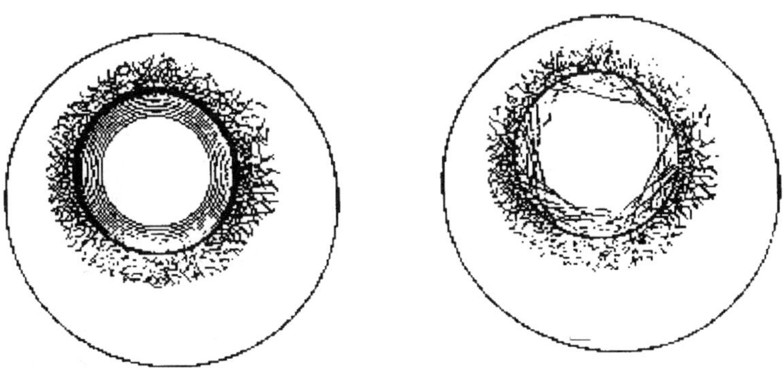

Figure 11.5. Circumferential distribution of collagen fibril at the limbus.

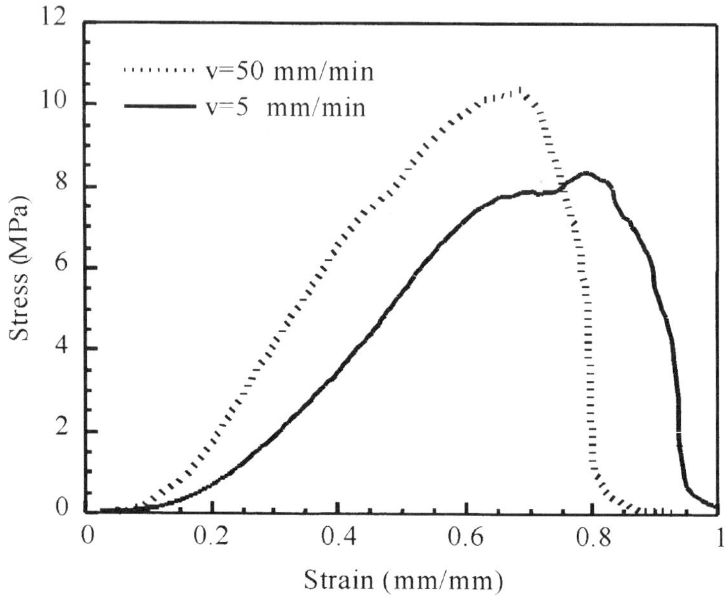

Figure 11.6. Stress–strain behavior of rabbit cornea.

stress in the fibers with a low elastic modulus (Figure 11.6). This behavior is typical of various natural structures. It could be related to the intrinsic properties of the straightening due to the progressive recruitment of collagen fibrils, reflecting viscoelastic properties compatible with the shock-absorbing function of the cornea. The sudden increase in the elastic modulus, which occurs after further specimen elongation, is related to the response of the collagen fibrils within stromal lamellae lying parallel to the strain axis. As more and more fibrils are straightened, the response stiffens, due to the tension being developed in the collagen fibers. These fibers react to strain by developing increased tension, which is reflected by the increased slope of this segment of the stress–strain curve (Figure 11.6). This critical region is indicative of the composite behavior of stromal elements and intercellular cohesive forces. The slope constant for this region has been regarded as representative of the elastic modulus for intact rabbit cornea stretched at 5mm/min (Nucci *et al.*, 1996).

Data acquired from these studies can be utilized to better understand subsequent modification of corneal structure and geometry induced after surgical procedures aimed at adjusting the refractive power of the eye.

11.3. The Sclera

Together with the cornea, the sclera forms the outer tunic of the eye (Figure 11.1). The anterior part of the sclera is covered by conjunctiva, while the remainder has an outer layer called Tenon's capsule. It is lined internally by the choroid, which contains blood vessels, and by the retina, that provides the phototransduction.

The major functions are to give the eye its shape, providing a protective coat, and to withstand the expansive force generated by the intraocular pressure.

The sclera is a fibrous connective tissue. The chemical composition of the sclera is similar to that of the corneal stroma. Water content ranges from 65% to 75%; collagen (75% of the dry weight) provides the main structural component, while GAGs represent a smaller fraction than the corneal stroma (Foster and Sainz de la Maza, 1994).

In mammals, the sclera can be considered as viscoelastic fibrous connective tissue consisting of isolated and flattened fibroblast embedded in an extracellular matrix. This matrix is composed of collagen and elastic fibrils interspersed with proteoglycan molecules. The geometry of the collagen fibers in the sclera differs significantly from the cornea: the diameter is much more variable (ranging from 30 to 300 nm) than in the corneal stroma and their center-to-center spacing ranges between 250 and 280 nm. The boundaries of collagen fibrils show no plate-like arrangement and they are interwoven in a more irregular and complex pattern than those of the cornea. The collagen lamellae run parallel, roughly anterior to posterior, and cross each other increasingly as they travel posteriorly (Fatt and Hedbys, 1970). The fiber distribution is strictly related to the stress exerted on the eye shell. In this, optic fibers are oriented to face the mechanical action of the extraocular muscle, to guarantee resistance against trauma in the anterior part of the eye shell (limbus in particular), and, finally, to ensure the distensibility needed at the posterior pole during the eye growth. The orientation of the scleral collagen fibers in fact, shows regional differences: where a high tensile strength is required (limbus), the number of fibers is increased and their direction is related to the prevailing forces (Figure 11.7). The arrangement of collagen boundaries also differs in the various layers: superficially fibers are further apart, while they become closer in the deeper layers. Deeper fibers are continuous with those of the cornea and condense in a ring, which forms the scleral spur. In this region fibers increase in size from 40 nm in the trabecular sheets to 80 nm close to the sclera, so that the scleral spur feels hard and rigid when surgically incised.

The stress–strain curve of the sclera shows the same profile of the cornea, confirming that a similar structure can result in similar mechanical

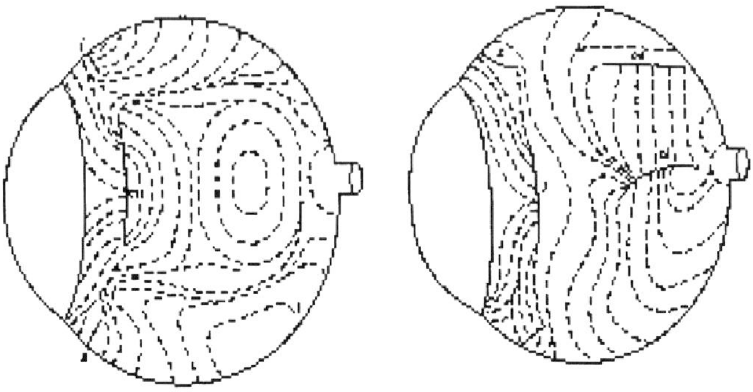

Figure 11.7. Direction of collagen fiber in the sclera. Extraocular muscle insertions are outlined.

behavior. Different sclera zones have in fact different mechanical properties (Figure 11.8). Higher modulus and maximum stress, observed in some scleral region, are probably related to the much more interwoven structure of the scleral collagen lamellae (Lepore *et al.*, 1996a). The distensibility of the limbar scleral region in the fast growing youngest rabbit (10 days old) is similar to that observed for the posterior pole (Figure 11.9), while adult rabbit sclera is much more rigid (Lepore *et al.*, 1996b). These data allows one to hypothesize an active role of the sclera in the eye emmetropization

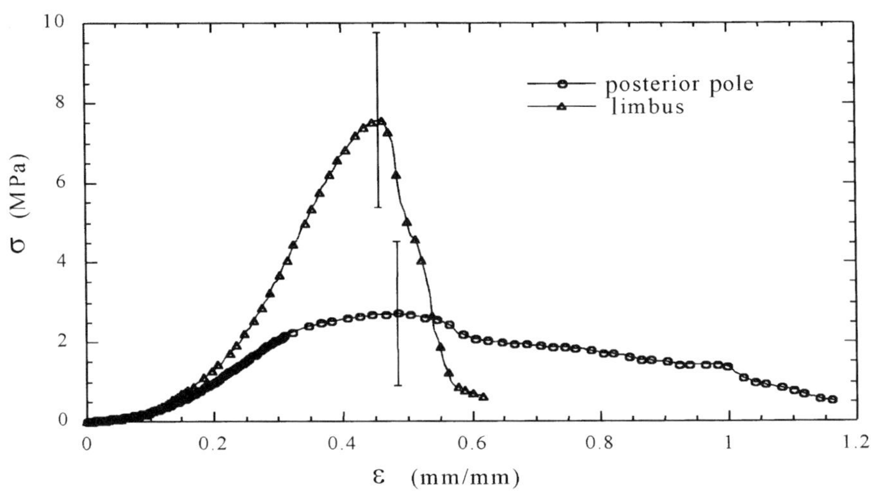

Figure 11.8. Stress–strain behavior of adult rabbit sclera.

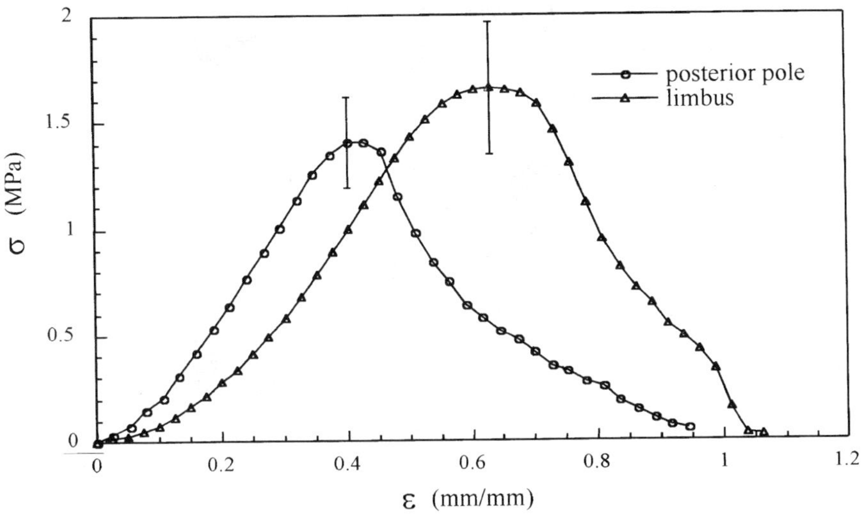

Figure 11.9. Stress–strain behavior of 10-day-old rabbit sclera.

and to explain, at least in part, pathogenesis of the axial myopia, based on the higher distensibility of the posterior pole.

11.4. The Vitreous

The vitreous body fills the center of the eye and, with its 4 ml volume, constitutes about 80% of the globe. It is bounded anteriorly by the lens and its zonular fibers and more posteriorly by ciliary body, retina, and optic disk (Figure 11.10). This particular connective tissue has a spherical shape with a diameter of 16.5 mm and provides an adequate support for the retina, allows the diffusion of metabolitic solutes, and allows the light to reach the retina.

Looking at the vitreous as a material, it can be considered as a hydrogel with high water content. The "vitreous gel," is in fact, essentially formed by water (about 97%) and by an ordered network of fine collagen fibrils (diameter about 10 nm) immersed in a matrix composed mainly of highly hydrated HA macromolecules (Figure 11.11), a glycosaminoglycan (GAG) consisting of residues of D-glucoronic acid, and *N*-acetyl-D-glucosamine (Denlinger and Balasz, 1989). The collagen fibrils run approximately parallel in small bundles. Some bundles of fibrils are orthogonal to others. The protein cores of proteoglycans are regularly associated with

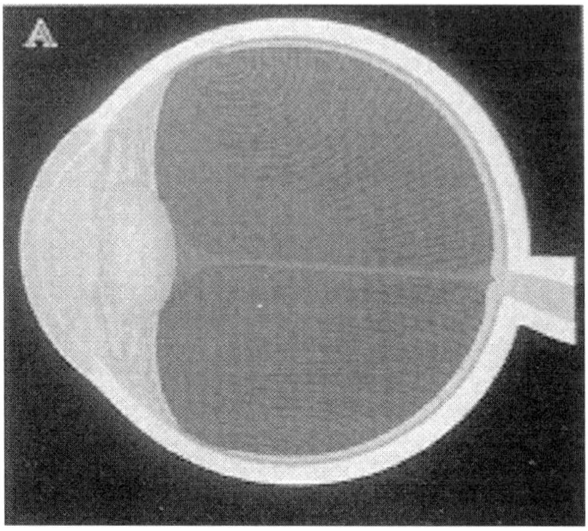

Figure 11.10. Vitreous body.

collagen fibrils at binding sites separated by about 60 nm. The glycosaminoglycan chains (hyaluronan and chondroitin sulfate) are aggregated, making bridges between the bundles of fibrils. This structure permits the vitreous body to be a transparent medium, to maintain an ocular shape, to serve as a mechanical buffer to any movements and impacts (Bettelheim and Wang, 1976), finally, to help keep the retina in its position. The spatial distribution of collagen and hyaluronic acid is not homogeneous: the ratio of hyaluronic acid to collagen is approximately 2 in the anterior portion near the lens, grows to 10 in the center of the eye, and is about 20 in the posterior near the retina.

From the mechanical point of view, the vitreous is a natural composite material formed by a viscoelastic matrix of highly hydrated HA macromolecules reinforced with a network of water-insoluble rigid gel-forming collagen fibrils (Mayne *et al.*, 1991). In aqueous medium it behaves as an expanded random coil molecule occupying a large hydrodynamic volume overlapping with other HA macromolecules, even at low concentration and molecular weight (MW), probably through physical interactions such as polymer "entanglements" responsible for its transient network structure. The viscoelasticity of HA solutions depends mainly on its concentration, molecular weight, and molecular weight distribution (MWD); moreover, owing to its polyelectrolyte nature HA rheological properties depend also on ionic strength, pH, proteins, and other substances present in living tissues. In the vitreous HA macromolecules account for water-retaining, and provide a stabilizing effect on the collagen network. The collagen fibrils

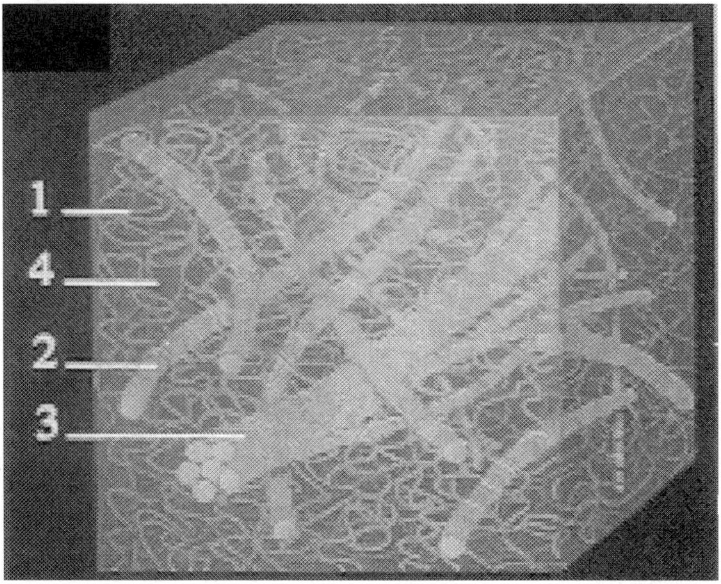

Figure 11.11. Vitreous structure: (1) hyaluronic acid; (2) collagen fibrils; (3) collagen bundles; (4) liquid vitreous.

(diameter about 10 nm) are tied together by PG bridges and run in approximately parallel bundles. The PG bridges can interact through their glycosaminoglycan chains with HA matrix via noncovalent bonds.

Gel vitreous composition changes with age and species, because of variations in collagen content and in HA concentration, MW and MWD. In fact there is a significant variation among different species in collagen fibril concentration, and hence in their network density, because all the species have about the same fibril thickness. Human gel vitreous has a low-density network of collagen fibrils, while rabbit gel vitreous (a model widely used in ophthalmic research) has a very dense collagen network. Moreover, hyaluronate in human vitreous has a weight-average molecular weight of $3–4.5 \times 10^6$, in rabbit vitreous $2–3 \times 10^6$, while this value drops to about 5×10^5 in old bovine. On the other hand, in newborn calf vitreous HA has a corresponding weight of about 3×10^6.

The rheological properties of goat (caprine), sheep (ovine), pig (suine), calf (bovine), and rabbit vitreus bodies, investigated with parallel-plate geometry through frequency sweep tests, strain sweep tests, and steady shear viscosity tests at $T = 37\,^{\circ}\mathrm{C}$, show a linear decrease in steady shear viscosity η and complex viscosity η^* with the imposed shear rate. This is typical of shear thinning (pseudoplastic) behavior (Mensitieri *et al.*, 1994). The values of η^* are one to two orders of magnitude higher than those of η in the investigated range, indicating that vitreous structure is very sensitive to deformations and that simple viscosity is not a correct measure of energy dissipation for this system. In fact, small amplitude oscillatory tests, determining only a slight periodic deformation in the proximity of the rest state of the sample, are more representative of vitreous motions than steady-state viscosity measurement implying large deformations of the material. The strain sweep tests at fixed frequency show a linear behavior of G' and G'' versus g_0 up to about 0.01 strain, then decaying due to destructuration of the material. The rheological behavior is qualitatively similar for all the analyzed vitreous gels. Even if different in absolute value, it behaves as a solid-like rubbery gel (Mensitieri *et al.*, 1994), with the dynamic elastic modulus G' always higher than the dynamic viscous modulus G'' throughout the frequency range investigated (0.05–10 Hz) and both moduli almost parallel to each other. Moreover G', G'', and tan δ do not vary significantly with frequency. It is noteworthy that tan δ varies for the different species in a restricted range (between 0.2 and 0.5 at 1 Hz).

As a result of these peculiar viscoelastic properties, vitreous is essential for the mechanical properties of the eye. In fact, these observations confirm that, apart from its biological and optical role, the vitreous gel plays a key role in maintaining the ocular shape and keeping the retina in position, acting as a mechanical shock absorber for neighboring tissues.

The vitreous body may lose its structural or functional properties due to the presence of opacities, bands, and membranes produced by various diseases. Some relevant eye diseases, such as diabetic proliferative retinopathy and retinal detachment, are directly related to vitreous body anomalies and degeneration. Often, a retinal detachment with or without retinal break is associated with pathological vitreous. Therefore, in many important eye diseases substitution of altered vitreous becomes an urgent need.

Several materials have been tested as vitreous substitutes: saline solutions, silicone oils, hyaluronic acid, air, gas, etc., but none of them has satisfactorily proved to be an ideal substitute. A permanent vitreous substitute should have appropriate properties: biocompatibility, transparency, permanency, refractive index, and viscoelasticity approximating those of natural vitreous. Moreover, these materials should tamponade retinal breaks, whenever present, and push the retina against the choroid. A substance has tamponade properties when it is insoluble in vitreous humor, is able to obstruct or reduce markedly the flow of preretinal fluid toward subretinal space through breaks, and has a poor tendency to diffuse into subretinal space.

Moreover, the relationships between structure and viscoelasticity of a vitreous body of animal origin is of primary importance, because an ideal permanent vitreous substitute must match primarily the mechanical properties of the natural one. It must possess a rheological behavior compatible with the surrounding tissues, protecting them from translatory and especially rotatory eye movements, body movements, vibrations, and indirect and direct traumas. The rheological analysis will therefore be a very useful tool in understanding the structural–mechanical property relationships of these materials and provides interesting information concerning the design of proper vitreous substitutes.

References

Axelsson I., Heinegard, D. 1977. Characterization of the keratan sulphate proteoglycans from bovine corneal stroma, *Biochem. J.* **169**, 517–530.

Bettelheim, F.A, Wang, T.J. 1976. Dynamic viscoelastic properties of bovine vitreous, *Exp. Eye Res.* **23**, 435–441.

Bryant, M.R., Szerenyi, K., Scmotzer, H., McDonnell, P.J. 1995. Corneal tensile strength in fully healed radial keratotomy wounds, *Invest. Ophthalmol. Vis. Sci.*, **35**, 3022–3031.

Denlinger, J.L., Balasz, E.A. 1989. Viscoelastic materials, in: *Vision and Visual Health Care*, Vol. 2 (E.S. Rosen, ed.), Pergamon Press, Oxford.

Eliason, J., Maurice, D. 1981. Stress distribution across the in vivo human cornea, *Invest. Ophthalmol. Vis. Sci.* **26**, 869–872.

Fatt, I., Hedbys, B.O. 1970. Flow of water in the sclera, *Exp. Eye Res.* **10**, 243–249.

Fatt, I., Weissman, J. 1992. *Physiology of the Eye. An Introduction to the Vegetative Functions*, 2nd edn., Butterworth-Heinemann, Boston.

Foster, C.S., Sainz de la Maza, M. 1994. The Sclera, Springer-Verlag, New York.

Gallagher, B., Maurice, D. 1977. Striations of light scattering in the corneal stroma, *J. Ultrastruct. Res.* **61**, 100–114.

Lepore, D., De Santis R., Pagliara, M.M., Borzacchiello, A., Molle, F., Minicucci, G., Ambrosio, L. 1996a. Biomechanical behaviour of human sclera, *Exp. Eye Res.* **63**, Suppl. 1, 719.

Lepore, D., Pagliara, M.M., Nucci, C., Molle, F., DeSantis, R., Ambrosio, L. 1996b. Biomechanical properties of rabbit sclera and cornea, *Vis Res.* **36**, 319.

Maurice, D.M. 1988. Mechanics of the cornea, in: *The Cornea: Transactions of the World Congress on Cornea III* (H.D. Cavanagh, ed.), Raven Press, New York.

Mayne, R., Brewton, R.J., Wright D.W., Ren, Z.X. 1991. Biochemistry of the eye, *Biochem. Soc. Trans.* **19**, 319–340.

Mensitieri, M., Lepore, D., Ambrosio, L., Balzano, L., Nicolais, L. 1994. The rheological behaviour of vitreal substitutes and its comparison with vitreous of animal origin, *J. Mater. Sci., Materials in Medicine* **5**, 743–747.

Nucci, C., Lepore, D., De Santis, R., Ambrosio, L. 1996. Biomechanical properties of rabbit cornea, *Invest. Ophthalmol. Vis.* **37**(3), 379.

Scott, J.E., Haigh, M. 1985. Small proteoglycan: collagen interactions: Keratan sulphate proteoglycan associates with rabbit corneal collagen fibrils at the "a" and "c" bands, *Biosci. Rep.* **5**, 765.

12

Articular Cartilage

Paolo A. Netti and Luigi Ambrosio

12.1. Introduction

Articular cartilage is a 0.5 to 5 mm thick layer of hydrated soft tissue that covers the articulating extremities in diarthrodial joints. The main biomechanical function of articular cartilage is to sustain and transmit loads between bones, allowing the joint to have relative motion along multiple axes. During a normal walking cycle these loads can be as large as six times that of body weight (Mow *et al.*, 1992) . To fulfil its biomechanical functions, the articular cartilage must have a set of unique mechanical and physiochemical properties. The assortment and variety of these properties make the articular cartilage a material which presents a real challenge to modern materials science. Indeed, from an engineering point of view, these tissues are very extraordinary materials: they are able to function effectively for more than 80 years in a nearly frictionless and wear-resistant manner. The macroscopic mechanical properties of articular cartilage are determined by the composition of the tissues, mainly collagen and proteoglycans, their assembly at ultramolecular level, and their interactions with the interstitial fluids. Fluid flow through the interstitial space plays an important role not only in determining the mechanical functions of the articular cartilage, but also in regulating the trafficking of nutrients and waste within the tissue.

If the composition and assembly of the extracellular matrix regulates the load-bearing features of the articular cartilage, the mechanical stresses within the tissue affect the biosynthesis and organization of the matrix. In this sense articular cartilage is a self-adaptive material. Significant

---

Paolo A. Netti and Luigi Ambrosio • Institute of Composite Materials Technology C.N.R., and C.R.I.B., University of Naples "Federico II", Piazzale Tecchio 80, 80125 Naples, Italy.

Integrated Biomaterials Science, edited by R. Barbucci. Kluwer Academic/Plenum Publishers, New York, 2002.

mechanoelectrochemical transduction occurs within the extracellular matrix which affects and modulates chondrocyte metabolic activities. These activities include biosynthesis, assembly, and degradation of the macromolecular components of the extracellular matrix. Thus the appropriate balance between all these activities results in a maintenance of the cartilage matrix and its biological function providing the long-lasting properties of this tissue. Significant progress has been made over the past two decades for the comprehension of the biomechanical function of the articular cartilage (Mow *et al.*, 1984, 1992, 1993; Simon 1992). Seminal work carried out by Mow and co-workers (Mow *et al.*, 1992, 1993; Woo *et al.*, 1987) and other groups (Frank and Grodzinsky, 1987a,b; Simon 1992) has elucidated the link between the composition and structure of the tissue and its biomechanical functions. This work is beneficial for both engineers, who can learn from nature's design how to develop synthetic materials with the same extraordinary long-lasting properties, and biomedical researchers, who can better understand the joint function and origin of cartilage pathology. In this chapter we present a summary of the intrinsic mechanical properties of the articular cartilage and discuss these in terms of the composition and hierarchical structure of the tissue.

12.2. Composition and Structure

12.2.1. Composition

Articular cartilage consists of a liquid phase, composed of fluids and electrolytes, and a solid phase, composed of cells (chondrocytes), collagen, proteoglycans, and hyaluronic acid. In healthy tissue, the cellular content is very modest ($<5\%$ by volume) and does not contribute significantly to the mechanical properties of the cartilage, although it plays an active role in biosynthesis and remodeling. The major constituent of the organic phase is the collagen present in fibrillar form with a composition of about 50–80% of the dry weight or about 15–22% of the wet weight. In healthy cartilage, the predominant type of collagen in cartilage is type II with traces of other types, including type IX and XI (Eyre *et al.*, 1987; Kuettner *et al.*, 1986; Nimni 1988; Van de Rest and Mayne, 1988). An amount of collagen type I has been reported in degenerated cartilage (Ratcliffe and Mow, 1996). Proteoglycans (PGs) represent the second largest portion of the organic phase. The major PGs present in articular cartilage are the high molecular weight (range 1×10^6 to 4×10^6) aggregating and not aggregating type (about 90%) with a small percentage of low molecular weight PGs (Mow *et al.*, 1992). The interstitial space is filled with water and dissolved electrolytes. The fluid content in cartilage ranges from 60 to 85% by weight (Mow *et al.*, 1984; Torzilli, 1985).

12.2.2. Structure

As other soft tissues, articular cartilage has a hierarchical structure at various scale lengths: the molecular scale (nanoscale, 1–100 nm), the ultramolecular scale (microscale, 0.1–100 mm), and the tissue scale (0.1–10 mm). At each hierarchical level, the structure has a significant role in determining the physical and physiological properties of cartilage.

At the molecular scale collagen is present as tropocollagen, which is a rod-like molecule of approximately 1.4 nm diameter and 300 nm long. These tropocollagen molecules are formed by three collagen polypeptide chains coiled into left-handed helices, which are coiled on each other into right-handed triple helices. Tropocollagen is produced intracellularly and then secreted into the extracellular space, where the basic tropocollagen units assemble together to form collagen fibrils whose diameter ranges from 20 to 200 nm with a length that can reach also some millimeters (Nimni, 1988). Collagen fibers further cross-link together to form a stable network (Figure 12.1). The collagen network thus provides the high tensile stiffness and strength of the tissue.

PGs are composed of a core protein to which glycosaminoglycan (GAG) units (chondroitin sulfate and keratin sulfate) are covalently bound (Figure 12.1). Chondroitin sulfate is composed of repeating units of glucuronic acid and N-acetyl-galactosamine with a sulfate group (SO_4) and a carboxyl group (COOH) per disaccharide, while keratin sulfate is composed of repeating disaccharide units of galactose and N-acetyl-glucosamine with one SO_4 group per disaccharide. These carboxylic and sulfate groups are partially hydrolyzed, leading to fixed charges on PGs chains (Figure 12.1). The presence of these fixed charges on the GAG chains provides important physiochemical properties to cartilage, as we shall see in the next section. Depending on molecular weight and the type of GAG units attached to the core protein, the PGs are classified as high and low molecular weight and aggregating and nonaggregating. These different kinds of PGs have different physiological functions. High molecular weight PGs are highly ordered structures with dimensions ranging from 10 to 1000 nm. PGs often form large aggregates by binding to a long filament chain of hyaluronate. The size of these aggregates is variable and can reach 350 mm. The molecular weight of PGs, the relative amount of different GAG that form the PGs, the fixed charge density on a PG chain, the length of core

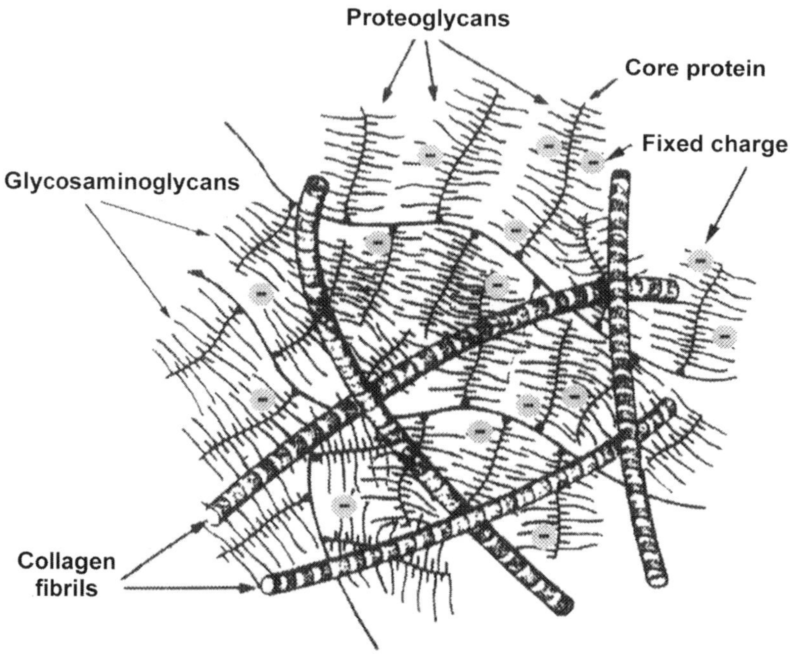

Figure 12.1. Schematic representation of extracellular matrix structure at a microscale level. The fibrillar component is mainly constituted by collagen fibrils whose diameters range from 20 to 200 nm and have length up to some millimeters. The hydrophilic chains of proteoglycans are anchored to the collagen network, helping to stabilize the collagen network. The hydrophilic groups on the proteoglycan chains are partially hydrolyzed, leading to fixed negative charges which are balanced by counterions present in the interstitial fluids.

protein, and the degree and size of aggregates all contribute to the mechanical properties of the tissue.

At tissue level, the collagen network and PGs should not be considered as two separate phases of the extracellular matrix but rather as a single phase similar to an interpenetrated polymer network (IPN). Indeed, although covalent bonds are not possible between collagen and PGs, there is evidence to indicate the existence of collagen–proteoglycan mechanical and electrostatic interactions. The negatively charged groups on the PGs can interact with the positively charged groups along the collagen fibrils (Muir, 1981; Nimni, 1988), and it has been shown that hyaluronates interact with collagen type II, IX and X (Poole *et al.*, 1982). Furthermore, it has been reported that there is strong mechanical friction between PGs and collagen fibers (Schmidt *et al.*, 1990) and this leads to strong physical entanglements. The collagen and PG content in cartilage varies from the surface to the deep zone. In particular, collagen content is highest in the surface zone and decreases by approximately 15% in the middle and deep zone (Mow *et al.*, 1992) . Conversely, the PG content is lowest at the surface and increases by 15% in the middle and deep zone (Mow *et al.*, 1992). Also, the orientation of the collagen fibers changes from the surface to the deep zone. At the surface, collagen fibers are aligned parallel to the articular surface; in the middle zone the fibers have a larger diameter and are arranged randomly; in the deep zone the fibers are woven in bundles and aligned perpendicular to the surface (Clark, 1985; Poole *et al.*, 1984; Redler *et al.*, 1975).

Also, the water content in cartilage is variable. It reflects the change measured for collagen, being highest at the surface (about 80%) and lowest in the deep zone (about 65%).

Interspersed with the collagen–PG network is the cellular phase constituted by chondrocytes. Chondrocytes have dimensions of the order of tens of microns and are anchored to both collagen and PGs. They are responsible for matrix molecule biosynthesis, organization, and remodeling. It has been suggested that the inhomogeneity in extracellular matrix composition and structure found in cartilage correlates with the different biosynthetic activity of cells.

Another important structural aspect of the articular cartilage is the dimension of the interspace between the macromolecular component of the tissue (i.e., pore size) and the distribution of interstitial water. About 70% of the interstitial water is entrapped in the solution domain of proteoglycans molecules (Katz *et al.*, 1986; Torzilli, 1985) while the remainder is within the intrafibrillar compartment of collagen. The total amount of interstitial water depends mainly on the number of hydrophilic groups present on the PG chains and their degree of hydrolysis, the ionic strength of the interstitial fluid, and the organization and mechanical strength of the collagen–PG network. The size of the pores between the macromolecular component controls both convective and diffusive transport of fluids and macromolecules within the tissues. As we shall see, resistance to fluid transport plays an important role not only in controlling the dynamical-mechanical response of articular cartilage but is also important for many other biological functions of the tissues. Interstitial fluid percolates through the interfibrillar space (2 to 6 nm) of the matrix (Mow *et al.*, 1984) driven by hydrostatic and osmotic pressure gradients. Fluids movements controls the transport of nutrients and metabolic waste to and from the cells, the tissue homeostasis, and regulates the mechanical response of the articular cartilage.

12.3. Mechanical Properties

The macroscopic behavior of cartilage depends on its complex microscopic structure, specifically, the synergistic interactions among the various components of the extracellular matrix. As discussed in the previous section, articular cartilage as well as other biological tissues is a nonisotropic and nonhomogeneous composite material. Therefore, also its properties will be anisotropic and inhomogeneous, as has been well documented in the literature (Mow *et al.*, 1990b; Roth and Mow, 1980; Schmidt *et al.*, 1990; Woo *et al.*, 1987). In the following, experimental methods commonly used to measure the static and dynamical mechanical properties will be presented along with a discussion of the most peculiar mechanical behavior of articular cartilage.

12.3.1. Static Properties

Typical static load–strain curves of articular cartilage are represented in Figure 12.2. These curves, which are also typical of others soft tissues (Fung, 1993; Netti *et al.*, 1996), show the nonlinear and anisotropic behavior of the tissue. In tension, the curve presents an initial upward curvature (toe region) followed by a progressive increase in modulus up to a "linear" region. Conversely, in compression the curve presents an initial linear region followed by a downward curvature. Furthermore, the slope at the origin is not continuous, going from compression to tension. The nonlinear behavior in tension can be explained as follows: The low strain region is associated with the stretching or uncrimping of collagen bundles, while the linear region results from the alignment of the collagen fibers in the direction of stretch. Therefore, the modulus of the low region is characteristic of the PG phase while the higher modulus of the linear region is characteristic of the collagen network (Fung, 1993; Roth and Mow, 1980; Woo *et al.*, 1987). This nonlinear behavior has been usually described with a fiber-recruitment model in which the progressive alignment of the collagen fibers along the direction of the load is modeled by an exponential constitutive equation:

$$\sigma = E(e^{\alpha\varepsilon} - 1)$$

which gives an expression for Young's modulus:

$$\frac{d\sigma}{d\varepsilon} = \alpha\sigma + \alpha E$$

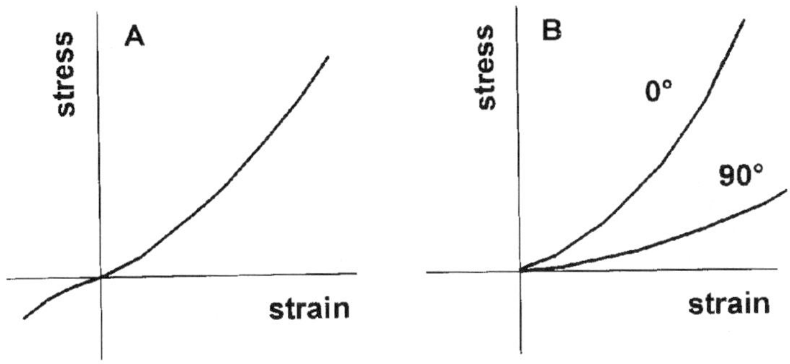

Figure 12.2. Typical static stress–strain curves of articular cartilage. Figure 12.2A shows the nonlinear behavior of the tissue; at low strain the curve presents the initial toe regions (low modulus) followed by a progressive increase of the modulus in both compression and tension. The stress–strain curve is not symmetric with respect to the origin, indicating a difference of the response in compression and tension. Figure 12.2B shows the nonisotropic behavior of the tissue; the specimens taken parallel to the split line (0°) are stiffer than the specimens taken perpendicular (90°). Rearranged from Mow *et al.* (1992).

The exponential law is suggested by the experimental data and leads to the result that the elastic modulus increases linearly with the stress as more and more collagen fibers become stretched, according to the concept of fiber recruitment (Fung, 1993).

In compression, articular cartilage withstands static load with an even more intriguing mechanism. Tissue proteoglycans are immobilized within the collagen network through electrostatic and mechanical constraints. The presence of these constraints prevents the free swelling of the PGs, leading to an osmotic pressure on the interstitial water. Furthermore, a Donnan contribution to the osmotic pressure also arises due to the presence of fixed negative charge on the PG chains. Indeed, the ionized sulfated and carboxyl groups (SO_3^- and COO^-) on keratin and chondroitin sulfated GAGs generate an imbalance between the total ion concentration within the tissue and that of the outside fluid. This imbalance of ions brings about an osmotic pressure known as the Donnan pressure. The presence of an osmotic pressure, also referred to as swelling pressure, ensures that the cartilage is constantly maintained in a swollen state while loaded. The osmotic pressure contributes significantly to the overall mechanical stiffness of the cartilage in static compression. Another important effect is due to repulsive forces between the charged groups of PGs. These charged groups are very close to each other (1.0 to 1.5 nm) and this distance is within the Debye length. Therefore, there is a strong charge-to-charge repulsive force acting between charged groups which also contributes significantly to the rigidity of the tissue in compression.

In conclusion, the behavior of cartilage in compression depends not only on the intrinsic elasticity of the macromolecular component, but also on the electromechanical effects due to the presence of fixed charges. Mow and co-workers (1990a) have reported that the contribution of this charge effect to the overall compressive stiffness can be up to 50%.

Figure 12.2b shows the anisotropy of the articular cartilage: specimens cut along different directions exhibit different behavior. In particular, specimens harvested perpendicularly to the surface are stiffer than those harvested along the direction of the surface. Furthermore, the mechanical properties also change from the surface to the deep zone. According to the collagen distribution, the elastic modulus in tension decreases passing from the surface to the deep zone (Mow *et al.*, 1992). The linear-region elastic modulus of articular cartilage ranges from 42 to 1.1 MPa while the toe-region modulus ranges from 60 to 0.4 MPa depending on the orientation and position (Roth and Mow, 1980).

12.3.2. Time-Dependent Properties

The most relevant loading mode in articular cartilage is dynamic. To discuss viscoelastic properties of the articular cartilage it is convenient to separate the shear from the compression properties. This is because there are two distinct contributions to the time-dependent behavior of articular cartilage, namely, (a) the intrinsic viscoelastic properties of the macromolecular network and (b) the *flow-dependent* viscoelastic properties. The former are related to macromolecular rearrangement induced by stress, while the latter are related to the frictional drag due to interstitial fluid flow. Interstitial fluid redistribution occurs as a result of an external applied compressive load. In a pure deviatoric strain field (i.e., shear), no volumetric change of the tissue occurs and thus no fluid flow results. Hence, shear experiments are useful to evaluate the intrinsic viscoelastic tissue properties.

12.3.3. Viscoelastic Shear Properties

The stress relaxation test indicates that articular cartilage is a relatively high-compliant tissue having a shear modulus ranging from 0.2 to 0.4 MPa (Mow *et al.*, 1992). These values are comparable to the modulus in the toe region in tension. The stress relaxation follows a quasi-linear viscoelastic behavior (Fung, 1993) with one relaxation time.

Viscoelastic shear properties of articular cartilage have also been determined in dynamics. These properties are characterized by two parameters, the storage modulus (G') and the loss modulus (G'') (Jenkins and Little, 1974). The former is associated with the elastic energy stored in the material, while the latter is associated with the dissipation of energy caused by structural rearrangements within the material. Experimentally, it is possible to measure these two moduli by imposing a sinusoidal perturbation on the material, either in load or strain, and measuring the elastic (in-phase) and viscous (out-of-phase) components of the response (Christensen, 1971; Fung, 1993). The moduli G' and G'' are only rigorously defined in the limit of linear viscoelasticity, and thus G' and G'' are functions only of time or frequency. However, in the case of nonlinear viscoelastic behavior (as in cartilage), it is still possible to approximate the quantities G' and G'' at a given level of stress with a local linearization of stress vs. strain [quasi-linear viscoelastic solid (Fung, 1993)]. The ratio between G'' and G' indicates the energy dissipated during the shearing, which is related to the phase shift angle between the solicitation and the response. Applying a sinusoidal strain with a frequency ω [$\varepsilon = \varepsilon_o \sin(\omega t)$], the material properties are defined:

$$G^* = G' + iG'' = \sigma_0(\cos\delta + i\sin\delta), \ \tan\delta = \frac{G''}{G'}$$

where $i = \sqrt{-1}$, and σ_0 is the response stress amplitude. The magnitude of the complex shear modulus ($|G^*| = \sqrt{G'^2 + G''^2}$) increases monotonically from 0.2 to 2.5 MPa with increasing frequency from 0.01 to 20 Hz (Mow *et al.*, 1992), indicating a strong strain-rate dependence of the collagen–proteoglycan matrix. Within the same frequency range, the phase shift varies between 9° and 22°. Comparing these results with those of proteoglycan solution, it could be concluded that the shear stiffness of articular cartilage is mainly controlled by the collagen network. Indeed, the complex modulus of proteoglycan solution is low by about 3 orders of magnitude (10 Pa) and the phase shift lies between 40° and 85°, indicating a more viscous behavior (Mow *et al.*, 1992). Furthermore, this conclusion is supported by the strong statistical correlation found between $|G^*|$ and the collagen content of the tissue. However, since the PGs in the tissues are anchored to the collagen scaffold, their role in controlling the shear modulus of the tissue can be more important than that suggested by the data of PG solutions.

12.3.4. Viscoelastic Properties in Compression

The compressive behavior of articular cartilage, as well as many other soft hydrated tissues, depends not only on the intrinsic mechanical stiffness of the macromolecular components, but also on the fluid transport properties of the tissue. This concept is better described if we consider the tissue as being a sponge-like material, i.e., a biphasic material made up of a fluid phase (water and electrolytes) and a porous–solid phase (collagen and proteoglycans). When a sponge is compressed, fluid movement takes place as a result of the solid deformation. The fluid percolates through the pores of the sponge and oozes out from the surface driven by a pressure gradient, which is generated by the deformation of the sponge. The percolating fluid, on the other hand, induces a deformation of the solid matrix. The resulting process is governed by the fluid transport and the mechanical properties of the sponge. To squeeze the sponge, it is necessary to overcome both the stiffness of the solid phase and the fluid flow resistance. The stiffness of the solid phase depends on the rigidity of the network, while the flow resistance is mainly controlled by the pore size and the fluid properties. Therefore, to describe the mechanical properties in compression of cartilage it is necessary to characterize its fluid transport properties.

12.3.5. Hydraulic Conductivity of Cartilage

Interstitial fluid movement is involved in many important biological processes and contributes to the mechanical behavior of articular cartilage. Fluid movement is driven by tissue hydrostatic pressure gradients (Fung, 1990) and is controlled by the composition and structure of the extracellular matrix. The physical parameter that measures how easily fluid moves through the interstitium is the hydraulic conductivity (K), defined as

$$K = q/\nabla p$$

where q is Darcy's fluid flux (m/s) and ∇p is the hydrostatic pressure gradient. Experimentally, the hydraulic conductivity can be measured by applying a given pressure gradient across a tissue slab and measuring the resulting fluid flow. Results from these experiments showed that the hydraulic conductivity for articular cartilage ranges from 10^{-14} to 10^{-16} $m^4/N/s$ (Lai and Mow, 1980; Mansour and Mow, 1976). It has been shown that the hydraulic conductivity depends strongly on tissue hydration (Levick, 1987a, b; Mow *et al.*, 1984, 1992). On compressing the articular cartilage, a compaction of the tissue will result as a consequence of fluid exudation. This compaction leads to a significant decrease in hydraulic conductivity. Usually an exponential function is used to describe this hydration dependence behavior (Lai and Mow, 1980; Levick, 1987a; Winlove and Parker, 1995):

$$K = K_0 e^{b(\phi - \phi_0)}$$

where ϕ is the actual tissue hydration and ϕ_0 is the hydration of the tissue in its unstrained state; K_0 is the hydraulic conductivity of the unstrained tissue and b is a fitting parameter.

It has been suggested by several authors (Lai and Mow, 1980; Levick, 1987a; Mow *et al.*, 1984; Winlove and Parker, 1995) that the resistance to fluid transport is mainly controlled by the proteoglycan component of the extracellular matrix. Indeed, PGs are highly hydrophilic polymers and thus have a large excluded volume that hinders fluid movement. This hypothesis has also been supported by experimental observations that there is a strong correlation between the hydraulic conductivity and the GAG content of a tissue (Levick, 1987a; Winlove and Parker, 1995) and that collagen network *in vitro* provides a resistance to fluid transport which is orders of magnitude lower that of PG solutions (Barocas and Tranquillo, 1997; Maroudas *et al.*, 1987; Saltzman *et al.*, 1994).

The very low values of hydraulic conductivity of articular cartilage indicate that the tissue poses a strong resistance to fluid transport and thus very large pressure gradients are required to move fluid through the interstitium or, equivalently, a large amount of energy is dissipated by frictional forces between water and solid matrix during loading. During daily activities, the contact stress acting on the cartilage surface is within the range of 3 to 10 MPa (Hodge *et al.*, 1986). This stress is distributed between the solid and the fluid component of the matrix according to their volume fraction. Assuming an average volume fraction of fluid of 75%, the interstitial fluid pressure at the articular surface would be within the range of 0.22 to 7.5 MPa. Thus assuming a 2-mm-thick layer of cartilage, at the highest value of surface stress the fluid flux across the cartilage surface would be very modest (within 5 to 50 m/s). Since the bone side of cartilage is impermeable to fluids, the exudate from the surface is pressurized. This fluid pressurization plays an important role in the load-bearing features of articular cartilage and also causes a cyclic fluid flow in and out the cartilage as the joint moves, providing the required film of fluid for lubrication (Mow and Lai, 1980b; Mow and Soslowsky, 1991).

12.3.6. Compressive Behavior of Articular Cartilage

Two continuum models are commonly used to describe the mechanics of soft tissues: biphasic and poroelasticity theory. The former considers soft tissue as an intimate mixture of solid and fluid phases (a concentrated macromolecular solution) while the latter simulates soft tissue to be a fluid-saturated poroelastic solid (a sponge-like material). The poroelastic theory was originally formulated by Biot for the analysis of wet soil consolidation (Biot, 1941, 1955) and then applied to soft tissue mechanics

(Simon *et al.*, 1983). The mixture theory as developed by Truesdell and Toupin (1960), Bowen (1976, 1980), and others was applied to soft tissue mechanics by Mow *et al.* (1980) who first developed a linear biphasic model for articular cartilage (Mow *et al.*, 1980, 1984, 1990b; Mow and Lai, 1980).

The theory assumes that the total stress acting on the tissue is the sum of the stress acting on the elastic solid and the stress acting on the interstitial fluid:

$$\boldsymbol{\sigma}' = \boldsymbol{\sigma}^s + \boldsymbol{\sigma}^f$$

where the fluid phase can be described by the hydrostatic pressure within the tissue (Netti *et al.*, 1997), i.e., $\boldsymbol{\sigma}^f = -\phi^f p\mathbf{I}$. The momentum balance for the tissue under the hypothesis of negligible inertial forces is

$$\nabla \cdot \boldsymbol{\sigma}^T = \mathbf{0} \tag{12.1}$$

For the momentum balance of the fluid phase it is assumed that the divergence of the fluid stress is balanced by the frictional drag force, i.e.,

$$\nabla \cdot \boldsymbol{\sigma}^f = \zeta(\mathbf{v}^f - \mathbf{v}^s)$$

where ζ is the drag coefficient; $\mathbf{v}^f$ and $\mathbf{v}^s$ are the local velocities of the fluid and solid phase, respectively. This equation can be also be written as

$$\phi^f(\mathbf{v}^f - \mathbf{v}^s) = -K\nabla p \tag{12.2}$$

where $K = (\phi^f)^2/\zeta$ is the tissue hydraulic conductivity. This equation can also be seen as a generalized Darcy's law, where the hydrostatic pressure gradient acts on the relative velocity between the solid and liquid phases, and it expresses the basic concept of the biphasic theory, i.e., the coupling between stress and fluid movement. Indeed, if the divergence of the solid stress tensor $(\nabla \cdot \sigma^s)$ is not zero, then a hydrostatic pressure gradient arises leading to a relative motion between the solid and fluid phase. Equations (12.1) and (12.2) along with the mass balance equations for the solid and fluid phase and the constitutive equation for the solid network can be solved together in the variables $\mathbf{v}^f$, $\mathbf{v}^s$, $\boldsymbol{\sigma}^f$, p, and $\boldsymbol{\sigma}^s$.

In the case of infinitesimal strain, linearly elastic solid, and constant hydraulic conductivity, the theory takes a simple form known as KLM biphasic theory for cartilage (Mow *et al.*, 1980, 1984, 1990b; Mow and Lai, 1980). The linear biphasic theory has also been extended to include nonlinearities corresponding to strain-dependent permeability (Holmes *et al.*, 1985; Lai and Mow, 1980), finite deformation (Holmes, 1986; Mow *et al.*, 1986; Simon and Gaballa, 1988a, 1988b), and viscoelasticity (Mak, 1986). This model successfully describes the load-bearing behavior of articular cartilage (Mow and Lai, 1979; Spilker and Suh, 1990; Spilker *et al.*, 1992), as well as other soft hydrated tissues such as intervertebral discs (Simon, 1992; Simon *et al.*, 1983), artery walls (Jain and Jayaraman, 1987; Kenyon, 1979; Simon and Gaballa, 1988a), brain tissue (Basser, 1992; Nagashima *et al.*, 1987, 1990), hydrogels and other tissues (Barocas *et al.*, 1995; Barocas and Tranquillo, 1997; Grimshaw *et al.*, 1989; Netti *et al.*, 1995, 1997).

Using the biphasic theory, creep and stress relaxation behavior in compression of articular cartilage can be accurately described. The time-dependent features of the tissue result from a coupling between fluid transport and macromolecular rearrangement of the solid matrix. Experimentally, the material properties in compression are usually determined by tests of creep or stress relaxation in confined compression or unconfined geometry.

12.3.7. Confined Compression

In this test, the surface of a small cylindrical plug of cartilage is loaded with a rigid fitted porous platen as shown schematically in Figure 12.3. The plug is mounted in an impermeable confining chamber which prevents both radial deformation and fluid leakage from the lateral surface of the tissue. The porous platen allows interstitial fluid to flow freely between the tissue

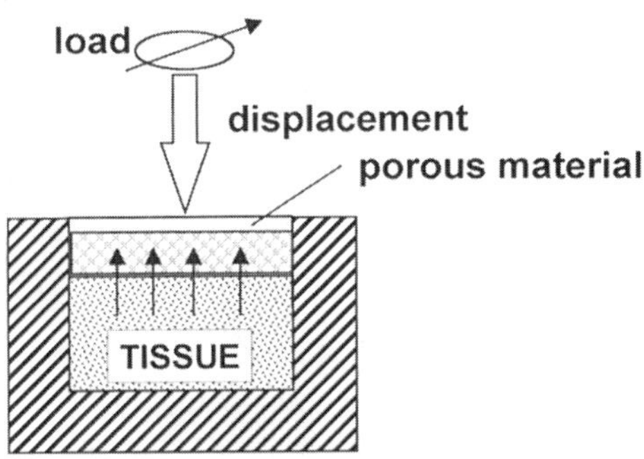

Figure 12.3. Confined compression experiment chamber. A small cylindrical plug of tissue is placed in an impermeable confining chamber which prevents both radial deformation and fluid leakage from the lateral surface of the tissue. The surface of the cartilage specimen is loaded with a rigid fitted porous platen which allows interstitial fluid to flow freely to and from the tissue during the experiment. Depending on the experiment, a load (creep) or a displacement (stress relaxation) is applied to the sample.

and the saline reservoir during the experiment. Depending on the experiment, a load (creep) or a displacement (stress relaxation) is applied to the sample. The confinement of the sample guarantees that fluid flow and strain field are uniaxial.

Figure 12.4 shows schematically the fluid and stress distribution within an articular cartilage sample during a stress relaxation experiment. In this experiment a displacement ramp is imposed on the sample. To allow the deformation of the tissue, fluid is forced out of the sample through the porous platen (point a). Owing to the low values of the tissue hydraulic conductivity, large loads are needed to compress the tissue (point b). At the end of the displacement ramp, fluid redistribution occurs within the tissue to dissipate the hydrostatic pressure gradient within the tissue generated during the compression (point c). When the hydrostatic pressure gradient is completely dissipated, fluid flow stops and a new equilibrium condition is attained (point d). The stress measured at this final equilibrium can be used to estimate the elastic modulus of the tissue, while the time constant of the relaxation process can be used to estimate the hydraulic conductivity. The characteristic time for the relaxation process is

$$\tau = h^2/HK$$

where h is the specimen thickness, H the elastic modulus, and K the hydraulic conductivity. A more accurate determination of parameters H and K can be obtained by fitting the stress relaxation curve to the analytical solution of the biphasic model (Mow *et al.*, 1980).

Extensive tests have been performed on several kinds of human cartilage using confined compression analysis (Woo *et al.*, 1987). The materials properties obtained have been correlated with age (Armstrong and Mow, 1982b), water content (Armstrong and Mow, 1982b), and GAG and collagen content (Armstrong and Mow, 1982a; Mow *et al.*, 1992). These data show that the articular cartilage is a very soft material in compression, having an equilibrium elastic modulus of about 1MPa (Woo *et al.*, 1987). The apparent stiffness of articular cartilage in compression is thus mainly controlled by the high resistance that this tissue poses to fluid movement. The very low hydraulic conductivity ensures a high interstitial fluid pressurization during loading, so that articular cartilage can work at relatively modest deformation suitable for long-lasting performances.

12.4. Electromechanical Transduction

We have already discussed the effect of the fixed charges on the PG chains upon the equilibrium swelling pressure of articular cartilage. In

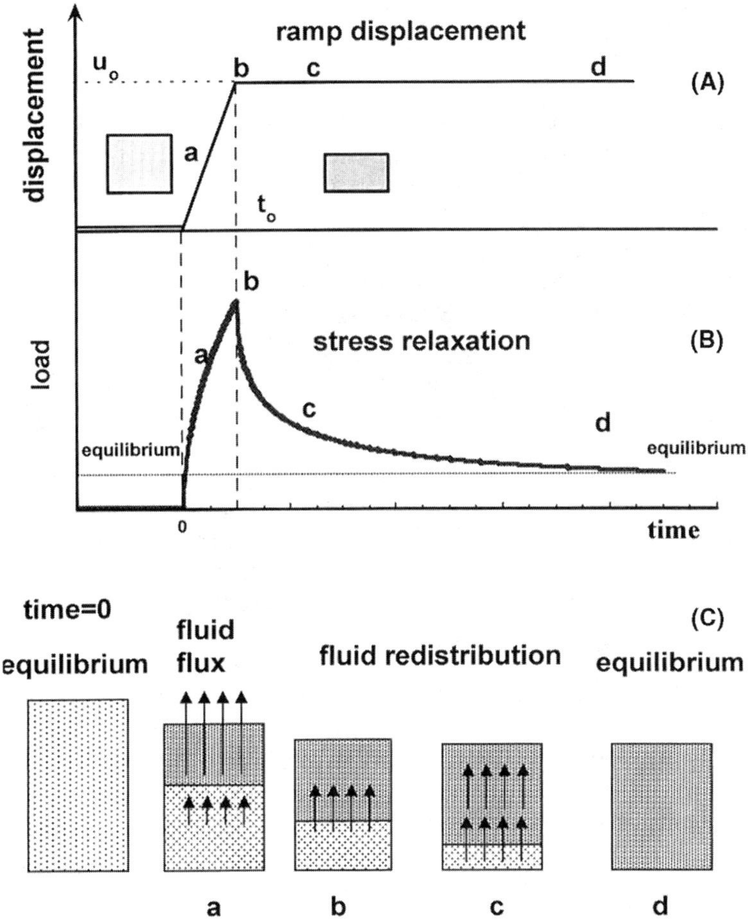

Figure 12.4. Confined compression stress relaxation test. Figure 12.4A and B show the imposed ramp displacement (A) and the resulting stress relaxation response (B). Figure 12.4C shows the fluid distribution within the sample during the experiment. During the ramp diplacement, fluids are squeezed out of the tissue; the stress increases due to the low values of the tissue hydraulic conductivity. At the end of the ramp displacement, fluid redistribution occurs within the tissue to dissipate the hydrostatic pressure gradient within the tissue generated during the compression (point c). When the hydrostatic pressure gradient is completely dissipated, fluid flow stops and a new equilibrium condition is attained (point d). Rearranged from Woo *et al.* (1987).

dynamic situations, such as that of a physiological loading cycle, the presence of fixed charges and mobile counterions gives rise to an important phenomenon of mechanoelectrochemical transduction, which is of fundamental importance in the biomechanical function of articular cartilage and may play an important role in controlling chondrocyte metabolism and tissue homeostasis.

When cartilage is compressed, fluid exudates from the surface. Mobile ions in solution are carried by fluid, leading to a transient perturbation in the electrical neutrality of the tissue. This charge separation phenomenon induces a streaming potential, i.e., an electrical field along the fluid streamlines and proportional to the local fluid velocity. Deformation-induced potential in articular cartilage and other soft tissues has been reported over the past twenty-five years (Bassett and Pawluk, 1972; Fukada, 1974; Grodzinsky *et al.*, 1978; Lotke *et al.*, 1974). Furthermore, not only are currents generated during deformation of the matrix but applied current, in turn, can generate deformation (Frank and Grodzinsky, 1987a,b). This streaming potential effect has an important biomechanical role in controlling the dynamical stiffness of the articular cartilage (Grodzinsky, 1983). Indeed, since the mechanical properties of the tissue depends on the ionic strength of the interstitial fluid, the transient change of ion concentration induced by dynamic loading induces changes in the tissue stiffness (Grodzinsky *et al.*, 1981). The charged PGs are mainly responsible for the streaming potential effect. Collagen has a negligible net fixed electric charge near neutral pH, i.e., the number of ionized positive and negative groups along the collagen chains are about the same near the neutral pH. Therefore, the collagen stiffness is insensitive to change in ionic strength. In contrast to collagen, PGs have a high fixed charge at neutral pH and are highly sensitive to the ionic strength of the interstitial fluid.

Besides its role in the biomechanical properties of the articular cartilage, the streaming potential may also be very important in tissue remodeling and repair. The hypothesis that a mechanically induced electric field may modulate tissue remodeling has been put forward by several investigators, although there is no direct evidence of these phenomena.

12.5. Remodeling and Repair

One of the most important characteristics of biological tissues is their ability to self-remodel and self-repair in response to external stimuli. The continuous process of extracellular matrix production, assembly, and breakdown ensures the long-lasting properties of the articular cartilage. This maintenance process is the result of a delicate balance between fluid flow, mechanical stress, and cellular metabolism. The chondrocytes in cartilage maintain the mechanically functional matrix by regulating synthesis, assembly, and degradation. The mechanical stress, on the other hand, stimulates the biological activities of the chondrocytes. During loading, mechanical compression of cartilage can lead to matrix consolidation, cell deformation, hydrostatic and osmotic pressure gradients, fluid flow, streaming potentials and currents; all these can serve as signals to alter chondrocyte behavior. It has been shown that mechanical stimuli modulate cartilage matrix metabolism and turnover. Reducing the static load on cartilage by immobilizing the joint leads to a decrease in PG synthesis (Bayliss *et al.*, 1986; Gray *et al.*, 1988, 1989) and to an increase in PG degradation (Beherens *et al.*, 1989), while applying moderate dynamic loads leads to an increase in PG synthesis (Bayliss *et al.*, 1986). These results have also been confirmed with *in vitro* models: static compression inhibits PG synthesis while dynamic loads upregulate the synthesis (Jones *et al.*, 1982; Palmosky and Brandt, 1984; Parkkinen *et al.*, 1992; Sah *et al.*, 1989, 1990; Schneiderman *et al.*, 1986). However, Valhmu *et al.* (1998) have shown that the effect of static compression on chondrocyte biosynthesis depends upon the duration of the stress application and upon the level of the applied load. At low compression stress (0.1 MPa) the biosynthesis of aggrecan was transiently upregulated, resulting in a 2–3-fold higher than baseline value at 1 hour. After a longer time (>4 h) aggrecan synthesis returned to baseline values. The effect of stress-induced aggrecan upregulation decreased with the applied stress. At 0.5 MPa the aggrecan mRNA level was lower than that at 0.1 MPa, suggesting a reversal of the stimulatory effect of aggrecan gene expression at higher loads.

Beside stress, fluid flow, hydrostatic and osmotic pressure, and streaming potential also have an effect on chondrocyte bioactivity. Kim *et al.* (1988) have shown that fluid flow can dramatically change matrix biosynthesis. In particular, PG synthesis was highly enhanced in the region where fluid flow was the highest. Besides this direct implication on chondrocyte activity, interstitial fluid flow also regulates the transport of macromolecules within the tissues. Indeed, since healthy cartilage is an avascular tissue, chondrocyte biosynthetic activity must rely on interstitial transport of metabolites and metabolic waste from and to the synovial fluids. Transport of large molecular weight molecules (e.g., growth factors, metalloproteinase, and proteinase inhibitors) occurs principally by convection, which is controlled by fluid flow induced by mechanical loading. Hydrostatic pressure can stimulate or suppress PG synthesis depending on the loading conditions (Hall *et al.*, 1991; Parkkinen *et al.*, 1993; Schmidt *et al.*, 1990).

In conclusion, experimental evidence indicates that the physiological function of articular cartilage is the result of a delicate and intimate balance between physiochemical properties of the tissue, loading, and biosynthetic activity of chondrocytes. The study and identification of the mechanoelectrochemical signals that chondrocytes perceive *in vivo* during cartilage loading and the mechanisms by which these signals are transduced in biological stimuli represent a challenge to the several researchers involved in this area.

References

Armstrong, G.C., Mow, V.C. 1982a. Biomechanics of normal and osteoarthrotic articular cartilage, in: *Clinical Trends in Orthopaedics* (P.D. Wilson, L.R. Straub, eds.), pp. 189–197, Thieme-stratton, New York.

Armstrong, G.C., Mow, V.C. 1982b. Variation of the intrinsic mechanical properties of human cartilage with age, degeneration, and water content, *J. Bone Jt. Surg.* **64-A**, 88–94.

Barocas, V.H., Tranquillo, R.T. 1997. An anisotropic biphasic theory of tissue-equivalent mechanics: the interplay among cell traction, fibrillar network deformation, fibril alignment, and cell contact guidance, *J. Biomech. Eng.* **119**, 137–145.

Barocas, V.H., Knapp, D.M., Tranquillo, R.T. 1995. Biphasic mechanical theory of fibrillar gels, Beaver Creek (Colorado): ASME, BED-29, pp. 309–310.

Basser, P.J. 1992. Interstitial pressure, volume and flow during infusion into brain tissue, *Microvasc. Res.* **44**, 143–165.

Bassett, C.A.L., Pawluk, R.J. 1972. Electrical behavior of cartilage during loading, *Science* **178**, 982–983.

Bayliss, M.T., Urban, J.P.G., Jhonstone, B., Holm, S. 1986. In vitro method for measuring synthesis rates in the intervertebral disc, *J. Orthop. Res.* **4**, 10–17.

Beherens, F., Kraft, E.L., Oegema, T.R. 1989. Biochemical changes in articular cartilage after joint immobilization by casting or external fixation, *J. Orthop. Res.* **7**, 335–343.

Biot, M.A. 1941. General theory of three-dimensional consolidation, *J. Appl. Phys.* **12**, 155–164.

Biot, M.A. 1955. Theory of elasticity and consolidation for a porous anisotropic solid, *J. Appl. Phys.* **26**, 182–185.

Bowen, R.M. 1976. Theory of mixtures, in: *Continuum Physics III* (A.C. Eringen, ed.), pp. 1–127, Academic Press, New York.

Bowen, R.M. 1980. Incompressible porous media models by use of the theory of mixtures, *Int. J. Eng. Sci.* **18**, 1129–1148.

Christensen, R.M. 1971. *Theory of Viscoelasticity: An Introduction*, Academic Press, New York.

Clark, J.M. 1985. The organization of collagen in cryofractured rabbit articular cartilage: a scanning electron microscopic study, *J. Orthop. Res.* **3**, 17–29.

Eyre, D.R., Apone, S., Wu, J.J., Ericson, L.H., Walsh, K.A. 1987. Collagen type IX: evidences for covalent linkages to type II collagen in cartilage, *FEBS Lett.* **220**, 337–341.

Frank, E.H., and Grodzinsky, A.J. 1987a. Cartilage electromechanics—I. Electrokinetic transduction and the effect of electrolyte pH and ionic strength, *J. Biomech.* **20**, 615–627.

Frank, E.H., and Grodzinsky, A.J. 1987b. Cartilage electromechanics—II. A continuum model of cartilage electrokinetic transduction and correlation with experiments. *J. Biomech.* **20**, 629–639.

Fukada, E. 1974. Piezoelectric properties of biological macromolecules, Adv. Biophys. **6**, 121.

Fung, Y.C. 1990. *Biomechanics: Motion, Flow, Stress and Growth*, Springer, New York.

Fung, Y.C. 1993. *Biomechanics: Mechanical Properties of Living Tissues*, Springer-Verlag, New York.

Gray, M.L., Pizzanelli, A.M., Grodzinsky, A.J., Lee, R.C. 1988. Mechanical and physiochemical determinants of the chondrocyte biosynthetic response. *J. Orthop. Res.* **6**, 777–792.

Gray, M.L., Pizzanelli, A.M., Lee, R.C., Grodzinsky, A.J., Swan, D.A. 1989. Kinetics of the chondrocyte biosynthetic response to compressive load and release. *Biochim. Biophys. Acta* **991**, 415–425.

Grimshaw, P.E., Grodzinsky, A.J., Yarmush, M.L., Yarmush, D.M. 1989. Dynamic membranes for protein transport: Chemical and electrical control, *Chem. Eng. Sci.* **44**, 827–840.

Grodzinsky, A.J. 1983. Electromechanical and physiochemical properties of connective tissue, *CRC Crit. Rev. Biomed. Eng.* **9**, 133–199.

Grodzinsky, A.J., Liphitz, H., Glimcher, M.J. 1978. Electromechanical properties of articular cartilage during compression and stress relaxation, *Nature* **275**, 448–450.

Grodzinsky, A.J., Roth, V., Myers, E.R., Grossman, W.D., Mow, V.C. 1981. The significance of electric and osmotic forces in the non-equilibrium swelling behavior of articular cartilage in tension, *J. Biomech. Eng.* **103**, 221–231.

Hall, A.C., Urban, J.P., Gehl, K. A. 1991. The effects of hydrostatic pressure on matrix synthesis in articular cartilage, *J. Orthop. Res.* **9**, 1–10.

Hodge, W.A., Fijan, R.S., Carlson, K.L., Burgess, R.G., Harris, W.H., Mann, R.W. 1986. Contact pressure in the human hip joint measured in vivo, *Proc. Natl. Acad. Sci. USA* **83**, 2879–2883.

Holmes, M.H. 1986. Finite deformation of soft tissue: analysis of a mixture model in uniaxial compression, *J. Biomech. Eng.* **108**, 372–381.

Holmes, M.H., Lai, W.M., Mow, V.C. 1985. Singular perturbation analysis of the nonlinear, flow-dependent, compressive stress-relaxation behavior of articular cartilage. *J. Biomech. Eng.* **107**, 206–218.

Jain, R., Jayaraman, G. 1987. A theoretical model for water flux through the arterial wall, *J. Biomech. Eng.* **109**, 311–317.

Jenkins, R.B., Little, R.W. 1974. A constitutive equation for parallel-fibered elastic tissue, *J. Biomech.* **7**, 397.

Jones, I.L., Klamfeld, D.D.S., Sandstrom, T. 1982. The effect of continuous mechanical pressure upon the turnover of articular cartilage proteoglycans in vitro, *Clin. Orthop. Relat. Res.* **165**, 283–289.

Katz, E.P., Watchel, E.J., Maroudas, A. 1986. Extrafibrillar proteoglycans osmotically regulate the molecular packing of collagen in cartilage, *Biochim. Biophys. Acta* **882**, 136–139.

Kenyon, D.E. 1979. A mathematical model of water flux through aortic tissue, *Bull. Math. Biol.* **41**, 79–90.

Kim, Y.J., Sah, R.L., Doong, J.Y., Grodzinsky, A.J. 1988. Fluorometric assay of DNA in cartilage explants using Hoechst 33258. *Anal. Biochem.* **174**, 168–176.

Kuettner, K.E., Schleyerbach, R., Haschall, V.C. 1986. *Articular Cartilage Biochemistry*, Raven Press, New York.

Lai, M.W., Mow, V.C. 1980. Drag-induced compression of articular cartilage during a permeation experiment, *Biorheology* **17**, 111–123.

Levick, J.R. 1987a. Flow through interstitium and other fibrous matrices. *Q. J. Exp. Physiol.* **72**, 409–437.

Levick, J.R. 1987b. Relation between hydraulic resistance, composition of the interstitium, in: *Interstitial-Lymphatic Liquid and Solute Movement* (N.C. Staub, J.C. Hogg, A.R. Hargens, eds.), pp. 124–133, Karger, Basel.

Lotke, P.A., Black, J., Richardson, S.J. 1974. Electromechanical properties in human articular cartilage. *J. Bone J. Surg.* **56A**, 1040–1046.

Mak, A.F. 1986. The apparent viscoelastic behavior of articular cartilage—the contributions from the intrinsic matrix viscoelasticity, interstitial flows, *J. Biomech. Eng.* **108**, 123–130.

Mansour, J.M., Mow, V.C. 1976. The permeability of articular cartilage under compressive strain, at high pressures, *J. Bone J. Surg.* **58A**, 509–516.

Maroudas, A., Mizrahi, J., Ben Haim, E., Ziv, I. 1987. Swelling pressure in cartilage, in: *Interstitial-Lymphatic Liquid and Solute Movement* (N.C. Staub, J.C. Hogg, A.R. Hargens, eds.), pp. 203–212, Karger, Basel.

Mow, V.C., Lai, W.M. 1979. Mechanics of animal joints, *Annu. Rev. Fluid Mech.* **11**, 247–288.

Mow, V.C., Lai, W.M. 1980. Recent developments in synovial joint biomechanics, *SIAM Rev.* **22**, 275–317.

Mow, V.C., Soslowsky, L.J. 1991. Friction, lubrication and wear of diarthrodial joints, in: *Basic Orthopaedic Biomechanics* (V.C. Mow, W.C. Haynes, eds.), pp. 254–291, Raven Press, New York.

Mow, V.C., Kuei, S.C., Lai, W.M., Armstrong, C.G. 1980a. Biphasic creep, stress relaxation of articular cartilage in compression, theory, experiments, *J. Biomech. Eng.* **102**, 73–84.

Mow, V.C., Holmes, M.H., Lai, W.M. 1984. Fluid transport, mechanical properties of articular cartilage: a review, *J. Biomech.* **17**, 377–394.

Mow, V.C., Kwan, M.K., Lai, W.M., Holmes, M.H. 1986. A finite deformation theory for nonlinearly permeable soft hydrated biological tissues, in: *Frontiers in Biomechanics* (S. Schmid-Schonbein, L.-Y. Woo, B.W. Zweifach, eds.), Springer-Verlag, New York.

Mow, V.C., Lai, W.M., Hou, J.S. 1990a. A triphasic theory for the swelling properties of hydrated charged soft biological tissues, *Appl. Mech. Rev.* **43**, 134–141.

Mow, V.C., Ratcliffe, A., Woo, S.L.-Y. 1990b. *Biomechanics of Diarthrodial Joints, I & II*, Springer-Verlag, New York.

Mow, V.C., Ratcliffe, A., Poole, R.A. 1992. Cartilage, diarthrodial joints as paradigms for hierarchial materials, structures, *Biomaterials* **13**, 67–97.

Mow, V.C., Ateshian, G.A., Spilker, R.L. 1993. Biomechanics of diarthrodial joints: a review of twenty years of progress, *J. Biomech. Eng.* **115**, 460–467.

Muir, H. 1981. Proteoglycans as organizer of the intercellular matrix, *Biochem. Soc. Trans.* **9**, 1983.

Nagashima, T., Tamaki, N., Matsumoto, S., Horwitz, B., Seguchi, Y. 1987. Biomechanics of hydrocephalus: a new mathematical model, *Neurosurgery* **21**, 898–904.

Nagashima, T., Horwitz, B., I., R.S. 1990. A mathematical model for vasogenic brain edema, *Adv. Neurol.* **52**, 317–326.

Netti, P.A., Baxter, L.T., Boucher, Y., Skalak, R., Jain, R.K. 1995. Time-dependent behavior of interstitial fluid pressure in solid tumors: implication for drug delivery, *Cancer Res.* **55**, 5451–5458.

Netti, P.A., D'Amore, A., Ambrosio, L., Ronca, D., Nicolais, L. 1996. Structure-mechanical properties relationship of natural tendons and ligaments, *J. Mater. Sci., Materials in Medicine* **7**, 525.

Netti, P.A., Baxter, L.T., Boucher, Y., Skalak, R., Jain, R.K. 1997. Macro and microscopic fluid transport in living tissues: application to solid tumors, *AIChE J.* **43**, 818–834.

Nimni, M.E. 1988. *Collagen Biochemistry, I, II & III*, CRC Press, Boca Raton.

Palmosky, M.J., Brandt, K.D. 1984. Effects of salicylate, indomethacin on glycosaminoglycan, prostaglandin E2 synthesis in intact canine knee cartilage ex vivo, *Arthritis Rheum.* **27**, 398–403.

Parkkinen, J.J., Lammi, M.J., Helminen, H.J., Tammi, M. 1992. Local stimulation of proteoglycan synthesis in articular cartilage explants by dynamic compression in vitro, *J. Ortho. Res.* **10**, 610–620.

Parkkinen, J.J., Ikonen, J., Lammi, M.J., Laakkonen, J., Tammi, M., Helminen, H.J. 1993. Effects of cyclic hydrostatic pressure on proteoglycan synthesis in cultured chondrocytes and articular cartilage explants, *Arch. Biochem. Biophy.* **300**, 458–465.

Poole, A.R., Pidoux, I., Rosemberg, L.C. 1982. An immuno electron microscope study of the organization of proteoglycans monomer, link protein, and collagen in the matrix of articular cartilage, *J. Cell Biol.* **93**, 921–937.

Poole, C.A., Flint, M.H., Beaumont, B.W. 1984. Morphological and functional interrelationships of articular cartilage matrix, *J. Anat.* **138**, 113–138.

Ratcliffe, A., Mow, V.C. 1996. Articular cartilage, in: *Extracellular Matrix* (W.D. Comper, ed.), pp. 234–302, OPA, Harwood Academic Publisher, Amsterdam.

Redler, I., Zimny, M.L., Mansell, J., Mow, V.C. 1975. Significance of the tidemark of articular cartilage, *Clin. Orthop. Relat. Res.* **112**, 357–362.

Roth, V., Mow, V.C. 1980. The intrinsic tensile behaviour of the matrix of bovine articular cartilage, its variation with age, *J. Bone Jt. Surg.* **62A**, 1102–1117.

Sah, R.L., Kim, Y.J., Doong, J.Y., Grodzinsky, A.J., Plaas, A.H., Sandy, J.D. 1989. Biosynthetic response of cartilage explants to dynamic compression, *J. Orthop. Res.* **7**, 619–636.

Sah, R.L., Grodzinsky, A.J., Plaas, A.H., Sandy, J.D. 1990. Effects of tissue compression on the hyaluronate-binding properties of newly synthesized proteoglycans in cartilage explants, *Bioch. J.* **267**, 803–808.

Saltzman, W.M., Radomsky, M.L., Whaley, K.J., Cone, R.A. 1994. Antibody diffusion in human cervical mucus, *Biophys. J.* **66**, 508–515.

Schmidt, M.B., Mow, V.C., Chun, L.E., Eyre, D.R. 1990. Effect of proteoglycan extraction on the tensile behavior of articular cartilage, *J. Orthop. Res.* **8**, 353–363.

Schneiderman, R., Keret, D., Maroudas, A. 1986. Effects of mechanical and osmotic pressure on the rate of glycosaminoglycan synthesis in the human adult femoral head cartilage: an in vitro study, *J. Orthop. Res.* **4**, 393–408.

Simon, B.R. 1992. Multiphase poroelastic finite element models for soft tissue structure, *Appl. Mech. Rev.* **45**, 191–218.

Simon, B.R., Gaballa, M. 1988a. Finite strain poroelastic finite element models for large arterial cross sections, in: *Computational Methods in Bioengineering* (R.L. Spilker, B.R. Simon, eds.), pp. 325–331, ASME, New York.

Simon, B.R., Gaballa, M. 1988b. Poroelastic finite element models for the spinal motion segment including ionic swelling, in: *Computational Methods in Bioengineering* (R.L. Spilker, B.R. Simon, eds.), pp. 93–99, ASME, New York.

Simon, B.R., Wu, J.S.S., Evans, J.H. 1983. Poroelastic mechanical models for the intervertebral disc, in: *Advances in Bioengineering* (D. Bartel, (ed.), ASME Winter Annual Meeting, Boston, pp. 106–107.

Spilker, R.L., Suh, J.K. 1990. Formulation and evaluation of a finite element model for the biphasic model of hydrated soft tissue, *Comput. Struct.* **35**, 425–439.

Spilker, R.L., Suh, J.K., Mow, V.C. 1992. A finite element analysis of indentation stress-relaxation response of linear biphasic articular cartilage, *J. Biomech. Eng.* **114**, 192–201.

Torzilli, P.A. 1985. Influence of cartilage conformation on its equilibrium water partition, *J. Orthop. Res.* **3**, 473–483.

Truesdell, C., Toupin, R.A. 1960. The classical field theories, in: *Handbuck der Physik III/I*, Springer, Berlin.

Valhmu, W.B., Stazzone, E.J., Bachrach, N.M., Saed-Nejad, F., Fischer, S.G., Mow, V.C., Ratcliffe, A. 1998. Load-controlled compression of articular cartilage induces a transient stimulation of aggrecan gene expression, *Arch. Biochem. Biophys.* **353**, 29–36.

Van de Rest, M., Mayne, R. 1988. Type IX collagen proteoglycan from cartilage is covalently cross-linked to type II collagen, *J. Biol. Chem.* **263**, 1615–1618.

Winlove, C.P., Parker, K.H. 1995. The physiological function of the extracellular matrix, in: *Interstitium, Connective Tissue and Lymphatics* (R.K. Reed, G.A. Laine, J.L. Bert, C.P. Winlove, N. McHale, eds.), pp. 137–165, Portland Press, London.

Woo, S. L.-Y., Mow, V.C., Lai, W.M. 1987. Biomechanical properties of articular cartilage, in: *Handbook of Bioengineering* (R. Skalak, S. Chien, eds.), McGraw-Hill, Inc., New York.

13

The Material and Mechanical Properties of the Healthy and Degenerated Intervertebral Disc

Ron Alkalay

13.1. Introduction

The intervertebral disc is an essential part of the basic functional spinal unit (FSU), defined as the disc and two vertebrae with their associated ligamentous structures. The biomechanical performance of the spine throughout its length is the sum of the properties of the individual FSUs. The main functions of the intervertebral disc are to allow motion between adjacent vertebrae while being able to resist compressive and bending loads and, to a lesser degree, torsional and shear loads. The disc provides dynamic load attenuation as a result of its viscoelastic mechanical properties and, through its mechanical interaction with the vertebral body, it may have a role in the regulation of cancellous bone structure. In the succeeding sections the anatomy of the disc, the material and mechanical properties of its various structures, its overall mechanical behavior, and the effects of degeneration on these properties will be described. The chapter culminates with a discussion on past and current approaches in the design of artificial disc replacement implants.

Ron Alkalay • Orthopaedic Biomechanics Laboratory, Beth Israel Deaconess Medical Centre, Boston, Massachusetts, 02215, United States.

Integrated Biomaterials Science, edited by R. Barbucci. Kluwer Academic/Plenum Publishers, New York, 2002.

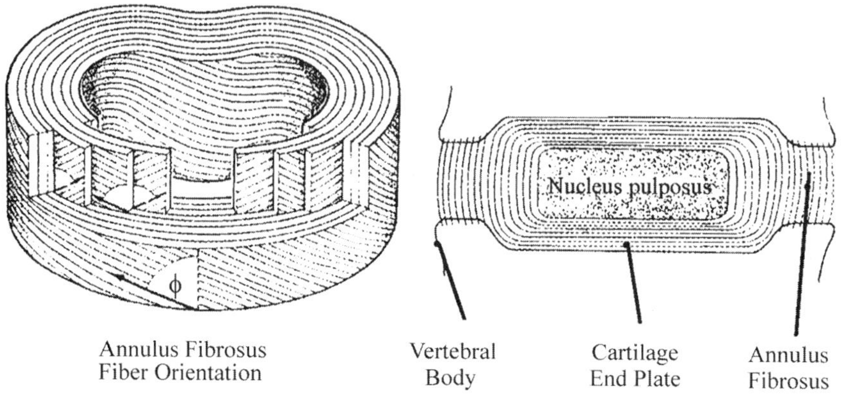

Figure 13.1. Intervertebral disc anatomy: ϕ represents the angle of fibers within a single lamina. Reproduced from Panjabi and White (1990), with permission.

13.2. Anatomy

The disc is composed of three histologically different, yet functionally and physically interdependent, elements: the nucleus pulposus, the annulus fibrosus, and the cartilaginous end plates (Figure 13.1).

13.2.1. Nucleus Pulposus

The nucleus is situated at the center of the disc occupying 30–50% of its cross-sectional area. It is composed of an irregular network of collagen fibers, 0.10–0.15 mm in diameter, embedded in a granular gel with 70–90% water (Buckwalter, 1982). This extracellular tissue, the framework being a complex matrix of proteoglycan macromolecule aggregates, is composed of central hyaluronate filaments and multiple attached aggrecan molecules, with the complex stabilized by link proteins (Buckwalter, 1982; Buckwalter *et al.*, 1989; Eyre *et al.*, 1989). The cells of the nucleus are generally large, round, chondrocyte-type cells, which produce mainly collagen type II (Table 13.1).

The proteoglycan network of macromolecules is responsible for the considerable potential for swelling of the nucleus by up to more than 200% of its initial volume (Urban and Maroudas, 1981). Experimental and theoretical work on related tissues, particularly knee (Mow *et al.*, 1990; Holmes *et al.*, 1990), has demonstrated that the proteoglycan network, through its interaction with both the collagen fibers and the interstitial water, play a major role in the static and dynamic mechanical properties of the intervertebral disc (Best *et al.*, 1994; Iatridis *et al.*, 1997).

Table 13.1. Typographical Distribution of Collagen Types in the Vertebral Disc[a]

Collagen[b]	Tissue	Overall collagen fraction
Type I*	Inner and outer annulus and transition zone	Decreases from about 80% at outer annulus to 0% at the nucleus
Type II*	Nucleus, transition zone, and inner annulus	Increases from about 0% at outer annulus to 80% at the nucleus
Type III*	Small quantities throughout the disc tissue	
Type V*	Inner and outer annulus	Approximately 3%
Type XI*	Nucleus pulposus	Approximately 3%
Type VI‡	Annulus fibrosus and nucleus pulposus	Approximately 10 and 15% respectively
Type IX‡	Throughout the disc	Maximum 2%

[a] Data from Eyre *et al.* (1989) and Buckwalter (1982).
[b] * or ‡ symbols indicates fibrillar or a short helix type.

13.2.2. Annulus Fibrosus

The annulus, which encloses the nucleus pulposus, is formed from a series of concentric collagenous laminae embedded in a ground substance (Figure 13.1). In contrast to the nucleus pulposus, the annulus cell population consist of long, thin, fibroblast-type cells (Buckwalter, 1982; Butler, 1989), with the gradual replacement of collagen type I at the periphery by weaker collagen type II in the inner layers (Eyre *et al.*, 1989) (Table 13.1). The inner laminar fibers are connected to the vertebral end plates, while the outer laminar fibers, known as Sharpey's fibers, are connected to the outer rim of the vertebra. Previously, the fibers of each lamina were described as being inclined at about $\pm 30^\circ$ with respect to the vertebral transverse plane with fibers from successive laminae perpendicular to each (Galante, 1967; Brown *et al.*, 1957) (Figure 13.1). However, recent studies have suggested that, depending on the topographical location and the locations of laminar irregularities, the angle of the fibers shows considerable departure from this 30° orientation (Marchand and Ahmad, 1990; Tsuji *et al.*, 1993). The annulus structure was observed to be highly irregular circumferentially with many of the layers, up to 40% at any sector of 20°, being noncontinuous with the laminae exhibiting sharp discontinuities at their termination or initiation. Similarly, the mean thickness of the lamellae, ranging from 0.14 to 0.52 mm, was noted to vary with increasing thickness toward the inner layers. It is noteworthy that both the observed irregularities and the highest fiber orientation, up to 70°, were most common posterolaterally. These structural irregularities expose the posterolateral areas of the disc to early failure and may serve as the underlying cause for the increased pattern of annular tears observed in these regions (Farfan *et al.*, 1972). With age, the number of distinct laminae underwent a significant reduction, while both the thickness and the spacing of intercollagen bundles within an individual layer increased (Marchand and Ahmad, 1990).

13.2.3. End Plate

The cartilaginous end plates, separating the disc from the adjacent vertebrae, play an important role in disc metabolism (Buckwalter, 1982; Ogata and Whiteside, 1981), in the growth of the vertebrae (Brenick *et al.*, 1980) and in transferring the stresses to the vertebral cancellous bone (Keller *et al.*, 1987). In the young (under 10 years), the end plates are composed of an inner growth plate zone, an articular region bordering the intervertebral disc, and a thin calcified articular cartilage layer adjacent to the diaphyseal bone trabeculae (Brenick and Caillet, 1982). With maturation (10 to 20 years of age), there is a gradual reduction in the width of the growth plate and thickening of the cartilaginous layer. In the adult, the cartilaginous layer is composed of 0.6 to 1 mm thick hyaline- and fibro-cartilage with a very tight collagen framework arranged parallel to the vertebral bodies (Roberts *et al.*, 1989). They possess a relatively low water content, 58%, and a high collagen content, up to 71% of dry tissue (Roberts *et al.*, 1989; Setton *et al.*, 1993). With increasing age, there is a resorption of the cartilage layer being replaced by bone, with the blood vessels at the endplate–vertebral bone border becoming partially or completely blocked (Brenick and Caillet, 1982).

13.3. Material Properties of the Structures of the Disc

13.3.1. Nucleus Pulposus

The material properties of the nucleus have been widely described as those of incompressible fluid, i.e., the material is unable to sustain applied stress when not confined. Thus the main thrust of research has been to elucidate the hydrostatic pressure developed in the material *in vivo* (Nachemson, 1960) and *in vitro* (McNally *et al.*, 1992), or the swelling pressure *in vitro* (Urban and Maroudas, 1981; Urban and McMullin, 1988). However, in recent years, results from several experimental studies have suggested the material to exhibit a more complex behavior. Panagiotacopulos *et al.* (1987), although employing a limited sample size due to the difficulties encountered in gripping the specimens, found that the tensile

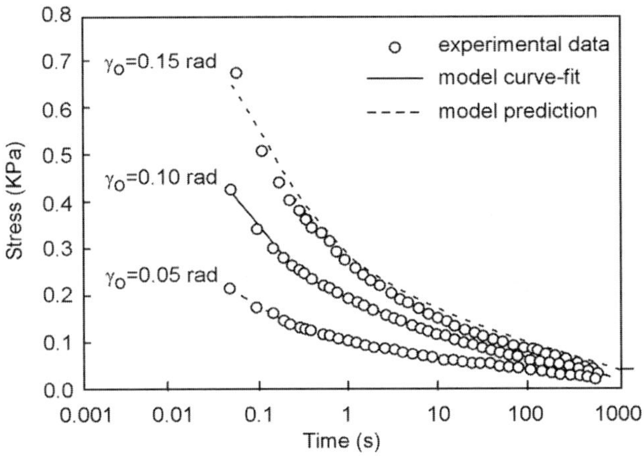

Figure 13.2. The stress-relaxation behavior of the nucleus pulposus as a function of applied stress rate. (Adapted from Iatridis *et al.* (1997) with permission.

relaxation modulus of a nondegenerated material ranges from 30 to 40 kPa (Figure 13.2). Similarly, both the complex dynamic shear modulus ($|G^*|$), derived by dividing the peak shear stress, σ_0, by the peak shear strain, γ_0 (Figure 13.3), found to range from 10–50 kPa, and the material energy dissipation, δ, measured by the phase angle between the loading and response curves, were noted to increase with increasing loading frequency (Iatridis *et al.*, 1997; Bodine *et al.*, 1982). It is noteworthy that the tests

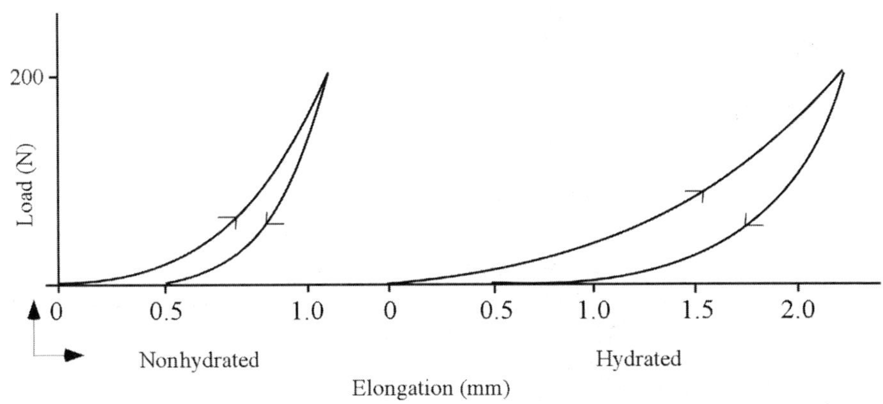

Figure 13.3. A schematic diagram of the dynamic shear test detailing the viscoelastic parameters.

revealed the phase angle to remain below 45°, indicating more solid-like behavior. For a material exhibiting a fluid-like behavior, this angle would approach 90°. However, when subjected to a fast ramp-relaxation test, the nucleus exhibited an extremely rapid relaxation to less than 50% of the peak stress in less than one second. This rapid relaxation is then followed by a gradual relaxation with the material stress approaching zero at $t = 600$ s (Bodine *et al.*, 1982). This behavior is indicative of that of a fluid. Despite experimental drawbacks which include the need to maintain appropriate hydration levels and significant alterations in the boundary conditions which these materials are likely to experience *in vivo*, these observations suggest a rate-dependent behavior for the nucleus. At high loading rates, the nucleus behaves as a viscoelastic material, while at low loading rates, it possesses a more "fluid-like" behavior.

13.3.2. Annulus Fibrosus

The mechanical properties of the annulus have been studied extensively using experimental (Best *et al.*, 1994; Galante, 1967; Brown *et al.*, 1957; Ebara *et al.*, 1996; Skaggs *et al.*, 1993, 1994; Acaroglu *et al.*, 1995; Kirsmer *et al.*, 1996), theoretical (Broberg, 1983, 1993), and computational (Shirazi-Adl, 1989, 1991). The great interest in the mechanical properties of the annulus stems from its role in the overall mechanical behavior of the disc, its involvement in disc herniation, and its potential role in the aetiology of low back (Eyre *et al.*, 1989; Kelsly, 1980; White *et al.*, 1981). The annulus tissue could be regarded as a complex porous fiber-reinforced composite material consisting of a dense network of collagen fibers with its composition dependent on the radial location of the lamellae (Table 13.1). The matrix is made from a dense ground substance, having a heterogeneous structure made from a wide distribution of constituents, with water its most abundant component comprising 65–75% by weight (Kraemer *et al.*, 1985).

Galante (1967) showed the annulus fibrosus tissue to be anisotropic with tissue strength directly dependent on fiber orientation and location about the disc. Tissue samples oriented parallel to the main axis of the fibers exhibited a tensile stiffness threefold greater than those along the transverse plane. The stress–strain tensile behavior of single (Skaggs *et al.*, 1994) and whole lamellae (Galante, 1967; Ebara *et al.*, 1996) exhibit nonlinear behavior (Figure 13.4a). The stress–strain behavior is best described by a cubic relationship given in equation (13.1) (Ebara *et al.*, 1996; Skaggs *et al.*, 1994; Araroglu *et al.*, 1995),

$$\sigma = A\varepsilon + B\varepsilon^3 \tag{13.1}$$

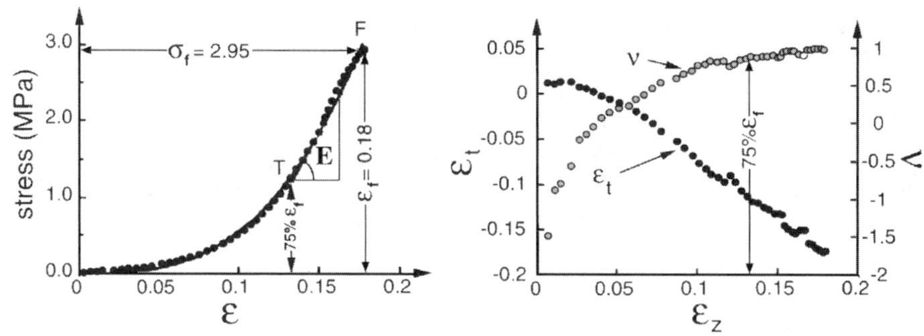

(a) (b)

Figure 13.4. (a) Typical stress–strain curve for a specimen from a peripheral laminae. σ_f and ε_f represent stress and strain at failure. (b) Plot of the transverse strain, ε_t, and Poisson's ratio, ν, as a function of axial strain, ε_z. Adapted from Acaroglu *et al.* (1995) with permission.

where the constant A corresponds to the tensile modulus of the material at zero strain and the constant B is a measure of the nonlinear dependence of the stress–strain curve. The tensile modulus for the tissue along the major axis of the collagen fibers, as estimated from the linear portion of the stress–strain curve, ranges from 60 to 140 MPa for single layer specimens (Skaggs *et al.*, 1994) and 1 to 50 MPa for whole lamellae (Ebara *et al.*, 1996; Acaroglu *et al.*, 1995). The failure stress and the failure strain of whole lamellar specimens were reported to range from 1 to 3 MPa (Ebara *et al.*, 1996; Acaroglu *et al.*, 1995) and 10 to 18% (Ebara *et al.*, 1996), respectively. In contrast, the tensile modulus for the tissue perpendicular to the major axis of the collagen fibers was observed to be as low as 0.2 to 0.5 MPa (Fujita *et al.*, 1995; Marchand and Ahmed, 1989). The tissue Poisson's ratio was estimated to range from 0.46 to 1.63 (Acaroglu *et al.*, 1995) clearly showing the tissue to be anisotropic (Figure 13.4b).

An important finding of the above-mentioned studies was the significant dependence of the estimated parameters, apart from Poisson's ratio, on the radial and, to a lesser extent, the anterior versus posterior location of the tissue. Tissue specimens taken from the outer annulus exhibited significantly higher modulus and failure strength than those from the inner lamellae (Skaggs *et al.*, 1993; Acaroglu *et al.*, 1995). Conversely, the tissue strain to failure was lower in specimens from the outer and anterior annulus than those from the inner and posterior annulus. In contrast, the tensile properties of adjacent laminae with alternating fiber orientation from similar locations did not differ distinctly, suggesting the lamina to be the basic structural unit of the annulus (Skaggs *et al.*, 1994). These marked differences may also reflect the higher content of collagen type I in the outer lamellae as compared to the higher content of type II collagen content in the inner lamellae (Eyre *et al.*, 1989).

The high tensile modulus of the outer lamellae limits the tensile (hoop) stresses created in the disc due to the swelling of the tissue and as a result of the external loads applied to the disc. Indeed, experimental studies have shown the outer fibers to undergo relatively small circumferential strains, less than 5% (Shah *et al.*, 1978; Stokes and Greenapple, 1985). The high tensile strength of the outer lamellae, when combined with the inner lamellas lower modulus and higher strain to failure, allows the tissue to create a more uniform stress distribution across the disc *in situ*.

A significant determinant of tissue properties was the level of tissue hydration with, at equilibrium, the inner layers being significantly more hydrated than the outer layers (Acaroglu *et al.*, 1995). It is noteworthy that several studies reported the dependence of the tensile (Galante, 1967; Panagiotacopulos, 1987) and compressive (Best *et al.*, 1994) properties on water content (Figure 13.5). This dependency reflects the reduction in the tissue resistance to solute motion with increasing water content and highlights the role of the proteoglycan interaction with the collagen fibers in maintaining the latter spatial orientation, thus affecting the mechanical behavior of the tissue (Lai *et al.*, 1991). Furthermore, the interaction of the inner lamellae with the nucleus through the transport of fluids resulting in flow-induced dissipation and changes in fluid volume are thought to provide considerable energy dissipation within the tissue (Best *et al.*, 1994). This mechanism, involving both flow dependent and independent viscoelastic phenomena with frictional drag caused by the

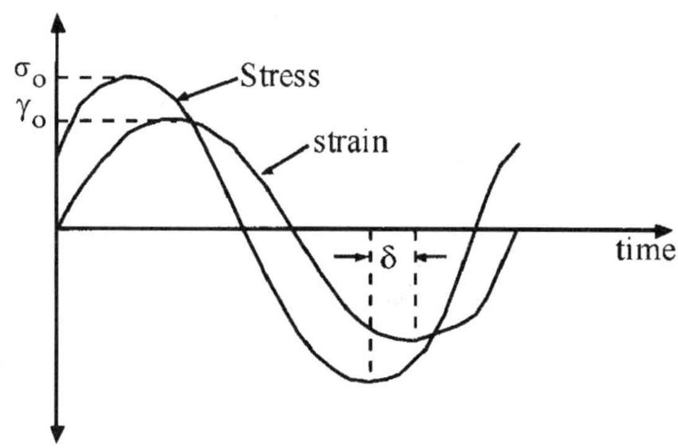

Figure 13.5. The effect of hydration level on the load-deformation response of an annulus specimen under tensile load. Adapted from Galante (1967) with permission.

interactions between the matrix macromolecules and the interstitial water, has been coined the "biphasic behavior" of the tissue (Mow *et al.*, 1990).

13.3.3. End Plate

A recent study on the end plates of baboons (Setton *et al.*, 1993) showed the end plate to exhibit a coefficient of permeability, k, of $14 \times 10^{-14} \mathrm{m}^4/\mathrm{N \cdot s}$, nearly three orders of magnitude higher than that reported for human annulus fibrosus, $0.03 \times 10^{-14} \mathrm{m}^4/\mathrm{N \cdot s}$ (Best *et al.*, 1989). This high level of permeability underlies their role in the transport of water and solutes from blood vessels at the border of the vertebral bone and end plates into the avascular disc. The end plate tissue demonstrated a high compressive creep rate, characterized by the sudden and rapid deformation on the application of load, followed by slower but continuous creep with the tissue failing to reach equilibrium by 10^5 seconds (Setton *et al.*, 1993). By contrast, the annulus fibrosus reaches equilibrium at 10^5 seconds (Best *et al.*, 1994). It has been suggested that the increased permeability of the tissue with consequent high creep rate allows for the rapid pressurization of the tissue (Setton *et al.* 1991). This rapid pressurization, when combined with the relatively impermeable adjacent vertebral structures, may lead to a uniform stress distribution across the end plate. This uniform stress distribution, being resisted by the tight collagen framework (Roberts *et al.*, 1989), could act to facilitate load transfer between the vertebral bodies and the intervertebral discs.

13.4. Mechanical Behavior of the Intervertebral Disc

In term of its *in vitro* characteristics, the disc exhibits a nonlinear load-displacement curve with two distinct phases similar to that of its components (Figure 13.4a) (Brown *et al.*, 1957). The first phase is characterized by large displacements for relatively low axial or bending loads, resulting in minimum energy expenditure required by the muscles to initiate and maintain physiological motion. The second phase is characterized by decreasing levels of displacement in response to increasing loads until a maximum is achieved. This behavior is the result of the increase in the load carried by the solid constitutes of the matrix, i.e. the collagen fibers. A similar response is seen when the disc is loaded in torsion (Farfan *et al.*, 1970). Estimated disc stiffness under several load conditions is presented in Table 13.2.

Table 13.2. Estimated Stiffnesses for Adult Lumbar Intervertebral Discs

Loading mode	Estimated stiffness	Reference
Compression	0.7–2.5 MN/m	Brown *et al.* (1957); Virgin (1951)
Tension	1.0 MN/m	Markolf (1972)
Shear	0.26 MN/m	Markolf (1972)
Torsion	2.0 Nm/deg	Virgin (1951)

Throughout the day, the disc in a normal subject is exposed to alternating periods of static and dynamic loading. However, due to the relative inaccessibility of the disc to external measurements, little is known about both the type and magnitude of such loads *in vivo*. Nachemson (1960), employing a pressure-sensitive needle inserted into the disc of live volunteers, estimated the compressive loads occurring at the L3-4 disc level to range from 0.6 times body weight (BW) in standing and sitting to 3.0 BW in a subject holding a weight of 20 kg in the hands. However, as the pressure measurements were calibrated against the results from cadaver spinal segments with their discs likely to have been superhydrated, these results may not portray an accurate picture. There exists a large body of research which has used noninvasive modeling techniques, including electromyography (McGill and Norman, 1986; Granata and Marras, 1993) and link segment models (McGill and Norman, 1985; Trafimow *et al.*, 1993) in an attempt to predict the loads occurring on the disc under flexion/extension and torsional moments. Although these models produce widely varying predictions of possible loads, they do suggest that the disc tissue is exposed to complex stresses in response to both single and multiple external and internal loads. At present, such models still await a more direct experimental validation.

The effect of both the duration and the frequency of the applied loads on the mechanical properties of the disc is well documented, suggesting that the response of the disc as a whole is governed by its viscoelastic properties (Burns *et al.*, 1984; Kalpes *et al.*, 1984; Kazarian, 1975; Markolf and Morris, 1974; Virgin, 1951). Viscoelastic models composed of ideal Hookian (spring) elements and Newtonian (dashpot) elements and their combinations have been successfully employed to model the gross creep and stress-relaxation behavior of the disc. The former represents the instantaneous elastic response of the material with the latter representing the time-dependent response of the material. For example, the three-parameter model (Keller *et al.*, 1987) represents the time-dependent strain behavior of the disc via the following characteristic equation:

$$\varepsilon(t) = \frac{\sigma_0}{E_1} + \frac{\sigma_0}{E_2}(1 - e^{-1/\tau}) \tag{13.2}$$

where $\varepsilon(t)$ is the time-dependent strain, σ_0 is the applied stress, E_1 is the mean compressive viscous modulus, (E_2) is the mean compressive modulus of the disc, and t is the relaxation time constant. The model fitted to the experimental data yielded a mean(SD) value of 6.3 (2.7) MPa and 1.6 (0.9) MPa for E_1 and E_2, respectively (Keller *et al.*, 1987; Kalpes *et al.*, 1984). The coefficient of viscosity (η), obtained from the relationship (13.3) between t, E_2, and σ_0, was found to have a mean (SD) value of 5.4 (3.9) GPa.s.

$$\eta = \frac{\tau E_2}{\sigma_0} \tag{13.3}$$

Although successful in modeling the experimental creep and stress-relaxation behavior of the disc, these models cannot account either for the contribution and time-dependent deformation of individual disc structures or the effects of interstitial fluid flow. The effect of the latter could be observed most clearly in the disc response to compressive loads. Initially, the hydrostatic pressure generated at the nucleus caused the disc to bulge simultaneously radially via the deformation of the annulus and axially through the deformation of the vertebral end plates into the vertebral bodies (Brinckmann *et al.*, 1983; Holmes *et al.*, 1993). It has been suggested that this mechanism allows the disc to resist compression while reducing the radial bulge of the disc, thereby minimizing the likelihood of neural cord compression. However, with time, the nucleus experiences a loss in pressure due to water transport through the end plates, which causes the disc to lose up to 20% of its volume (Broberg, 1983; Kraemer *et al.*, 1985; Adams and Hutton, 1983; Botsford *et al.*, 1994). Of this 20%, up to 25% is due to creep of the collagen fibers in the annulus. The diurnal changes in the hydration state of the disc, manifested externally by the 15–25 mm change in stature (Krag *et al.*, 1993), could lead an increasing proportion of the inner annulus to lose up to 36% of its stress-carrying ability (McNally *et al.*, 1992; Adams *et al.*, 1996).

Further insight into the mechanical function of the disc has been obtained by the use of an instrumented pressure needle to map the pressure distribution across the disc (McNally and Adams, 1992). In the non-degenerated disc (Figure 13.6), the nucleus and the inner regions of the annulus were observed to act as a "functional nucleus" exhibiting a relatively uniform stress distribution.

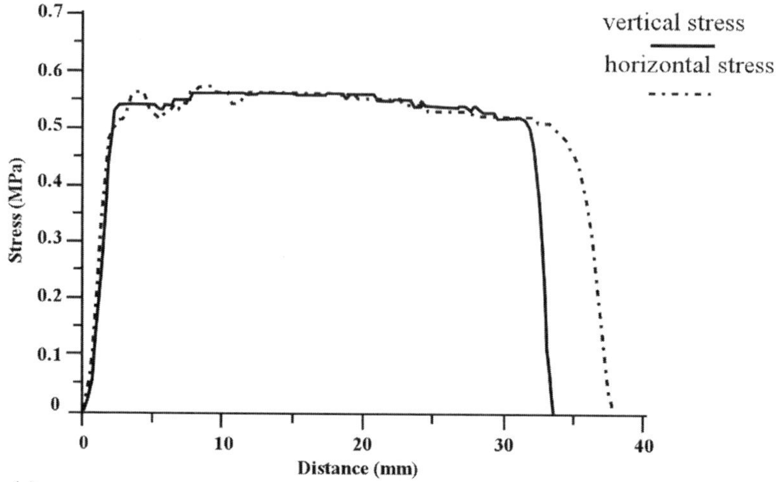

(a)

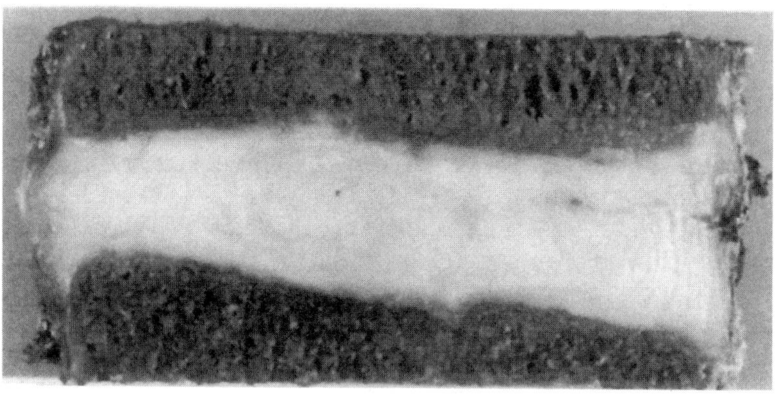

(b)

Figure 13.6. Pressure profile obtained for a nondegenerated lumbar disc (a) with the sagittal section of the disc presented in (b). Adapted from McNally *et al.* (1992) with permission.

The middle and outer layers of the annulus acted as a "functional annulus" with the posterior region registering higher compressive stress values. Under flexion/extension moments and constant loading conditions stress, gradients were seen in the pressure profile with high peaks noted for the posterior annulus and the nucleus pressure decreasing markedly. These changes indicate stress shielding by the annulus and the osseous structures of the vertebra. Under cyclical loads, likely to exist in daily activities such as driving, the hysteresis demonstrated by the disc was dependent on age, spinal level, and the magnitude and frequency of loading (Kazarian, 1975; Markolf and Morris, 1974).

13.5. The Effect of Degeneration on the Mechanical Properties of the Disc

With age, the intervertebral disc undergoes remarkable changes in its shape, volume, structure, and composition, causing the alteration of the disc material properties and mechanical behavior (Jhonstone and Bayliss, 1995). These alterations are directly related to the changes in the biology of the disc. Subsequent to the maturation of the spine, the disc exhibits loss of height, a gradual replacement of the nucleus with fibrocartilaginous tissue through the expansion of the inner annulus, and the appearance of fissures and cracks in the annulus (Vernon-Roberts, 1987). These gross structural changes are accompanied by a sharp decrease in the concentration of viable cells, with the highest reduction observed at the central regions (Buckwalter, 1982; Trout *et al.*, 1982a, b) and by a decrease in water and proteoglycan concentration (Urban and McMullin, 1988). At the same time, the noncollagenous protein concentration increases (Dickson *et al.*, 1967) while dense granular material, likely to contain degraded matrix molecules (Buckwalter *et al.*, 1993), accumulates throughout the matrix (Buckwalter, 1982; Trout *et al.*, 1982a, b). The outcome of these processes in conjunction with both the reduced vascularization of the outer annulus and the ossification of the end plates (Repanti *et al.*, 1998), results in the reduction of the diffusion rate of solutes across the disc (Maroudas *et al.*, 1975; Urban, 1993), further compromising cell nutrition. In the elderly, almost the entire disc tissue turns into fibrocartilage with additional loss of height and evidence of deep fissures at the center of the disc (Vernon-Roberts, 1987).

Several studies investigating the effect of degeneration on the mechanical properties of the annulus fibrosus tissue reported conflicting results. Galante (1967) and Best *et al* (1994), reported the tissue tensile and compressive modulus to exhibit weak correlation with the grade of degeneration. However, recent studies suggested that the material properties of the tissue, including compressive and tensile modulus, failure strength, Poisson's ratio, and strain energy, were strongly affected by the grade of disc degeneration (Ebara *et al.*, 1996; Acaroglu *et al.*, 1995; Iatridis *et al.*, 1998). Age, although found to affect the tensile properties of the tissue (Galante, 1967; Ebara *et al.*), has far less influence than that of disc degeneration (Best *et al.*, 1994; Ebara *et al.*, 1996; Skaggs *et al.*, 1994; Acaroglu *et al.*, 1995). These material changes affect the gross behavior of the disc, namely, the reduction in the energy dissipation of the disc (Kazarian, 1975), increased creep rate (Keller *et al.*, 1987; Virgin, 1951), and the increase in tissue stresses under dynamic loads (Kasra *et al.*, 1982). The changes in tissue properties, as reflected by the changes in the overall mechanical behavior of the disc, indicate the transference of tissue loading from a uniform "fluid pressurized" mechanism to an alternative nonuniform mechanism which predominately loads the solid matrix. Further evidence of this transference could be observed by the reported decrease in radial swelling pressure with degeneration and by the significant changes in the pressure distribution across the disc (McNally and Adams, 1992) (Figure 13.7).

These changes could cause local buckling and, ultimately, separation of the laminae with the inner laminae buckling toward the nucleus (Adams *et al.*, 1993), a phenomenon observed in degenerated and failed discs (Gunzburg *et al.*, 1992; Tanaka *et al.*, 1993). This structural disruption and the accompanying changes in hydrostatic pressure, demonstrated to cause cell-mediated degenerative changes (Osti *et al.*, 1990; Pfeiffer *et al.*, 1994), are likely to have a marked effect on chondrocyte metabolism and proteoglycan synthesis in the annulus (Bayliss *et al.*, 1988; Hall *et al.*, 1991). The increased loading of the solid matrix, when combined with the changes in tissue properties, may explain the increased predisposition of the annulus tissue to premature failure.

13.6. Intervertebral Disc Prostheses

At present, treatment for a severally degenerated disc with neurological involvement ranges from a removal of nucleus material for the bulging disc to a complete removal of the disc and the creation of bone fusion between the two bounding vertebrae in the case of a severally ruptured disc. These procedures, although relatively effective in alleviating pain, predispose the adjacent segments to early degeneration due to increased functional demands (Lee and Langrana, 1984; Leong *et al.*, 1983). In order for an articulating device to present a significant advantage over spinal fusion, a suitable design needs to comply with a stringent set of safety, functional, dynamical, and material based requirements for up to 40 years of operation. Kostuik (1997) and Lemaire *et al.*, (1997) provide a detailed discussion of some of these requirements. Clearly, due to the intimate relationships between the disc space and the neural cord and major blood vessels, the operational safety of these devices is of utmost importance.

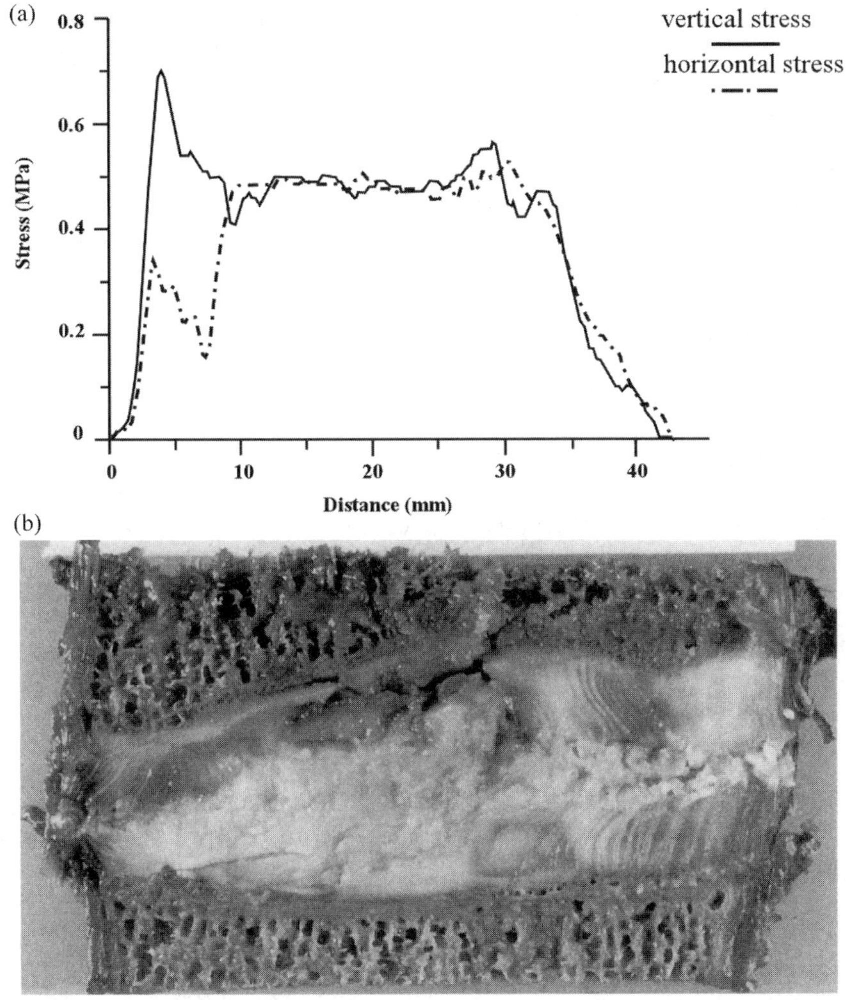

Figure 13.7. Pressure profile obtained for a degenerated lumbar disc (a) with the sagittal section of the degenerated disc presented in (b). Adapted from McNally *et al.* (1992) with permission.

For the past 35 years, large numbers of alternative designs for total disc replacement have been proposed. Low friction designs, composed of sliding congruent surfaces made from either metal (Patil, 1982) and/or a combination of metal and polymeric materials (Salib and Pettine, 1989), although providing a degree of flexibility, lack inherent kinematical constraints. This results in reduced "stability" to the affected spine and, ultimately, may cause early failure due to wear. An all-metal spacer with a posterior "floating" hinge connecting two cobalt chromium platens with two interposed coiled titanium springs was proposed by (Hedman *et al.*, 1988, 1991). This device possesses high fatigue strength, primary flexion/extension, and a degree of lateral bending motion, and was shown in a sheep model to perform successfully in the short term with no evidence of fibrous tissue growth (Kostuik, 1997). However, no clinical application of this device has been reported.

The majority of these alternative designs have employed single or multiple components made from a combination of polymeric elastomers with or without metal components and have a geometry closely related to that of the natural disc (Stubstad *et al.*, 1975; Edeland, 1989). Examples of composite disc designs included end plates made of silicone elastomer with a fluid filled core element bonded by Dacron fibers (Stubstad *et al.*, 1975) and two polyurethane end plates with an interposing porous silicone (Edeland, 1989). In an attempt to replicate disc structure, Lee *et al.* (1990) and Parsons *et al.* (1992) proposed a design with a soft elastomer core which was encircled by reinforced fiber sheets. These fiber sheets have alternating fiber orientation arranged in six to fifteen lamellae, are embedded in a second polymer, and are capped by two metal end plates. A similar principle was employed by Steffee (1991), using a hexene-based, carbon-black-filled polyolefin, rubber core, vulcanized to two titanium end plates. Currently, the most successful design, known as the SB Charite'III, combines two concave end plates made of cobalt chromium, with a bi-convex contoured polyethylene oval spacer (Büttner-Janz *et al.*, 1989; Zippel, 1991). In a clinical multicenter retrospective study, Griffith (1994) found that up to 70% of patients reported a resolution or a reduction in preoperative lag pain.

A second approach, particularly in the case of an early degenerated disc with structurally intact annulus, has been to develop a prosthesis to replace the degenerated nucleus. This approach has the advantage of being less invasive and, depending on the degenerative state of the disc, may restore the function of the annulus. Past endeavors attempted to fill the nucleus void ether with polymeric materials such as self-curing silicon (Scheider and Oyen, 1974; Roy-Camille *et al.*, 1978; Fassio and Ginestie, 1978) and contained systems made from either a polymer sac filled with an incompressible medium (Baumgartner, 1992) or a fiber wave based material filled with thixotropic gel (Ray and Corbin, 1990). Bao and Higham (1993), in an attempt to mimic the fluid transport in a disc, in addition to its mechanical performance, employed a hydrogel-based material having 70% water content. Although this design resulted in a biomechanical behavior similar to that of a natural disc (Odrdway *et al.*, 1994), no clinical application has been reported. Recently, a novel bioelastic polymer manufactured using genetic engineering methods, which is able to imbibe up to 25% water thus causing it to swell, was employed to restore the mechanical function and anatomical relationship of a denucleated lumbar disc (Alkalay *et al.*, 2001) Preliminary tests, which suggested that the material restored the axial compressive stiffness and hysteresis to that of the intact disc, indicated that the use of such a polymer could provide immediate restoration of disc function and anatomy while exhibiting excellent long term biocompatibility. In recent years, the rapid development, in tissue engineering and tissue regenerative methods, is being increasingly explored for the treatment of early degenerated disc. These methods use sophisticated three-dimensional scaffolds, seeded with cells and growth factors, and employ viral vectors to transfect disc cells to stimulate the production of necessary proteins to affect the regeneration of disc tissue. Although these methods face many difficult challenges with respect to their effective delivery, integration, and regeneration of the tissue, and their short- and long-term viability, ultimately they hold great promise.

13.7. Summary

In this chapter, the anatomy and material properties of the intervertebral disc as a whole and its individual structural components were reviewed. The contribution of each of these structures to the mechanical behavior of the intervertebral disc was discussed, with the effects of degeneration on these structures highlighted. The state of hydration and the interaction of charged structural macromolecules with the interstitial fluid flow were demonstrated to critically affect the compressive viscoelastic creep stress-relaxation and dynamic load attenuation of the disc. These mechanisms, in conjunction with the intrinsic nonlinear properties of the collagen proteoglycan matrix, which form the structures of the annulus and vertebral end plates, underlie the anisotropic properties of the disc. Thus, the varied functions of the intervertebral disc are intimately related to its biomechanical composition and architectural arrangements. The process of disc degeneration was found to affect significantly the biology and structure of the intervertebral disc, thereby leading to marked changes in its mechanical behavior. Similarly, mechanical fatigue was demonstrated to cause a breakdown of the tissue, thus altering the state of stress–strain in the disc. Both of these mechanisms were suggested to disrupt the nutritional pathways and to accelerate tissue catabolism, culminating in the failure of the disc. The efforts to devise a whole intervertebral disc or nucleus prosthesis have, to a large extent, met with limited success.

At present, our knowledge pertains predominantly to the *in vitro* quasi-static behavior of the intervertebral disc. Such a condition seldom occurs in daily life. New developments in noninvasive techniques, particularly MRI imaging, may prove valuable in extending our knowledge of the function of the intervertebral disc *in vivo* and the effect of degeneration on these functions. The use of such techniques may well point to possible treatments of some of the underlying causes of disc degeneration and spinal back pain. When combined with new materials and biologically based engineering methods, the developmental effort to design intervertebral disc prosthesis and to reverse the effects of degeneration directly could show greater success than that which has been achieved thus far.

References

Acaroglu, E.R., Setton, L.A., Iatridis, J.C., Weidenbaum, M., Foster, R.J., Mow, V.C. 1995. Degeneration and aging affect the tensile behavior of human lumbar annulus fibrosus, *Spine* **20**(24), 2690–2701.

Adams, M.A., Hutton, W.C. 1983. The effect of posture on the fluid content of lumbar intervertebral discs, *Spine* **8**, 665–671.

Adams, M.A., McNally, D.S., Wagstaff, J., Goodship, A.E. 1993. Abnormal stress concentrations in lumbar intervertebral discs following damage to the vertebral body: a cause for disc failure, *Eur. Spine J.* **1**, 214–221.

Adams, M.A., McMillan, D.W., Green, J.P., Dolan, P. 1996. Sustained loading generates stress concentrations in lumbar intervertebral discs, *Spine* **21**(4), 434–438.

Alkalay, R.N., Patenick, A., Urry, D., Glazer, P.A. 2001. The use of a novel bio-elastic polymer for the restoration of the function of partially denucleated intervertebral disc: experimental study, in press.

Bao, Q.B., Higham, P.A. 1993. Hydrogel intervertebral disc nucleus, *US Patent 5,192,326*.

Baumgartner, W. 1992. Intervertebral prosthesis, *US Patent 5,171,280*.

Bayliss, M.T., Jhonstone, B., O'Brien, J.P. 1988. Proteoglycan synthesis in the human intervertebral disc: variation with age, region and pathology, *Spine* **13**, 972–981.

Best, B.A., Setton L.A., Guilak, F., Ratcliffe, A., Weidenbaum, M., Mow, V.C. 1989. Permeability and compressive stiffness of annulus fibrosus: variation with site and composition, 35th Annual Meeting Orthopaedic Research Society, p. 354.

Best, B.A., Guilak, F., Setton, L.A., Zhu, W., Saed-Nejed, F., Ratclifte, A. 1994. Compressive mechanical properties of the human annulus fibrosus and their relationship to biochemical composition, *Spine* **19**(2), 212–221.

Bodine, A.J., Ashany, D., Hayes, W.C., White, A.A. 1982. Viscoelastic shear modulus of the human intervertebral disc, 28th Annual Meeting Orthopaedic Research Society, p. 330.

Botsford, D.J., Esses, S.I., Ogilvie-Harris, D.J. 1994. In vivo diurnal variation in intervertebral disc volume and morphology, *Spine* **19**, 935–940.

Brenick, S., Caillet, R. 1982. Vertebral end plate changes with aging of the human vertebrae, *Spine* **7**(2), 97–102.

Brenick, S., Caillet, R., Levy, B.M. 1980. The maturation and aging of the vertebrae of marmosets, *Spine* **5**, 519–524.

Brinckmann, P., Frobin, W., Hierholzer, E., Horst, M. 1983. Deformation of the end-plate under axial loading of the spine, *Spine* **8**, 851–856.

Broberg, K.B. 1983. On the mechanical behavior of intervertebral discs, *Spine* **8**(2), 151–161.

Broberg, K.B. 1993. Slow deformation of intervertebral discs, *J. Biomech.* **26**(4,5), 501–512.

Brown, T., Hansen, R.J., Yorra, A.J. 1957. Some mechanical test on the lumbosacral spine with particular reference to the intervertebral discs, *J. Bone Jt. Surg.*, **39A**(7), 1135–1164.

Buckwalter, J.A. (ed.). 1982. Fine structural studies of human intervertebral discs, in: *Idiopathic Low Back Pain* (A.A. White, S.L. Gordon, eds.), pp. 108–143, C.V. Mosby, St Louis.

Buckwalter, J.A., Smith, K.C., Kazarien, L.E., Rosenberg, L.C. 1989. Articulator cartilage and intervertebral proteoglycans differ in structure, *J. Orthop. Res.* **7**, 146–151.

Buckwalter, J.A., Woo, S.L.Y., Goldberg, V.M. 1993. Soft tissue aging and musculoskeletal function, *J. Bone Jt. Surg.* **75**, 1533–1548.

Burns, M.L., Kalpes, I., Kazarian, L.E. 1984. Analysis of compressive creep beahviour of the intervertebral unit subjected to uniform axial loading using exact parametric solution equations of Kelvin-solid models: Part I. Human intervertebral joints, *J. Biomech.* **17**, 113–130.

Butler, W.F. (ed.) 1989. Comparative anatomy and development of mammalian disc, in: *The Biology of the Intervertebral Disc* (P. Ghosh, ed.), pp. 84–108, CRC Pres, Boca Raton.

Büttner-Janz, K., Schellnack, K., Zipple, H. 1989. Biomechanics of the SB Charité lumbar intervertebral disc endoprosthesis, *Int. Orthop.* (*SICOT*) **13**, 173–176.

Dickson, I.R., Happey, F., Pearson, C.H. 1967. Variations in protein components of the human intervertebral disc with age, *Nature* **215**, 50–53.

Ebara, S., Iatridis, J.C., Setton, L.A., Foster, R.J., Mow, V.C., Weidenbaum, M. 1996. Tensile properties of nondegenerated human lumbar annulus fibrosus, *Spine* **21**(4), 452–461.

Edeland, H.G. 1989. Some additional suggestions for an intervertebral disc prosthesis, *J Biomed. Mater. Res., Appl. Biomater.* **23**, 189–194.

Eyre, D.R., Benya, P., Buckwalter, J.A., Gatersion, B., Heinegard, D., Oegema, T., *et al.*, (eds.). 1989. Basic science perspectives. Part B. Intervertebral disc, in: *New Perspective on Low Back Pain* (J.W. Frymoyer, S.L. Gordon, eds.), pp. 147–207, American Academy of Orthopaedic Surgeons, Park Ridge, IL.

Farfan, H.F., Cossette, J.W., Robertson, G.H., Wells, R.V., Kraus, H. 1970. The effects of torsion on the lumbar intervertebral joints: the role of torsion in the production of disc degeneration, *J. Bone Jt. Surg.* **52** (Am. Ed), 468–497.

Farfan, H.F., Huberdeau, R. M., Dubow, H.I. 1972. Lumbar intervertebral disc degeneration: The influence of geometric features on the pattern of disc degeneration—A postmortem study, *J. Bone Jt. Surg.*, **54-A**(3), 492–510.

Fassio, B., Ginestie, J.F. 1978. Disc prosthesis made of silicone. Experimental study and first clinical cases, *Nouv. Presse Med.* **21**, 207.

Fujita, Y., Lotz, C., Soejima, O. 1995. Site specific radial tensile properties of the lumbar annulus fibrosus, 37th Annual Meeting Orthopaedic Research Society, p. 673.

Galante, J.O. 1967. Tensile properties of the human lumbar annulus fibrosus, *Acta Orthop. Scand.*, **100** (suppl.).

Granata, K.P., Marras, W.S. 1993. An EMG-assisted model of loads on the lumbar spine during asymmetric trunk extensions, *J. Biomech.* **26**(12), 1429–1438.

Griffith, S.L., *et al.* 1994. A multicenter retrospective study of the clinical results of the LINK SB Charite intervertebral prosthesis, *Spine* **19**, 1842–1949.

Gunzburg, R., Parkinson, R., Moore, R. 1992. A cadaveric study comparing discography, MRI, histology, and mechanical behavior of the human lumbar disc, *Spine* **17**, 417–423.

Hall, A.C., Urban, J.P.G., Gehl, K.A. 1991. The effects of hydrostatic pressure on matrix synthesis in articular cartilage, *J. Orthop. Res.* **9**, 1–10.

Hedman, T.P., *et al.* 1988. Artificial spinal disc, *US Patent 4,759,769*.

Hedman, T.P., *et al.* 1991. Design of an intervertebral disc prosthesis, *Spine* **16**, S256–S260.

Holmes, H.M., Lai, W.M., Mow, V.C. 1990. The nonlinear characteristics of soft gels and hydrated connective tissue in ultra-filtration, *J. Biomech.* **23**, 1145–1156.

Holmes, A.D., Hukins, D.W.L., Freemont, A.J. 1993. End-plate displacement during compression of lumbar vertebra-disc-vertebra segments and mechanisms of failure, *Spine* **18**(1), 128–135.

Iatridis, J.C., *et al.* 1997. The viscoelastic behavior of the non-degenerated human lumbar nucleus pulposus in shear, *J. Biomech.*, **30**(10), 1005–1013.

Iatridis, J.C., *et al.* 1998. Degeneration affects the anisotropic and nonlinear behaviors of human anulus fibrosus in compression, *J. Biomech.* **31**(6), 535–544.

Jhonstone, B., Bayliss, M.T. 1995. The large proteoglycans of the human intervertebral disc: changes in their biosynthesis and structure with age, topography, and pathology, *Spine* **20**(6), 674–684.

Kalpes, I., Kazarian, L.E., Burns, M.L. 1984. Analysis of compressive creep beahviour of the intervertebral unit subjected to uniform axial loading using exact parametric solution equations of kelvin-solid models-Part I. Rhesus monkey intervertebral joints, *J. Biomech.* **17**, 131–136.

Kasra, M., Shirazi-Adl, A., Drouin, G. 1982. Dynamics of human lumbar intervertebral joints: Experimental and finite element investigations, *Spine* **17**(1), 93–101.

Kazarian, L.E. 1975. Creep characteristics of the human spinal column, *Orthop. Clinics North America* **6**(1), 3–18.

Keller, T.S., Spengler, D.M., Hansson, T.H. 1987. Mechanical behavior of human lumbar spine I. Creep analysis during static compressive loading, *J. Orthop. Res.* **5**, 467–478.

Kelsly, J.L. 1980. Epidemiology and impact of low back pain, *Spine* **5**, 133–142.

Kirsmer, M., Hiad, C., Rabi, W. 1996. The contribution of annulus fibers to torque resistance, *Spine* **21**(22), 2551–2557.

Kostuik, J.P. 1997. Intervertebral disc replacement: experimental study, *Clin. Orthop. Relat. Res.* **337**, 27–41.

Kraemer, J.D., Kolditz, M., Gowin, R. 1985. Water and electrolyte content of the human intervertebral disc under variable load, *Spine* **10**, 69–71.

Krag, M.H., *et al.* 1993. Effect of denucleation and degeneration grade on intervertebral disc stress relaxation, 39th Annual Meeting, Orthopaedic Research Society.

Lai, W.M., How, J., Mow, V.C. 1991. A triphasic theory for the swelling and deformation behavior of cartilage tissue, *J. Biomech. Eng.* **113**, 145–158.

Lee, C.K., Langrana, N.A. 1984. Lumbosacral spinal fusion. A biomechanical study, *Spine* **9**, 574–581.

Lee, C.K., Langrana, N.A., Alexander, H., Clemow, A.J., Chen, E.H., Parsons, J.R. 1990. Functional and biocompatible intervertebral disc spacer, *US Patent 4,911,718*.

Lemaire, J.P., Skalli, W., Lavaste, F., Templier, A., Mendes, F., Diop, A., *et al.* 1997. Intervertebral disc prosthesis. Results and prospects for the year 2000, *Clin. Orthop. Relat. Res.* **337**, 64–76.

Leong, J.C., Chun, S.Y., Grange, W.J., Fang, D. 1983. Long term results of lumbar intervertebral disc prolapse, *Spine* **8**(7), 793–799.

Marchand, F., Ahmed, A.M., 1989. Mechanical properties and failure mechanisms of the lumbar disc annulus, in: *35th Annual Meeting, Orthopaedic Research Society.*

Marchand, F., Ahmad, A. M. 1990. Investigation of the laminate structure of lumbar disc annulus fibrosus, *Spine* **15**(5), 402–408.

Markolf, K.L. 1972. Deformation of the thoracolumbar intervertebral joint in response to external loads: a biomedical study using autopsy material, *J. Bone Jt. Surg.* **54A**: 511–533.
Markolf, K.L., Morris, J.M. 1974. The structural components of the intervertebral disc: A study of their contribution to the ability of the disc to withstand compressive forces, *J. Bone Jt. Surg.* **56A**(4), 675–684.
Maroudas, A., *et al.* 1975. Factors involved in the nutrition of the human lumbar intervertebral disc: cellularity and diffusion of glucose in vitro, *J. Anat.* **120**, 113–130.
McGill, S.M., Norman, R.W. 1985. Dynamically and statically determined low back moments during lifting, *J. Biomech.* **18**(12), 877–885.
McGill, S.M., Norman, R.W. 1986. Partitioning of the L4-L5 dynamic moment into disc, ligamentous, and muscular components during lifting, *Spine* **11**(7), 666–677.
McNally, D.S., Adams, M.A. 1992. Internal intervertebral disc mechanics as revealed by stress profilometry, *Spine* **17**(1), 66–73.
McNally, D.S., Adams, M.A., Goodship, A.E. 1992. Measurement of stess distribution within intact loaded intervertebral disc, in: *Experiemental Mechanics* (E.G. Little, ed.), pp. 139–150, Elsevier Science Publishers B.V. Amsterdam.
Mow, V.C., *et al.*, (eds.). 1990. Biphasic and quasi-linear viscoelastic theories for hydrated soft tissue, in: *Biomechanics of Diarthrodial Joints* (V.C. Mow, A. Ratcliffe, S.L.Y. Woo, eds.), pp. 215–260, Springer-Verlag, New York.
Nachemson, A.L. 1960. Lumbar interdiscal pressure, *Acta Orthop. Scand.* **43** (Suppl), 1–104.
Ogata, K., Whiteside, L.A. 1981. Nutritional pathways of the intervertebral disc: An experimental study using hydrogen washout technique, *Spine* **6**(3), 211–216.
Ordway, N.R., Han, Z.H., Bao, Q.B. 1994. Biomechanical evaluation for the intervertebral hydrogel nucleus, 9th Annual Meeting of the North American Spine Society, Minneapolis, MN.
Osti, O.L., Vernon-Roberts, B., Fraser, R.D. 1990. Annulus tears and intervertebral degeneration: an experimental study using animal models, *Spine* **15**, 762–767.
Panagiotacopulos, N.D., Pope, M.H., Krag, M.H., Bloch, R.A. 1987. Mechanical model for the human intervertebral disc, *J. Biomech.* **20**(9), 839–850.
Panjabi, M.M., White, A.A. (eds.). 1990. *Clinical Biomechanics of the Spine*, J.B. Lippincott Company, Philadelphia.
Parsons, J.R., *et al.* 1992. Functional and biocompatible intervertebral disc spacer containing elastomeric material of varying hardness, *US Patent 5,171,281.*
Patil, A. 1982. Artificial intervertebral disc, *US Patent* 4,309,777.
Pfeiffer, M., Griss, P., Franke, P. 1994. Degeneration model of the porine lumbar motion segment: effect of various interdiscal procedures, *Eur. Spine J.* **5**, 8–16.
Ray, C.D., Corbin, T.P. 1990. Prosthetic disc containing therapeutic material, *US Patent 4,904,280.*
Repanti, M., Korovessis, P.G., Stamatakis, M.V., Spastris, P., Kosti, P. 1998. Evaluation of disc degeneration in lumbar spine: A comparative histological study between herniated postmortem retrieved disc specimens, *J Spinal Disorders* **11**(1), 41–45.
Roberts, S., Menage, J., Urban, J.P.G. 1989. Biomechanical and structural properties of cartilage end-plate and it relation to the intervertebral disc, *Spine* **14**, 166–174.
Roy-Camille, R., Saillant, G., Lavaste., F. 1978. Experimental study of lumbar disc replacement, *Rev. Chir. Orthop. Repar. Appar. Mot.* **64** (Suppl II), 106–107.
Salib, R.M., Pettine, K. A. 1989. Intervertebral disk arthroplasty, *US Patent 5,258,031.*
Scheider, P.G., Oyen, R. 1974. Plastic surgery on intervertebral disc. Part I: intervertebral disc replacement in the lumbar region with silicone rubber. Theoretical and experimental studies, *Z. Orthop.* **112**, 1078–1086.
Setton, L.A., Zhu, W.B., Mow, V.C. 1991. Compressive viscoelastic properties of cartilaginous endplates of lumbar intervertebral discs, 37th Annual Meeting, Orthopaedic Research Society.

Setton, L.A., *et al.* 1993. Compressive properties of cartilaginous end plate of the Babon lumbar spine, *J. Orthop. Res.* **11**, 228–239.

Shah, J.S., Hampson, W.G.J., Jayson, M.I.V. 1978. The distribution of surface strain in cadaveric lumbar spine, *J. Bone Jt. Surg.* **60**(Br), 246–251.

Shirazi-Adl, A. 1989. On the fibre composite material models of disc annulus-comparison of predicted stresses, *J. Biomech.* **22**(4), 357–365.

Shirazi-Adl, A. 1991. Mechanical role of disc annulus fibers and matrix in poroelastic creep response of a human lumbar disc, 37th Annual Meeting, Orthopaedic Research Society, p. 241.

Skaggs, D.L., Gibbons, J.C., Richardson, L.C., Foster, R.J., Weidenbaum, M. 1993. Regional variations in the tensile properties and biochemical compositions of single lamellae of human annulus fibrosus, 39th Annual Meeting, Orthopaedic Research Society, p. 420.

Skaggs, D.L., *et al.* 1994. Regional variation in tensile properties and biochemical composition of the human lumbar anulus fibrosus, *Spine* **19**(12), 1310–1319.

Steffee, A.D. 1991. Artificial disc, *US Patent 5,071,437.*

Stokes, I., Greenapple, D.H. 1985. Measurement of surface deformation of soft tissue, *J. Biomech.* **18**, 1–7.

Stubstad, J.A., Urbaniak, J.R., Khan, P. 1975. Prosthesis for spinal repair, *US Patent 3,867,728,25.*

Tanaka, M., Nakahara, S., Inoue, H. 1993. A pathologic study of discs in the elderly, *Spine* **18**, 1456–1462.

Trafimow, J.H., *et al.* 1993. The effects of quadriceps fatigue on technique of lifting, *Spine* **18**(3), 364–367.

Trout, J.J., Buckwalter, J.A., Moore, K.C. 1982a. Ultrastructure of human intervertebral disc I. Cells of the nucleus pulposus, *Anat. Rec.* **204**, 307–314.

Trout, J.J., *et al.* 1982b. Ultrastructure of human intervertebral disc II. Changes in notocordal cells with age, *Tissue Cell* **14**, 359–369.

Tsuji, H., Hirano, N., Ohsima, H., Ishihara, H., Terahata, N., Motoe, T., 1993. Structural variation of the anterior annulus fibrosus in the development of human lumbar intervertebral disc, *Spine*, **18**(2), 204–210.

Urban, J.P.G. (ed.). 1993. The effect of physical factors on disc cell metabolism, in: *Musculoskeletal Soft Tissue Aging: Impact on Mobility* (J.A. Buckwalter, V.M. Goldberg, S.L.Y. Woo, eds.), American Academy of Orthopeadic Surgeons, Rosemont, IL.

Urba, J.P.G., Maroudas, A., Swelling of the intervertebral disc in vitro, *Connect. Tissue Res.* **9**, 1–10.

Urban, J.P.G., McMullin, J.F. 1988. Swelling pressure of the lumbar intervertebral discs: Influence of proteoglycan and collagen contents, *Biorheology* **13**, 179–187.

Vernon-Roberts, B. (ed.). 1987. The pathology and interrelation of intervertebral disc lesions, osteoarthrosis of apophyseal joints, lumbar spondylosis and low back pain, in: *The Lumbar Spine and Back Pain* (M.D.V. Jayson, ed.), pp. 83–114, Churchill Livingstone, New York.

Virgin, W. 1951. Experimental investigations into the physical properties of intervertebral discs, *J. Bone Jt. Surg.* **33B**(4), 607–611.

White, A.A., Edwards, W.T., Liberman, D., Hayes, W.C., Lewinnek, E.G., (eds.). 1981. Biomechanics of lumbar spine and sacroiliac articulation: relevance to idiopathic low back pain, in: *Symposium on Idiopathic Low Back Pain* (A.A. White, S.L. Gordon, pp. 296–322, C.V. Mosby, St. Louis.

Zippel, H. (ed.). 1991. "Charité modular": concept, experience and results, in: *The Artificial Disc* (M. Brock, H.M. Mayer, K. Weigel, eds.), pp. 69–77, Springer, Berlin.

14

Soft Tissue Replacement

Matteo Santin, Luigi Ambrosio, Andrew W. Lloyd, and Stephen P. Denyer

14.1. Introduction

There is a wide range of applications for soft tissue replacement in the biomaterials field. Vascular grafts and stents, heart valves, artificial skin, and intraocular devices are among the most important since they tackle widespread pathologies of the vascular system, cosmetic needs, and ocular surgery (Silver and Doillon, 1989). In addition, other applications can also been framed in the context of the substitution of soft tissues. Ureteral stents, catheters, artificial sphincters, and penile implants constitute important tools in urology (Wironen *et al.*, 1997), while hernias are routinely repaired by polymer meshes (Alexandre and Bouillot, 1996; Bebawi *et al.*, 1997). Other materials have important applications as intervertebral disc prostheses, replacement ligaments, tendons, and as artificial skin materials.

Although materials have been produced which fulfill the mechanical requirements for these applications, improvements in biocompatibility still have to be achieved. In fact, failure of the surrogate soft-tissue-replacing implants is generally linked to an adverse response of the host tissues toward the foreign material (Anderson, 1988). The physicochemical properties of a material surface present a challenge to the surrounding biological environment. Regardless of the tissue into which the implant is inserted, the material surface will undoubtedly contact those body fluids which permeate that particular body district (Wahlgren and Arnebrant, 1991). This leads to

---

Matteo Santin, Andrew W. Lloyd and Stephen P. Denyer • School of Pharmacy and Biomolecular Sciences, University of Brighton, Cockcroft Building, Lewes Road, Brighton, BN2 4GJ, UK. **Luigi Ambrosio** • Institute of Composite Materials Technology C.N.R., and C.R.I.B., University of Naples "Federico II", Pizazzale Tecchio 80, 80125 Naples, Italy.

Integrated Biomaterials Science, edited by R. Barbucci. Kluwer Academic/Plenum Publishers, New York, 2002.

interactions between the material surface and selected components of the body fluid with a consequent formation of an organic layer completely masking the nascent material surface (Anderson, 1988; Santin *et al.*, 1999). Biomolecules such as proteins and proteoglycans, which are present in this organic film and frequently involved in the regulation of metabolism, govern the subsequent host response. Surface biocompatibility, therefore, ultimately reflects the composition of this organic layer and the design of novel products cannot disregard the need to achieve appropriate interactions between the implant surface and the adsorbing biological molecules (Ratner, 1993). In a recent publication, we have demonstrated the similarity in protein composition of some of the body fluids contacting implanted biomaterials and the almost identical profile of proteins able to adsorb onto different polymeric surfaces (Santin *et al.*, 1997). We have also recently shown that a material surface may influence the orientation of an adsorbed protein leading to preferential expression of activity (Martin *et al.*, 1999). These data suggest that the involvement of protein adsorption is an important aspect which requires consideration in the development of new biomaterials. The presence of specific proteins from a particular body fluid may also influence the performance of the implant (Anderson and Anderson, 1991; Bueler *et al.*, 1995). This emphasizes the importance of producing biomaterials with surface characteristics suitable for a particular application. Furthermore, in some cases protein adsorption has to be minimized in order to reduce the degree of interaction of the prosthesis with the tissue (Franklin *et al.*, 1993).

For these reasons, the overview of soft tissue replacement by biomaterials given in this chapter will be framed in the context of the biological processes occurring at the material/tissue interface. Performance of the biomaterials and guidelines for the synthesis of novel products will be discussed as a consequence of these early interactions.

14.2. Cardiovascular Devices

Cardiovascular diseases are a primary cause of mortality in the western world (Silver and Doillon, 1989). In particular, stroke and heart valve defects constitute a threat to the longevity and quality of life of the aged population. Treatment of such patients relies strongly on the availability of new biomedical devices able to support or substitute the damaged tissue. Therefore, considerable efforts in the biomaterial field have been directed toward producing implants able to satisfactorily replace these damaged tissues. Of these devices, vascular grafts and stents and heart valves (Silver and Doillon, 1989) are the most important. Improvement of the performance of these devices continues to be pursued to address the aggressive biological response which occurs on implantation.

14.2.1. Vascular Grafts

Vascular grafts are mainly made from synthetic materials which are processed into woven and nonwoven fabrics (Silver and Doillon, 1989). The arrangement of the fibers in different geometries produces final products with a high stiffness and strength and low extensibility. Furthermore, the porosity of the fabric facilitates effective tissue in-growth with minimal lateral permeation of blood. Poly(ethylene terephthalate) (Dacron^{TM}) and poly(tetrafluoro ethylene) (Teflon^{TM}) are the most used polymers for the production of vascular grafts. These materials are used to replace large and small diameter vessels, respectively, reflecting their different textures and elicited host responses.

14.2.1.1. Biocompatibility of Vascular Grafts

In a recent study, the inflammatory and neovascularization of vascular stents manufactured in a variety of designs from both Dacron^{TM} and Teflon^{TM} were compared. This study demonstrated that the degree of interaction of these materials with the surrounding tissues depended more on their morphology than on their material chemistry (Salzmann *et al.*, 1999). This study also demonstrated different performances of the same material at different implantation sites and an inverse relationship was found between inflammation and neovascularization. These observations are supported by other studies carried out on a particular Dacron^{TM} fabric geometry (Velour^{TM}), in which the fibers are knitted into bundles to form loops perpendicular to the surface of the artificial vessel (Silver and Doillon, 1989). Dacron grafts incorporating this design feature on the outer surface were shown to have reduced clotting time in the preclotting procedures usually carried out before implantation and had enhanced tissue in-growth on implantation.

These findings highlight the main goals in the production of effective vascular grafts: the need to achieve a high degree of integration of the outer surface with the surrounding tissues and minimal interactions of the inner surface of the device with blood components. As mentioned earlier, both processes ultimately depend on the formation of an organic film which conditions the surface of the material.

In the case of the preclotting technique, the adsorption of proteins induces the integration of the prosthesis with the surrounding connective tissue. Fibrin deposition triggers hemostasis (Linares, 1996), a process in which adhering platelets contribute to the formation of the initial clot, "the pseudo-intima," which reduces the permeation of blood throughout the polymer mesh. Likewise in the normal wound healing processes, the fibrin network, generated by the preclotting practice, also facilitates the migration of fibroblasts into the wall of the artificial vessel, thus inducing the gradual replacement of the pseudo-intima with collagen-rich fibrous connective tissue.

Fibrin network formation is a consequence of a cascade of interconnected zymogen–enzyme conversions triggered by the surface (Vogler *et al.*, 1995a, b). The early interaction of factors of the blood coagulation system, such as Factor XII, prekallikrein, and high molecular weight kininogen with the surface and their conversion to activated forms (i.e., Factor XIIa), leads to the formation of the thrombus (Figure 14.1). Therefore, on the inner surface of the vascular grafts the adsorption of these factors has to be

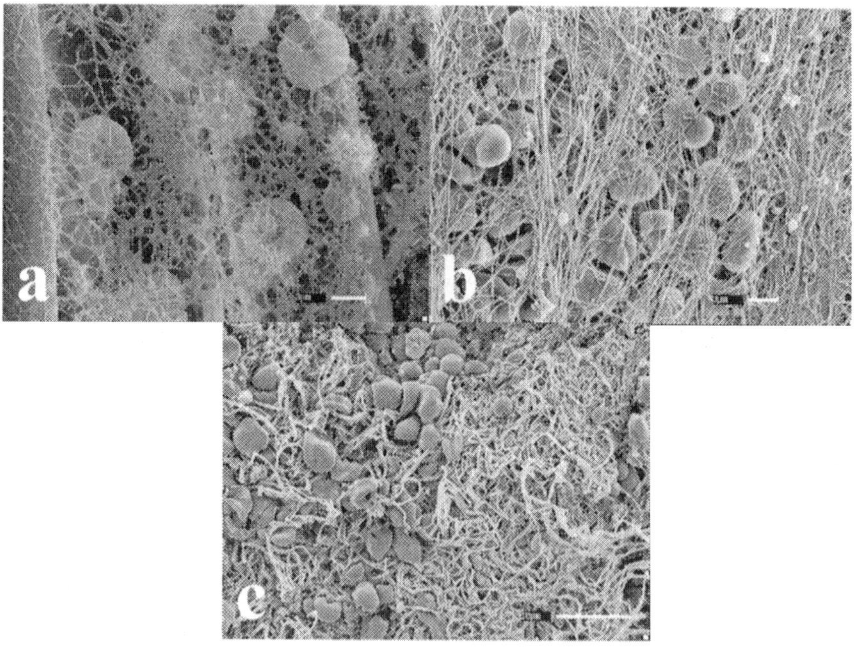

Figure 14.1. Thrombus formation on the surface of the Venticular Assist Device: (a) day 15; (b) day 30; (c) day 40. The fibrin network progressively grew on the material fibers entrapping red blood cells and platelets. Photos by Dr Antonella Motta, University of Trento, Italy. C.I.R.M.I.B. Masters Thesis.

minimized to reduce the risks of partial or complete occlusion of the artificial vessel.

Another important aspect of the compatibility of polymers used for vascular grafts is their potential to elicit the inflammatory response (Anderson, 1988). The adsorption of proteins of the complement system, such as the C3 and C5 fragments, appears fundamental to activation of the complement cascade (Liu and Elwing, 1994, 1996; Gemmell, 1997) and to adhesion and activation of the inflammatory cells. Other proteins (e.g., fibrinogen) can also adsorb onto surfaces and increase the level of adhesion and activation of the monocytes/macrophages (Yun *et al.*, 1995).

14.2.1.2. Strategies for the Production of Hemocompatible Vascular Grafts

Several strategies have been adopted to avoid activation of the blood coagulation system and the inflammatory response at the polymer surface. Blood compatibility has been pursued by the polymer surface modification, essentially using four approaches.

a. Hydrophilic Materials. Increased surface hydrophilicity seems to be the best solution to the problem of material thrombogenicity. The rationale to this approach assumes that protein adsorption is minimized on water-wettable surfaces (Morra and Cassinelli, 1995). However, in an elegant study, Vogler *et al.* (1995a,b) clearly demonstrated that the coagulation cascade was activated more by certain hydrophilic surfaces than by non-wettable materials. Furthermore, hydrophilic materials, despite their potential to diminish protein adsorption and cell adhesion, induce the activation of the complement C3 fragment on their surface due to the presence of the hydroxyl groups which are able to covalently bind one of the C3 subunits by a nucleophilic reaction (Payne and Horbett, 1987; Elwing *et al.*, 1988). This reaction induces cleavage of the fragment and its activation with the related release of anaphylatoxin (Porter and Reid, 1978) enabling inflammatory cells to be recruited at the surface (Anderson, 1988).

b. Grafting of Biologically Active Molecules. The chemical grafting of anticoagulants (Becquemin *et al.*, 1997; Dempsey *et al.*, 1998; Phaneuf *et al.*, 1998), platelet aggregation inhibitors (Markou *et al.*, 1998), or plasminogen activators (able to dissolve the thrombus) (Sundell *et al.*, 1997) has been considered. The most common approach is the heparinization of polymer surfaces (Taylor and Fletcher 1995).

c. Inert Materials. Surfaces have also been "passivated" with the use of albumin to block the adsorption of other blood proteins involved in the host response to foreign bodies (Osada *et al.*, 1999). In a recent study, albumin-heparin conjugates for polymer surface modification have been synthesized with the goal of combining the effects of both the molecules (Bos *et al.*, 1999). Surfaces have also been made inert toward blood coagulation by the grafting of phosphorylcholine to the surface (Courtney *et al.*, 1994). The rationale of using this molecule is that it is naturally present in the membrane of the endothelial cells and should not precipitate the formation of thrombi. Polymers containing these zwitterionic functional groups in their structure seem to markedly reduce the adsorption of fibrinogen and the adhesion of platelets to the surfaces (Ishihara *et al.*, 1992; Iwasaki *et al.*, 1997). Both extremely hydrophilic biomimetic phosphorylcholine-based biomaterials as well as very hydrophobic materials such as fluorinated polymers seem to minimize protein adsorption (Ishihara *et al.*, 1992; Ueda *et al.*, 1995) making the surface inert toward biointeractions (DeFife *et al.*, 1995; Chinn *et al.*, 1998). For these reasons a fluorinate polymer such as Teflon is considered as the material of choice for the production of small-diameter grafts where the risks of occlusion are enhanced (Silver and Doillon, 1989; Ariyoshi *et al.*, 1997). Even so, the percentage of obstruction in Teflon grafts is still high (Bos *et al.*, 1998) and evidence has accumulated to support the defluorization of this material by the oxidative burst of macrophages (Hauptmann *et al.*, 1996). Finally, in a recent publication, the grafting of poly(ethylene glycol)-diisocyanate to fibrinogen pre-adsorbed onto Dacron has been suggested to produce a precoating of inert material which can inhibit the adsorption of plasma proteins upon implantation (Deible *et al.*, 1998).

d. Endothelium-Scaffolding Materials. Polymers have been functionalized with the intent of favoring the growth of endothelial cells on the inner surface of the device, thus restoring the natural environment of the vessel (Pollara *et al.*, 1999). Materials containing surface-based cell receptor amino acid sequences have been reported to favor the growth of endothelial cells (Chinn *et al.*, 1998). However, these receptors are also recognized by cells of the inflammatory response, thus posing doubts concerning their efficiency *in vivo*. These concerns have been strongly supported in the same study; an increase in the inflammatory response on Dacron modified with the Arg-Gly-Asp tripeptide receptor has been shown (Chinn *et al.*, 1998). Endothelial cell growth on nonfunctionalized Dacron has also been shown to depend on both the surface morphology of the single fibers and the geometry of the fabrics (Tunstall *et al.*, 1995).

14.2.1.3. Other Biomaterials for the Production of Vascular Grafts

a. Polyurethanes. Stimulation of the inflammatory response (Zhao *et al.*, 1990; Kao *et al.*, 1995), as well as the thrombogenic potential (van der Kamp *et al.*, 1995), have limited the use of the polyurethanes in vascular graft production. Degradation of these materials has also been detected upon implantation with cracking appearing throughout the exposed surface (Petillo *et al.*, 1994). However, the synthesis of novel polycarbonate polyurethanes resistant to degradation and with a generally improved hemocompatibility has recently been performed (Edwards *et al.*, 1998; Jeschke *et al.*, 1999). This achievement, together with the promising results obtained by the functionalization of other polyurethanes with anticoagulants (Barbucci and Magnani, 1994) and other functional groups (Inoue *et al.*, 1997) create new opportunities for the use of these polymers.

b. Autologous Materials. The replacement of small-diameter vessels can be performed with the use of autograft materials. Veins from other body regions are removed and used to substitute for the damaged vessel (Purcell *et al.*, 1997). However, the surgical procedure for removing the vein from its original location and to graft it at the new site often induce damage which can lead to the failure of the implant. Furthermore, the limited availability of autograft material and the problems related to the transmission of diseases in the use of allografts (Desgranges *et al.*, 1998) significantly reduce the opportunities for this approach in the substitution of large-diameter vessels and in large-scale production.

14.2.2. Vascular Stents

Vascular stents are devices used in coronary angioplasty, a medical practice that decreases restenosis following vessel lesions (Bertrand *et al.*, 1998). The production of biocompatible vascular stents relies on the same principles required for vascular grafts. Early thrombus formation and late neo-intima development must be avoided following insertion of these devices in order to keep the lumen of the blood vessel patent. In general, stents are made from materials able to fulfil precise mechanical properties, the main characteristics of a stent being the ability to expand when deployed and to preserve this expansion against the pressure exerted by the vessel wall.

14.2.2.1. Metals for the Production of Vascular Stents

Early attempts in the production of vascular stents used surgical grades of stainless steel or tantalum (Bertrand *et al.*, 1998). These materials have the correct mechanical properties required of a stent; they can be easily compressed and expanded and retain the final diameter when inserted into the vessel. However, from a biocompatibility perspective, although stainless steel is shown resistant to oxidation and is not cytotoxic, it is thrombogenic (Bertrand *et al.*, 1998). It has been suggested that the oxide layer which forms on the surface of tantalum should minimize protein adsorption, however clinical studies have demonstrated that this material does not offer any particular advantages with respect to thrombogenesis. Nitinol, an alloy composed of nickel (55%) and titanium (45%), provides superelasticity and thermal shape memory properties (Hurlstone, 2000). Although this alloy shows good biocompatibility in the short-term, no long-term follow-up data is available and concerns have been raised regarding the potential release of nickel particles which may induce cytotoxic and immunological problems.

14.2.2.2. Coating of Metal Surfaces with Biocompatible Polymers

To improve the biocompatibility of these metals, a variety of polymeric coatings have been evaluated.

a. Stable Synthetic Polymers. The success of synthetic polymeric coatings improving stent biocompatibility is dependent on the same factors outlined under the previous discussion of their use in coating vascular grafts. Dacrons and polyurethanes give rise to the same problems encountered when used in that thrombi and immunocompetent cells accumulate on the surface (Bertrand *et al.*, 1998). The use of silicone-based materials has also been investigated, albeit with poor results. Similar to vascular grafts, phosphorylcholine-based polymers' significant success has been achieved using a pig coronary model (Malik *et al.*, 1997) and the recent evaluation of this technology in the clinic has demonstrated improved clinical outcome.

b. Biodegradable Synthetic Polymers. The opportunity of supporting the integration of the stent in the vessel wall by biodegradable polymers has been offered by a series of co-polymers such as poly(glycolic/polylactic acid), poly(hydroxy-butyrate/valerate), and poly(ethyleneoxide)/poly(butylene terephthalate) (Bertrand *et al.*, 1998). To these, polycaprolactone, polyorthoester, and poly-l-lactic acid (PLLA) must also be added. PLLA has been evoked as a biodegradable highly biocompatible polymer, since its degradation leads to the formation of CO_2 and water. Although in general this material elicits a reduced inflammatory response compared to other biodegradable polymers, severe inflammation has been observed when low molecular weight polymers are implanted, suggesting that some degree of caution is required in considering the use of this polymer (Lam *et al.*, 1995).

c. Natural Polymers. In vivo tests carried out on fibrin-coated metallic and polymeric stents improved the performances of these devices (Holmes *et al.*, 1994), with respect to occlusion and foreign body reaction. Furthermore, fibrin induced an increase in the rate of endothelization of the stent surface (Kipshidze *et al.*, 1994). Since fibrin is a protein involved in the hemostasis, forming a network that entraps platelets for the clot formation, it is surprising to find an improvement of the material hemocompatibility in its presence. A reduction of the platelet adhesion has been shown following short-term incubation of fibrin-coated titanium balloon expandable stents *in vitro* (Baker *et al.*, 1996). Although to our knowledge no study has been conducted on plasma protein adsorption on fibrin coatings, it seems reasonable to assume that interactions on fibrin with blood components follow a natural path leading to the formation of a conditioning film recognized as "self" by the immunocompetent cells. This film would be expected to closely resemble the composition of the newly formed extracellular matrix upon re-endothelization. As fibrin represents the bridge element dictating the end of the hemostasis and the beginning of tissue regeneration (Linares 1996), it is likely that its surface is recognized by structural proteins of the extracellular matrix more than by blood components involved in the coagulation and complement cascades.

d. Alternative Approaches. The use of polymers as core materials has been also considered. For example, Murphy *et al* (1992) have described the use of self-expanding Dacron meshes. *In vivo* biocompatibility studies using this system gave contradictory results, from which it is not possible to draw conclusions about their potential clinical use (Bertrand *et al.*, 1998). However, as the inflammatory response of this material is expected to resemble that encountered in their use as vascular grafts, their clinical application may be limited. Polyglycolic acid and PLLA devices have also been produced, the latter having a particularly good biocompatibility and appropriate degradation rate (Bertrand *et al.*, 1998). The undesired body reactions toward stent implants may also be reduced by using the device as carriers for thrombolytic agents (Bertrand *et al.*, 1998). However, the use of such technologies is limited by the desire to avoid regulatory classification of devices as drug delivery systems.

14.2.3. Substitute Heart Valves (SHV)

Degenerative processes, infections, and congenital morphological defects of heart valves require their substitution with artificial devices, produced using synthetic or animal-derived materials.

14.2.3.1. Mechanical Valves

Various synthetic devices have been produced with differing designs. In general, mechanical valves have a support which can be sewn to the surrounding natural tissue (Silver and Doillon, 1989). The support provides a framework to which is attached the occluder. The most famous mechanical valves have balls (Starr-Edwards; Figure 14.2b) and tilting discs (Bjork-Shiley) (Figure 14.2a, c). These designs inevitably alter the natural hemodynamics. Such alterations, in addition to the physicochemical properties of the material employed, can activate the blood coagulation cascade necessitating the associated life-long use of anti-thrombolytic agents (Stein *et al.*, 1995). In addition, device deterioration under the continuous mechanical stresses can lead to the failure of the implant and release of degradation products into the circulation. (Schoen and Levy, 1994; Bernacca *et al.*, 1997). Titanium alloys are commonly forged in the form of rings and cages to support and guide disks and balls, which are normally made of polymers and pyrolytic carbon. The latter has been shown to result in less wear and reduced fibrous tissue formation when compared to that usually found on the surface of polymer-based systems (Silver and Doillon, 1989). Furthermore, pyrolytic carbon appears to reduce the activation of

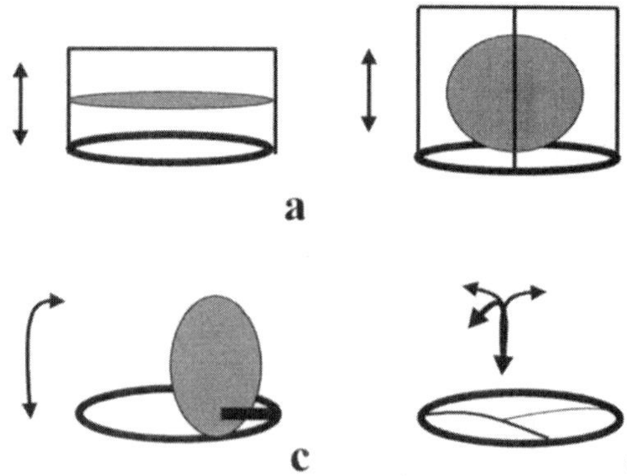

Figure 14.2. Main types of SHV: (a) disk in cage; (b) ball in cage; (c) tilting disk; (d) bioprosthetic valve. Arrows indicate the direction of the occluder or leaflet motion.

complement (Cenni *et al.*, 1997), although, *in vitro* platelet adhesion has been highlighted (Goodman *et al.*, 1996).

14.2.3.2. Bioprosthetic Valves

Allografts can be used for the production of SHV with bovine pericardium and porcine cusp valves being the main sources of material (Schoen and Levy, 1994). After being obtained from the donor, the tissue is generally fixed and stored in glutaraldehyde and subsequently sewn onto a polymeric ring before implantation (Figure 14.2d); on implantation, the construct is sutured into the surrounding tissues. In developing the surgical technique, these devices have also been implanted, without annulus, direct to the aorta wall (Sidiropoulos *et al.*, 1999). Although these valves offer hemodynamics similar to that of the natural valves, they often undergo calcification (Schoen and Levy, 1994). The main "intrinsic calcification" theory explaining this formation of mineral deposits proposes the devitalization of the tissue by the fixative which then transforms the entrapped cells into potential sites for crystal formation (Schoen and Levy, 1994). In this process, the calcium channels in the plasmalemma are unable to pump actively out calcium ions from the cells, thus raising the calcium concentration inside the phosphate-rich cytoplasm resulting in subsquent nucleation of calcium phosphate crystals. The growth of these crystals eventually disrupts the cells and invades the collagen-rich tissue. The potential to minimize the calcification processes by the use of an alternative fixative to glutaraldehyde and the discovery of some permanent or temporary inhibitors of calcification does suggest that other mechanisms are involved in this phenomenon, however (Santin *et al.*, 1998c). The alternative "extrinsic calcification" theory suggests that, in addition to cell-based nucleation, the adsorption of plasma proteins also leads to the precipitation of the mineral phase. Recent publications strongly support this hypothesis (Gura *et al.*, 1997; Santin *et al.*, 1999). Calcium-binding proteins have been found to adsorb onto the surface of plasma-incubated tissues (Gura *et al.*, 1997) and different protein adsorption profiles have been found to occur on cellular glutaraldehyde-cross-linked collagen sponges before and after their treatment with calcification inhibitors (Santin *et al.*, 1998b).

14.2.3.3. Guidelines for the Development of New SHV

In a meeting held in Washington DC in 1996, a group of scientists gathered to assess the state of the art in SHV production and to indicate the future directions for research in this sector (Edmunds *et al.*, 1997). The necessity of a new generation of valves was outlined with a particular emphasis on the design of new materials, tissue engineering approaches, and new strategies to reduce thromboembolism especially in mechanical valves. Furthermore, it was recognized that new *in vitro* and animal models must be established to predict the performance of the SHV. Among the suggestions made was the development of *in vitro* models to study the role of protein adsorption in the processes of calcification and thrombus formation on the material surfaces.

14.3. Intraocular Devices

The maintenance of vision is important for both our general quality of life and for healthy aging in an increasingly aged population. Two key structural components of the eye that are subject to deterioration are the transparent cornea, which allows the passage of light into the eye, and the lens, which focuses the light onto the retina at the back of the eye (Figure 14.3). Opacification of the natural crystalline lens or cataract formation in the aged is the commonest treatable form of blindness worldwide. Treatment involves the surgical removal of the cataract and replacement with an artificial intraocular lens (IOL). Artificial corneas, or keratoprosthesis (Kpro), are used to treat patients with chronic corneal surface inflammation, chemical burns, and Stevens-Johnson syndrome where corneal transplanta-

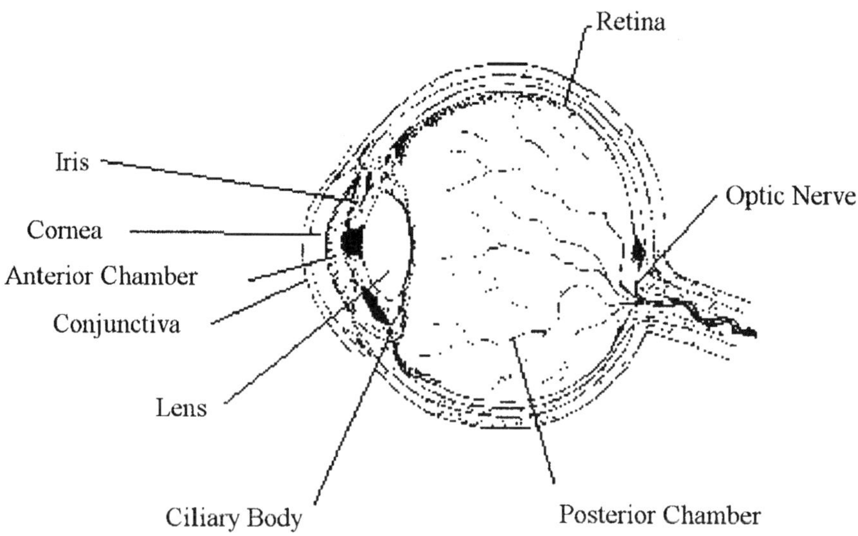

Figure 14.3. The structure of the eye showing the essential physiological features.

tion by penetrating keratoplasty has a poor prognosis (Chirila, 1997). In such cases implantation of an artificial cornea that provides a transparent window offers a means of restoring some degree of visual acuity. The following describes the recent advances in the development of both IOLs and Kpros.

14.3.1. Intraocular Lenses

The first intraocular lens was manufactured from poly(methyl methacrylate) (PMMA) by Rayners Ltd. and implanted by Harold Ridley in 1949 (Ridley, 1951). The material was selected on the basis of its ocular compatibility, refractive properties, and ease of manufacture. This implant revolutionized the treatment of cataract, providing patients with good visual acuity following surgery. Although PMMA IOLs are still widely used today, there have been marked changes in lens design and surgical procedures in the intervening years. Various lens manufacturers have also introduced new materials based on silicone and hydrogel-based technologies (Obstbaum, 1994). Initially, procedures involved the removal of the natural lens followed by the implantation of an intraocular lens in the posterior chamber (Ridley, 1951). Several clinicians later explored the use of anterior chamber IOLs. Although these were generally easier to implant than posterior chamber lenses, problems with corneal endothelial cell damage due to contact with the anterior IOL limited their use to specialist cases. The traditional posterior chamber IOL consists of a central optic and peripheral haptics, which serve to centralize the IOL within the capsular bag (Figure 14.4). The procedure for insertion requires a 5–6 mm incision in the cornea in order to allow both the removal of the lens fragments and the insertion of the IOL. This large incision contributes to increased visual astigmatism following surgery and a significant postoperative inflammatory response (Obstbaum,

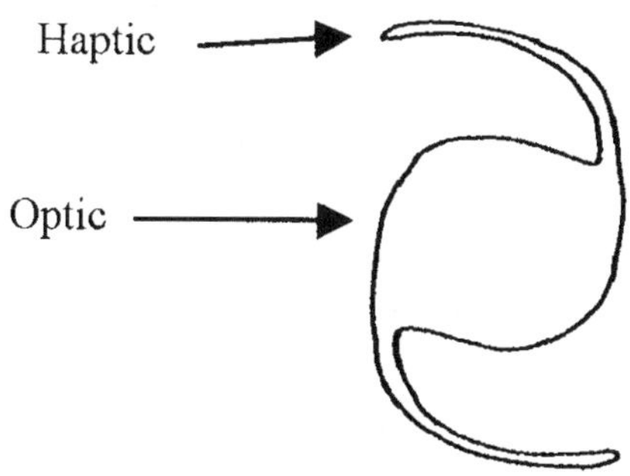

Figure 14.4. A typical intraocular lens.

Table 14.1 Examples of Intraocular Lens Materials (Modified from Kohnen, 1996)[a]

Lens type	Material	Refractive index	Water content	Comment
PMMA	MMA	1.49	<1%	Rigid
Alcon Acrylsof	PEA/PEMA	1.55	<1%	Foldable
Allergan Clariflex	EA/EMA/TFEMA	1.47	<1%	Foldable
ORC MemoryLens	HEMA/MMA	1.47	20%	Foldable
Storz Hydroview	HEXMA/HEMA	1.47	18%	Foldable
Alcon HydroSof	HEMA	1.44	38%	Foldable
Chiron C10UB				
Adatomed 90D				
Staar AA-4203				
Allergan SI-18NGB/SI-26NB	PDMS	1.41	<1%	Foldable
Iolab Soflex				
Domilens Silens				
Pharmacia Cee ON 920				
Allergan SI-30NB/SI-40NB	PDMDPS	1.43/1.46	<1%	Foldable

[a] PMMA, poly(methyl methacrylate); MMA, methyl methacrylate; PEA, 2-phenethyl acrylate; PEMA, 2-phenethyl methacrylate; EA, ethyl acrylate; EMA, ethyl methacrylate; TFEMA, 2,2,2-trifluoroethyl methacrylate; HEXMA, 6-hydroxyhexyl methacrylate; HEMA, 2-hydroxyethyl methacrylate; PDMS, poly(dimethylsiloxane); PDMDMS, poly(dimethyldiphenylsiloxane)

1994). In recent years, the development of the technique of phacoemulsification for cataract removal has allowed surgery to be performed through a smaller incision (Rosen, 1993). This technique involves the use of an ultrasonic probe which may inserted through a 3 mm incision into the anterior chamber to break up the natural lens so it can be removed by aspiration. The development of this surgical technique has led to the use of a new generation of foldable IOL which may be implanted through a small incision. These IOLs have been manufactured from a range of silicones and acrylate-based materials (Table 14.1) (Kohnen, 1996).

There are four principal clinical complications of intraocular surgery: corneal decompensation, postoperative inflammation, bacterial endophthalmitis, and posterior capsule opacification.

14.3.1.1. Corneal Decompensation

The corneal endothelium is responsible for ensuring the maintenance of corneal clarity. As corneal endothelial repair is limited by the slow turnover of these cells, corneal endothelial cell damage rapidly results in corneal decompensation, through water logging of the corneal stroma with an associated impairment of vision (Kaufman and Katz, 1976). The degree of damage that occurs on IOL contact with the endothelium is dependent on the nature of the IOL material. For example, materials with more hydrophobic surfaces, such as poly(methyl methacrylate), generally cause significantly greater damage to endothelial cells than those with more hydrophilic surfaces such as poly(2-hydroxyethyl methacrylate) (Mareo and Ratner, 1989). In present-day surgery, corneal decompensation is minimized by the use of viscoelastic agents such as carboxymethyl cellulose and hyaluronan, during both surgery and the implantation of posterior IOLs.

14.3.1.2. Postoperative Inflammation

Surgical intervention and implant biocompatibility contribute to the clinical outcome of IOL implantation (Obstbaum, 1994). Surgical intervention inevitably results in an acute inflammatory response as part of the natural wound healing process; this is often short term and results in the infiltration of proteins and inflammatory cells into the anterior chamber. Although the aqueous humor does contain various proteins, the surface activation of the inflammatory cascade results primarily from the adsorption of plasma proteins to the IOL following breach of the blood-ocular barrier (Obstbaum, 1994). Any inflammatory process within the eye tends to lead to increased postoperative anterior flare and to the adhesion of inflammatory cells to implant surfaces as evidenced by, for example, the deposition of diffuse cells on implanted intraocular lenses. These diffuse cells, which are primarily macrophage-like in nature, ultimately coalesce to form multinucleated giant cells. However, unlike implantation in other tissues, fibrosis of the implant fails to occur since the inflammatory response occurs within the anterior chamber rather than in tissue. The surgically-induced postoperative inflammatory response has been reduced over the years by the use of anti-inflammatory agents during surgery and the development of less invasive surgical techniques. Various approaches have been adopted in order to minimize the biomaterial-associated inflammatory response, including the use of surface passivation (Balyeat *et al.*, 1989; Amon and Menapace, 1994), heparin coatings (Larsson *et al.*, 1989), and more recently biomimetic phosphorylcholine (PC)-based coating of PMMA lenses (Hanlon *et al.*, 1997). A recent study in the rabbit model has shown that the PC-coatings significantly reduce the adhesion of diffuse cells and subsequent formation of giant cells on the IOL surface following implantation (Filipec *et al.*, 1997; Lloyd *et al.*, 1999). This technology has also been extended to the development of a foldable PC-based bulk material for use in small incision surgery (Lloyd *et al.*, 1997).

14.3.1.3. Bacterial Endophthalmitis

Although the incidence of postoperative bacterial endophthalmitis following refractive surgery is infrequent, the severe consequences of endophthalmitis are such that every precaution must be taken to minimize the potential transfer of particular skin organisms into the anterior chamber of the eye (Egger *et al.*, 1994). Although this transfer may be a consequence of the surgical procedure, the implant surface can play a key role in the establishment of any infection by providing an adherent surface for circulating bacteria in the anterior chamber. Recent evidence has shown that the adsorption of proteins to certain implant surfaces may facilitate the attachment of specific bacteria by causing conformational changes in the sorbed protein resulting in presentation of bacterial binding domains on the surfaces of the material (Martin *et al.*, 1999). In addition, the formation of bacterial biofilms on biomaterial surfaces protects the organisms from the host's natural defences, allowing the ultimate establishment of a localized focus of infection. Various clinical groups have investigated the relationships between IOL materials and the incidence of bacterial endophthalmitis (Bainbridge *et al.*, 1998). These data suggest that the material from which the haptics are manufactured may influence the frequency of bacterial endophthalmitis, with a particularly high incidence in patients implanted with IOLs possessing polypropylene haptics (Raskin *et al.*, 1992). Others have shown that the use of very hydrophilic materials, such as PC-coated devices, may reduce the incidence of bacterial endophthalmitis (Dropcova *et al.*, 1995; Ng *et al.*, 1996).

14.3.1.4. Posterior Capsule Opacification

Posterior capsule opacification (PCO) following extracapsular cataract extraction and intraocular lens implantation is primarily caused by the migration of lens epithelial cells across the posterior capsular bag (Apple *et al.*, 1992). This condition is also referred to as secondary cataract and is the major postoperative complication of modern-day intraocular surgery. PCO normally requires secondary postoperative surgery in which a YAG laser is employed to destroy the posterior capsular bag at the site of PCO. Although this technique has been widely used in a large patient population, there are complications associated with damage to the IOL surface during the laser treatment which can lead to impaired vision and the need for further invasive surgery (Ram *et al.*, 1999). As a consequence, various groups have attempted to develop IOLs which reduce PCO. One approach is to coat the IOL with a slow-releasing cytotoxic agent, such as thapsigargin, to kill the migrating epithelial cells (Duncan *et al.*, 1997). However, this may be limited by low level toxicity to iris and retinal cells. Recent clinical studies have shown that specific acrylate-based IOLs significantly reduce the occurrence of PCO (Ursell *et al.*, 1998). Although these results were initially attributed to the formation of a seal against the posterior capsular wall thereby preventing lens epithelial cell migration between the posterior capsular bag and the posterior surface of the IOL, recent data suggest that lens design may be the key parameter rather than the biomaterial *per se* (Nishi and Nishi, 1999).

It is anticipated that the new generation of IOLs will be fabricated from foldable, hydrophilic materials to minimize corneal decompensation, postoperative inflammatory response, and bacterial endophthalmitis of designs which serve to eliminate posterior capsule opacification.

14.3.2. Keratoprostheses

In comparison to IOLs, the development of kPros is still embryonic. Despite this there have been a number of clinical successes using a wide range of devices (Doane *et al.*, 1996). Ideally a Kpro should provide a clear visual window while supporting sufficient cellular integration to ensure the device is retained in the cornea. Kpro extrusion is the most common problem resulting from a failure to promote wound healing at the implant margins (Girard, 1983).

The original Kpros designed by Cardona and co-workers in the 1960s employed a “nut and bolt” manufactured from high quality PMMA (Figure 14.5) (Cardona, 1969). Following surgical removal of the epithelial layer, the underlying corneal stroma and endothelium were excised and the implant secured to the extracted tissue by means of a trepanned “bolt hole.” The tissue containing the keratoprosthesis was then sutured back into the eye. In addition to the visual problems arising from the use of a fixed implant

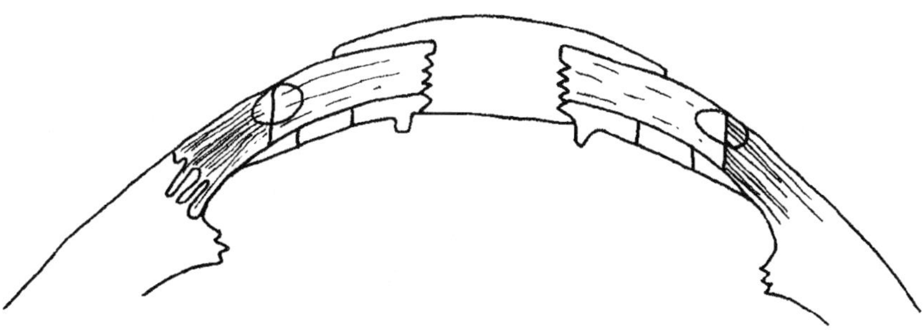

Figure 14.5. A schematic diagram showing a keraprosthesis implanted in the cornea.

size and a fixed surgical position, these devices had a failure rate of over 30% as a result of tissue erosion and subsequent extrusion of the implant (Catroveijo *et al.*, 1969). More recently, Doane *et al.* have demonstrated clinical success with a similar twin-plate keratoprosthesis manufactured from PMMA but with design modifications which permit their use in very dry eyes. Although attempts have been made to improve the retention of these Kpros by, for example, coating with collagen, PMMA Kpros have yet to find general acceptance as a result of their high failure rates (Kirkham and Dangle, 1991).

An alternative device, the osteo-odonto-keratoprosthesis (OOKP), was developed in Italy by Strampelli (1963). This device uses a lamina prepared from a single-root tooth extracted from the patient. A PMMA optic is cemented into the center of the lamina and the device implanted in a subcutaneous pocket below the eye in the patient's cheek. After 3 months the device is removed from the subpalpebral pocket, the optic is placed through a hole trephined in the cornea into the anterior chamber, and the device is sutured over the cornea below a covering of buccal mucosa. These devices have been used in both Italy and the UK for the last 30 years with reasonable success (Marchi *et al.*, 1994). More recently, the focus has turned to the development of biointegrative Kpros comprised of a central optic with a porous peripheral skirt to facilitate cell migration and stromal integration (Chirila, 1997).

It is clear that the base material of any Kpro should have refractive and mechanical properties as close as possible to the natural cornea in order to obtain appropriate refraction with sufficient strength to resist the internal pressures of the eye (Lee *et al.*, 1996). In order to achieve a skirt material which will support keratocyte integration, Kpros have been fashioned from a range of materials including melt-blown polyolefins (Trinkaus-Randall *et al.*, 1991), poly(HEMA) (Hicks *et al.*, 1998), and a range of polytetrafluoroethylene (PTFE) fabrics, Impra, Gore-tex, and Proplast (Legeais *et al.*, 1992). The porous skirt of the poly(HEMA) Kpros are fabricated using phase separation during polymerization of HEMA in water (Chirila, 1997). The central optically transparent poly(HEMA) core is attached to the skirt through an interpenetrating network. The clinical studies of these devices at this time are limited and variable (Hicks *et al.*, 1997; Chirila, 2001). Another hydrogel-based device fabricated from a polyvinyl alcohol–collagen composite material led to rejection of the keratoprosthesis after four weeks (Trinkaus-Randall *et al.*, 1988). *In vitro* studies indicate that pore size is a key factor for effective cell integration (Legeais *et al.*, 1997). Pores of less than 20 μm diameter are simply too small to allow keratocytes to enter. Although hydrogels with pore sizes in excess of 20 μm are readily invaded by stromal cells, the limited cellular adhesion of keratocytes to poly(HEMA) may prevent the ultimate synthesis of stromal matrix. In an attempt to improve cell adhesion to the HEMA skirt, material studies are presently in progress to employ other copolymer systems which demonstrate enhanced keratocyte adhesion (Sandeman *et al.*, 2000).

Hydrophobic materials such as PTFE tend to support cell adhesion more readily. This is confirmed by a recent study in rabbits of keratocyte invasion of custom-made Impra PTFE with a 50 μm pore size (Drubaix *et al.*, 1996). This study demonstrated a steady increase in the quantity of collagen laid down in the implanted materials and a transition toward those collagen subtypes and arrangement typical of untraumatized stroma. However, studies using the commercial PTFE, Proplast, demonstrated over 50% implant extrusion after four months (Legeais *et al.*, 1995).

There is considerable debate as to whether the external surface of the implant needs to allow ready epithelialization or not. A nonepithelialized surface would need to support the normal blink reflex and minimize the risk of protein and lipid deposition, minimize any surface-associated inflammatory response, and prevent bacterial endophthalmitis. The ideal material would therefore be exceptionally hydrophilic and extremely biocompatible—PC-coating technology may therefore have an application in this field. Furthermore, the design of any such device should suppress epithelial downgrowth, which has been shown to contribute to extrusion of PMMA devices in the past. Any device which does not undergo re-epithelialization must also eliminate downgrowth of epithelial cells.

Any re-epithelialized surface will need to allow adequate nutrient to reach any encroaching or overlying cells and must permit intercellular communication between the surviving cell layers of the cornea, which control the normal epithelial wound healing response, since de-epithelialization of the cornea results in apoptosis of the underlying keratocytes. Previous studies aimed at achieving epithelialization have involved the glow-discharge grafting of poly(HEMA) onto silicone base materials (Lee *et al.*, 1996). In modifying the surface concentration of poly(HEMA) the group were able to modulate the extent of colonization by epithelial cells. Although tolerated well in animal studies over several months, the workers reported a tendency for high concentrations of poly(HEMA) and to encourage invasion of the implant skirt by epithelia.

Finally, the internal surface of the Kpro, which lies within the anterior chamber of the eye, is subject to similar challenges as are IOL surfaces. It is unlikely that the internal surface of the implant will support the reestablishment of an endothelial cell layer given the slow turnover of these cells *in vivo*. The surface will therefore have to be highly biocompatible to minimize postoperative inflammation and associated protein and cell deposition, which will compromise visual clarity.

The development of clinically effective Kpros offers a greater challenge than that presented by IOLs, since the device is exposed to two different surface environments, the aqueous humor on the inside and the tear film on the outside, and it requires specific physicochemical surface properties in the skirt component to achieve long-term stromal integration. The control of specific protein deposition on both of these surfaces will undoubtedly feature significantly in the future development of suitable materials for Kpro fabrication. This is unlikely to be achieved through the use of a single biomaterial, but through the development of hybrid biofunctional materials of specifically designed molecular architectures needed to address each of these challenges.

14.4. Other Applications in Soft Tissue Replacement

14.4.1. Artificial Skin

The substitution of damaged skin areas with fabricated materials requires development of a complex structure able to simulate the extracellular matrix of the dermis. For this reason the main emphasis in skin replacement involves the use of tissue engineering to permit the reconstitution of the complex environment of the dermis and its covering with natural epidermis (Bonassar and Vacanti, 1998; Pomach *et al.*, 1998; Hafemann *et al.*, 1999). Nevertheless, the use of biomaterials able to support the regeneration of the tissue *in vivo* has also been pursued (Santin *et al.*, 1996; Kim *et al.*, 1999; Pieper *et al.*, 1999). With few exceptions, skin reconstruction has been attempted with the aid of natural polymers such as glycosaminoglycans (Poggi *et al.*, 1999) and collagen (Pachence, 1996), which are among the most abundant components in skin. Polysaccharide hydrogels such as chitosan (Biagini *et al.*, 1991; Bhaskara and Sharma 1997; Kim *et al.*, 1999) and alginate (Kim *et al.*, 1999) have also been employed. Sponges have been prepared where each of these polymers is present alone (Biagini *et al.*, 1991) or in combination with others (Butler *et al.*, 1999; Choi *et al.*, 1999; Pieper *et al.*, 1999). Composite materials have been produced combining synthetic materials such as poly(HEMA) with collagen (Jeyanthi and Panduranga Rao, 1990) and gelatin (Santin *et al.*, 1996). Amino acid sequences with receptor activity for the cells have also been prepared to increase the rate of tissue in-growth throughout the mesh of the hydrogels (Grzesiak *et al.*, 1997; Tschopp *et al.*, 1998). Polyurethanes, silicone, and poly(vinyl alcohol) foams have been employed as templates for skin regeneration (Jayasree *et al.*, 1995), sometimes associated with other polymers in a laminated form (Silver and Doillon, 1989).

14.4.2. Hernia Repair

Meshes of poly(tetrafluoro ethylene) (ePTFE, GORE-TEX), poly(ethylene terephthalate) (Dacron), and polypropylene have been used to repair inguinal and paracolostomal hernias (Alexandre and Bouillot, 1996; Bebawi *et al.*, 1997). Similar to the materials used for skin regeneration, the polymeric mesh for hernia repair must facilitate tissue in-growth to achieve a complete integration of the membrane with the surrounding tissues. This improves the mechanical properties of the mesh and its long-term stability on implantation. A certain degree of clotting potential is considered an appropriate prerequisite in this kind of application in order to obtain a new extracellular matrix; the design of new materials will therefore need to focus on this aspect.

14.4.3. Urological Devices

14.4.3.1. Catheters and Stents

The main area of application for biomaterials in urology is the production of ureteral stents and urethral catheters, which can alleviate the occlusion problems associated with pathologies of the lower urinary tract (Wironen *et al.*, 1997) such as urolithiasis and tumor occlusions caused by calculi and growing tissue, respectively (Stevens and Lowe, 1995). These devices are not free from drawbacks, however. Bacterial adhesion and encrustation on the lumens surface can soon lead to occlusion or fracture of the device as well as to infections of the urinary tract (Elves and Feneley, 1997). Various groups have sought to synthesize polymers which are able to reduce the conditioning of the surface by organic molecules present in the urine, since both bacterial adhesion and crystal nucleation and growth are enhanced by early formation of an organic layer on the polymer surface (Elves and Feneley, 1997). Minimization of the deposition of urine organic macromolecules, such as receptor proteins for microorganisms (Wassall *et al.*, 1998) or with affinity for the crystals (Santin *et al.*, 1998a,b,c) is a main target in the improvement of device performance.

Silicone, latex (natural polyisoprene rubber), and polyurethanes are the most commonly used polymers in these applications. However, all these materials are susceptible to encrustation and bacterial adhesion and they can induce inflammation of the mucosa (Wironen *et al.*, 1997). Hydrogel coatings have been used in attempts to reduce the formation of the conditioning layer (Gorman *et al.*, 1997; Wironen *et al.*, 1997). Recently we have demonstrated that the presence of a hydrophilic coating may be insufficient since a stable protein-rich film is still able to form and induce crystal growth both *in vitro* and *in vivo* (Santin *et al.*, 1999). A reduction in the organic conditioning layer has also been pursued using fluorinated materials such as poly(tetrafluoro ethylene) (Wironen *et al.*, 1997). In the specific case of urological implants, the use of fluorinated polymers appears to minimize urine protein adsorption (Santin, 2000). Although there was early interest in the poly(vinyl chloride), this has subsequently been abandoned since this material lacks the mechanical properties required for this kind of application (Wironen *et al.*, 1997).

14.4.3.2. Other Urological Implants

Penile implants, testicular implants, and artificial urinary sphincters are among other applications for biomaterials in the replacement of damaged parts of the urinary tract (Wironen *et al.*, 1997).

Silicones, acrylic, and polyethylene rods have been used for penile implants; silicone/stainless steel constructs have been employed as artificial sphincters; and poly(methyl methacrylate), glass marbles, Dacron, and polyethylene are the materials of choice for testicular implants. Fracture, infection, erosion, and pain are associated with the penile implant, while the use of silicones in the production of testicular implants has been discouraged by the American Urological Association due to possible links between the implant of silicone gels and systemic diseases. In addition, unless textured, silicone implants usually lead to the formation of a fibrotic capsule.

14.4.4. Ligament and Tendon Prostheses

The use of artificial ligaments and tendons to surgically repair or augment ruptured natural tissue has been introduced mainly to reduce the long rehabilitation time associated with the traditional technique of using autologous repair.

The first description of the use of an artificial ligament replacement material occurred in 1906. However, it is only in the last twenty years that a number of the experimental materials used in the field of vascular applications were implemented to design structures for tendon and ligament prostheses. These include polyethylene, polypropylene, aramide, polytetrafluoroethylene (PTFE), polyester (Dacron), carbon, absorbable polymer/carbon, polyester carbon, polyester/silicon, polyamide/PTFE composites, and xenografts. Different forms and fiber technologies have been applied to optimize the performance of these devices intra-articularly and intraosseously.

Clinical and biomechanical studies have shown that most of the commercial braided, woven, and knitted ligament prostheses undergo mechanical failure as a consequence of their weak resistance to bending and friction (Turner *et al.*, 1990; Durselen *et al.*, 1996). Improved mechanical and biological properties are therefore necessary to reduce the number of implant failures due to either foreign body reactions or to poor biomechanical properties. The aggressive *in vivo* environment and the effects of cyclic loading conditions can act synergistically, resulting in a decrease of the mechanical performances which dramatically affects the life of the prosthesis (Ambrosio *et al.*, 1996). As a consequence, except for augmentation or in cases where no autologous tissue is available, these devices are no longer used clinically to repair tendon and ligament failure.

The primary purpose of the prosthetic replacement of ligaments and tendons is to replace a damaged tissue with an artificial device that will mimic the function of the original tendon and ligament as well as possible.

New prostheses' designs, that more effectively emulate the complex aspects of these systems, may improve the success rate of the replacement surgery (O'Connor *et al.*, 1993). The reproduction of the mechanical and viscoelastic features of the natural systems is therefore necessary. This can be done by imitating the composite structure of natural tendons and ligaments. Good functional reproduction of these properties is impossible to obtain with a single material, as a consequence of the many functions of the tissue which affect mechanical behavior, and may therefore only be achieved using composite prosthesis (Pradas *et al.*, 1991; Migliaresi *et al.*, 1981).

A development of a semibiodegradable composite artificial tendon prosthesis, composed of water-swollen poly(2-hydroxyethylmethacrylate)/poly(caprolactone) blend hydrogel matrix reinforced with poly(glycolic acid) fibers, was presented by Davis *et al.* (1991). The latter is constituted by fibers wound in a matrix of hydrogel and oriented in such a way as to obtain the desired mechanical behavior. The nonlinear behavior of the mechanical response of such a system has been correlated with the deformation mechanism associated with the geometrical variations of the composite structure during a loading process. The mechanical behavior of such soft composite structures have been shown to resemble closely the natural tissue (Ambrosio *et al.*, 1998). Recently, the advanced technique of tissue engineering has been applied to design scaffolds and cellular devices which may lead to the ultimate production of nature-like ligaments and tendons (Goulet *et al.*, 1997).

14.4.5. Intervertebral Disc Prostheses

Low back pain is one of the most common medical conditions in the world. Disc degeneration, an inevitable process of aging, is one of the major causes of low back pain. Currently, there are two major surgical interventions for treating conditions related to the degenerative disc: discectomy and fusion. Altough discectomy and fusion produce a relatively good short-term clinical result in relieving pain, both these surgical treatments alter the biomechanics of the spine, possibly leading to further degeneration of the surrounding tissue and the discs at adjacent levels (Qi-Bin Bao *et al.*, 1996).

The primary purpose of discectomy is to excise any disc material compressing the spinal nerve causing pain. The surgery requires removal of a small portion of lamina and ligament with an incision in the posterior annulus. Discectomy is successful in relieving the radical pain caused by a herniated disc. However, such surgery alone is unable to restore the nucleus to its original load-bearing capacity and makes long-term results more questionable (Weber, 1993). Disc degeneration and its sequelae are allowed to continue leading to alterations in spine stability (Goel *et al.*, 1985; Tribewal *et al.*, 1985).

Fusion means eliminating a motion segment between the two vertebrae by using bone graft and internal fixation. This procedure is performed for gross instability of a motion segment resulting from traumatic surgery or degeneration. The success rate of spinal fusion is poorly defined in the literature and varies in the very wide range between 32% and 98%. Biomechanical studies also show that fusion alters the biomechanics of the spine and causes increased stresses at the junction between fused and unfused segments (Lee and Langrana, 1984).

Over the past 35 years, a tremendous effort has been made to develop an artificial disc to replace the degenerated disc. An alternative to the use of disrupted or degenerative discs involves the utilization of artificial discs. Two types of intervention are possible: (a) total disc replacement (nucleus and annulus) and (b) a nucleus pulposus substitute. Both methods require duplication of the natural durable structure (Hellier *et al.*, 1992), and an easy and safe means of implant replacement or removal.

The currently available intervertebral disc prostheses are made of metals, metallic-polymer systems, and polymers. They include a low friction sliding surface like the ball and socket, spring and hinge systems, fluid-filled chamber, and discs of rubber and other elastomer (Salib and Pettine, 1993; Lee *et al.*, 1990; Enker *et al.*, 1993). In order to reproduce mechanical and transport properties of an intervertebral disc, a composite hydrogel structure has been proposed (Ambrosio *et al.*, 1996).

Rather than replacing the entire disc, several investigators have described prostheses that simply replace the nucleus when no failure of the annulus is present. Several materials and methodology have been proposed. *In situ* polymerization of silicone or polyurethane (Garcia *et al.*, 1995) based materials has been used to replace the nucleus. To obtain a nucleus with more appropriate properties (nutrition and mechanical) a hydrogel system has also been used (Qi-Bin Bao and Higham, 1993).

14.5. Conclusions

Regardless of the site of implantation, the formation of an organic layer conditioning the surface of any implant from the earliest phase of body fluid contact is a common feature. This organic layer is rich in blood components, which are key factors in the host response toward foreign bodies. In particular, proteins play a role in regulating the two principal systems of this host reaction, which are coagulation and inflammation (Linares, 1996).

The activation of the coagulation cascade emerges as a competing event in the context of the biocompatibility of biomaterials. Although it appears absolutely detrimental when triggered on the lumen surfaces of vascular grafts and stents, it is the foundation for building a structural continuity between the surface of the implant and the regenerating new tissue. This continuity is pivotal for the complete integration of the implant in the host environment and the consequent fulfilment of the device's mechanical performance. In this role, a new generation of biointegrative materials has to be produced which is able to support the adsorption of, and promote activation of the enzymatic factors in their native state. Chemical groups have already been identified which are able to trigger the coagulation cascade (Vogler *et al.*, 1995a). Carboxylic groups showed a particularly high procoagulant potential making them first choice candidates for activating relevant plasma factors. The activity of these functional groups is even greater than that predicted by theoretical models based on surface wettability. This suggests that specific chemical interactions may also be involved in generating a thin layer of active factors at the interface. It has been suggested that such a layer would not be bound to the material surface, but floats on the material in a material-bound water film (Vogler *et al.*, 1995b). Therefore, it can be postulated that modulation of the procoagulant potential of materials relies on the formation of a loosely interacting protein film in which the native conformation of the constituents is preserved. On this basis, strategies can be developed to modulate biological stimulation through the use of a range of carboxylic-acid terminated lateral chains protruding from the polymer surface. Different lengths of the spacing arm may modulate the degree of interaction of the biomaterial with its biological environment. The surface density of these functional groups can also be considered another parameter of choice to temper enzyme activation at the interface. The procoagulant activity of different functional groups has been shown to be exponentially related to their surface density (Vogler *et al.*, 1995b).

A review of this literature suggests that the production of polymers suitable for lumen coating in vascular and urological devices has to focus on two main options: (i) grafting of biological molecules (e.g., phosphorylcholine, heparin, fibrin, albumin), and (ii) protein-repellent functional groups (e.g., fluorinated polymers).

In the first class of compounds, fibrin is highly regarded since it seems to bring with it many of the advantages required in the production of vascular devices, such as low thrombogenicity and endothelium-growth-supporting potential (Baker *et al.*, 1996). The synthesis of polypeptides with a structure resembling that of fibrin fragments and with specific biological properties represents an example of more sophisticated biomimetic approaches whereby material scientists can capitalize on approaches used in nature.

The second category favors certain fluorinated materials due to their general ability to minimize protein adsorption (Ishihara *et al.*, 1992) and their extremely low procoagulant activity (Chinn *et al.*, 1998). These polymers may be used to solve coagulation and inflammatory problems in temporary vascular implants where re-endothelialization is not required. They certainly represent, in our opinion, one of the better candidates for the coating surfaces of urological catheters and stents.

Looking at the complexity of biological structures and at the multiple functions of soft tissues, specific applications will require the use of functionalizing moieties in unique combinations. For instance, vascular grafts and keratoprostheses contact different environments but their surfaces have to perform related functions. Tissue integration and inertness are both required in these devices. Vascular grafts have to stimulate the integration of its external surface and suppress blood coagulation in the lumen; keratoprostheses require a biointegrating skirt surrounding a nonbiofouling optic. Novel devices, incorporating both properties, will undoubtedly be developed in the near future providing a bridge linking the biomaterials field to the developing area of tissue engineering.

References

Alexandre, J.H., Bouillot, J.L., 1996. Recurrent inguinal hernia: surgical repair with a sheet of Dacron mesh by the inguinal route, *Eur. J. Surg.* **162**, 29–33.

Ambrosio, L., De Santis, R., Iannace, S., Netti, P.A., Nicolais, L. 1998. Viscoelastic behaviour of composite ligament prostheses, *J. Biomed. Mater. Res.* **42**, 6–12.

Ambrosio, L., Netti, P.A., Iannace, S., Huang, S.J., Nicolais, L. 1996. Composite hydrogels for intervertebral disc prostheses, *J. Mater. Sci., Materials in Medicine* **7**, 251–254.

Amon, M., Menapace, R. 1994. *In vivo* documentation of cellular reactions of lens surfaces for assessing the biocompatibility of different intraocular implants, *Eye* **8**, 649–656.

Anderson, J. M. 1988. Inflammatory response to implants, *Asaio* **11**(2), 101–107.

Anderson, N.L., Anderson, N.G. 1991. A two-dimensional gel database of human plasma proteins, *Electrophoresis* **12**, 883–906.

Apple, D.J., Solomon, K.D., Tetz, M.R., Assia, E.I., Holland, E.Y., Legler, U.F.C, Castaneda, V.E., Hoggatt, J.P., Kostick, A.M.P. 1992. Posterior capsule opacification, *Surv. Ophthalmol.* **37**, 73–116.

Ariyoshi, H., Okuyama, M., Okahara, K., Kawasaki, T., Kambayashi, J., Sakon, M., Monden, M. 1997. Expanded polytetrafluoroethylene (ePTFE) vascular graft loses its thrombogenicity six months after implantation, *Thromb. Res.* **88**(5), 427–433.

Bainbridge, J.W.B., Teimory, M., Tabandeh, H., Kirwan, J.F., Dalton, R., Reid, F., Rostron, C.K. 1998. Intraocular lens implants and risk of endophthalmitis, *Br. J. Ophthalmol.* **82**, 1312–1315.

Baker, J., Horn, J., Nikolaychik, N., Kipshidze, N. 1996. Fibrin stent coatings, in: *Endoluminal Stenting* (U. Sigwart, ed.), pp. 84–89, W.B. Saunders, London, Philadelphia, Toronto, Sidney, Tokyo

Balyeat, H.D., Nordquist, R.E., Lerner, M.P., Gupta, A. 1989. A comparison of endothelial cell damage produced by control and surface modified poly(methyl methacrylate) intraocular lenses, *J. Cataract Refract. Surg.* **15**, 491–494.

Bao Qi-Bin, Higham P.A. 1993. Hydrogel intervertebral disc nucleus, *US Patent* 5,192,326,9 March 93.

Bao Qi-Bin, McCullen, G.M., Higham P.A., Dumbleton J.H., Yuan H.A. 1996. The artificial disc: theory, design and materials, *Biomaterials* **17**, 1157–1167.

Barbucci, R., Magnani, A. 1994. Conformation of human plasma proteins at polymer surfaces: the effectiveness of surface heparinization, *Biomaterials* **15**, 955–962.

Bebawi, B. A., Moqtaderi, F., Vijay, V. 1997. Giant incisional hernia: staged repair using pneumoperitoneum and expanded polytetrafluoroethylene. *Am. Surg.* **63**, 375–381.

Becquemin, J.P., Riff, Y., Kovarsky, S., Ardaillou, N., Benhaien-Sigaux, N. 1997. Evaluation of a polyester collagen-coated heparin bonded vascular graft, *J. Cardiovasc. Surg.* **38**, 7–14.

Bernacca, G.M., Mackay, T.G., Wilkinson, R., Wheatley, D.J. 1997. Polyurethane heart valves: fatigue failure, calcification, and polyurethane structure, *J. Biomed. Mater. Res.* **34**, 371–379.

Bertrand, O.F., Sipehia, R., Mongrain, R., Rodes, J., Tardif, J-C., Bilodeau, L., Coté, G., Bourassa, M.G. 1998. Biocompatibility aspects of new stent technology, *J. Am. Coll. Cardiol.* **32**, 562–571.

Bhaskara Rao, S., Sharma, C.P. 1997. Use of chitosan as biomaterial: studies on its safety and hemostatic potential, *J. Biomed. Mater. Res.* **34**, 21–28.

Biagini, G., Bertani, A., Muzzarelli, R., Damadei, A., DiBenedetto, G., Belligolli, A., Riccotti, G., Zucchini, C., Rizzoli, C. 1991. Wound management with N-carboxybutyl chitosan, *Biomaterials* **12**, 281–286.

Bonassar, L.J., Vacanti, C.A. 1998. Tissue engineering: the first decade and beyond, *J. Cell. Biochem.* **S30-31**, 297–304.

Bos, G.W., Poot, A.A., Beugeling, T., van Aken, W.G., Feijen, T. 1998. Small-diameter vascular graft prostheses: current status, *Arch. Physiol. Biochem.* **106**(2), 100–115.

Bos, G.W., Scharenborg, N.M., Poot, A.A., Engbers, G.H.M., Beugeling, T., vanAken, W.G., Feijen, T. 1999. Proliferation of endothelial cells on surface-immobilized albumin-heparin conjugate loaded with basic fibroblast growth factor, *J. Biomed. Mater. Res.* **44**, 330–340.

Bueler, M.R., Wiederkehr, F., Vondershmitt, D.J. 1995. Electrophoretic, chromatographic and immunological studies of human urinary proteins, *Electrophoresis* **16**, 124–134.

Butler, C.E., Yannas, I.V., Compton, C.C., Correia, C.A., Orgill, D.P. 1999. Comparison of cultured and uncultured keratinocytes seeed into a collagen-GAG amtrix for skin replacements, *Br. J. Plastic Surg.* **52**, 127–132.

Cardona, H. 1969. Mushroom transcorneal keratoprosthesis, *Am. J. Ophthalmol.* **68**, 604–612.
Catroveijo, R., Cardona, H., DeVoe, A.G. 1969. Present state of prosthokeratoplasty, *Am. J. Ophthalmol.* **68**, 613–625.
Cenni, E., Granchi, D., Ciapetti, G., Stea, S., Verri, E., Gamberini, S., Gori, A., Pizzoferrato, A., Zucchelli, P. 1997. In vitro complement activation after contact with pyrolytic carbon-coated and uncoated polyethylene terephthalate, *J. Mater. Sci., Materials in Medicine* **8**, 771–774.
Chinn, J.A., Sauter, J.A., Phillips, R.E., Kao, W.Y.J., Anderson, J.M., Hanson, S.R., Ashton, T. R. 1998. Blood and tissue compatibility of modified polyester: thrombosis, inflammation, and healing, *J. Biomed. Mater. Res.* **39**, 130–140.
Chirila, T. 1997. Artificial cornea with a porous polymeric skirt, *Trends Polym. Sci.* **5**(11), 346–348.
Chirila, T.V. 2001. An overview of the development of artificial cornea with porous skirts and the use of PHEMA for such an application. *Biomaterials* **22**, 3311–3317.
Choi, Y.S., Hong, S.R., Lee, Y.M., Song, K.W., Park, M.H., Nam, Y.S. 1999. Study on gelatin-containing artificial skin: I. Preparation and characteristics of novel gelatin-alginate sponge, *Biomaterials* **20**, 409–417.
Courtney, J.M., Lamba, N.M.K., Sundaram, S., Forbes, C.D. 1994. Biomaterials for blood-contacting applications, *Biomaterials* **15**, 737–743.
Davis, P.A., Huang, S.J., Ambrosio, L., Ronca, D., Nicolais, L., 1991. A biodegradable composite artificial tendon. *J. Mater. Sci.: Materials in Medicine* **3**, 359–364.
DeFife, K., Yun, J.K., Azeez, A., Stack, S., Ishihara, K., Nakabayashi, N., Colton, E., Anderson, J. M. 1995. Adhesion and cytokine production by monocytes on poly(2-methacryloyloxyethyl phosphorylcholine-co-alkyl methacrylate)-coated polymers, *J. Biomed. Mater. Res.* **29**, 431–439.
Deible, C.R., Petrosko, P., Johnson, P.C., Beckman, E.J., Russell, A.J., Wagner, W.R. 1998. Molecular barriers to biomaterial thrombosis by modification of surface proteins with polyethylene glycol, *Biomaterials* **19**, 1885–1893.
Dempsey, D.J., Phaneuf, M.D., Bide, M.J., Szycher, M., Quist, W.C., Logerfo, F.W. 1998. Synthesis of a novel small diameter polyurethane vascular graft with reactive binding sites, *ASAIO J.* **44**, M506–M510.
Durselen, L., Claes, L., Ignatius, A., Rubenacker, S. 1996. Comparative animal study of three ligament prostheses for the replacement of the anterior cruciate and medial collateral ligament, *Biomaterials* **17**, 977–982.
Desgranges, P., Beaujan, F., Brunet, S., Cavillon, A., Qvafordt, P., Melliere, D., Becquemin, J.P. 1998. Cryopreserved arterial allografts used for the treatment of infected vascular grafts, *Ann. Vasc. Surg.* **12**, 583–588.
Doane, M.G., Dohlman, C.H., Bearse, G. 1996. Fabrication of a keratoprosthesis, *Cornea* **15**, 179–184.
Dropcova, S., Bowers, R.W.J., Denyer, S.P., Faragher, R.G.A., Gard, P.R., Hall, B, Hanlon, G.W., Jones, S.A., Lloyd, A.W., Mikhalovsky, S.M., Olliff, C.J., Riding, M., Rosen, P.H. 1995, The effect of adsorbed phosphorylcholine based biomimetic copolymers on bacterial adhesion to poly(methyl methacrylate) intraocular lens materials, *J. Pharm. Pharmacol.* **47**, (Suppl.), 1072.
Drubaix, I., Legeais, J.M., Malek-Chehire, N., Savoldelli, M., Menasche, M., Robert, L., Renard, G., Pouliquen, Y. 1996. Collagen synthesized in fluorocarbon polymer implant in the rabbit cornea, *Exp. Eye Res.* **62**, 367–376.
Duncan, G., Wormstone, I.M., Liu, C.S.C., Marcantonio, J.M., Davies, P.D. 1997. Thapsigargin-coated intraocular lenses inhibit human lens cell growth, *Nat. Med.* **3**, 1026–1028.
Edmunds, L.H., Mckinlay, S., Anderson, J.M., Callahan, T.H., Chesebro, J.H., Geiser, E.A., Makanani, D.M., McIntire, L.V., Meeker, W.Q., Naughton, G.K., Panza, J.A., Schoen,

F.J., Didisheim, P. 1997. Directions for improvement of substitute heart valves, National Heart, Lung, and Blood Institute's working group report on heart valves, *J. Biomed. Mater. Res.* **38**, 263–266.

Edwards, A., Carson, R.J., Szycher, M., Bowald, S. 1998. In vitro and in vivo biodurability of a compliant microporous vascular graft, *J. Biomat. Appl.* **13**, 23–45.

Egger, S.F., Huberspitzy, V., Scholda, C., Schneider, B., Grabner, G. 1994. Bacterial-contamination during extracapsular cataract-extraction—prospective-study on 200 consecutive patients, *Ophthalmologica* **208**, 77–81.

Elves, A.W.S., Feneley, R.C.L. 1997. Long-term urethral catheterization and the urine-biomaterial interface, *Br. J. Urol.* **80**, 1–5.

Elwing, H., Nilsson, B., Svenson, K-E., Askendahl, A., Nilsson, U.R., Lundstrom, I. 1988. Conformational changes of a model protein (complement factor 3) adsorbed on hydrophilic and hydrophobic solid surfaces, *J. Coll. Interf. Sci.* **125**, 139–145.

Enker P., Steffe A.D., McMillen C., Keppler L., Biscup R., Miller S. 1993. Artificial disc replacement, *Spine* **18**, 1067–1070.

Filipec, M., Bowers, R.W.J., Dropcova, S., Denyer, S.P., Faragher, R.G.A., Gard, P.R., Hall, B, Hanlon, G.W., Jones, S.A., Lloyd, A.W., Muir, A., Olliff, C.J., Rosen, P.H., Riding, M. 1997. *In vivo* evaluation of novel biomimetic intraocular lenses, *Invest. Ophthalmol. Vis. Sci.* **38**, S178.

Franklin, V.J., Bright, A.M., Tighe, B. 1993. Hydrogel polymers and ocular spoilation processes, *Trends Polym. Sci.* **1**, 9–16.

Garcia A., Lavignolle B., Baquey C. 1995. Intervertebral disc prostheses with intradiscal polymerisation *Rachis* **7**, 51–62.

Gemmell, C.H. 1997. A flow cytometric immunoassay to quantify adsorption of complement activation products (iC3b, C3d, SC5b-9) on artificial surfaces, *J. Biomed. Mater. Res.* **37**, 474–480.

Girard, L.J. 1983. Keratoprosthesis, *Cornea* **2**, 207–224.

Goel V.K., Goyal S., Clark C., Nishyama K., Nye T. 1985. Kinematics of the whole lumbar spine, effect of discectomy, *Spine* **10**, 543–554.

Goodman, S.L., Tweden, K.S., Albrecht, R.M. 1996. Platelet interaction with pyrolytic carbon heart-valve leaflets, *J. Biomed. Mater. Res.* **32**, 249–258.

Gorman, S.P., Tunney, M.M., Keane, P.F., van Bladel, K., Bley, B. 1997. Characterization and assessment of a novel poly(ethylene oxide)/polyurethane composite hydrogel (Aquavene) as a ureteral stent biomaterial, *J. Biomed. Mater. Res.* **39**, 642–649.

Goulet, F., Germain, L., Rancourt, D., Caron, C. Normand, A., Auger, F.A. 1997. Tendons and ligaments, in: *Principles of Tissue Engineering* (R.P. Lanza, R. Langer, W.L. Chick, eds.), pp. 633–644, R.G. Landes Company, Austin, TX.

Grzesiak, J.J., Piershbacher, M.D., Amodeo, M.F., Malaney, T.I., Glass, J.R. 1997. Enhancement of cell interactions with collagen/glycosaminoglycan matrices by RGD derivatization, *Biomaterials* **18**, 1625–1632.

Gura, T.A., Wright, K.L., Veis, A., Webb, C.L. 1997. Identification of specific calcium-binding noncollagenous proteins associated with glutaraldehyde-preserved bovine pericardium in the rat subdermal model, *J. Biomed. Mater. Res.* **35**, 483–495.

Hafemann, B., Ensslen, S., Erdmann, C., Niedballa, R., Zuhlke, A., Ghofrani, K., Kirkpatrick, C.J. 1999. Use of a collagen/elastin-membrane for the tissue engineering of dermis, *Burns* **25**, 373–384.

Hanlon, G.W., Bowers, R.W.J., Dropcova, S., Denyer, S.P., Faragher, R.G.A., Gard, P.R., Hall, B, Jones, S.A., Lloyd, A.W., Muir, A., Olliff, C.J., Rosen, P.H., Riding, M. 1997. In vitro evaluation of a novel biocompatible intraocular lens coating, *Invest. Ophthalmol. Vis. Sci.* **38**, S179.

Hauptmann, S., Klosterhalfen, B., Mittermayer, C., Ruhlmann, K. U., Kaufmann, R., Hocker, H. 1996. Evidence for macrophage-mediated defluorization of a Teflon vascular graft, *J. Mater. Sci., Materials in Medicine* **7**, 345–348.

Hellier W.G., Hedman T.P., Kostuik J.P. 1992. Wear studies for the development of an intervertebral disc prostheses, *Spine* **17**, S86–S96.

Hicks, C., Lou, X., Platten, S., Clayton, A., Vijayasekaran, S., Fitton, H., Chirila, T., Crawford, G., Constable, I. 1997. Keratoprosthesis results in animals: an update, *Aust. N. Z. J. Ophthalmol.* **25** (Suppl. 1), S50–S52.

Hicks, C., Chirila, T., Clayton, A., Fitton, J., Vijayasekaran, S., Dalton, P., Lou, X., Platten, S., Ziegelaar, B., Hong, Y., Crawford, G., Constable, I. 1998. Clinical results of implantation of the chirila keratoprosthesis in rabbits, *Br. J. Ophthalmol.* **82**(1), 18–25.

Holmes, D., Camrud, A., Jorgenson, M., Edwards, W., Schwartz, R. 1994. Polymeric stenting in the porcine coronary artery model: differential outcome of exogenous fibrin sleeves versus polyurethane-coated stents, *J. Am. Coll. Card.* **24**, 525–531.

Hurlstone, C.J. 2000. Working with nitinol shape. Memory Alloys II Medical Device Technology. November 24–29.

Inoue, H., Fujimoto, K., Uyama, Y., Ikada, Y. 1997. Ex vivo and in vivo evaluation of the blood compatibility of surface-modified polyurethane catheters. *J. Biomed. Mater. Res.* **35**, 255–264.

Ishihara, K., Oshida, H., Endo, Y., Ueda, T., Watanabe, A., Nakabayashi, N. 1992. Hemocompatibility of human whole blood on polymers with a phospholipid polar group and its mechanism, *J. Biomed. Mater. Res.* **26**, 1543–1552.

Iwasaki, Y., Mikami, A., Kurita, K., Nobuhiko, Y., Ishihara, K., Nakabayashi, N. 1997. Reduction of surface-induced platelet activation on phospholipid polymer, *J. Biomed. Mater. Res.* **36**, 508–515.

Jayasree, R.S., Rathinam, K., Sharma, C.P. 1995. Development of artificial skin (template) and influence of different types of sterilization procedures on wound healing pattern in rabbits and guinea pigs, *J. Biomat. Appl.* **10**, 144–162.

Jeschke, M.G., Hermanutz, V., Wolf, S.E., Koveker, G.B. 1999. Polyurethane vascular prostheses decreases neointimal formation compared with expanded polytetrafluoroethylene, *J. Vasc. Surg.* **29**, 168–176.

Jeyanthi, R., Panduranga Rao, K. 1990. In vivo biocompatibility of collagen-poly(hydroxyethyl methacrylate) hydrogels. *Biomaterials* **11**, 238–243.

Kao, W.Y.J., McNally, A.K., Hiltner, A., Anderson, J.M. 1995. Role for interleukin-4 in foreign body giant cell formation on a poly(etherurethane urea) in vivo, *J. Biomed. Mater. Res.* **29**, 1267–1275.

Kaufman, H.E., Katz, J.I. 1976. Endothelial damage from intraocular lens insertion, *Invest. Ophthalmol.* **15**, 996–1000.

Kim, H.J., Lee, H.C., Oh, J.S., Shin, B.A., Oh, C.S., Park, R.D., Yang, K.S., Cho, C.S. 1999. Polyelectrolyte complex composed of chitosan and sodium alginate for wound dressing application, *J. Biomater Sci., Polym. Ed.* **10**, 543–556.

Kipshidze, N., Baker, J., Nikolaychik, N. 1994. Fibrin coated stents as an improved vehicle for endothelial cell seeding, *Circulation* **90**, I-597.

Kirkham, S., Dangle, M. 1991. The keratoprosthesis: improved biocompatibility through design and surface modification, *Ophthal. Surg.* **22**(8), 455–461.

Kohnen, T. 1996. The variety of foldable intraocular lens materials, *J. Cataract Refract. Surg.* **22**, 1255–1258.

Lam, K.H., Schakenraad, J.M., Groen, H., Esselbrugge, H., Dijkstra, P.J., Feijen, J., Nieuwenhuis, P. 1995. The influence of surface morphology and wettability on the inflammatory response against poly(L-lactic acid): a semi-quantitative study with monoclonal antibodies, *J. Biomed. Mater. Res.* **29**, 929–942.

Larsson, R., Selen, G., Bjorklund, H., Fagerholm, P. 1989. Intraocular PMMA lenses modified with surface immobilized heparin: evluation of biocompatibility in vitro and in vivo, *Biomaterials* **10**, 511–516.

Lee, C.K., Langrana, N.A. 1984. Lambrosacral spinal fusion. A biomechanical study, *Spine*, **9**, 574–581.

Lee, C.K., Langrana, N.A., Alexander, H., Clemow, A.J., Chen, E.H., Parsons, J.R. 1990. Functional and biocompatible intervertebral disc spacer, *US Patent* 4,911,718, 27 March 1990.

Lee, S.D., Hsiue, G.H., Kao, C.Y., Chang, P. 1996. Artificial cornea: surface modification of silicone rubber membrane by graft polymerization of pHEMA via glow discharge, *Biomaterials* **17**, 587–595.

Legeais, J.M., Rossi, C., Renard, G., Salvoldelli, M., D'Hermies, F., Pouliquen, Y.J. 1992. A new fluorocarbon for keratoprosthesis, *Cornea* **11**, 538–545.

Legeais, J., Renard, G., Parel, J., Savoldelli, M., Pouliquen, Y. 1995. Keratoprosthesis with biocolonizable microporous fluorocarbon haptic. *Arch. Ophthalmol.* **113**, 757–763.

Legeais, J.M., Renard, G., Parel, J.M., Serdarevic, O., Mei Mui, M., Pouliquen, Y. 1997. Expanded fluorocarbon for keratoprosthesis cellular ingrowth and transparency, *Exp. Eye Res.* **58**, 41–52.

Linares, H.A. 1996. From wound to scar, *Burns* **22**, 339–352.

Liu, L., Elwing, H. 1994. Complement activation on solid surfaces as determined by C3 deposition and hemolytic consumption. *J. Biomed. Mater. Res.* **28**, 767–773.

Liu, L., Elwing, H. 1996. Complement activation on thiol-modified gold surfaces. *J. Biomed. Mater. Res.* **30**, 535–541.

Lloyd, A.W., Bowers, R.W.J., Dropcova, S., Denyer, S.P., Faragher, R.G.A., Gard, P. R., Hall, B, Hanlon, G.W., Jones, S.A., Muir, A., Olliff, C.J., Rosen, P.H., Riding, M. 1997. In vitro evaluation of novel biomimetic intraocular lens materials, *Invest. Ophthalmol. Vis. Sci.* **38**, S178.

Lloyd, A.W., Dropcova, S., Faragher, R.G.A., Gard, P.R., Hanlon, G.W., Mikhalovsky, S.M., Olliff, C.J., Denyer, S.P., Letko, E., Filipec, M. 1999. The development of in vitro biocompatibility tests for the evaluation of intraocular materials. *J. Mater. Sci., Materials in Medicine* **10**, 621–627.

Malik, N., Gunn, J., Sheperd, L., Newman, C., Crossman, D., Cumberland, D. 1997. Phosphorylcholine-coated stents in porcine coronary arteries: angiographic and morphometric assessment, *Eur. Heart J.* **18**, 52.

Marchi, V., Ricci, R., Pecorella, I., Ciardi, A., Tondo, U. 1994. Osteo-Odonto-Keratoprosthesis, *Cornea* **13**(2), 125–130.

Mareo, N.B., Ratner, B.D. 1989. Relating surface properties of intraocular lens materials to endothelial cell adhesion damage, *Invest. Ophthalmol. Vis. Sci.* **30**, 853–860.

Markou, C.P., Brown, J.E., Pursley, M.D., Hanson, S.R. 1998. Boundary layer drug delivery using a helical catheter, *J. Contr. Rel.* **53**, 281–288.

Martin, J., Faragher, R.G.A., Cederholm-Williams, S., Hanlon, G.W., Lloyd, A.W. 1999. Do biomaterial surfaces influence the conformation of adsorbed fibrinogen and the subsequent adhesion of bacteria? *Int. J. Artif. Organs* **22**, 430.

Migliaresi, C., Kolaric, J., Stol, M., Nicolais, L. 1981. Mechanical properties of model synthetic tendons. *J. Biomed. Mater. Res.* **15**, 147–157.

Morra, M., Cassinelli, M. 1995. Surface field of forces and protein adsorption behavior of poly(hydroxyethylmethacrylate) films deposited from plasma, *J. Biomed. Mater. Res.* **29**, 39–45.

Murphy, J., Schwartz, R., Edwards, W., Camrud, A., Vliestra, R., Holmes, D. 1992. Percutaneous polymeric stents in porcine coronary arteries, *Circulation* **86**, 1596–1604.

Ng, E.W.M., Barrett, G.D., Bowman, R. 1996. In vitro bacterial adherence to hydrogel and poly(methyl methacrylate) intraocular lenses, *J. Cataract Refract. Surg.* **22**, 1331–1335.

Nishi, O., Nishi, K. 1999. Preventing posterior capsule opacification by creating a discontinuous sharp bend in the capsule, *J. Cataract Refract. Surg.* **25**, 521–526.

Obstbaum, S.A. 1994. Another look at hydrogel intraocular lenses, *J. Cataract Refract. Surg.* **20**, 219–231.

O'Connor, J.J., Zavatsky, A. 1993. Anterior cruciate ligament forces in activity, in: *The Anterior Cruciate Ligament* (D.W. Jackson, ed.), pp. 131–140, Raven Press Ltd., New York.

Osada, T., Yamamura, K., Fujimoto, K., Mizuno, K., Sakurai, T., Ohta, M., Nabeshima, T. 1999. Prophylaxis of local vascular graft infection with levofloxacin incorporated into albumin-sealed Dacron graft (LVFX-ALB graft), *Microb. Immun.* **43**, 317–321.

Pachence, J.M. 1996. Collagen-based devices for soft tisue repair, *J. Biomed. Mater. Res.* **33**, 35–40.

Payne, M.S., Horbett, T.A. 1987. Complement activation by hydroxyethylmethacrylate-ethylmethacrylate copolymers, *J. Biomed. Mater. Res.* **21**, 843–859.

Petillo, O., Peluso, G., Ambrosio, L., Nicolais, L., Kao, W.Y.J., Anderson, J.M. 1994. In-vivo induction of macrophage IA-antigen (MHC Class-II) expression by biomedical polymers in the cage implant system, *J. Biomed. Mater. Res.* **28**, 635–646.

Phaneuf, M.D., Dempsey, D.J. Bide, M.J., Szycher, M., Quist, W.C., Logerfo, F.W. 1998. Bioengineering of a novel small diameter polyurethane vascular graft with covalently bound recombinant hirudin, *ASAIO J.* **44**, M653–M658.

Pieper, J.S., Oosterhof, A., Dijkstra, P.J., Veerkamp, J.H. 1999. Preparation and characterization of porous crosslinked collagenous matrices containing chondroitin sulphate, *Biomaterials* **20**, 847–858.

Poggi, M.M., Klein, M.B., Chapo, G.A., Cuono, C.B. 1999. Effects of cryopreservation and deconstruction on the dermal glycosaminoglycan content of human skin, *J. Burn Care Rehabil.* **20**, 201–206.

Pollara, P., Alessandri, G., Bonardelli, S., Simonini, A., Cabibbo, E., Portolani, N., Tiberio, G.A. M., Giulini, S.M., Turano, A. 1999. Complete in vitro prosthesis endothelialization induced by artificial extracellular matrix, *J. Invest. Surg.* **12**, 81–88.

Pomach, B., Svensjo, T., Yao, F., Brown, H., Eriksson, E. 1998. Tissue engineering of skin, *Crit. Rev. Oral Biol. Med.* **9**, 333–344.

Porter, R.R., Reid, K.B.M. 1978. The biochemistry of complement, *Nature* **275**, 699–704.

Pradas, M.M., Calleja, R.D. 1991. Reproduction in a polymer composite of some mechanical features of tendons and ligaments, in: *High Performance Biomaterials* (M. Szycher, ed.), pp 519–526. Technomic Publishing Co., Inc., Lancaster, PA.

Purcell, C., Tennant, M., McGeachie, J. 1997. Neo-intimal hyperplasia in vascular grafts and its implications for autologous arterial grafting, *Ann. R. Coll. Surg. Eng.* **79**, 164–168.

Ram, J., Apple, D.J., Peng, Q., Visessook, N., Auffarth, G.U., Schoderbek, R.J., Ready, E.L. 1999. Update on fixation of rigid and foldable posterior chamber intraocular lenses. Part II—Choosing the correct haptic fixation and intraocular lens design to help eradicate posterior capsule opacification, *Ophthalmology* **106**, 891–900.

Raskin, E., Speaker, M., Peltonhenrion, K., Wong, D., McCormick, S. 1992. Polypropylene haptics increase bacterial adherence to intraocular lenses, *Invest. Ophthalmol. Vis. Sci.* **33**, 1420–1424.

Ratner, B.D. 1993. New ideas in biomaterial science: a path to engineered biomaterials. *J. Biomed. Mater. Res.* **27**, 837–850.

Ridley, H.L. 1951. Intra-ocular acrylic lenses, *Trans. Ophthalmol. Soc. U.K.* **71**, 617–621.

Rosen, E.S. 1993. Intraocular lenses, *Curr. Opinion Ophthalmol.* **4**, 44–53.

Salib R.M., Pettine K.A. 1993. Intervertebral disc arthroplasty, *U.S. Patent* 5,258,031, 2 November 1993.

Salzmann, D.L., Kleinert, L.B., Berman, S.S., Williams, S.K. 1999. Inflammation and neovascularization associated with clinically used vascular prosthetic materials, *Cardiovasc. Pathol.* **8**, 63–71.

Sandeman, S., Faragher, R.G.A., Allen, M.C.A., Liu, C.S.C., Lloyd, A.W. 2000. Novel materials to enhance keratoprosthesis integration, *Br. J. Ophthalmol.*, **84**, 640–644.

Santin, M. 2000. The role of urine components in clinical complications associated with urological devices. British PhD thesis.

Santin, M., Huang, S.J., Iannace, S., Ambrosio, L., Nicolais, L., Peluso, G. 1996. Synthesis and characterization of a new interpenetrated poly(2-hydroxyethylmethacrylate)-gelatin composite polymer, *Biomaterials* **17**, 1459–1467.

Santin, M., Wassall, M.A., Peluso, G., Denyer, S.P. 1997. Adsorption of alpha-1-microglobulin from biological fluids onto polymer surfaces, *Biomaterials* **18**, 823–827.

Santin, M., Cannas, M., Wassall, M.A., Denyer, S.P. 1998a. Adsorption of serum alpha 1-microglobulin onto biomaterials, *J. Mater Sci., Materials in Medicine* **9**, 135–140.

Santin, M., Motta, A., Cannas, M. 1998b. Changes in serum conditioning profiles of glutaraldehyde-crosslinked collagen sponges after their treatment with calcification inhibitors, *J. Biomed. Mater. Res.* **40**, 434–441.

Santin, M., Motta, A., Cannas, M. 1998c. Changes in the composition of the surface conditioning of calcium crystals treated with physiological and alkaline urine, *Br. J. Urol.* **82**, 97–103.

Santin, M., Motta, A., Denyer, S.P., Cannas, M. 1999. Effect of the urine conditioning film on ureteral stent encrustation and characterization of its protein composition, *Biomaterials* **20**, 1245–1251.

Schoen, F.J., Levy, R.J. 1994. Pathology of substitute heart valves: new concepts and developments, *J. Cardiovasc Surg.* **9**, 222–227.

Sidiropoulos, A., Rombeck, B., Hotz, H., Liu, J., Konertz, W. 1999. Hemodynamic benefits after total root replacement with stentless bioprostheses, *Artif. Organs* **23**, 669.

Silver, F., Doillon, C. 1989. in: *Biocompatibility: Interactions of Biological and Implantable Materials.* VHC Publishers, Stuttgart.

Stein, P.D., Alpert, J.S., Copeland, J., Dalen, J.E., Goldman, S., Turpie, A.G.G. 1995. Antithrombotic therapy in patients with mechanical and biological prosthetic heart valves, *Chest* **108**, 371S–379S.

Stevens, A., Lowe, J. 1995. in: *Pathology*, Ch. 2, C.V. Mosby Co., St. Louis.

Strampelli, B. 1963. Osteo-odonto-keratoprosthesis. *Ann. Ophthalmol. Clin. Ocul.* **89**, 1039–1044.

Sundell, I.B., Marzec, U.M., Kelly, A.B., Chronos, N.A.F., Petersen, L.C., Hanson, S.R., Hedner, U., Harker, L.A. 1997. Reduction in stent and vascular graft thrombosis and enhancement of thrombolysis by recombinant Lys-plasminogen in nonhuman primates, *Circulation* **96**, 941–948.

Taylor, A., Ao, P., Fletcher, J. 1995. Inhibition of intimal hyperplasia and occlusion in Dacron graft with heparin and low molecular weight heparin, *Int. Angiol.* **14**, 375–380.

Tribewal S.B., Pearcy M.J., Portek I., Spivey J. 1985. A prospective study of lumbar spinal movements before and after disectomy, *Spine* **10**, 455–459.

Trinkaus-Randall, V., Capecchi, J., Newton, A., Vadasz, A., Leibowitz, H., Franzblau, C. 1988. Development of a biopolymeric keratoprosthetic material, *Invest. Ophthalmol. Vis. Sci.* **29**(3), 393–400.

Trinkaus-Randall, V., Bansatt, R., Capecchi, J., Leibowitz, H.M., Fransblau, C. 1991. In vivo fibroplasia of a porous polymer in the cornea, *Invest. Ophthalmol. Vis. Sci.* **32**(13), 3245–3251.

Tschopp, J.F., Chan, F., Pierschbacher, M.D. 1998. RGD-enhanced INTEGRA(TM) artificial skin (IAS), *Abstr. Pap. Am. Chem. Soc.* **216**, 415.

Tunstall, A., Eberhart, R.C., Prager, M.D. 1995. Endothelial cells on Dacron vascular prostheses: adherence, growth, and susceptibility to neutrophils, *J. Biomed. Mater. Res.* **29**, 1193–1199.

Ueda, T., Ishihara, K., Nakabayashi, N. 1995. Adsorption-desorption of proteins on phospholipid polymer surfaes evaluated by dynamic contact angle measurement, *J. Biomed. Mater. Res.* **29**, 381–387.

Ursell, P.G., Spalton, D.J., Pande, M.V., Hollick, E.J., Barman, S., Boyce, J., Tilling, K. 1998. Relationship between intraocular lens biomaterials and posterior capsule opacification, *J. Cataract Refract. Surg.* **24**, 352–360.

van der Kamp, K.W.H.J., Hauch, K.D., Feijen, J., Horbett, T.A. 1995. Contact activation during incubation of five different polyurethanes or glass in plasma, *J. Biomed. Mater. Res.* **29**, 1303–1306.

Vogler, E.A., Graper, K.C., Harper, G.R., Sugg, H.W., Lander, L.M., Brittain, W.J. 1995a. Contact activation of the plasma coagulation cascade. I. Procoagulant surface chemistry and energy, *J. Biomed. Mater. Res.* **29**, 1005–1016.

Vogler, E.A., Graper, K.C., Sugg, H.W., Lander, L.M., Brittain, W.J. 1995b. Contact activation of the plasma coagulation cascade. II. Protein adsorption to procoagulant surfaces, *J. Biomed. Mater. Res.* **29**, 1017–1028.

Wahlgren, M., Arnebrant, T. 1991. Protein adsorption to solid surfaces. *TIB* **9**, 201–208.

Wassall, M.A., Santin, M., Peluso, G., Denyer, S.P. 1998. Possible role of alpha-1-microglobulin in mediating bacterial attachment to model surfaces, *J. Biomed. Mater. Res.* **40**, 365–370.

Weber, H. 1993. Lumbar disc herniation: a controlled prospective study with ten years observation, *Spine* **8**, 131–140.

Wironen, J., Marotta, J., Cohen, M., Batich, C. 1997. Materials used in urological devices, *J. Long-Term Effects Med. Implants* **7**, 1–28.

Yun, J.K., DeFife, K., Colton, E., Stack, S., Azeez, A., Cahalan, L., Verhoeven, M., Cahalan, P., Anderson, J.M. 1995. Human monocyte/macrophage adhesion and cytokine production on surface-modified poly(tetrafluoroethylene/hexafluoropropylene) polymers with and without protein preadsorption, *J. Biomed. Mater. Res.* **29**, 257–268.

Zhao, Q., Agger, M.P., Fitzpatrick, M., Anderson, J.M., Hiltner, A., Stokes, K., Urbanski, P. 1990. Cellular interactions with biomaterials: in vitro cracking of pre-stressed Pelethane 2363-80A, *J. Biomed. Mater. Res.* **24**, 621–637.

15

Mechanics of Hard Tissues

Arturo N. Natali and Richard T. Hart

15.1. Introduction

The study of the biomechanics of biological tissues has a long and rich history, dating back to at least Galileo's time and his interest in the proportional sizing of bone (Galilei, 1744; Treharne, 1981).

Recent studies in biomechanics have been motivated by the desire to quantitatively describe the mechanical behavior of biological materials. Much progress has been made in experimental studies that use traditional mechanical measurement techniques to characterize the mechanical response of *in vitro* tissues. However, these characterizations are often more difficult than for traditional engineering materials, because of steps needed to prevent degradation of material properties due to drying, detachment from adjacent tissues, temperature and chemical environment changes, etc., and because the material properties can change depending upon the specific bone being studied, a specimen's location (bone is inhomogeneous), and upon a specimen's orientation (bone is anisotropic).

The experimental studies that have characterized the behavior of biological materials have served to provide the required prerequisite information for many current studies that seek to predict the mechanical behavior of biological structures. The methodology for many of these studies is to combine information about the mechanical behavior of the constituent biological materials with further descriptions of the considered biological structure, including geometry, mechanical loading details, and boundary conditions, to predict the response of the structure. Considerable

Arturo N. Natali • Centre of Mechanics of Biological Materials, Dipartimento di Costruzioni e Trasporti, Università di Padova, Via F. Marzolo 9, 35131 Padova, Italy. **Richard T. Hart** • Department of Biomedical Engineering, Boggs Center, Suite 500, Tulane University, New Orleans, Louisiana 70118, United States.

Integrated Biomaterials Science, edited by R. Barbucci. Kluwer Academic/Plenum Publishers, New York, 2002.

success has been achieved with these studies, usually numerical analyses such as the finite element method, with a variety of applications. For example, recent progress has been made with quantitative predictions of the phenomena occurring in the interaction process between implants and cortical or trabecular bone tissue, or to determine the response of spinal motion segment under static or dynamic loading, or to simulate the evolutionary response of the tissue in time.

"Hard tissue" is the label used to differentiate calcified tissues, including teeth and bone, from other structural tissues (cartilage, ligaments, tendons, etc.). This chapter focuses exclusively upon bone which Katz (1995) describes as "one of the most interesting materials known in terms of structure–property relationships."

The complexity of the relationship between structure and properties necessitates a hierarchy of scale to describe bone's structural organization (Cowin, 1989; Katz, 1995). At the macroscopic level, that of the whole bone or a large sample of bone, material tests reveal the sensitivity of mechanical properties to sample location, and also reveal the dependence of properties upon specimen orientation and environment and handling (dryness, temperature, chemical environment, method of storage, etc.). These macroscopic properties are determined primarily by the next smaller scale, that of the microstructural level. The microstructural, or tissue, level reveals the two primary architectures of bone as shown in Figure 15.1. The hard outer shell

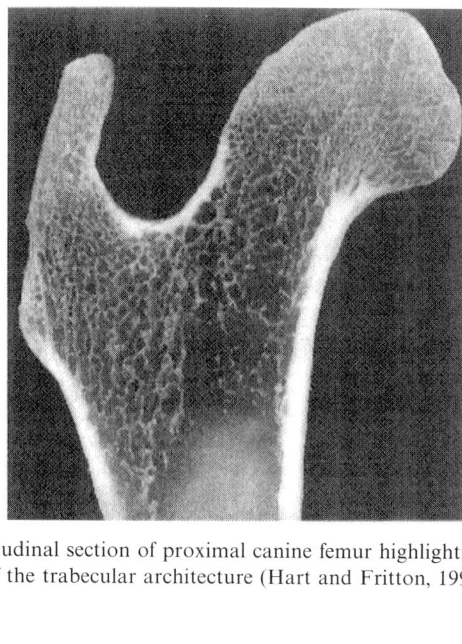

Figure 15.1. Longitudinal section of proximal canine femur highlighting the inhomogeneity and the complexity of the trabecular architecture (Hart and Fritton, 1997).

of bone is composed of cortical (compact) bone, which is itself classified as primary bone when composed of well-organized lamellar sheets or as secondary bone when there is evidence of the disruption of the organized sheets due to the tunneling of osteons centered about a Haversian canal. Inside the hard cortical shell, and especially near the ends of long bones, is a porous network of calcified tissue variously called trabecular, spongy, or cancellous bone. Most biomechanics studies have concentrated upon characterizing material properties of bone at this tissue level, which in turn depends upon the quantification of material and structural (architectural) properties. Increasingly, there is an awareness of the role of bone's smaller structural levels and its influence upon cellular processes that in turn determine the material and structural properties measured at the tissue level.

Bone is a structural history of bone cell activity. Bone contains three primary types of cells: osteoblasts are mainly responsible for producing new bone tissue; osteoclasts are large multinucleated cells that are associated with resorption of bone tissue; osteocytes are the most numerous cell type and their wide distribution within bone tissue is supported by an intricate network of connecting cellular processes. Clearly, the distribution and activity of the bone cells are responsible for bone material and architectural properties and via the process of functional adaptation, discussed subsequently, the mechanical demands upon bone are one of the factors that influence the cellular behavior. Clinical identification of bone disease can now be diagnosed at the ultrastructural level which reveals bone as a composite of fibers (3–5 μm thick) which are in turn composed of mineralized collagen microfibrils. The next smaller level, the molecular level, reveals that the microfibrils are composed of the three left-handed helical peptide chains coiled into a triple helix forming the tropocollagen molecule (approximately 1.5×280 nm) (Katz, 1995). Associated with the tropocollagen molecule is bound apatite crystallite ($4 \times 20 \times 60$ nm) (Katz, 1995).

The ultimate complexity of bone, and its lasting fascination, is as a living structural material. Most spectacularly, bone can heal itself following fracture. However, bone can also change at the macroscopic scale as a result of age, disease, and functional demands. Crucial to understanding these macroscopic changes is characterization of changes at the smaller structural organizational levels, and upon understanding the interactions between the various levels. The multidisciplinary biomechanics studies of the near future will be able to build upon previous studies that quantitatively describe and predict mechanical behavior to be able to manipulate the mechanical behavior of biological tissues. Traditional engineering techniques and methods will be supplemented by genetics and molecular biology techniques to lead a new era of tissue engineering that holds the promise of manipulating living tissues and providing therapeutic intervention. In the specific field of biomechanics, particular attention is paid to the techniques in the area of physics of solid state and in chemical investigation over the configuration of material that interact with biological tissue.

This chapter aims to introduce the methods, results, and interpretation of bone mechanics studies at the macroscopic and tissue levels. It assumes a base knowledge of elementary mechanics and emphasizes the experimental and numerical studies that contribute to our current and future understanding of bone as a living structure.

The following section provides an overview of some results from experimental testing of bone. The methods for determining the experimental results are briefly discussed, and the results are used to motivate some of the theories for describing the mechanics of bone that are introduced in a subsequent section.

15.2. Experimental Methods and Results: Determination of Mechanical Properties and Structural Configuration

15.2.1. Mechanical Testing

In order to determine how bone specimens behave when loaded mechanically, methods from mechanical testing of traditional engineering materials have been adapted for use with bone. In order to obtain *in vitro* results that are thought to be close to *in vivo* behavior, care must be taken to maintain hydration during handling and while appropriate test specimens are prepared. Freezing has only a small influence upon properties, but use of embalmed bone should generally be avoided (Ashman, 1989).

For mechanical testing of cortical bone, regularly sized "dumbbell shaped" specimens of circular or square cross-section are machined from pieces of bone stock large enough to obtain specimens of approximately $5\,mm \times 5\,mm \times 15\,mm$ (Ashman, 1989; Reilly *et al.*, 1974). For cancellous bone, specimens of similar size may be prepared, often with the ends "potted" in acrylic. In the sections that follow, examples of the observed behavior of cortical and trabecular bone are presented following a brief description of the test method.

15.2.1.1. Cortical Tensile Tests

a. Cortical Tensile Tests: Influence of Hydration. Figure 15.2 shows a plot of stress vs. strain for two cortical bone specimens. The tensile tests were performed at a strain rate of just 10^{-3}, so slow that inertial effects are negligible and these tests are classified as "quasi-static." In the graphs

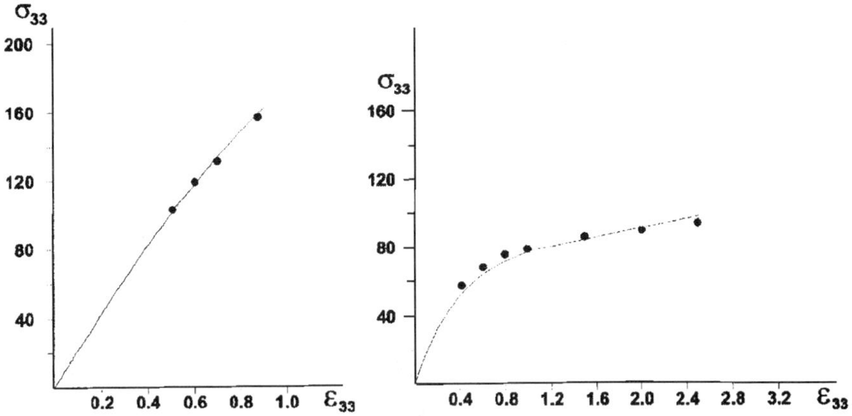

Figure 15.2. Stress versus strain at 2.5% and 10.5% moisture level and 10^{-5} strain rate.

reported units are: for stress, MPa; for elasticity, GPa; for time, seconds; for density, grams per cubic centimeter; deformation is given in percentage. In both tests, the initial portion of the stress–strain curve is nearly linear until strain levels of up to 0.3%. Strains up to this level are termed the "physiological range" because studies have shown that vigorous physical activities generate strains that are less than 0.3% (Rubin and Lanyon, 1984). The slopes of the linear portions from both specimens are similar, indicating little influence of bone's modulus of elasticity upon hydration. However, the dryer specimen ($w = 2.5\%$) maintains the linear behavior until failure, indicative of brittle response. Conversely, the hydrated specimen can be approximated as two linear portions, the initial portion typical of the physiological range. The sudden decrease in slope for the second linear portion indicates damage that is followed by a long "plastic" portion of the stress–strain curve, similar to failure of ductile metals.

b. Cortical Tensile Tests: Influence of Specimen Location and Age. Figure 15.3 shows the location of various bone specimens around the cortex of the tibia. The modulus of bone was found to depend upon the specimen location in a predictable pattern around the tibia. Figure 15.3 also shows that the pattern of modulus around the tibia may form a predictable pattern that depends upon the age of the subject.

c. Cortical Tensile Tests: Loading Rate and Hydration. Figure 15.4 shows that the stiffness of cortical bone is dependent upon the rate of loading, with higher loading rates typically resulting in larger resistance to deformation (stiffness). This effect is shown to be particularly sensitive to the

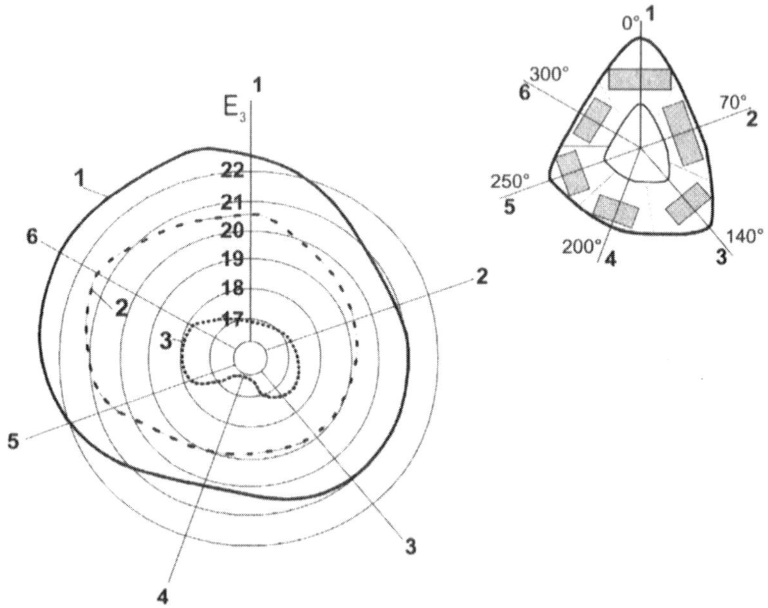

Figure 15.3. Elasticity modulus as a function of age and of zones of tibia cross-section. Age groups: 25–34 years (1); 35–59 years (2); 60–95 years (3).

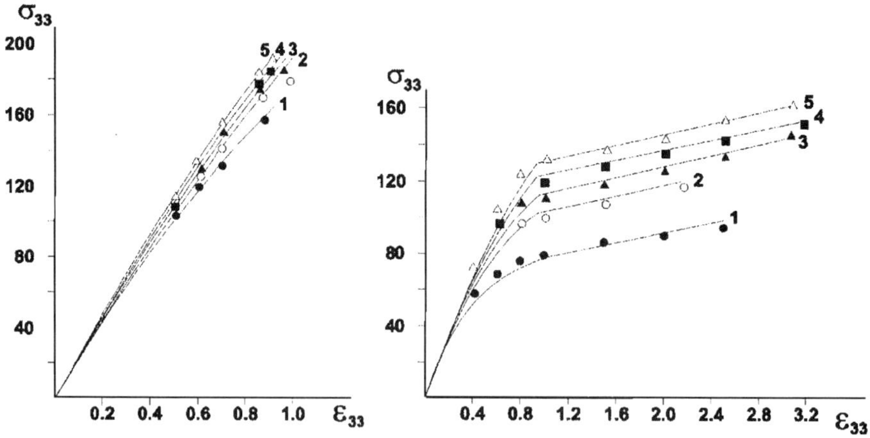

Figure 15.4. Stress versus strain curves at different moisture levels for different strain rates, as 10^{-5} (1); 10^{-4} (2); 10^{-3} (3); 10^{-2} (4); 10^{-1} (5).

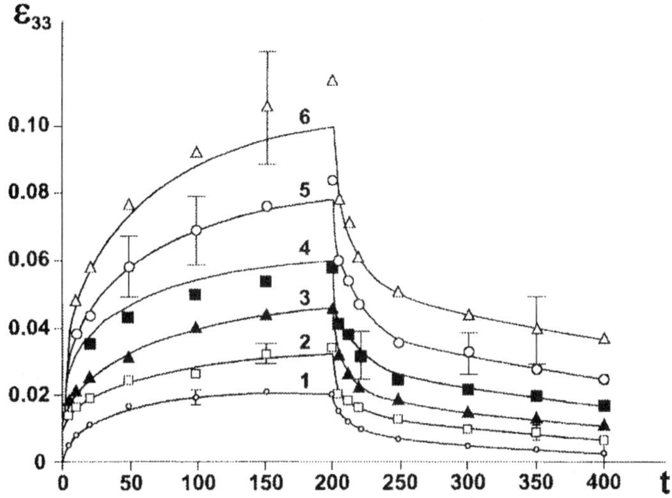

Figure 15.5. Dependence of average values of active and passive creep over stress levels σ_{33}/σ_{33u}, as 0.2 (1); 0.3 (2); 0.4 (3); 0.5 (4); 0.6 (5); 0.7 (6).

water content in the bone, with increased water content generally increasing the bone stiffness. The influence of water content, already noted in Figure 15.2, is again evident, with the dryer specimens showing brittle failure and the hydrated specimens showing pronounced "plastic" regions before failure, with generally larger strain at failure than for the dry specimens.

d. Cortical Tensile Tests: Load Duration. Figure 15.5 shows the influence of maintaining constant loads upon the measured strain. The initial portion of the curves is generated by the sudden load application and monitoring the axial strain for 200 minutes. The strain continues to depend upon time, as active creep, which the multiple curves show to be time-dependent and also dependent upon the magnitude of the axial stress applied. The second portion of the curves show the strain history following the removal of the loads, as passive creep, with strain that tends toward zero resulting in a return to the original size. Large initial stress magnitudes are shown to result in significant residual strain after 200 minutes of passive creep: this indicates a permanent deformation that is symptomatic of damage to the specimen.

e. Cortical Tensile Tests: Strength and Loading Mode. Figure 15.6 reveals data about the strength (stress at failure) for cortical bone specimens. The failure is dependent upon the mode of loading: tensile strength is shown

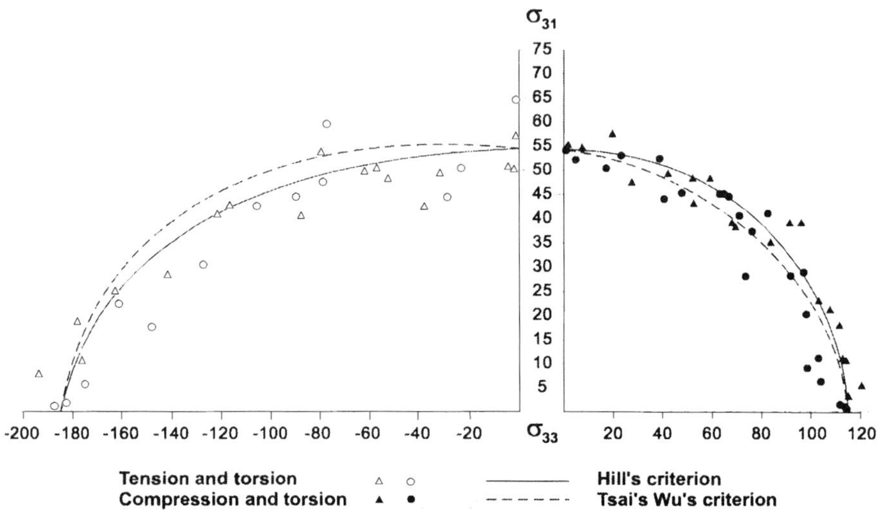

Figure 15.6. Yield stress for human femur. Comparison between experimental data and values obtained with different criteria.

to be approximately 120 MPa (in the right-hand side of the horizontal axis); compressive strength is shown to be approximately 185 MPa (left-hand side of the horizontal axis); and the torsional strength is shown to be approximately 55 MPa (on the vertical axis). In addition to these simple loading modes, the influence of combined loading, axial and torsional, is shown by the majority of the data points shown in the figure. The collection of all the data points reveals the shape of the "failure surface" for the cortical bone specimens tested.

f. Cortical Uniaxial Test Specimens: Influence of Fatigue. In addition to failure of cortical bone with loading that exceeds the tensile strength of bone, damage can occur with repeated loading with lower magnitudes. This damage is observed by a decreased stiffness following repeated loading, and microscopic examination of bone that must be subjected to repeated loading can also reveal the existence of "microcracks" in the bone. Figure 15.7 (Carter *et al.*, 1981) shows data from several studies and reveals the dramatic loss of strength with increasing loading cycles. With one million loading cycles (estimated to be the loading rate on the leg bones during a year) the stress at failure is less than one-third of the cortical bone strength that is loaded once to failure. As a consequence, some of the bone cellular activity involved in bone remodeling, discussed subsequently, is thought to be a continuous repair process to heal fatigue damage.

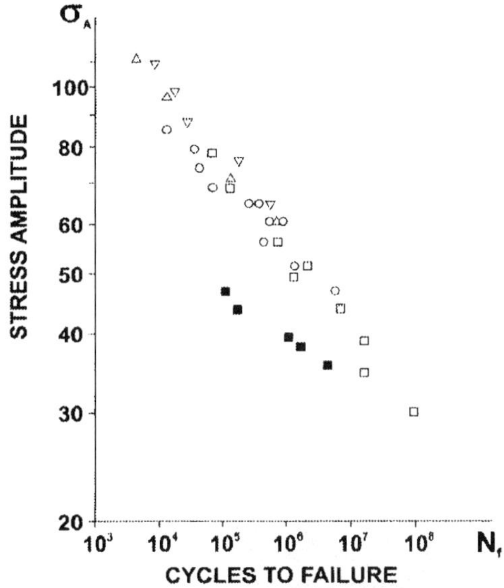

Figure 15.7. Stress-related behavior of *in vitro* bone with completely reversed loading from data reported in several studies. Reprinted from Carter *et al.* (1981), with permission from Elsevier Science.

15.2.1.2. Cancellous Uniaxial Test Specimens

Cancellous Uniaxial Test Specimens: Influence of Density and Loading Direction. Cancellous bone is visibly porous, and it is to be expected that the mechanical behavior of a specimen of cancellous bone is dependent on the porosity. The amount of bone tissue contained within a given volume of bone may be termed the "structural density" (sometimes called the "apparent density") as measure of the volume of a cancellous bone specimen minus the volume of the pores. Tensile test results are summarized in Figure 15.8 with the solid points representing the modulus of cancellous specimens plotted as a function of the structural density. As expected, there is a clear dependence of the modulus upon the structural density. The open points in the figure show the measured modulus from tests in compression. Again, there is a clear dependence of the modulus upon the structural density. Also, the cancellous modulus is shown to depend on the mode of loading. Cancellous bone is generally less stiff when loaded in tension than when loaded in compression. Some references on bone mechanical properties are reported (Ashman and Rho, 1988; Bowman *et al.*, 1994; Dalstra *et al.*, 1993; Ford and Keaveny, 1996; Fyhrie and Schaffler, 1994; Goldstein, 1987; Goulet *et al.*, 1994; Kuhn *et al.*, 1987; Mente and Lewis, 1987).

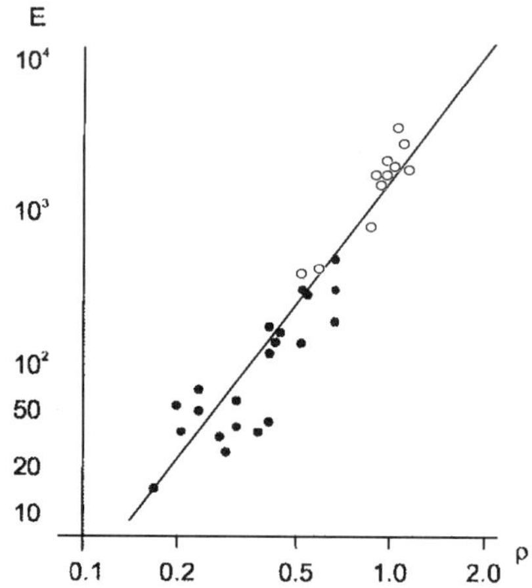

Figure 15.8. Elastic modulus in compression versus density of bone.

15.2.2. Ultrasound Analysis

Several studies have attempted to examine the potential of ultrasound for evaluation of bone characteristics *in vivo* and *in vitro*. The studies examined mainly the relationship between ultrasonic velocity and attenuation, and bone density with regard to cortical bone and mostly to trabecular bone. A significant development of ultrasound attenuation measurements in cancellous bone can be observed after the work of Langton *et al.* (1996). Influence of anisotropy of cancellous bone architecture on ultrasonic parameters measurements was also investigated. Gluer *et al.* (1993) demonstrated the close dependence of ultrasound broad-band attenuation on the direction of trabeculae alignment. Nicholson *et al.* (1994) showed differences in ultrasonic velocity and attenuation for waves propagating in three main anatomical directions in human vertebral bone specimens. Ashman *et al.* (1989) showed the anisotropy of velocity of ultrasound in proximal tibia. However, the influence of number, thickness, and orientation of trabeculae on the ultrasound attenuation and velocity values in cancellous bone remains to be investigated (Natali and Trebacz, 1999).

Mechanical properties of bone tissue depends upon both density and architecture. A typical example is given in Figure 15.9 where velocity is reported versus density for vertebral and calcaneus. The different architecture of trabeculae influences the responses at the same ash density level.

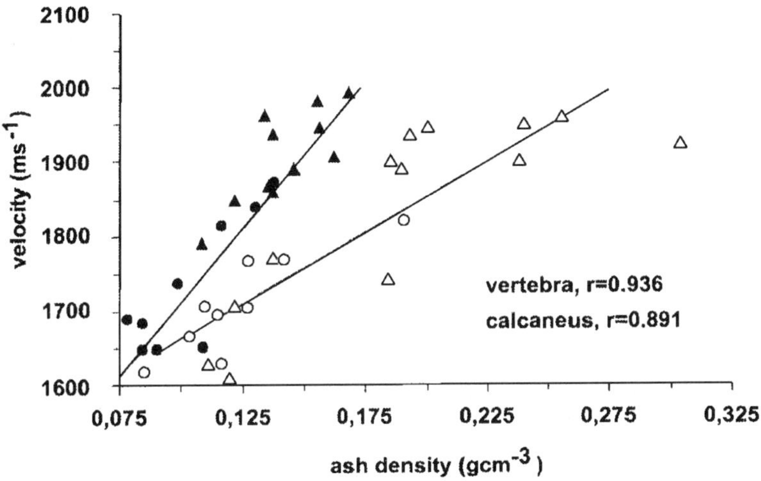

Figure 15.9. Velocity of ultrasound versus ash density in human cancellous bone samples from vertebrae L1 (filled symbols), and in calcanei (open symbols): triangles—male, circles—female.

15.3. Mechanics of Bone

15.3.1. Material Properties

As a starting point for describing the material behavior of bone, understanding linear elastic behavior is most useful. Although idealized, the behavior of bone may often be approximated using linear elasticity theory if bone is loaded within "physiological conditions." For this limited range of forces and displacements, "Hooke's Law" applies, so that doubling the applied force would double the resultant displacements. This relationship can be used to describe the behavior of a structure, or normalized so that it represents the material behavior by using stress and strain relationships.

The linear relationship between the six stress components, σ, and the six strain components, ε, may be generally written as:

$$\begin{Bmatrix} \sigma_{11} \\ \sigma_{22} \\ \sigma_{33} \\ \sigma_{23} \\ \sigma_{31} \\ \sigma_{12} \end{Bmatrix} = \begin{bmatrix} D_{11} & D_{12} & D_{13} & D_{14} & D_{15} & D_{16} \\ D_{21} & D_{22} & D_{23} & D_{24} & D_{25} & D_{26} \\ D_{31} & D_{32} & D_{33} & D_{34} & D_{35} & D_{36} \\ D_{41} & D_{42} & D_{43} & D_{44} & D_{45} & D_{46} \\ D_{51} & D_{52} & D_{53} & D_{54} & D_{55} & D_{56} \\ D_{61} & D_{62} & D_{63} & D_{64} & D_{65} & D_{66} \end{bmatrix} \begin{Bmatrix} \varepsilon_{11} \\ \varepsilon_{22} \\ \varepsilon_{33} \\ \varepsilon_{23} \\ \varepsilon_{31} \\ \varepsilon_{12} \end{Bmatrix} \tag{15.1}$$

However, because the relationship is symmetric ($D_{ij} = D_{ji}$), the 36 material constants above reduce to 21. Further, depending upon the observed symmetry of the material response, the 21 constants may not be unique. In particular, if the material is completely symmetric in its load-deformation response the material is said to be isotropic, and there are only 2 unique constants needed to describe the material behavior. Although many materials are isotropic (e.g., metals), biological materials are rarely isotropic. If the material's load-deformation response is symmetric with respect to rotation about a unique "material axis," then there are 5 unique constants, and the material is classified as transversely isotropic. Less symmetry is characterized by independence with respect to mirroring the material about two orthogonal planes of symmetry, and requires 9 independent constants, and is said to be an orthotropic material. Less symmetric still is a monoclinic material that is characterized with 13 unique constants which describe the material's independence with respect to mirroring the material about a single plane of symmetry. Lack of symmetry, so that the load-deformation response is always dependent upon the loading direction, requires all 21 of the material constants to characterize the material's load-response behavior.

Experimental measures of cortical bone tissue properties, already described as being dependent upon the hydration, age, location, loading rate, and loading duration, have been shown to be well described using orthotropic symmetry, requiring 9 constants, when loaded in the "physiologic" range. The following shows the orthotropic material description with the material stiffness constants represented by combinations of three Young's moduli, E, three Poisson's ratios, v, and three shear moduli, G:

$$\begin{Bmatrix} \sigma_{11} \\ \sigma_{22} \\ \sigma_{33} \\ \sigma_{23} \\ \sigma_{31} \\ \sigma_{12} \end{Bmatrix} = \begin{bmatrix} \frac{1}{E_1} & -\frac{v_{12}}{E_2} & -\frac{v_{13}}{E_3} & 0 & 0 & 0 \\ -\frac{v_{21}}{E_1} & \frac{1}{E_2} & -\frac{v_{23}}{E_3} & 0 & 0 & 0 \\ -\frac{v_{31}}{E_1} & -\frac{v_{32}}{E_2} & \frac{1}{E_3} & 0 & 0 & 0 \\ 0 & 0 & 0 & \frac{1}{G_{23}} & 0 & 0 \\ 0 & 0 & 0 & 0 & \frac{1}{G_{31}} & 0 \\ 0 & 0 & 0 & 0 & 0 & \frac{1}{G_{12}} \end{bmatrix} \begin{Bmatrix} \varepsilon_{11} \\ \varepsilon_{22} \\ \varepsilon_{33} \\ \varepsilon_{23} \\ \varepsilon_{31} \\ \varepsilon_{12} \end{Bmatrix} \tag{15.2}$$

As shown in Figures 15.2–15.7, loading outside the envelope of normal physiologic conditions is also important because these data regarding

Table 15.1. Average Elastic Constants of Corpus Mandibular Bone in Inferior, Lingual, and Buccal Zones

	Inferior	Lingual	Buccal
E_1 (GPa)	10.63	10.85	11.04
E_2 (GPa)	12.51	16.39	15.94
E_3 (GPa)	19.75	18.52	18.06
G_{12} (GPa)	3.89	4.59	4.31
G_{13} (GPa)	4.85	5.45	5.2
G_{23} (GPa)	5.84	6.49	6.45
ν_{12}	0.313	0.138	0.138
ν_{13}	0.246	0.338	0.322
ν_{23}	0.226	0.332	0.294
ν_{21}	0.368	0.178	0.257
ν_{31}	0.465	0.572	0.518
ν_{32}	0.356	0.357	0.326

damage and failure of bone contribute to our understanding of the material. However, a description of the theoretical nonlinear techniques to handle these conditions is beyond the scope of this chapter.

Experimental data are reported to show data pertaining to the mechanical characteristics of cortical and trabecular bone tissue. As already mentioned, the mechanical properties of bone tissue depend on specific bone and on location.

In Table 15.1 average elastic constants of cortical bone in mandible are reported, with reference to corpus area in inferior, lingual, and buccal zones.

In Table 15.2 data pertaining to trabecular bone tissue are reported, showing analytical and experimental data that refer to different types of bone.

In Table 15.3, the ultimate strength and strain for cortical bone in human femur are reported.

15.3.2. Structural Properties

The inherent pertaining to the mechanical response of a structure depends upon the material properties and also upon the geometrical arrangement of material to form the structure. However, the word "bone" is used with multiple meanings: it describes an organ, a material, and a structure. Unfortunately, this usage of "bone" that encompasses both material and structure in the same word can mask the intended meaning. Consequently, when describing gross properties of a "chunk" of bone tissue,

Table 15.2. Estimates and Determinations of the Elastic Modulus of Individual Trabecular of Cancellous Bone

Source	Type of bone	Estimate of trabeculae elastic modulus
Wolff (1986)	Human	17 to 20 GPa (wet)
	Bovine	18 to 22 GPa (wet)
Pugh *et al.* (1973)	Human, distal femur	Concluded that the modulus of the trabeculae was less than that of compact bone
Townsend *et al.* (1975)	Human, proximal tibia	11.38 GPa (wet), 14.13 GPa (dry)
Ashman and Rho (1988)	Bovine femur	10.90 ± 1.60 GPa (wet)
	Human femur	12.7 ± 2.0 GPa (wet)
Runkle and Pugh (1975)	Human, distal femur	8.69 ± 3.17 GPa (dry)
Mente and Lewis (1987)	Dried human femur	5.3 ± 2.6 GPa
	Fresh human tibia	
Khun *et al.* (1987)	Fresh frozen human tibia	3.17 ± 1.5 GPa
Williams and Lewis (1982)	Human, proximal tibia	1.30 GPa
Rice *et al.* (1988)	Bovine	1.17 GPa
Ryan and Williams (1986)	Fresh bovine femur	0.76 ± 0.39 GPa
Rice *et al.* (1988)	Human	0.61 GPa

Table 15.3. Effects of Age on the Mechanical Properties of Cortical Bone from the Human Femur

	Age (years)						
Property	10–20	20–30	30–40	40–50	50–60	60–70	70–80
Ultimate strength (MPa)							
Tension	114	123	120	112	93	86	86
Compression	—	167	167	161	155	145	—
Bending	151	173	173	162	154	139	139
Torsion	—	57	57	52	52	49	49
Ultimate strain (%)							
Tension	1.5	1.4	1.4	1.3	1. 3	1.3	1.3
Compression	—	1.9	1.8	1.8	1.8	1.8	—
Torsion	—	2.8	2.8	2.5	2.5	2.7	2.7

some authors use the prefixes "apparent" or "structural" to clarify the intended meaning as being a structural description rather then a material one. For example, a measure of "bone density" would imply a material meaning, namely the density of the mineral matrix of bone, while a measure of "apparent bone density" (or "structural bone density") would imply a measure that includes both the matrix material and also voids in the structure. The distinction is particularly acute in discussions of trabecular bone, where the "volume fraction" of bony material is low.

In 1977, a relationship relating bone's "structural density" to its stiffness was reported by Carter and Hayes, and showed that the stiffness was strongly dependent upon the structural density, ρ, and weakly dependent upon the rate of loading, as measured by the strain rate, $\dot{\varepsilon}$. Empirically, they found that pooled data for the compressive stiffness of human and bovine bone tissue, including cortical and trabecular tissues, was described by the relationship:

$$E = 3790\dot{\varepsilon}^{0.06}\rho^3 \tag{15.3}$$

where E is the elastic modulus (MPa), ρ is the structural density (g/cm^3), and $\dot{\varepsilon}$ is the strain rate (inverse seconds). Rice *et al.* (1988) found that when the cortical and cancellous bone values were separated and when human and bovine data were separated, the dependence of the stiffness depended upon the square of the "structural density" rather than the cubic power.

Carter and Hayes (1977) also reported a similar relationship to describe the axial compressive strength (the stress at failure) of cancellous bone, with a squared dependence upon the "structural density" as follows:

$$S^- = 68\dot{\varepsilon}^{0.06}\rho^2 \tag{15.4}$$

where S^- is the axial compressive strength(MPa), ρ is the structural density (g/cm^3), and $\dot{\varepsilon}$ is the strain rate (inverse seconds). A quadratic relationship for the strength of cancellous bone was maintained even when bovine and human data were separated (Rice *et al.*, 1988).

Although the "structural density" is a strong determinant of the modulus and strength of cancellous bone, the arrangement of the individual trabeculae are also important determinants of the structure's stiffness and strength (Figure 15.10). As recently reported, studies have shown that the "structural density" may account for 31% of the variance of the modulus of cancellous bone near the knee joint, but that when a measure of the local trabecular architecture is also included, the two measures can account for 72% of the variation (Turner, 1997).

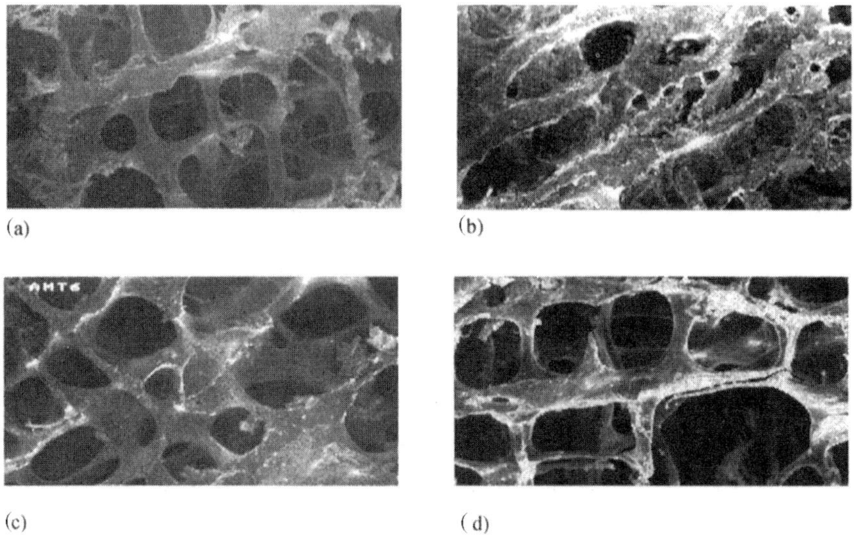

Figure 15.10. Configuration of trabecular structure for 24-year-old man, in: (a) vertebra L1; (b) calcaneus. Trabecular arrangement of vertebrae: (c) 36-year-old woman; (d) 74-year-old woman.

There are several local measures of the local architecture of trabecular bone. They have been shown to be highly correlated to one another, and highly correlated to the elastic anisotropy of trabecular bone (Odgaard *et al.*, 1997). One method leads to a second-rank tensor, called the "fabric tensor," based on stereological measurements of local trabecular architecture called the mean intercept length (MIL). The process is illustrated in Figure 15.11. In Figure 15.11(a) a two-dimensional grayscale image of trabecular bone is shown. That image can be "thresholded" and gives a pure black and white image in which all bone material is seen as white, and everything else shown as black. Then, in Figure 15.11(b), a series of parallel test lines, oriented at some angle, θ, is introduced into the image. The "intercept length" of any one of the parallel lines is equal to the length of the line, divided by the number of "intercepts" along that line, defined as the number of transitions between bone and the surrounding area. The "mean intercept length" for a given angle, θ, is the average intercept length for all of the parallel test lines. If these measures are made for a range of angles between 0° and 180° and plotted as a polar plot with the MIL shown as a function of the angle, θ, the result is well characterized as an ellipse (Whitehouse, 1974). Extending these 2-D measures to 3-D results in a geometric representation of the architecture as an ellipsoid, and the math-

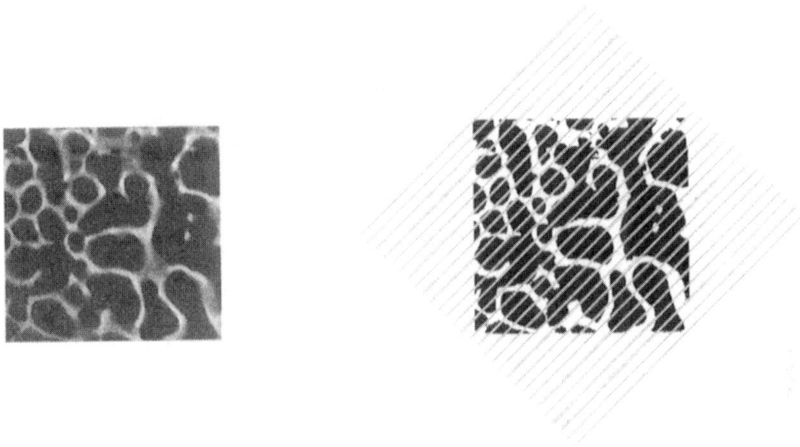

Figure 15.11. Fabric tensor scheme. Photo courtesy of S. Fritton.

ematical description is a second-rank tensor: the fabric tensor as described by Cowin (1989).

15.4. Bone Physiology

The biology and physiology of bone is a complex topic that is reviewed comprehensively in a 9 volume series, *Bone*, edited by Hall (1990–1994).

However, for the purposes of this overview, it is necessary to be aware of the process of "remodeling" which describes a constant renewal of bone tissue that results in the replacement of primary bone by the formation of osteonal (or secondary) cortical bone in the adult. The coordinated activity of the resorption and formation of bone is carried out by the BMU (basic multicellular unit) (H. A. Frost, 1964). First is the appearance and activation of osteoclasts at a (cortical or trabecular) bone site that begin to resorb bone by digging a tunnel at a variable rate (as high as 40 μm/day in the canine) with a diameter of 200 μm at the base and a length of 4000 μm (Eriksen and Kassem, 1992) (Figure 15.12). There is a concurrent development of vascularization in the cavity that provides for needed cell nutrients while removing resorbed bone constituents. The resorptive phase lasts from 30–50 days and the void is refilled centripitally with osteoid (unmineralized bone) that is deposited by osteoblasts, with the formation period lasting approximately 100–150 days (Eriksen and Kassem, 1992). Osteoblasts that are

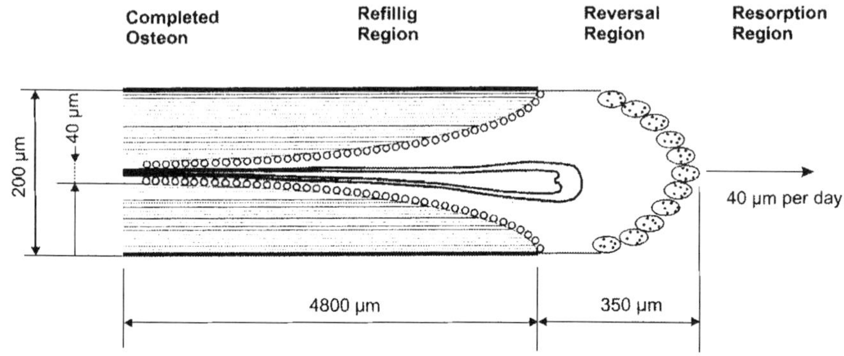

Figure 15.12. Diagram showing an osteonal BMU in longitudinal section view. Redrawn after Martin, R.B., Burr, D.B., *Structure, Function, and Adaptation of Compact Bone*, Raven Press, 1989.

trapped in the new osteoid material change appearance and function, becoming osteocytes, but remain connected to neighboring osteoblasts via their cellular processes in small channels called canniculi. The osteoid surrounding the blood vessel (in what is called the Haversian canal) is gradually mineralized, nearly replacing the volume of bone that was resorbed.

Curiously, the mechanical properties of the secondary bone results from the normal remodeling process is mechanically inferior to the primary bone that is replaced. However, the remodeling process seems to be important in maintaining calcium balances in the blood, and is also responsible for the repair of accumulated microdamage that would otherwise accrue in mature bone (Figure 15.13).

15.5. Functional Adaptation of Bone

This section is adapted from an overview of functional adaptation presented at BIOMED 95 meeting in Milan, Italy (Hart, 1995).

The ability of living bone to adapt to its mechanical use is a well-known example linking biological form and function. In the 1800s a number of investigators made observations about bone form and function (e.g., Ward, von Meyer, Culman, Roux) as described in Julius Wolff's classic book *Das Gesetz der Transformation der Knochen* (Wolff, 1892). The most concise statement of "Wolff's law" is that "Every change in the... function

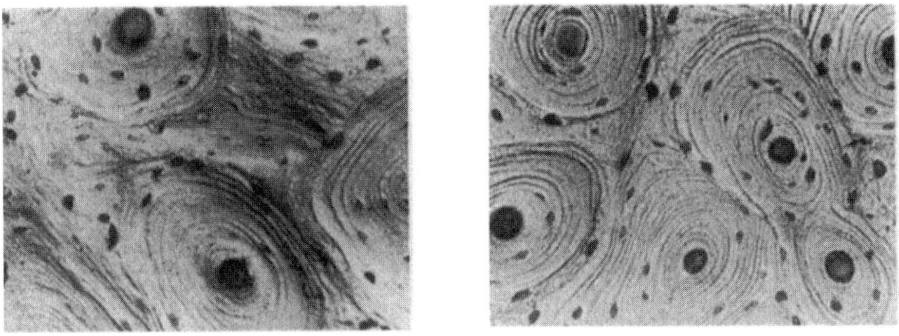

Figure 15.13. Reflected light photomicrographs showing the lamellar structure of secondary osteons. Original magnification $\times 35.2$. Reproduced courtesy of M. Shaffler.

of bone...is followed by certain definite changes in...internal architecture and external conformation in accordance with mathematical laws," Roesler (1981). Thus, there are two distinct portions to "Wolff's law." The law that pertains to trabecular bone architecture relies on the observed similarity of the predominant alignment of trabecular bone struts found internally near the ends of long bone and the approximate principal stress trajectories. The second portion of Wolff's law is that the external form of bone is dependent upon its function (Figure 15.14).

For over a century, these observations by Julius Wolff about bone form and function have presented fertile ground for further investigation and criticism; see, Roesler (1981), Cowin and Hegedus (1976), Cowin *et al.* (1985), Cowin (1997), and Currey (1997). His claim that there are mathematical rules that described the coordinated loss or addition of bone tissue as a result of functional (mechanical) needs has guided much of the experimental, theoretical, and computational studies in bone mechanics ever since.

Models to describe functional adaptation may be classified as phenomenological or mechanistic. The phenomenological models attempt to simulate cause and effect (e.g., changed mechanical loading leading to changed bone architecture) without much attention to the physical mechanisms involved. These models can allow for conveniently testing the consequences of different hypotheses about bone adaptation.

This "what-if" environment may be useful for eliminating some assumptions that don't match experimental or clinical results and observations (e.g., only compressive static loading leads to bone formation) or stimulate further investigations (e.g., strain rates and spatial gradients may regulate adaptation). The mechanistic models start instead with parameters

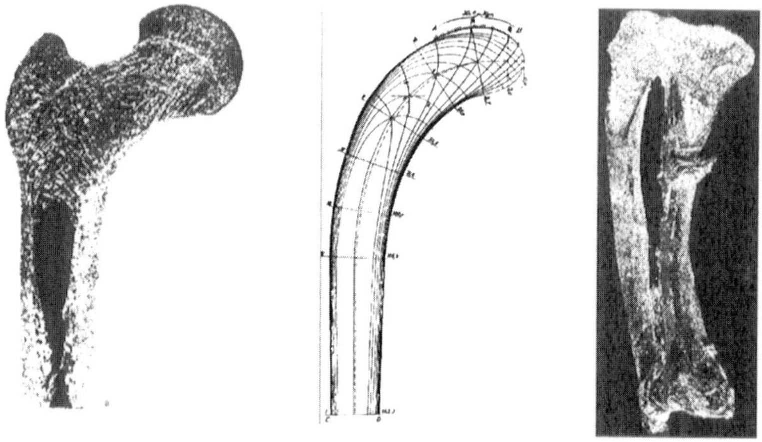

(a) (b) (c)

Figure 15.14. (a) Thin longitudinal section of a human femur; (b) patterns of principal stresses in the Fairbairn crane, used as a model for the proximal end of the femur; (c) specimen that Wolff obtained from Prof. Roux of Innsbruck with gross hypertrophy of the fibula following the development of a pseudo-arthrosis in the tibia (Wolff, 1986).

(e.g., bone cell activities, distributions) that are linked to portions of the biological processes involved in bone maintenance, turnover, and repair. These models, currently less developed than some of the phenomenological models because they are more complex, may lead to successfully linking mechanical and biological causes and effects. These models offer the promise of not only extending the descriptive and predictive capabilities of phenomenological models, but may offer insights into manipulation of the bone response, and development of pharmacological therapeutic agents. Many of the phenomenological and mechanistic models for cortical and cancellous bone adaptation have recently been reviewed (Hart, 1995; Hart and Fritton, 1997). The models are still being actively developed and tested, with fundamental questions about their utility and validity being discussed (Huiskes, 1995; Currey, 1995).

15.5.1. Phenomenological Models

Examples of some of the phenomenological model developments are summarized in the following. Although this review is not all inclusive, the selected models are illustrative of the range of ideas that have been proposed.

a. Frost. Beginning in the early 1960s, Frost developed the descriptive "flexure-neutralization theory" to formalize some of the clinical observations of bone realignment (Frost, 1964). He stated that repeated nontrivial dynamic bending loads cause strains that cause bone formation drifts to build up upon concave-tending surfaces, while resorption drifts tend to erode convex-tending surfaces (Frost, 1986, 1990). In addition to many observations of the biology and mechanics of bone adaptation, Frost has recently been quantified in his "3-way rule," which symbolically represents the observations of the flexure neutralization theory.

b. Cowin and Co-Workers. Of key interest among many investigators has been Cowin's theory of adaptive elasticity (Cowin, 1981). The grounding of the adaptive theory in elasticity theory has also led to its computational implementation (Hart *et al.*, 1984; Cowin *et al.*, 1985; Sadegh *et al.*, 1993). One key feature is the use of an assumed error signal to drive the remodeling process. The error signal is the difference between the mechanical state in its equilibrium configuration (a quiescent state with no net remodeling) and the current mechanical state (following some perturbation to the bone such as a changed mechanical load). The error signal is then used to drive the net remodeling process. The theory has three major parts: one for the shape change of cortical bone (net surface remodeling), one for the density changes of cortical bone (net internal remodeling), and one for changes in the density and the orientation of continuum representations of trabecular bone tissue.

For net surface remodeling, Cowin and Van Buskirk (1979) proposed the following equation:

$$U = C_{ij}(Q)[(\varepsilon_{ij}(Q) - \varepsilon_{ij}^{0}(Q)] \tag{15.5}$$

where U is the "velocity" (change in position over time) of the bone's external bone surface at point Q, C_{ij} are remodeling rate parameters, $\varepsilon_{ij}(Q)$ is the strain at point Q, and $\varepsilon_{ij}^{0}(Q)$ is the remodeling equilibrium strain at point Q.

For net internal remodeling, Cowin and Hegedus (1976) proposed:

$$\dot{e} = a(e) + tr[A(e)\varepsilon] \tag{15.6}$$

where $\dot{e}$ is the rate of change in solid fraction of bone, $a(e)$ are constitutive constants, A is a remodeling rate parameter, and ε is the strain tensor.

For the trajectoral theory of trabecular orientation, Cowin (1986) develops a continuum model that segregates changes in the density of the trabecular bone from changes in the predominant orientation of the struts of trabecular bone as measured by a "fabric tensor" (defined as the inverse square root of the mean intercept length, easily measured steriologically). By describing the elastic material properties, **D**, as a function of the solid volume fraction, **v**, and the fabric tensor, **H**, the stress, **T**, is written as: $\mathbf{T} = \mathbf{T}(\mathbf{v}, \mathbf{E}, \mathbf{H})$. He then presents a mathematical expression of Wolff's trajectoral theory (Cowin, 1986) as the commutative multiplication property of the relevant tensors: $\mathbf{T}^*\mathbf{H}^* = \mathbf{H}^*\mathbf{T}^*$ and $\mathbf{T}^*\mathbf{E}^* = \mathbf{E}^*\mathbf{T}^*$ and $\mathbf{H}^*\mathbf{E}^* = \mathbf{E}^*\mathbf{H}^*$, where the symbol * indicates a remodeling equilibrium value. Cowin *et al.* (1992) has also written trabecular rate equations for the evolution of the fabric tensor reorientation back to the remodeling equilibrium configuration (assumed dependent on the deviatoric portion of the strain), simultaneously with the change of the density (assumed dependent upon the dilatational portion of the strain). The process is illustrated in Figure 15.15.

c. Huiskes and Co-Workers. An approach similar to Cowin's has been developed by Huiskes *et al.* (1987). One difference was implemented to model the observed bone behavior which shows that some threshold of mechanical stimulus is required to start the process of net remodeling, sometimes referred to as a "lazy zone" or a "dead zone." In addition, the mechanical stimulus is not taken to be the strain tensor, but a scalar, the strain energy density, $U = 1/2E_{ij}T_{ij}$.

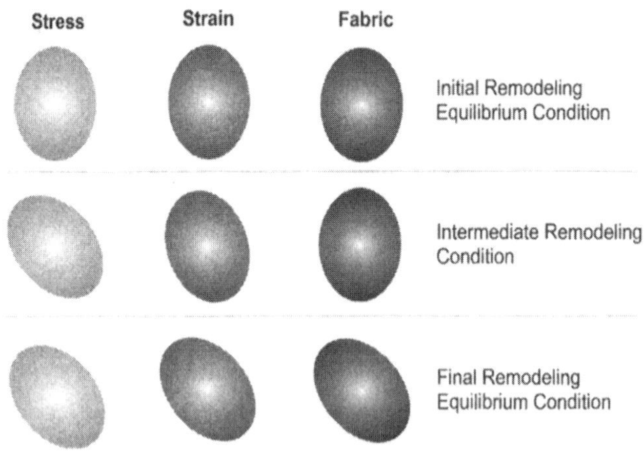

Figure 15.15. Ellipsoidal representations of the stress, strain, and fabric tensors that geometrically represent the adaptation of trabecular bone. In the initial remodeling equilibrium condition, the ellipsoids are aligned. Following a simulated change in loading, the stress ellipsoid and the strain ellipsoid have changed instantaneously, but the fabric tensor that represents the trabecular structure has not changed. The result of the adaptation is to have all three tensors realigned into a new remodeling equilibrium configuration (Hart and Fritton, 1997).

Then the rate equation is written as

$$\frac{dX}{dt} = \begin{cases} C_x[U - (1+s)U_n]; & U > (1+s)U_n \\ 0; & U_n < U < (1+s)U_n \\ C_x[U - (1-s)U_n]; & U < (1+s)U_n \end{cases} \tag{15.7}$$

where X is the surface growth, C_x is the remodeling rate coefficient, $2s$ is the width of the "lazy zone," and U_n is a homeostatic strain energy density.

d. Beaupré, Orr, and Carter. Similar to the models of Cowin and Huiskes is the model proposed by Beaupré *et al.* (1990). However, it uses a "daily tissue level stress stimulus" defined as $\varphi_b = (\Sigma\, n_i \sigma_{bi}^m)^{1/m}$, where n_i is the number of cycles of load type i, σ_{bi} is a true bone tissue level effective stress, and m is an empirical constant, summed over one day. Then,

$$\frac{dr}{dt} = \begin{cases} c(\varphi b - \varphi_{bAS}) + c \cdot w; & \varphi_\beta - \varphi_{bAS} < -w \\ 0; & -w \leqslant \varphi_\beta - \varphi_{bAS} \leqslant w \\ c(\varphi b - \varphi_{bAS}) - c \cdot w; & \varphi_\beta - \varphi_{bAS} > \mathrm{w} \end{cases} \tag{15.8}$$

e. Mattheck. A somewhat different approach has been taken by Mattheck and Huber-Betzer (1991) in developing the "CAO," a computer aided optimization hypothesis. Mattheck makes the observation that: "A good mechanical design is characterized by a homogeneous stress distribution at its surface." As a result, a computerized implementation of CAO was developed and has been used to simulate shape change of bone (and plants). The governing equation is

$$\dot{\varepsilon}_n = k(\sigma_M - \sigma_{ref}) \tag{15.9}$$

where $\dot{\varepsilon}_n$ is defined as the volumetric swelling rate and σ_M is the von Mises equivalent stress.

15.5.2. Mechanistic Models

The second broad class of models are mechanistic models that try to incorporate portions of the biological processes. The chief advantage from this approach will come from successful linkage between mechanical and biological causes and effects, but the chief disadvantage is the complexity of the models, and uncertainty about which of the many mechanical and biological parameters are most important to measure and track.

Of course, the bone cells must somehow sense the need to either add new bone material or remove it. This implies the need for a mechanicobiological transducer. An excellent 1981 review article by Treharne summarizes a number of suggested transducers. Although the nature of the transducer is ignored here, such a biological transducing mechanism must exist or else the observed functional adaptation could not occur.

a. McNamara, Prendergast, and Taylor. The first of the models presented here may be considered as a mechanistic model because of the hypothesis that bone adaptation is activated by accumulated damage, although it stops short of directly addressing the biological processes. McNamara *et al.* (1992) assume that there is some damage at RE (Remodeling Equilibrium), and that the rate of repair is associated with the damage rate. Mathematically, at RE, $\dot{\omega}_{\text{eff}} = 0$ and $\dot{\omega} = \omega_{\text{RE}}$, where ω_{eff} is the effective damage, ω is the current rate of damage production, and ω_{RE} is the rate of damage production at RE. Then,

$$\frac{dX}{dt} = C \cdot \omega_{\text{eff}} \tag{15.10}$$

b. Davy, Hart and Heiple. In an effort to begin to tie the mechanics and the biology into the net remodeling rate equations, a model based upon observable cellular measures was developed (Davy and Hart, 1983; Hart *et al.*, 1984). The net remodeling was regarded as a manifestation of competing cellular activities and numbers, following the work of Martin (1972). Then the rate equation was written as

$$\dot{d} = \lambda_b a_b n_b - \lambda_c a_c n_c \tag{15.11}$$

where the subscript b refers to osteoblasts and c refers to osteoclasts, λ is the surface area fraction available, a is a measure of cellular activity, and n is a measure of cellular number. Further equations were then written to relate each of the parameters in equation (15.7) to measures of the strain history. The theory has recently been used to make a priori predictions of experimentally induced net surface remodeling with encouraging results (Oden *et al.*, 1995).

15.6. Numerical Approach

A short note is reported on a numerical approach to bone mechanics. In fact the numerical simulation proves to be a very powerful and reliable tool and should contribute in turn with experimental analysis in the investigation of the mechanics of hard tissues. The methods used are usually the finite element or the geometric element method. These approaches allow for a reduction in terms of cost and time, in comparison with experimental analysis, but also depend upon the appropriate theoretical formulation of the problem. A deep knowledge of tissue mechanics is essential, together with specific competence in numerical methods. One should point out the possibility, by this way, of accessing a large field of simulation conditions within the investigated problem, varying the characteristics of the leading variables. Examples are reported just to show, by means of specific applications, some of the possibilities offered by this approach.

In Figure 15.16 the analysis of the interaction phenomena occurring between a dental implant and the surrounding trabecular and cortical bone tissue (lower jaw) is shown, in different conditions of full integration of the implant or considering detachment at the bone–implant interface. This latter case refers to the simulation of inflammatory process or inappropriate surgical procedure (Natali, 1999; Natali *et al.*, 1997a, b, 1998; Natali and Meroi, 1996).

The results of a different formulation are reported in Figure 15.17, where the intervertebral segment, as vertebra and disc, is simulated by using a poroelastic approach. In this formulation, the real multiphase medium is modeled as the superposition of different continuous phases: solid, liquid, and gas, by imposing properly the linear momentum and mass balance equations. With reference to an axial compressive loading, the pressure distribution is given over a deformed configuration at subsequent steps of the analysis to show the evolutionary trend of the phenomenon (Meroi *et al.*, 1998; Natali *et al.*, 1997a, b; Natali and Meroi, 1990, 1993, 1997, 1998).

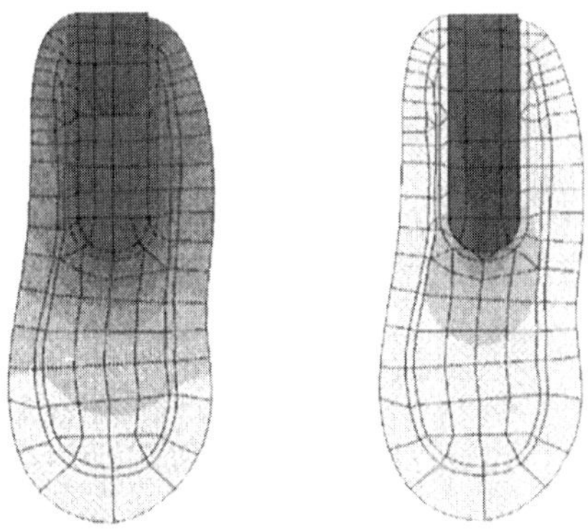

(a) (b)

Figure 15.16. Contour displacement for cylindrical smoothed implant in: (a) integrated condition; (b) condition of detachment occurring at bone–implant interface.

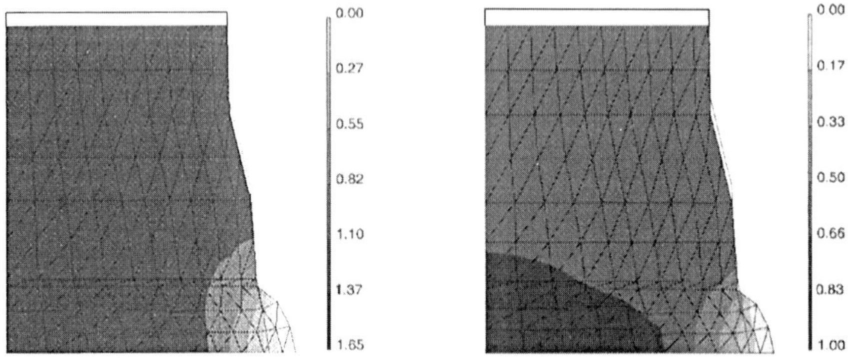

(a) (b)

Figure 15.17. Pressure field distribution within a segment at subsequent steps of the analysis in a condition of axial load.

Computer simulations have been used to study bone's functional adaptation using the phenomenological and mechanistic models discussed previously. Most of the simulations are based on using the finite element method for solution of the structural elasticity problem, and then coupling that solution to a method for changing the shape and/or density of the bone model to simulate functional adaptation. Often the process is implemented in a time-stepping procedure, and results in a solution that starts from a given initial configuration and, due to changed loading, materials, or shape, evolves to a new solution for bone geometry and material properties.

Net remodeling simulations have been used to simulate the changes in bone due to implants (Huiskes *et al.*, 1987), due to loading changes such as an osteotomy (Oden *et al.*, 1995), and due to changed bone shape, such as a fracture that has healed with a malalignment (Hart and Rust-Dawicki, 1995). Simulations have also started with a uniform distribution of bone material, and applied functional loading to test whether different theories of adaptation can predict the appropriate inhomogeneous distribution of bone material (Carter *et al.*, 1987).

As a simple example, an early simulation of bone addition following an osteotomy is shown in Figure 15.18 (Hart *et al.*, 1990). The computational simulation is based on an experiment on sheep in which an ulnar osteotomy was performed, and the pattern of cortical bone response, primarily addition of new bone on the radius, was observed (Lanyon *et al.*, 1982). The simulations were based on using the measured strain on the radius at two locations before and following the ulnar osteotomy (Lanyon

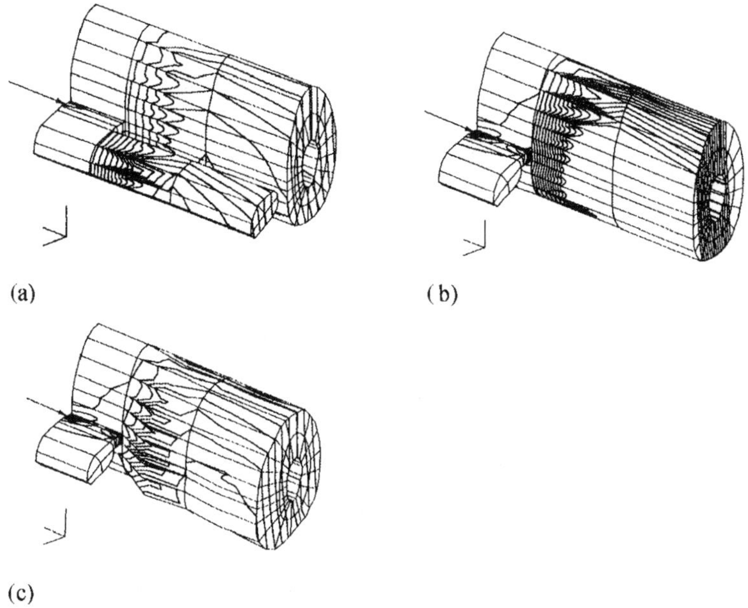

Figure 15.18. (a) The initial configuration showing the radius and intact ulna, with contours mapping the axial remodeling equilibrium strain. (b) The forelimb at the start of the remodeling simulation, immediately following the ulnar osteotomy. (c) The simulated radius shape and strain distribution after 9 months which mirror the experimental results observed by Lanyon (Hart *et al.*, 1990).

et al., 1982), and estimating the remodeling rate constants for use with Cowin's adaptive elasticity theory, as expressed in equation (15.5) (Cowin et al., 1985). Figure 15.18a shows the axial strain distribution calculated for the initial, intact sheep forelimb, and matches the measured peak strains (Lanyon *et al.*, 1982). Immediately following the osteotomy, Figure 15.18b shows calculated axial strains that have now increased in magnitude, because the radius is alone supporting the forelimb loads that had previously been shared with the ulna. Figure 15.18c shows the simulated adaptation in which the cortical additions are similar to what was observed in the experimental animals nine months following the osteotomy (Lanyon *et al.*, 1982).

Increasingly sophisticated computational methods and simulation theories hold the promise of being able to predict bone response to a variety of changed loading conditions, including in the proximity of an orthopedic implant.

15.7. Conclusions

The goal of this introduction to the mechanics of bone tissue has been to show the need for interdisciplinary approaches to understanding skeletal mechanics. In the first section, the experimental results were highlighted to demonstrate some of the complexities of bone tissue, including its structural complexity, its sensitivity to moisture, its inhomogeneity, its dependence upon loading rate, its viscoelastic response, its strength dependence upon loading type, and its response to repeated loading. In addition to complexity in mechanical behavior, some of the purely biological aspects of skeletal tissue were introduced with a focus upon the role of the bone cells in changing the material behavior and geometric structure of bone.

These complex mechanical and biological behaviors were employed to motivate the theoretical descriptions that are used to quantify bone's behavior, although only the simplest linear elastic behavior was included. A number of ideas about how to simulate the adaptive response of bone tissue was introduced, and the role of numerical simulations in the study of bone and implants and in the study of the adaptive response was highlighted.

Despite the required brevity, this introduction has highlighted the need for a multidisciplinary approach to the study of skeletal mechanics that requires a team with competencies in clinical, mechanical, chemical, experimental, and numerical approaches. Future progress will be increasingly dependent upon collaboration, and hold the promise of prediction of bone responses, study of skeletal disease, and development and manipulation of therapeutic agents to repair, and to perhaps avoid, skeletal disease.

References

Ashman, R.B. 1989. Experimental techniques, in: *Bone Mechanics* (S.C. Cowin, ed.), pp. 75–96, CRC Press, Inc., Boca Raton.

Ashman, R.B., Rho, J.Y. 1988. Elastic moduli of trabecular bone material, *J. Biomech.* **21**, 177.

Ashman, R.B., Rho, J.Y., Turner, C.H. 1989. Anatomical variation of orthotropic elastic moduli of the proximal human tibia, *J. Biomech*, **22**, 895–900.

Beaupré, G.S., Orr, T.E., Carter, D.R. 1990. An approach for time-dependent bone modeling and remodeling—theoretical development, *J. Orthop. Res.* **8**(5), 651–661.

Bowman, S.M., Keaveny, T.M., Gibson, L.J., Hayes, W.C., McMahon, T.A. 1994. Compressive creep behavior of bovine trabecular bone, *J. Biomech.* **27**, 301–310.

Carter, D.R., Hayes, W.C. 1977. The compressive behavior of bone as a two-phase porous structure, *J. Bone Jt. Surg., Am. Vol.* **59**(7), 954–962.

Carter, D.R., Caler, W.E., Spengler D.M., Frankel, V.H. 1981. Uniaxial fatigue of human cortical bone. The influence of tissue physical characteristics, *J. Biomech.* **14**(7), 461–470.

Carter, D.R., Fyhrie, D.P., Whalen, R.T. 1987. Trabecular bone density and loading history: regulation of connective tissue biology by mechanical energy, *J. Biomech.* **20**(8), 785–794.

Cowin, S.C. 1981. *Mechanical Properties of Bone*, Presented at the Joint ASME–ASCE Applied Mechanics, Fluids Engineering, and Bioengineering Conference, Boulder, Colorado, June 22–24, 1981, New York, N.Y. (345 E. 47th St., New York 10017), American Society of Mechanical Engineers.

Cowin, S.C. 1986. Wolff's law of trabecular architecture at remodeling equilibrium, *J. Biomech Eng*, **108**(1), 83–88.

Cowin, S.C. 1989. The mechanical properties of cortical bone tissue, in: *Bone Mechanics* (S.C. Cowin, ed.), pp. 97–128, CRC Press, Inc., Boca Raton.

Cowin, S.C. 1997. The false premise of Wolff's law, *Forma* **12**, 247–262.

Cowin, S.C., Hegedus, D.H. 1976. Bone remodeling I: Theory of adaptive elasticity, *J. Elast.* **6**(3), 313–326.

Cowin, S.C., Van Buskirk, W.C. 1979. Surface bone remodeling induced by a medullary pin, *J. Biomech*, **12**(4), 269–276.

Cowin, S.C., Balser, J.R., Hart, R.T., Kohn, D.H. 1985. Functional adaptation in long bones: establishing in vivo values for surface remodeling rate coefficients, *J. Biomech.* **18**(9), 665–684.

Cowin, S.C., Sadegh, A.M., Luo, G.M. 1992. An evolutionary Wolff's law for trabecular architecture, *J. Biomech. Eng.* **114**(1), 129–136.

Currey, J.D. 1995. The validation of algorithms used to explain adaptive remodelling in bone, in: *Bone Structure and Remodelling* (A. Odgaard, H. Weinans, eds.), pp. 9–13, World Scientific, Singapore.

Currey, J.D. 1997. Was Wolff correct?, *Forma* **12**, 263–266.

Dalstra, M., Huiskes, R., Odgaard, A., van Erning, L. 1993. Mechanical and textural properties of pelvic trabecular bone, *J. Biomech.* **26**, 523–535.

Davy, D.T., Hart, R.T. 1983. *A Theoretical Model for Mechanically Induced Bone Remodeling*, American Society of Biomechanics, Rochester, MN.

Eriksen, E.F., Kassem, M. 1992. Editorial, The cellular basis of bone remodeling, *Triangle, Sandoz J. Med. Sci.* **31**, 45–57.

Ford, C.M., Keaveny, T.M. 1996. The dependence of shear failure properties of trabecular bone on apparent density and trabecular orientation, *J. Biomech.* **29**, 1309–1317.

Frost, H.A. 1964. Dynamics of bone remodeling, in: *Bone Biodynamics* (H.A. Frost, ed.), pp. 315–333, Little, Brown, Boston.

Frost, H.M. 1964. *The Laws of Bone Structure*, C.C. Thomas, Springfield, IL.

Frost, H.M. 1986. *Intermediary Organization of the Skeleton*, CRC Press, Boca Raton.

Frost, H.M. 1990. Skeletal structural adaptations to mechanical usage (SATMU): 1. Redefining Wolff's law, the bone modeling problem, *Anat Rec.* **226**(4), 403–413.

Fyhrie, D.P., Schaffler, M.B. 1994. Failure mechanisms in human vertebral cancellous bone, *Bone* **15**, 105–109.

Galileo Galilei, 1744, *Opere di Galileo Galilei divise in 4 tomi*, Dialogo delle scienze nuove, Volume 3, pp. 63 and 87, Stamperia del Seminario, Padova.

Gluer, C.C., Wu, C.Y., Genant, H.K. 1993. Broadband ultrasound attenuation signals depend on trabecular orientation: an in vitro study, *Osteoporosis Int.* **3**, 185–191.

Goldstein, S.A. 1987. The mechanical properties of trabecular bone: dependence on anatomic location and function, *J. Biomech.* **20**, 1055–1061.

Goulet, R.W., Goldstein, S.A., Ciarelli, M.J., Kuhn, J.L., Brown, M.B., Feldkamp, L.A. 1994. The relationship between the structural and orthogonal compressive properties of trabecular bone, *J. Biomech.* **27**, 375–389.

Hall, B.K. (ed.). 1990–1994, *Bone*, Volumes 1–9, The Telford Press, Inc., Caldwell, N.J., and CRC Press, Inc., Boca Raton.

Hart, R.T. 1995. Review and overview of net bone remodeling, in: *Computer Simulations in Biomedicine* (H. Power, R.T. Hart, eds.), pp. 267–276, Computational Mechanics Publications, Southampton, Boston.

Hart, R.T., Rust-Dawicki, A.M. 1995. Computational simulation of idealized long bone re-alignment, in: *Computer Simulations in Biomedicine* (H. Power, R.T. Hart, eds.), pp. 341–350, Computational Mechanics Publications, Southampton, Boston.

Hart, R.T., Fritton, S.P. 1997. Introduction to finite element based simulation of functional adaptation of cancellous bone, *Forma* **12**, 277–299.

Hart, R.T., Davy, D.T., Heiple, K.G. 1984. A computational method for stress analysis of adaptive elastic materials with a view toward applications in strain-induced bone remodeling, *J. Biomech. Eng.* **106**, 342–350.

Hart, R.T., Hennebel, V.V., Thongpreda, N., Dulitz, D.A. 1990. Computer simulation of cortical bone remodeling, in: *Science and Engineering on Supercomputers* (E.J. Pitcher, ed.), pp. 57–66, 565–566, Computational Mechanics Publications, Southampton, Boston.

Huiskes, R. 1995. The law of adaptive bone remodelling, A case for crying Newton?, in: *Bone Structure and Remodelling* (A. Odgaard, H. Weinans, eds.), pp. 15–24, World Scientific, Singapore.

Huiskes, R., Weinans, H., Grootenboer, H.J., Dalstra, M., Fudala, B., Slooff, T.J. 1987. Adaptive bone-remodeling theory applied to prosthetic-design analysis, *J. Biomech.* **20**(11–12), 1135–1150.

Katz, J.L. 1995. Mechanics of hard tissue, in: *The Biomedical Engineering Handbook* (J.D. Bonzino, ed.), CRC Press, Inc., Boca Raton.

Kuhn, J.L., nee Ku, J.L., Goldstein, S.A., Choi, K.W., Landon, M., Herzig, M.A., Matthews, L.S. 1987. The mechanical properties of single trabeculae, pp. 12–48, Trans. 33rd Annu. Meet. Orthop. Res. Soc.

Langton, C.M., Njeh, C.F., Hodgskinson, R., Currey, J.D. 1996. Prediction of mechanical properties of the human calcaneus by broadband attenuation, *Bone* **18**, 495–503.

Lanyon, L.E., Goodship, A.E., Pye, C.J., MacFie, J.H. 1982. Mechanically adaptive bone remodelling, *J. Biomech.* **15**(3), 141–154.

Martin, R.B. 1972. The effects of geometric feedback in the development of osteoporosis, *J. Biomech.* **5**(5), 447–455.

Mattheck, C., Huber-Betzer, H. 1991. CAO: Computer simulation of adaptive growth in bones and trees, in: *Computers in Biomedicine* (K.D. Held, C.A. Brebbia, R.D. Ciskowski, eds.), pp. 243–252, Computational Mechanics Publications, Southampton, Boston.

McNamara, B.P., Prendergast, P.J., Taylor, D. 1992. Prediction of bone adaptation in the ulnar-osteotomized sheep's forelimb using an anatomical finite element model, *J. Biomed. Eng.* **14**(3), 209–216.

Mente, P.L., Lewis, J.L. 1987. Young's modulus of trabecular bone tissue, pp. 112–149, Trans. 33rd Annu. Meet. Orthop. Res. Soc.

Meroi, E.A., Natali, A.N., Schrefler, B.A. 1998. A porous media approach to finite deformation behaviour in soft tissues, *Comp. Meth. Biomech. Biomed. Eng.* **2**(2), 157–170.

Natali, A.N. 1999. The simulation of load bearing capacity of dental implants, in: *Computer Technology in Biomaterials Science and Engineering*, John Wiley & Sons, New York.

Natali, A.N., Meroi, E.A. 1990. Nonlinear analysis of intervertebral disk under dynamic load, *ASME J. Biomech Eng.* **112**, 358–363.

Natali, A.N., Meroi, E.A. 1993. The mechanical behaviour of bony endplate and annulus in prolapsed disc configuration, *J. Biomed. Eng.* **15**, 235–239.

Natali, A.N., Meroi, E.A. 1996. Biomechanical analysis of dental implant in its interaction with bone tissue, in: *Ceramics, Cells and Tissues — Bioceramic Coatings for Guided Bone Growth*, pp. 223–240, Irtec CNR, Faenza.

Natali, A.N., Meroi, E.A. 1997. Numerical formulation of intervertebral joint with regard to ageing problems of soft and hard tissues, in: *Ceramics, Cells and Tissues*, pp. 101–108, Irtec CNR, Faenza.

Natali, A.N., Meroi, E.A. 1998. Numerical formulation for biomechanical analysis of spinal motion segment, Proc. Mathematical Theory of Networks and Systems MTNS98 — 13th Int. Symp. on Math Theory of Networks and Systems, pp. 1051–1054.

Natali, A., Trebacz, H. 1999. The ultrasound velocity and attenuation in cancellous bone samples from lumbar vertebra and calcaneus, *Osteoporosis Int.* **9**(2), 99–105.

Natali, A.N., Meroi, E.A., Donà, S. 1997a. Tissue-implant interaction phenomena for dental implants: a numerical approach, in: *Ceramics, Cells and Tissues*, pp. 93–100, Irtec CNR, Faenza.

Natali, A.N., Meroi, E.A., Trebacz, H. 1997b. The influence of ageing on mechanical behaviour of intervertebral segment, Proc. 3rd Int. Symp. on Computer Methods in Biomechanics & Biomedical Engineering, pp. 323–330.

Natali, A.N., Meroi, E.A., Williams, K.R., Calabrese, L. 1998. Investigation of the integration process of dental implants by means of a numerical analysis of dynamic response, *Dent. Mater.* **13**(5), 325–337.

Nicholson, P.H.F., Haddaway, M.J., Davie, M.W.J. 1994. The dependence of ultrasonic properties on orientation in human vertebral bone, *Phys. Med. Biol.* **39**, 1013–1024.

Oden, Z.M., Hart, R.T., Forwood, M.R., Burr, D.B. 1995. A priori prediction of functional adaptation in canine radii using a cell based mechanistic approach, Trans. 41st Orthop. Res. Soc.

Odgaard, A., Kabel, J., van Rietbergen, B., Dalstra, M., Huiskes, R. 1997. Fabric and elastic principal directions of cancellous bone are closely related, *J. Biomech.* **30**(5), 487–495.

Pugh, J.W., Rose, R.M., Radin, E.L. 1973. Elastic and viscoelastic properties of trabecular bone: dependence of structure, *J. Biomech.* **6**, 475.

Reilly, D.T., Burstein, A.H., Fankel, V.H. 1974. The elastic modulus for bone, *J. Biomech.* **7**, 271–275.

Rice, J.C., Cowin, S.C., Bowman, J.A. 1988. On the dependence of the elasticity and strength of cancellous bone on apparent density, *J. Biomech.* **21**, 155–161.

Roesler, H. 1981. Some historical remarks on the theory of cancellous bone structure (Wolff's law), in: *Mechanical Properties of Bone* (S.C. Cowin, ed.), pp. 27–42, American Society of Mechanical Engineers, New York.

Rubin, C.T., Lanyon, L.E. 1984. Dynamic strain similarity in vertebrates: an alternative to allometric limb bone scaling, *J. Theor Biol.* **107**(2), 321–327.

Runkle, J.C., Pugh, J.W. 1975. The micromechanics of cancellous bone. II. Determination of the elastic modulus of individual trabeculae by buckling analysis, *Bull. Hosp. Jt. Dis.* **36**, 2.

Ryan, S.D., Williams, J.L. 1986. Tensile testing of individual bovine trabeculae, Proc. 12th NE Bio-Engineering Conference, 35.

Sadegh, A.M., Luo, G.M., Cowin, S.C. 1993. Bone ingrowth, an application of the boundary element method to bone remodeling at the implant interface, *J. Biomech.* **26**(2), 167–182.

Townsend, P.R., Rose, R.M., Radin, E.L. 1975. Buckling studies of a single human trabecula, *J. Biomech.* **8**, 199.

Treharne, R.W. 1981. Review of Wolff's law and its proposed means of operation, *Orthop. Rev.* **10**(1), 35–47.

Turner, C.H. 1997. The relationship between cancellous bone architecture and mechanical properties at the continuum level, *Forma* **12**, 225–233.

Whitehouse, W.J. 1974. The quantitative morphology of anisotropic trabecular bone, *J. Microsc.* **101**, 153–168.

Williams, J.L., Lewis, J.L. 1982. Properties and an anisotropic model of cancellous bone from the proximal tibial epiphysis, *J Biomech. Eng.* **104**, 50.

Wolff, J. 1892. *Das Gesetz der Transformation der Knochen*, Hirschwald, Berlin.

16

Hip Joint Prosthesis

Giuseppe Guida and Dante Ronca

16.1. Introduction to Joint Replacements

The functional deficits consequent to joint affections of various types of etiology can from a remarkable entity and determine serious impairments. The most frequently involved joints are the hip and the knee and, in the superior limbs, the finger joints and the shoulder. Since the end of 19th century, but mostly in the first years of the 20th century, the interest of many orthopedic surgeons and their research have been directed toward the development of surgical procedures able to restore the joint function. The first attempts at arthroplasty were performed on the hip and, after an initial period of substituting only the joint head (endoprosthesis), the era of total joint substitution began in 1960 with John Charnley. Subsequently arthroplasties of the knee (Gunston, 1971; Coventry *et al.*, 1972), of the ankle (Stauffer and Segal, 1981), of the fingers of the hand (Swanson, 1973), of the shoulder (Neer, 1955, 1964, 1974; Neer *et al.*, 1982), of the wrist (Cooney *et al.*, 1984) and elbow followed.

The development of prosthetic joint substitution is closely related to knowledge of the joint biomechanics and to the technological developments in the field of biomaterials. The implant of a prosthetic element into a bone determines important alterations in the normal distribution of strengths on the bone, with consequent architectural changes in the bone itself. The change of the bone structure, following changes of the mechanical condition due to the presence of a rigid extraneous element, is called bone remodeling.

The nature and extension of the remodeling also depend on the form and rigidity of the implanted element, for which the importance of a deep knowledge of joint biomechanics and of the characteristics of biomaterials

---

Giuseppe Guida and Dante Ronca • Istituto di Clinica Ortopedica, Università di Napoli, via S. Andrea delle Dame 4, 80138 Napoli, Italy.

Integrated Biomaterials Science, edited by R. Barbucci. Kluwer Academic/Plenum Publishers, New York, 2002.

that technology makes available for us becomes evident in the planning of a joint prosthesis. The crucial point is, therefore, to try to prolong the duration of the arthroprostheses to the longest possible term. This can be obtained thanks to the ability of an implant to induce in the host bone an answer which determines an adaptation to the change in the load conditions (Zong-Ping Luo, 1996).

16.2. History

The hip joint can be affected by numerous pathological conditions (primitive and secondary arthritis, rheumatoid arthritis, aseptic osteonecrosis, results of trauma, etc.) that determine an important functional deficit due to pain and stiffness. One can therefore easily understand why the possibility of a surgical treatment able to eliminate pain and restore joint mobility has always fascinated orthopedic surgeons. The first attempts were made by a biological arthroplasty which consists of the interposition of a biological material (muscle, skin, fascia lata) between the modeled joint surfaces. The first arthroplasty with the use of a biomaterial was performed 60 years ago, when Smith-Petersen (1939) interposed a metallic cup of chrome–cobalt alloy (vitallium) between the head of the femur and the cotyle (Figure 16.1). After the experience of Moore and Bohlman (1943), the first substitution of the femoral head on a large scale is owed to the Judet brothers (1946), who used a femoral head in polymethylmethacrylate linked to a stem that was inserted in the femoral neck as far as the lateral cortex (Judet and Judet, 1950) (Figure 16.2).

All these implants were failures, from either the biomechanical (collapse of the zone of implant and serious problems of wear) or the biological

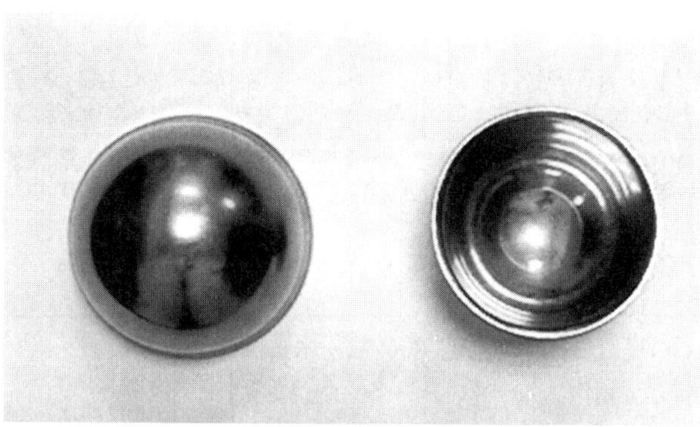

Figure 16.1. A Smith-Peterson cup.

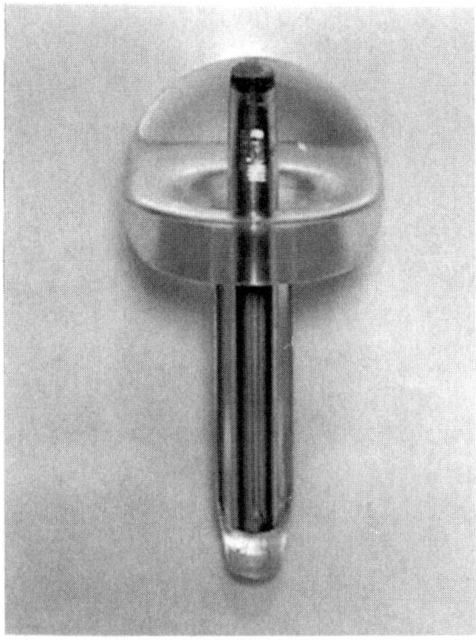

Figure 16.2. The prosthesis of Judet.

point of view (persistence of pain and functional limitation of the mobility of the prosthetic head in a cotyle, which is also the object of the pathological process). Subsequent to these failures, the prosthesis was made of chrome–cobalt alloy. After other experience in substituting the femoral head using different kinds of materials (Bakelite, ivory, stainless steel), the first endoprosthesis with endomedullar stem is owed to Austin Moore (1943). His prosthesis, which was afterward widely used, was of chrome–cobalt alloy, with a holed-in stem to allow bone growth and a collar to be placed on the femoral calcar (Figure 16.3). A change in the prosthesis of Moore was made by Thompson (1954) (Figure 16.4).

The first total substitution of the coxofemoral articulation was due to McKee and Farrar, when in 1956 they began the era of prosthetic substitution of the hip. The prosthesis of McKee and Farrar (1966) was of chrome–cobalt alloy and constituted by a large head (40 mm) linked to a stem similar to Thompson's, to be inserted in the medullar canal and articulated with a cotyle, also made of chrome–cobalt alloy. Originally the prosthesis was fixed with screws, then it was cemented with acrylic cement, thanks to the research of Charnley (1970) (Figure 16.5). The prosthesis of McKee and Farrar has been modified by Postel with the insertion, into the acetabular cup, of the so-called "bandes de glissement," in order to reduce friction and favor lubrication (Figure 16.6).

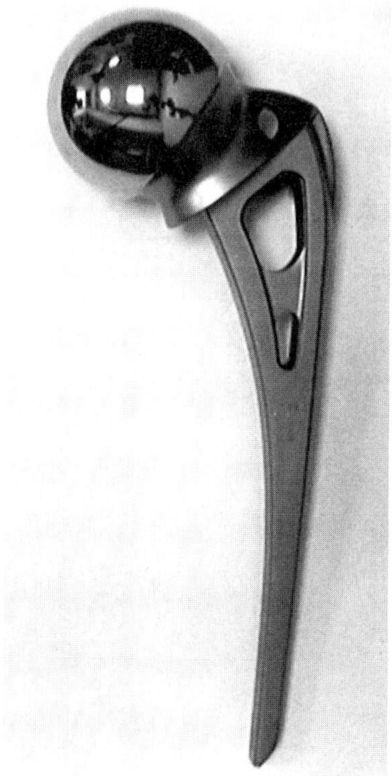

Figure 16.3. The prosthesis of Moore.

However, the development and extensive spread of the total prosthesis of the hip is owed to John Charnley (1961, 1979), who introduced low friction arthroplasty and the routine use of acrylic cement as means to fix the prosthetic stem to the femoral canal and the acetabular cup to the pelvis. The prosthesis of Charnley (Figure 16.7) was used on a large scale and is still in use today, even if small changes have been made to the original model (Figure 16.8). It is made of a stainless steel stem with a small head (22 mm); the stem is inserted in the medullar canal of the femur, previously modeled with a broach of corresponding form, and fixed to the bone with acrylic cement (PMMA). The cotyle was originally made of Teflon, but afterward it was given up because of numerous failures due to rapid wear and consequent tissue reaction. After numerous attempts and research the best material was shown to be ultrahigh molecular weight polyethylene (UHMWPE). The cementation of the prosthetic component and the metal–polyethylene coupling allowed one to obtain a high rate of success. The

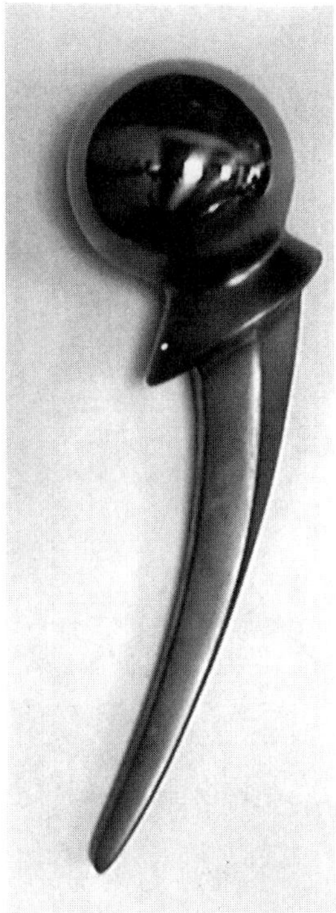

Figure 16.4. The prosthesis of Thompson.

resulting prostheses with these characteristics were numerous, but all with heads of larger diameter: the prosthesis of Muller (Figure 16.9) with a head diameter of 32 mm, the prosthesis of Bucholz with 38 mm, the trapezoidal prosthesis of Amstutz with 28 mm, and several others.

The aim of reducing bone resections to a minimum and preserving the bone patrimony brought up the idea of the resurfacing prosthesis (Muller, 1970; Paltrinieri and Trentani, 1971; Gérard *et al.*, 1974; Amstutz *et al.*, 1977; Freeman, 1978; Wagner, 1978) (Figure 16.10), but the high rate of failures, both numerous and precocious, made them give up.

With the passing of time and the increasing spread of the prosthesization of the hip, it became evident that one of the more frequent problems of joint prostheses was the stability of the fixation of the prosthetic component to the bone.

The observation of long-term prosthetic failures due to mobilization of the prosthesis–cement complex, to mechanical collapse of the acrylic cement and the formation of osteolysis, brought Jones and Hungerford

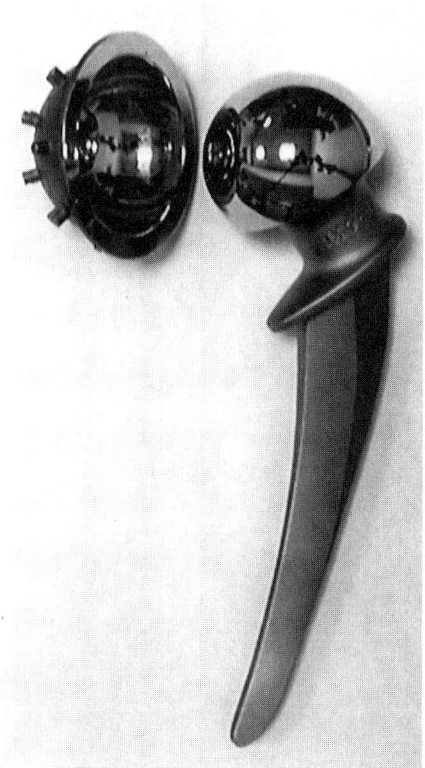

Figure 16.5. The prosthesis of McKee and Farrar.

(1987) to consider the cement as the cause for those failures, and they coined the term "cement disease." The interest of researchers therefore focused on searching for some kind of biological direct fixation of the prosthetic component to the bone.

To achieve this, prostheses whose surface could allow bone growth which would fix the prosthetic component firmly to the bone were constructed. The noncemented prosthesis, as far as it concerns shape, dimensions, and technique of application, must be able to guarantee "primary stability," a necessary condition to develop the bone growth that will definitely fix the prosthesis to the bone, that is, "secondary stability."

In order to obtain the first condition (primary stability) it is necessary to have a number of prostheses of different size available at the operating table, and to use the one that better fits the dimensions of the bone. The

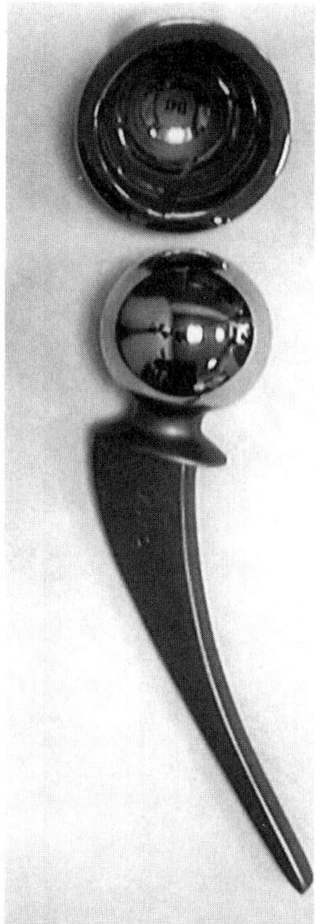

Figure 16.6. The prosthesis of Postel.

cavity in the bone must be prepared with tools (broaches, drills) with form and dimensions exactly matching the prosthesis to be implanted in order to guarantee the best possible filling (fill) and adherence (fit), which are the conditions for a good primary stability.

To get bone growth, the prostheses are made of biomaterials that assure biocompatibility and allow or, if possible, favor bone ingrowth; besides, the surfaces are made irregular by different techniques (porous metal, sintering of spheres of varied diameter, plasma spray, etc.).

The middle- and long-term results of a noncemented prosthesis, however, were no better than those of the cemented prosthesis, especially after the improvement of the cementation techniques. Aseptic loosening is also present in a noncemented prosthesis and seems to be caused by the reaction of the organism to the debris of wear, especially of polyethylene.

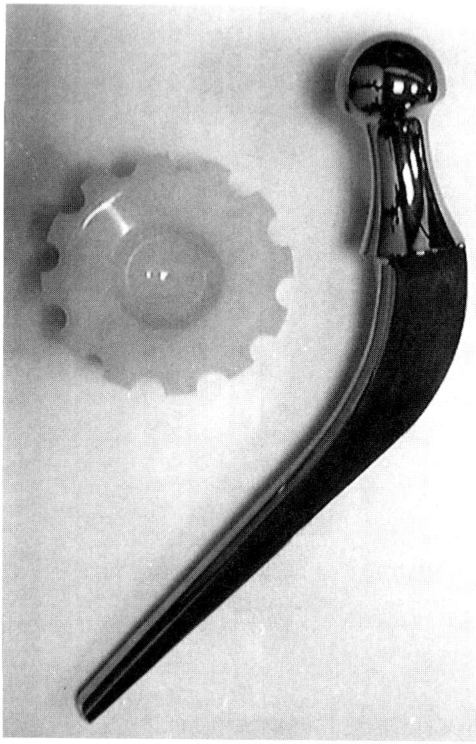

Figure 16.7. The prosthesis of Charnley.

16.3. Cemented Prostheses

16.3.1. Femoral Stem

The femoral part is made by a stem that is inserted in the remaining part of the cut femoral neck and in the medullar canal and that, in its upper extremity, has a sphere of varying dimensions according to the type of prosthesis, from 32 mm to 22 mm. The axis of the endomedullar portion of the stem and the axis of the head and the neck form an angle, also varying with reference to the type of prosthesis, from 117° to 142. Most prostheses anyhow introduce an angle similar or correspondingly to the normal angle of inclination of the femoral neck (125°–128°). In the first types of prostheses (McKee and Farrar, 1966; Charnley, 1961; Muller, 1970) the stems were in one piece, a monoblock, but currently almost all are made in two parts: one includes the stem and the neck and the other the head. The

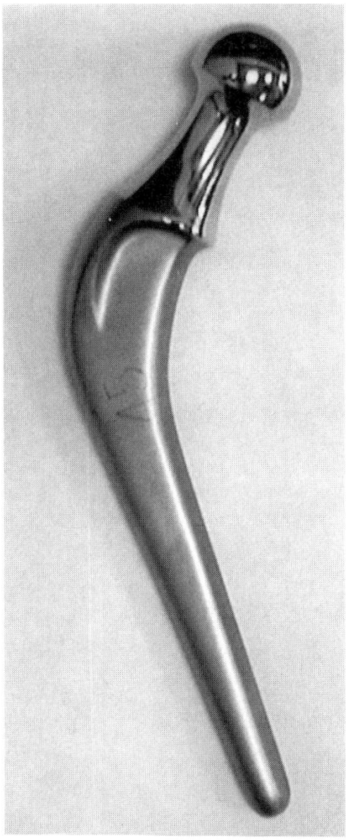

Figure 16.8. The modified prosthesis of Charnley.

extremity of the neck is conformed to a morse cone to which is applied the head that, according to the depth of the mold cone, allows one to obtain different neck lengths. Monoblock prostheses still exist today (Charnley, Kerboull, Muller, CAD, etc.); these, while on the one-hand avoid formation of deposits due to the modularity, can on the other hand oblige one to have a greater number of prostheses available at the time of surgery.

The stems exist in different measures to better adapt to the dimensions of the femur. As far as the length of the stem is concerned, despite several different opinions, currently the optimal length seems to be between 100 and 130 mm (Berry and Chao, 1996). The cavity is prepared with broaches of increasing dimensions, matching the size of the prosthesis.

The surface of the cemented stems is extremely variable according to the type of prosthesis and can be schematized in two kinds of surface: (1) smooth surface, without collar (Exeter-like stem); (2) irregular surface, rough or coated, with or without collar.

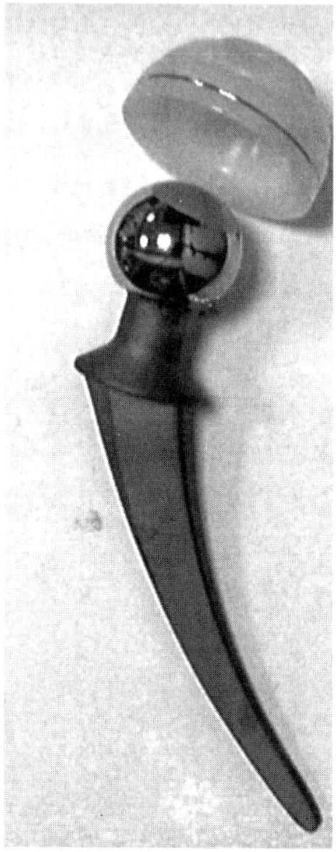

Figure 16.9. The prosthesis of Charnley and Muller.

The two types of surface correspond to two different schools of thought. The first (Figure 16.11), which uses prostheses with a double cone design, with smooth shiny surfaces, and without bumps or dents, thinks that the prosthesis should not be tightly bound to the cement but should have the possibility, throughout the years, of small movements (sinking) on the inside of the polymethylmethacrylate shell, without fracturing the layer of cement as a result of its plastic deformation. (Fowler *et al.*, 1988; Ling, 1992).

To facilitate sinking of the implant and to avoid a situation in which the apex of the stem comes in contact with the cement, a mold centering device of polymethylmethacrylate is applied to the distal extremity of the stem. The sinking of the stem in the cement determines an increase of the tear and wear force and a decrease of the shear stress on the cement–bone interface, and also causes a proximal transmission of the loads (Lee and Ling, 1974; Crowninshield *et al.*, 1978; Linder and Hansson, 1983; Weightman *et al.*, 1987; Lee *et al.*, 1992).

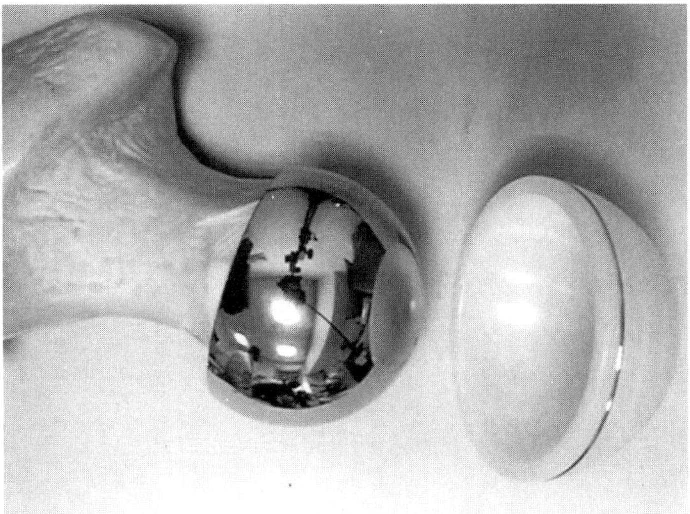

Figure 16.10. The Wagner resurfacing prosthesis.

The second school of thought, instead, thinks that the first collapses which bring on the loosening occur on the cement–prosthesis interface (Crowninshield *et al.*, 1985; Miller and Ahmed, 1985; Harris, 1985) and therefore the prosthesis–cement link must be extremely stable. For this reason the surfaces of the femoral stem are engraved, only in the proximal part, to avoid the phenomenon of stress shielding, with dents and bumps, spallette, sanding, plasma spray (Figure 16.12), and coating of materials such as polymethylmethacrylate to create a closer implant–cement contact. The favorable effects have been shown by numerous researchers (Raab *et al.*, 1981; Crowninshield and Tolbert, 1983).

Distal centering devices and proximal spacing collars, usually of polyethylene, are used to optimize the centering of the prosthesis in the cement and hence to obtain a uniform thickness of the cement.

a. Design. The cemented stem is shaped to give the smallest possible stress to the cement, eliminating sharp edges and transmitting mostly forces of compression (Crowninshield *et al.*, 1980).

The cemented stems were created as straight stems and most of them still possess this characteristic today. Currently, in order to optimize the distribution of the loads, to avoid concentration of stress, to improve the interfaces, and to maintain the thickness of the cement at the maximum, prostheses with a so-called anatomical curve have been introduced (Figure

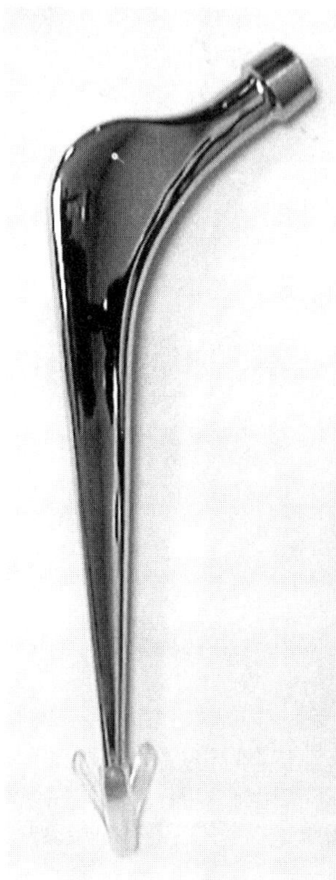

Figure 16.11. The Exeter prosthesis.

16.13). These stems allow a reduction in stress on the interface from 30% to 70% (Huiskes and Boeklagen, 1989).

b. Material. Cemented stems can be made of several different materials, such as stainless steel, chrome–cobalt alloy (vitallium, Protasul 10), or titanium alloy (Ti-6A-4V-Ti6A17Nb: Protasul® 100). For cemented implants it is preferable to use Co–Cr stems that possess double the coefficient of elasticity compared to alloys of titanium and transmit a smaller amount of stress to the cement (Crowninshield *et al.*, 1980).

c. Collar. The presence of the collar represents, in cemented prostheses, a useful element and a complication at the same time. The utility of the collar is related to the contribution it gives to the pressurization of the cement in the last phases of introducing the stem. It also improves the

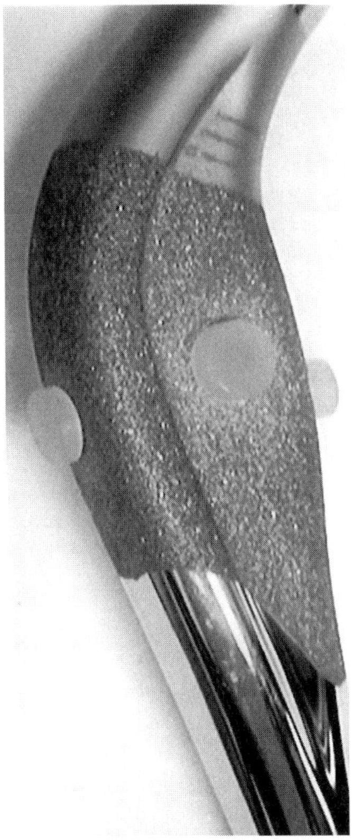

Figure 16.12. Plasma-spray coating of a cemented stem.

distribution of loads on the proximal part of the femur (Andriacchi *et al.*, 1976; Crowninshield *et al.*, 1980; Markolf *et al.*, 1980; Lewis *et al.*, 1984).

However, when the removal of a prosthesis is indicated, the collar represents an obstacle to the introduction of the chisels, which have to penetrate close and parallel to the surface of the stem. Obviously Exeter-like stems are always collarless.

16.3.2. Cotyle

The cemented cotyles currently in use and more commonly used are essentially of two types: (1) ultrahigh molecular weight polyethylene cotyles (UHMWPE); (2) cotyles with metal backing and internal insert of polyethylene. Actually, other types exist (cotyles of ceramics; cotyles with metal backing, insert of ceramics, and intermediary insert of polyethylene; cotyles

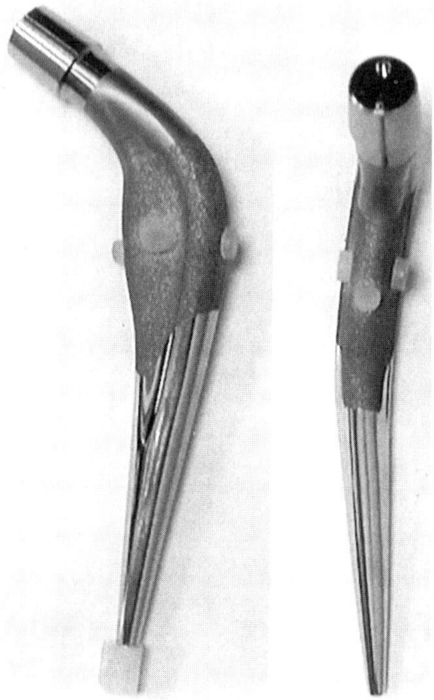

Figure 16.13. A curved cemented stem (SHP).

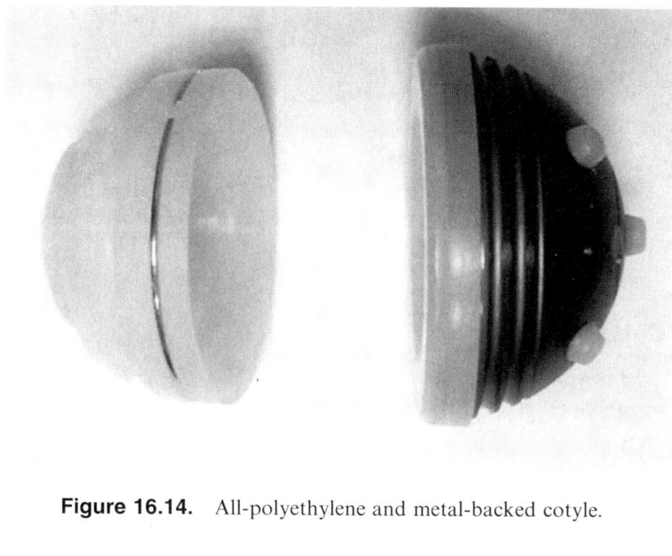

Figure 16.14. All-polyethylene and metal-backed cotyle.

with metal backing, insert of metal, and intermediary insert of polyethylene) but they have not yet entered into current use because they lack follow-up.

The most diffused cotyles are made of polyethylene with or without metal backing (Figure 16.14). The cotyles made of polyethylene were in fact created without metal backing (Charnley, Muller, etc.). Subsequently, numerous authors showed that metal-backed cotyles distributed the stress better in the region of the acetabulum (Carter *et al.*, 1982; Pedersen *et al.*, 1982; Van Syckle and Walker, 1980; Vasu *et al.*, 1982; Harris, 1985).

Such theoretical premises, however, did not produce any evidence in the clinical practice, because numerous demonstrations showed early wear in metal-backing cotyles (Morrey and Adams, 1996), with the result that they have been completely discarded and currently there is a return to the cemented cotyle of polyethylene. The all-polyethylene cotyle also allows one to obtain greater thickness, which reduces the stress on the cement and on the subchondral bone (Pedersen *et al.*, 1982).

16.4. The Noncemented Prostheses

Noncemented prostheses are based on the principle of obtaining the fixation of the prosthesis to the bone through a biological bond, determined from bone growth around the implant. To obtain this, it is essential that the prosthesis comes perfectly dimensioned and adapted to the opportunely prepared bone shell, in order to assure primary stability, which is a necessary condition to allow bone ingrowth and therefore secondary stability.

In noncemented prostheses, the design and characteristics of the surface are again of fundamental importance.

16.4.1. Femoral Stem

As far as the design is concerned, numerous models of the femoral stem exist; however, they can be divided into three fundamental types: straight stems, curved stems, and modular stems. Custom-made stems and so-called isoelastic stems also exist.

a. Straight Stems. These do not introduce curves on the sagittal plan, but only on the frontal plan, with inclinations between the axis of the neck and the axis of the stem (Figure 16.15). The straight stems, considering the physiological curve of the proximal and middle femur (anti-version and pro-curvature), obtain primary stability thanks to a fixation that is predominantly above three points.

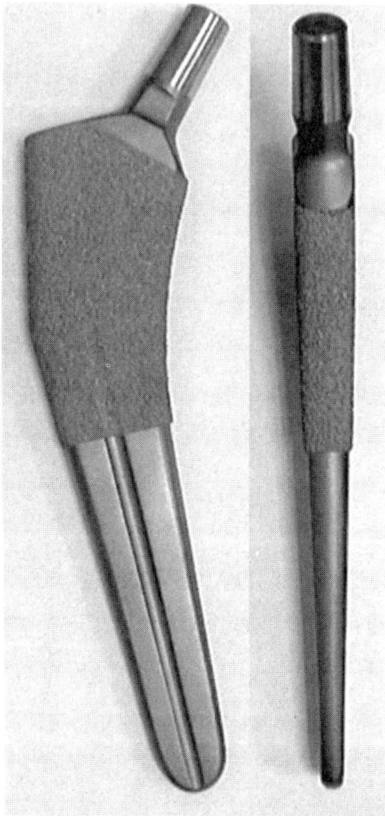

Figure 16.15. A straight uncemented stem.

b. Curved Stems. These are called "anatomical stems" and reproduce the morphology of the femur, either for the anti-version or the pro-curvature (Figure 16.16). Thanks to their curves they better match the morphology of the bone, with consequent better fixation, adherence, and distribution of the loads.

c. Collar. Both types of stems, straight or anatomical, can be equipped with collars that can be fixed or modular. Modular collars can be applied after the introduction of the stem and, in case of removal of the prosthesis, they can be taken out first and do not represent an obstacle to the removal (Figure 16.17).

For prostheses with very short stems, when a large part of the femoral neck has to be preserved, the collar represents an essential element for primary stability and for the transfer of the loads.

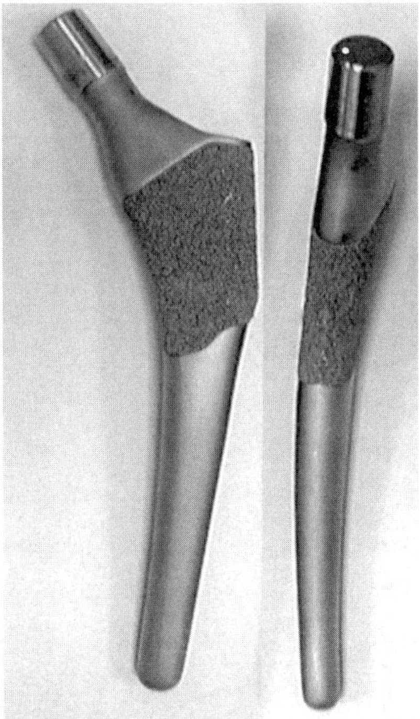

Figure 16.16. A curved uncemented stem.

The femoral stem must find its fit and its optimal fill as soon as it penetrates the medullar canal. The collar will therefore find support on the calcar before the stem has completed its penetration and, in this case, it will perform a perfect adherence; otherwise, if the stem has reached the maximum penetration, it will not yet find any support on the calcar and the result will be entirely useless.

We do not think that the application of collars gives real advantages after the complete insertion of the stem has been performed and the neck has been modeled with special broaches. The collar also represents an obstacle to any small further penetration of the stem which occurs in the first moments of the load and represents a mechanism of ulterior stabilization.

d. Modular Stems. These consist of different components, each available in numerous sizes that, assembled together, allow a perfect match to the host bone (Figure 16.18). This type of stem is particularly useful in cases of both dysplastic femurs and reimplants, where the morphology of the bone

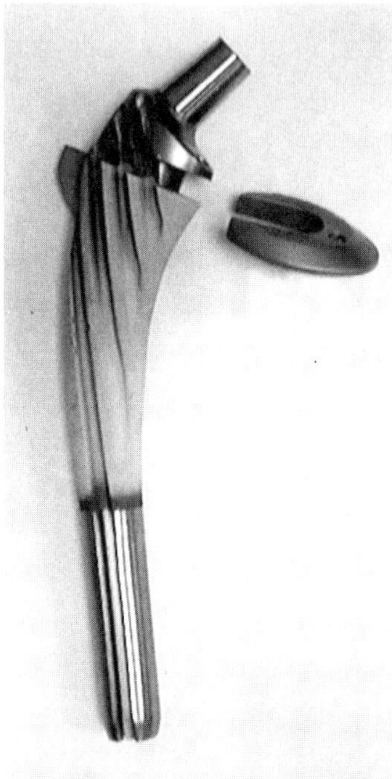

Figure 16.17. A collared stem.

has been markedly altered by the periprosthesic osteolysis processes. Naturally, the modularity gives the inconvenience of a greater formation of metallic deposits and development of osteolysis (Bobyn *et al.*, 1980; Mathiesen *et al.*, 1991; Collier *et al.*, 1992a, b, c; Cook *et al.*, 1994; Chmel *et al.*, 1995; Jacobs *et al.*, 1995).

e. Custom-Made Stems. These are made with a morphology which perfectly matches that of the bone which must host them. Their use should be required only in case of serious deformities of the proximal femur. They are realized with technical CAD/CAM (computer aided design and computer aided manufacture), but their results have not proven as good as those of prefabricated prosthesis. Moreover, the high cost, the inevitable defects of construction, and the inadequacy of the instrumentation (Balderston *et al.*, 1992), as well as the possibility to increase the phenomenon of stress shielding for the dimensions of the implant (Engh and Bobyn, 1987; Engh *et al.*, 1987), have increasingly limited their use.

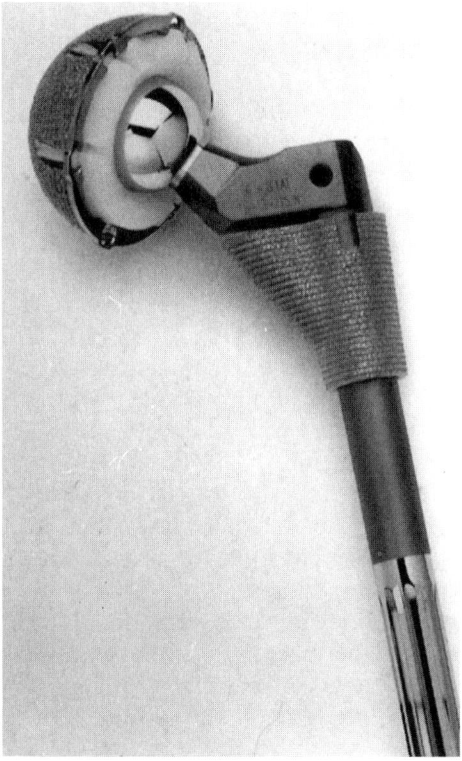

Figure 16.18. Modular stem.

f. Materials. The materials used for the femoral stems are essentially the same as those used for the cemented stems: stainless steel, but mostly chrome–cobalt alloys and titanium alloys. In theory, the titanium alloy should be preferred for noncemented prosthesis, its coefficient of elasticity being about half that of the Cr–Co alloy, and therefore closer to the elasticity of the bone, thus allowing a better transfer of the loads from the implant to the bone (Huiskes, 1987; Huiskes *et al.*, 1992). This problem is particularly felt in cases of large femoral canals, when stems of big dimensions and with elevated flexional rigidity are required.

These theoretical presuppositions are not borne out by the results of the different series, because a superiority of the results of titanium alloy prostheses compared with those with cobalt–chrome alloy has not been actually shown. As far as bone growth is concerned, both the Co–Cr and Ti-6Al-4V porous-coated alloys are involved in an equivalent manner. Some authors report a certain superiority of the titanium alloy while many others formed equivalent results with the Co–Cr alloy (Collier *et al.*, 1992a, b, c; Cook *et al.*, 1988a, b, 1991).

g. Coatings. Primary stability and consequent biological fixation can be obtained according to two fundamental principles: that of the press fit and that of the press fit associated with porous coating.

With time it became evident that the press-fit technique, using femoral stems with smooth surfaces, with or without bumps, i.e., the prosthesis of Mittelmeier (1974), modified by Muller (1978), Parhofer and Monch (1984), Zweymüller and Semlitsch (1982), did not give satisfactory results (Duparc and Massin, 1992; Coventry, 1991) (Figure 16.19). This gave birth to the idea of fixing the prosthesic stem to the bone through bone ingrowth, which could be obtained with the use of porous coatings.

The first prosthesis coated with pores of big diameter (1 mm or more) were Judet *et al.*'s in porous metal (1978) and Lord *et al.*'s madreporique (1979) (Figure 16.20). The extension of the porous coating to the whole stem, determining the fixity of the stem from the distal end to the apex, provoked the stress-shielding phenomenon with consequent bony reabsorption at the level of the metaphysis.

This problem, together with the serious difficulty occurring in cases of removal, led to limiting the extension of the porous coating only to the proximal portion of the stem. Currently, the optimal dimension of the pore seems to range between 100 and 500 μm (Bobyn *et al.*, 1980; Robertson *et*

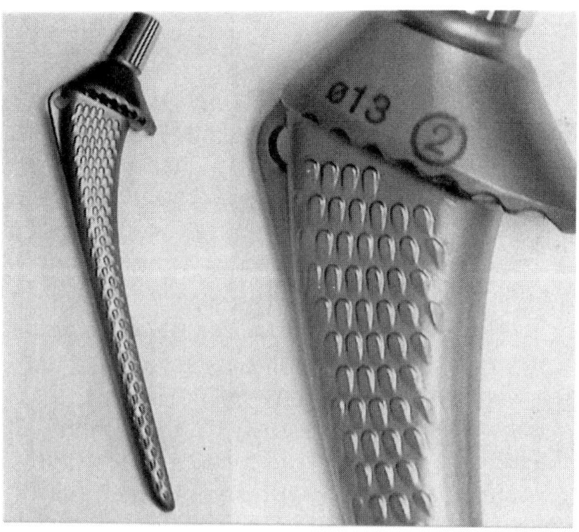

Figure 16.19. The stem of Parhofer.

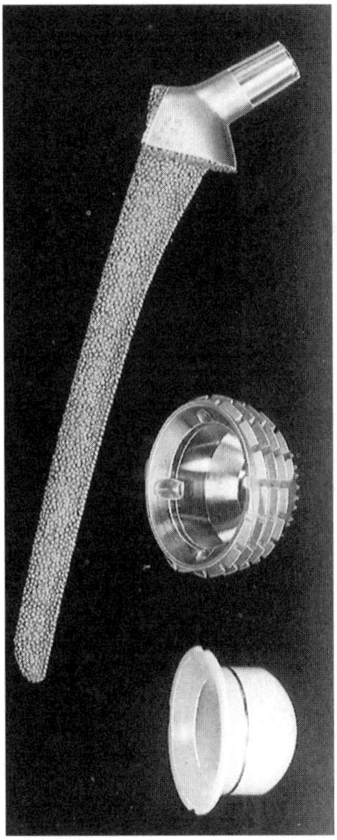

Figure 16.20. The stem of Lord.

al., 1976; Pilliar *et al.*, 1975; Kang *et al.*, 1991; Bobyn *et al.*, 1996). The pores are obtained with different types of coatings. The most common coatings consist of:

1. Several layers of sintered microspheres of Co–Cr alloy of about 500 μm diameter (PCA, Meridien, Citation) (Figure 16.21).
2. Titanium wire nets (Galante *et al.*, 1971) (Figure 16.22).
3. Plasma spray (Hahn and Palich, 1970) (Figure 16.23).
4. Hydroxyapatite. The coating with hydroxyapatite (HA) is employed for accelerating and improving the osteointegration; it has been proposed and used for coating smooth, press-fit, and porous surface prostheses (porous coating). The coating of HA has been introduced and studied by Geesink *et al.* (1987). These and other authors have shown that the HA facilitates and accelerates the process of osteointegration (Thomas *et al.*, 1989; Oonishi *et al.*, 1989; Cook *et al.*, 1991; D'Antonio *et al.*, 1992; Jasty *et al.*, 1992) and reduces the migration of the implant (Sobelle *et al.*,

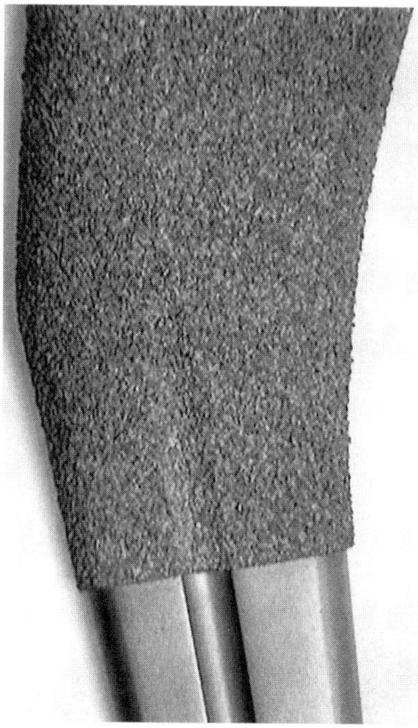

Figure 16.21. Sintered microsphere (left) and plasma spray (right).

1993). Nevertheless, some well-known problems, related to the separation of particles whose migration can cause wear to three bodies (Howie, 1990), have so far limited the large-scale use of the coatings of HA.

Currently, the stems to a large extent present a distal portion perfectly smooth and shiny, to avoid both fixation in this part and the phenomenon of stress shielding. Some of them present an opening at their distal end (diapason extremity) to reduce distal rigidity and to avoid tight pain (Meridien, Citation, S.Rom and other).

16.4.2. Cotyle

As for the femoral stems, so also for the noncemented cotyles the pursuit of a good biological fixation has determined the increase in the numerous models of cotyles. Except for the cemented cotyle, which can be entirely made of polyethylene, the noncemented cotyle, apart from some trials with polyethylene (Knahr *et al.*, 1984; Morscher *et al.*, 1982), currently consists of a metal back, generally porous coated, to obtain primary stability and subsequent biological fixation and including an insert of polyethylene.

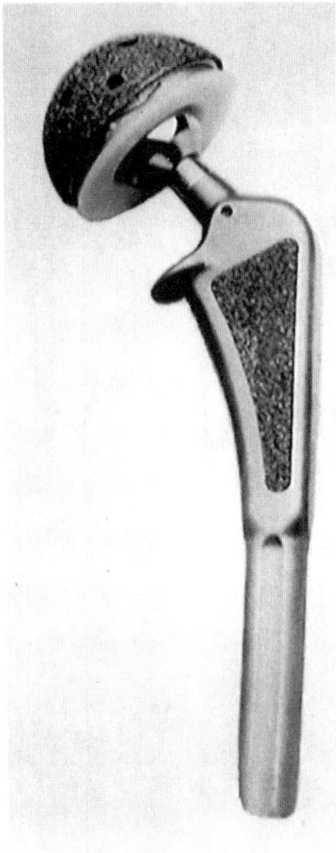

Figure 16.22. Wires of titanium.

The principal models of cotyles consist of three fundamental types:

- threaded cotyles, hemispheric or trunk-conic;
- hemispheric cotyles, with or without holes for screws, with pegs, spikes, and lugs;
- cotyles with double geometry.

a. Threaded Cotyles (Figure 16.24). Despite an apparent excellent initial stability, the screwed cotyles, particularly trunk-conic ones, have shown bad results for the middle and long term. Several authors (Cook *et al.*, 1988a, b; Apel *et al.*, 1989; Shaw *et al.*, 1990; Thomas *et al.*, 1991; Tallroth *et al.*, 1993) reported a high rate of failures. Trousdale and Cabanela (1996) affirm that biological fixation does not occur well and the implant has the tendency to loosen. Moreover, an excessive removal of bone is necessary for the implant and the orientation can be difficult.

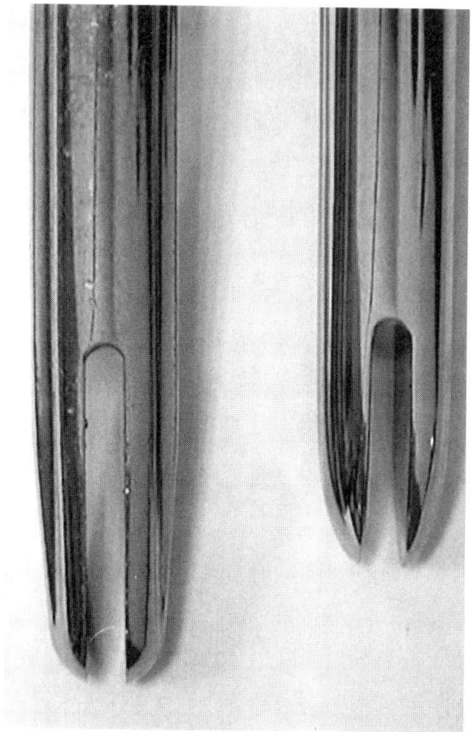

Figure 16.23. Diapason extremity.

b. Hemispheric Cotyles. Hemispheric cotyles are those more commonly used today. The coating of the metal back is made, as for the femoral stem, of synthesized spheres (synthesized beads), wire net, and plasma spray (wire mesh). The materials used are Co–Cr alloy and Ti-6Al-4V alloy.

The hemispheric cotyles can be without prominences or holes, or can show some kind of appendixes to increase their primary stability: pegs, lugs, or spikes (Figures 16.25 and 16.26). Also, holes for the introduction of screws can be present. It is preferable, according to anatomical conditions, to apply a cotyle without appendixes and without holes. The appendixes can cause great difficulty in the orientation of the cup which, once the impact begins, can no longer be modified. The holes for the screws represent ways for migration of the polyethylene and metallic debris, produced by the micromovements of the polyethylene insert in the metallic shell between screw and hole. Currently, the manufacturers are trying to reduce the production of debris by shining the internal surface of the metal backing, or by reducing to a minimum the movement between metallic shell and

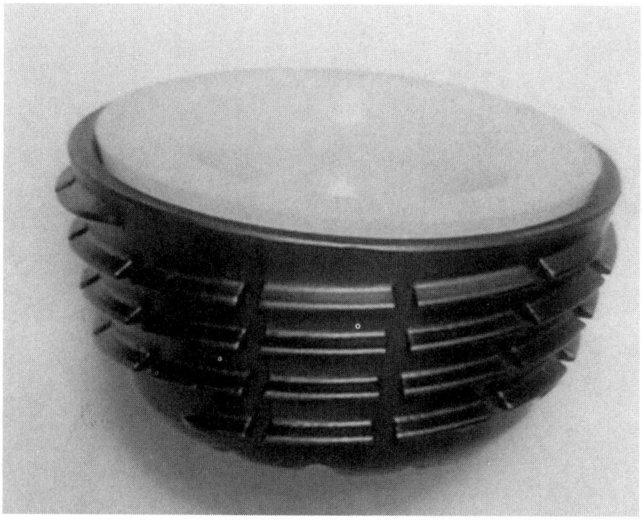

Figure 16.24. Threaded cotyle.

polyethylene and improving the cavity of the screw heads in the holes. The screws holes, particularly if they are numerous, also reduce the porous coated surface of the implant, with consequent decrease in bone ingrowth.

Cotyles without prominences and without screws must be inserted in a cavity whose diameter has been broached 2 mm smaller than that of the

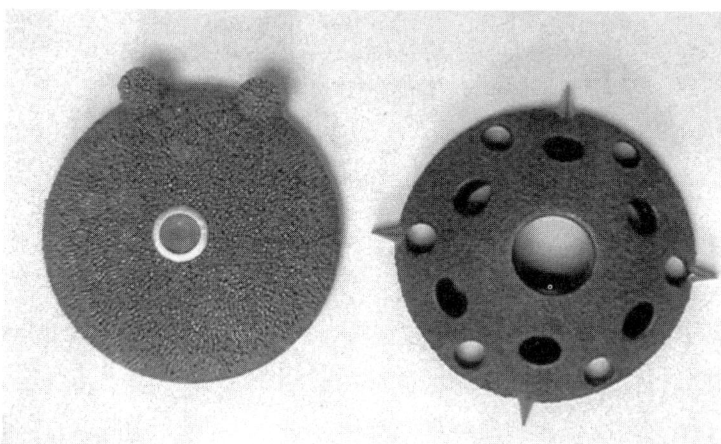

Figure 16.25. Hemispheric cotyle with pegs and spikes.

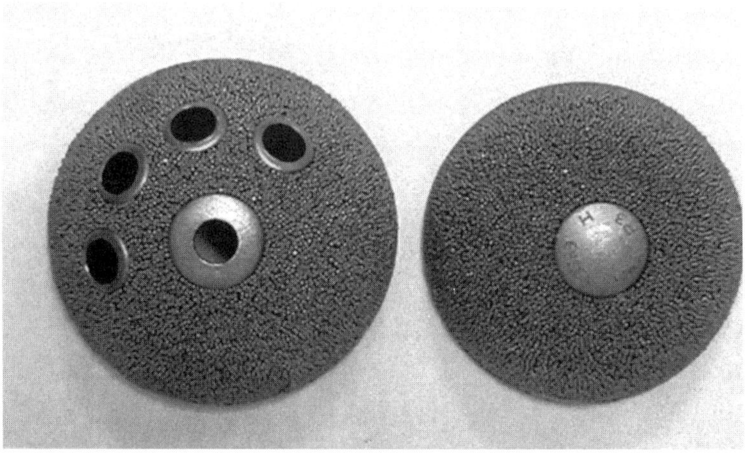

Figure 16.26. Hemispheric cotyle with and without holes for screws.

cup to be installed. A broaching of diameter equal to that of the cotyle causes exposure to precarious primary stability. A broached cavity with a diameter 3 mm smaller than the cotyle's causes instead exposure to the risk of fracture of the acetabulum.

When anatomical conditions (dysplastic cotyles, necessity of application of bone grafts, etc.) do not guarantee a sufficient primary stability, cotyles with appendixes or, preferably, with screws must be used.

The inserts made from polyethylene are available with inside diameters from 32, 20, 26, and 22 mm; they can be both neutral or with a sloped roof that increases the inclination of 10°, 15°, 20° and can be placed differently according to necessity.

c. Cotyles with Double Geometry. These are not currently used. Owing to their design they can be used only for implants in bone cotyles with perfect morphology (Trousdale and Cabanela, 1996). Double geometry can also determine imperfect contact between the whole surface of the implant and the bone, even if the bone ingrowth surface represents about 30–40% of the total surface (Pidhorz *et al.*, 1993; Engh *et al.*, 1995).

In conclusion, the noncemented implants (both the stem and the porous coated cotyle) have shown good qualities to obtain a biological fixation. They can achieve good osteointegration, which guarantees good stability over some period of time, if some fundamental principles are observed:

1. Good primary stability: too ample movements, wider than 150°, inhibit the formation of bone tissue and determine the formation of fibrous tissue (Pilliar *et al.*, 1986).

2. Contact between the implant and the host bone must be as close as possible, and empty spaces must be avoided. The gap between the bone and the implant, even if it cannot be completely eliminated, must be reduced to as little as possible (Bobyn *et al.*, 1981; Sandborn *et al.*, 1988). It has been shown that a gap smaller than 0.5 mm determines a good bone growth (bone ingrowth), while gaps over 2 mm slow down or stop the bone ingrowth (Sandborn *et al.*, 1987).

Equally, expectations about the use of the so-called isoelastic prostheses have not been fulfilled (Mathys and Mathys, 1984).

The use of composite materials for the realization of articular prostheses represents a vast and promising field of research.

Experimentation in this field has yielded a stem of hip prosthesis (Figure 16.27) of composite material (PEI, continuous fibers of carbon and fiberglass) with mechanical properties (coefficient of elasticity) varying along the axis of the prosthetic stem in a way corresponding to the variation in the same mechanical properties along the axis of the bone femur (Ambrosio *et al.*, 1987, 1996); see Table 16.1.

16.5. Friction and Wear

The main problems affecting the long-time endurance of a total prosthesis of the hip are aseptic loosening and formation of periprosthetic osteolysis. It is known that these phenomena result from the tissue reaction to debris, especially to those of polyethylene. The debris, especially those of small dimensions, cause a foreign body reaction of about 1 micron (Lee *et al.*, 1992; Schmalzried *et al.*, 1992) with presence of macrophages and fybroblastes and with production of factors determinant for bone reabsorption (IL-1, IL-6, TNF-, PGE2) (Howie, 1990; Ohlin *et. al.*, 1990; Santavirta *et al.*, 1990; Haynes *et al.*, 1993).

It is therefore evident that the problems of friction and wear are of fundamental importance for the long-term endurance of a joint prosthesis, particularly for that of the hip. In the prosthetic couplings a primary role is therefore represented on the one hand by the head, and on the other by the cotyle. The problems concern both the materials used for the head and for the cotyle and the dimensions either of the head or of the cotyle.

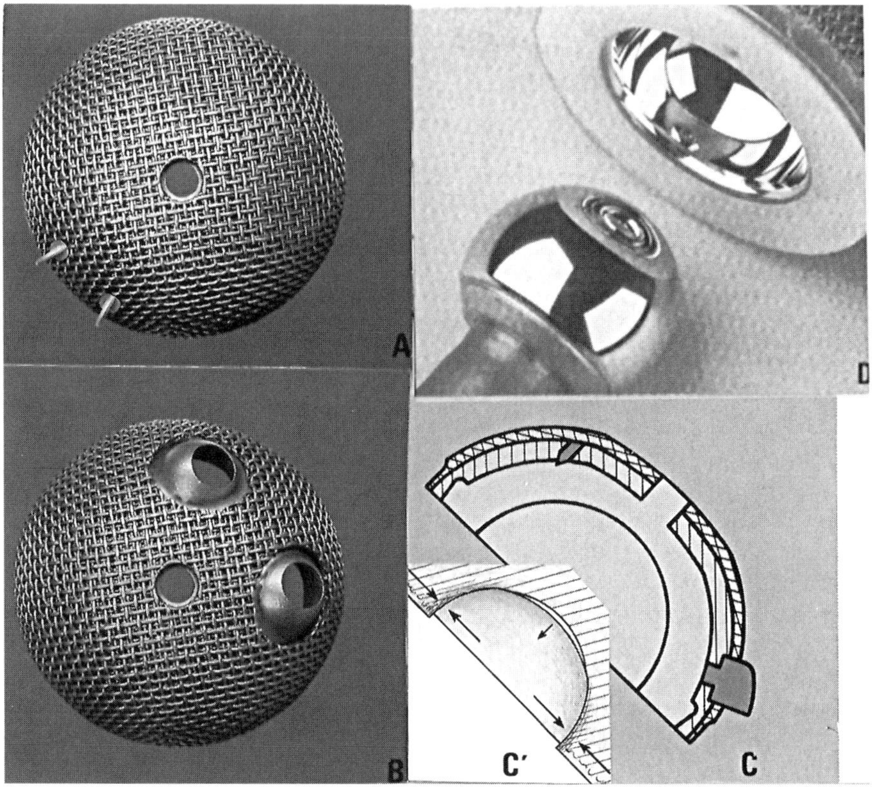

Figure 16.27. Stem in composite material.

16.5.1. Femoral Head Materials

The materials used to construct a prosthetic head must have two main characteristics: hardness and wettability. The degree of superficial finishing also assumes remarkable importance.

The materials used for prosthetic heads are chrome–cobalt alloys, ceramics, zirconium, Ti-6Al-4V, and stainless-steel 316L. Those more widely used are generally the Co–Cr alloys, by far the most used, and the ceramics. The heads of titanium alloy and especially those of stainless steel introduce insufficient hardness, for which they can be easily scratched with consequent increase in wear and the possibility of three-body wear (McKellop *et al.*, 1995; Isaac *et al.*, 1992). For the same reason, apart from the stems of titanium, heads are generally assembled in Co–Cr or in ceramics.

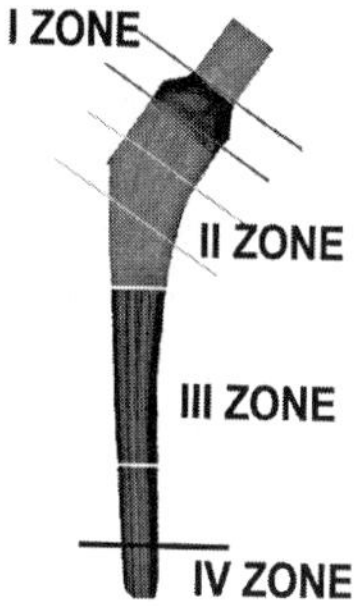

Table 16.1. Composite Prosthesis

Property	Zone I	Zone II	Zone III	Zone IV
I (mm^4)	3842	1400	1017	598
$E \cdot I \cdot 10^{-6}$ ($kg \cdot mm^2$)	15.72	5.87	4.08	0.71
M_{fu} ($kg \cdot mm$)	33,681	14,029	11,072	2114

Certainly ceramics and zirconium have the greatest hardness and thus the smallest possibility of being scratched. Both these materials also have good qualities as far as concerns their wettability (Cuckler *et al.*, 1995). Despite these good theoretical qualities, the heads in Co–Cr, which present the best characteristics of hardness and wettability among the metallic ones, remain the most widely used. The limit to the use of ceramic heads is represented by the risk of fracture, which notably rises with reduction in the diameter, so dissuading the use of heads below 32 mm in diameter.

As for heads of zirconium, even if there are good expectations, they have not yet passed the clinical long-term follow-ups.

16.5.2. Dimensions of the Head

The heads currently in use are produced with diameters of 22, 26, 28, and 32 mm. It is known, after the research of Charnley (1979), that the 22-mm head produces a smaller attrition compared to those of greater dimension. Further experience has shown that a diameter of 26–28 mm is optimal, because it represents the best compromise between attrition and linear wear. Attrition is, in fact, inversely proportional to diameter while the contrary is true for linear wear. However, the diameter of the head must also be chosen according to the dimensions of the cotyle. In fact if small cotyles are inserted, it is necessary to reduce the dimension of the head to avoid the layer of polyethylene becoming too thin, a condition that causes a more rapid wear (Berry and Chao, 1996; Trousdale and Cabanela, 1996).

16.5.3. Cotyle Materials

The material used for the cotyle is in most cases ultrahigh molecular weight polyethylene (UHMWPE). The couplings used more are therefore heads of Co–Cr alloy and UHMWPE and, frequently, heads of ceramics and cotyles of polyethylene.

The thickness of the polyethylene must be not less than 8 mm. Insufficient thickness contributes to a more rapid wear. The polyethylene certainly represents a point of weakness, but since a biomaterial with better characteristics has not been found yet, prostheses manufacturers try to improve their qualities and make them more wear-resistant. Improvements in the qualities of the polyethylene have been obtained both for the preparation of the prosthetic components and for their sterilization.

The polyethylene, produced in bars, can be treated to obtain the final product by two methods: "machined," which previews the modeling of the piece to the lathe, and "molded," which instead obtains the prosthetic element with a pressure stamp. It has been shown that the "molded" method allows one to realize elements with better characteristics of wear resistance and therefore smaller production of debris. Another well-known problem is that some oxidation of the polyethylene markedly alters its characteristics, making it less resistant. The oxidation is produced during the phase of sterilization, which usually was obtained in the atmosphere by gamma rays. The problem of oxidation has been resolved by using vacuum sterilization or sterilization in an atmosphere of inert gas.

Different couplings with low production of debris have been realized: ceramic–ceramic coupling and metal–metal coupling. Ceramic–ceramic coupling possesses notable problems related to hardness and brittleness of the material, and to the impossibility of realizing cotyles and heads of small dimension.

The metal–metal coupling represents in a certain sense a return to the past: the first total prosthesis, the one of McKee and Farrar, was with metal–metal coupling (Co–Cr). Metal–metal couplings have been realized with a particularly evolved technology (Muller, Marchetti, Wagner). The material is the Co–Cr alloy and Mo, and thanks to perfect polishing of the surfaces and perfect matching of the dimensions and curve between the head and cavity, the quantity of debris seems to be highly reduced. A shell of polyethylene is interposed between the metal backing and metallic cavity to make the complex more elastic. The results seem promising, but they must still pass the "sieve" of long clinical follow-ups to judge some as yet unresolved matters, such as the reaction of the tissues to metallic deposits, the effects on the organism of the metallic ions, and the possibility of developing cancers.

References

Ambrosio, L., Caprino, G., Nicolais, L., Nicodemo, L., Huang, S.J., Guida, G., Ronca, D. 1987. Composite materials for bone fracture fixation, *Compos. Struct.* **4**, 2337–2344.

Ambrosio, L., De Santis, R., Nicolais, L., Ronca, D., Guida, G. 1996. Protesi d'anca in materiale composito, *G.I.O.T.* **22** (suppl. 1), 475–480.

Amstutz, H.C. 1981. Materials and stem design of total hip replacement, *Orthop. Trans.* **3**, 357–364.

Amstutz, H.C., Clarke, I.C., Christie, J., Graff-Radford, A. 1977. Total hip articular replacement by internal eccentric shells, *Clin. Orthop.* **128**, 261–284.

Andriacchi, T.P., Galante, J.O., Belytschko, T.B., Hampton, S. 1976. A stress analysis of the femoral stem in total hip prostheses, *J. Bone Jt. Surg.* **58A**, 618–628.

Apel, D.M., Smith, D.G., Schwartz, C.M., Paprosky, W.G. 1989. Threaded cup acetabuloplasty: early clinical experience, *Clin. Orthop.* **241**, 183–189.

Balderston, R.A., Rothman, R.H., Booth, R.E., Hozack, W.J. 1992. *The Hip,* Lea & Febriger, Malvern, PA.

Berry, D.J., Chao, E.Y.S. 1996. Cemented femoral components, in: *Reconstructive Surgery of the Joints* (B.F. Morrey, ed.), pp. 943–960, Churchill Livingstone, New York.

Bobyn, J.D., Pilliar, R.M., Cameron, H.V., Weatherly, G.C. 1980. The optimum pore size for the fixation of porous-surfaced metal implants by the ingrowth of bone, *Clin. Orthop.* **150**, 263–270.

Bobyn, J.D., Pilliar, R.M., Cameron, M.U., Weatherly, G.C. 1981. Osteogenic phenomena across endosteal bone implant spaces with porous-surfaced intramedullary implants, *Acta Orthop. Scand.* **52**, 145–153.

Bobyn, J.D., Jacobs, J.J., Tanzer, M., Urban, R.M., Aribindi, R., Summer, D.R., Turner, T.M., Brooks, C.E. 1995. The susceptibility of smooth implant surfaces to perimplant fibrosis and migration of polyethylene wear debris, *Clin. Orthop.* **311**, 21–39.

Bobyn, J.D., Tanzer, M., Miller, J.E. 1996. Fundamental principles of biologic fixation, in: *Reconstructive Surgery of the Joints* (B.F. Morrey, ed.), pp. 75–94, Churchill Livingstone, New York.

Capello, W.N. 1989. Fit the patient to the prosthesis. An argument against the routine use of custom hip implants, *Clin. Orthop.* **249**, 56–59.

Carter, D.R., Vasu, R., Harris, W.H. 1982. Stress distributions in the acetabular region-II. Effects of cement thickness and metal backing of the total hip acetabular component, *J. Biomech.* **15**, 165–170.

Charnley, J. 1961. Arthroplasty of the hip: a new operation, *Lancet* **1**, 1129.

Chmel, M.J., Rispler, D., Poss, R. 1995. The impact of modularity in total hip arthroplasty, *Clin. Orthop.* **319**, 77–84.

Collier, J.P., Bauer, T.W., Bloebanm, R.D. 1992a. Results of implant retrieval from post-mortem specimens in patients with well-functioning, long-term total hip replacement, *Clin. Orthop.* **274**, 97–112.

Collier, J.P., Mayor, M.B., Chae, J.C. 1992b. Mechanism of failure of modular prostheses, *Clin. Orthop.* **285**, 129–139.

Collier, J.P., Surprenant, V.A., Jensen, R.E. 1992c. Corrosion between the components of modular femoral hip prostheses, *J. Bone Jt. Surg.* **74B**, 511–517.

Cook, S.D., Barrack, R.L., Thomas, K.A., Haddad, R.J. 1988a. Quantitative analysis of tissue growth into human porous total hip components, *J. Arthroplasty* **3**, 249–262.

Cook, S.D., Thomas, K.A., Haddad, R.J. Jr. 1988b. Histologic analysis of retrieved human porous-coated total joint components, *Clin. Orthop.* **234**, 90–101.

Cook, S.D., Barrack, R.L., Thomas, K.A. 1991. Tissue growth into porous primary and revision femoral stems, *J. Arthroplasty* **6** (suppl.), 37–46.

Cook, S.D., Barrack, R.L., Gregory, C.B. 1994. Wear and corrosion of modular interfaces in total hip replacements, *Clin. Orthop.* **298**, 80–88.

Cooney, W.P. III, Beckenbauen, R.D., Linscheid, R.L. 1984. Total wrist arthroplasty, *Clin. Orthop.* **187**, 121–128.

Coventry, M.B. 1991. Historical perspective of hip arthroplasty, in: *Reconstructive Surgery of the Joints* (B.F. Morrey, ed.), pp. 875–882, Churchill Livingstone, New York.

Coventry, M.B., Finermann, G.A.M., Riley, L.N., Turner, R.H., Upshaw, J.E. 1972. A new geometric knee for total knee arthoplasty, *Clin. Orthop.* **83**, 157–162.

Crowninshield, R.D., Tolbert, J.R. 1983. Cement strain measurement surrounding loose and well-fixed femoral component stems, *J. Biomat. Res.* **17**, 819–828.

Crowninshield, R.D., Johnston, R.C., Andrews, J.G., Brand, R.A. 1978. A biomechanical investigation of the human hip, *J. Biomech.* **11**, 75–85.

Crowninshield, R.D., Brand, R.A., Johnston, R.C., Milroy, J.C. 1980. The effect of femoral stem cross-sectional geometry on cement stresses in total hip reconstruction, *Clin. Orthop.* **146**, 71–77.

Crowninshield, R.D., Hawkins, M., Price, H. 1985. Poly(methylmethacrylate) precoating of orthopaedic implants, in: *Advanced Concepts in Total Hip Replacement* (W.H. Harris, ed.), pp. 67–78, Slack Inc., Thorofare, N.J.

Cuckler, J.M., Bearcroft, J., Asgian, C.M. 1995. Femoral head technologies to reduce polyethylene wear in total hip arthroplasty, *Clin. Orthop.* **317**, 57–63.

D'Antonio, J.A., Capello, W.N., Jaffe, W.L. 1992. Hydroxyapatite-coated hip implant: multicenter three-year clinical and roentgenographic results, *Clin. Orthop.* **285**, 102–115.

Duparc, J., Massin, P. 1992. Results of 203 total hip replacement using a smooth, cementless femoral component, *J. Bone Jt. Surg.* **74B**, 251–256.

Engh, C.A., Bobyn, J.D. 1987. The influence of stem size and extent of porous coating on femoral bone resorption after primary cementless hip arthroplasty, *Clin. Orthop.* **231**, 7–28.

Engh, C.A., Bobyn, J.D., Glassman, A.H. 1987. Porous coated hip replacement, *J. Bone Jt. Surg.* **69B**, 45–55.

Engh, C.A., Hooten, J.P., Zettl-Schaffer, K.F., Ghaffarpour, M., McGovern, T.F., Bobyn, J.D. 1995. Evaluation of bone ingrowth in proximally and extensively porous-coated anatomic medullary locking prostheses retrieved at autopsy, *J. Bone Jt. Surg.* **77A**, 903–910.

Fowler, J.L., Gie, G.A., Lee, A.J.C., Ling, R.S.M. 1988. Experience with the Exeter total hip replacement since 1970, *Orthop. Clin. North Am.* **19**, 477–489.

Freeman, M.A.R., Cameron, H.U., Brown, G.C. 1978. Cemented double cup arthroplasty of the hip: a 5 year experience with ICLH prosthesis, *Clin. Orthop.* **134**, 45–52.

Galante, J.O., Rostoker, W., Lueck, R., Ray, R.D. 1971. Sintered fiber metal composites as a basis for attachment of implant to bone, *J. Bone Jt. Surg.* **53A**, 101–114.

Geesink, R.G.T., De Groot, K., Klein, C.P.A.T. 1987. Chemical implant fixation using hydroxyl-apatite coatings: the development of a human total hip prothesis for chemical fixation to bone using hydroxyl-apatite coatings on titanium substrates, *Clin. Orthop.* **225**, 147–170.

Gérard, Y., Ségal, P., Bedoucha, J.S. 1974. L'arthroplastie de la hanche par cupules couplées, *Rev. Chir. Orthop.* **60** (suppl. 2), 281–289.

Gunston, F.H. 1971. Polycentric knee arthroplasty: prosthetic simulation of normal knee movement, *J. Bone Jt. Surg.* **53B**, 272–277.

Hahn, H., Palich, W. 1970. Preliminary evaluation of porous metal surfaced titanium for orthopedic implants, *J. Biomed. Mater. Res.* **4**, 571–577.

Harris, W.H. 1985. The Harris precoat total hip replacement system, in: *Advanced Concepts in Total Hip Replacement* (W.H. Harris, ed.), pp. 85–98, Slack Inc., Thorofare, N.J.

Haynes, D.R., Rogers, S.D., Ha, Y.S. 1993. The differences in toxicity and release of bone-resorbing mediators induced by titanium and cobalt-chromium alloy wear particles, *J. Bone J. Surg.* **75A**, 825–834.

Howie, D.W. 1990. Tissue response in relation to type of wear particles around failed hip arthroplasties, *J. Arthroplasty* **5**, 337–348.

Huiskes, R., Weinans, H., van Rietbergen, B. 1992. The relationship between stress shielding and bone resorption around total hip stems and the effect of flexible materials, *Clin. Orthop.* **274**, 124–134.

Isaac, G.H., Wroblewsky, B.M., Atkinson, J.R., Dowson, D. 1992. A tribological study of retrieved hip prostheses, *Clin. Orthop.* **276**, 115–125.

Jacobs, J.J., Urban, R.M., Gilbert, J.L., Skipor, A.K., Black, J., Jasty, M., Galante, J.O. 1995. Local and distant products from modularity, *Clin. Orthop.* **319**, 94–105.

Jasty, M., Rubash, H.E., Paiement, G.D., Bragdon, C.R., Parr, J., Harris, W.M. 1992. Porous-coated uncemented components in experimental total hip arthroplasty in dogs: effect of plasma-sprayed calcium phosphate coatings on bone ingrowth, *Clin. Orthop.* **280**, 300–309.

Jones, L.C., Hungerford, D.S. 1987. Cement disease, *Clin. Orthop.* **225**, 192–206.

Judet, J., Judet, R. 1950. The use of an artificial femoral head for arthroplasty of the hip joint, *J. Bone Jt. Surg.* **32B**, 166–173.

Judet, R., Siguier, M., Brumpt, D., Judet, Th. 1978. Prothèse totale de hanche en poro-metal sans ciment, *Rev. Chir. Orthop.* **64** (suppl. 2), 14–21.

Kang, J.D., McKerman, D.J., Kruger, M. 1991. Ingrowth and formation of bone in defects in an uncemented fiber-metal total hip replacement model in dogs (Review), *J. Bone Jt. Surg.* **73A**, 93–105.

Knahr, M., Salzer, M., Frank, P. 1984. Experience with uncemented polyethylene acetabular prostheses, in: *The Cementless Fixation of Hip Endoprostheses* (E.W. Morscher, ed.), pp. 205–210, Springer-Verlag, Heidelberg.

Lee, A.J.C., Ling, R.S.M. 1974. A device to improve the extrusion of bone cement into the bone of the acetabulum in the replacement of the hip joint, *Biomed. Eng.* **9**, 522–524.

Lee, J.M., Salvati, E.A., Betts, F. 1992. Size of metallic and polyethylene debris particles in failed cemented total hip replacements, *J. Bone Jt. Surg.* **74B**, 380–384.

Lewis, J.L., Askew, M.J., Wixson, R.L., Kramer, G.M., Tarr, R.R. 1984. The influence of prosthetic stem stiffness and a calcar collar on stresses in the proximal end of the femur with a cemented femoral component, *J. Bone Jt. Surg.* **66A**, 280–286.

Lexer, E. 1908. Uber Gelenktransportation, *Med. Klin.* **4**, 817–820.

Linder, L., Hansson, H.A. 1983. Ultra-structural aspects of the interface between bone and cement in man, *J. Bone Jt. Surg.* **65B**, 646–649.

Ling, R.S.M. 1992. Clinical experience with primary cemented total hip arthroplasty, *Chir. Org. Mov.* **77**, 373–381.

Lord, G.A., Hardy, J.R., Kummer, F.J. 1979. An uncemented total hip replacement experimental study and review of 300 madreporique arthroplasties, *Clin. Orthop.* **141**, 2–16.

Luo Zong-Ping. 1996. Finite element analysis theoretical prediction of bony response to joint replacement, in: *Reconstructive Surgery of the Joints* (B.F. Morrey, ed.), pp. 13–18, Churchill Livingstone, New York.

Markolf, K.L., Amstutz, H.C., Hirscholwitz, D.L. 1980. The effect of calcar contact on femoral component micromovement, *J. Bone Jt. Surg.* **62A**, 1315–1323.

Mathiesen, E.B., Lingren, J.U., Blomgren, G.G. 1991. Corrosion of modular hip prostheses, *J. Bone Jt. Surg.* **73B**, 569–575.

Mathys, R., Mathys, R. Jr. 1984. The use of polymers for endoprosthetic components, in: *The Cementless Fixation of Hip Endoprostheses* (E.W. Morscher, ed.), pp. 71–80, Springer-Verlag, Heidelberg.

McKee, G.K., Watson-Farrar, J. 1966. Replacement of arthritic hips by the McKee-Farrar prosthesis, *J. Bone Jt. Surg.* **48B**, 245–259.

McKellop, H.A., Campbell, P., Sang-Hyun, P. 1995. The origin of submicron polyethylene wear debris in total hip arthroplasty, *Clin. Orthop.* **311**, 3–20.

Miller, J., Ahmed, A.M. 1985. Precoating-concept and results of testing, in: *Advanced Concepts in Total Hip Replacement* (W.E. Harris, ed.), pp. 79–84, Slack Inc., Thorofare, N.J.

Mittelmeier, H. 1974. Zementlose verankerung von Endoprothesen nach dem Tragrippemprinzip, *Z. Orthop.* **112**, 27–33.

Moore, A.T., Bohlman, H.R. 1943. Metal hip joint: a case report, *J. Bone Jt. Surg.* **25**, 688–693.

Morrey, B.F., Adams, R.A. 1996. The elbow: Semiconstrained devices, in: *Reconstructive Surgery of the Joints* (B.F. Morrey, ed.), Churchill Livingstone, New York.

Morscher, E.W., Dick, W., Kermen, V. 1982. Cementless fixation of polyethylene acetabular component in total hip arthroplasty, *Arch. Orthop. Surg.* **99**, 223–230.

Muller, M.E. 1970. Total hip prosthesis, *Clin. Orthop.* **72**, 46–68.

Muller, M.E. 1995. The benefits of metal on metal total hip replacements, *Clin. Orthop.* **311**, 54–59.

Neer, C.S. II. 1955. Articular replacement for the humerale head, *J. Bone Jt. Surg.* **37A**, 215–228.

Neer, C.S. II. 1964. Articular replacement for the humerale head, *J. Bone Jt. Surg.* **46A**, 1607–1610.

Neer, C.S. II. 1974. Replacement arthroplasty for glenohumeral osteo-arthritis, *J. Bone Jt. Surg.* **56A**, 1–13.

Neer, C.S. II, Watson, K.L., Stanton, F.J. 1982. Recent experience in total shoulder replacement, *J. Bone Jt. Surg.* **64A**, 319–337.

Ohlin, A., Johnel, O., Lerner, U.H. 1990. The pathogenesis of loosening of total hip arthroplasties. The production of factors by periprosthetic tissues that stimulate in vitro bone resorption, *Clin. Orthop.* **253**, 287–296.

Oonishi, H., Yamamoto, M., Ishimaru, H. 1989. The effect of hydroxyapatite coating on bone growth into porous titanium alloy implants, *J. Bone Jt. Surg.* **71B**, 213–216.

Paltrinieri, M., Trentani, C.A. 1971. Variante di artroprotesi d'anca, *Chir. Org. Mov.* LX, Fasc. II **60**, 85–95.

Parhoferf, R., Monch, W. 1984. Experience with revision arthroplastics for failed cemented total hip replacements using uncemented Lord and PM prostheses, in: *The Cementless Fixation of Hip Endoprostheses* (W.H. Harris, ed.), pp. 275–278, Slack Inc., Thorofare, N.J.

Pedersen, D.R., Crowninshield, R.D., Brand, R.A., Johnston, R.C. 1982. An axisymmetric model of acetabular components in total hip arthroplasty, *J. Biomech.* **15**, 305–315.

Pidhorz, L.E., Urban, R.M., Jacobs, J.J. 1993. A quantitative study of bone and soft tissues in cementless porous-coated acetabular components retrieved at autopsy, *J. Arthroplasty* **8**, 213–225.

Pilliar, R.M., Cameron, H.U., Macnab, I. 1975. Porous surface layered prosthetic devices, *Biomed. Eng.* **10**, 126–131.

Pilliar, R.M., Lee, J.M., Maniatopolous, S.C. 1986. Observation on the effect of movement on bone ingrowth into porous-surfaced implants, *Clin. Orthop.* **208**, 108–113.

Raab, S., Ahmed, A.M., Provan, J.W. 1981. The quasistatic and fatigue performance of the implant/bone cement interface, *J. Biomat. Res.* **15**, 159–182.

Robertson, D.M., Pierre, L.M., Chahal, R. 1976. Preliminary observations of bone ingrowth into porous materials, *J. Biomed. Mater. Res.* **10**, 335–344.

Sandborn, P.M., Cook, S.D., Anderson, R.C. 1987. The effect of surgical fit on bone growth into porous-coated implants, *Trans. Orthop. Rec. Soc.* **12**, 217–222.

Sandborn, P.M., Cook, S.D., Spires, S.W., Kester, M.A. 1988. Tissue response to porous-coated implants lacking initial bone apposition, *J. Arthroplasty* **3**, 337–346.

Santavirta, S., Konttinen, Y.T., Bergroth, V., Eskola, A., Tallroth, K., Lindholm, T.S. 1990. Aggressive granulomatous lesions associated with hip arthroplasty. Immunopathological studies, *J. Bone Jt. Surg.* **72A**, 252–258.

Schmalzried, T.P., Jasty, M., Harris, W.H. 1992. Periprosthetic bone loss in total hip arthroplasty: Polyethylene wear debris and the concept of the effective joint space, *J. Bone Jt. Surg.* **74A**, 849–863.

Shaw, J.A., Bailey, J.H., Bruno, A., Greer, R.B. 1990. Threaded acetabular components for primary and revision total hip arthroplasty, *J. Arthroplasty* **5**, 201–215.

Smith-Petersen, M.N. 1939. Arthroplasty of the hip: a new method, *J. Bone Jt. Surg.* **21**, 269–288.

Sobelle, K., Toksvig-Larsen, S. Gelineck, J. 1993. Migration of hydroxyapatite coated femoral prostheses: a roentgen stero-photogrammetric study, *J. Bone Jt. Surg.* **75B**, 681–687.

Stauffer, R.N., Segal, N.M. 1981. Total knee arthroplasty: four years' experience, *Clin. Orthop.* **160**, 217–221.

Swanson, A.B. 1973. *Flexible Implant Resection Arthoplasty in the Hand and Extremities*, C.V. Mosby, St. Louis.

Tallroth, K., Slätis, P., Ylien, P. 1993. Loosening of threaded acetabular components, *J. Arthroplasty* **8**, 581–584.

Thomas, B.J., Amstutz, H.C., Campbell, P. 1991. Cementless acetabular reconstruction, in: *Hip Arthroplasty* (H.C. Amstutz, ed.), pp. 271–283, Churchill Livingstone, New York.

Thomas, K.A., Cook, S.D., Haddad, R.J., Kaj, J.F., Jarcho, M. 1989. Biologic response to hydroxyapatite coated titanium hips: a preliminary study in dogs, *J. Arthroplasty* **4**, 43–53.

Thompson, F.R. 1954. Two and a half years experience with a vitallium intramedullary hip prosthesis, *J. Bone Jt. Surg.* **36A**, 489–502.

Trousdale, R.T., Cabanela, M.E. 1996. Uncemented acetabular components, in: *Reconstructive Surgery of the Joints* (B.F. Morrey, ed.), pp. 961–978, Churchill Livingstone, New York.

Van Syckle, P.B., Walker, P.S. 1980. Parametric analysis of design criteria for acetabular components of surface replacement hip design, *Trans. Orthop. Res. Soc.* **5**, 292–298.

Vasu, R., Carter, D. R., Harris, W.H. 1982. Stress distribution in the acetabular region-I before and after total hip joint replacement, *J. Biomed.* **15**, 155–164.

Wagner, H. 1978. Surface replacement arthroplasty of the hip, *Clin. Orthop.* **134**, 102–130.

Weightman, B., Freeman, M.A.R., Revell, P.A., Braden, M., Albrektsson, B.E.J., Carlson, L.V. 1987. The mechanical properties of cement and loosening of the femoral component of hip replacements, *J. Bone Jt. Surg.* **69B**, 558–564.

Zweymüller, K., Semlitsch, M. 1982. Concept and material properties of a cementless hip prosthesis system with Al_2O_3 ceramic balls heads and wrought Ti-6Al-4V Stems, *Arch. Orthop. Trauma Surg.* **100**, 229–236.

17

Knee Joint Replacements

Dante Ronca and Giuseppe Guida

17.1. Introduction

Total knee prostheses have evolved over the last 25 years from the hinged prostheses to the current mechanically superior anatomic designs. Initially, a hinge replacement appeared to be a simple and efficacious solution; but the lack of rotation and abduction–adduction produces excessive forces at the bone–cement interface, which can lead to loosening of the implant. However, this type of prosthesis represented the first step in the knee joint arthroplasty, which is still utilized in case of severely damaged knees. The interest in total knee prostheses has resulted in a proliferation of prosthetic designs. At present, there is a multitude of implants, whose majority is a modification of the total condylar prosthesis. Modern prosthetic designs cover the cut surfaces of the femur, tibia, and patella, transferring joint loads to the underlying cancellous bone such as that which occurs in a normal knee (Figure 17.1). Unlike the hip joint, which is relatively favorable for prosthetic design, the complexities of motion and stability at the knee provide a different and more demanding challenge. The total hip arthroplasty (THA) design has a concave-down cup and a completely congruent ball. Muscular forces and resultants about the hip cause the joint to move in a quite simple nonseparating fashion. On the contrary, due to the absence of a unique center of rotation, the total knee arthroplasty (TKA) design has a highly incongruent metal femoral condylar component which articulates with a planar or mildly concave-up polymeric tibial component. Like other joint prostheses, TKA poses many problems such as wear and corrosion; but, in addition, there is a greater possibility of infection, because the prosthesis is near the skin. Therefore, the prosthetic

Dante Ronca and Giuseppe Guida • Istituto di Clinica Ortopedica, Università di Napoli, via S. Andrea delle Dame 4, 80138 Napoli, Italy.

Integrated Biomaterials Science, edited by R. Barbucci. Kluwer Academic/Plenum Publishers, New York, 2002.

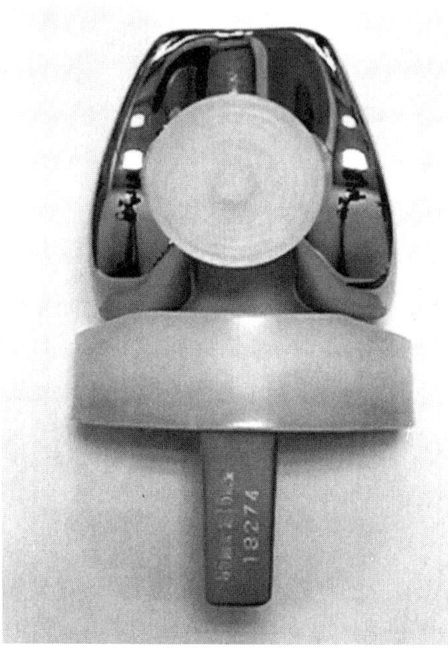

Figure 17.1. The anatomically graduated components (AGC) total knee prosthesis.

joint must not only be able to provide the motions and to transmit functional loads that occur in a normal knee, but also it must have long life. In other words, it needs to avoid disruption of the interface between the implant and the bone and also to minimize articulating surface damage. This event generates debris, whose accumulation in the soft tissue surrounding the joint may be responsible for late infection and implant loosening. Formal gait analysis has been used to analyze gait patterns after TKA. Most authors concur that arthroplasty results in improvement of gait function but does not return normal joint kinematics (Andriacchi *et al.*, 1982). It is widely accepted that knee arthroplasty, such as hip arthroplasty, does not restore normal gait, but simply replaces an abnormal arthritic joint with an abnormal artificial joint which just makes the patient free of pain (Li and Ritter, 1995). Nevertheless, considerable progress has been made. In the last 25 years, total knee prosthesis has proven to be an efficacious procedure not only to relieve pain due to arthritis, but also to restore the stability and mobility of a damaged knee (Font-Rodriguez *et al.*, 1997).

17.2. History

17.2.1. Total Knee Arthroplasty

In 1890, Glück (Glück, 1890) described a system of total joint arthroplasty with prosthetic units made of ivory and stabilized by cement made of colophony, pumice, and plaster of Paris (gypsum). Although the concept was fascinating, the materials of prosthetic components and cement necessary for their fixation to bone were absolutely inadequate and unsuitable. In 1958, MacIntosh (MacIntosh, 1958) placed an acrylic tibial plateau prosthesis similar to that of Jansen in Denmark (Riley, 1976). Metal tibial plateau replacement prostheses were used by McKeever in 1960 (McKeever, 1960) and by MacIntosh in 1966 (MacIntosh, 1966). In 1964, Aufranc, Jones, and Kermond performed the first replacement of the distal femur, using a bicondylar cap anchored to the shaft by a long metal intramedullary stem (Jones *et al.*, 1967). The greatest advances in knee arthroplasty and the development of nonhinged total knee replacement were due to the work of John Charnley and G.K. McKee in using methylmethacrylate to fix the prosthetic components to the bone and utilizing the high-density polyethylene, stainless steel, and chrome–cobalt alloys as suitable materials for total joint replacement prostheses (Charnley, 1960; McKee and Watson-Farrar, 1966; Charnley, 1970). In 1968, Gunston designed and performed the first nonhinged total knee that was the first polycentric knee arthroplasty simulating normal knee movement (Figure 17.2). This polycentric knee arthroplasty consisted of two semicircular runners of stainless steel (or chrome–cobalt alloy) cemented into slots in the femoral condyles articulating with two grooved tracks of high-density polyethylene cemented into the tibial plateau (Gunston, 1973). In 1969, the "St Georg unit" was first used. It was a four-piece unit in which the metal femoral component contoured the femoral condyles and articulated with a flat polyethylene tibial block which replaced the articular surface of the tibia (Engelbrecht and Zippel, 1973). In 1970, Freeman and Swanson performed their first knee arthroplasty, using a metal on polyethylene bearing with cemented components. This prosthesis represented the first two-component condylar type of arthroplasty (Freeman *et al.*, 1973). In 1971, the geometric total knee arthroplasty, designed by Coventry, Riley, Finerman, Turner, and Upshaw (Coventry *et al.*, 1972), was first utilized (Figure 17.3). The plastic tibial component, consisting of two halves connected by an anterior bar, had an articular curvature designed to mate with the femoral component. In 1971, Insall, Ranawat, and Walker implanted two different kinds of prostheses for treating arthritis: the unicondylar prosthesis and the duocondylar prosthesis. The unicondylar prosthesis was an

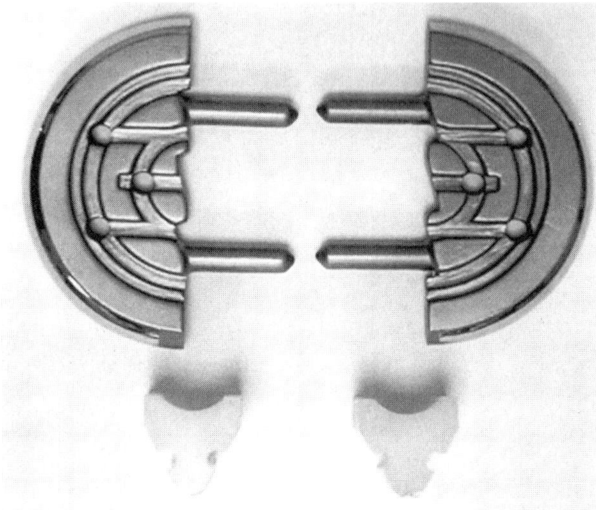

Figure 17.2. The polycentric knee prosthesis.

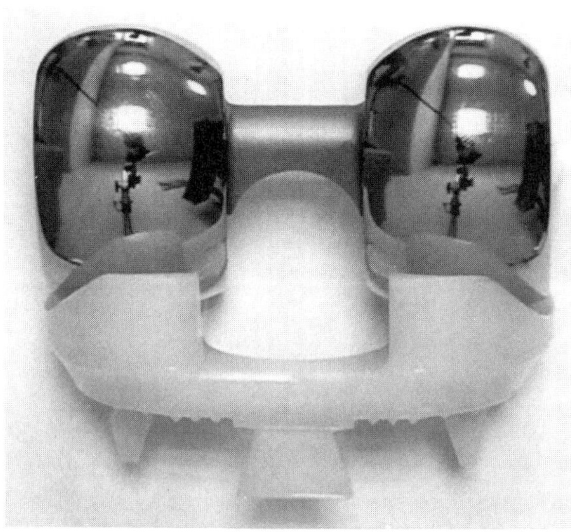

Figure 17.3. The geometric prosthesis.

anatomically designed replacement for either the medial or the lateral femoral tibial articulation. The femoral component was made of vitallium; the tibial component was made of polyethylene (Insall and Walker, 1976). The duocondylar prosthesis had the femoral component similar in shape to that of the unicondylar model, except that there was no anterior flange and instead the halves were connected by an anterior cross bar. The two separate tibial components were identical to those of the unicondylar prosthesis. In 1973, the first modified duocondylar prosthesis was implanted. This new prosthesis, the Total Condylar Knee (Insall *et al.*, 1976a), required four flat bone cuts (three in the femur and one in the tibia), cruciate resection, and was provided with a new patellar component to articulate with the femoral component (Figure 17.4). In 1973, Marmor reported his preliminary experience in 39 patients with the "modular knee" arthroplasty. The basic idea of the femoral component was to replace the articular cartilage that has been

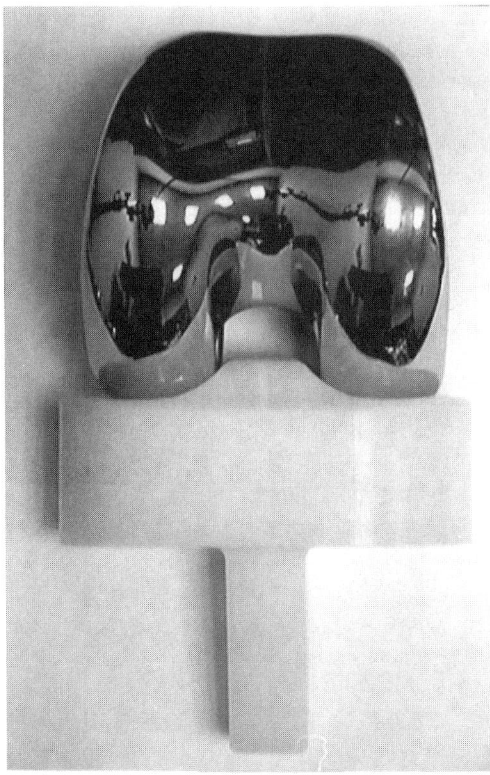

Figure 17.4. The total condylar prosthesis.

lost without destroying the strong cortical bone over the femoral condyle (Marmor, 1973). In 1973, Mattheus presented the spherocentric knee, designed to allow triaxial rotation and minimize torsional loading at the prosthesis–cement–bone interface. This prosthesis had a contained ball-and-socket joint that represented an attempt to achieve the stability of a hinge joint without the disadvantage of a fixed hinge (Matthews *et al.*, 1973). In 1977, Freeman implanted his first uncemented tibial component in which polyethylene was in direct contact with bone (Blaha *et al.*, 1982). In 1978, after combined studies between Goodfellow and O'Connor, the "Oxford knee" prosthesis was implanted, consisting of two separate spherical metal femoral components fixed with cement. The tibial components were flat metal plates. Between the femoral and tibial components, sliding polyethylene menisci were free to move anteroposteriorly on the tibial component and rotationally on the femoral component. The resultant articulation permitted flexion/extension at the bearing between the meniscus and the femur and axial tibial rotation between the menisci and the tibial component (Goodfellow and O'Connor, 1978). In 1980, Freeman, in conjunction with Samuelson, modified his implant (then known as the ICLH prosthesis) to form the Freeman–Samuelson prosthesis.

17.2.2. Hinged Knee Arthroplasty

In 1947, Judet and co-workers (Judet *et al.*, 1947) designed the first hinged knee replacement made of acrylic, which was never applied in clinical practice.

In 1951, Walldius (Walldius, 1954) performed his first acrylic hinged knee replacement which, made of metal since 1958, had a good clinical success. These fixed hinge joints frequently loosened or broke because of heavy mechanical strain in a joint such as the knee with multicentric axes of motion. The hinge prosthesis replaces both the femoral and tibial articular surface and has great intrinsic stability. However, unlike a normal knee, mechanical hinges allow no motion in the frontal plane (abduction–adduction) and no torsional motion. Therefore, forces which tend to produce torsion or abduction–adduction are entirely transmitted to the implant–bone interface with great possibility of loosening, bone resorption, and implant failure. The hinge prosthesis has stops at the end of flexion and extension, which generate high peaking impact loads, so contributing to implant–bone interface breakdown. This is in contrast to the behavior of total hip prostheses, which allow free rotation in all directions without mechanical motion stop. A prosthetic joint which permits only flexion–extension cannot reproduce the complex knee function, but remains merely a hinge. Moreover, the hinge prosthesis causes an unphysiological flexion

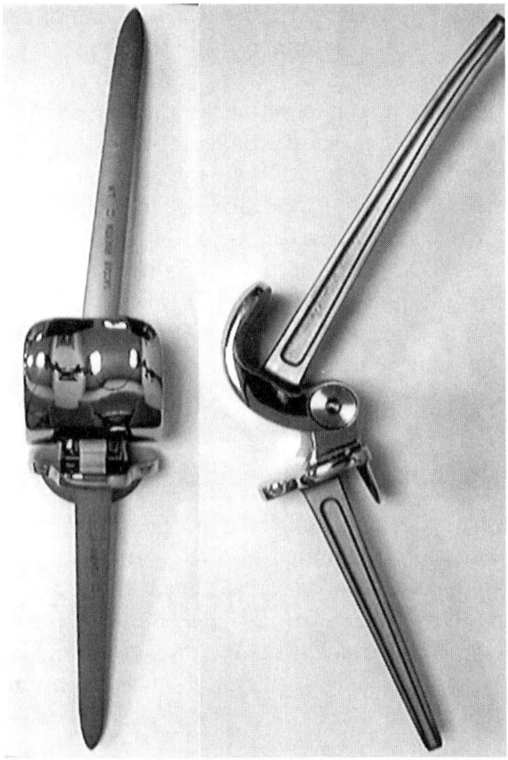

Figure 17.5. The Guepar prosthesis, sagittal (left) and lateral (right) view.

arc and prevents the axial rotational adjustments which occur normally during motion of the knee and gait. This anomaly increases the forces at the patellofemoral joint during motion and may be responsible for the high incidence of patellar-tracking problems reported with the use of constrained hinge prostheses. In 1970, the Guepar hinged prosthesis was used. It was a fully constrained prosthesis, developed in Paris by a group of orthopedic surgeons, providing motion in a fixed axis without rotation (Figure 17.5). The axle is placed posteriorly in a rough approximation of the axis of rotation of the normal knee. The intramedullary stems are about fifteen centimeters long, and the femoral component is provided by a patellar surface. It has a 7° offset between the femoral and tibial stems to provide physiologic valgus alignment. A Sylastic buffer lessens the impact in full extension. The femoral and tibial components are articulated after insertion with an axle which is secured by spreading flanges on the lateral side by means of a special c-clamp. There are left and right prostheses, but only one size. All models must be fixed to the bone by means of cement. The hinge designs of total knee replacements routinely sacrifice the collateral ligaments, whose function is replaced with a linked component. The hinge prosthesis itself provides absolute stability in all planes without reliance on the soft tissues. Due to the rigidity of metal-to-metal hinge, much of the torsional load is transferred directly to the interfaces between the bone, cement, and prosthesis. As a consequence, the intramedullary stems must be long and fixed with cement; therefore, such an implant is not conservative of bone stock. These aspects can lead to a high complication rate, including loosening and implant failure (Jones *et al.*, 1979; Ranawat *et al.*, 1976). Today, this prosthesis continues to be implanted everywhere in the world, in case of both malignant diseases and arthritis, having been modified from the original in few details.

17.2.3. Unicompartmental Knee Arthroplasty

The first implants introduced to treat unicompartmental disease were, in 1958, the MacIntosh (MacIntosh, 1958) and McKeever (McKeever, 1960), in which only the tibia was resurfaced. Since that time, numerous prosthetic designs have been introduced and unicompartmental knee arthroplasty has demonstrated satisfactory results in those patients who fit its narrow indications: age over 55, competent ligament, arthritis involving only one compartment, light weight, and low demand (Figure 17.6).

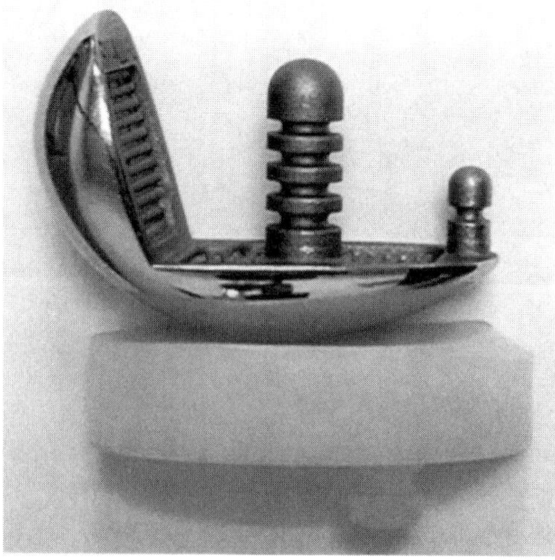

Figure 17.6. Unicompartmental knee prosthesis (Duracon, UNI).

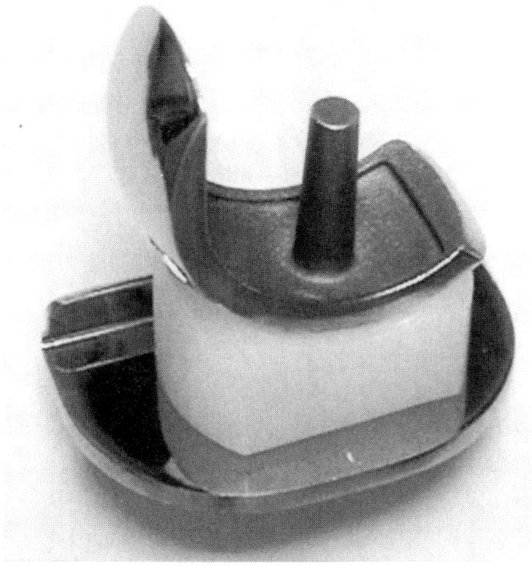

Figure 17.7. The Unicompartmental Oxford Meniscal Knee prosthesis.

In 1972, Marmor expanded the unicompartmental implant to one replacing both the proximal tibial and distal femoral articular surfaces. He reported 70% satisfactory results with an average 11-year follow-up period in 60 patients. The failures were due to progression of disease to the other compartments and tibial component failure. The initial tibial tray was thin polyethylene, which resulted in a high rate of fragmentation and subsidence because of poor load transfer properties. To eliminate this complication the thickness of the polyethylene of the tibial tray was increased from 6 to 8 mm and metal backing was added (Marmor, 1988). Loosening of femoral component is rare. Various designs have been used, most with multiple fixation pegs and a curved bone–implant interface.

In 1978, Goodfellow and O'Connor implanted a new original knee prosthesis, called "Oxford knee," consisting of two separate spherical metal femoral components fixed with cement (Figure 17.7). The tibial components were flat metal plates also fixed with cement. Interposed between the metal femoral and tibial components were high-density-polyethylene meniscal bearings, which were concave superiorly and flat inferiorly, creating two joints which reproduce the rolling and sliding components of free movement, respectively. The natural menisci move backward and forward during flexion and extension, as do the meniscal bearings of the prosthesis. This prosthesis requires the presence of all ligamentous structures and removes very little of the skeleton (Goodfellow and O'Connor, 1978). The problem of excessive wear in the noncongruent components of two-part prostheses is avoided by having articulating surfaces which are congruent, with large areas of contact and low rate of wear. The unique feature of the design is that it provides an entirely unconstrained joint in which rotation and translation are completely unrestricted but at the same time achieves perfect congruity between the articular components in all positions.

17.3. The Knee: Anatomical, Functional, and Structural Considerations

The knee is the largest and most complex of the human joints, whose purpose is not only to accept and transfer loads among the femur, tibia, and patella, but even to dissipate loads generated at the end of the long mechanical lever arms of the femur and tibia (Winter, 1983). Due to the design of tibial plateaus and femoral condyles, asymmetrical moving parts, the knee is an unsteady joint which needs a complex peripheral system of stabilization; this is represented by various ligaments and muscles, which act as nonrigid, adaptive, passive linkages and active control mechanisms, respectively. The knee presents two kinds of movement: flexion–extension, in the sagittal plane, that reaches about 150°; rotation, in the horizontal plane, that reaches 10°–15° in full extension. During flexion and extension, the knee shows its typical combined gliding and rolling movements. The tibial plateaus are relatively flat, so the contact between the femoral condyles and the tibial plateaus occurs over a small area. The medial area is larger than the lateral area with an average medial to lateral ratio of 1.6 (Kettelkamp and Nasca, 1973). The articular cartilage and menisci represent bearings with the transmission. For functions of daily living, such as walking and ascending or descending stairs, the value of contact forces between the femur and the tibia has been estimated to range from 2.7 to 4.9 times the body weight (Paul, 1976; Walker, 1978).

As a consequence, for an individual who weighs 70 kilograms the femoral–tibial contact force varies from 280 to 450 kilograms. The patella with respect to the femur moves in the sagittal plane and its motion is determined by the geometry of its articulating surfaces and the patellar groove of the femur. The distal femur and the proximal tibia consist of cancellous bone and an outer cortical shell. The properties (density and elastic modulus) of cancellous bone vary according to the transmission of the loads. Presently, the components of total knee prostheses are designed to cap the cut surfaces of the femur, tibia, and patella; in other words, they are surface replacements and do not rely on intramedullary stems for fixation (Figure 17.8). So, joint loads are transferred directly

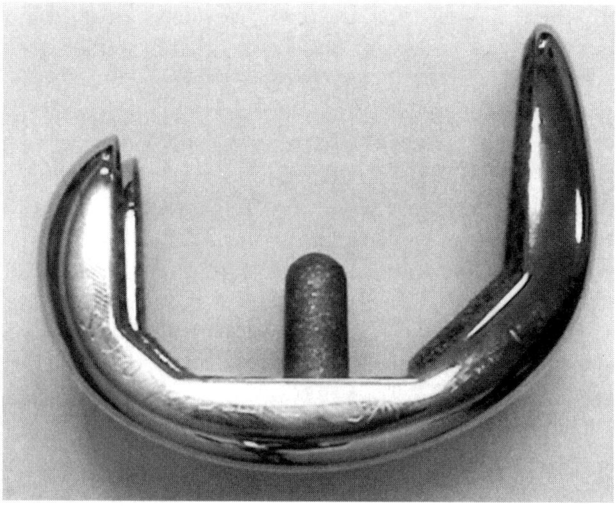

Figure 17.8. Contemporary metal femoral component designed to cap the cut surfaces of the femur.

to the underlying cancellous bone of the distal femur and proximal tibia. This situation is very similar to the distribution of joint loads in the normal knee.

17.4. Polyethylene

17.4.1. Contact Stress, Congruency, and Conformity

While the high-density polyethylene (HDPE) shows excellent wear resistance when used to fabricate total hip replacements, it undergoes much more rapid deterioration in the form of abrasive wear and creep when employed in TKA. The ball and socket configuration of the hip is highly conforming, and load transfer occurs over a large contact area, which results in small stresses. Experimental and theoretical studies have shown that contact stresses are greater for nonconforming surfaces such as knee prostheses than for conforming surfaces such as hip prostheses. In the much less conforming knee prostheses, the contact areas are smaller; consequently, the stresses are greater. Therefore, the surface damage on total knee components has been found to be greater than that observed on total hip components (Wright *et al.*, 1985). As a consequence of contact stress between the metal and polyethylene components, several damage modes including wear, permanent deformation (creep), and fracture in the polyethylene components may occur. Debris resulting from damage to the surface of a polyethylene implant has been demonstrated to contribute to loosening of total joint arthroplasty (Wroblewski, 1979).

The layer of polyethylene in contact with the metal component undergoes compressive stress in a direction perpendicular to the surface, whose maximum value occurs at the center of the contact area. Near the edge of contact, the polyethylene is stretched and undergoes tensile stress. Moreover, the indentation of the metal component causes distortion of the polyethylene in directions that are tangent to the surface. These observations suggest that surface damage is related to the cyclic contact stresses on the polyethylene and that the pits and delamination seen in tibial components are due to fatigue loading, resulting from the movement on the contact area between the femoral and tibial components during functional loading of the knee. During one gait cycle, a point on the surface is subjected to a cyclic stress sequence consisting of both compressive stresses and tensile stresses. Recent results for fatigue tests of ultrahigh molecular weight polyethylene (UHMWHD-PE) foretold failure in fewer than 1,000,000 cycles for such a range of stress. This predicted number of cycles shrinks to 100,000 in case the load is borne by one condyle (Weightman and Light, 1985). Most contemporary designs of TKA have articulating surfaces that are nonconforming, particularly some cruciate-retaining implants. Tibial surfaces of these implants are nearly flat to allow the posterior cruciate ligament to function properly. Since the contact stresses increase with decreasing conformity, in these nonconforming implants they would be greater than those reported in more conforming prostheses. Many studies showed less surface damage in the posterior stabilized designs than the less congruent posterior cruciate ligament-retaining implants (Feng *et al.*, 1995; Hirakawa *et al.*, 1996). Results of recent clinical and radiological evaluations demonstrated the least failure rate with a survival rate of >98% at 10 years in a nonconforming posterior cruciate ligament-sparing prosthesis (Knutson *et al.*, 1994). The tibial component of this prosthesis was compression-molded high molecular weight polyethylene; its surfaces had a slight dish anterior to posterior but were basically flat. Investigators hypothesized that the success of this kind of prosthesis depended on the quality and preparation of the polyethylene utilized for the tibial component (Ritter *et al.*, 1995).

Pitting and delamination are the main modes of surface damage (Figure 17.9). Pits are caused by surface or subsurface cracks, which later propagate into the material and toward the surface, respectively. Delamination is due to subsurface cracks, which continue to propagate tangent to the surface. Propagation of surface cracks would be associated with cyclic tensile and compressive stresses acting tangent to the surface, while propagation of subsurface cracks would be associated with shear stresses (Bartel

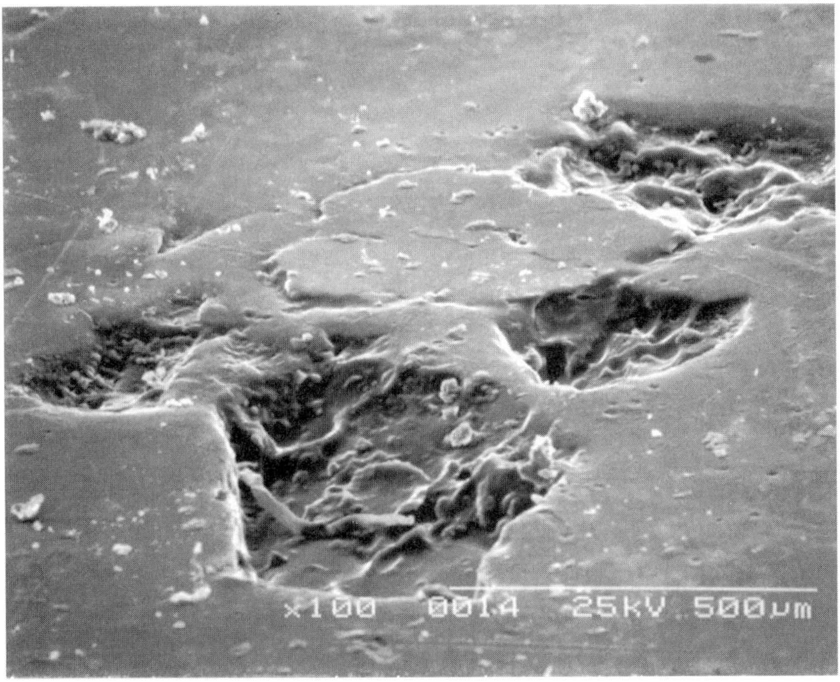

Figure 17.9. Pits and delamination of articular surface of a retrieved polyethylene tibial plateau (scanning electron photomicrograph).

et al., 1986, 1995). Contact stress could be reduced by increasing the conformity between the femoral and tibial components in both the anteroposterior and the lateromedial directions, but completely conforming surfaces may not be advantageous. In the normal knee, rotational loads are shared by the menisci, joint surfaces, and the surrounding soft tissue. Complete conformity would eliminate rotational motion about the long axis of the tibia; in such a case the greater portion of torsional load applied to the knee will be carried by the prosthesis and the smaller portion by the surrounding soft tissue. The fixation interface will be subjected to higher stresses and loosening could be more likely. The contact stress is relatively insensitive to changes in conformity in the anteroposterior direction. So, to avoid high stresses at the fixation interface and have little rotational constraint the articulating surfaces could be completely flat in the mediolateral direction; but if a varus or valgus motion occurs between the femur and tibia, higher contact stresses will occur between the edge of the femoral component and the tibial plateau. There is considerable controversy about

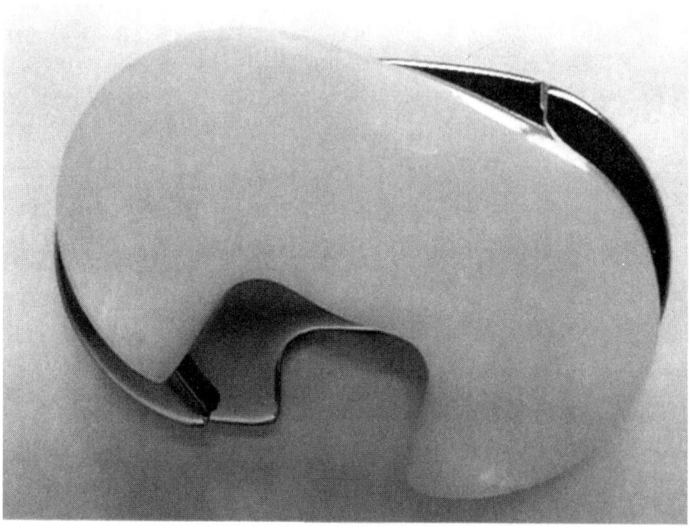

Figure 17.10. Tibial component of a mobile bearing total knee prosthesis.

the optimum congruency for knee prostheses. Congruent bearing surfaces are widely accepted as desirable to limit wear debris. In fact, components with low conformity, and thus high contact stresses, undergo the highest amount of wear (Bartel *et al.*, 1995; Blunn *et al.*, 1991). Designs of high conformity, and therefore high contact area, may reduce the amount of wear but, on the other hand, may also be associated with posterior impingement during knee flexion. Limiting the extent of implant conformity allows femoral roll back without impingement but, unfortunately, reduces contact area and increases contact stress. Mobile bearing prostheses have been created to optimize wear through highly congruent matched surfaces, replicating the meniscal function, while removing constraint in rotation by allowing the components to slide with each other (Figure 17.10). Sliding meniscal bearing surfaces reduce contact stress between the femoral component and the tibial polyethylene and allows femoral roll back, but at the cost of more complexity of sliding between the polyethylene and the metal base of the tibia (Whiteside, 1986). Therefore, minimizing contact stresses and minimizing prosthesis–bone interface stresses are competing objectives.

17.4.2. Thickness

The stress associated with crack propagation, the maximum principal stresses, and the maximum shear stresses are affected not only by the conformity of articulating surfaces, but also by the thickness of the component and by the elastic modulus of the polyethylene. The contact stresses on the tibial component depend on the thickness of the layer of polyethylene. The relationship of ultrahigh molecular weight polyethylene bearings to wear in TKAs is widely accepted. In previous studies the amount of contact stress was noted to increase rapidly with decreasing thickness; very thin polyethylene components are associated with high contact stresses in nonconforming designs. Surface damage of polyethylene is more severe in thin (<4–6 mm) components and in components with relatively flat tibial articulating surfaces. As the thickness decrease, the stresses increase since the structural stiffness of the polyethylene component increase even though the elastic modulus of the material remains constant. Analyzing compressive contact stresses and the relationship between thickness and contact stress for metal-backed tibial components, it was shown that a thickness of more than 8 to 10 mm should be maintained when feasible (Bartel *et al.*, 1986). Similarly, greater wear in thinner components than in thicker implants of the same design was noted. As the polyethylene thickness decreases, the stress associated with wear and surface damage of the polyethylene increases; so, very thin polyethylene components, with thickness less than 8 mm, are associated with high contact stresses, particularly in nonconforming designs.

17.4.3. Metal Backing

Prior to the advent of metal-backed tibial trays, aseptic loosening was the main mode of failure of TKAs. Aseptic loosening was due to the all-polyethylene tibial tray flexibility. A metal backing placed between the polyethylene portion of the tibial component and the cancellous bone allows for more uniform distribution of the loads (Figure 17.11). The applied loads are distributed over a larger area of trabecular bone, reducing the compressive stresses occurring in the cancellous bone beneath the tibial component. The reduction in stresses, due to the increased stiffness of the component, is relative if the loads are distributed symmetrically over the tibial plateaus. However, a significant reduction occurs when the loads are applied asymmetrically (Bartel *et al.*, 1982). On the other hand, even though the presence of a metal backing leads to reduce compressive stresses occurring in cancellous bone, it increases the tensile stresses; so, when an asymmetric load is applied to one plateau, the opposite plateau tends to lift off from the trabecular bone. As a consequence, the prosthesis–bone interface requires greater tensile strength, which can be obtained by dovetails or undercuts to allow better cement intrusion into the metal back or by screws or by pegs provided with special configuration from the backing to the underlying

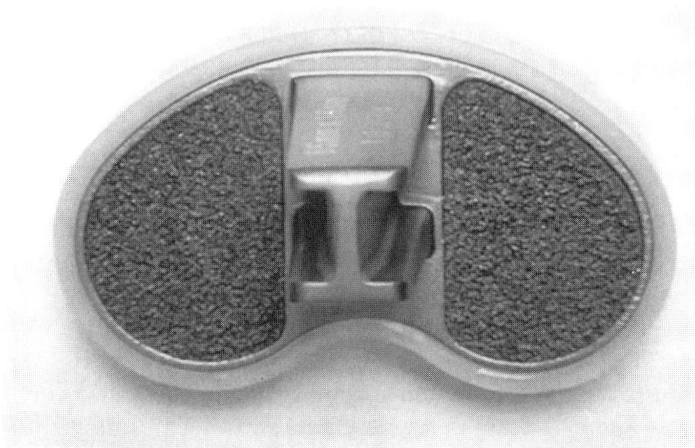

Figure 17.11. Porous coating metal-backed tibial component. The I-beam stem provides additional resistance to shear and torsional loads between the implant and the bone.

cancellous bone (Figure 17.11). However, the presence of metal backing requires the polyethylene to be attached strongly to the metal tray. For this purpose tabs, dovetails, and direct molding of the polyethylene over the metal tray have been employed. When metal-backed components are utilized and the overall thickness of the components is to be maintained, the thickness of polyethylene may be reduced. So, it must be made clear that labeling usually refers to the total thickness of the tibial implant, not to the thickness of ultrahigh molecular weight polyethylene. The tibial component has to be as wide as possible to cover the entire area of the tibia, because with a wider plateau the intercondylar distance is increased and the loads imposed in the collateral ligaments and the surface stress are reduced. Nevertheless, it is not necessary to extend the tibial component so that it makes contact with the cortical shell at the outer edge of the tibia, since the mechanical properties of the cortical shell and cancellous bone are very similar (Murray *et al.*, 1984).

17.4.4. Strength

Many attempts have been made to reduce surface damage by increasing the strength of the polyethylene. Addition of carbon fibers was advocated on the basis of improved mechanical strength and increased wear resistance (Ainsworth *et al.*, 1977). Unfortunately, they have not been successful since they have resulted in stiffer materials. Many studies demonstrated that addition of carbon fibers substantially reduced the resistance of the polyethylene to fatigue crack propagation, because of higher contact stresses resulting from increased stiffness of components made from the fiber-reinforced material. Stresses in knee components made from carbon-fiber-reinforced polyethylene may be as much as 40% greater than in components made from plain polyethylene. When the elastic modulus of a polymeric material increases, the compressive stresses acting on the surface also increase; that is, as the stiffness increases, the contact area decreases, and the stresses with surface damage also increase (Bartel *et al.*, 1985). Therefore, the carbon-fiber-reinforced material does not offer any advantage over the plain polyethylene (Bartel *et al.*, 1986; Wright *et al.*, 1981; Connelly *et al.*, 1984).

Moreover, the elastic modulus of the polyethylene may increase because of the manufacturing processing or *in vivo* degradation. The structural stiffness of the component is increased and the contact stress will increase, since the metal component cannot indent as far as it would in a less stiff material. As previously mentioned, the contact area is decreased and the contact stresses are increased.

17.4.5. Degradation

Wear of the UHMWHD-PE component remains a major cause of failure in long-term joint replacements, particularly in TKAs. In recent years, several clinical problems relating to degradation of UHMWHD-PE have become apparent and therefore the polymer degradation is of increasing importance in the production and use of medical devices. The surface damage is related to the contact stresses on the polyethylene and it may be caused by a fatigue mechanism. This process is certainly promoted by the various oxidation processes that can occur in the bulk and on the surface during the prosthesis lifetime. The modes of surface damage occurring on polyethylene joint components which can produce changes in the physical properties of the polyethylene can be related to the fabrication techniques, sterilization, and *in vivo* degradation. The UHMWHD-PE components are subjected to hot pressing during the fabrication; this technique has been shown to influence the physical properties of the polyethylene material near the articulating surface. The hypothesis of the formation of an oxidation layer on the polyethylene which results from the high temperature compression sintering of the as-synthesized draw UHMWHD-PE powder has been proposed (Miller, 1991). Also, the gamma radiation process used to sterilize the UHMWHD-PE components has been cited as a main factor affecting the microstructural and mechanical properties of the polyethylene (Batheja *et al.*, 1989; Tanner *et al.*, 1995). The gamma radiation sterilization process is a widespread method used to sterilize polyethylene; 2.5 Mrad is sufficient to kill most microorganisms. However, the radiation sterilization can significantly affect the physicochemical and toxicological properties of the devices. The primary active species created by this irradiation are radicals and ions. Most of the radicals formed during irradiation remain trapped in the material and they can be converted in peroxidic radicals that further recombine, inducing cross-links and material degradation. The introduction of cross-links between polymer chains and chain scission which increases crystallinity are the two main effects of the gamma radiation sterilization on polyethylene (Rimnac *et al.*, 1994; White *et al.*, 1996). The presence of an oxidized surface layer on the periphery in polyethylene components has been reported too. Components sterilized with gamma radiation have shown a granular structure with fusion defects and large subsurface cracks. These findings are significant because, during gait, the rolling and sliding motion of the knee causes high shear stresses on the polyethylene of the tibial component and can cause wear of the articular surface. The presence of these defects can significantly alter the resistance of the polyethylene to high shear stresses. It seems that ethylene oxide sterilized components have not shown evidence of a granular structure or subsurface cracking, and show a higher ultimate tensile strength, elongation to failure, and toughness (White *et al.*, 1996). Moreover, when implants are inserted into living tissue, an inflammatory response caused by the surgical trauma follows. The experimental observations of retrieval polyethylene tibial components showed that both chemical and physical changes take place in UHMW-PE during the implantation time. Particularly, microscopic examination of the articulating surfaces revealed burnishing, scratching, pitting, and delamination as the most common modes of surface damage. The gamma radiation produces changes in mechanical properties and a low oxidation (predamage), but the chemical modification of the UHMWPE occurs principally during the implantation time and it consists of an oxidation of the prosthesis surface. A large quantity of hydroxyl and carbonyl functions is produced during the *in vivo* oxidation on the exterior surface of the prostheses. The increase of the crystallinity on the articulating surface confirms the progression of the aging of UHMWPE due to the synergism effect of the described phenomena (Ambrosio *et al.*, 1996).

17.4.6. Debris

Polyethylene wear debris and associated granulomatous response are frequently cited as the cause of bone loss and implant failure (Nolan and Bucknill, 1992; Robinson *et al.*, 1995). The extent of wear and consequent production of debris particles is influenced by many factors, including overall implant design, polyethylene thickness, surface finish of articulating bearings, implant alignment, patient activity or weight, and physiochemical properties of the polyethylene. It seems that particles produced by TKAs have a larger range of sizes than those of explanted total hip prostheses (Hirakawa *et al.*, 1996). The tibial insert to femoral component articulation is the principal source of polyethylene debris generated in TKAs; the source of debris causing femoral and tibial osteolysis are both the articular and nonarticular surfaces. Severe wear on the undersurface of tibial inserts is related to the occurrence of tibial metaphyseal osteolysis and to osteolysis around transfixation screws. Many studies on the insert retrievals have shown that wear was occurring at both the main and undersurface articulations. These insert retrievals frequently move visibly into their respective tibial trays. This motion may explain the observed severe wear on the undersurface of retrieved tibial insert (Lewis *et al.*, 1995). These findings suggest that the locking mechanism should be carefully designed to decrease relative micromotion between the insert and respective tibial tray. Laboratory studies have demonstrated that under physiologic loading modular insert designs have motion at the metal backing to insert articulation regardless of the insert fixation mechanism. This motion occurs, since normal physiologic loads cause elastic deformation of the polyethylene insert with the insert returning to its preload configuration after the load is removed. When this motion is great enough, it may cause deformation of the polyethylene insert by cold flow mechanism. Retrieval analysis of mobile bearing designs that polish the tibial try have not shown excessive wear of the back insert surface. These studies suggest that wear of the undersurface of the insert could be minimized by polishing tibial trays. Decreasing the polyethylene wear debris may delay osteolytic processes and improve implant longevity (Buechel, 1994; Wasielewski *et al.*, 1997).

17.5. Alignment

Long-term success after TKA is dependent on proper intraoperative component positioning (Bargren *et al.*, 1983; Tew and Waugh, 1985). Several authors are convinced that TKA malalignment is a major cause of component loosening and subsequent failure (Windsor *et al.*, 1989; Bargren *et al.*, 1983). On an anteroposterior long-leg radiograph, a line from the center of the femoral head to the center of the body of the talus normally passes through the middle third of the knee (Maquet, 1967). If this does not occur after TKA, compression forces on the concave side and tensile force on the convex side of the joint may lead to loosening (Denham and Bishop, 1978). So, methods of alignment which enable the surgeon to restore the normal tibiofemoral angle are required. Two major categories of TKA alignment systems for determining femoral bone cuts exist: intramedullary and extramedullary. Intramedullary femoral alignment systems are considered by several authors to be the most reliable method of producing a distal-femoral valgus resection angle of 7°, because they are easy to use and minimize operative steps (Cates *et al.*, 1993).

17.6. Fixation

Fixation of total knee components with bone cement is considered the current "gold standard." Many studies have reported excellent long-term results with cemented total arthroplasty and loosening of cemented components is a rare complication in most large clinical series (Ranawatt *et al.*, 1994; Ritter *et al.*, 1994). Despite excellent results, concern about the long-term survival of cemented prostheses still continues. Moreover, many surgeons are reluctant to use cemented prostheses in young active patients. This has led to the development of other fixation methods, such as press-fit and porous-coated total knee replacements, with the aim of achieving stable biological interlock, not susceptible to long-term fatigue cracking such as cement. Stable initial fixation must be achieved for adequate tissue ingrowth to occur. Relative motion between the implant and bone must be minimized to allow ingrowth to occur. The exact amount of repetitive motion that inhibits bone ingrowth is not known, even though it is in the range of 100 to 150 μm (Pillar *et al.*, 1986). Unfortunately, the relationship between the way loads are transferred in the initial period after implantation and the subsequent extent and distribution of tissue ingrowth is still unknown. Many studies have shown proliferation of fibrous or fibrocartilaginous tissue at the interface between the porous layer and the bone because of the repetitive motions that can occur at this interface. Probably, biological ingrowth is not a prerequisite for successful cementless TKAs. These prostheses are implanted so as to maximize the area of intimate bone to prosthesis contact, with better initial stabilization due to press fit and increased chance for biological bony ingrowth. Implant designs that rely on ingrowth into a porous metal layer must have a metal backing. In this case, the bond between the beads or fiber mesh that make up the porous layer and the underlying metal substrate must be strong to avoid fracture of both the porous layer from substrate and the metal substrate itself (Manley *et al.*, 1987; Morrey and Chao, 1988). Devices to supply this initial fixation consist of screws, pegs, and porous coated knee implants, stabilized by virtue of their inherent geometry. The pegs employed in many contemporary cementless designs can be fabricated from metal or polyethylene. Generally, they are centrally located between the plateaus; so, they are connected with less stiff cancellous bone. Therefore, they provide additional resistance to shear and torsional loads between the implant and the bone, but can bear and transmit little load.

Tibial component stems are used with various knee arthroplasty systems for both cemented and uncemented applications. These tibial trays incorporate built-in short central stems or posts. Generally, the built-in stems do not enter the tibial medullary canal, but extend a few centimeters distal to the tray surface. The longer intramedullary stems are used in revision knee arthroplasty or in case the tibial plateau bone stock is insufficient. The tibial component intramedullary stems enter the tibial medullary canal and contact the inner surface of the cortical shell, transferring load down the shaft of the tibia, away from the tibial plateau.

17.7. Patellofemoral Joint

In the earliest knee replacement designs, the patellofemoral joint was not resurfaced. In most of these designs, condylar or hinge-type prostheses replaced the medial and lateral tibiofemoral articulations, but the patellar groove was not replaced. Disabling anterior knee pain was a frequent clinical problem with all of these early designs (Insall *et al.*, 1976b). About 15% of knee replaced without resurfacing the patella have persistent patella pain (Lavai *et al.*, 1983). Contemporary TKA designs include surface replacements for both the femoral groove and the posterior surface of the patella. The anatomical femoral groove is replaced by a concave groove on the extended flange of the metal femoral components. Patellar surface is replaced by a dome-shaped implant made of polyethylene. There is one spherical radius for the patellar component as there is one mediolateral radius for the femoral groove. Conforming contact is achieved only near full extension, since during flexion the convex patellar surface articulates against the convex inner surface of the condyles on the femoral component. A central peg or smaller peripheral pegs provide resistance to shear stress. Usually, the patellar component is fixed by bone cement. The variety of patellar prostheses currently marketed reflects the lack of consensus with respect to ideal design. Prostheses vary considerably in size, shape, number, and location of pegs, and presence or absence of metal backing. Even though the clinical results with dome-shaped implants were good, many retrieval studies showed that the component were worn and deformed, resulting in a more conforming shape.

To improve load transfer, metal backing in patellar components was introduced, such as in tibial components (Figure 17.12). Metal backing of a

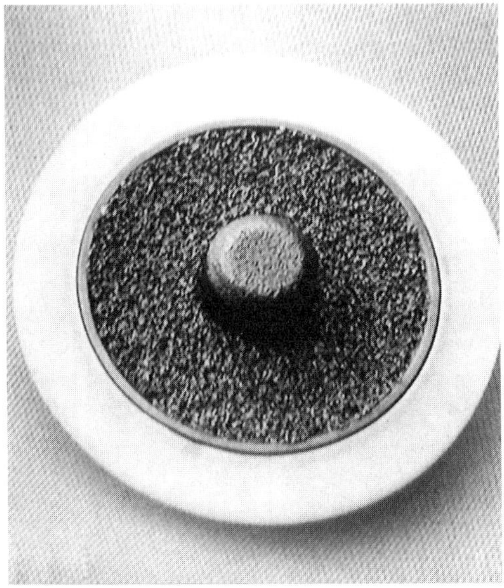

Figure 17.12. Single peg metal reinforced UHMWPE patellar component.

patellar component significantly reduces cement stresses. To be effective, the metal backing should support the peripheral portions of polyethylene, since predicted displacements in the loaded patella are $6\frac{1}{2}$ times greater in this region. Unfortunately, metal backing of components predispose to failure related to wear or fatigue failure of the thin polyethylene present at the peripheral margins of the metal backing. Early results with metal-backed patellar components were poor. Many failures due to components wearing through the polyethylene layer and dissociation of the polyethylene layer from the metal backing were reported. In many cases, the polyethylene of metal-backed patellar prostheses has worn or split allowing metal-on-metal contact. This contact between the metal backing of the patellar component and the trochlear surface of the femoral component has caused wear debris and a resultant synovitis (Bayley *et al.*, 1988; Stulberg *et al.*, 1988). Because of these failures, metal-backed patellar component has been nearly abandoned. More anatomic articulating surfaces have been introduced to create a more conforming articulation between the patellar component and the femoral groove, and to minimize the contact stresses. The spherical convex dome is maintained to articulate against the femoral groove near the extension, but a concave surface near the circumference has been included to provide a more conforming surface to articulate against the femoral condyles during flexion. The indication for resurfacing the patella remains controversial. Patellar resurfacing during TKA is still a dilemma for the orthopedic surgeon, who has no convincing scientific study available dealing with the issue of patellofemoral resurfacing. Unfortunately, it is not possible to predict before operation which knee will be painful. There are absolute or relative indications for patellar resurfacing. Absolute indications would include rheumatoid arthritis and a joint replacement primarily done for patellofemoral arthrosis; relative indications might include moderate to severe arthritis and a nonanatomic patellofemoral joint in the total knee implant.

Patellar fracture, patellar loosening, and instability are the principal problems associated with resurfacing of patella (Mochizuki and Schurman, 1979; Tria *et al.*, 1994; Ranawat, 1986). Patellar fractures have become the most common complication of the extensor mechanism of TKA. The incidence of fracture of the patella is reported in the literature as 1%–11% (Ranawat and Rose, 1983). A common location of the fracture is in the superior pole or through the middle substance of the patella. Proposed causes of this complication include avascular necrosis of the patella secondary to lateral release, component design, component malalignment and increased tension in the quadriceps caused by improper selection of the size of the femoral component, especially in the sagittal plane, and increased patellar thickness. Fractures may occur with a fixed fulcrum prosthesis which displaces the femoral condyle anteriorly as the knee is flexed, increasing the tension in the quadriceps. Therefore, much attention has been paid to normalizing patellofemoral function, and the importance of placing tibial and femoral components within a neutral range, so that the position of the joint line is unaltered and the quadriceps mechanism can function more efficiently, has been emphasized (Figgie *et al.*, 1989). Several authors have implicated the disruption of the bloody supply to the patella during surgery as a factor in eventual patellar fracture.

The most common cause of dislocation of the patella is malalignment of the quadriceps muscle system. The findings in studies reported in the literature suggested certain factors which predispose to lateral dislocation, including errors in surgical technique, trauma, and prosthetic design. Patellae with tilt and displacement are at greater risk for cold flow and wear of the polyethylene. Creep, independent of wear in patellar component polyethylene, which permits adaptation to the tracking position, has been reported (Wright, 1991). Moreover, tilt could be one of the reasons for the high failure rate of metal-backed patellae, because of the increased loading at the periphery of the component where most metal-backed prostheses have thin polyethylene (Bindelglass *et al.*, 1993).

Knee implant design is a less frequent cause of dislocation. Implants with greater sagittal width than the anatomic sagittal width of the femoral condyle and a shallow patellofemoral groove in flexion can displace the patella forward with increased tension in quadriceps muscle in flexion, so causing dislocation.

17.8. Conclusion

Due to the absence of a unique center of rotation, the knee requires more complex geometry in its prosthetic replacement. The relative motions of the components are a combination of rolling and sliding, so causing a much more complex wear, whose debris remain trapped between articulating surfaces, producing three-body wear. Contact areas smaller than in total hip prosthesis can lead to more pronounced creep and greater possibility of local fatigue cracks developing. Where there is severe loss of articular cartilage but the normal bony structure is preserved, procedures that involve lowest resection of bone from both the femur and the tibia must be utilized, because the implant designs that require a great deal of excavation, so producing large cavities in the femur and in the tibia, leave relatively insufficient bone stock for revision or arthrodesis. Long stems require a large amount of intramedullary cement for fixation that may create difficulties in case of infection. If a prosthetic component becomes loose, the cement attached to it may abrade and destroy the surrounding bone and create an even larger cavity, which makes revision impossible or arthrodesis difficult to achieve. Finally, it is essential to restore the normal tibiofemoral valgus angle, because an eccentrically loaded tibial component on either the medial or lateral aspect can produce uneven wear and early loosening. So, jigs and guides which make it as easy as possible to resect the bone surfaces with precision have to be available. At present, there is a multitude of implants on the market. The selection of a prosthesis depends on many factors, including the surgeon's preference and his familiarity with the device.

References

Ainsworth, R., Farling, G., Bardos, D. 1977. An improved bearing material for joint replacement prostheses: Carbon fiber reinforced UHMW polyethylene, *Trans Orthop. Res. Soc.* **2**, 120.

Ambrosio, L., Carotenuto, G., Nicolais, L., Ronca, D. 1996. Degradation of explanted UHMW-PE components prostheses. *Biomaterials* **10(1-2)**, 15–23.

Andriacchi, T.P., Galante, J.O., Fermier, B.S. 1982. The influence of total knee replacement design on walking and stair climbing, *J. Bone Jt. Surg.* **64A**, 1328–1335.

Bargren, J.H., Blaha, J.D., Freeman, M.A.R. 1983. Alignment in total knee arthroplasty: correlated biomechanical and clinical observations, *Clin. Orthop.* **173**, 178–183.

Bartel, D.L., Burstein, A.H., Santavicca, E.A., Insall, J.N. 1982. Performance of the tibial component in total knee replacement, *J. Bone Jt. Surg.* **64A**, 1026–1033.

Bartel, D.L., Burstein, A.H., Toda, M.D, Edwards, D.L. 1985. The effects of conformity and plastic thickness on contact stress in metal-backed plastic implants, *J. Biomech. Eng.* **107**, 193–199.

Bartel, D.L., Bicknell, V.L., Wright, T.M. 1986. The effect of conformity, thickness and material stresses in ultra-high molecular weight components for total joint replacement, *J. Bone Jt. Surg.* **68A**, 1041–1051.

Bartel, D.L., Rawlinson, J.J., Burstein, A.H., Ranawatt, C.S., Flynn, W.F. 1995. Stresses in polyethylene components of contemporary total knee replacements, *Clin. Orthop.* **317**, 76–82.

Batheja, S.K., Andrews, E.H., Yarbrough, S.M. 1989. Radiation induced crystallinity in linear polyethylenes: Long term aging effects, *Polym. J.* **21**, 739–750.

Bayley, J.C., Scott, R.D., Ewald, F.C, Holmes, G.B. Jr. 1988. Metal-backed patellar component failure following total knee replacement, *J. Bone Jt. Surg.* **70A**, 668–674.

Binderglass, D.F., Cohen, J.L., Dorr, L.D. 1993. Patellar tilt and subluxation in total knee arthroplasty. Relationship to pain, fixation and design. *Clin. Orthop.* **286**, 103–109.

Blaha, J.D., Insler, H.P., Freeman, M.A.R. 1982. The fixation of a proximal tibial polyethylene prosthesis without cement, *J. Bone Jt. Surg.* **64B**, 326–335.

Blunn, G.W., Walker, P.S., Joshi, A., Hardinge, K. 1991. The dominance of cyclic sliding in producing wear in total knee replacements, *Clin. Orthop.* **273**, 253–260.

Cates, H.E., Ritter, M.A., Keating, E.M., Faris, P.M. 1993. Intramedullary versus extramedullary femoral alignment systems in total knee replacement. *Clin. Orthop.* **286**, 32–39.

Charnley, J. 1960. Anchorage of the femoral head prosthesis to the shaft of the femur, *J. Bone Jt. Surg.* **42B**, 28–30.

Charnley, J. 1970. Low friction arthroplasty, *Clin. Orthop.* **72**, 7–21.

Connelly, G.M., Rimnac, C.M., Wright, T.M., Hertzberg, R.W., Manson, J.A. 1984. Fatigue crack propagation behavior of ultrahigh molecular weight polyethylene, *J. Orthop. Res.* **2**, 119–125.

Coventry, M.B., Finerman, G.H., Riley, L.H., Turner, R.H., Upshaw, J.E. 1972. A new geometric knee for total knee arthroplasty, *Clin. Orthop.* **83**, 157–162.

Denham, R.A, Bishop, R.E.D. 1978. Mechanics of the knee and problems in reconstructive surgery, *J. Bone Jt. Surg.* **60B**, 308–309.

Engelbrecht, E., Zippel, J. 1973. The sledge prosthesis "Model St. Georg." *Acta Orthop. Belg.* **39**, 203–209.

Feng, E.L., Stulberg, D.S., Wixon, R.S. 1995. Progressive subluxation and polyethylene wear in total knee replacements with flat articular surfaces, *Clin. Orthop.* **205**, 43–48.

Figgie, H.E., Goldberg, V.M., Heiple, K.G., Moller, H.S., Gordon, N.H. 1989. The influence of tibial-patellofemoral location on function of the knee in patients with posterior stabilized condylar knee prostheses, *J. Bone Jt. Surg.* **68A**, 1035–1040.

Font-Rodriguez, D.E., Scuderi, G.R., Insall, J.N. 1997. Survivorship of cemented total knee arthroplasty, *Clin. Orthop.* **345**, 79–86.

Freeman, M.A.R., Swanson, S.A., Tood, R. 1973. Total replacement of the knee using the Freeman-Swanson knee prosthesis, *Clin. Orthop.* **94**, 153–170.

Glück, T. 1890. Die invaginationsmethode der osteo-und arthroplastik, *Berl. Klin. Wochenschr. Circulation* **33**, 752.

Goodfellow, J., O'Connor, J., 1978. The mechanics of the knee and the prosthesis design, *J. Bone Jt. Surg.* **60B**, 358–369.

Gunston, F.H. 1973. Polycentric knee arthroplasty, *Clin. Orthop.* **94**, 128–135.

Hirakawa, K., Bauer, T.W., Stulberg, B.N., Wilde, A.H., Borden, L.S. 1996. Characterization of debris adjacent to failed knee implants of 3 different designs, *Clin. Orthop.* **331**, 151–158.

Insall, J.N., Walker, P. 1976. Unicondylar knee replacement, *Clin. Orthop.* **120**, 83–85.

Insall, J.N., Ranawat, C.S., Scott, W.N., Walker, P. 1976a. Total condylar replacement—Preliminary report, *Clin. Orthop.* **120**, 149–154.

Insall, J.N., Ranawat, C.S., Aglietti, P., Shine, J. 1976b. A comparison of four models of total knee-replacement prostheses, *J. Bone Jt. Surg.* **58A**, 754–765.

Jones, E.C., Insall, J.N., Inglis, A.E., Ranawat, C.S. 1979. GUEPAR knee arthroplasty results and late complications, *Clin. Orthop.* **140**, 145–152.

Jones, W.N., Aufranc, O.E., Kermond, W.L. 1967. Mould arthroplasty of the knee, *J. Bone Jt. Surg.* **49A**, 1022.

Judet, J., Judet, R., Crepin, G.T. 1947. Essais de prothèse ostéoarticulaire, *Presse Med.* **52**, 302.

Kettelkamp, D.B., Nasca, R. 1973. Biomechanics and knee replacement arthroplasty, *Clin. Orthop.* **94**, 8–14.

Knutson, K., Lewold, S., Robertsson, O., Lidgren, L. 1994. The Swedish knee arthroplasty register, *Acta Orthop. Scand.* **65**, 375–386.

Lavai, J.P., McLeod, H.C., Freeman, M.A.R. 1983. Why not resurface the patella? *J. Bone Jt. Surg.* **65B**, 448–451.

Lewis, P.L., Rorabeck, C.H., Bourne, R.B. 1995. Screw osteolysis after cementless total knee replacement, *Clin. Orthop.* **321**, 173–177.

Li, E., Ritter, M.A. 1995. Total knee arthroplasty, *J. Arthroplasty* **10**, 560–563.

MacIntosh, D. 1958. Hemiarthroplasty of the knee using a space occupying prosthesis for painful varus and valgus deformities, *J.Bone Jt. Surg.* **40A**, 1431.

MacIntosh, D.L. 1966. Arthroplasty of the knee, *J. Bone Jt. Surg.* **48B**, 179.

Manley, M.T., Kotzar, G., Stern, L.S., Wilde, A. 1987. Effects of repetitive loading on the integrity of porous coatings, *Clin. Orthop.* **217**, 293–302.

Maquet, P. 1967. Biomechanique du genou et gonarthrose, *Rev. Chir. Orthop.* **53**, 111–138.

Marmor, L. 1973. The modular knee, *Clin. Orthop.* **94**, 242–248.

Marmor, L. 1988. Unicompartmental arthroplasty of the knee with a minimum ten-year follow-up period, *Clin. Orthop.* **228**, 171–177.

Matthews, L.S., Sonstengard, D.A., Kaufer, H. 1973. The spherocentric knee, *Clin. Orthop.* **94**, 234–241.

McKee, G.K, Watson-Farrar, J. 1966. Replacement of arthritic hips by the McKee–Farrar prosthesis, *J. Bone Jt. Surg.* **48B**, 245–249.

McKeever, D. 1960. Tibial plateau prosthesis, *Clin. Orthop.* **18**, 86–95.

Miller, R.C. 1991. UHMW polyethylene, *Modern Plastic*, Mid-October Encyclopaedia Issue **67**.

Mochizuki, R.M., Schurman, D.J. 1979. Patellar complications following total knee arthroplasty. *J. Bone Jt. Surg.* **61A**, 879–883.

Morrey, B.F., Chao, E.Y.S. 1988. Fracture of the porous-coated metal tray of a biologically fixed knee prosthesis: Report of a case, *Clin. Orthop.* **228**, 182–189.

Murray, R.P., Hayes, W.C., Edwards, W.T., Harry, J.D. 1984. Mechanical properties of the subchondral plate and the metaphyseal shell, *Trans. 30th Orthop. Res. Soc.* **9**, 197.

Nolan, J.F., Bucknill, T.M. 1992. Aggressive granulomatous from polyethylene failure in an uncemented knee replacement. *J. Bone Jt. Surg.* **74B**, 23–24.

Pillar, R.M., Lee, J.M., Maniatopoulos, C. 1986. Observations on the effect of movement on bone ingrowth into porous-surfaced implants, *Clin. Orthop.* **208**, 108–113.

Ranawat, C.S. 1986. The patellofemoral joint in total condylar knee arthroplasty. Pros and cons based on five- to ten-year follow-up observations, *Clin. Orthop.* **205**, 93–99.

Ranawat, C.S., Rose, H.A. 1983. Total-condylar knee arthroplasty—A three to eight year follow-up, Proceedings of the American Academy of Orthopaedic Surgeons, Annual Meeting, Los Angeles, California.

Ranawat, C.S., Wilde, A.H., Rover, G.D. 1976. Experience with the GUEPAR total knee prosthesis, *Orthop. Rev.* **5**, 47–53.

Ranawat, C.S., Flynn, W.F., Deshmukh, R.G. 1994. Impact of modern technique on long-term results of total condylar knee arthroplasty, *Clin. Orthop.* **309**, 131–135.

Riley, L.H. Jr. 1976. The evolution of total knee arthroplasty, *Clin. Orthop.* **120**, 7–10.

Rimnac, C.M., Klein, R.W., Betts, F., Wright, T.M. 1994. Post-irradiation aging of ultra-high molecular weight polyethylene, *J. Bone Jt. Surg.* **76A**, 1052–1056.

Ritter, M.A., Herbst, S.A., Keating, E.M., Faris, P.M., Meding, J.B. 1994. Long term survival analysis of a posterior cruciate retaining total condylar total knee arthroplasty, *Clin. Orthop.* **309**, 136–145.

Ritter, M.A., Worland, R., Saliski, J., Helphenstine, J.V., Edmondson, K.L., Keating, E.M., Faris, P.M, Meding, J.B. 1995. Flat-on-flat, nonconstrained compression molded polyethylene total knee replacement, *Clin. Orthop.* **321**, 79–85.

Stulberg, S.D., Stulberg, B.N., Hamati, Y., Tsao, A. 1988. Failure mechanism of metal-backed patellar component, *Clin. Orthop.* **236**, 88–105.

Tanner, M.G., Whiteside, L.A., White, S.E. 1995. Effect of polyethylene quality on wear in total knee arthroplasty, *Clin. Orthop.* **317**, 83–88.

Tew, M. and Waugh, W. 1985. Tibiofemoral alignment and results of knee replacement. *J. Bone Jt. Surg.* **67B**, 551–556.

Tria, A.J., Harwood, D.A., Alicea, J.A., Cody, R.P. 1994. Patellar fractures in posterior stabilized knee arthroplasty, *Clin. Orthop.* **299**, 131–138.

Walker, P.S. 1978. *Human Joints and Their Artificial Replacements*, Charles C. Thomas, Springfield, Illinois.

Walldius, B. 1954. Arthroplasty of the knee joint using an acrylic prosthesis, *Acta Orthop. Scand.* **23**, 121–131.

Wasielewski, R.C., Parks, N., Williams, I., Surprenant, H., Collier, J.P., Engh, G. 1997. Tibial insert undersurface as a contributing source of polyethylene wear debris, *Clin. Orthop.* **345**, 53–59.

Weightman, B., Light, D.A. 1985. A comparison of RCH 1000 and Hi-Fax 1900 ultra-high molecular weight polyethylene, *Biomaterials* **6**, 177–183.

White, S.E., Paxson, R.D., Tanner, M.G., Whiteside, L.A. 1996. Effects of sterilisation on wear in total knee arthroplasty, *Clin. Orthop.* **331**, 164–171.

Whiteside, L.A. 1986. Wear in total knee arthroplasty, in: *Biological Material and Mechanical Consideration of Joint Replacement* (B.F. Morrey, ed.), pp. 253–260, Raven Press, New York.

Windsor, R.E., Scuderi, G.R., Moran, M., Insall, J.N. 1989. Mechanism of failure of the femoral and tibial components in total knee arthroplasty, *Clin. Orthop.* **248**, 15–23.

Winter, D.A. 1983. Energy generation and absorption at the ankle and knee during fast, natural and slow cadences, *Clin. Orthop.* **175**, 147–154.

Wright, T.M. American Association of Orthopaedic Surgeons course. 1991. Total Knee Arthroplasty, Orlando, Florida, October.

Wright, T.M., Fukubayashi, T., Burstein, A.H. 1981. The effect of carbon fiber reinforcement on contact area, contact pressure and time dependent deformation in polyethylene tibial components, *J. Biomed. Mater. Res.* **15**, 719–730.

Wright, T.M., Burstein, A.H., Bartel, D.L. 1985. Retrieval analysis of total joint replacement components: a six-year experience, in: *Proceedings of Second Symposium on Corrosion and Degradation of Implant Materials*, pp. 415–428, American Society for Testing and Materials, Philadelphia.

Wroblewski, B.M. 1979. Wear of high-density polyethylene on bone and cartilage, *J. Bone Jt. Surg.* **61B**, 498–500.

18

Biomaterial Applications: Elbow Prosthesis

Luigi Celli

18.1. Introduction

The first elbow prostheses were created in an artisan way and with a custom design, usually derived from the contralateral elbow. In conditions of extensive bone loss (traumatic, neoplastic, or degenerative) it was preferred to carry out an arthroplasty resection or an arthrodesis of the elbow. Custom prostheses were made of a constrained hinge, in metal acrylic material or in nylon, with prosthetic components stabilized in the bone through press fit, with or without screws.

Since 1970 the use of acrylic cement, introduced by Sir John Charnley for hip prostheses, has allowed an improvement in fixing the prosthesis to the bone. Despite this technical development elbow prostheses with a constrained hinge still showed a high loosening rate in a short period of time (3–5 years) equal to 14–40% (Dee, 1973; Garrett, 1977; Morrey *et al.*, 1981a, b).

The biomechanical studies by Morrey *et al.*, 1981a,b, Volz (1979), and Inglis (1977) broaden our knowledge of the distribution of loads and articular kinematics, enabling a more physiologic prosthetic design. Following this, prostheses with no intra-articular hinge resurfacing (covering prosthesis) (Souter, 1977; Wadswort, 1980; Kudo, 1980; Roper and Tuke, 1986) and semiconstrained prostheses with intra-articular laxus bonds (Coonrad-Morrey and GSB) were made.

Luigi Celli • Clinica Ortopedica e Traumatologica, Università degli Studi di Modena e Reggio Emilia, Dipartimento delle Discipline Chirurgiche e delle Emergenze, Policlinico: Largo del Pozzo 71, 41100 Modena, Italy.

Integrated Biomaterials Science, edited by R. Barbucci. Kluwer Academic/Plenum Publishers, New York, 2002.

18.2. The Prosthetic Design

The design of constrained (custom or noncustom) elbow prostheses simply reproduces a uniaxial hinge made of metal—two metal surfaces sliding one on the other during the flexion–extension movement. Recent biomechanical studies have underscored the fact that the movement occurring in the ulno-humeral articulation is not a simple uniaxial movement with the hinge perpendicular to the diaphysis humeral axis, but is a helicoid movement of the trochlear groove. The axis on which this movement occurs is the result of various axes contained in a small area of 2.5–7.8 mm (Morrey and Chao, 1976). With respect to the epicondylian anatomic axis, this ulno-humeral rotation axis presents a 6°–8° valgus inclination and a 5°–7° internal rotation. For these reasons, the forearm, passing from extension to flexion, creates a complicated rotation movement called "carrying angle," which carries the forearm from a valgus position in extension to a varus position in flexion. The axis rotation movement is about 5° internal rotation in flexion and 5° extra-rotation in extension (Morrey and Chao, 1976). This functional necessity, which is dependent on the skeletal morphology, also requires integrity and a different tension in ligamental structures for its realization. The medial collateral ligament varies in tension according to the different positions of the elbow; in fact it is completely tight during flexion and gradually relaxes during extension, thus enabling the elbow to reach a valgus position. Vice versa the side collateral ligament is isometric, i.e., it does not modify its tension during the movements of the elbow, contributing to the brachial–antebrachial axis variations. Therefore, it is evident that the elbow undergoes varus, valgus, and rotation stresses, due to the articular morphology, the muscle activity, and the ligament tension.

The experience gained with the first constrained prostheses underscores its tendency to loosen early at the top level of the humeral shaft. The biomechanical premises described above clearly justify this clinical complication: in fact, the tension strengths present at the articulation level and not neutralized by a relative elasticity of the hinge were transferred along the humeral shaft until they were localized in the bone–cement and bone–prosthesis interfaces in the early models, causing them to loosen early. From 1975 onward, the changes introduced in the various prosthesis designs were made with the purpose of increasing the rotation tolerance, in an effort to reproduce the articular kinematics as accurately as possible. As a result, resurfacing prostheses and semiconstrained prostheses with loose hinges have been realized.

Resurfacing prostheses try to reproduce in a more or less accurate way the shape of the ulno-humeral (Souter, 1977, Kudo, 1980, Roper-Tuke,

1986) or radio-ulno-humeral (condylar capital) articular surfaces. They do not present any intra-articular hinge, and their stability depends on an intramedullary or condylar fixation, while the articulation stability is entrusted to the ligaments, muscles, and tendinous structures. For this type of prosthesis design, ligamentous structures must be present and saved from surgical access.

However, a distinction must be made between resurfacing prostheses that do not reproduce the articular surface and those that, on the contrary, reproduce the trochlear surface. The prostheses that do not reproduce the articular surface can be made of a covering shell with diaphyseal stem (Kudo, 1998) or without diaphyseal stem (Kudo, 1980, Roper-Tuke, 1986).

The prostheses that reproduce the trochlear surface can be fixed inside the medullary channel with a cemented stem (Guepar, condylar capital) or with an epiphyseal anchorage with flanges (Souter). In a revision of the literature it is pointed out that the average rate of the loosening effect has decreased considerably to about 4% (0.9–12%) in 2–10 years (Kudo, Souter, Davis, Roper-Tuke, and others).

The constrained prostheses have maintained the intra-articular hinge, but changes have been introduced to try and get a functional condition closer to the physiological one. The hinges between the humerous and the ulna become looser with the possibility of varus-valgus (about 10%) and rotation (about 10%) movement, and presents low friction (metal–polyethylene).

The prosthesis components are fixed to the humeral and ulnar diaphyseal axis with acrylic cement along the intramedullary shaft. A semiconstrained prosthesis with a loose hinge can re-establish normal kinematics of the elbow during the flexion–extension movement with a sharp reduction of stresses in the bone–cement interface (O'Driscoll *et al.*, 1992).

This has been confirmed by clinical experience, since the revised literature (Morrey and Adams, 1992, Inglis and Pellicci, 1980, Gschwend *et al.* 1988, etc.) highlights the fact that the average loosening rate for these prostheses is about 3–4% in 2–5 years. In current semiconstrained prostheses (Coonrad-Morrey and GSB III) the presence of the hinge makes anatomical ligaments unnecessary, as their stability is ensured by the prosthetic design. In addition, the state of the host bone is less important, as in these last models the number of bone-fixing points has been increased. In fact, besides the intramedullary humeral and ulnar stem, five flanges are present with front metaphyseal humeral support (Coonrad-Morrey) and lateral condylian support (GSB III), which increase resistance to torsion and front–back stresses.

18.3. Cases in which the Elbow Prosthesis Is Advisable

Pain and serious elbow instability force a patient to undergo prosthetic implantation. Rheumatoid arthritis is the main pathology that requires the use of a prosthesis, while in primary and secondary post-traumatic osteoarthritis the use of prostheses is less frequent. In the rheumatoid patient it is important to maintain a usable function of the hand and sufficient mobility of the shoulder, especially in extra-rotation. In case of post-traumatic elbow, on the contrary, it is necessary to be very careful when advising an elbow prosthesis, as patients suffering from this problem are often young, without pain, and with high functional requirements. In such cases the patient tolerates a rigid, not painful elbow more than a prosthetic implantation, which if stressed excessively is a high risk for its survival.

Finally, we wish to reiterate that in the choice of prosthetic implantation the following points must be taken into consideration:

- Resurfacing prostheses are advisable for young patients with preserved bone stock and with good residual articular stability.
- Semiconstrained prostheses are advisable in elderly patients with a scarce bone stock and with articular instability.

In conclusion, we think that the elbow arthroprosthesis must currently be considered a reliable surgical procedure, able to re-establish good articular function. Nonetheless, the advice given to patients with an elbow arthroprosthesis implanted at the Mayo Clinic (1994) must be reiterated: You can no longer carry more than 5 kg at a time, carry more than 2.5 kg repeatedly, or push or pull something with strength. Such activities may cause wear of the prosthetic components and of the bone where the prosthesis is implanted.

References

Dee, R. 1973. Total replacement of the elbow joint, *Orthop. Clinc. North Am.* **4**, 415.

Garrett, J.C., Ewald, F.C., Thomas, W.H., Sledge, C.B. 1997. Loosening associated with GSB hinge total elbow replacement in patients with rheumatoid arthritis, *Clin. Orthop.* **127**, 170

Gschwend, N., Loehr, J., Ivosevic-Radovanovic, D., Scheier, H., Muzinger, U. 1988. Semiconstrained elbow prosthesis with special reference to the GSB III prosthesis, *Clin. Orthop.* **232**, 104.

Inglis, A.E., Pellicci, P.M. 1980. Total elbow replacement, *J. Bone Jt. Surg.* **62A**, 1252.

Inglis, A.E. Jr., Figgie, M.M., Asnis, L. 1997. Total elbow arthoplasty for flaiul and unstable elbows, *J. Shoulder Elbow Surg.* **6**, 29.

Kudo, H. 1980. Total replacement: the rheumatoid elbow with a hingeless prosthesis, *J. Bone Jt. Surg.* **62A**, 277.

Kudo, H., Iwano, K. 1998. Total elbow arthroplasty with a non-constrained surface replacement prosthesis in patients who have rheumatoid arthritis, *J. Bone Jt. Surg.* **80B**, 234.

Kudo, H., Iwano, K., Watanabe, S. 1980. Total replacement of the rheumatoid elbow with a hingeless prosthesis, *J. Bone Jt. Surg.* **62A**, 277.

Morrey, B.F., Adams, R.A. 1992. Semi-constrained arthroplasty for treatment of rheumatoid arthritis of the elbow. *J. Bone Jt. Surg.* **74A**, 479.

Morrey, B.F., Chao, E.Y. 1976. Passive motion of elbow joint. *J. Bone Jt. Surg.* **58A**, 501.

Morrey, B.F., Askew, L.J., An, K.N., Chao, E. 1981a. A biomechanical study of normal functional elbow motion, *J. Bone Jt. Surg.* **63A**, 872.

Morrey, B.F., Bryan, R.S., Dobyns, J.H., Linscheid, R.L. 1981b. Total elbow arthroplasty: a five-year experience at the Mayo Clinic, *J. Bone Jt. Surg.* **63A**, 1050.

O'Driscoll, S.W., An, K.N., Korinek, S., Morrey, B.F. 1992. Kinematics of semi-constrained total elbow arthroplasty, *J. Bone Jt. Surg.* **74B**, 297.

Roper, B.A., Tuke, M. 1986. A new constrained elbow: a prospective review of 60 replacements, *J. Bone Jt. Surg.* **68B**, 560.

Roper, B.A., Tuke, M., O'Riordan, S.M., Bulstrode, C.J. 1986. A new unconstrained elbow, *J. Bone Jt. Surg.* **68B**: 566.

Souter, W.A. 1977. Total replacement arthroplasty of the elbow in joint replacement in the upper limb, *Inst. Mech. Eng. Conference Publications.*

Volz, R.G. 1979. Development and clinical analysis of a new semiconstrained total elbow prosthesis, in: *Upper Extremity Joint Replacement Symposium on Total Elbow Joint Replaement of the Upper Extremity* (A.E. Inglis, ed.), C.V. Mosby Co., St. Louis.

19

Biomaterial Applications: Shoulder Prosthesis

Luigi Celli

19.1. Introduction

After the first custom-made shoulder prosthesis was created and implanted by Pean in 1893 for a tubercular osteoarthritis, thanks to Neer, in 1951 a noncustom prosthesis of the humeral head was created. This prosthesis was made of a head-shaft monobloc in a chromium–cobalt alloy with a head bend radius of 44 mm, obtained by an average of measurements carried out on cadavers. In 1970, Neer introduced the high-density glenoid prosthesis in polyethylene favored by the possibility of using cement, which had been introduced by Charley in the fixing of the hip prosthesis. In the last 28 years many authors have underscored the advantages, but also the secondary problems, arising from the use of the prosthesis. On the basis of these experiences, we now know that the success of a shoulder prosthesis depends on the possibilities that the prosthetic design and the surgical techniques will re-establish a normal anatomy of the shoulder, able to bear stabilization and movement strengths applied on the scapula-humeral articulation. For these reasons we do not consider constrained or semiconstrained (nonanatomic) prostheses, but only nonconstrained (anatomic) prostheses, when analyzing the problems of the prosthetic design and implantation.

Luigi Celli • Clinica Ortopedica e Traumatologica, Università degli Studi di Modena e Reggio Emilia, Dipartimento delle Discipline Chirurgiche e delle Emergenze, Policlinico: Largo del Pozzo 71, 41100 Modena, Italy.

Integrated Biomaterials Science, edited by R. Barbucci. Kluwer Academic/Plenum Publishers, New York, 2002.

19.2. The Prosthetic Design

The prosthetic design must try to re-establish the size and shape of a bone surface in order to allow good control of muscular strength. This aim can be achieved if the prosthesis is able to re-establish an equal bend radius and thickness for the humeral head, and, for the glenoid prosthesis, an equal bend radius and size (front-back and upper-lower size) of the bone surfaces to which the prosthesis must be applied. In an anatomic study performed on 140 shoulders, Iannotti *et al.* (1992) determined that the average bend radius for the humeral head is 24 ± 2.1 mm and the average thickness is 20 ± 2.0 mm, while the bend radius for the glenoid is 29 ± 3.1 mm. Taking the size of the glenoid into consideration, important differences have been observed between the maximum front-back distance (average 29 ± 3.1 mm) and upper-lower distance (average 39 ± 3.7 mm). The glenoid bend radius can generally be considered to be 2 mm (Soslowsky *et al.*, 1992) to 4 mm (Harryman *et al.*, 1995) wider than that of the humeral head. However, there may be important individual anatomic variations between the humeral and the glenoid bend radius. These conditions of mismatch can be counterbalanced by the extent of the humeral head translation on the glenoid. The humeral translation, which depends on the tension of capsulo-ligamental structures, has an average value of 10–12 mm of front and upper displacement of the humeral head when the limb is 90° abducted in maximum extra-rotation.

After a shoulder endo- or arthroprosthesis, the preservation of the humeral head rotation and translation must be evaluated, with the presence of anterior or posterior drawer or sulcus of at least 15 mm. A drawer movement of only 9 mm (Matsen *et al.*, 1994) reduces the physiological articular relaxation by about 50%; this involves a reduction in the width of the articular movement. The glenoid shape and size condition the translation. In the shoulder movement, the necessary presence of the translation in a glenoid surface with an equal bend radius of the humeral head may cause an overload of the edges with possible loosening of the glenoid prosthesis. On the contrary, if the glenoid bend radius is wider, the rotation determines an increase in the load strengths in the central zone of the glenoid surface, while the translation causes the "rocking horse" phenomenon of the humeral head on the glenoid, with its consequent mobilization. In addition, it has also been accepted that an excessive translation can cause an internal (back and upper) glenoid impingement just as occurs with the hyperlaxed shoulders of throwers. According to these observations, for a correct prosthetic design of the shoulder the following points must be taken into consideration:

(a) A slightly elliptical humeral head (spherical only in its central portion). This conformation improves not only the rotation, but also the translation of the humeral head on the glenoid.

(b) A slightly concave glenoid both on the front-back and on the upper-lower axis, with a bend radius 2–4 mm wider than that of the humeral head.

(c) A great number of prosthetic humeral heads and glenoids available with different bend radius and thickness (modular components), so that they can be adapted to the various anatomical conditions and can reduce an excessive mismatch. In addition, the modularity of the prosthetic components (humeral shaft, neck, head, and glenoid) allow changing a hemi-arthroplasty into an arthroplasty.

19.3. The Prosthetic Implantation

Nonconstrained anatomical prostheses require the integrity of the periarticular muscular structures and, in particular, the integrity of the rotator cuff muscles. Normal mobility and stability are possible only when the scapula-humeral articulation is able to transfer and cancel the different loads on the hand and on the elbow. The direction of strength varies according to the position of the limb: at 0° abduction it is directed downward, at about 60° abduction it goes upward, and at 150° it goes downward again. In addition, these strengths are often not perpendicular to the glenoid surface and their control depends closely on the activity of the rotator cuff muscles.

Poppen and Walker (1978), in a mathematical model, calculated the strengths applied on the glenoid with the integrity of the muscles. The maximum compression strength is equal to 0.89 times the body weight at 90° abduction, while it decreases to 0.4 times at 150° elevation of the limb. In these situations a defect of orientation or a mismatch of the prosthetic components or a greater retraction of periarticular soft parts may be the conditions that lead to erroneous loads on the glenoid with loosening or secondary mobilizations. The analysis of the strengths that are transferred through the glenoid-humerus articulation is very important, not only for the re-establishment of the mobility and stability of the implantation but also for its survival. Therefore, when a surgeon makes a prosthetic implantation of the shoulder, he has to take the following biomechanical necessities into consideration:

(a) Re-establish an adequate conformity of the articular surfaces.
(b) Avoid the increase in articular or periarticular resistances.
(c) Restore the active control role of the muscles.

19.4. Conforming Design of the Articular Surfaces

Adequate contact between the articular surfaces is the necessary premise to re-establish a wide mobility without instability. This can be achieved with an implantation that presents a correct retroversion and inclination of the prosthetic shaft, an adequate articular conformity between the head and the glenoid without an exaggerated back offset. The retroversion angle is measured between the transepicondyliar or trochlear axis and the axis perpendicular to the plane of the articular surface (central radius of the humeral head). Anatomical studies, XR, CAT, and other more sophisticated methods of three-dimensional analysis (Randelli and Gambrioli, 1986; Boileau and Walch, 1997; Pearl and Wolk, 1995) have determined an average retroversion value of 25° to 40°. However, individual variability is high and can go from 10° to 50° in the same series of cases observed (Pearl and Wolk, 1995). Many surgical techniques in the implantation of the humeral prosthesis recommend the resection of the head with a plane retroverted from 30° to 50° with respect to the one including the elbow. To this end the surgeon must simply bend the elbow and rotate the arm toward the exterior, correcting the retroversion of the humeral head. If the limb is not sufficiently extra-rotated, the resection of the humeral head is performed on a slanting plane, as the back tendinous fibers of the rotator cuff may be damaged. For these reasons and because of the individual variability, the surgeon must use simpler intraoperatory methods in order to obtain a retroversion angle closer to the individual value. At an intraoperatory level we think it useful to refer to the following points:

(a) The plane including the pericephalic sulcus. With the extrarotation of the limb, when cutting, this must be orthogonal to the plane of the humeral diaphyseal axis.

(b) The section plane must be perpendicular to the central radius of the humeral head, considering that there is a precise relationship between this axis and the bicipital groove. The central radius of the humeral head can be obtained by a line linking the point of maximum convexity of the humeral head with a point located at about 9 mm from the back edge of the bicipital groove.

The inclination angle obtained between the humeral diaphyseal axis and the epiphyseal axis is generally 130°–145°. There are individual variations that are also important.

To perform an osteotomy of the humeral head on a plane inclined at 45° to the humeral diaphysis in an individual who possesses a smaller inclination angle of only 30°–35°, one must place the prosthetic head in varus. In these conditions the medial translation of the rotation center (smaller lateral offset) decreases the right tension of the cuff muscles. The same condition can be attained when the shaft is inserted in a place that is too medial with respect to the center of the bend radius of the humeral head. This inconvenience occurs in cemented prostheses with scarce press fit. Fischer (1977) and his colleagues emphasized that in a humeral head with an average radius of 25 mm, if the bend center of the humeral head is moved 5 mm, the strength of the shoulder muscles is reduced by about 20%. Therefore, it is evident that the section level and the orientation of the osteotomy of the humeral epiphysis determine the final varus-valgus, front-back, and medial-lateral position of the humeral prosthesis. The surgeon uses the orthopedic axis for the penetration point of the prosthetic shaft in the humeral medullary canal. This point does not correspond to the bend radius of the humeral head (head diameter); in fact, it is about 3–5 mm more medial and more at the back than the orthopedic axis (Matsen *et al.*, 1994). The front-back distance between the center of the humeral head and the orthopedic axis is defined as "anterior-posterior offset." The orthopedic axis, the center of the diameter of the humeral head, and the axis of the prosthetic shaft represent the three possible variables that can modify the position of the prosthetic head. These three variables can have consequences for the prosthesis stability and for the extent of the movement recovery. The clinical consequences may be an anterior–posterior subluxation, a reduction in the intra- and extra-rotation, or a possible anterior–posterior or superior impingement. Due to the retroversion reduction or to the excessive front translation of the head, the coracoidal impingement occurs with pain and with the prosthetic head tending to subluxate at a front-superior level under the acromio-coracoidal arch.

This condition becomes even more clear when it is associated with the rupture of the rotator cuff. The back glenoid impingement, due to excessive retroversion, can cause pain, but it mainly determines a back overload of the glenoid component, which is often at the origin of a secondary mobilization. It is possible to avoid these errors in the implantation, if one can:

(a) Vary the head size, having at one's disposal a prosthesis with a different size in order to avoid an excessive medial translation of the bend center.

(b) Use a shaft suited to the size of the humeral channel placed laterally near the tuberosities.

(c) Avoid implanting the prosthesis with an excessive retroversion or antiversion, nevertheless having the secondary possibility, even after the implantation of the shaft, of correcting the defect of the prosthetic rotation.

For these reasons new-generation prostheses must enable the surgeon to correct possible errors, making available particular eccentric heads with different size and bend radius, and necks and shafts with different length and size in order to obtain an appropriate humeral press fit.

19.5. Articular and Periarticular Resistances

The necessary condition to re-establish the mobility in a shoulder arthroprosthesis is to avoid maintaining or realizing a rigid shoulder. This purpose can be achieved with an accurate surgical release of periarticular retracted soft tissues and not by an overstuffing in the implantation due to oversized prosthetic components. The subscapularis must have the right length and excursion, the retracted capsule must be completely excised, in particular the lower and posterior one. In the release of the soft parts, particular attention must be paid in order not to damage the cuff muscles and tendons and not to injure the axillary nerve. The degree of functional limitation, especially in extra-rotation, must be estimated before the operation, and this factor will condition the lysis extension of periarticular soft tissues and the choice of the prosthesis to implant.

The articular overstuffing (overstuffed articulation) can be avoided when, after the release of the soft parts, a modular prosthesis is used which, adapting to the tension of the tissues, allows one to control the thickness and size of the humeral head and the glenoid. The test prosthesis enables the orthopedist to choose the right components to re-establish the right muscular tension. This must allow passive intraoperatory movement with the possibility to make a 140° elevation, a 40° extra-rotation, and a 70° intra-rotation of the limb, with a 90° abducted arm, after having replaced the subscapularis in its seat. In addition to the test prosthesis there must be a back drawer with at least 15-mm translation and a pumping effect both downward and laterally. To maintain an overstuffing means considerably reducing the articular mobility: 3–4 degrees for each millimeter overstuffing (Matsen *et al.*, 1994). The most frequent causes of overstuffing are the use of a very thick glenoid and the erroneous positioning of the humeral shaft. A glenoid with thick polyethylene or with "metal-backed" stuffing, although it can ensure better anchorage in the bone, can cause the risk of making an articular overstuffing. In the same way, if the humeral shaft is inserted in varus and in too low a position, the overstuffing effect occurs when the arm is adducted, while if it is inserted in too high a position, this effect occurs when the limb abducts. Both conditions limit the elevation of the upper limb.

19.6. The Active Role of Periarticular Muscles

The re-establishment of movement and strength in shoulder endo-arthroprosthesis depends on the integrity and activity of the muscles controlling the scapula-humerus and the scapula-thoracic articulations. In the abduction movement of the arm, the scapula rotation with the elevation of the acromion-coracoidal vault encourages the deltoid action which lets the humeral head rotate on the glenoid elevating it (spinning and rolling). In order to avoid a conflict between the great tuberosity and the humeral vault, the supraspinal-subscapular system lowers and centers it (sliding). At about 60° abduction the lower glenoid-humeral ligament enhances the activity of the subspinal muscles and determines an extra-rotation of the humeral head. That way the great tuberosity can get over the acromion and position itself backward, so that the limb is able to reach the maximum elevation.

The deltoid is the most important muscle responsible for movement in a shoulder with a prosthesis. The paralysis of this muscle is a contraindication for the arthroprosthesis. If the rotator cuff is intact, it can be damaged during the surgical operation (in humeral osteotomy, in periarticular release, etc.), but even worse, it can become insufficient when the application of the prosthesis modifies the physiological tension of the muscles. To achieve this it is necessary to re-build a correct lateral offset. The humeral lateral offset measures the distance between the coracoid and the humeral tuberosity and is strictly bound to the tension status to which the cuff muscles are subjected. It is evident that an excessive increase in the lateral offset means that the prosthesis used is oversized or the glenoid is too thick. In these conditions the excessive stretching of the cuff muscles reduces their physiological shortening in the muscular contraction and consequently their function, but can also encourage their rupture. This can occur when prostheses are implanted in elderly people with a chronic pathology of the shoulder, in which the tendinous tissue is often very thin and fragile. The average lateral offset value measured by Iannotti *et al.*, (1992), in an anatomical study carried out on 140 shoulders, was 56 ± 5.7 mm. To improve the deltoid function, it is also important to re-establish the right distance between the acromium lateral edge and the humeral big tuberosity. The function of the cuff muscles, and in particular of the supraspinal muscle, depends also on the greater height of the articular surface compared to the big tuberosity. The average distance (Iannotti *et al.*, 1992) between the top of the articular surface and the top of the big tuberosity surface is 8 ± 3.2 mm. This distance must be absolutely respected in order to avoid a conflict and to enable the supra- and infraspinatus muscles to lower and extra-rotate the prosthetic head.

In conclusion, we think that the knowledge and respect of basic biomechanical problems is the necessary condition to re-establish, through an arthroprosthesis intervention of the shoulder, a normal articular function which can enable the patient to make a sufficient movement with appropriate strength and without pain. This fundamental aim can be achieved when the surgeon selects the patients carefully and carries out an accurate surgical technique in the re-building of the normal skeletal anatomy. The patient will then focus on an adequate rehabilitation program.

References

Boileau, P., Walch, G., 1997. The three-dimensional geometry of proximal humerus, *J. Bone Jt. Surg.* **79A**, 857–865.

Fischer. 1977. Kinematisch Organische Gelenke, Braunschweig.

Harryman, D.T., Sidles, J.A., Harris, S.L., Lippit, S.B., Matsen, F.A. III. 1995. The effect of articular conformity and the size of humeral head component on laxity and motion after glenohumeral arthroplasty: a study in cadavera, *J. Bone Jt. Surg.* **77A**, 555–563.

Iannotti, J.P., Gabriel, J.P., Schnek, S.L., Evans, B.G., Misra, S. 1992. The normal glenohumeral relationships: an anatomical study of the one hundred and forty shoulders, *J. Bone Jt. Surg.* **74A**, 491–500

Matsen, F.D.M., Lippitt, S.B., Sidles, J.A., Harryman, D.T.M. 1994. *Practical Evaluation and Management of the Shoulder*, W.B. Saunders, Philadelphia.

Neer, C.S. 1955. Articular replacement for the humeral head, *J. Bone Jt. Surg. (Am)* **46**, 1607–1610.

Pearl, M., Wolk, A.G. 1995. Retroversion of the proximal humerus in the relationship to prosthetic replacement arthroplasty, *J. Shoulder Elbow Surg.* **4**, 286–289.

Poppen, N.K., Walker, P.S. 1978. Forces at the glenohumeral joint in abduction, *Clin. Orthop. Relat. Res.* **135**, 165–170.

Randelli, M., Gambrioli, P.L. 1986. Glenohumeral osteometry by computed tomography in normal and instable shoulders, *Clin. Orthop. Relat. Res.* **208**, 151–156.

Soslowsky, L.J., Flatow, E.L., Bigliani, L.U., Mow, V.C. 1992. Articular geometry of the glenohumeral joint, *Clin. Orthop. Relat. Res.* **285**, 181–190.

20

Acrylic Bone Cements

Maria-Pau Ginebra, Francisco-Javier Gil, and Josep-Anton Planell

20.1. Introduction

In the early sixties Sir John Charnley presented the preliminary results of a new method for the fixation of joint prostheses to bone (Charnley 1964a, b, 1970). The idea was to distribute the contact stresses between the implant and the bone over a large area by means of a filler material, called bone cement and consisting in self-curing polymethylmethacrylate (PMMA). This idea represented an important breakthrough in the field of orthopedics and led to the development of a worldwide successful technique.

The main advantages of the cemented prostheses lay in the excellent primary fixation, in the even load distribution between the implant and the bone, and in the fact that the technique allows a fast recovery of the patient. However, the main disadvantage is that about 10% of the patients may need revision in less than 10 years after implantation. The observed aseptic loosening which appears with time is attributed to causes such as the lack of secondary fixation, the mechanical failure of the cement, the initial formation of a fibrous tissue between the cement and the bone, partly due to the necrosis of bone induced by the heat liberated during the setting stage, and the osteolysis caused by the foreign body reaction induced by wear particles and debris, part of which could come from the bone cement. The toxicity of the liquid monomer of the cement should also be mentioned as another disadvantage. The balance which can be carried forward shows, however, that acrylic bone cements have still a long way to go and a future ahead, mainly when the moderate success of other fixation techniques such

Maria-Pau Ginebra, Francisco-Javier Gil, and Josep-Anton Planell • CREB (Biomedical Engineering Research Center), Department of Materials Science and Metallurgical Engineering, Universitat Politècnica de Catalunya, Av. Diagonal 647, 08028 Barcelona, Spain.

Integrated Biomaterials Science, edited by R. Barbucci. Kluwer Academic/Plenum Publishers, New York, 2002.

as metallic porous coatings and plasma sprayed hydroxyapatite coatings is taken into account.

20.2. Chemistry of Acrylic Bone Cements

20.2.1. Chemical Composition: Powder and Liquid

Acrylic bone cements are based in PMMA which is accepted as a biocompatible polymer when cured. The bone cement is usually prepared by mixing the two components of the dose: a transparent liquid and a white powder. The main properties of each component are [for an excellent review, see Lautenschlager *et al.* (1984)]:

(a) Liquid component: the liquid is transparent, volatile, and has a characteristic penetrant smell. Its viscosity is low and its boiling temperature is approximately 100 °C at 760 mm Hg. Its density is 0.94 g/cm^3. It contains three basic ingredients:

(1) MMA monomer ($CH_2C(CH_3)COOCH_3$): 97% v/v approximately,
(2) *N*,*N*-Dimethyl-*p*-toluidine (p-$N(CH_3)C_6H_4CH_3$): 2.7% v/v approximately,
(3) Hydroquinone (OHC_6H_4OH): 750 ppm.

The *N*,*N*-dimethyl-*p*-toluidine (DMT) acts as accelerant of the polymerization reaction, which activates the initiator mixed with the powder. The hydroquinone is an inhibitor, which prevents the premature polymerization of the monomer. The volume of liquid is usually 20 ml.

(b) Solid component: the basic ingredients of the powder are:

(1) PMMA ($[CH_3C(CH_2)COOCH_3]_n$): 89% w/w approximately. In some instances, instead of PMMA beads, other polymers or copolymers are used.
(2) Benzoil peroxide ($COC_6H_5OOCC_6H_5O$), BP: 0.75% w/w approximately.
(3) Barium sulfate ($BaSO_4$) or zirconium dioxide (ZrO_2): 10% w/w.

The BP acts as initiator, producing free radicals when it reacts with the amine (DMT). $BaSO_4$ or ZrO_2 are added in order to obtain a radio-opaque cement. The diameter of most of the PMMA particles in the cement ranges between 30 and 150 μm and their shape depends on the manufacturing process used. Figure 20.1 shows the morphology of the powder of acrylic bone cement. Both PMMA beads and $BaSO_4$ particles are clearly visible.

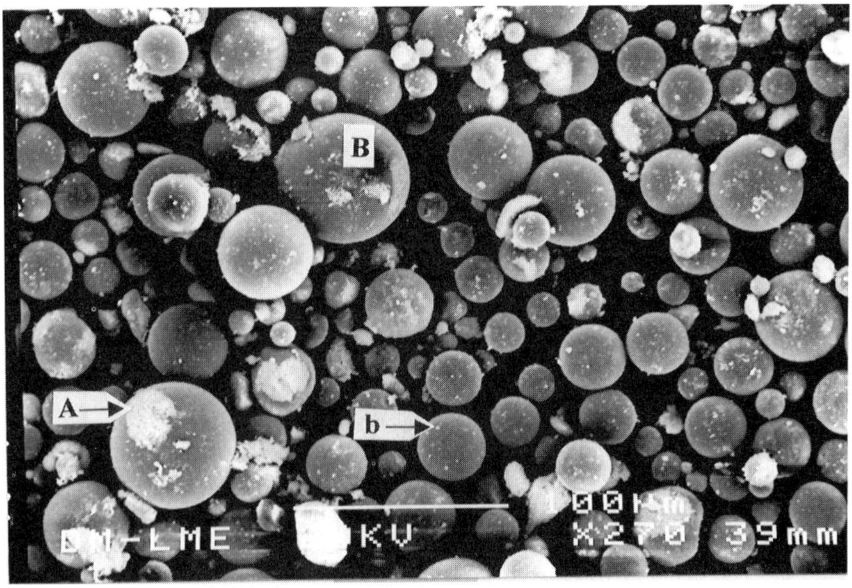

Figure 20.1. Morphology of the powder of an acrylic bone cement. Small barium sulfate particles (b) distributed on the surface of the PMMA beads (B), and forming in certain cases larger agglomerates (A), are clearly visible.

20.2.2. Chemical Reactions and Setting Process

At the moment of the mixing of the two components, solid and liquid, the polymerization of the liquid monomer starts as a typical reaction of addition polymerization. Figure 20.2 represents schematically the reactants and the product obtained after the polymerization reaction. Both physical and chemical phenomena take place simultaneously, which will affect the setting process as well as the microstructure and the mechanical properties of the set material, and which depend on variables such as the chemical composition and concentration of the initial powder and liquid components, the physical mixing method, and the chemical environment.

The time elapsed from the moment at which the powder and liquid components are mixed until the cement is set is known as the *setting time.* If the evolution of the temperature with time is recorded, the setting time is the time when the temperature of the polymerizing mass is: $T_{amb} + (T_{max} - T_{amb})/2$, where T_{amb} is the ambient temperature, taken as $23 \pm 1\,^{\circ}C$, and T_{max} is the maximum temperature reached by the polymerizing cement in °C (ASTM Standard, 1986; Meyer *et al.*, 1973). The maximum

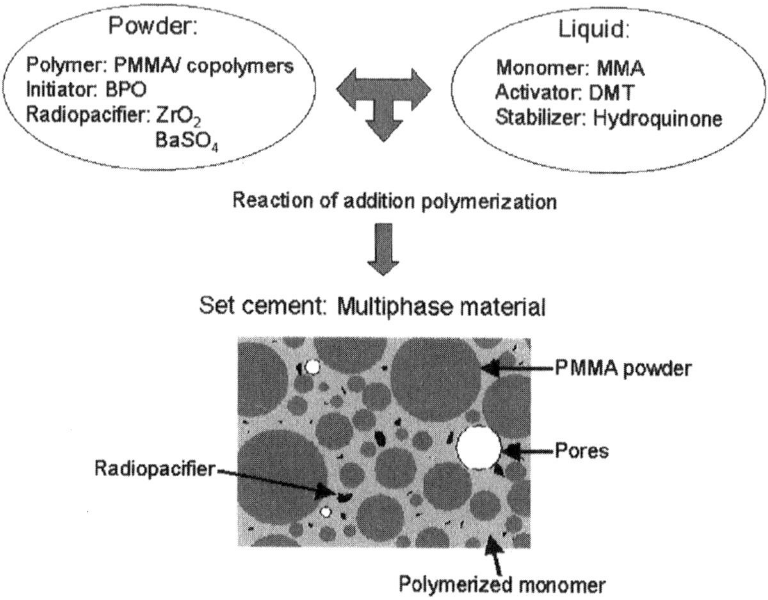

Figure 20.2. Polymerization process of an acrylic bone cement.

temperature or peak temperature is produced by the exothermic propagation reactions which take place during polymerization. The cement sets before the peak temperature is reached. The time at which the mixed cement mass does not adhere to a surgically gloved finger is known as the *dough time*. Finally, the difference between the setting time and the dough time is called the *handling time*, and it corresponds to the period of time during which the cement is workable and has to be implanted (or molded). The leaflets of the commercial brands of bone cements usually give the working time of the cement in terms of environmental temperature.

For the cement to be produced, it is necessary that the liquid monomer wet the powder particles of PMMA, which should then swell and allow the diffusion of the liquid into the organic matrix of the particles. Simultaneously, it is necessary that a component such as BP is completely diluted into the liquid. Monomer evaporation during these early stages of mixing is well known, and the clinical consequences have been considered (Bayne *et al.* 1977; Gentil *et al.*, 1993). The good adhesion between the polymerized monomer and the PMMA particles in the set cement means that chain entanglement of the polymer powder and the polymerized monomer should exist at the interface. Consequently, it should be expected that the physical processes of swelling of the powder, diffusion of the monomer, dilution of the BP into the liquid, and polymer–polymer interdiffusion will affect the setting dynamics.

The BP-DMT reactions may produce other free radicals or by-products different from the benzoyl peroxide free radical. The kinetics of the free radicals and their slow decay have been well studied (Turner, 1984). It has been suggested that unreacted radicals and residual components in the set mass may affect the biocompatibility of the cement and its eventual degradation (Trap *et al.*, 1992).

A very important residual component is the monomer left unpolymerized after the setting of the cement, excluding the unreacted monomer evaporated before the cement sets and cools down to its environmental temperature. The amount of residual monomer left in the cement mass depends on the type of cement, since different commercial brands give different results, but in all cases it decreases with time. The actual values reported depend also on the environment in which the specimens are kept, ranging between 0.05, and 1.3% after 21 days in water at 37 °C degradation (Trap *et al.*, 1992).

The polymerization process is strongly dependent upon the environmental temperature at which the reaction takes place (Haas *et al.*, 1975; Noble, 1983). Both dough time and setting time depend not only on chemical composition and concentration of the liquid, but also on the size and size distribution of the powder (Pascual *et al.*, 1996) and on environmental factors such as relative humidity or kneading frequency of the mix. In order to be able to compare, the ASTM Standard on acrylic bone cements imposes that the dough time and the setting time evaluation should be conducted at a room temperature of 23 °C $\pm$ 1 °C and a relative humidity of 50% $\pm$ 10%, and it allows a maximum dough time of 5 minutes and a setting time ranging from 5 to 15 minutes. The idea to accelerate the polymerization process has been proposed and the use of preheated implants considered (Dall *et al.*, 1986).

A parameter that has a very strong effect on the working time of the cement and that is under the control of the manufacturer is the powder-to-liquid ratio of the product, which is taken as the ratio between the weight of the powder in g and the volume of the liquid in ml. As the powder-to-liquid ratio increases, the peak temperature decreases (Lautenschlager *et al.*, 1984; Haas *et al.*, 1975; Meyer *et al.*, 1973). These results can be understood in terms of the relative amounts of initiator and monomer present in the various powder-to-liquid ratios and the role played by unreactive particles in absorbing heat.

There is extensive discussion in the literature about the role of the exotherm in the necrosis of the surrounding bone. The amount of heat released depends on the weight of reacting monomer in the mixture.

However, the peak temperature reached depends also on the volume of cement and its surface-to-volume ratio, in other words its thickness in service. This is the reason why the ASTM Standard defines very clearly the geometry of the mold and the place where to introduce the thermocouple in the cement for the evaluation of the maximum temperature.

More important than the temperature reached by the cement is the temperature at the bone–cement interface, since bone necrosis will be possible if such temperature reaches values over 56 °C, which corresponds to the onset of coagulation of albumin (Lehnartz, 1959). However, it seems that this temperature should not be taken as a threshold, since cell damage is not only a question of temperature but also of time. A wide variety of temperatures at the bone–bone cement interface have been reported depending on the thickness and the position of the thermocouple.

20.2.3. Molecular Weight

It is well known that the molecular weight and the molecular weight distribution of linear polymers play a very strong role on their mechanical properties. It is usually accepted for PMMA that most mechanical properties are practically independent of molecular weight when this is higher than 1 to 1.5×10^5, although even then the molecular weight distribution may play a strong role (Brauer *et al.*, 1977; Kusy, 1978; Ward, 1983). It is known that fracture surface energy of PMMA is closely related to molecular weight (Berry, 1964), although for high molecular weights (MV over 10^5) it becomes practically independent (Kusy and Katz, 1976).

It should be noted that in most cases the molecular weight of the cement is higher than that of the PMMA powder. This means that the polymerized monomer forms longer molecular chains than those present in the PMMA initial powder (Bayne *et al.*, 1975).

20.3. Mechanical Properties

Bone cement in service performs mainly a mechanical task, by distributing evenly the contact forces and transferring them from the prosthesis to the bone. This is the reason why mechanical properties of bone cements have been measured and reported by many authors. Since acrylic bone cements are based on PMMA polymers, with a glass transition temperature $T_g \approx 110\,^\circ\mathrm{C}$, their mechanical properties will be very sensitive to the environmental temperature, and strain rate will deeply affect their mechanical

Table 20.1. Range of Values of Some Mechanical Properties of Acrylic Bone Cements Reported in the Literature (Data from Lewis, 1997)

Tensile properties	
Ultimate tensile strength (MPa)	24–49
Elastic modulus in tension (MPa)	1580–4120
Compressive properties	
Ultimate compressive strength (MPa)	73–117
Elastic modulus in compression (MPa)	1940–3180
Flexural properties	
4-Point bending strength (MPa)	12–74
Elastic modulus in bending (MPa)	1950–3160
Shear strength (MPa)	32–69

behavior due to their viscoelastic nature. Finally, fracture and fatigue mechanisms have to be carefully analyzed. Bone cement is a self-cured multiphase material when compared to industrial PMMA. These microstructural and process differences explain their poorer mechanical properties. Good reviews of the mechanical properties of acrylic bone cements can be found in Saha and Pal (1984) and Lewis (1997).

20.3.1. Strength and Elastic Modulus

The strength and modulus of elasticity of bone cements has been measured using different kinds of tests such as tension, compression, bending, torsion, and shearing, and controlling different parameters such as temperature, environment, crosshead speed of the testing machine, and specimen geometry and size. Consequently, a wide variety of results is available. Moreover, the results reported refer to different commercial cement brands. Other factors related with the manufacture of the specimens contribute to the scatter of results. Examples of the ranges reported for the strength and the elastic modulus for different mechanical tests can be seen in Table 20.1 (Lewis, 1997).

20.3.2. Viscolelastic Behavior

Due to their polymeric nature, they exhibit a viscoelastic behavior and consequently the mechanical properties of acrylic bone cements are strongly dependent on temperature and strain rate. From a practical point of view, creep and stress relaxation will be very important parameters when assessing the life in service of acrylic bone cements.

The creep behavior seems to be correlated with the molecular weight distribution and the glass transition temperature. It has been shown that creep resistance increases with density and large PMMA powder particle size, and residual monomer, radio-opaque fillers and a plasticizing environment like water decrease it (Treharne and Brown, 1975). Creep will also depend upon the polymerizing process of the cement and the temperature at which the test is carried out (Oysaed and Ruyter, 1989). Different models to represent creep behavior of bone cements have been proposed (Norman *et al.*, 1995; Verdonschot and Huiskes, 1995).

20.3.3. Fracture Toughness

The fracture features of bone cements have been deeply studied, although some fracture mechanisms have not been well explained yet. The bone cements are taken as linear elastic solids, since PMMA behaves as a brittle material, and K_{IC} can be easily evaluated. An excellent review on the fracture toughness of acrylic bone cements is available (Lewis, 1989). Fracture toughness has been evaluated using different kinds of specimens. The results reported range between 1.03 to 2.32 $MPa \cdot m^{1/2}$ (Lewis, 1997). The brittleness of acrylic bone cements is apparent since the K_{IC} are even lower than those of ceramic materials. It can be noted that the highest fracture toughness reported is about double the lowest one. This means that the type of cement, the preparation and the molding conditions, and the type of test conducted will play a major role in the values obtained.

20.3.4. Fatigue

Among the causes of loosening of cemented joint prostheses, fatigue failure of the cement is currently understood as one of the most important. A good review of the fatigue properties of acrylic bone cements was published in 1988 (Krause and Mathis, 1988).

The most common approach taken when studying the fatigue failure of acrylic bone cements has been to assess the fatigue endurance at a given number of cycles. S–N curves have been obtained in rotating bending fatigue (Freitag and Cannon, 1977; Topoleski *et al.*, 1990), in tension–tension (Krause *et al.*, 1988; Johnson *et al.*, 1989), in tension–compression (Davies *et al.*, 1989), in three-point bending (Topoleski *et al.*, 1990), in four-point bending (Soltész and Ege, 1992), and even in compression (Jaffe *et al.*, 1974), usually under load control. Tests have been also carried out in tension–compression under strain control (Carter *et al.*, 1982). Most of the authors carry out their tests in sinusoidal loading, although this information is not always reported.

Taking fatigue endurance at 10^6 cycles, values of 6 to 20 MPa (Jaffe *et al.*, 1974; Freitag and Cannon, 1977; Krause and Mathis, 1988), and for a fatigue endurance at 10^7 cycles 15 to 26 MPa bending (Soltész and Ege, 1992) have been reported for different commercial bone cements. Such a wide scatter of results will depend not only on the type of cement used, but also on its preparation process and its final microstructure. Since fatigue has a statistical nature and the probability that two specimens of a same batch exhibit a different behavior is high, a possible approach is to analyze the fatigue results using the Weibull distribution of survival probability, the failure probability or reliability at a given number of cycles, for a constant stress amplitude and a defined frequency (Topoleski *et al.*, 1990; Krause *et al.*, 1988). Here again there is also a scatter of results because different authors use different fatigue tests, the type and geometry of the specimens is different, and the maximum stresses and frequencies used are also different.

All the tests reported have been conducted with unnotched specimens, which means that the fatigue failure process has required a crack nucleation stage and a crack propagation stage. The number of cycles spent in the nucleating stage will depend on the smoothness and lack of porosity of the surface. In fact when the cement will set in service, it should be expected that its surface will not be smooth and porosity and voids at the metal–cement and bone–cement interfaces should be expected. This means that surface flaws exist and will be responsible for a fast crack nucleation. Therefore, the fatigue behavior of bone cement in service may be dominated by the crack propagation behavior (Wright and Robinson, 1982; Vila, 1992; Molino and Topoleski, 1996; Lewis, 1997) as in most engineering structural components. Fatigue crack propagation in bone cements behaves according to the Paris law: $da/dN = A(\Delta K)^m$, where da/dN is the crack propagation rate in one cycle, ΔK is the amplitude of the stress intensity factor which depends on the load applied, the crack length, and the geometry of the crack, while A and m are constants which depend on the material and the environment. Some results reported in the literature for the Paris law parameters A and m are summarized in Table 20.2.

Table 20.2. Paris–Erdogan Parameters Reported in the Literature for Barium-Sulfate-Containing Cements

Cement	m	A (m/cycle)
Wright and Robinson (1982)	6.5	2.5×10^{-6}
Liu *et al.* (1987)	6.8	6.6×10^{-7}
Nguyen *et al.* (1997)	5.5	4.6×10^{-7}
Ginebra *et al.* (2000a, b)	6.15	5.09×10^{-6}

The fractographic analysis of acrylic bone cement explanted from patients at their revision operation has shown that fatigue crack growth is most likely the leading *in vivo* failure mechanism (Topoleski *et al.*, 1990). The fracture surfaces of the explanted specimens compare very well with those obtained from *in vitro* fatigue tests.

20.4. Factors Affecting the Microstructure and the Microstructure–Mechanical Properties Relationship

The microstructure of acrylic bone cements can be interpreted as multiphase materials consisting in PMMA beads, polymerized monomer, and radiopacifying agent particles, as can be observed in Figure 20.3. Moreover, there are factors related with the mixing technique, the presence of blood, grease or body fluids, the laminations produced when introducing the cement in the bone cavity, the interfaces with the old cement, with the metallic prosthesis, or with the cancellous bone, the

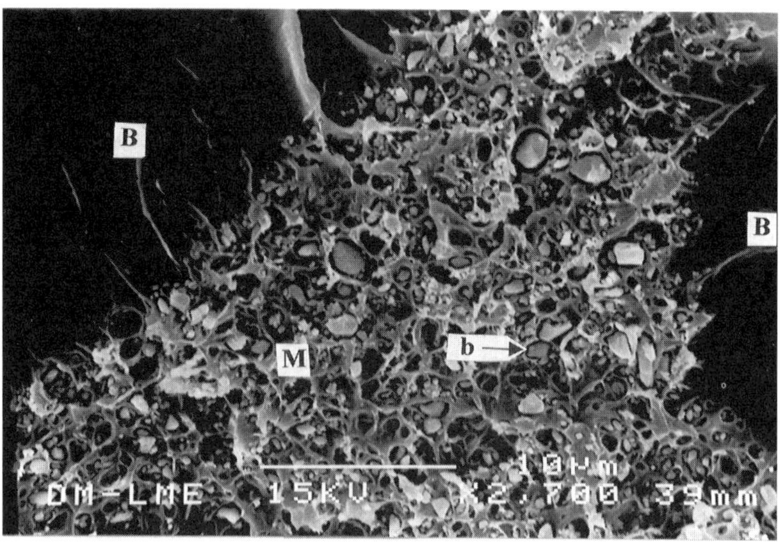

Figure 20.3. Scanning electron micrograph of a fracture surface of acrylic bone cement, which contains 10 wt% of barium sulfate, showing the cement matrix (M) between two PMMA beads (B). It can be seen that very good continuity exists between the beads and the PMMA matrix. In contrast, the barium sulfate particles (b) do not adhere to the surrounding polymeric matrix.

thickness of the cement and the water sorption, which will affect the bulk or the interfacial microstructure of the cements and consequently their mechanical behavior.

20.4.1. Porosity

The presence of porosity in bone cements has always been detected, with a volume fraction usually ranging between 2 and 8% (Kusy, 1978). The discussion about the real influence of porosity on the mechanical properties goes on, although it is clear to every one that it is always convenient to reduce the porosity of bone cements. Consequently, the improvement in mixing techniques has undergone a fast and spectacular evolution.

The techniques used to reduce porosity include the improvement of hand mixing, mechanical or ultrasound mixing, pressurization of the cement, centrifugation of the mixture, and vacuum mixing. All these techniques result in a reduction of porosity from about the 8% which is achieved by conventional hand mixing to values below 1% for vacuum mixing. Good revisions and discussions about the results on the fight against porosity have been published (Wang and Pilliar, 1989; Wixson, 1992).

Most of the reported results show that mechanical properties improve as porosity is decreased. However, certain authors find that certain mechanical properties do not improve at all, mainly fracture toughness and the fatigue crack propagation rate published (Wang and Pilliar, 1989; Rimnac *et al.*, 1986). The main argument used to explain the detrimental effect of porosity is that pores act as a stress concentrator. However, it has to be borne in mind that under a tensile state of stress polymers have a maximum inherent flaw size which will control the fracture load of the material. On the other hand, the main deformation mechanism of PMMA in tension is crazing and therefore the crack will propagate with a Dugdale plastic region ahead of it, which will account for the crazed region. This model of crack propagation in bone cements would explain that more important than porosity is the size of the largest pore in the plane of the advancing crack. A pore will or will not blunt the tip of the crack, depending on the Dugdale zone size and the size of the pore.

20.4.2. *In Vivo* Environment

The influence of body fluids and body temperature (37 °C) properties is significant in different properties of the cement. Uptake of liquids has been shown to affect some of the properties of the cement after implantation. Sorption of water generally lowers its mechanical properties (Bargar *et al.*, 1986; Looney and Park, 1986). However, fracture mechanics studies show that the crack velocity is slower in water than in air, and that fracture toughness is about 15 to 20% higher in water than in air (Beaumont and Young, 1975). Other results show that the work to fracture increases with the time of storage of the cement in liquids such as water, Ringer's solution, and lipids, although in each case the work to fracture after storage at 21 °C is higher than after storage at 37 °C (Hailey *et al.*, 1994). Water in bone cement acts as a plasticizer.

20.4.3. Additives

The main additives usually found in bone cements are radiopacifier particles such as $BaSO_4$ and ZrO_2, and antibiotics.

Recent studies have shown that the addition of radio-opaque agents to PMMA enhance the macrophage–osteoclast differentiation and therefore they may contribute to the bone resorption and aseptic loosening (Sabokbar *et al.*, 1997). Furthermore, these agents evoke a significant pathological response in the surrounding tissue. Barium sulfate has been shown to intensify the release of inflammatory mediators in response to PMMA particles (Lazarus *et al.*, 1994). There is also evidence that the release of the radiopacifier particles in the surrounding tissues can cause damage to the articulating surfaces and a marked increased in the production of polyethylene wear debris if they enter the joint space (Isaac *et al.*, 1987; Caravia *et al.*, 1990; Cooper *et al.*, 1991).

On the other hand, it can be stated that the radiopacifying agents have a significant effect on the mechanical properties of acrylic bone cements, which depend on their size and morphology. Indeed, it has been shown that while the addition of $BaSO_4$ produces a decrease in the tensile strength of about 10% (Haas *et al*, 1975; Kusy, 1978; Ginebra *et al.*, 1999), the addition of ZrO_2 does not affect this parameter. On the other hand, it has been reported that the fracture toughness, which is unaffected by the inclusion of $BaSO_4$, is increased around 20% by the addition of ZrO_2 (Ginebra *et al.*, 2000a). Moreover, it has been shown that both inorganic radiopacifiers enhance the fatigue crack propagation resistance of the cement (Molino and Topoleski, 1996; Ginebra *et al.*, 2000a, b). This behavior can be explained in terms of the microstructure of the radiopacifying agents and their interaction with the polymeric matrix, which is illustrated in Figure 20.4a, b). Since there is no chemical adhesion between the inorganic particles and the PMMA (cf. also Figure 20.3), it could be interpreted that the filler particles behave like pores when a tensional state of stress is applied to the cement. However, at this point the morphology of the particles plays a determinant role with respect to the mechanical behavior of the cement. Indeed, the ZrO_2 particles, which have a cauliflower-like shape, can anchor mechanically to

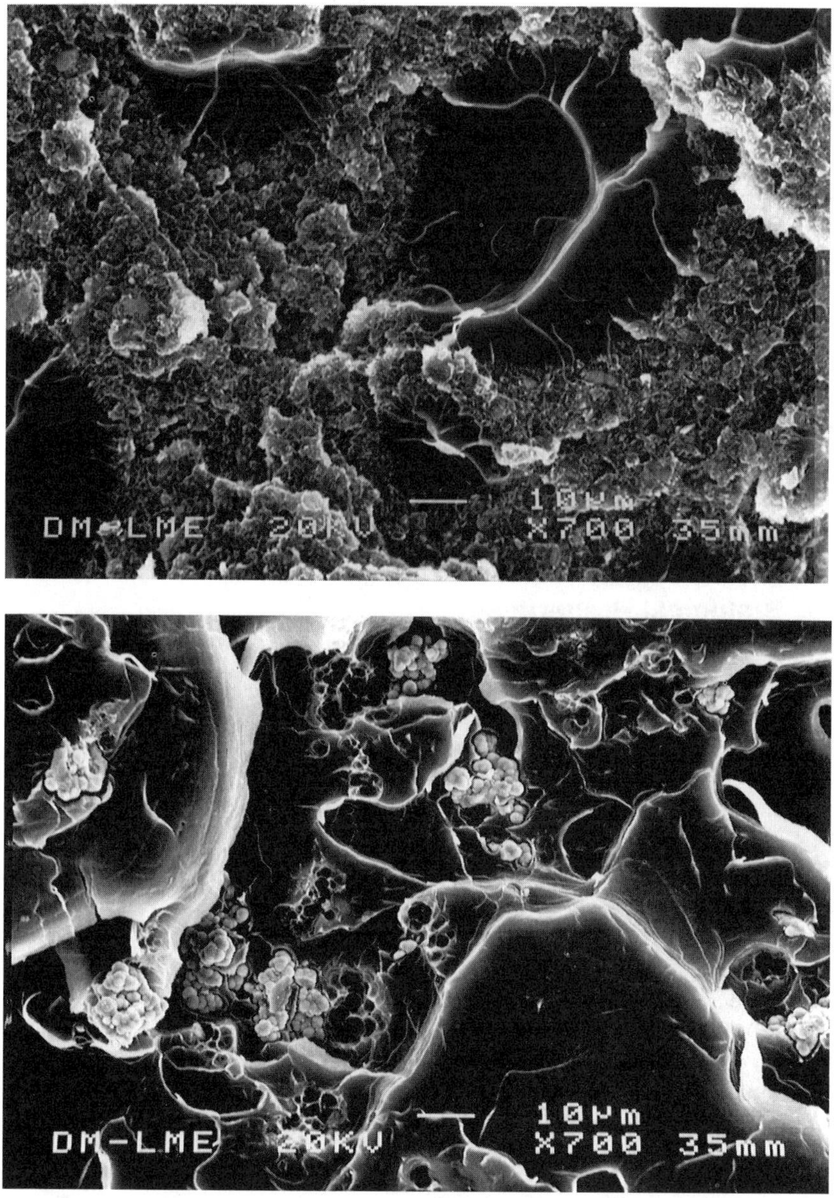

Figure 20.4. Fracture surfaces of acrylic bone cements containing different radiopacifying agents: (a) barium sulfate and (b) zirconium dioxide. Neither the barium sulfate nor the zirconium dioxide particles bond to the polymeric matrix. In the barium-sulfate-containing cement, the interbead matrix has a much rougher appearance due to the small size of the inorganic particles. In the cement containing zirconium dioxide, the characteristic cauliflower-like morphology allows a mechanical anchorage of the inorganic particles to the polymeric matrix, which can be responsible for the enhancement of the mechanical properties.

the matrix, reinforcing it to a certain extent. This effect does not take place in the case of the smaller and more regular $BaSO_4$ particles.

At present, some iodine-containing monomers are being investigated as potential substitutes for the inorganic radiopacifying agents with improved biological and mechanical characteristics (Vázquez *et al.*, 1999; Ginebra *et al*, 1999, 2000a, b).

The need to tackle the problem of postoperative infections led to the idea of mixing antibiotics with the bone cement and allowing them to leach out into the surrounding tissues. A great research effort was devoted to the study of the effect of antibiotic addition on the mechanical properties of bone cements, and a very good review was published (Nelson *et al.*, 1978). It seems clear that the addition of antibiotics to bone cements reduces its mechanical properties, although the reduction depends very strongly on the amount of antibiotic added (Davies *et al.*, 1989; Lautenschlager *et al.*, 1976; Davies and Harris, 1991).

20.5. Biological Properties

Certain clinical complications have been associated with the use of bone cement and particularly with monomer release. A very good review on the peroperative complications and those during anesthesia was published some years ago (James, 1987). An extensive amount of information regarding hypotension, hazards, local tissue damage, and even the burn of the sciatic nerve caused by bone cements has been reported by different authors, some of which can be found in Newens and Volz (1972), Milne (1973), Linder and Romanus (1976), and Birch *et al.* (1992).

On the other hand, some studies show that the products of wear and fracture or fragmentation of bone cement, as well as wear debris of polyethylene from the articulating surface, may cause a foreign body response consisting in a macrophage, a giant cell foreign body granulomatous reaction. This tissue can produce a variety of chemical mediators of inflammation and eventually bone resorption. This process of osteolysis induced by bone cement fragmentation may be the biological cause for the loosening of the cemented joint prostheses (Jasty *et al.*, 1992; Willert *et al.*, 1990).

20.6. Modification of Acrylic Bone Cements

At present, a wide variety of possible modifications of conventional bone cements are being investigated, focusing on the improvement of either the mechanical or the biological properties. They are summarized in Figure

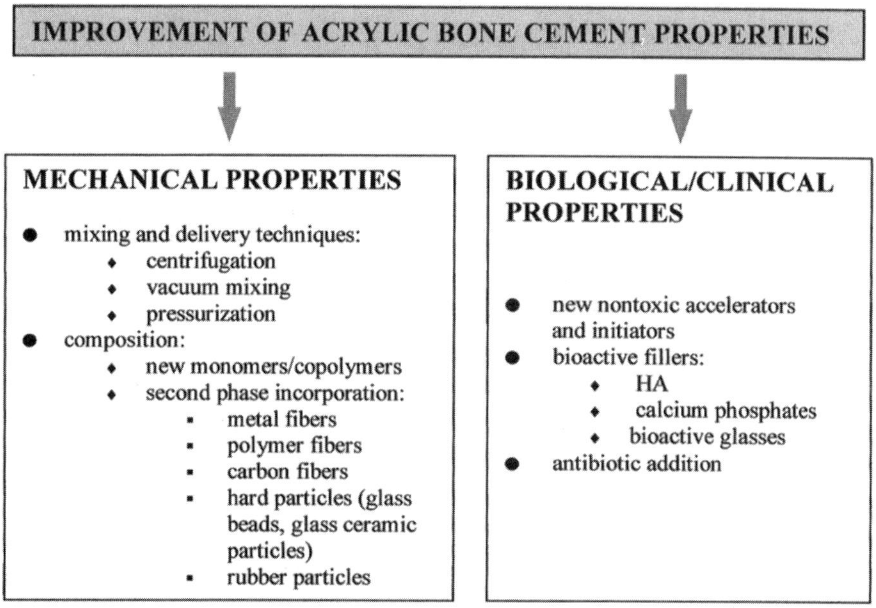

Figure 20.5. Recent trends in the search for the improvement of some mechanical and biological properties of acrylic bone cements.

20.5. Some of them have already been described since they refer to the improvement of the preparation techniques, such as porosity reduction, or of surgical techniques, such as reaming and cleaning the bone cavity or pressurization.

The main path followed to improve the mechanical properties of conventional bone cements has been the reinforcement of the matrix either with particles or with fibers. In relation to particle addition, three main directions can be described: First, reinforcement with hard particles such as glass beads (Beaumont, 1977; Guida *et al.*, 1984) or glass ceramic particles (Henning *et al.*, 1979), second, the reinforcement with tough or rubber toughened particles (Vila, 1992; Vila *et al.*, 1999a, b; Murakami *et al.*, 1988), and finally reinforcement with bioactive particles, such as inorganic bone and demineralized bone matrix (Liu *et al.*, 1987; Henrich *et al.*, 1993) and hydroxyapatite (Low *et al.*, 1993; Dandurand *et al.*, 1990) which could improve both the mechanical properties of the bulk cement and the interfacial bone–cement strength.

The fiber reinforcement of bone cements has followed two main paths: reinforcement with metallic fibers (Fishbane and Pond, 1997; Topoleski *et al.*, 1991, 1992) and reinforcement with polymeric fibers, including carbon fibers (Saha and Pal, 1986; Pourdeyhimi and Wagner, 1989; Buckley *et al.*, 1991; Pilliar *et al.*, 1976).

Alternative chemical modifications of the bone cement matrix, such as the substitution of initiatiors, accelerators (Brauer *et al.*, 1986; Tanzi *et al.*, 1991; Vázquez *et al.*, 1997), or radiopacifying agents (Vazquez *et al.*, 1999; Ginebra *et al.*, 1999, 2000a, b) by more biocompatible compounds, or the addition of other monomers to the liquid phase (Migliaresi and Capuana, 1990; Davies and Harris, 1992; Pascual *et al.*, 1999a, b; Oysaed, 1990, Brauer *et al.*, 1986), improve other physical, chemical, and biological properties.

References

ASTM Standard, 1986. *Medical Devices*, Section 13, **13.01**, Philadelphia.

Bargar, W.L., Brown, S.A., Paul, H.A., Voegli, T., Hseih, Y., Sharkey, N. 1986. In vivo versus in vitro polymerization of acrylic bone cement: effect on material properties, *J. Orthop. Res.* **4**, 86.

Bayne, S.C., Lautenschlager, E.P., Compere, C.L., Wildes, R. 1975. Degree of polymerization of acrylic bone cement, *J. Biomed. Mater. Res.* **9**, 27.

Bayne, S.C., Lautenschlager, E.P., Greener, E.H., Meyer, P.R. 1977. Clinical influences on bone cement monomer release, *J. Biomed. Mater. Res.* **11**, 859.

Beaumont, P.W.R. 1977. The strength of acrylic bone cements and acrylic cement-stainless steel interfaces. Part I, The strength of acrylic bone cement containing second phase dispersions, *J. Mater. Sci.* **12**, 1845.

Beaumont, P.W.R., Young, R.J. 1975. Slow crack growth in acrylic bone cement, *J. Biomed. Mater. Res.* **9**, 423.

Berry, J. 1964. Fracture processes in polymeric materials. V. Dependence of the ultimate properties of polymethylmethacrylate on molecular weight, *J. Polym. Sci. A*, **2**, 4069.

Birch, R., Wilkinson, M.C.P., Vijayan, K.P., Gschmeissner, S. 1992. Cement burn of the sciatic nerve, *J. Bone Jt. Surg.* **74B**, 731–733.

Brauer, G.M., Termini, D.J., Dickson, G. 1977. Analysis of the ingredients and determination of the residual components of acrylic bone cements, *J. Biomed. Mater. Res.* **11**, 577.

Brauer, G.M., Steinberger, D.R., Stansbury, J.W. 1986. Dependence of curing time, peak temperature, and mechanical properties on the composition of bone cement, *J. Biomed. Mater. Res.* **20**, 839.

Buckley, C.A., Lautenschlager, E.P., Gilbert, J.L. 1991. High strength PMMA fibers for use in a self-reinforced acrylic cement, fiber tensile properties and composite toughness, *Proceedings of the 17th Annual Meeting of the Society for Biomaterials*, p. 45.

Caravia, L., Dowson, D., Fisher, J., Jobbins, B. 1990. The influence of bone and bone cement debris on counterface roughness in sliding wear tests of ultra-high molecular weight polyethylene on stainless steel, *Proc. Inst. Mech. Eng.* **204**, 65–70.

Carter, D.R., Gates, E.I., Harris, W.H. 1982. Strain-controlled fatigue of acrylic bone cement, *J. Biomed. Mater. Res.* **16**, 647.

Charnley, J. 1964a. Anchorage of the femoral head prosthesis to the shaft of the femur, *J. Bone Jt. Surg.* **42B**, 28.

Charnley, J. 1964b. Bonding of prosthesis to bone by cement, *J. Bone Jt. Surg.* **46B**, 518.

Charnley, J. 1970. *Acrylic Cement in Orthopaedic Surgery*, E.& S. Livingstone, London.

Cooper, J.R., Dowson, D., Fisher, J., Jobbins B. 1991. Ceramic bearing surfaces in total artificial joints: resistance to third body wear damage from bone cement particles, *J. Med. Eng. Technol.* **15**, 63–67.

Dall, D.M., Miles, A.W., Juby, G. 1986. Accelerated polymerization of acrylic bone cement using preheated implants, *Clin. Orthop. Relat. Res.* **211**, 148.

Dandurand, J., Delpech, V., Lebugle, A., Lamure, A., Lacabanne, C. 1990. Study of the mineral-organic linkage in an apatitic reinforced bone cement, *J. Biomed. Mater. Res.* **24**, 1377.

Davies, J.P., Harris W.H. 1991. Effect of hand-mixing tobramycin on the fatigue strength of Simplex P, *J. Biomed. Mater. Res.* **25**, 1409.

Davies, J.P., Harris, W.H. 1992. The effect of the addition of methylene blue on the fatigue strength of simplex P bone-cement, *J. Appl. Biomat.* **3**, 81.

Davies, J.P., O'Connor, D., Burke, D., Harris, W. 1989. Influence of antibiotic impregnation on fatigue life of Simplex P and Palacos R acrylic bone cements with and without centrifugation, *J. Biomed. Mater. Res.* **23**, 379.

Fishbane, B.M., Pond, R.B. 1977. Stainless steel fiber reinforcement of polymethylmethacrylate, *Clin. Orthop. Relat. Res.* **128**, 194.

Freitag, T.A., Cannon, S.L. 1977. Fracture characteristics of acrylic bone cements. II. Fatigue, *J. Biomed. Mater. Res.* **11**, 609.

Gentil, B., Paugam, C., Wolf, C., Lienhart, A., Augereau, B. 1993. Methylmethacrylate plasma levels during total hip arthroplasty, *Clin. Orthop. Relat. Res.* **287**, 112.

Ginebra, M.P., Aparicio, C., Albuixech, L., Fernández-Barragán, E., Gil, F.J., Planell, J.A., Morejón, L., Vázquez, B., San Román, J. 1999. Improvement of the mechanical properties of acrylic bone cements by substitution of the radio-opaque agent, *J. Mater. Sci., Materials in Medicine* **10**, 733–737.

Ginebra, M.P., Albuixech, L., Fernández-Barragán, Aparicio, C., Gil, F.J., San Román, J., Vázquez, B., Planell, J.A. 2000a. Mechanical performance of acrylic bone cements containing different radiopacifying agents, *Biomaterials*, in press.

Ginebra, M.P., Albuixech, L., Fernández-Barragán, Clément, J., Gil, F.J., Planell, J.A. 2000b. Effect of different radiopacifying agents on the fatigue crack propagation of acrylic bone cements, *Proceedings of the 9th International Conference on Polymers in Medicine and Surgery*, pp. 288–295, IOM Communications Ltd, London.

Guida, G., Riccio, V., Gatto, S., Migliaresi, C., Nicodemo, L., Nicolais, L., Palomba, C. 1984. A glass bead composite acrylic bone cement, in: *Biomaterials and Biomechanics* (P. Ducheyne, G. Van der Perre, A.E. Aubert, eds.), p. 19, Elsevier Science Publ., Amsterdam.

Haas, S.S., Brauer, G.M., Dickson, G. 1975. A characterization of polymethylmethacrylate bone cement, *J. Bone Jt. Surg.* **57A**(3), 380.

Hailey, J.L., Turner, I.G., Miles, A.W., Price, G. 1994. The effect of post-curing chemical bone changes on the mechanical properties of acrylic bone cement, *J. Mater. Sci. Materials in . Medicine*, **5**, 617–621.

Henning, W., Blencke, B.A., Brömer, H., Deutscher, K.K., Gross, A., Ege W. 1979. Investigations with bioactivated polymethylmethacrylates, *J. Biomed. Mater. Res.* **13**, 89.

Henrich, D.E., Cram, A.E., Park, J.B., Liu, Y.K., Reddi, H. 1993. Inorganic bone and demineralized bone matrix impregnated bone cement: A preliminary in vivo study, *J. Biomed. Mater. Res.* **27**, 277.

Isaac, G.H., Atkinson, J.R., Dowson, D. Kennedy P.D., Smith M.R. 1987. The causes of femoral head roughening in explanted Charnley hip prostheses, *Eng. Med.* **16**, 167–173.

Jaffe, W.L., Rose, R.M., Radin, E.L. 1974. On the stability of the mechanical properties of self-curing acrylic bone cement, *J. Bone Jt. Surg.* **56A**(8), 1711.

James, M.L. 1987. Complicaciones anestésicas y metabólicas, in: *Complicaciones de las artroplastias totales de cadera* (R.S.M. Ling, ed.), Salvat Editores, Barcelona.

Jasty, M., Jiranek, W., Harris, W. 1992. Acrylic fragmentation in total hip replacements and its biological consequences, *Clin. Orthop. Relat. Res.* **285**, 116.

Johnson, J.A., Provan, J.W., Krygier, J.J., Chan, K.H., Miller J. 1989. Fatigue of acrylic bone cement: effect of frequency and environment, *J. Biomed. Mater. Res.* **23**, 819.

Krause, W., Mathis, R. 1988. Fatigue properties of acrylic bone cements: review of the literature, *J. Biomed. Mater. Res.* **22**, 37.

Krause, W., Mathis, R., Grimes, L. 1988. Fatigue properties of acrylic bone cement: S-N, P-N and P-S-N data, *J. Biomed. Mater. Res.* **22**(A3), 221.

Kusy, R.P. 1978. Characterization of self-curing acrylic bone cements, *J. Biomed. Mater. Res.* **12**, 271.

Kusy, R.P., Katz, M.J. 1976. Effect of molecular weight on the fracture surface energy of poly(methyl methacrylate) in cleavage, *J. Mater. Sci.* **11**, 1475.

Lautenschlager, E.P., Jacobs, J.J. Marshall, G.W., Meyer, P.R. 1976. Mechanical properties of bone cements containing large doses of antibiotic powders, *J. Biomed. Mater. Res.* **10**, 929.

Lautenschlager, E.P., Stupp, S.I., Keller, J.C. 1984. Structure and properties of acrylic bone cement, in, *Functional Behaviour of Orthopaedic Biomaterials. Volume II. Applications* (P. Ducheyne, G.W. Hastings, eds.), pp 88ff., CRC Press Inc., Boca Raton.

Lazarus, M.D., Cuckler, J.M., Schumacher, H.R., Ducheyne, P., Baker, D.G. 1994. Comparison of the inflammatory response to particulate polymethylmethacrylate debris with and without barium sulphate, *J. Orthop. Res.* **12**, 532–541.

Lehnartz, E. 1959. *Chemical Physiologie*, S. 87, Springer-Verlag, Berlin.

Lewis, G. 1989. The fracture toughness of biomaterials: I. Acrylic bone cements, *J. Mater. Educ.* **11**, 429–479.

Lewis, G. 1997. Properties of acrylic bone cement: state of the art review, *J. Biomed. Mater. Res.* (*Appl. Biomater.*) **38**, 155–182.

Linder, L., Romanus, M. 1976. Acute local tissue effects of polymerizing acrylic bone cement, *Clin. Orthop. Relat. Res.* **115**, 303.

Liu, Y.K., Park, J.B., Njus, G.O., Steinstra, D. 1987. Bone particle impregnated bone cement I. In vitro studies, *J. Biomed. Mat. Res.* **21**, 247.

Looney, M.A., Park, J.B. 1986. Molecular and mechanical property changes during aging of bone cement in vitro and in vivo, *J. Biomat. Mater. Res.* **20**, 555.

Low, R.F., Hulbert, S.F., Sogal, A. 1993. Mechanical properties of hydroxyapatite-polymethylmethacrylate bone cement composite: hydroxyapatite embedded on surface and throughout cement matrix, in: *Bioceramics Vol. 6* (P. Ducheyne, D. Christiansen, eds.), p. 339, Butterworth-Heinemann, London.

Meyer, P.R., Lautenschlager, E.P., Moore, B.K., 1973, On the setting properties of acrylic bone cement, *J. Bone Jt. Surg.* **55A**(1), 149.

Migliaresi, C., Capuana, P. 1990. 2-Hydroxyethylmethacrylate modified bone cement, in: *Clinical Implant Materials, Advances in Biomaterials Vol. 9*, p. 141, Elsevier, Amsterdam.

Milne, I.S. 1973. Hazards of acrylic bone cement, *Anaesthesia* **28**, 538.

Molino, L.N., Topoleski, L.D.T. 1996. Effect of $BaSO_4$ on the fatigue crack propagation rate of PMMA bone cement, *J. Biomed. Mater. Res.* **31**, 131–137.

Murakami, A., Behiri, J.C., Bonfield, W. 1988. Rubber-modified bone cement, *J. Mater. Sci.* **23**, 2029.

Nelson, R.C., Hoffman, R.O., Burton, J.A. 1978. The effect of antibiotic addition on the mechanical properties of acrylic cement, *J. Biomed. Mater. Res.* **12**, 473.

Newens, A.F., Volz, R.G. 1972. Severe hypotension during prosthetic hip surgery with acrylic bone cement, *Anesthesiology* **36**, 298.

Nguyen, N.C., Maloney, W.J., Dauskardt, R.H. 1997. Reliability of PMMA bone cement fixation, fracture and fatigue crack-growth behaviour. *J. Mater. Sci., Materials in Medicine* **8**, 473–483.

Noble, P.C. 1983. Selection of acrylic bone cements for use in joint replacement, *Biomaterials* **4**, 94.

Norman, T.L., Kisch, V., Blaha, J.D., Gruen, T.A., Hustosky, K. 1995. Creep characteristics of hand and vacuum mixed acrylic bone cement at elevated stress levels, *J. Biomed. Mater. Res.* **29**, 495–501.

Oysaed, H. 1990. Dynamic mechanical properties of multiphase acrylic sistems, *J. Biomed. Mater. Res.* **24**, 1037.

Oysaed, H., Ruyter, I.E. 1989. Creep studies of multiphase acrylic systems, *J. Biomed. Mater. Res.* **23**, 719.

Pascual, B., Vázquez, B., Gurruchaga, M., Goñi, I., Ginebra, M.P., Gil, F.J., Planell, J.A., Levenfeld,B., San Román, J. 1996. New aspects of the effect of size and size distribution on the setting parameters and mechanical properties of acrylic bone cement, *Biomaterials* **17**, 509–516.

Pascual, B., Goñi, I., Gurruchaga, M. 1999a. Characterization of a new acrylic bone cement based on a (methyl methacrylate/1-hydroxypropyl methacrylate) monomer, *J. Biomed. Mater. Res. Appl. Biomater.* **48**, 447–457.

Pascual, B., Gurruchaga, M., Ginebra, M.P., Gil, F.J., Planell, J.A., Vázquez, B., San Román, J., Goñi I. 1999b. Modified acrylic bone cement with high amounts of ethoxytriethyleneglycol methacrylate, *Biomaterials* **20**(5), 453–463.

Pilliar, R.M., Blackwell, R., MacNab I., Cameron, H.V. 1976. Carbon fiber-reinforced bone cement in orthopaedic surgery, *J. Biomed. Mater. Res.* **10**, 893.

Pourdeyhimi, B., Wagner, H.D. 1989. Elastic and ultimate properties of acrylic bone cement reinforced with ultra-high-molecular weight polyethylene fibers, *J. Biomed. Mater. Res.* **23**, 63.

Rimnac, C., Wright, T., McGill, D. 1986. The effect of centrifugation on the fracture properties of acrylic bone cements, *J. Bone Jt. Surg.* **68A**, 281.

Sabokbar, A., Fujikawa, Y., Murray, D.W., Athanasou, N.A. 1997. Radio-opaque agents in bone cement increase bone resorption, *J. Bone Jt. Surg., Br. Vol.* **79B**, 129–134.

Saha, S., Pal, S. 1984. Mechanical properties of bone cement: a review, *J. Biomed. Mater. Res.* **18**, 435.

Saha, S., Pal, S. 1986. Mechanical characterization of commercially made carbon-fiber-reinforced polymethylmethacrylate, *J. Biomed. Mater. Res.* **20**, 817.

Soltész, U., Ege, W. 1992. Fatigue behavior of different acrylic bone cements, *Proceedings of the 4th World Biomaterials Congress*, p. 90.

Tanzi, M.C., Sket, I., Gatti, A.M., Monari, E. 1991, Physical characterization of acrylic bone cement cured with new accelerator system, *Clin. Mater.* **8**, 131.

Topoleski, L.D.T., Ducheyne, P., Cuckler, J.M. 1990, A fractographic analysis of in vivo poly(methyl methacrylate) bone cement failure mechanisms, *J. Biomed. Mater. Res.* **24**, 135.

Topoleski, L.D.T., Ducheyne, P., Cuckler J.M. 1991. Fatigue properties and failure mechanisms of titanium fiber reinforced and pore reduced polymethylmethacrylate bone cement, *Proceedings of the 17th Annual Meeting of the Society for Biomaterials*, p. 48.

Topoleski, L.D.T., Ducheyne, P., Cuckler, J.M. 1992. The fracture toughness of titanium-fiber reinforced bone cement, *J. Biomed. Mater. Res.* **26**, 1599.

Trap, B., Wolff, P., Jensen, J.S. 1992. Acrylic bone cements: residuals and extractability of methacrylate monomers and aromatic amines, *J. Appl. Biomater.* **3**, 51.

Treharne, R.W., Brown, N. 1975. Factors influencing the creep behavior of Poly(methyl methacrylate) cements, *J. Biomed. Mater. Res. Symp.* **6**, 81.

Turner, R.C. 1984. Free radical decay kinetics in PMMA bone cement, *J. Biomed. Mater. Res.* **18**, 467.

Vázquez, B., Elvira, C., Levenfeld, B., Pascual, B., Goñi, I., Gurruchaga, M., Ginebra, M.P., Gil, F.X., Planell, J.A., Liso, P.A., Rebuelta, M., San Román, J. 1997. Application of new tertiary amines with reduced toxicity to the curing process of acrylic bone cements, *J. Biomed. Mater. Res.* **34**, 129–136.

Vázquez, B., Ginebra, M.P., Gil, F.J., Planell, J.A., López Bravo, A., San Román, J. 1999. Radiopaque acrylic cements prepared with a new acrylic derivative of iodo-quinoline, *Biomaterials* **20**, 2047–2053.

Verdonschot, N., Huiskes, R. 1995. Dynamic creep behavior of acrylic bone cement, *J. Biomed. Mater. Res.* **29**, 575–581.

Vila, M. M. 1992, Ph.D. Thesis, Universitat Politècnica de Catalunya.

Vila, M.M., Ginebra, M.P., Gil, F.J., Planell, J.A. 1999a. Effect of porosity and environment on the mechanical properties of acrylic bone cement modified with acrylonitrile-butadiene-styrene particles: Part I. Fracture toughness, *J. Biomed. Mater. Res.* (*Appl. Biomater.*) **48**, 121–127.

Vila, M.M., Ginebra, M.P., Gil, F.J., Planell, J.A., 1999b, Effect of porosity and environment on the mechanical properties of acrylic bone cement modified with acrylonitrile-butadiene-styrene particles: Part II. Fatigue crack propagation, *J. Biomed. Mater. Res.* (*Appl. Biomater.*) **48**, 128–134.

Wang, C.T., Pilliar, R.M. 1989. Fracture toughness of acrylic bone cements, *J. Mater. Sci.* **24**, 3725.

Ward, I.M. 1983. Mechanical properties of solid polymers, 2nd edn., John Wiley & Sons, Bristol.

Willert, H.G., Bertram, H., Buchhorn, G.H. 1990. Osteolysis in alloarthroplasty of the hip: the role of bone cement fragmentation, *Clin. Orthop. Relat. Res.* **258**, 108.

Wixson, R.L. 1992. Do we need to vacuum mix or centrifuge cement?, *Clin. Orthop. Relat. Res.* **285**, 84.

Wright, T.M., Robinson, R.P. 1982. Fatigue crack propagation in polymethylmethacrylate bone cements, *J. Mater. Sci.* **17**, 2463–2468.

21

Mechanical Properties of Tooth Structures

Roberto De Santis, Luigi Ambrosio, and Luigi Nicolais

21.1. Introduction

Enamel, dentine, cementum, and pulp are the dental tissues. These four materials are joined as shown in Figure 21.1 and characterize the external and internal junctions, CEJ and DEJ, respectively (cementum–enamel and dentine–enamel junctions). The enamel, dentine, and cementum mineralized structures with the bone structure are the connective hard tissues.

Dentine is the bulk of a tooth and, as compact bone material, is formed by an inorganic mineral part (hydroxyapatite) and an organic matrix (mainly formed by collagen). Type I fibrillar collagen is the main constituent of bone and the dentine extracellular matrix. However, chromatography tests suggest a different cross-link distribution between bone and dentine collagen (Kuboky and Mechanic, 1982). Dentinal tubules across dentine (Veis, 1996) and the intertubular and intratubular dentine is distinguished (ITD and PTD, respectively).

Dentinal tubules course through dentine following an S-shaped curvature and change their diameter. Lateral branches of tubules with smaller diameter complete the tubules' network beside the DEJ (Cagidiaco and Ferrari, 1995). There is a different distribution of dentinal tubules and diameters in the P-DEJ direction (Garberoglio and Brannstrom, 1976). Tubules are wider and more numerous near the pulp.

Enamel covers the crown of the tooth and its structure consists of a tightly packed mass of hydroxyapatite crystals which are organized in highly

---

Roberto De Santis, Luigi Ambrosio, and Luigi Nicolais • Institute of Composite Materials Technology C.N.R., and C.R.I.B., University of Naples, "Federico II", Piazzale Tecchio 80, 80125 Naples, Italy.

Integrated Biomaterials Science, edited by R. Barbucci. Kluwer Academic/Plenum Publishers, New York, 2002.

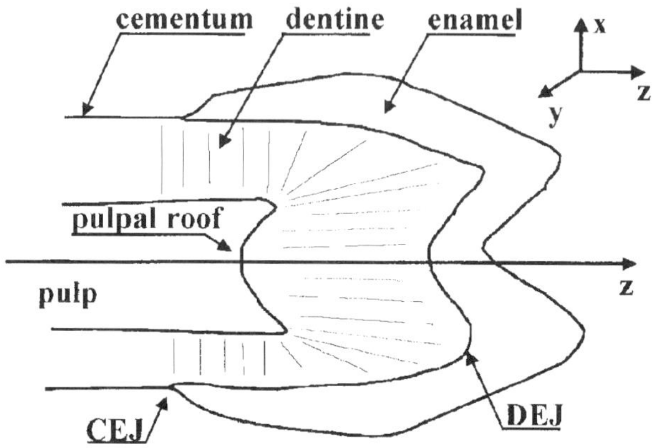

Figure 21.1. Arrangement of the dental tissues.

oriented patterns (enamel rods). Rods, which extend from the DEJ to the surface of the enamel, are arranged in circumferential rows around the main axis of a tooth. Figure 21.2 shows a scanning electron microscopy (SEM) of enamel and etched enamel (etched with 37% phosphoric acid for 30 s).

The pulp is the soft tissue of a tooth which is richly innervated. It occupies the central portion of the tooth which is divided into a coronal pulp chamber and a radicular root canal. The principal cells of the pulp are the odontoblasts, whose processes extend into dentine, fibroblast,

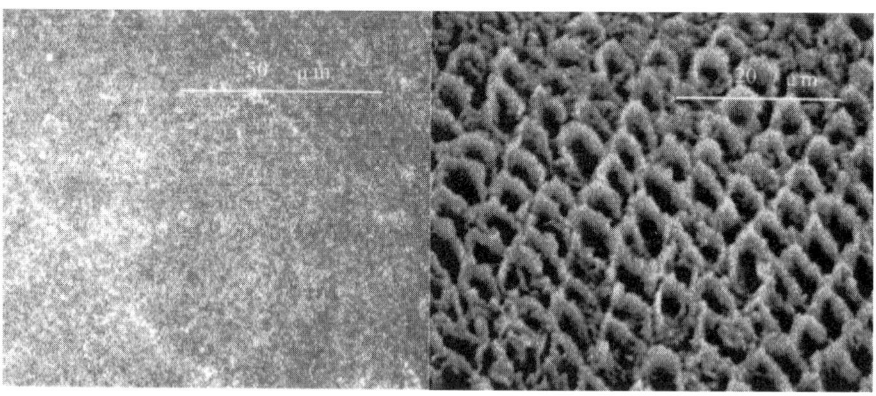

Figure 21.2. SEM of enamel and etched enamel.

mesenchymal cells and cells of connective tissue related to the neural, vascular, and immune systems. Vessels enter into the pulp through the apical foramina.

Cementum is the mineralized tissue which covers the root of a tooth; it is a bone-like structure. This tissue is deposited as a thin layer from the CEJ to the apex of the tooth; the thickness of this layer is higher at the apex. Cementoblasts and cementocytes are the cells of cementum which are similar to the osteoblasts and osteocytes of bone; however, unlike bone, cementum is avascular and incapable of remodeling. Cementum anchors the tooth to the surrounding alveolar bone through the periodontal ligament.

The periodontal ligament system is the soft connective tissue made of fibers spanning from the cement of the root to the alveolar bone following an obliquely cervical direction. The periodontal ligament characterizes the articulation between the tooth and bone; during the masticatory functions the periodontal ligaments act as a natural shock absorbing system.

Physical Properties. Table 21.1 shows physical properties of connective hard tissues. The values of densities (Berghash and Hodge, 1940) increase in the bone–teeth structure direction, reflecting the mineral content increase in the same direction. Dentine and enamel are 65% and 95–98% mineralized, respectively (mature enamel is not a living tissue). This density distribution is consistent with homogeneous model structures and mechanical properties.

Thermal properties suggest that enamel has a higher heat transfer rate than dentine. The overall natural organization of dentine and enamel reflects the best way of joining two materials, working in a hostile environment (the oral environment), in order to optimize their thermomechanical functions.

Table 21.1. Physical Properties of Connective Hard Tissues

Structure \ Property	Density (g/cm^3)	Specific heat ($cal/g \cdot °C$)	Thermal conductivity [$mcal/(sec) \cdot (cm^2) \cdot (°C/cm)$]
Bone			
spongy	1.3	0.44	1.4
cortical	1.3	0.44	1.4
Tooth			
cementum	2.03		0.50–1.51
dentine	2.14	0.28–0.38	1.36
enamel	2.97	0.18	1.84–2.23
Hydroxyapatite	3.1	0.21	3.0

Heterogeneity of natural tissue and the anisotropy in their mechanical behaviors are a fact regarded as a source for high-performance engineering designs. However, modes of failure and bond strengths depend on the mode of testing, and this is a problem that needs to be resolved if strength and bond strength data are to be believed (Stanley, 1990; Drummond *et al.*, 1996; van Noort, 1998).

21.2. Mechanical Properties

Dentine, as compact bone, is a heterogeneous multiphase material which exhibits a multiscale composite structure; thus mechanical properties depend on the testing conditions. Classical mechanical tests (macroscopic tests in tension, compression, torsion, flexion, etc.) on connective tissue specimens suggest a minimum cross-sectional area of 4 mm^2. Such specimens contain various Haversian systems (Reilly *et al.*, 1974) and thus provide significant data. Unfortunately this cross-sectional value is high if compared to the average of overall dentine dimensions, preventing the distinguishing of material properties.

Human third molars and the diaphyses of femoral compact bone have been the main source for material research because of their geometrical constraints.

Reductions in cross-sectional values lead to micromechanical tests whose results suggested that there is no relation between the applied load and the cross-sectional area (Sano *et al.*, 1994).

Indentation tests, by means of atomic force microscopes (AFM), are an alternative to classical micromechanical testing (Xu *et al.*, 1998). Using AFM it has been possible to apply loads in the range of 1 μN to 100 N through the tip of the indenter (Balooch *et al.*, 1998).

21.2.1. Static Mechanical Properties

Figure 21.3 presents typical stress–strain curves of dentine and compact bone. Young's moduli of hydroxyapatite and collagen are 114 GPa and 1.2 GPa, respectively, so upper and lower bounds of the elastic modulus of hard tissues may be derived from composite models where the mineral crystal is the reinforcement while the surrounding collagen is the matrix phase.

The averaged values of the elastic modulus of dentine (Craig *et al.*, 1961) and enamel (van Meerbeek *et al.*, 1993; Willems *et al.*, 1993) are 10–20 GPa and 75–90 GPa, respectively.

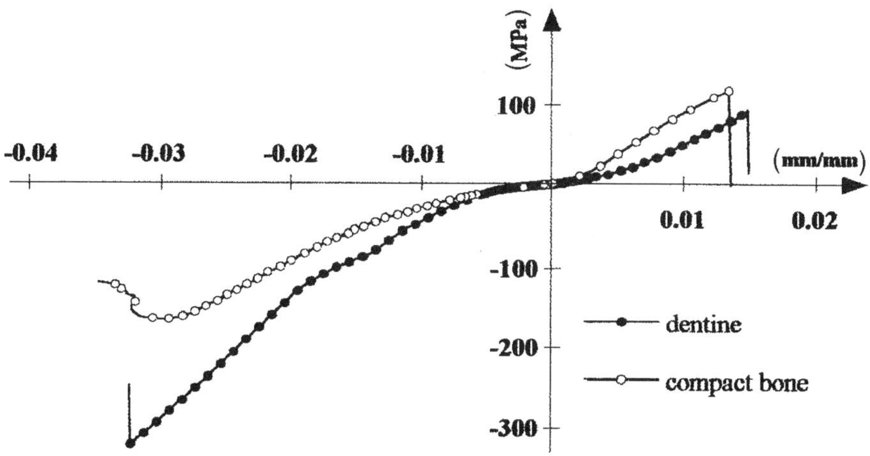

Figure 21.3. Typical stress–strain curves of dentine and compact bone.

The anisotropy in the mechanical properties of bone derives from the ultrastructural organization of collagen fibrils and mineral crystals within the osteons and the lamellar microstructure. The partial alignment of the osteons in the longitudinal direction of long bones makes this the stiffer and stronger axis of the material. This microstructure organization controls the relationship between loading conditions and fracture patterns in bone. The elastic modulus of femoral compact bone (Bonfield and Grypass, 1977) varies from 14 GPa to 17 GPa (measured in the longitudinal direction of the femur). The average mechanical properties of compact femoral bone and dentine (Table 21.2) show that the elastic modulus of dentine is similar to that of cortical bone. However, the different hydroxyapatite–collagen network grants higher compression performances to dentine and higher tensile performances to compact bone (Figure 21.3).

The collagen contribution to the elastic modulus of enamel is negligible; even viscoelastic properties do not change in the pulp DEJ direction. Instead, dentine strength, toughness, and bonding performances are dependent on the collagenic network properties.

Based on measured Young's moduli of 30 GPa for PTD and 15 GPa for ITD and the tubule density in dentine, a slight variation was found in the axial and transverse shear moduli with position in the tooth and the mean values were 16 GPa and 6.2 GPa for the Young's modulus and shear modulus, respectively (Kinney *et al.*, 1999).

Figure 21.4 presents the effect of tubule organization (Garberoglio and Brannstrom, 1976) on shear strength (measured with dentine specimens of

Table 21.2. Mechanical Properties of Hard Connective Tissues

Structure \ Property	Elastic modulus (GPa)	Compression strength (MPa)	Tensile strength (MPa)	Shear strength (MPa)	Poisson ratio
Bone					
spongy	0.49	9.4–25.2	2–20		0.30
cortical	14–17	167	121	71	0.30
Tooth					
dentine	15	297	105	134	0.31
enamel	75–90	384	10–20	90	0.33
Hydroxyapatite	110				0.28
Amalgam	50–60	200–400	27–55	188	0.33
Titanium	117		550–930	122	0.33
Composite polymers	5–21	280–390	32–63		0.24–0.35

$5 \times 1 \times 1$ mm) (Watanabe *et al.*, 1996), where the x, y, and z directions are shown in Figure 21.1. It can be seen that the shear strength increases in the pulp–enamel direction while tubule density and diameter decrease in the same direction.

Microtensile tests assess local variation in dentine bonding strength (van Noort, 1998). These tests showed that bond strength to root dentine is lower than that to coronal dentine (Yoshiyama *et al.*, 1996). Micromechanical tests are important, especially when the specimen sizes are constrained.

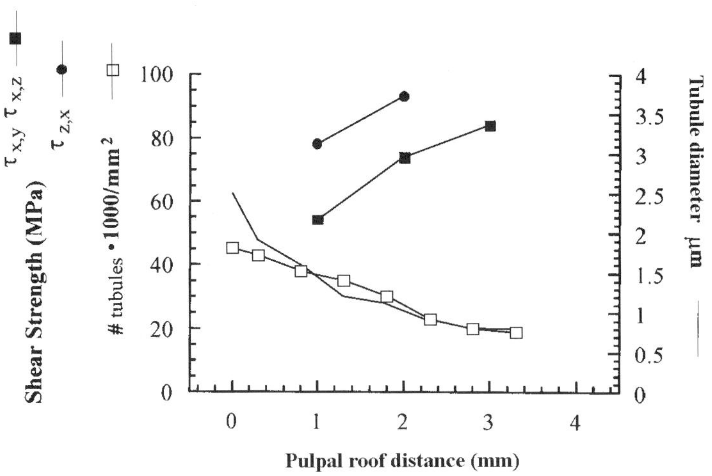

Figure 21.4. Effect of dentine organization on shear strength.

21.2.2. Hardness

Investigations using a modified atomic-force microscope suggest that the hardness of hydrated PTD and ITD is 2.3 $\pm$ 0.3 GPa and 0.5 $\pm$ 0.1 GPa, respectively (Kinney *et al.*, 1996a). The hardness of ITD increased in the pulp–DEJ direction (0.15$\pm$0.03 to 0.50$\pm$0.02 GPa, respectively) while that of PTD had a homogeneous distribution (Kinney *et al.*, 1996b).

The impression size in dentine using loads of the order of 10 mN is similar to heterogeneities such us enamel rods or dentinal tubules, preventing one from distinguishing material properties (Xu *et al.*, 1998). This load, applied through a nano-indentator, suggested an elastic modulus of 19.3$\pm$2.3 GPa and 90.6$\pm$16.1 GPa for dentine (van Meerbeek *et al.*, 1993) and enamel (Willems *et al.*, 1993), respectively. By using higher loads (2 to 50 N) the resulting elastic modulus of dentine was 20$\pm$2 GPa and the anisotropy in the mechanical properties of enamel were related to microstructural organization: the crack propagating toward the DEJ arrests at DEJ (Xu *et al.*, 1998).

The averaged values of Vickers' hardness of dentine and enamel are 57–60 kg/mm^2 and 294–408 kg/mm^2, respectively (Willems *et al.*, 1992; Forss *et al.*, 1991).

21.2.3. Fracture Toughness

Linear elastic fracture mechanics (LEFM) have been applied to bone and dentine in order to characterize its resistance to fracture. The stress intensity factor K characterizes the stress amplification at the crack tip of a loaded material. According to LEFM each material has a critical stress intensity factor K_c, also known as fracture toughness. Fracture occurs when K reaches the value K_c.

The fracture toughness reflects the ability of a material to resist crack initiation and propagation. The critical value K_C is a material characteristic, which provides a basis for predicting the onset of unstable crack propagation as a function of stress and crack dimensions (Suresh, 1991; Rooke, 1993).

In the last decades LEFM and mechanical tests have been used to evaluate the fracture toughness of cortical bone and dentine according to mode I fracture (crack extension in which the tensile stresses, acting normal to crack faces, are responsible for crack propagation). Toughness was evaluated in the direction parallel to the long axis of a long bone (longitudinal direction) and in the direction parallel to dentinal tubules according to a variety of precracked specimens: the compact tension specimen (CT)

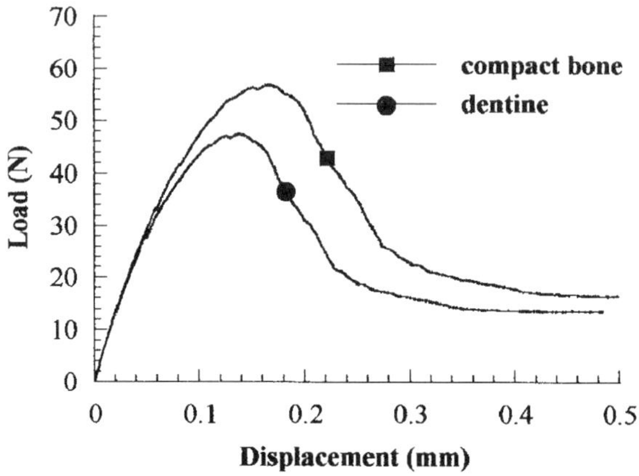

Figure 21.5. Mechanical behavior of CNT short-rod specimens of dentine and bone.

(Bonfield and Datta, 1976; Behiri and Bonfield, 1984; Vashishth *et al.*, 1997; Norman *et al.*, 1995, 1996), the single edge notched specimen (SEN) (Melvin and Evans, 1973; Moyle and Gavens, 1986), the center notched cylindrical specimen (CNC) (Bonfield, 1987), the compact sandwich specimens (Wang and Agrawal, 1996), and the 3-point bending specimen (Robertson *et al.*, 1978). The aim of these investigations is propagation rather than initiation of the crack.

The CT geometry has proven to be the most useful for studying bone fracture mechanics in the longitudinal direction, even if the dimension requirement (ASTM E 399-72, 1983) was difficult to match with connective tissues specimens. Plane strain fracture toughness (K_{IC}) using CT specimens of coronal dentine, with DT parallel to the notch plane, suggested a value of 3.08 $MN/m^{1.5}$ (standard deviation 0.33) (El Mowafy and Watts, 1986).

The main features of the CNT specimen are its geometry and the V-shaped notch. The latter constrains the crack to a steady-state propagation in the chevron-notch ligament (ASTM B 771-87, 1987) while the former allows a diameter 40% smaller than the thickness of a standard CT (Barker, 1997). These features are essential to distinguish the anisotropy in the fracture properties of a material like bone and dentine. Moreover, by using the CNT geometry, fracture toughness is computed as a function of the maximum load (F_c) and the specimen's geometry:

$$K_{IC} = A \cdot F_c / [B^{3/2} \cdot (1 - \upsilon^2)^{1/2}]$$

where A is a CNT constant ($A = 20.8$ for ASTM specimens), B is the diameter, and υ is Poisson's ratio. Figure 21.5 shows the mechanical behavior of CNT short-rod specimens of dentine and bone.

A CNT short-bar bovine specimen (with the notch tip in enamel) suggested that the lower boundary value of K_{IC} and G_{IC} (critical strain energy release), in the direction perpendicular to the DEJ, are 3.38 ± 0.40 MN/m$^{1.5}$ and 988 ± 231 J/m^2, respectively (Lin and Douglas, 1994a); G_{IC} of the bonding system–dentine interface is one order of magnitude lower (Lin and Douglas, 1994b).

The value of K_{IC} measured by using CNT short-rod specimens of a dentine–bonding system, with the interface positioned in the notch plane, suggests a range of 0.20 to 0.80 MN/m$^{1.5}$ (a significant lower limit of fracture toughness is reached in a deep dentine–bonding system interface) (Tam and Yim, 1997).

The fracture toughness of dentine is midway in the range (0.23–6.56 MN/m$^{1.5}$) observed for cortical bone and is at least one order of magnitude greater than the value for dentine-restorative materials.

References

ASTM Standards E 399-72. 1983. *Standard Method of Test for Plane-Strain Fracture Toughness of Metallic Materials.*

ASTM Standards B 771-87. 1987. *Standard Test for Short Rod Fracture Toughness of Cemented Carbides.*

Balooch, M., Wu-Magidi, I.C., Balazs, A., Lundkvist, A. S., Marshall, S.J., Marshall, G.W., Siekhaus, W.J., Kinney, J.H. 1998. Viscoelastic properties of demineralised human dentin measured in water with atomic force microscope (AFM)-based indentation, *J. Biomed. Mater. Res.* **40**, 539–544.

Barker, L.M. 1997. http ://www.terratek.com7fracto_2.htm

Behiri, J.C., Bonfield, W. 1984. Fracture of bone: the effect of density, specimen thickness and crack velocity on longitudinal fracture, *J. Biomech.* **17**, 25–34.

Berghash, S.R., Hodge, H.C. 1940. http://www.lib.umich.edu/libhome/Dentistry.lib/Dental_tables/intro.html.

Bonfield, W. 1987. Advances in the fracture mechanics of cortical bone, *J. Biomech.* **20**, 1071–1081.

Bonfield, W., Datta, P. K. 1976. Fracture toughness of compact bone, *J. Biomech.* **9**, 131–134.

Bonfield, W., Grynpass, M.D. 1977. Anisotropy of the Young's modulus of bone, *Nature* **270**, 453–454.

Cagidiaco, M.C., Ferrari, M. 1995. Dentinal tubules, in: *Bonding to Dentin*, O. Debatte & F. Ed., Livorno.

Craig, R.G., Peyton, F.A., Johnson, D.W., 1961. Compressive properties of enamel, dental cements and gold, *J. Dent. Res.* **40**, 936–945.

Drummond, J.L., Sakaguchi, R.L., Racean, D.C., Wozny, J., Steinberg, A.D. 1996. Testing mode and surface treatment effects on dentin bonding, *J. Biomed. Mater. Res.* **32**, 533–541.

El Mowafy, O.M., Watts, D.C. 1986. Fracture of human dentin, *J. Dent. Res.* **35**, 677–681.

Forss, H., Seppa, L., Lappalainen, R. 1991. In vitro abrasion resistance and hardness of glass-ionomer cements, *Dent. Mater.* **7**, 36–39.

Garberoglio, R., Brannstrom, M. 1976. Scanning electron microscopic investigation of human dentinal tubules, *Arch. Oral Biol.* **21**, 355–362.

Kinney, J. H., Balooch, M., Marshall, S.J., Marshall, G.W., Weihs, T.P. 1996a. Atomic force microscope measurements of the hardness and elasticity of peritubular and intertubular human dentin, *J. Biomech. Eng.* **118**, 133–135.

Kinney, J.H., Balooch, M., Marshall, S.J., Marshall, G.W., Weihs, T.P. 1996b. Hardness and Young's modulus of human peritubular and intertubular dentine, *Arch. Oral Biol.* **41**, 9–13.

Kinney, J. H., Balooch, M., Marshall, G. W., Marshall, S. J. 1999. A micromechanics model of the elastic properties of human dentine, *Arch. Oral Biol.* **44**, 813–822.

Kuboky, Y., Mechanic, G.L. 1982. Comparative molecular distribution of cross-link in bone and dentine collagen: structure-function relationship, *Calcif. Tissue Int.* **34**, 306–308.

Lin, C.P., Douglas, W.H. 1994a. Structure–property relations and crack resistance at the bovine dentin–enamel junction, *J. Dent. Res.* **73**, 1072–1078.

Lin, C.P., Douglas, W.H. 1994b. Failure mechanism at the human dentin–resin interface: a fracture mechanism approach, *J. Biomech.* **27**, 1037–1047.

Melvin, J.W., Evans, F.G. 1973. Crack propagation in bone, pp. 87–88, Biomechanics Symposium, ASME New York.

Moyle, D.D., Gavens, A.J. 1986. Fracture propeties of bovine tibial bone, *J. Biomech.* **19**, 919–927.

Norman, T.L., Vashishth, D., Burt, D. 1995. Fracture toughness of human bone under tension, *J. Biomech.* **28**, 309–320.

Norman, T.L., Vashishth, D., Burt, D. 1996. Resistance to crack growth in human cortical bone is greater in shear than in tension, *J. Biomech.* **29**, 1023–1031.

Reilly, D.T., Burstein, A.H., Frankel, V.H. 1974. The elastic modulus for bone, *J. Biomech.* **7**, 271–275.

Robertson, D.M., Robertson, D., Barret, C.G. 1978. Fracture toughness, critical crack length and plastic zone size in bone, *J. Biomech.* **11**, 359–364.

Rooke, D.P. 1993. Development of fracture mechanics, in: *Static and Dynamic Fracture Mechanisms* (M.H. Aliabad, C.A. Brebbia, V.Z. Parton, eds.), pp. 3–35, Computational Mechanics Publications, Portland.

Sano, H., Shono, T., Sonoda, H., Takatsu, T., Ciucchi, B., Carvalho, R., Pashley, D.H. 1994. Relationship between surface area for adhesion and tensile bond strength — evaluation of a micro-tensile bond test. *Dent Mater*, **10**, 236–40.

Stanley, H.R. 1990. Pulpal responses to ionomer cements — biological characteristics, *J. Am. Dent. Assoc.* **120**, 25–29.

Suresh, S. 1991. Principles of fracture mechanics and their implication for fatigue, in: *Fatigue of Materials* (D.R. Clarke, ed.), Cambridge University Press.

Tam, L.E., Yim, D. 1997. Effect of dentine depth on the fracture toughness of dentine–composite adhesive interfaces, *J. Dent.* **25**, 339–346.

van Meerbeek, B., Willems, G., Celis, J.P., Roos, J.R., Braem, M. 1993. Lambrechts. Assessment by nano-indentation technique of the hardness and elasticity of the resin dentin bonding area, *J. Dent. Res.* **72**, 1434–1442.

van Noort, R. 1998. Dental Materials: 1996. Dentine bonding, *J. Dent.* **26**, 191–207.

Vashishth, D., Behiri, J.C., Bonfield, W. 1997. Crack growth resistance in cortical bone: Concept of microcrack toughness, *J. Biomech.* **30**, 763–769.

Veis, A. 1996. in: *Dentin. Extracellular Matrix. Tissue Function* (Wayne D. Comper, ed.), Vol. 1, Amsterdam.

Wang, X., Agrawal, C.M. 1996. Fracture toughness of bone using a compact sandwich specimen: effect of sampling sites and crack orientations, *J. Biomed. Mater. Res.* **33**, 13–21.

Watanabe, L.G., Marshall, G.W., Marshall, S.J. 1996. Dentin shear strength: effects of tubule orientation and intratooth location, *Dent. Mater.* **12**, 109–115.

Willems, G., Lambrechts, P., Braem, M., Celis, J.P., Vanherle, G.A. 1992. Classification of dental composites according to their morphological and mechanical characteristics, *Dent. Mater.* **8**, 310–331.

Willems, G. Celis, J.P., Lambrechts, P., Braem, M. 1993. Hardness and Young's modulus determined by nano-indentation technique of filler particles of dental restorative materials compared with human enamel, *J. Biomed. Mater. Res.* **27**, 747–755.

Xu, H.H.K., Smith, D.T., Jahanmir, S., Romberg, E., Kelly, J.R., Thompson, V.P., Rekow, E.D. 1998. Indentation damage and mechanical properties of human enamel and dentin, *J. Dent. Res.* **77**, 472–480.

Yoshiyama, M., Carvalho, R.M., Sano, H., Horner, J.A., Brewer, P.D., Pashley, D.H. 1996. Regional bond strengths of resins to human root dentine, *J. Dent*, **24**, 435–442.

22

Dental Materials and Implants

Maria Rosa Pinasco, Arturo Natali, Patrizia Loria, Marc Bolla, and Franck J. Hagege

22.1 Introduction

Biomaterials are widely used in stomatologic dentistry therapy because of the great number of stomatognatic apparatus functions and the frequent appearance of pathologies that injure the dental arch, maxillary bones and other biological structures that compose that apparatus. Odontostomatologic biomaterials are used for dental restoration both for fixed and removable prostheses and for endosteal implants. The latter are useful when a partial or total prosthetic rehabilitation of the masticatory function is necessary.

Oral surgery, besides, often requires materials that can substitute for bone, or substances that aid the regeneration of the original tooth-supporting structures that have decayed. Owing to the extent and variability of the necessity to improve functions, repair structural defects, or replace lost teeth (extremely important for mastication, phonation, social life) (Bradley, 1981), odontostomatologic biomaterials used nowadays are many and varied from the point of view of composition as well as structure. Thus they represent a "research field" apart, while obviously taking into consideration the several biological needs connected with the entire organism.

Maria Rosa Pinasco • Dipartimento di Chimica e Chimica Industriale, Università degli Studi di Genova, via Dodecaneso 31, 16146 Genova, Italy. **Arturo Natali** • Center of Mechanics of Biological Materials, Dipartimento di Costruzioni e Trasporti, University of Padova, via F. Marzolo 9, 35131 Padova, Italy. **Patrizia Loria** • Department of Biophysical, Medical and Odontostomatological Sciences and Technologies, University of Genova, Corso Europa 30, 16132 Genoa, Italy. **Marc Bolla and Franck J. Hagege** • Laboratoire de biomatériaux dentaires, UFR Odontologie, Université de Nice Sophia Antipolis, 24, avenue des Diables Bleus, 04537 Nice Cedex 05, France.

Integrated Biomaterials Science, edited by R. Barbucci. Kluwer Academic/Plenum Publishers, New York, 2002.

Owing to the breadth of the topic and the space limitations only some functions and materials will be detailed here.

22.2. Stomatognatic Apparatus: Some Considerations

Various anatomic structures form the oral cavity, i.e., maxillary bones, teeth, masticatory muscles, tongue, salivary glands, lips, and cheeks. Moreover, the oral cavity is covered by a mucous tissue, which acts as a defensive barrier against possible physical and chemical exogenous damage. The temporomandibular joint, thanks to a remarkable musculature, allows, besides the opening and shutting of the mouth, a rather complicated series of spatial relations between the dental arches. These relations enable chewing by both the meisal action of the front teeth and the grinding action of the cusps and fossa back teeth (Rouviere, 1978; Sicher and Du Brul, 1970). This articular structure together with the oral cavity forms the stomatognatic apparatus.

Teeth show a crow and a radicular area (Figures 22.1 and 21.2). They are made of mineralized tissues: enamel, dentine, and cement which give the necessary mechanical properties to mastication (Ten Cate, 1989). Dental pulp, enclosed in the pulp chamber and root canal, ensures sensitivity and trophism (Figure 22.2).

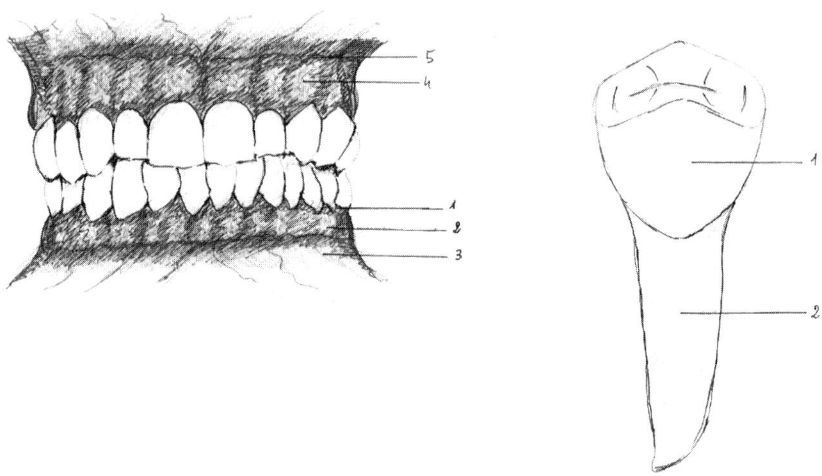

Figure 22.1. Schematic picture of dental arches and parodontal structures in the oral cavity: (1) free gingiva, (2) attached gingiva, (3) oral mucosa, (4) orange peel feature, (5) mucosal-gingival line. Right: Schematic picture of removed premolar tooth: (1) crown, (2) root.

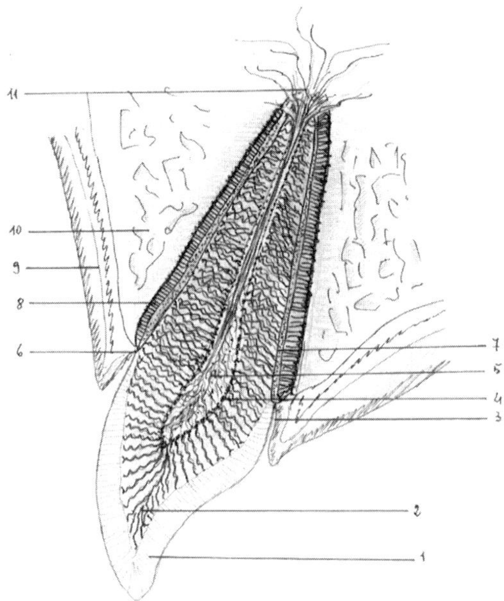

Figure 22.2. Schematic picture of the incisor tooth longitudinal section: (1) enamel and prisms, (2) dentine, (3) gingival sulcus, (4) odontoblast layer, (5) dental pulp, (6) epithelial attachment, (7) cement, (8) periodontal ligament (not in scale), (9) gingiva, (10) alveolar bone, (11) apical forearm for nerves and vessels.

Enamel, i.e., the extremely hard tissue covering the crow, is 94% composed of rod-shaped hydroxyapatite crystals which pack together closely. They constitute the "enamel prisms" regarded today as the histological unit of the very tissue visible through the optical and electronic microscope (Ten Cate, 1989). They oppose as a barrier against possible mechanical and chemical damage. Should the enamel be affected by traumatic lesions or carious processes caused by acid demineralizing action or by acid substances repeatedly introduced, it will not regenerate; moreover, it has no cellular element.

Dentine is located under both the crown enamel and radicular cement; it gives to every dental element the specified morphology according to its presence in the dental arch. It contains about 26% of organic substance and the calcified component is made of hydroxyapatite. Through the microscope the presence of a thick collagen fiber net can be seen. Dentine is crossed by a centrifugal canaliculus structure which contains an odontoblast cellular prolongation (Ten Cate, 1989) (Figure 22.2). Odontoblasts are cells which originate during dentinogenesis; after setting dental tissue odontoblasts occupy the external pulp, keeping their citoplasmatic prolongations inside the teeth canaliculus. This explains the possible toxic action of dental restoration. With time they ensure a slow and constant flow of a new dentine, called secondary dentine. Odontoblasts also prevent mechanical and toxic-infective injury creating a reaction tissue acting as a barrier against endogenous damage. This new tissue is called tertiary dentine (Ten Cate, 1989).

Besides allowing the grinding of food resisting to a compression strength up to 180 kg, dentine protects dental pulp housing it in the pulpar cavity (Figure 22.2). Dentine can be exposed to carious lesions or to chemical-physical injuries (thermal stress, trauma, exogenous and endogenous toxic substances) as well as to alterations due to imperfections occurring while being formed. Dentine like enamel cannot regenerate.

Mechanical, chemical, and thermal stimuli cause a subjective sensation due to movements produced by the fluids contained in the canaliculus after contraction, expansion, and also after the rather complex hydrodynamic ratio such as osmotic strength and dehydrogenating defects. Thanks to the above-mentioned transmission mechanism, dental pulp can stimulate nerve endings free from pulp (Brannstrom, 1986) so that biomaterials with high thermal conductivity can cause high sensitivity.

Dental pulp is an organ housed in the pulp chamber and bound by dentine inside every tooth. The pulp chamber spatial configuration varies according to the outer tooth morphology and to its specific function. It consists of a connective tissue containing living cells having different functions, a basic intercellular substance rich in collagen fibers, vessels, and nerve fibers. The pulp chamber extends into the root canal and its vascular nerve bundle crosses the root apex jointly with a terminal nerve vascular mass of periodontium (Ten Cate, 1989).

Periodontal structures are formed of root cement, periodontal membrane, alveolar bone, and gingiva (Figures 22.1 and 22.2). Cement is a calcified tissue lying on the root making up an interface between the root dentine and the connective tissue which form the periodontal membrane. Its matrix is calcified and rich in collagen fibers. The cement has the aim of tying periodontal membrane fibers to the radicular area and repairing occurred damage through a new production of tissue. The periodontal membrane, also called periodontal ligament, is structured by collagen fibers bundles, its own cells, blood and lymphatic vessels, and essential substance. It surrounds the root and penetrates the cement and the alveolar bone through a complex system of oriented fibers giving stability to the tooth. Fibers, also called Sharpey fibers (Figure 22.2), have the function of a softening structure which is lost together with the tooth. Up to now implants can substitute root but not periodontal membrane.

Gingiva is named "free," "attached," or "interdental" according to its position and the extent of its connections to the tooth and to the periostium placed below. The extreme gingiva edge is called "free gingiva." The junction between attached gingiva and marginal gingiva forms the "gingival sulcus." The surface of the attached gingiva is so firmly joined by fibers to the underlying periostium as to look like "orange peel"; this is due to the traction made by the fibers themselves. The under-placed mucogingival junction turns to alveolar mucosa (Figure 22.1, point 5). Histologically, gingiva is made up of keratinized stratified epithelium; the epithelium "junctional" ring firmly binds gingiva to the tooth collar under gingiva sulcus, giving the dental crown perfect isolation from deep periodontal structures (see Figure 22.2, point 6). The epithelium ring is known as the epithelial attachment; it cannot be completely reformed by implant therapy (Ten Cate, 1989; Rouviere, 1978; Sicher, 1970).

The alveolar bone surrounds the dental roots and forms the interdental alveolar ridge. Histologically, the alveolar bone looks more solid around the roots forming the so-called interdental "duralamina." The periodontium bears the whole chewing function and gives the indispensable sensory perceptions regulating the masticatory movements.

For physical and mechanical properties of dental tissues, see Chapter 21, "Mechanical Properties of Tooth Structures."

The mouth is constantly wet with saliva. Saliva represents the whole of the oral cavity secretions coming from the production of larger and lesser salivary gland fluids and from the gingival discharges. The quantity of saliva secreted during 24 h is about 1000 to 2000 ml. Saliva is an electrolyte solution formed by 90% of water and 10% inorganic ions and organic substances such as amino acid and protein. Among organic components immunoglobulins support the defense system, enzymes contribute to the digestive function, and the complex mucoproteins accomplish a lubricating and protective action on dental surfaces being then absorbed into hydroxyapatite of the enamel in order to develop the "salivate film." In the salivate fluid there are also urea, uric acid, and ammonia bicarbonate of sodium as a buffer function. Among inorganic substances, calcium and phosphorus represent the larger quantities, while sodium, potassium, magnesium, chlorine, sulfates, and thiocyanates represent the smaller ones. The total carbon dioxide in the saliva contains also carbon acid and H^+ and HCO_3^- dissociated from it; this dissociation differs according to pH value variations. Saliva microscopic analysis shows the existence of oral mucosa "flaking cells," leukocytes, and several bacteria.

Its composition fluctuates according to the rhythm of secretion and depending on what one eats and on the condition of the microbial metabolism, so pH would also vary appreciably.

Moreover, the steady-state temperature in the mouth equals that of normal body temperature (37 °C) but it may range from 0°–70 °C depending on what one is eating. Thus dental restoration works in a strange corrosive environment: complicated saliva composition, constantly fluctuating chemical and physical conditions, differing from one person to another (Endo *et al.*, 1993). It is evident, therefore, that it is not easy to reproduce every possible condition in artificial saliva biomaterials tests.

Saliva has digestive functions and performs an antitoxic and antiseptic activity.

The above-mentioned anatomic structures are essential in performing the oral cavity functions: grinding, swelling, phonation, swallowing. In particular, grinding coordinates the different parts forming the oral cavity; it in fact includes cutting, grinding food, and mixing saliva together with bolus before swallowing.

Bacterial plaque is an attached and structured formation which rests on teeth or prostheses, or on restoration not sufficiently cleaned. Its deposit is supported by salivate mucoproteins (salivate film), absorbing and so helping the adhesion of germs living in the oral cavity. In fact, bacterial plaque is formed by germs that, if not removed, grow in colonies on the dental enamel surface localized where food passage is less frequent. The interbacterial plaque component is formed mainly by polysaccharides (produced for the larger quantity by germs), bacterial proteins and enzymes, and mineral salts (Leach, 1980).

Bacterial plaque may or may not have any pathogen possibility. When in the oral cavity suitable conditions for salt precipitation inside the plaque are developed, the plaque can calcify, so sticking to the enamel or to cementum (tartar). Restoration biomaterials must be refractory to the plaque bacterial layer. Caries development is related to plaque formation.

Carious pathology is widespread all over the world; it starts from childhood and its successive development during adult life seems due to many congenital and gained predisposing causes (Newbrun, 1990; Thylstrup and Fejerskov, 1986). More renowned pathogenic theories identify in a series of constitutional causes the predisposing condition necessary to the genesis of caries, while a microbic population harbored in the bacterial plaque, able to produce acids which cause a critical drop in pH, is responsible for dissolving dental enamel hydroxyapatite crystals. One of the bacteria present in plaque is *Streptococcus mutans*, which takes up sugars and breaks them down to organic acids such as methanoic, ethanoic, butanoic, propanoic, and 2-hydroxypropanoic acid. The drop in pH caused by these acids results in a big change in the solubility of calcium phosphate.

Hydroxyapatite is converted to a more soluble salt, calcium hydrogen phosphate:

$$Ca_{10}(PO_4)_6(OH)_2 + 8H^+ \Leftrightarrow 6CaHPO_4 + 4Ca^{2+} + 2H_2O.$$

Its constituent ions (Ca^{2+} and HPO_4^{2-}), which gradually develop by dissociation, can be lost in the saliva. If the surface of the teeth becomes neutral again (i.e., plaque removing), the calcium, hydrogen phosphate is converted back to hydroxyapatite. However, if the acid attack is continuous and prolonged, a permanent loss of calcium and phosphate ions occurs, causing a demineralized zone of calcified teeth tissue. Bacterial invasion follows and plaque forms, beginning a vicious circle: more acid attack develops and more enamel is destroyed. This is known as carious lesion. When bacterial invasion digs deeper until the dental enamel is penetrated, the dentine is exposed and a process of demineralization causes the destruction and a varying loss of tissue. If the caries continues, reaching the living pulp, it becomes inflamed, causing toothache.

Sucrose being present in the diet has an important function in helping the survival and breeding of the cariogenous microbes harbored inside the bacterial plaque (Nikiforuk, 1985).

Enamel caries develop slowly and at first it shows with the appearance of white demineralization stains which, according to circumstances, can be found on the bottom of the occlusal groove, close to the cervical area and interdental faces of deciduous teeth and successional ones (Figure 22.3) (Newbrun, 1990).

Carious lesion, or dental decay as it is more colloquially known, must be stopped through prompt action to extirpate irremediably lost structures and to substitute them through restoring biomaterials (Nikiforuk, 1985; Newbrun, 1990)

The periodontal disease field includes several pathologies such as gingivitis, initial or light periodontitis, and periodontitis at a later stage of development (Sluger *et al.*, 1997). Pathogenic causes are due to bacterial plaque germs harbored in the gingival sulcus. These germs develop according to complex conditions, both congenital and acquired. Such lesions can achieve a progressive destruction of periodontal structures through strong instability of the teeth themselves till their ejection (Sluger *et al.*, 1977; McGhee *et al.*, 1982).

Therapy can bc medical as well as surgical and it can keep the bacterial plaque under control or, when necessary, regenerate or substitute injured tissues through biomaterials called membranes or artificial bones.

Inside the oral cavity many other different pathologies can develop owing to abnormal embryogenesis, bacterial, toxic, traumatic, degenerative

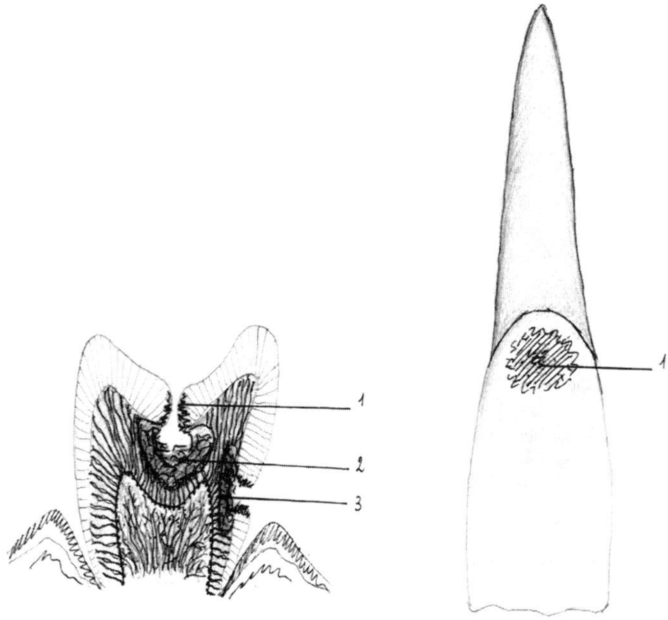

Figure 22.3. Right: Schematic picture of an incisor tooth: cervical carious lesion of enamel at the first stage of developing: (1) demineralization area. Left: Schematic picture of longitudinal section of a tooth with different carious lesions: (1) caries on enamel, (2) caries on dentine, (3) caries in cervical position.

and neoplastic causes, affecting all tissues forming the mouth, tongue, peridontium, and maxillary bones.

We can clearly understand that the use of biomaterials in odontology therapy is usually suggested in order to substitute tissues belonging to the oral cavity which have been seriously injured or lost owing to specific pathologies. Such substitution implies not only that the material has all the characteristics necessary to replace the specific damaged function, but also the requisites for a compulsory integration with large and complex biological functions both local and systemic.

Moreover, the use of biomaterials must take into consideration the patient's general health as well as the local physiological or pathological conditions. All this can have great influence on biomaterial properties. Consideration must be given to the kind of teeth, whether primary teeth or successional ones, strength used in grinding according to age and sex, qualitative and quantitative saliva variations, pH variations, the presence of substances or drugs ejected via saliva, temperature changes, physical characteristics, and food composition, as well as oral hygienic conditions. Dentists must choose according to the different local or pathological conditions what kind of treatment to use, i.e., reconstructive or rehabilitative.

22.3. Dental Materials for Hard and Plastic Restorative Treatment

22.3.1. Tooth Restoration: Filling, Inlay, and Onlay

When we talk of restoration, we mean conservative dentistry treatment which allows biomaterials to replace lost or decayed dental tissue.

Indirect restoration is called "inlay" or "onlay" according to its extension; besides, we can say it is made up of biomaterial hardened outside the patient's mouth and then inserted into a well-prepared cavity. It is first necessary to prepare, through different techniques, the filling on a plaster model, reproducing a part or the whole arch of the patient obtained through a negative impression. The inlay and onlay can be located in the cavity using a system of cementing.

We refer to plastic material restoration or direct restoration when the filling gets hard directly in the oral cavity and modeling and adaptation take place in the patient's mouth. The soft filling paste is inserted into the tooth cavity, thus taking the shape of the cavity itself. Direct restoration is faster and allows the saving of still healthy dental tissue, as technically it requires the preparation of a less large tooth cavity.

Restorative materials must possess many characteristics, allowing their use without spoiling either the therapy with the passage of time or the patient's health. Biocompatibility ensures that biomaterials can be used without any damage to dental tissues and organs located in the oral cavity as well as to the whole organism. Chemical or physical interaction with food and the oral sphere must not develop. No production of toxic substances which could be absorbed owing to solubilization, wear, and corrosion phenomena of biomaterials must arise. Dentists clearly know that the material must be biocompatible. They take special care to get rid of the waste or substances produced and let in; in fact it is very important that the material be highly ecological.

Mechanical properties are essential in re-establishing the masticatory function and preserving the restoration over a period of time. Restoration must resist push, wear, and corrosion, and also have a good volumetric stability not only during the passage from plastic to hard conditions but also to temperature variations in the oral cavity.

The electric and thermal conductivity must be in accordance with the biological needs and as close as possible to those of dental tissues. During hardening in the oral cavity materials must not develop any heat. Both hard or plastic materials must easily fit the cavity walls with no empty space.

A chemical or physical adhesion to enamel or dentine is important in preventing recurring caries, to avoid marginal breakdown and infiltration, and in saving the healthy tissue.

Radio-opaqueness in the oral picture is advisable to check the state of the restoration over time and show up demineralization areas in case of development of recurring lesions.

Easy restoration and easily-handled materials to reduce any discomfort to the patient and to limit prices are necessary.

Esthetics is very important in restorative treatment of the front teeth, while function is more important in back teeth. Anyway, restoration should be very similar to dental enamel not only for esthetic reasons, but also to help food sliding, autocleaning, and a better reproduction of morphological details.

It is useful to obtain restoration biomaterials able to insert therapeutic or prophylactic active principles which are released over a period of time.

22.3.2. Restorative Materials: Metals and Alloys, Composite Resins, Glass Ionomers

22.3.2.1. Metal Materials

Nowadays metals are used both for inlay, onlay, or direct restorations. They have a proper surface easily polished to avoid bacterial plaque. Such materials can restore damage due to weighty lesions or large tissue losses while keeping the precise morphofunctional details and resisting biting force action for their toughness, high resistance to brittle fracture, and high impact strength.

For direct restoration a soft metallic paste is inserted into the tooth cavity. Sometimes, this cavity is previously isolated through the application of acrylic paints or thin cement coats on dental tissue in order to avoid possible damage to odontoblasts and pulp. This could be caused by direct toxic action or by the high thermal conductivity of metal materials.

Metals for direct or indirect restoration can be used only in the back of the mouth because of esthetic reasons. These materials cannot stick to calcified tissues; as a result it is necessary not only to remove the decay, but also to shape the tooth cavity so that the filling cannot fall out. So they need large cavities and it may be necessary to sacrifice still healthy dental tissues.

It may happen that the presence of different metal materials in the mouth (i.e., gold alloys and silver amalgam) determines galvanic currents.

Direct metal materials are mainly silver amalgam or gold for filling.

Direct restoration with gold filling is formed by 99.99% chemically pure gold in the cohesive gold technique (Rapson, 1978; Horibe and Fukuoka, 1986; Brown, 1988).

Restorative gold is available in three forms: (1) gold foil, which is crumpled into small pellets before use; (2) mat gold, a structure of fine packed dendritic crystals prepared by electrodeposition, compressed, and sintered to form thin cylinders or strips; (3) gold powder, prepared by atomization of molten pure gold as well as by chemical precipitation.

Before use, all three forms of gold are annealed at least at 315 °C to remove surface contamination, and to ensure cold welding and cohesive bonding when they are condensed incrementally in the tooth cavity. A hand mallet as well as a mechanical condenser is used. During placement of cohesive gold its Knoop hardness value rises up to 75 and the tensile strength up to 45,000 psi (Rapson, 1978) due to cold working.

This kind of restoration, despite its high corrosion resistance, is little used owing to its complexity, time-consumption, and few clinical indications. Pure gold is used in very small caries lesions, in simple cavities with good access, in sites where very little wear is expected, or to repair gold inlay small fractures.

The term "dental amalgam" refers to the silver–tin–mercury alloy (see the chapter dealing with the structure of metals and alloys). Its use is widespread in the world. The reasons for the popularity of amalgams are mainly the following: (i) they possess a surprising ability to withstand the stresses and corrosive conditions that occur during chewing; (ii) they are relatively inexpensive (Waterstrat and Okabe, 1994).

At their service temperature (about 37 °C) amalgams, though composed of relatively brittle intermetallic compounds, show a compressive strength close to that of cast iron and a corrosion resistance that can be compared with that of pure silver (Waterstrat and Okabe, 1994). Restorations of gold foil or gold alloy castings have higher stress and corrosion resistance, but the cost of a skilled laboratory and the greater time needed to fabricate a gold restoration make dental amalgam restoration less expensive.

Dental amalgam is prepared as a plastic metallic paste by mixing silver alloy particles with approximately 45% of liquid mercury. The mixture hardens directly in the tooth cavity at a rate that allows the dentist to construct desired anatomical contours before the amalgam "set" and becomes too rigid. The hardening is related to a diffusion reaction in which the liquid mercury is replaced by solid intermetallic compounds. Amalgam results in a particle reinforced composite material: the unconsumed alloy particles are embedded in a matrix which is composed of the new developed reaction phases. Composition of alloy powder and its internal stresses, as well as the methods used to mix and pack it, control the dimensional change of amalgam during hardening (Waterstrat and Okabe, 1994).

Silver amalgam is still discussed owing to its Hg content, which may be damaging to the patient's health, the dentist, and the environment (Dodes, 1988; Ahmad and Standard, 1990).

However, because of the low price, rapidity and ease of application, as well as suitable mechanical properties, this material continues to be used in social dentistry.

Ekstrand *et al.* (1998) summarized some recent reports on toxicological aspects of the release and systemic uptake of mercury from dental amalgam. In a series of studies on subjects with amalgam restorations, the released mercury levels were followed in saliva, fecal excretion, blood, and plasma. In addition, mercury released from amalgam filling and its possible effect on the resistance pattern in normal oral and intestinal microflora, as well as its relation with the renal function, were discussed. They concluded, according to the final results of independent evaluations from different state health agencies, that the release of mercury from amalgam restorations does not present any "non-acceptable risk to the general population."

Some gallium alloys melting at temperatures lower than room temperature and able to react with metallic powders like mercury have been studied (Horibe and Fukuoka, 1986; Hero and Hokabe, 1994).

Two gallium alloys are present on the market: Gallium Alloy GF (Japan) and Galloy (Australia). The first alloy has been approved by the Japanese government for clinical use. The latter has met the requirement of ANSI-ADA Specification No. 1 for amalgam and has been granted the ADA Seal of Acceptance (Venugopalan *et al.*, 1998).

Alloy powders with compositions similar to those for amalgam alloys are triturated with a liquid gallium alloy (see Table 22.1). The mix can be condensed into a prepared cavity in the same way as for amalgam. The handling characteristic, inferior to that of amalgam, can be overcome by special techniques and placement instruments.

Some properties (compressive and tensile strength, hardness, creep, wear resistance) have been found to be similar to those of leading high copper amalgams. Gallium may decrease environmental risks due to its lower vapor pressure than mercury (Oshida and Moore, 1993) and it has been found to be less cytotoxic. However, *in vitro* and *in vivo* studies have expressed concern in relation to the corrosion resistance of Ga alloys (Hero *et al.*, 1997; Venugopalan *et al.*, 1998).

Also, these alloys can exhibit too much expansion or slight contraction upon setting, and clinical studies have shown surface roughness, marginal breakdown, and loss of luster of restoration.

Optimization of the properties of Ga alloys involves adequate knowledge of their structure. Ga alloy GF has been found to be composed of unconsumed spherical alloy particles surrounded by a reaction layer of $CuGa_2$ and Cu_9Ga_4 phases and embedded in a matrix of grains of Ag_9In_4, Ag_2Ga, and β-Sn phases (Hero *et al.*, 1996).

To carry out indirect inlay and onlay metal restoration, the same casting precious alloys used for dental fixed prostheses can be employed. The technique involves the forming of the precious alloy through the "lost wax casting technique."

22.3.2.2. Composite Resins

To produce a soft material hardening in the mouth, it is possible to use substances able to polymerize inside the cavity. The first addition polymer used was polymethylmethacrylate. However, like most polymers (see the chapter on the structure and properties of polymeric materials), it shrinks as the monomers link together. Polymerization shrinkage is of critical importance, causing adhesive or cohesive failure and interfacial gap formation between the filling and the tooth in which saliva, bacteria, and carbohydrates can crowd and promote secondary caries. By conserving adhesion, deformation of the residual tooth structure may develop. Moreover, the thermal expansion coefficient of the polymethylmethacrylate is about ten times that of enamel and dentine, so that in the presence of hot or cold food and drink the filling contracts and expands much more than the tooth. A pumping action results at the interface between enamel and filling, making the leakage problem worse. The first-used polymer, neither strong nor stiff and with poor wear resistance, was soon replaced with a more suitable material: the composite resins or polymer–ceramic composites. Their evolution over the last 25 years follows two basic developments:

(i) The development of dimethacrylate polymers, shrinking much less on polymerization than methylmethacrylate and having superior mechanical properties. However, their thermal expansion coefficient was still greater than that of the tooth.

(ii) The addition of particles of inert filler (SiO_2, Al_2O_3, and various types of glass, improving dental composite strength and reducing polymerization shrinkage simply because less monomer is present to react. Due to its inertness, the filler did not bond to the polymer so that it could wear away greatly, owing to particle loss. To promote bond formation the filling particles were coated with a silane bonding agent able to link with the polymer at one end and with ceramic filler at the other.

The basic monomer mainly used today is BIS-GMA (aromatic dimethacrylate monomer 2,2-bis[4-(2-hydroxy-3-methacryloyloxypropoxy)-phenyl] propane) having high molecular size and low shrinkage, hardening quickly and developing stronger and stiffer resins. Its high viscosity is lowered by thinning BIS-GMA with other monomers such as DEGMA (diethylene glycol dimethacrylate) and TEGDMA (triethylene glycol dimethacrylate) to improve the capacity of embedding fillers. Alternatively, some other monomer systems are proposed to lower viscosity and water sorption and improve toughness: (i) the total or partial replacement of BIS-GMA by aliphatic or aromatic urethane dimethacrylate; and (ii) the synthesis of a BIS-GMA analogue free from the hydroxyl group in the structure.

With respect to fillers, silica in fused quartz form and lithium aluminum silicate glasses having a zero or negative thermal expansion coefficient were selected in order to equalize the thermal dimensional change of the composite to that of tooth tissues. Radio-opaque glasses with barium, strontium, and zinc have partially or totally replaced the early silica to obtain a refractive index of filler matching the organic monomer, thus improving composite translucence and esthetic requirements ($n \cong 1.5$ for methacrylate resins). In fact, optical properties of restorative materials should be equal, especially in color and translucency, to those of hard tooth tissues.

Filler particles can have the form of spheres, but they are often irregularly shaped to promote mechanical retention in the resin and better mechanical properties. They range in size from 0.04 to 10 μm. The original composite resins generally had a filler size ranging from 50 to 100 μm and were difficult to finish and polish. At the lower limit in size range there are very fine particles (0.05 μm) of pyrolytic silica which are present in the microfilled composites. Sometimes pyrolytic silica is incorporated into monomer, which is then polymerized, ground, and used as "organic filler" to make the composite with further monomer. The so-called hybrid composites contain mainly silica or glass fillers with consistent amounts of microfine material and a great variety of sizes, shapes, and size distributions of fillers. They try to combine the advantages of micro- and macro-particles.

The arrangement of the particles in the matrix is a semirandom distribution. Porosity may frequently arise from air incorporation during mixing.

The surface profile of composites changes in use, owing to degradation and wear processes. Surface smoothness and polishability are clinically important and are determined principally by particle size and type.

Several studies reviewed by Watts (1992) showed that compressive strength, stiffness, and abrasion resistance of composite resins increase with the amount of filler, also depending upon the largest size of filler, size distribution, and particle packaging. Smith (1985) suggested that a filler separation distance of less than 0.1 μm enhanced wear resistance, defending softer resin from abrasion. Studies on paste rheology and improvement in the grinding and filler incorporation technology made it possible to achieve highly filled composites (87 mass%) to be used in posterior restoration.

Initiators and activators of polymerization reaction are incorporated in the organic monomers. The initiator is generally benzoyl peroxide (a few percent) in the two-paste or self-cure systems supplied by the market. It is contained in one paste; the other paste includes a tertiary amine (usually di-hydroxyethyl-*p*-toluidine) as activator. On mixing the two pastes the polymerization process starts, and the dentist has to work quickly to get the mixed paste into the cavity before it becomes too stiff.

Over the last ten years one-paste light-activated systems have developed (VLC visible light-cured composite). These contain a free-radical photoinitiator, usually α-1,2 diketone such as benzil or camphorquinone, either of which is used in combination with an amine reducing agent (dimethylaminoethyl methacrylate or dimethyl-*p*-toluidine). The polymerization reaction starts when the initiator is exposed to intense visible blue light, the ideal wavelength being 470 nm. The intensified radicals produced in the process greatly improve the standard of treatment. The polymerization mechanism and kinetics of these composites as well as light transmission and depth of treatment have recently been reviewed (Watt, 1992).

Despite extensive cross-linking of dimethacrylate monomers on polymerization, some degree of residual unsaturation remains in the polymer network, either as a residual monomer or mainly as a pendant side chain having reacted at only one end of the difunctional molecule. It has deleterious effects on the mechanical properties and dimensional stability of the restoration. The degree of conversion (DC) ranges from 55 up to 75%. It is possible that a low conversion degree reduces material biocompatibility.

Polymer–ceramic composites in more than sixty different formulations are today available on the world market. Their development and properties have been recently summarized (Watts, 1992; Smith, 1985).

Composite resin adhesion to dental tissue can be obtained by means of two systems:

(i) The first system involves an acid etching carried out by putting 37% solutions of orthophosphoric acid on enamel for about 30 seconds. This produces an irregular and superficial prism demineralization with microcavity development. A bonding fluid resin chemically similar to that of composite resin, spread further, gets into the above-mentioned microcavities. By the bonding polymerization a micromechanic adhesion is obtained on the enamel while the filling sticks chemically to the bonding.

(ii) The second system involves the dentine treatment through orthophosphoric acid generally at 10%, which gives rise to emerging superficial collagen fibers.

The further bonding application achieves a partially mechanical and a partially chemical adhesion as the fluid resin links chemically with the collagen and, polymerizing, gets into the same fibers and inside the canaliculus with a thickness of a few microns, making the so-called "hybrid stratum." At the moment of the further filling, adhesion of the composite resin to the bonding of the hybrid stratum takes place.

The fringe fissure development is more frequent when polymerization is executed with chemical activation; as a matter of fact, the photoactivation allows a polymerization of further material coats introduced gradually into the cavity. All this limits the shrinking phenomena compared to the polymerization of the whole filling compound all at once. Adhesive techniques are not always able to prevent the material being removed from the cavity walls.

Composite resins are used also for indirect restoration with heat filling polymerization carried out in the laboratory according to the cavity impression. In such a case a cementing system is necessary; this indirect restoration allows a more homogeneous material polymerization and a more correct repairing of anatomic detail reconstruction. Cementing through adhesive acrylic resins or C.V.I. makes it possible to obtain good adaptation to the cavity walls, limiting the marginal fissures. However, a certain degree of shrinkage, a rather complicated procedure, and the necessity of cavities which preserve to a lesser extent the healthy tissue to allow the fitting of inlay, restrict the use of these materials to limited clinical medication.

22.3.2.3. Glass Ionomers

Glass-ionomer cements (GICs) or glass-polyalkenoate cements (Wilson and McLean, 1988) are traditionally a group of materials which undergo setting through an acid–base reaction between an ion-leachable glass and an aqueous polyacid. They have multiple uses in dentistry (such as luting or restorative or lining or base cement) and they exhibit a high degree of biocompatibility to the pulp and surrounding soft tissues. Outside dentistry, glass ionomers have begun to find uses that exploit their good biocompatibility, such as artificial ear ossicles and bone substitute plates for craniofacial reconstruction, for orthopedics, and for ENT surgery as bioac-

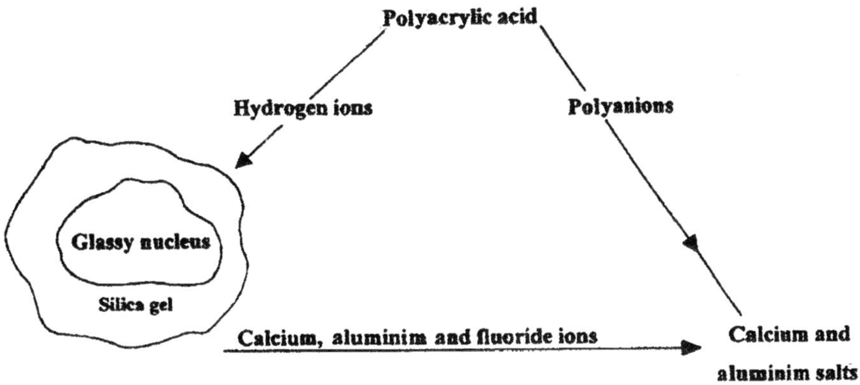

Figure 22.4. Hardening scheme of glass ionomers.

tive implant material, as fixation of coclear implants, and for sealing defects in the skull (Nicholson *et al.*, 1998).

Glass-polyalkenoate cements were introduced into the dental profession by Wilson and McLean in 1975. The original GICs consisted of an aqueous solution of polyacrylic acid which was made to react with a powder consisting of calcium fluoroaluminosilicate glass. The setting reactions are shown in Figures 22.4 and 22.5. The microstructure of modern glass-ionomer Alphafil is visible in Figure 22.6.

The traditional glass ionomers are characterized by adhesion, fluoride release, and brittleness (Wilson and McLean, 1988). The early materials set sluggishly, showed some sensitivity to moisture, and appeared to be rather opaque cements. Early on, the setting characteristics were improved by Wilson and co-workers with the addition of tartaric acid. Now it is added at a level of 5–10% in order to extend the working time, so delaying the setting stage and increasing ultimate compressive and tensile strengths. Since then a number of modifications have become available:

1. The use of more reactive polyacids (e.g., copolymers of acrylic and maleic acid) as polyacid components.
2. The use of dried polymer powders blended with the glass and activated by the addition of water.
3. The development of so-called cermets or metal-reinforced cements, performed (i) by sintering the glass together with metals, (ii) by adding a metal, such as silver–tin alloy (Figure 22.7) or stainless steel. In these materials, the metal part can absorb mechanical stress to some extent and subsequently reduce the brittleness of the cement system.

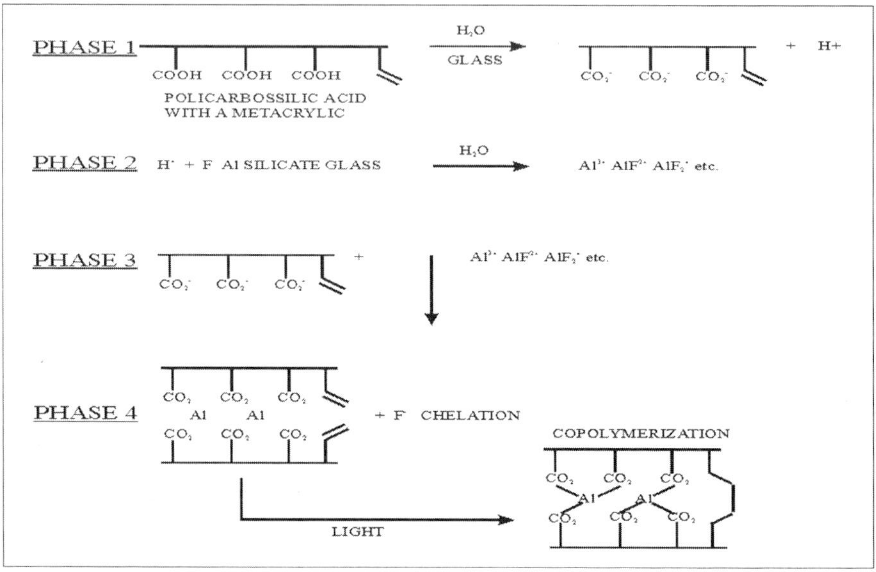

Figure 22.5. Setting reactions of glass ionomers.

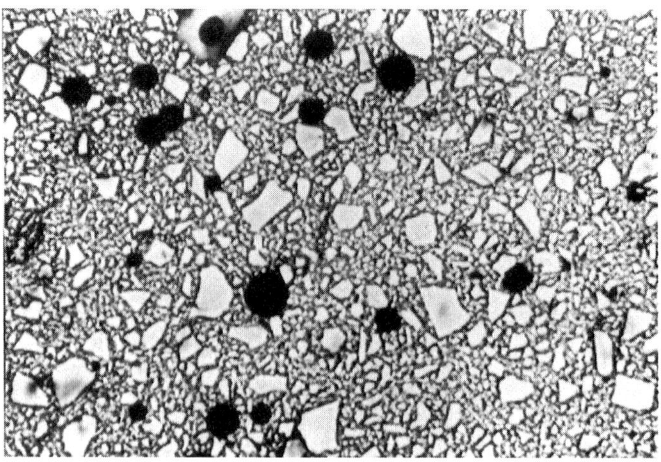

Figure 22.6. Microstructure (optical micrograph) of the glass-ionomer Alphafil: white glass particles of different size and black round pores in the matrix after setting reactions.

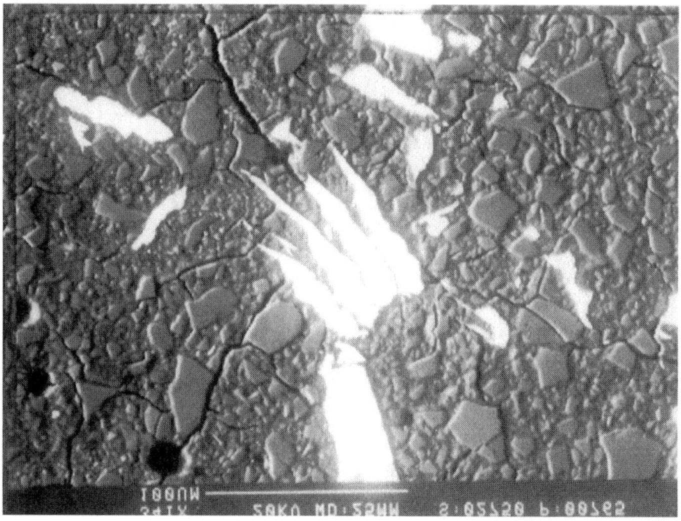

Figure 22.7. Microstructure (SEM-BSE) of the commercial cermet Alpha Silver. The metallic phase is a Ag–Sn–Cu alloy.

4. Performing resin-modified cement setting by both acid–base reaction and polymerization. The conventional acid–base components are added by monomers and initiators in order to allow photochemical polymerization and reduce moisture sensitivity and lack of "command cure."

With respect to point 4, in the early 1990s a couple of so-called "light-cured glass ionomers" that attempted to combine glass-ionomer chemistry with that of composite resin were released on the market (McCabe, 1998; Leyhausen *et al.* 1998). Two different chemical approaches toward these hybrid materials are possible: the first adapts the resin matrix to the GIC matrix so that the two different setting mechanisms lead to an interpenetrating network; the second approach modifies the polyacid partially by attaching polymerizable groups like 2-hydroxyethyl methacrylate (HEMA), the remaining carboxylic groups allowing an acid–base reaction with the glass filler. Guggenberger *et al.* (1998) suggest a simplified picture of all these materials where pure GICs and composites are the two extremes of a so-called "GIC composite continuum" as shown in Figure 22.8. The conventional GICs (an example is Ketac-Fil) are connected along an ideal line with the resin-modified GICs (typified by Fuji II LC, Vitremer, Photac-Fil), then with a second class of materials, the so-called "compomers" (such as Dyract,

Traditional GICs	⇔	Resin modified GICs	⇔	Polyacid modified composites	⇔	Composite resins

Figure 22.8. From conventional GICs to composite resins in a "continuum." Modified from Guggenberger *et al.* (1998).

Compoglass), which lie close to the composites (such as Pertac-Hibrid) localized at the end point of the line (Berg, 1998).

The compomers consist of an ion-leachable glass embedded in a polymeric matrix; their chemistry is almost identical to composite resin, so they are also called "polyacid modified composite resin" (Meyer *et al.*, 1998). They differ from the GICs because both the glass particles are partially silanized to provide a direct bond with the resin matrix, and the matrix is formed essentially during the light-activated radical polymerization reaction of monomers. These monomers are fundamentally modified methacrylates (UDMA, BisGMA,...) and new bifunctional monomers characterized by two carboxylic groups and two double-bond functions such as TCB or DCDMA. The latter should be able to react with both the pendant methacrylate groups of other monomers, by radical polymerization, and by means of an acid–base neutralization reaction with the cations liberated by the glass particles. Then the resulting three-dimensional network should be built with a covalent as well as ionic bond, but no water is present as an ingredient of the compomer so that the neutralization reaction is inhibited. A very limited reaction of this type is thought to occur later as the material absorbs water.

Many papers, monographs, and reviews are available on the development, chemistry, structure, properties, biocompatibility, clinical application, and new trends of GICs (Mount, 1998; De Barra and Hill, 1998).

There are two distinguishing (Smith, 1989, 1998) effective characteristics of the classical polyacrylate-based GICs: long sustained fluoride release and intrinsic adhesion to tooth tissues, enamel as well as dentine. Both in prevention and in treating caries the fluoride may act in different ways. The metabolism of the bacteria causing caries is inhibited and the resistance of enamel and dentine is increased; porous enamel and softened dentine can be remineralized in the presence of fluoride.

In general, the available literature data regarding the resin-modified glass ionomers refer to the debate on nomenclature pertaining to these products. To compare the results of the researchers is sometimes difficult, owing to the variety of the chemistry of GIC system materials and the many different names given to them. However, setting characteristics of resin-modified GICs (McCabe, 1998; Nicholson, 1998) seem to be similar in many respects to those of light-activated composites, although some products have a limited working time due to the influence of the acid–base setting reaction and sensitivity to ambient light. Water absorption and swelling are generally very high. The mechanical properties of most materials lie between those of the composites and conventional glass ionomers, depending upon the resin content of the matrix phase of the set material.

Some products demonstrate an inherent adhesion to enamel; however, etching may be required to make the bond clinically effective. The bonding mechanism to dentine may be more complex than that involved with traditional glass ionomers (Abate, 1997). The fluoride release rate and its clinical significance require clarification and standardization (Forsten, 1998).

It is also suggested in the literature that in some kind of resin-modified glass ionomers the improvement in strength, fracture toughness, and lower moisture sensitivity has been gained at the expense of increased overall dimensional change, reduced direct adhesion and fluoride release, reduced polyelectrolyte character, and a lesser biocompatibility (Kan *et al.*, 1997; Jumlongras and White, 1997).

Few reports can be found in the literature on the properties (Meyer *et al.*, 1998) and clinical evaluation of the compomers as they have only recently appeared on the market. Recently, Meyer *et al.* (1998) studied some physical properties of commercial polyacid-modified composite resins and compared them with composites and conventional and resin-modified glass-ionomer cements. They concluded that compomers behave more like composite resins than glass ionomers due to lack of setting in the absence of light, the very small quantity of sorbed water, the subsequent lesser effect of water on the material stiffness, the higher mechanical properties, and a severely reduced release of fluoride. However, the overall *in vitro* behavior of compomers tested by Meyer and co-workers had to be considered as somewhat inferior to that of the compared composite resins The manufacturers generally limit the use of the polyacid-modified composites to clinical situations where only low stress would be suffered, despite a recognized improvement in the handling characteristics of this material.

22.4. Materials for Complex Reconstructions

In restorative dentistry, it is sometimes necessary in the case of serious lesions to use accessory pins to restore the morphology of a large amount of dental tissue which will have long-term resistance and stability. The dentine pins are thin and threaded cylinders about 0.8 cm long and 0.3–0.8

gauge-caliber made of stainless steel or titanium. They are settled in healthy dentine through manual or mechanical screwing and thus grant stability and resistance to restoration, which would be impossible using plastic materials or by a direct technique. The abutment post pins have a wide head and a long body both of different morphology, gauge, and length (Craig, 1993; Shavel, 1980). These pins will be located inside the previously prepared root canal.

Screw pins having a helicoidal threading are generally made of steel, gold, brass, or titanium. Cylindrical pins with threading or lateral retention are made of these materials and also of carbon fiber. The latter are generally set in with dental cement. The abutment post pins allow a very durable application, thanks to the retention head shape. The abutment post pins are often used as a retentive bearing in hard restoration made in gold alloy cast together with the filling material.

22.5. Prosthetic Therapy Materials

Prosthetic therapy is used in the presence of dental loss and compromise phonation, masticatory and digestive functions, and also the esthetic appearance.

According to the kind of edentulousness, say partial or total, we can use a partial or a total prosthesis. The first can find anchorage in different ways on the remaining teeth and eventually on osteomucosa structures. The second can find anchorage or retention on the remaining osteomucosa structures belonging to the edentulous arch.

Prostheses can be fixed or moving (Figures 22.9 and 22.10) according to the anchorage, which may be only dental or both mucous and dental (Graber, 1986; Rosenstiel and Land, 1988).

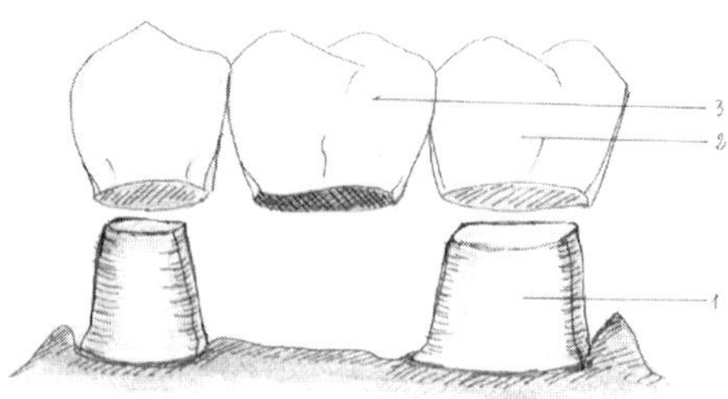

Figure 22.9. Schematic picture of a fixed prosthesis: (1) residual prepared tooth, (2) total coverage crown, (3) crown, to substitute the missing tooth, built together with other crowns through casting.

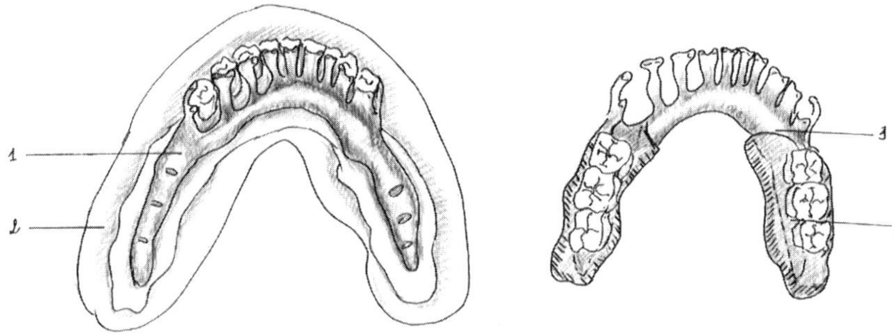

Figure 22.10. Picture of a moving skeleton prothesis: (1) skeleton of Co–Cr alloy, (2) gypsum model of the patient's dental arches, (3) connectors, (4) resin plate with resin or ceramic teeth.

Moving prostheses vary according to different kinds of anchorage; these can be completely removable or partly removable and partly fixed (mixed prosthesis).

22.5.1. Fixed Prosthesis Materials

Fixed prosthesis involves restoration by total coverage (crown) of a single damaged tooth, or substitution of missing teeth by anchorage to remaining teeth by total or partial coverage crowns of one or more residual elements. A replacement pontic for the missing tooth is connected to the anchorage through stiff or soft soldering.

The technique consists in the use of resins made of vinyl acrylic copolymers or polycarbonate, generally used only temporarily to make provisional prostheses which will be substituted after favorable clinical conditions occur.

Definitive work is performed according to the duly prepared plaster model of the patient's arch. Artificial teeth and their anchorage are built through casting and forming with lost wax. Nowadays, gold alloys or precious alloys are mostly used thanks to their biocompatibility.

Base metal alloys are very useful owing to their good mechanical properties which present a sufficient resistance even on critical bridge areas affecting (soldering, welding) anchorage, and also for their good biological properties which must allow a proper contact with periodontal tissues and the oral cavity.

Alloys have a good possibility of reproducing the morphofunctional characteristics of the replaced parts. Poor esthetic properties of metal alloys used for fixed prostheses are reduced by partial or total covering in resin or porcelain. Fixed prostheses are cemented to dental anchorage, with no possibility for the patient to remove them, using adhesive cement such as C.V.I. or cements made mainly of acrylic resins, or zinc oxide cements or carboxylic cements.

22.5.2. Moving Partial or Total Prosthesis Materials

Moving partial prostheses can be removable partial dentures in metal alloy when their standing structure is made by metal connectors (chromium cobalt alloy or gold alloy) obtained by casting on a plaster model from a patient's mouth. The connector system supports the resin saddles, which are strengthened by the metal itself. These saddles cover up the edentulous area where artificial dental members in resin or porcelain are soldered. In this case the anchorage can be made by metal claps on the remaining teeth, or by a more sophisticated hinge joint system, or with crowns or fixed bridge bearings (mixed prosthesis).

Moving partial prostheses can be totally constructed in acrylic resin when its use is temporary, or when the remaining teeth do not allow anchorage to be used for removable partial dentures in a metal alloy prosthesis. In such a case the resin collector dimensions are larger for reasons of mechanical resistance.

When anchorage consist in clasps, these are in soldered gold alloy, or in steel, or in soldered chromium–cobalt alloy, and partially included in the resin. Junction members articulated within the mixed prosthesis (connectors, attachments, shock absorbers) can be in gold alloy or in stainless steel. Obviously, the choice of materials used together must consider the possible problems that arise in coupling them.

The methacrylic resin used for saddles in partial dentures in metal alloy, in removable, and in total ones is hot polymerized in the laboratory. Methylmethacrylic (monomer) is a colorless liquid at room temperature while polymethacrylate (polymer) looks stiff and transparent. These materials possess rather good mechanical properties, but they have little abrasion resistance; they generally are thought to have little toxicological effect and to be chemically stable and inert in the mouth. Esthetic qualities are rather good because of their translucence, pigmentation facility, and color stability.

Artificial teeth can be made in polyacrylic resin, in polyvinylic ester, polystyrene, and copolymers as well as in porcelain. The latter must be soldered to the resin saddle through a mechanical retention system, while the other teeth link chemically.

Besides remaining unaltered, porcelain teeth maintain their esthetic qualities for a long time and resist abrasion, but they can easily break. Resin teeth have few esthetic qualities, as they lose their original color and are more elastic.

22.5.3. Precious and Nonprecious Alloys for Dental Prostheses

For restoration which is going to be subjected to both loading and abrasion during its time in a normal mouth, a resistance to deformation and wear is an obvious necessity. This restoration takes the form of inlays, crowns, or bridges and is suitably made of metal alloys.

Their close fit to the teeth is obtained by precision casting techniques (Brown, 1988). The first stage after the teeth have been prepared is to take an impression in a material which flows in a controlled way into the affected areas and then sets.

From this negative impression a positive model is made in hard plaster, and this is used by the dental technician to produce a wax pattern of the inlay, crown, or bridge. This pattern is then invested in a mixture of refractory silica and a binding agent, often gypsum. When it is set, the wax is burned away in a furnace and the appropriate dental alloy is forced by pressure into the space within the covering formerly occupied by the wax. It solidifies and can then be removed, cleaned, and polished before being sent to the dental surgeon, who cements it into or onto the prepared teeth.

The suitable alloy must have many different accompanying properties. Some of these depend on the need to facilitate alloy industrial production or prosthesis forming in the dental laboratory (castability, workability, ease of manipulation and welding, etc.); others are necessary to make the product suitable to perform its function in the oral cavity. So the material must have strength, stiffness, toughness, and resistance to wear in order to withstand daily masticatory stress. It must show long durability in use and appropriate esthetic qualities at a low cost. It must have high resistance to surface tarnish and corrosion to be neither toxic nor irritating.

For about 50 years noble metal alloys whose major constituent was gold have been preferred for their high chemical stability. In the 1920s the casting alloys were classified by the American Dental Association (ADA) according to their mechanical properties and chemical composition. They were known as Type I (A or soft), Type II (B or medium), Type III (C or hard), and Type IV (D or extra hard). The gold and platinum group metal content should exceed 75, 78, 78, and 83 wt% for types I–IV, respectively. These traditional systems were Au–Ag–Cu alloys. Manufacturers have achieved the alloy properties by means of a proper Cu/Ag ratio and by adding a certain amount of platinum and palladium, grain refiners, and other dedicated minor components.

Due to the high cost of raw material, alternatives to the classic type III and IV alloys have been developed. These new systems did not satisfy the ADA specification requirements concerning their chemical composition.

Table 22.2. Vrijhoef Classification of Precious Metal Alloys

Class	Gold content (wt%)
0, no gold	$0 \leqslant Au \leqslant 20$
1, low gold	$20 \leqslant Au \leqslant 40$
2, medium gold	$40 \leqslant Au \leqslant 60$
3, high gold	$Au > 60$

Therefore, on the basis of the gold amount another classification has been proposed by Vrijhoef (Table 22.2).

There has been a general trend to lower the gold content (Tuccillo, 1977). Silver and copper have been increased, while the amount of palladium has become greater and greater in order to obtain an acceptable tarnish and corrosion resistance (Mezger, 1989). At present, the rising price of palladium creates reverse problems: gold may become more economic than palladium.

The evolution of metal restoration regarding its esthetic aspects leads to alloys capable of ceramic veneering (Tuccillo and Cascone, 1983). Porcelain-fused-to-metal (PFM) restoration consists of a cast metal coping onto which a porcelain veneer is fired. With this technique low-fusing, high-expansion, highly vitreous porcelain powders (first, opaque layers; then, translucent layers) are stacked, fired, shaped, and glazed against the oxidized surface of the casting in order to mask the metal. A high oxide adherence is necessary to improve metal–ceramic bonding strength. The chemical composition of the alloys highly influences metal–ceramic compatibility because some components can modify color and opacity of the ceramic while improving oxide layer formation or lowering oxide adherence (Jones, 1992). PFM restoration may develop cracks during processing or while in use in mouth service, if the relative physical-mechanical properties (particularly the coefficient of thermal expansion) of the porcelain and alloy are highly mismatched. Many processing and property variations can affect the stress developed throughout a porcelain–alloy system (Asaoka, 1991; Gettleman, 1991).

The PFM alloys were introduced onto the market several years ago. Since 1958 Au–Pt–Pd alloys have been available containing 77–88% Au, considerable additions of Pt and Pd, and minor amounts of some other elements. In gold (45–75 wt%) lowered PFM alternative Au–Cu–Ag alloys, virtually no Pt, a Pd amount varying from 4 to 44 wt%, and an increased Ag content (up to 16 wt%) may be present.

At the end of the 1970s, silver-free modification of this system, the so-called Au–Pd alloys, were introduced and considered reliable. The fairly new Pd–Ag alloys hardly contain any gold. The Pd content varies from 50 to 60 wt%. The amount of Ag varies from 24 to 42 wt%.

The recently developed Pd-based alloys are moving to high-Pd alloys containing about 80 wt% Pd as well as other components, like Ga, Cu, Co, In, and Sn, to allow hardening and bonding to ceramic.

Composition limits for the different types of noble PFM alloys are shown in Figure 22.11. These alloys generally have a complex microstructure (Figure 22.12) owing to the presence of alloying elements such as Ga and In which can form intermetallics. The microstructure of these alloys is generally affected by the different casting conditions, deformation rate, and thermal treatments used in alloy industrial production and prosthesis manufacturing (Pinasco *et al.*, 1999; Angelini *et al.*, 1998). Despite this, they generally show great corrosion resistance in every metallurgical state (Angelini *et al.*, 1998, Angelini *et al.* 2000).

The different aspects of the corrosion behavior of dental casting alloys have been extensively studied and reviewed (Corso, 1985; Mezger, 1989; Mezger *et al.*, 1989; Meyer and Reclaru, 1995; Wataha and Malcom, 1996; Holland, 1992).

The majority of the current nonprecious base metal alloys belong to the Ni (60 up to 85 wt%)–Cr (5–22 wt%) type. Molybdenum is a third important component (Figure 22.13). Furthermore, a large variety of minor elements is used. Beryllium is sometimes added for castability, grain refining, and increasing hardness.

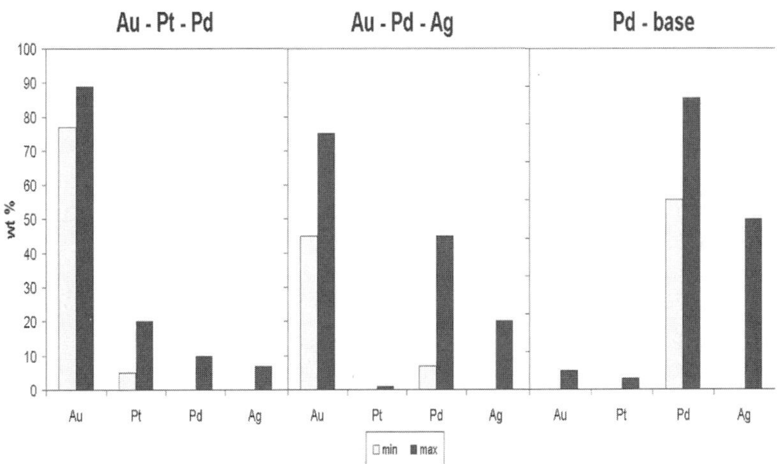

Figure 22.11. Composition limits (white = minimum, black = maximum) for the different types of precious PMF alloys. From data of Mezger (1989).

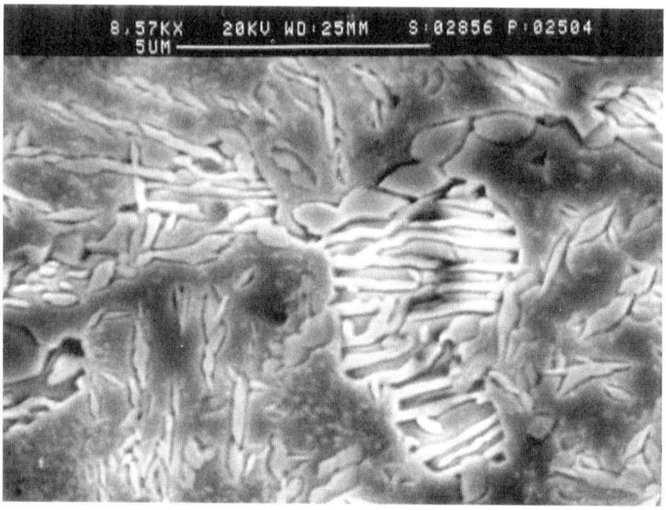

Figure 22.12. Microstructure (SEM-SE) of a Pd-based porcelain-fused-to-metal dental alloy in the metallurgical state characterizing the alloy in the oral cavity.

Ni–Cr–Be alloys are very popular. The relatively low density of Ni–Cr alloys is an advantage in certain clinical situations. In the 1980s, Co–Cr ceramic alloys derived from partial denture casting systems were introduced: the Co content varies from 52 to 70 wt%, Cr from 20–30 wt%, and Mo from 0–10 wt%. As usual, many minor elements are added to improve properties.

Most of the alternative base metal casting alloys have superior physical and mechanical properties, high-temperature sag resistance, are less expensive than precious metal alloys, but have some technique sensitivity. The principal deficiencies are the potential for hypersensitivity of the patient to nickel, chromium, or beryllium, difficulty in brazing or soldering, and a casting peculiarity. Report No. 34 from the Fédération Dentaire Internationale (1990) outlines the technical differences between noble and base metal alloys. The popularity of the base metal alloys for fixed partial dentures has increased greatly in the past decade due to their advantageous mechanical properties and the high cost of gold. One disadvantage of these alloys is the hard-to-control chromium oxide formation that results in lower porcelain–metal bond strength.

Titanium and Ti-6Al-4V alloy have many desirable properties that would recommend them for crown and bridgework, such as good corrosion resistance, low specific gravity, good mechanical properties, excellent biocompatibility, and low cost (see the chapter on the structure and properties

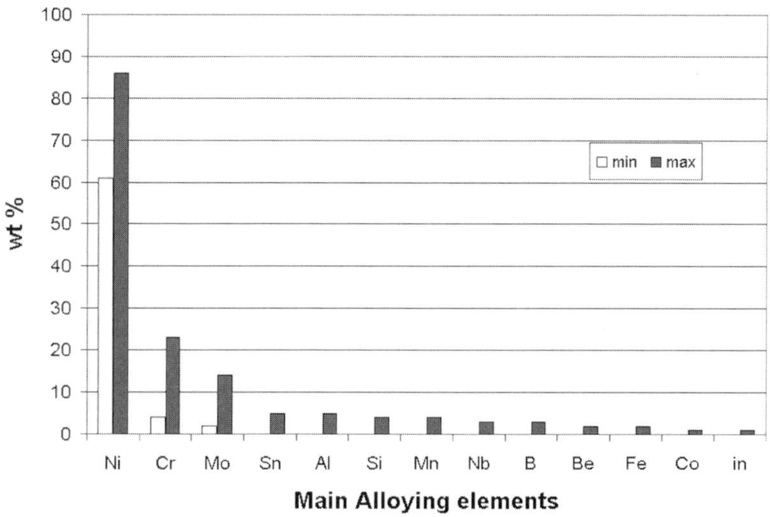

Figure 22.13. Composition limits (white as minimum, black as maximum) of the main alloying elements of PFM NiCr alloys. From data of Mezger (1989).

of metals). Nevertheless, the high melting temperature and violent chemical reactivity at high temperature of titanium and its alloys lead to many technical problems and difficulties with casting and porcelain bonding (Adachi *et al.*, 1990; Kvam *et al.*, 1995). Titanium requires ceramics compatible with its low thermal expansion. The $\alpha-\beta$ phase transformation temperature (880 °C) must be avoided; ceramics must have a lower firing temperature than traditional ceramics for veneering to metals.

There is current interest in titanium as a dental restorative material, and ceramics for veneering to titanium have been developed during the past few years (Kvam *et al.*, 1995).

22.6. Dental Implant Materials: A Few Considerations

Implants constitute an important system for prosthetic therapy in partial or total edentulousness. The subject has developed greatly during the last few years and involves so many aspects that lack of space has obliged us to provide only very little information.

This system involves teeth support apparatus substitution with metal or other kinds of systems belonging to different morphologies and formulations. These systems can allow an anchorage to the dental arch bone structures (Frank, 1970).

According to the kind of connection implants obtained with edentulous bone ridges, they are known as juxta osseous or under periosteum, or endosteal implants. The first involve the building of a biocompatible metal structure provided with a grate which adapts to the support structures (milohyoid ridges, mental symphysis, oblique ridges) inserted beneath the oral mucosa according to the bone impression. An abutment tooth for future prosthetic rebuilding projects in the oral cavity through a gap into the very same mucosa (Frank, 1970).

Endosteal implants can be divided into "immediate or fibrointegrated" when the prosthetic device is laid down just after the surgery to insert the implant. Implants are called osteointegrated when they are to be used as a prosthesis or rehabilitation. It is necessary to have integration with bone biological tissue, generally carried out 5 or 6 months after insertion. We can also classify them by the different types of implant morphology chosen to conform with edentulous ridges, clinical conditions, and with the entity and quality of the remaining tissue (endosteal needle implants, blade implants, spiral implants) (Von Fraunhofer and Estrange, 1971).

According to the materials employed we can have metal, ceramic, metal-ceramic, and vetrocarbonious implants. Metal implants are produced in pure titanium or in titanium alloys including aluminum (6%) and vanadium (4%); they are generally covered by a thin titanium oxide film or, using the "plasma spray" method, by a very thin pure titanium coat to make the osteointegration easier (Donley and Gillette, 1991; Keller, 1998; Pilliar, 1998).

Sintered ceramic implants have a porous surface to increase the biocompatibility qualities. Sometimes, porcelain is used as metal implant covering material. Both metal implants as well as ceramic ones can be covered with hydroxyapatite. This bioactive material reduces the time necessary for osteointegration, but it can give a certain fragility to the system.

Vetrocarbonious implants are generally used for the immediate insertion of substances into the socket of teeth which have just been removed in order that the alveolar bone should retain its physiological dimensions (Von Fraunhofer). They can be made in thick hydroxyapatite and polyethylene, or by glazed carbons obtained by means of controlled thermal degradation of organic polymers.

Recently, Glantz (1998) summarized biomaterials considerations in the use of metals and metal alloys, ceramics and carbons, and synthetic materials for implant therapy. He also discussed implant material selection, biomaterial aspects of bioadhesion and osseointegration, and hygiene-related biomaterial factors.

The choice of the most suitable implant system and its performance depend strongly on the patient's general and local clinical condition (Taylor,

1988). Whatever the method used for osteointegration and prosthesis execution, the system cannot reproduce a physiological periodontal membrane and an epithelial attachment (Klinge, 1991).

22.7. Biomaterials for Surgical Reconstitution

We distinguish among biomaterials used in periodontal regeneration, barrier membranes, and materials used as a filler of intrabony defects.

22.7.1. Periodontal Regeneration

Periodontal regenerative materials are used in situations where the treatment outcome is expected to improve the function and prognosis of periodontitis involved teeth. The objectives were always to accomplish a new attachment, however the regeneration remained controversial. Numerous investigations (Patur and Glickman, 1962; Yukna *et al.*, 1976) have indicated that the morphology of a periodontal bony defect was essential for the establishment of predictable clinical prognosis using opening curettage. However, several histologic studies in animals and humans indicated that formation of a new attachment is not predictable following curettage or flap surgery alone.

22.7.2. Goal of Osseous Grafting

The goals of osseous graft procedures have been described as being pocket elimination, restoration of alveolar process, and regeneration of a functional attachment apparatus.

22.7.3. Factors Influencing Graft Success

Oral hygiene, defect morphology (numbers of walls, narrow versus wide defects), furcation involvement, operator technique, and graft material as well as the size of the particles are influencing factors. For example, it was determined that a pore size of 100 μm is needed between particles to allow blood supply and bone formation. It was then concluded that the ideal particle size was about 380 μm for grafting materials.

22.7.4. Regenerative Materials

We can split implant materials utilized in periodontal bony defects for regeneration into four categories: autogenous grafts, allograft, xenografts, and alloplastic materials.

22.7.4.1. Autogenous Grafts

This type of graft, which is transferred from one body area to another within the same individual, is made of cortical bone or cancellous bone and marrow, and is harvested either from extraoral or intraoral donor sites.

a. Extraoral Autogenous Grafts. Hip marrow grafts (iliac crest marrow) has been used in the treatment of furcation and intrabony defects (Schallhorn, 1967, 1968). This autogenous bone is considered the most predictable method for osseous regeneration. It may be due to osteogenic, osteoinductive, and osteoconductive properties associated within the graft material itself, necrosis of the graft material and release of substances that may stimulate new bone formation, and nonviable cellular elements within the graft that may act as a scaffold for new host bone formation. Fresh and frozen cancellous bone and marrow from the illiac crest have been used; frozen specimens demonstrated the greatest mean bone opposition, which was believed to be due to cellular breakdown and release of an inductive substance. New attachment was observed at 3 months. However, Patur (1974) stated that even with fresh iliac crest marrow, bone regeneration is variable and unpredictable. Dragoo and Sullivan (1973a, b) evaluated fresh autogenous iliac bone graft clinically and histologically over a 2 to 8 month period. New cementum was present as early as 2 months, with a functionally oriented PDL noted at 3 months. Osteoblastic activity was greatest at 2 months, but persisted at 8 months. At 8 months, the PDL was completely mature and about 2 mm of supracretal new attachment had also formed. However, clinical evidence of root resorption was noted. In animal studies, Ellegaard *et al.* (1973, 1974) evaluated the healing of interradicular and intrabony lesions following placement of iliac crest marrow. They also observed ankylosis and root resorption. Viability of the marrow elements is thought to play a role in root resorption. Frozen marrow did not demonstrate any resorptive association. The decrease in the use of iliac crest marrow grafts in regenerative periodontal therapy today is related to the morbidity associated with the donor site and root resorption.

b. Intraoral Autogenous Grafts. The autogenous intraoral bone has also been used as donor material in osseous grafting. Generally, cancellous bone is preferred as graft material. Cortical bone, applied as small chips, and intraoral bone grafts mixed with blood prior to placement in the defects have also been reported to be effective. Hiatt *et al.* (1978) treated 166 intrabony lesions with intraoral autogenous cancellous bone. Measurements taken from 9 months to 7 years showed no significant difference between the three types of donor tissue. The largest bone fill was observed in defects with the highest number of bony walls, with histologic demonstration of new cementum, bone, and DPL. The marrow from the maxilla had the greatest probability of containing foci of red marrow with associated pleuripotential cells. Rivault *et al.* (1971) observed on monkeys that defects filled with osseous coagulum healed with new bone formation, but no more bone was found in such experimental defects than was observed in similar control defects treated with surgical curettage. The histologic evaluation of many studies suggests that the treatment of periodontal osseous defects with intraoral bone grafts may results in the formation of new connective tissue attachment; however, it is not always predictable.

c. Allograft Materials. Due to the fact that the use of autogenous grafts implies an additional surgical site, allografts were utilized in attempts to stimulate bone formation in intrabony defects or interradicular areas. However, the use of allografts involves a certain risk regarding antigenicity. In order to suppress foreign body reactions, the allografts are usually pretreated by freezing, radiation, or chemicals. Altiere (1979) treated 10 pairs of intraosseous defects. Irradiated FDBA was compared to control sites which received flap curettage only. No significant difference was found between the two groups with respect to pocket reduction and amount of new attachment. It was concluded that the irradiation of the bone may remove or compromise the inductive potential present in the graft material. However, the demineralization process of a cortical bone allograft (DFDBA) enhances its osteogenic potential by exposing the bone morphogenic proteins. Melloning *et al.* (1981) evaluated the osteogenic potential of four different grafting materials: FDBA, DFDBA, autogenous osseous coagulum, and autogenous bone blend. There was a significantly greater amount of new bone formation with the DFDBA than with any of the other materials. On the other hand, Rummelhart *et al.* (1989) found no statistical differences regarding attachment level changes and bone fill when comparing sites treated with FDBA and sites treated with DFDBA. Bowers (1989b, c) showed histological evidence of regeneration following grafting with DFDBA. About 80% of the original defect depth reported complete regeneration (new cementum, periodontal ligament, bone) at sites treated with DFDBA. The effect of allogenic DFDB matrix on regeneration of alveolar bone and periodontal attachment in dogs was recently evaluated. The results of this sudy suggested that the matrix implants may enhance cementum regeneration but have no apparent effect on alveolar bone regeneration. Moreover, the tissue blocks were harvested following a 4-week healing. This interval appeared to be insufficient for turnover of demineralized bone matrix.

22.7.4.2. Heterografts or Xenografts

Suprisingly, periodontal research studies show little interest in xenograft bone implants. Nielsen *et al.* (1981) evaluated the healing between defects treated with intraoral autogenous bone grafts and defects treated with kiel-bone® (i.e., defatted and deproteinized ox bone). Periodontal probing and radiographs showed no difference in the amount of clinical attachment gain between the two groups. In monkeys, Nielsen *et al.* (1980) demonstrated that the two types of bone graft displayed similar histologic features: connective tissue of healed defect showed isolated bone particules surrounded by a cementum-like substance. This material is compatible, noninflammatory, porous to allow conduction growth of bone into and around the implant, able to stimulate bone induction, resorbable with replacement by bone, easy to obtain, and inexpensive. However, xenografts are not radio-opaque, and doubts have been raised as to their risk of immunogenicity. In much of the osseous grafting literature, the lack of ungrafted controls has been criticized. The presence of bone fill subsequent to grafting procedures does not prove new attachment. To eliminate all doubts about healing with filling materials, Bowers (1983) compared the potential for regeneration in osseous defects associated with submerged and nonsubmerged roots, with and without DFDBA, in a 6-month human histologic study. Nongrafted, nonsubmerged sites were found to heal by long epithelium, while nongrafted but submerged defects healed by connective tissue attachment. Epithelium exclusion, obtained in submerged roots, is associated with a greater degree of regeneration and new connective tissue attachment in the absence of root resorption or ankylosis. However, it was demonstrated that granulation tissue derived from bone induces root resorption and ankylosis rather than a new connective tissue attachment. The concept of using bone graft in periodontal surgery has been questioned.

22.7.4.3. Membranes for Periodontal Defects

The connective tissue attachment would be predictably achieved if progenitor cells of the DPL populate the root surface during healing. Gottlow *et al.* (1984) strongly suggest that the exclusion of epithelial and gingival connective tissue cells from the healing area by the use of a physical barrier may allow periodontal ligament cells to repopulate the detached root surface. This observation provided the basis for the clinical application of *guided tissue regeneration* (GTR), which is defined as a procedure attachment to regenerate lost periodontal structures through differential tissues responses. In recent years, GTR has been applied in a number of clinical trials for the treatment of various periodontal defects such as intrabony defects, grade II and III furcations, and recession defects. GTR is not a procedure for the treatment of periodontitis, but rather a technique for regenerating defects which have developed as a result of periodontitis. Therefore, appropriate periodontal treatment should always be completed before GTR is initiated. In order for a barrier material to function, it has to encounter essential design criteria: (1) biocompatibility; (2) act as a barrier to maintain secluded space adjacent to the root surface, but also allowing the passage of nutrients and gases; (3) tissue integration: tissue may grow into the material without penetrating all the way through; the goal of tissue integration is to prevent rapid epithelial downgrowth on the outer surface of the material or encapsulation of the material, and also to provide stability to the overlying flap; (4) the design of material should be provided in configurations which are easy to trim and place.

a. Nucleopore/Millipore Filters. GTR was first attempted with a bacterial filter produced from cellulose acetate (Millipore®) used as an occlusive membrane. These membranes are nonresorbable, induce high inflammatory response, and are not ideal for clinical application.

b. Teflon/PTFE Membranes. Current studies have utilized membranes of expanded polytetrafluoroethylene specially designed for periodontal regeneration (GORE-TEX material®). They consist of two carbon–carbon bonds with four attached fluorine atoms to form a polymer. It is inert and does not result in any tissue reaction. They must be removed in a second-stage surgery, 4 to 6 weeks after insertion. They consist of two parts: an open microstructure collar to inhibit epithelial migration and an occlusive apron (25 μ pores) that isolates the root surface from the surrounding tissue.

c. Biobrane Membrane. Nonresorbable, it is a biological dressing primarily used in the treatment of skin burns.

d. Collagen. These membranes are biodegradable and do not require a second procedure for removal. Collagen membranes (type I or type III collagen) from different species and from different sites have been tested in animals and humans (Paul *et al.*, 1992; Blumenthal, 1993; Wang *et al.*, 1994). The material is chemotactic for DPL fibroblasts, a barrier for migrating epithelial cells, hemostatic, a fibrillar scaffold for early vascular and tissue ingrowth, and it exhibits a varying degree of immunogenicity. Furthermore, infectious agents from animal products can be transmitted to humans and autoimmunization is also a risk. Several complications have been observed, such as early degradation, epithelial downgrowth along the material and premature loss of collagen materials, difficult handling of the material at the time of placement, properties of the material at the time of placement, and properties of the material itself (Chung *et al.*, 1990). Degradation of the material depends on the host and is always initiated through the cell mediator process.

e. Polylactic Acid or Copolymer of Polylactic-Polyglycolic Acid. These materials are biocompatible, but by definition they are not inert. The materials are degraded by hydrolysis and eliminated from the organism through the KREBS cycle as carbon dioxide and water. A number of bioabsorbable membranes appeared to fit the requirements of a good barrier to varying extents (Vycril, Guidor, Resolut, Atrisorb). Several studies (Hugoson *et al.*, 1995; Cortellini, 1996b) have indicated that similar satisfactory results can be obtained with bioabsorbable barrier materials of polylactic–polyglycolic acid as with nonbioabsorbable materials. However, several factors can affect clinical outcomes of GTR whatever the barrier membrane used. Clinical improvement can be achieved with a membrane barrier placed during flap surgery, but complete resolution of the defects is observed in a minority of sites. A series of factors associated with clinical outcomes has been identified using multivariable approaches (Tonetti, 1993, 1996, Machte *et al.*, 1994):

1. Patient factors: Better clinical attachment level gain was observed in patients with optimal plaque control, nonsmokers, and with previous eradication of residual periodontal infection.

2. Defects factors: The deeper and narrower the defect, the greater the amount of clinical improvement (Garrett *et al.*, 1988; Tonetti, 1996). The number of residual walls also was related to variable outcomes in GTR. Mandibular grade II furcation in the first and second molars, buccal or lingual, with deep pockets and thick gingiva (>1 mm) showed excellent results from GTR procedures.

3. Technical factors: GTR is a very sensitive technique. Membrane exposure was reported to be a major complication with a prevalence in the range of 70–80% (Becker *et al.*, 1988; De Sanctis *et al.*, 1996a, b). The prevalence of exposure can be highly reduced by specifically designed flaps to preserve the interdental tissues. Membrane exposure will lead to bacterial contamination (Selvig, 1990; Nowzari, 1994, 1995; De Sanctis, 1996a, b), which may occur during surgery or during the postoperative healing phase. Contamination of exposed nonbioabsorbable and bioabsorbable membranes was associated with lower probing attachment level gains. However, despite the application of systemic antibiotics, postoperative wound infection was still noted. Another important issue with these clinical results is the coverage of the regenerated underlying tissue after removal of a nonbioabsorbable membrane (Cortellini, 1993; Tonnetti, 1993). This exposure will increase the risks of mechanical and infectious insults, which may prevent complete maturation of the regenerated tissue into a new connective tissue attachment. The question is whether the achieved attachment gain can be maintained over a long-term follow-up (Becker and Becker, 1993). Many recent studies (Cortellini, 1996a; Machtei, 1996) indicate that patient factors such as compliance with oral hygiene, smoking habits, and susceptibility to disease progression, rather than treatment modality, are the major determinants of stability of the treated sites.

22.7.4.4. Fillings of Bone Defects

Filling materials or implants are alloplastic materials that are surgically placed into the oral tissue beneath the mucosal or periosteal layer or within bone for functional, therapeutic, or esthetic purposes.

a. Nonceramic Implant. (i) Shaffer and App (1971) have used calcium sulfate (plaster of Paris), which is available, inexpensive, easy to handle, and sterilizable, but there is no evidence of its osteoinductive properties.

(ii) Hard tissue replacement (HTR) is a calcium layered composite of polymethyl methacrylate core (PMMA) with polyhydroxylethyl methacrylate (polyhema). It is microporous, nonresorbable, sterile and ready to use in granular or molded forms, strong, inexpensive, hydrophilic for easier handling, and electrically charged to promote osteogenesis (Ashman and Bruin, 1985; Ashman, 1990). It has been mostly used for bone maintenance, placed in extraction sockets to prevent bone loss, or for ridge augmentation (Leake, 1988). It has been placed into periodontal defects resulting in a greater decrease in probing depth and gain in clinical attachment compared to debridment alone (Yukna, 1990).

b. Bioactive Materials. Bioactive glass is a nonresorbable material whose medical use evolved 25 years ago due to various advantages: strong bond with living tissues and modulus of elasticity similar to that of bone. This bonding prevents fibrous encapsulation at the material interface. Hench (1986) used a dense form of bioglass in periodontal defect repair. Some authors (Shapoff *et al.*, 1997; Zameth, 1997) indicated that bioactive glass has potential as a bone replacement material and is effective in the treatment of intrabony defects in humans.

c. Ceramic Implant Materials. Ceramics are well documented because of their biocompatibility, chemical and physical resemblance to bone minerals, and ability to develop strong bonding to living bone by natural cementing mechanisms. Most calcium phosphate materials are radio-opaque, sterilizable, easy to obtain, and stable. The ceramics used today are composed of hydroxyapatite (HA, durapatite, tribasic calcium phosphate) or tricalcium phosphate (TCP or B-TCP).

(i) Tricalcium phosphate is a highly purified, multicrystalline, porous form of calcium phosphate. The calcium/phosphate ratio is 1.5 and is similar to that found in bone mineral (1.7), but it is not a natural component of bone mineral. TCP is compatible with host tissue, leads to no adverse reactions (McDavid *et al.*, 1979), and heals with a long functional epithelium tissue attachment (Caton, 1980a, b). In human studies, Hoexter (1983) showed that TCP has been well retained, provided flap support, reduced tooth mobility, and preserved function. Histological studies (Baldock *et al.*, 1985; Bowers *et al.*, 1985, 1986) failed to indicate any osteogenesis, cementogenesis, or new connective tissue attachment. Slow resorption of TCP particles became well encapsulated by gingival connective tissue. Defect fill and resorption of TCP varied and could take as long as 40 months to occur.

(ii) Bell and Beirne (1988) studied the composite TCP and collagen graft and found the material to be a biocompatible binder in periodontal defects.

(iii) Biphasic calcium phosphate (BCP) is composed of varying amounts of HA and TCP. It is considered to be partially resorbable (Nery *et al.*, 1992).

d. Hydroxyapatite (HA). HA is a nonresorbable material. It has a close crystal and chemical resemblance to vertebrate tooth and bone mineral (calcium/phosphate ratio = 1.7). HA is noninflammatory, nonantigenic, and highly biocompatible to human tissue. Two basics forms are available: nonporous and porous.

(i) Nonporous HA is extremely dense, pure, nonresorbable, and possesses great strength. It may help to stabilize the remaining structure, and stimulate formation of some new connective tissue attachment. Healing is generally by long junctional epithelium. Encapsulation of the crystals has been described and bone formation is not a predictable event.

(ii) Porous HA is a ceramic implant material formed by hydrothermal conversion of the calcium carbonate exoskeleton of coral into hydroxyapatite. This conversion yields a material similar to the natural bone microstructure. Fibrovascular ingrowth and subsequent bone formation have been observed between the channels within this material (190 to 230 μm interconnecting channels) (White *et al.*, 1975; White and Shors, 1986). In animal studies, Minegishi (1988) noticed a rapid surrounding of HA granules by fibrous connective tissue or new bone. At 1 year the bone defects were almost completely repaired. The granules were integrated with new bone and the PDL reformed between the thin cementum and the new bone. However, human studies have shown a reduction in probing depth, an increase in attachment levels, and good incorporation of surrounding bone into the implant, but failed to demonstrate new attachment. (Kenney *et al.*, 1986, 1987, 1988a, 1988b; Stahl and Froum, 1987). For the first time, Kenney (1986) observed evidence of this material's ability to stimulate osteogenesis within the porous structure. Carranza *et al.* (1987) exhibited new cementum opposite the implanted material (blocks sections at 6 months after implantation) but no new connective tissue attachment was expected. Closure of the wound treated with porous HA is always by long junctional epithelium and true regeneration is more likely with bone autograft or barrier membrane procedures.

22.8. Dental Implants and Biomechanics

22.8.1. Introduction

The aim of the present section is to report some notes on the biomechanical analysis of dental implants, paying peculiar attention to tissue–implant interaction phenomena. In dental biomechanics, relevant difficulties are found in performing experimental analysis because of complexity, heavy costs, and time-consuming procedures, while growing interest is shown for numerical simulation. On the other hand, this implies a deep knowledge of tissue mechanics, mostly trabecular and cortical bone. Special attention must be paid to the geometric definition of the anatomical site and implant device, to be in a position to offer an adequate representation of their biomechanical response, while also considering the effects of surgical procedures.

The literature reports the results of several computations performed by using different numerical techniques, but they seldom are associated with considerations on the reliability of the formulation developed and on the operational procedures. Using finite or geometric element method, different models can be obtained such as two-dimensional plane stress, plane strain, or axial-symmetric models, or three-dimensional models. Three-dimensional models should be used because they lead to the best definition of the problem treated. Two-dimensional models are currently adopted, but entails an approximation that must be carefully evaluated.

Some notes are reported on the procedure that leads to the configuration of the model, taking into account various aspects related to tissue mechanics, to definition of the geometrical configuration of the anatomical site, and to loading conditions. Results reported lead to the definition of the response of dental implants from a biomechanical viewpoint.

22.8.2. Tissue Mechanics

The investigation of interaction phenomena occurring with endosseous implants is faced with the problem of defining bone mechanical properties at different phases of the integration process (Ashman *et al.*, 1984; Bidez and Misch, 1992a, b; Brosh *et al.*, 1995; Friberg *et al.*, 1995; Murphy, 1995; Carter and Spengler, 1978; Natali, 1999; Natali and Meroi, 1989; Natali and Trebacz, 1996, 1999; Natali and Donà, 1999; Rohrer *et al.*, 1995; Terrier *et al.*, 1997; Throckmorton and Dechow, 1994; Vitins *et al.*, 1995).

Bone properties depend on different factors and certainly on age or presence of specific degenerative processes. With regard to a specific bone and to a specific region of the bone itself, mechanical characteristics depend upon liquid content, strain rate and creep, etc.

A numerical approach to dental biomechanics becomes more complex if soft tissues also have to be characterized. In this case, a Hookean material model is meaningless and a hyperelastic or porous media model must be regarded as a suitable constitutive formulation.

Bone tissue, as trabecular and cortical portions, presents different structural and macromechanical properties. Cortical bone is a highly organized tissue, while cancellous bone is a randomly oriented tissue. Such different configurations determine peculiar mechanical properties. Usually cortical tissue is represented using an orthotropic or transversely isotropic scheme, while for trabecular bone an equivalent isotropic scheme is used.

The configuration of human jaw is defined by cortical portion ranging from a very thin layer to a few millimeters, enclosing a core of trabecular bone. Trabecular bone assumes various configurations, with regard to the structural organization of trabecular net, in different zones of upper and lower jaw.

Specific elastic constants of cortical mandibular bone are reported in Table 22.3, such as elasticity modulus, shear modulus, and Poisson's ratio, according to an orthotropic scheme.

Values reported have also been estimated using an ultrasound technique, which makes it possible to calculate the mechanical properties by considering the velocity and/or the attenuation of the signal passing through the tissue. The mechanical characteristics depend upon both the density and the histologic and morphometric configuration of the tissue. Standard mechanical testing is also adopted for evaluation of the mechanical

Table 22.3. Average Elastic Constants of Corpus and Ramus of a Human Mandible

	Corpus	Ramus		Corpus	Ramus
E_1 (GPa)	10.93	11.77	ν_{12}	0.224	0.157
E_2 (GPa)	14.78	16.25	ν_{13}	0.295	0.292
E_3 (GPa)	18.89	20.42	ν_{23}	0.275	0.273
G_{12} (GPa)	4.24	4.8	ν_{21}	0.276	0.211
G_{13} (GPa)	5.13	5.72	ν_{31}	0.501	0.5
G_{23} (GPa)	6.27	6.67	ν_{32}	0.28	0.033

properties. On the basis of these techniques, average values of longitudinal and transversal elasticity moduli and Poisson's ratio for different regions of a human mandible cortical bone can be deducted.

The above constants vary as dependent on the anatomical region or tooth location. Table 22.4 illustrates elastic constant values at different anatomical regions.

As far as trabecular bone is concerned, it must be pointed out that the relevant complexity from a geometrical viewpoint entails employing the assumption of an equivalent isotropic scheme for the material. The mechanical constants are usually deduced from density measurements or, more properly, by adopting ultrasound testing, giving values that remain much lower in comparison with cortical bone.

Table 22.4. Average Elastic Constants of a Human Mandible by Tooth Location

	Wisdom tooth	Second molar	First molar	Second premolar	First premolar	Incisors	Average
E_1 (GPa)	11.59	11.66	11.65	10.14	10.13	10.64	10.97
E_2 (GPa)	13.22	15.13	13.61	13.38	12.81	13.49	13.95
E_3 (GPa)	17.66	19.82	20.44	16.4	17.42	19.6	18.3
G_{12} (GPa)	4.01	4.19	4.14	3.8	3.6	3.85	3.99
G_{13} (GPa)	4.23	4.98	4.97	4.43	4.72	4.93	4.83
G_{23} (GPa)	5.78	6.39	6.07	5.67	5.73	6.1	6.05
ν_{12}	0.357	0.27	0.319	0.229	0.288	0.271	0.264
ν_{13}	0.248	0.264	0.229	0.322	0.286	0.268	0.282
ν_{23}	0.229	0.235	0.211	0.291	0.256	0.238	0.255
ν_{21}	0.407	0.35	0.373	0.302	0.364	0.344	0.336
ν_{31}	0.378	0.449	0.402	0.521	0.492	0.486	0.471
ν_{32}	0.305	0.308	0.317	0.357	0.348	0.346	0.334

22.8.3. Implant Mechanics and Loading

A great variety of endosseous dental implants are nowadays present on the market. The most common implant shapes are cylindrical or conical, smoothed, or threaded. Examples of three different implant configurations are reported in Figure 22.14.

The material adopted for manufacturing dental implants is usually commercially pure titanium, thanks to its biocompatibility and the possibility of its complete integration with living bone during the healing phase. Experimental tests made on a classical implant demonstrate that, after a correct surgical procedure and favorable healing process, there is no evidence of lack of continuity between implant and bone (Bidez *et al.*, 1992a, b; Mericske *et al.*, 1992; Patterson *et al.*, 1995).

The mechanical properties of titanium consist on a Young's modulus of about 110,000 MPa and a Poisson's ratio of 0.3. As far as the implant configuration is concerned, different solutions can be suitable on the basis of the specific patient's problem. Single or multiple implant configurations can be adopted. For example, in case of complete edentulism, usually four or five implants can be inserted in mandible and connected with bars in order to adapt upper prosthesis. Such connecting bars have a complex geometry and are produced according to the specific patient configuration, and consequently they differ from case to case.

It is not easy to investigate how functional loads affect the bone in these different configurations. A various set of loading conditions can be considered. Loads can derive from functional or parafunctional activities, such as from masticatory and occlusal action or from bruxisme. The components of loads can be both horizontal and vertical. Vertical loads acting on teeth can also generate horizontal components on implants, as a consequence of inclined tooth surfaces. Different loading situations, with subsequent variation in bone stress distribution, originate by occlusion in

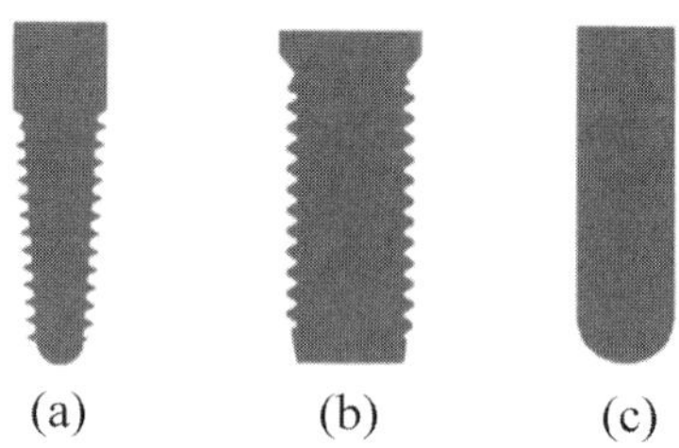

Figure 22.14. Examples of (a) a conical threaded implant, (b) a cylindrical threaded implant, (c) a cylindrical smoothed implant.

case of prosthesis with an opposing natural tooth, conventional complete denture, or tooth-supported fixed prosthesis. Moreover, implants can be perfectly osseointegrated or partially detached from peri-implant bone. Stress distribution on bone in these cases changes greatly. Some information can be given by reporting a few notes on numerical simulation of implant–bone interaction phenomena.

22.8.4. Numerical Formulation of Implant–Tissue Interaction Phenomena

Computer simulation is one of the most useful means used to investigate different configurations of the implant–bone interaction process. In fact, even if experimental analysis could give appropriate results, they are too expensive and time consuming and it is practically impossible to perform a wide range of tests on so many different configurations (Benzing *et al.*, 1995; Branemark *et al*, 1995; Chao *et al.*, 1995; Hart *et al.*, 1992; Hutton *et al.*, 1995; Kohn, 1992; Lewis, 1994; Liu *et al.*, 1995; Natali *et al.*, 1995, 1997, 1998; Natali and Donà, 1999; Natali, 1999; Wittkampf and Starmans, 1995).

Experimental results must be taken into account to have a comparison with the results obtained by numerical simulation, in order to have a reliability evaluation.

Different numerical models can be generated, both two and three dimensional. The first step to be performed in order to create an appropriate numerical model is geometry reconstruction. This process starts with data acquisition of the anatomical site by tomography. Then images of each bone section must be converted in order to be used for solid models and subsequent generation of finite element or geometric element models. Finally, the fixture's geometry must be defined in detail and its appropriate position within the anatomical site. As far as mechanical properties are concerned, they have to be assigned to each part of the bone and to the implant itself. It is not easy to find out the correct properties, as previously mentioned, and average values reported in the tables are considered. To take into account a gradual variation from cortical to trabecular properties, it may be also useful to define a transition zone, assigning to it intermediate mechanical characteristics. Transition zones between implant and cortical or trabecular bone can be provided in order to consider a zone in a healing phase or an altered layer due to a surgical procedure or to an inflammatory process. It has been demonstrated that corticalized bone develops all around the implant, as a consequence of the healing process. Different numerical analyses can be performed by consider-

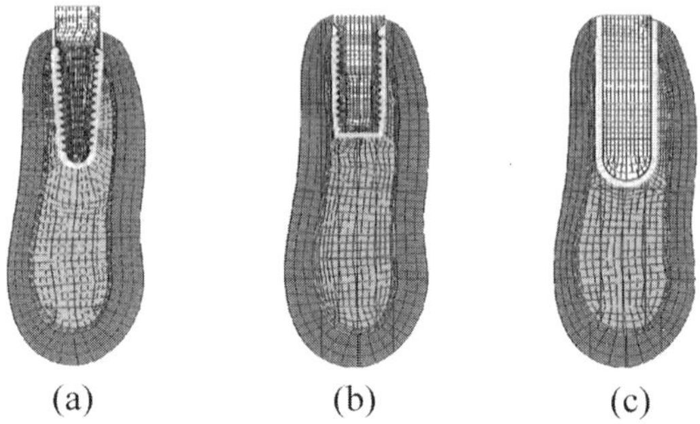

Figure 22.15. Transversal section of a mandible with (a) conical threaded implant, (b) cylindrical threaded implant, (c) cylindrical smoothed implant.

ing different mechanical properties of such transition zones, in order to simulate subsequent healing phases and to interpret the effects deriving from variations in properties.

Examples of models for the simulation of the interaction process between a single implant and bone are reported in Figure 22.15. Implant shapes are conical threaded, cylindrical threaded, and cylindrical smoothed. Both transition zones between implant and cortical and trabecular tissue are evident. Analyses have been performed to understand the effects of variations in the mechanical properties and also to evaluate bone behavior when the cortical layer changes its thickness.

A three-dimensional geometric model of a cylindrical smoothed implant is reported in Figure 22.16. It is possible to have a detailed view inside the anatomical region, in both longitudinal and transversal directions, leading to a clear definition of the response of the implant under vertical (200 N) and horizontal (20 N) loads.

A three-dimensional finite element model of a single implant is shown in Figure 22.17. The insight view clarifies the configuration of cortical and trabecular parts of the bone.

The displacement field in Figure 22.18 is the result of an analysis performed in osseointegrated conditions, under vertical and horizontal load. The fixture is supported by the surrounding bone, so that stress and strain are spread out in a uniform way.

Another situation pertains to the condition of unsuccessful integration in the cortical bone. Figure 22.19 shows displacement and pressure fields at the contact surface (the model's geometry is that reported in Figure 22.17).

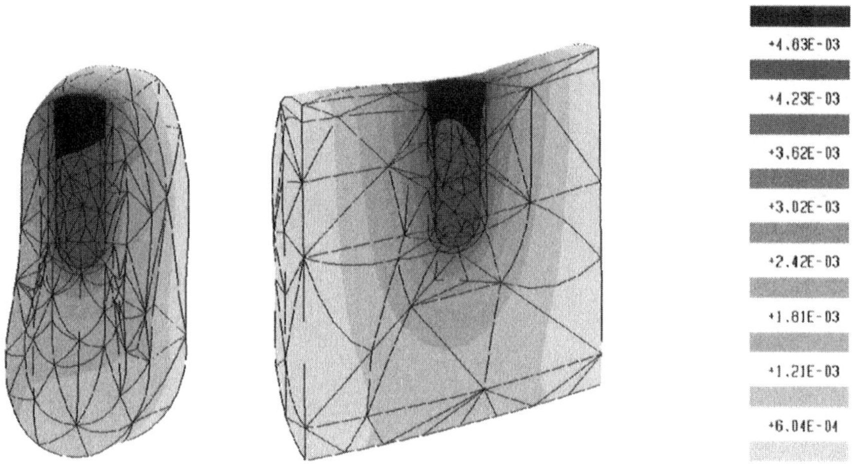

(a) (b)

Figure 22.16. Displacement magnitude fields by three-dimensional geometric element model: (a) transversal section, (b) longitudinal section.

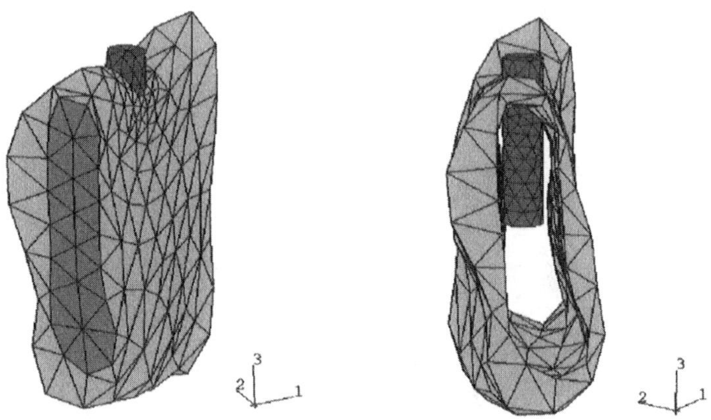

(a) (b)

Figure 22.17. Three-dimensional finite element model: (a) mandible with implant, (b) cortical bone portion and implant.

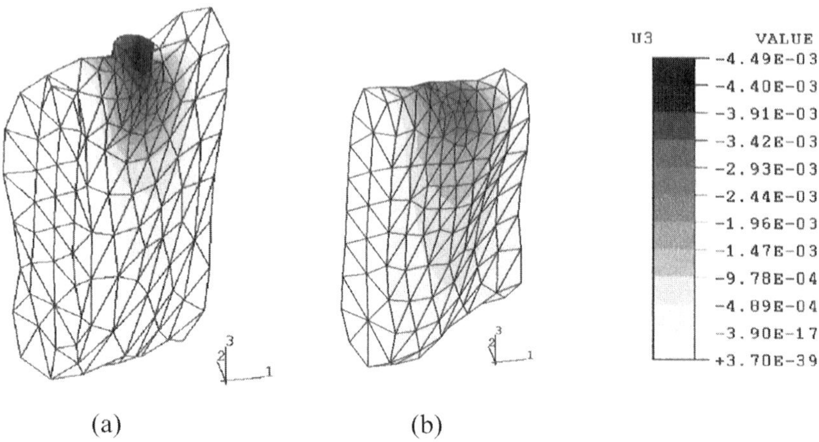

Figure 22.18. Displacement magnitude fields obtained by three-dimensional finite element model: (a) mandible with implant, (b) trabecular bone portion.

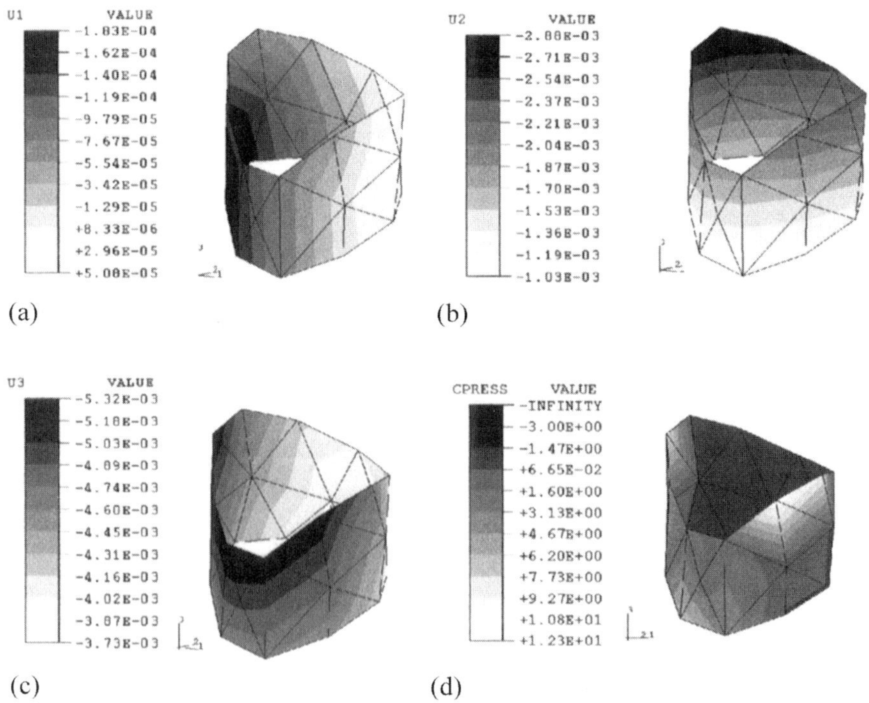

Figure 22.19. Three-dimensional analysis for a partially integrated implant. Magnitude fields at the contact surface between implant and bone: (a), (b), (c) displacement, (d) pressure.

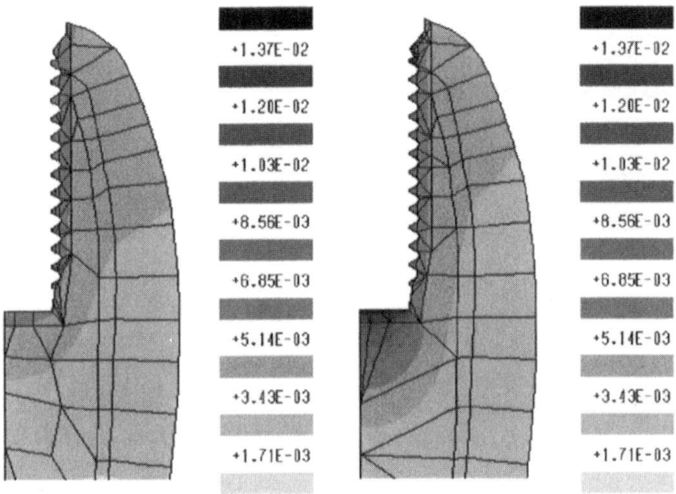

Figure 22.20. Cylindrical threaded implant: displacement magnitude field in (a) integrated condition, (b) detached condition.

A further example of detachment occurring between implant and surrounding cortical and trabecular tissue, because of inflammatory process or inappropriate surgical actions, is reported in Figures 22.20 by using geometric elements. Here, there is an axially symmetric model with a cylindrical threaded implant, assuming an average upper cortical thickness of 1.6 mm. The two images show in detail the considerable difference between an integrated and a detached condition.

In conclusion, the relevance of the numerical approach in investigating the biomechanics of dental implants by the possibility of a simulating various materials and the geometric configuration of parameters governing the problem is recalled. Particular competence is required owing to the necessity of having a deep knowledge of bone mechanics, geometrical survey, and numerical formulation of the problem.

References

Abate, P.F., Bertacchini, S.M., Polack, M.A., Macchi, R.L. 1997. Adhesion of compomer to dental structures, *Quintessence-Int.* **28**(8), 509–512.

Adachi, M., Mackert, J.R., Parry, E.E., Fairhurst, C.W. 1990. Oxide adherence and porcelain bonding to titanium and Ti-6Al-4V alloy, *J. Dent. Res.* **69**, 1230–1235.

Ahmad, L., Standard, J.G. 1990. Mercury release from amalgam: a study in vivo and in vitro, *Oper. Dent.* **15**, 207.

Altiere, E.T., Reeve, C.M., Sheridan, P.J. 1979. Lyophylised bone allografts in periodontal intraosseous defects, *J. Periodontol.* **50**(10), 510–519.

Angelini, E., Piccardo, P., Pinasco, M.R., Rosalbino, F. 1998. Relazioni tra microstruttura e resistenza alla corrosione e al tarnish di leghe auree utilizzate in odontoiatria protesica, *Metall. Ital.* **90**, 25–31.

Angelini, E., Cordano, E., Pinasco, M.R., Rosalbino, F. 2000. Reliability of Pd-based dental alloys regarding corrosion resistance and production processes, *J. Mater. Sci., Materials in Medicine* **11**, 1–9.

Asaoka, K. 1991. Transient and residual stress in porcelain-alloy strip for dental use as affected by tempering, *JSME Int. J. Ser. 1*, **34**, 156–162.

Ashman, A. 1990. Application of THR polymer in dentistry. *Compendium Continuing Educ. Dent.* **9** (suppl. 10), 330–336.

Ashman, A., Bruin, P. 1985. Prevention of alveolar bone loss post extraction with HTR grafting material, *Oral Surg., Oral Med. Oral Pathol.* **60**, 146–153.

Ashman, R.B., Cowin, S.C., Van Buskirk, W.C., Rice, J.C. 1984. A continuous wave technique for the measurement of the elastic properties of cortical bone, *J. Biomech.* **17**, 349–361.

Baldock, W.T., Hutchens, L.H., McFall, W.T., Simpson, D.M. 1985. An evaluation of tricalcium phosphate implants in human periodontal osseous defects in two patients, *J. Periodontol.* **56**, 1–7.

Becker, W., Becker, B.E. 1993. Clinical applications of guided tissue regeneration: surgical considerations, *Periodontol* **1**(2), 46–53.

Becker, W., Becker, B.E., Berg, L., Prichard, J., Caffesse, R., Rosenberg, E. 1988, New attachment after treatment with root isolation procedures: Report for treated class III and class II furcations and vertical osseous defects, *Int. J. Periodontol. Restor. Dent.*, **8**, 2–16.

Bell, R., Beirne, O. 1988. Effect of hydroxyapatite, tricalcium phosphate, and collagen on the healing of defects in the rat mandibule, *J. Oral. Maxillofac. Surg.* **46**, 589–594.

Benzing, U.R., Gall, H., Weber, H. 1995. Biomechanical aspects of two different implant-prosthetic concepts for edentulous maxillae, *Int. J. Oral Maxillofac. Implants* **10**, 188–198.

Berg, J.H. 1998. The continuum of restorative materials in pediatric dentistry—A review for the clinician, *Pediatr. Dent.* **20**(2), 93–100.

Bidez, M.W., Misch, C.E. 1992a. Force transfer in implant dentistry: basic concepts and principles, *J. Oral Implantol.* **18**, 264–274.

Bidez, M.W., Misch, C.E. 1992b. Issues in bone mechanics related to oral implants, *Implant-Dent.* **1** Winter, 289–294.

Blumenthal, N.M. 1993. A clinical comparison of collagen membranes with e-PTFE membranes in the treatment of human mandibular class II furcation defects, *J. Periodontol.* **64**, 925–933.

Bowers, G.-M., Granet, M., Steven, M., Emerson, J., Corio, R., Mellonig, J., Lewis, S.B., Pelzam, B., Romberg, E., Risom, L. 1985. Histologic evaluation of new attachment in humans. A preliminary report, *J. Periodontol.* **56**, 381–396.

Bowers, G.-M., Vargo, J.W., Lerg, B., Emerson, J.R., Bergquist, J.J. 1986. Histologic observations following the placement of tricalcium phosphate implants in human intrabony defects, *J. Periodontol.* **57**, 286–287.

Bowers, G.-M., Chadroff, B., Carnevale, R., Mellonig, J., Corio, R., Emerson, J., Stevens, M., Romberg, E. 1989a. Histologic evaluation of new human attachment apparatus in humans Part I, *J. Periodontol.* **60**, 664–674.

Bowers, G.-M., Chadroff, B., Carnevale, R., Mellonig, J., Corio, R., Emerson, J., Stevens, M., Romberg, E. 1989b. Histologic evaluation of new human attachment apparatus in humans Part II, *J. Periodontol.* **60**, 675–682.

Bowers, G.-M., Chadroff, B., Carnevale, R., Mellonig, J., Corio, R., Emerson, J., Stevens, M., Romberg, E. 1989c. Histologic evaluation of new human attachment apparatus in humans Part III, *J. Periodontol.* **60**, 683–693.

Bradley, R.M. *Basic Oral Phisiology*, Year Book Medical Publishers, Chicago, 1981.

Branemark, P.I., Svensson, B., Van Steenberghe, D. 1995. Ten-year survival rates of fixed prostheses on four or six implants ad modum Branemark in full edentulism, *Clin. Oral Implants Res.* **6**(4), 227–231.

Brannstrom, M. 1986. Hydrodynamic theory of detinal pain: sensation in preparation, caries, and the dentinal crack syndrome, *J. Endodon.* **12**, 453–457.

Brosh, T., Persovski, Z., Binderman, I. 1995. Mechanical properties of bone-implant interface: an in vitro comparison of the parameters at placement and at 3 months, *Int. J. Oral Maxillofac. Implants* **10**, 729–735.

Brown, D., 1988. Oral golds, *Gold Bull.* **21**, 24–28.

Carranza, F.A. Jr., Kenney, E.B., Lekovic, V., Talamante, E., Valencia, J., Dimitrijevic, B. 1987. Histologic study of healing of human periodontal defects after placement of porous hydroxylapatite implants, *J. Periodontol.* **58**, 682–688.

Carter, D.R., Spengler, D.M. 1978. Mechanical properties and composition of cortical bone, *Clin. Orthop.* **135**, 192.

Chao, Y.L., Meijer, H.J., Van Oort, R.P., Versteegh, P.A. 1995. The incomprehensible success of the implant stabilised overdenture in the edentulous mandible: a literature review on transfer of chewing forces to bone surrounding implants, *Eur. J. Prosthodont. Restor. Dent.* **3**(6), 255–261.

Chung, K.M., Salkin, L.M., Stein, M.D., Freedman, A.L. 1990. Clinical evaluation of a biodegradable collagen membrane in guided tissue regeneration, *J. Periodontol.* **61**, 732–736.

Corso, P.P., German, R.M., Simmons, H.D. 1985. Corrosion evaluation of gold-based dental alloys, *J. Dent. Res.* **64**, 854–859.

Cortellini, P., Clauser, C., Pini Prato, G. 1993. Histologic assessment of new attachment following the treatment of buccal recession by means of guided tissue regeneration procedure, *J. Periodontol.* **64**, 387–391.

Cortellini, P., Pini Prato, G., Tonetti, M. 1996a. Long term stability of clinical attachment following guided tissue regeneration and conventional therapy, *J. Clin. Periodontol.* **23**, 106–111.

Cortellini, P., Pini Prato, G., Tonetti, M. 1996b. Periodontal regeneration of human intrabony defects with bioresorbable membranes. A controlled clinical trial, *J. Periodontol.* **67**, 217–223.

Craig, R.G. 1993. *Restorative Dental Materials*, 9th edn., Mosby, St. Louis.

De Barra, E., Hill, R.G. 1998. Influence of alkali metal ions on the fracture properties of glass polyalchenoate (ionomer) cements, *Biomaterials* **19**, 495–502.

De Sanctis, M., Clauser, C., Zuchelli, G. 1996a. Bacterial colonization of resorbable barrier material and periodontal regeneration, *J. Periodontol.* **67**, 1193–1200.

De Sanctis, M., Zucchelli, G., Clauser, C. 1996b. Bacterial colonization and reorbable barrier material and periodontal regeneration, *J. Clin. Periodontol.* **23**, 1039–1046.

Dodes, J. 1988. Amalgam toxicity: a review of the literature, *Operat. Dent.* **13**, 32–40.

Donley, T.G., Gillette, W.B. 1991. Titanium endosseous implant–soft tissue interface: a literature review, *J. Periodontol.* **62**, 153–160.

Dragoo, M.R., Sullivan, H.C. 1973a. A clinical and histological evaluation of autogenous iliac bone grafts in humans. I. Wound healing 2 to 8 months, *J. Periodontol.* **44**, 599–613.

Dragoo, M.R., Sullivan, H.C. 1973b. A clinical and histological evaluation of autogenous iliac bone grafts in humans. II. External root resorption, *J. Periodontol.* **44**, 614–625.

Ekstrand, J., Bjorkman, L., Edlund, C., Sandborgh-Englund, G. 1998. Toxicological aspects on the release and systemic uptake of mercury from dental amalgam, *Eur. J. Oral. Sci.* **106**, 678–686.

Ellegaard, B., Karring, T., Davies, R., Loî, H. 1974. New attachment after treatment of intrabony defects in monkeys, *J. Periodontol.* **45**, 368–377.

Ellegaard, B., Karring, T., Listgarten, M., Loî, H. 1973. New attachment after treatment of interradicular lesions, *J. Periodontol.* **44**, 209–217.

Endo, K., Matsuda, K., Ohno, K. 1993. Corrosion of dental alloy in oral environment and its biological side effects, *Corros. Eng.* **42**, 913–925.

Fédération Dentaire Internationale. 1990. Technical Report No. 34, Alternative casting alloys for fixed prosthodontics, *Int. Dent. J.* **40**, 54–55.

Forsten, L. 1998. Fluoride release and uptake by glass-ionomers and related materials and its clinical effect, *Biomaterials* **19**, 503–508.

Frank, A. 1970. The endodontic endosseous implant, in: *Oral Implantology*. Charles C. Thomas Springfield.

Friberg, B., Sennerby, L., Roos, J., Lekholm, U. 1995. Identification of bone quality in conjunction with insertion of titanium implants. A pilot study in jaw autopsy specimens, *Clin. Oral Implants Res.* **6**(4), 213–219.

Garrett, S., Loos, B., Chamberlain, D., Egelberg, J. 1988. Treatment of intraosseous periodontal defects with a combined therapy of citric acid conditioning, bone grafting and placement of collagenous membranes, *J. Clin. Periodontol.* **15**, 383–389.

Gettleman, L. 1991. Noble alloys in dentistry, *Curr. Opinion Dent.* **2**, 218–221.

Glantz, P.O. 1998. Biomaterial considerations for the optimized therapy for the edentulous predicament, *J. Prosthet. Dent.* **79**(1), 90–92.

Gottlow, J., Nyman, S., Karring, T., Lindhe, J. 1984. New attachment formation of the result of controlled tissue regeneration, *J. Clin. Periodontol.* **11**, 494–503.

Graber, G. 1986. *Partielle Prothetik*, G.T. Verlag, Stuttgart.

Guggenberger, R., May, R., Stefan, K.P. 1998. New trends in glass ionomer chemistry, *Biomaterials* **19**, 479–483.

Hart, R.T., Hennebel, V.V., Thongprea, N., Van Buskirk, W.C, Anderson, R.C. 1992. Modelling the biomechanics of the mandible: a three-dimensional finite element study, *J. Biomech.* **25**, 261–286.

Hench, L. 1986. Ceramic implants for humans, *Adv. Ceramic Mater.* **1**, 306–324.

Hero, H., Hokabe, T., 1994. Gallium alloys as dental restorative materials: a research review, *Cells Mater.* **4**, 409–418.

Hero, H., Simensen, J.C., Jorgensen, R.B. 1996. Structure of dental gallium alloys, *Biomaterials* **17**, 1321–1326.

Hero, H., Hokabe, T., Wie, H. 1997. Corrosion of gallium alloy in vivo, *J. Mater. Sci., Materials in Medicine* **8**, 357–360.

Hiatt, W.H., Schallhorn, R.G., Aoronian, A.J. 1978. The induction of new bone and cementum formation. IV. Microscopic examination of the periodontium following human bone and narrow allograft, autograft and non-graft periodontal regenerative procedures, *J. Periodontol.* **49**, 495–512.

Hoexter, D.L. 1983. The use of tricalcium phosphate (synthograft). Part I: its use in extensive periodontal defects, *J. Oral Implantol.* **10**, 599–610.

Holland, R.I. 1992. Corrosion testing by potentiodynamic polarization in various electrolytes, *Dent. Mater.* **8**, 241–245.

Horibe, T., Fukuoka, J. 1986. Gallium alloys for dental resorations, *Dent. Coll.* **12**, 198.

Hugoson, A., Ravald, N., Fornell, J., Johard, G., Teiwik, A., Gottlow, J. 1995. Treatment of class II furcation involvements in human with bioresorbable and non-resorbable guided tissue regeneration barriers. A randomized multicenter study, *J. Periodontol.* **66**, 624–634.

Hutton, J.E., Heath, M.R., Chai, J.Y., Harnett, J., Jemt, T., Johns, R.B., McKenna, S., McNamara, D.C., Van Steenberghe, D., Taylor, R. *et al.* 1995. Factors related to success and failure rates at 3-year follow-up in a multicenter study of overdentures supported by Branemark implants, *Int. J. Oral Maxillofac. Implants* **10**, 33–42.

Jones, D.W. 1992. Materials for fixed and removable prosthodontic, in: *Medical and Dental Materials*, Vol. 14 (D.F. Williams, ed.), pp. 430–454, VCH, Cambridge.

Jumlongras, D., White, G.E. 1997. Bond strengths of composite resin and compomers in primary and permanent teeth, *J. Pediatr. Dent.* Spring **21**(3), 223–229.

Kan, K.C., Messer, L.B., Messer, H.H. 1997. Variability in cytotoxicity and fluoride release of resin modified glass-ionomer cements, *J. Dent. Res.* **76**, 1502–1507.

Keller, J.C. 1998. Tissue compatibility to different surfaces of dental implants: in vitro studies, *Implant Dent.* **7**, 331–337.

Kenney, E.B., Lekovic, V., Sa Ferreira, J.C., Han, T., Dimitijevic, B., Corranza, F.A. Jr. 1986. Bone formation within porous HA implants in human periodontal defects, *J. Periodontol.* **57**, 71–83.

Kenney, E.B., Lekovic, V., Han, T., Carranza, F.A. Jr., Dimitrijevic, B., Takei, H. 1987. Interpore 200 implants in interproximal periodontal defects—12 month results, *J. Dent. Res.* **66** (Spec. Issue), 196 (Abstr. 717).

Kenney, E.B., Lekovic, V., Carranza, F.A. Jr., Dimitrijevic, B., Han, T., Takei, H. 1988a. A comparative clinical study of solid and granular porous hydroxylapatite implants in human periodontal, *J. Biomed. Mater. Res.* **22**, 1233–1243.

Kenney, E.B., Lekovic, V., Elbaz, J.J., Kovacvic, K., Carranza, F.A. Jr., Takei, H. 1988b. The use of porous hydroxylapatite implants in periodontal defects. II. Treatment of class II furcation lesions in lower molars, *J. Periodontol.* **59**, 67–72.

Klinge, B. 1991. Implant in relation to natural teeth, *J. Clin. Periodontol.* **18** 482–487.

Kohn, D.H. 1992. Overview of factors important in implant design, *J. Oral Implantol.* **18**, 204–219.

Kvam, K., Derand, T., Austrheim, E.K. 1995. Fracture toughness and flexural strength of dental ceramics for titanium, *Biomaterials* **16**, 73–76.

Leach, 1980. *Dental Plaque and Surface Interactions in the Oral Cavity*, Information Retrieval Inc., S. A. ed., London.

Leake, D. 1988. HTR Polymer: Present and future applications, *Compendium Continuing Educ. Dent.* **9** (suppl. 10): S 328–S 329.

Lewis, G. 1994. A parametric finite element analysis study of the stresses in an endosseous implant, *Biomed. Mater. Eng.* **4**, 495–502.

Leyhausen, G., Abtahi, M., Karbakhsch, M., Sapotnick, A., Geutsen, W. 1998. Biocompatibility of various light-curing and one conventional glass-ionomer cement, *Biomaterials* **19**, 559–564.

Liu, H., Klein, C.P., Van Rossen, I.P., De Groot, K. 1995. A model for the evaluation of mandibular bone response to implant materials, *J. Oral Rehabil.* **22**, 283–287.

McCabe, J.F. 1998. Resin modified glass ionomers, *Biomaterials* **19**, 521–527.

Machtei, E.E., Grossi, S-G., Demford, R., Zambou, J.J., Genco, R.J. 1996. Long-term stability of class II furcation defects treated with barrier membranes, *J. Periodontol.* **67**(5), 523–527.

Machti, E., Cho, M., Dunford, R., Norderyd, J., Zambon, J., Genco, R. 1994. Clinical, microbiological, and histological factors which influence the success of regenerative periodontal therapy, *J. Periodontol.* **65**, 154–161.

McDavid, P.T., Bone, M.E., Kafrawy, A.H., Mitchell, D.F. 1979. Effect of autogenous marrow in the treatment of human periodontal osseous defects, *J. Periodontol.* **56**, 63–73.

McGhee, J.R., Micalek, S.M., Cassel, G.H. 1982. *Dental Microbiology*, Harper and Row, Philadelphia.

Mellonnig, J., Bowers, G., Bully, R. 1981. Comparison of bone graft materials. I. New bone formation with autografts and allografts determined by strontium-85, *J. Periodontol.* **52**, 291–296.

Mericske Stern, R., Geering, A.H., Burgin, W.B., Graf, H. 1992. Three-dimensional force measurements on mandibular implants supporting overdentures, *Int. J. Oral Maxillofac. Implants* **7**, 185–194.

Meyer, J. M., Reclaru, L. 1995. Electrochemical determination of the corrosion resistance of noble dental casting alloys, *J. Mater. Sci., Materials in Medicine* **6**, 534–540.

Meyer, J.M., Cattani-Lorente, M.A., Dupuis, V. 1998. Compomers: between glass-ionomer cements and composites, *Biomaterials* **19**, 529–539.

Mezger, P.R. 1989. *Corrosion Behaviour of Dental Casting Alloys*, ISBN 90-9002669-X, Drukkerij Benda BV, Nijmegen.

Mezger, P.R., Vrijhoef, M.M.A., Greener, E.H. 1989. The corrosion behaviour of high-palladium porcelain-bonding alloys, *J. Dent.* **17**, 33–37.

Minegishi, D., Lin, C., Noguchi, T., Ishikawa, I. 1988. Porous hydroxyapatite granule implants in periodontal osseous defects in monkeys, *Int. J. Periodon. Restor. Dent.* **8**(4), 50–63.

Mount, G.J. 1998. Clinical performance of glass ionomers, *Biomaterials* **19**, 573–579.

Murphy, W.M. 1995. Clinical and experimental bone changes after intraosseous implantation, *J. Prosthet. Dent.* **73**, 31–35.

Natali, A.N. 1999. The simulation of load bearing capacity of dental implants, in: *Computer Technology in Biomaterials Science and Engineering*, pp. 132–148, John Wiley & Sons, New York.

Natali, A.N., Donà S.A. 1999. Considerations on reliability of numerical models for bio-mechanical analysis of tissue-implant interaction, *Ceramics, Cells and Tissues*, pp. 81–89, IRTEC-CNR, Faenza.

Natali, A., Meroi, E. 1989. A review of the biomechanical properties of bone as a material, *J. Biomed. Eng.* **11**, 266–276.

Natali, A.N., Trebacz, A.J. 1996. Analysis of cancellous bone properties by using ultrasonic technique, *Ceramics, Cells and Tissues*, pp. 241–248, IRTEC-CNR, Faenza.

Natali, A.N., Trebacz, H.J. 1999. The ultrasound velocity and attenuation in cancellous bone samples from lumbar vertebra and calcaneus, *Osteoporosis Int.* **9**, 99–105.

Natali, A.N., Meroi, E., Hubsch, P., Middleton, J. 1995. An adaptive finite element approach for the analysis of bone prosthesis interaction, *J. Med. Biol. Eng. Comput.* **33**, 33–37.

Natali, A.N., Meroi, E.A., Williams, K.R., Calabrese, L.A. 1997. Investigation of integration proçess of dental implants by means of a numerical analysis of dynamic response, *Den. Mater.* **13**(5), 325–337.

Natali, A.N., Meroi, E.A., Donà, S.A. 1998. Tissue-implant interaction process of dental implant: a numerical approach, *Ceramics, Cells and Tissues*, pp. 93–100, IRTEC-CNR, Faenza.

Nery, E.B., Legeros, R.Z, Lynch, K.L. 1992. Tissue responses to biphasic calcium phosphate ceramic with different ratios of HA/BTCP in periodontal osseous defects, *J. Periodontol.* **63**, 729–735.

Nicholson, J.W. 1998. Chemistry of glass ionomer cements: a review, *Biomaterials* **19**, 485–494.

Nicholson, J.W., Brook, I.M., Hatton, P.V. 1998. Glass-ionomers: bioactive implant materials, *Biomaterials* **19**, 565–571.

Nielsen, I.M., Ellegaard, B., Karring, T. 1980. Kiel-bone® in healing interradicular lesions in monkeys, *J. Periodontol. Res.* **15**, 328–337.

Nielsen, I.M., Ellegaard, B., Karring, T. 1981. Kiel-bone® in new attachment attempts in humans, *J. Periodontol.* **52**, 723–728.

Newbrun, E. 1990. *Cariology*, Williams & Wilkins, Baltimore.

Nikiforuk, G. 1985. *Understanding Dental Caries: Etiology and Mechanism*, Karger, Basel.

Nowzari, H., Slots, J. 1994. Microorganisms in polytetrafluoroethylene barrier membranes for guided tissue regeneration. *J. Clin. Periodontol.* **21**(3), 303–310.

Oshida, Y., Moore, B.K. 1993. Anodic polarization behaviour and microstructure of a gallium based alloy, *Dent. Mater.* **9**, 234–241.

Patterson, E.A., Burguete, R.L., Thoi, M.H., Johns, R.B. 1995. Distribution of load in an oral prosthesis system: an in vitro study, *Int. J. Oral Maxillofac. Implants* **10**, 552–560.

Patur, B. 1974. Osseous defects. Evaluation, diagnostic and treatment methods, *J. Periodontol.* **45**, 523–541.

Patur, B., Glickman, I. 1962. Clinical and roentgenographics evaluation of the post-treatment healing of infrabony pockets, *J. Periodontol.* **33**, 164–171.

Paul, B.F., Mellonig, J.T., Towle, H.J., Gray, J.L. 1992. The use of collagen barrier to enhance healing in human periodontal furcation defects, *Int. J. Periodont. Rest. Dent.* **12**, 123–131.

Pilliar, R.M. 1998. Overview of surface variability of metallic endosseous dental implants: textured and porous surface-structured designs, *Implant Dent.* **7**, 305–314.

Pinasco, M.R., Cordano, E., Giovannini, M. 1999. X-ray diffraction and microstructural study of PMF precious metal alloys under different conditions, *J. Alloys Compd.* **289**, 289–298.

Rapson, W.S. 1978. *Gold Usage*, Academic Press Inc., New York.

Rivault, A.F., Toto, P.D., Levy, S., Gargiulo, A.W. 1971. Autogenous bone grafts: osseous coagulum and osseous retrograde procedures in primates, *J. Periodontol.* **42**, 787–788.

Rohrer, M.D., Bulard, R.A., Patterson, M.K. Jr. 1995. Maxillary and mandibular titanium implants 1 year after surgery: histologic examination in a cadaver, *Int. J. Oral Maxillofac. Implants* **10**, 466–473.

Rosenstiel, S.F., Land, M.F. 1988. *Contemporary Fixed Prosthodontics*, C.V. Mosby, St. Louis.

Rouviere, H. 1978. *Anatomie umane*, tome I, Masson, Paris.

Rummelhart, J.M., Mellonig, J.T., Gray, J.L., Towle, H.J. 1989. A comparison of freeze-dried bone allograft and demineralized freeze-dried bone allograft in human periodontal osseous defects, *J. Periodontol.* **60**, 655–663.

Schallhorn, R.G. 1967. Eradication of bifurcation defects utilizing frozen autogenous hip marrow implants, *Periodont. Abstr.* **15**, 101–105.

Schallhorn, R.G. 1968. The use of autogenous hip marrow biopsy implants for bony crater defects, *J. Periodontol.* **39**, 145–147.

Selvig, K.A., Nilvens, R.E., Fitzmorris, L. 1990. Scanning electron microscopy observations of cell populations and bacterial contamination of membranes used for guided periodontal tissue regeneration in humans, *J. Periodontol.* **61**(3), 303–310.

Shaffer, C.D., App, G.R. 1971. The use of plaster of Paris in treating infrabony periodontal defects on humans, *J. Periodontol.* **42**, 686–690.

Shapoff, C.A., Alexander, D.C., Clark, A.E. 1997. Clinical use of a bioactive glass particulate in the treatment of human osseous defects, *Compendium* **18**, 352–363.

Shavel H.M. 1980. The amalgam pin technique for complex amalgam restoration, *J. Calif. Dent. Assoc.* **8**, 48.

Sicher, H., Du Brul, E.L. 1970. *Oral Anatomy* C.V. Mosby, Saint Louis.

Sluger, S., Yuodelis, R.A., Page, R.C. 1977. *Periodontal Disease*, Lea and Febiger, Philadelphia.

Smith, D.C. 1985. Posterior composite resin, in: *Dental Restorative Materials* (G. Vanherle, D.C. Smith, eds.), pp. 47–60, Peter Szule, Amsterdam.

Smith, D.C. 1998. Development of glass ionomer cement systems, *Biomaterials* **19**, 467–478.

Stahl, S., Froum, S. 1987. Histologic and clinical responses to porous hydroxylapatite implants in human periodontal defects. Three to twelve months post implantation, *J. Periodontol.* **58**, 689–695.

Taylor, T.D. 1998. Prosthodontic problems and limitations associated with osseointegration, *J. Prosthet. Dent.* **79**(1), 74–78.

Ten Cate, A.R. 1989. *Dental Histology: Development, Structure and Function*, Mosby, St. Louis.

Terrier, R.L., Rakotomanana, R.N., Ramaniraka, T., Lyvraz, P.F. 1997. Adaption models of anisotropic bone, *Comput. Methods Biomech. Biomed. Eng.* **1**, 47–60.

Throckmorton, G.S., Dechow, P.C. 1994. In vitro strain measurements in the condylar process of the human mandible, *Arch. Oral. Biol.* **39**, 853–867.

Thylstrup, A., Fejerskov, O. 1986. *Texbook of Cariology*, Munksgaard, Copenhagen.

Tonetti, M., Pini Prato, G., Cortellini, P. 1993. Periodontal regeneration of human infrabony defects. IV. Determinants of the healing response, *J. Periodontol.* **64**, 934–940.

Tonetti, M., Pini Prato, G., Cortellini, P. 1996. Factors affecting the healing response of intrabony defects following guided tissue regeneration and access flap surgery, *J. Clin. Periodontol.* **23**, 548–556.

Tuccillo, J.J. 1977. Composition and functional characteristics of precious metal alloys for dental restorations, in: *Alternatives to Gold Alloys in Dentistry* (T.M. Valega, ed.), pp. 40–67, Dept. Health and Education and Welfare (NIH), Washington.

Tuccillo, J.J., Cascone, P.J. 1983. The evolution of porcelain to metal (PMF) alloy systems, in: *Dental Ceramics: Proceedings of the First International Symposium on Ceramics* (J.W. McLean, ed.), pp. 347–370, Quintesscence Publ. Co., Chicago.

Venugopalan, R., Broome, J.C., Lucas, L.C. 1998. The effect of water contamination on dimensional change and corrosion properties of a gallium alloy, *Dent. Mater.* **14**, 173–178.

Vitins, V., Laitzans, J., Knets, I., Natali, A.N. 1995. Analysis of mechanical response of healing bone tissue exposed to electromagnetic fields, in: *Bone Structure and Remodelling*, pp. 91–104, World Scientific, Singapore.

Von Fraunhofer, J.A., Estrange, P.R. 1971. Materials science in dental implantation and a promising new material: vitreous carbon, *Biomed. Eng.* **6**, 114.

Walls, A.W.G. 1986. *J. Dent. Res.* **14**, 231–246.

Wang, H., O'Neal, R., Thomas, C., Shyr, Y., MacNeil, R. 1994. Evaluation of an absorbable collagen membrane in treating class II furcation defects, *J. Periodontol.* **65**, 1029–1036.

Wataha, J.C., Malcom, C.T. 1996. Effect of alloy surface composition on release of elements from dental casting alloys, *J. Oral Rehabil.* **23**, 583–589.

Waterstrat, R.M., Okabe, T. 1994. Dental amalgam, in: *Intermetallics Compounds*, Vol. 2, *Practice* (J.H. Westbrook, R.L. Fleischer, eds.), pp. 575–590, John Wiley & Sons Ltd.

Watts, D.C. 1992. Dental restorative materials, in: *Medical and Dental Materials*, Vol. 14 (D.F. Williams, ed.), pp. 211–257, VCH, Cambridge.

White, E.W., Shors, E.C. 1986. Biomaterial aspects of interpore-200 porous hydroxyapatite, *Dent. Clin. North Am.* **30**, 49–65.

White, E.W., Weber, J.W., Roy, D.M., Owen, E.L., Chiraff, R.T., White, R.A. 1975. Replamineform porous biomaterials for hard tissue implant applications, *J. Biomed. Mater. Res. Symp.* **6**, 23–28.

Wilson, A.D., McLean, J.W. 1988. *Glass-Ionomer Cement*, Quintessence Publishing Co. Inc., Chicago.

Wittkampf, A.R., Starmans, F.J. 1995. Prevention of mandibular fractures by using constructional design principles. I. Computer simulation of human mandibular strength after segmental resections, *Int. J. Oral Maxillofac. Surg.* **24**, 306–310.

Yukna, R.A. 1990. HTR polymer grafts in human periodontal osseous defects. I. 6 month clinical results, *J. Periodontol.* **61**, 633–642.

Yukna, R.A., Bowers, G.M., Lawrence, J.J., Fedi, P.F. 1976. A clinical study of healing in humans following the excisional new attachment procedure, *J. Periodontol.* **47**, 696–700.

Zameth, J.S., *et al.* 1997. Particulate bioglass as a grafting material in the treatment of periodontal intrabony defects, *J. Clin. Periodontol.* **24**(6), 410–418.

23

Materials/Biological Environment Interactions

Orsolina Petillo, Alfonso Barbarisi, Sabrina Margarucci, Alfredo De Rosa, and Gianfranco Peluso

23.1. Introduction

The extracellular matrix (ECM), as a substrate capable of providing a stable structure for cell growth, is a fundamental precondition for the existence of multicellular organisms. In eukaryotes, all the central systems, such as neural or circulatory systems, evolved within and along with the ECM. In order to serve as a suitable scaffold for functional cellular elements, a huge set of ECM molecules (mainly proteins, proteoglycans, and glycosoaminoglycans) of unusual size and shape has evolved, and furnishes the tissue with its distinct features and anchors the cell in its surroundings. ECM components vary considerably in different tissues and this wide spectrum of expression provides a source of great diversity for cell matrix interaction. Again, the spatial relationships between cells and ECM differ between tissues. Cells can be completely surrounded by ECM, as in the case of chondrocytes, or can contact the ECM only at one surface, as exemplified by epithelial cells. In stratified epithelia, only a proportion of the cells is exposed to ECM. In all these cases, the ECM offers structural support for cells, and acts also as a physical barrier or selective filter to soluble factors. In addition to the above functions, the ECM plays a role in regulating the growth or the differentiated phenotype of cells. There are, at least, two main ways by which the ECM can affect cell behavior. One of these is the cell–ECM interaction which may directly regulate cell functions through

---

Orsolina Petillo, Alfonso Barbarisi, Sabrina Margarucci, Alfredo De Rosa, and Gianfranco Peluso • Istituto di Biochimica delle Proteine ed Enzimologia, Consiglio Nazionale delle Ricerche, Via Toiano 6, 0072 Arco Felice, Napoli, Italy.

Integrated Biomaterials Science, edited by R. Barbucci. Kluwer Academic/Plenum Publishers, New York, 2002.

receptor-mediated signaling. The other is that ECM can control the mobilization of growth or differentiation factors, thus modulating cell proliferation and controlling cell phenotype.

23.2. Cell–Extracellular Matrix Interactions

ECM glycoproteins influence intracellular events via their cell receptors, and thereby cell differentiation, migration, polarization, or growth. All the cell adhesion molecules (CAM) are protein receptors present on the external surface of cell membranes, but also extend across the membrane to the interior of the cell. The main groups of adhesion molecules are the integrins, the selectins, and the immunoglobulin superfamily. The cadherins, another CAM group, are receiving increased interest. Each group contains a number of individual subgroups, many of which have different functions and tissue specificity. Several studies have shown that the CAM-induced adhesive interactions mediate communication pathways that are critical for normal cell and organ function (Felsenfeld *et al.*, 1996).

In addition to generating their own signals, it is well known that molecules able to regulate cell adhesion to ECM can modulate the cellular response to other extracellular stimuli, such as soluble growth factors and differentiation-inducing agents (Schwartz and Baron, 1999). This means both that different ECM macromolecules may selectively stimulate specific types of signal transduction pathways, and that, for an efficient response to growth or differentiation factors, the cells need to interact with a matrix component in order that appropriate intracellular signal transduction cascades are triggered.

The ability to influence the downstream signaling of receptors that are activated by soluble growth and differentiation factors may be one of the most vital biological functions of ECM molecules and their cognate ligands.

Perhaps the clearest incarnation of this is anchorage-dependent growth, a phenomenon which has been studied for several years (Stoker *et al.*, 1968). By these studies it has been shown that the regulation of cellular events is through the coordinated effects of positive and negative signals, including those from soluble factors as well as those from the ECM and from adjacent cells (Schwartz and Lechene, 1992). It is this summation of signals conveying both biochemical and positional information which tells a cell when the time and place is right to conduct a particular activity. For example, there is compelling evidence that ECM and soluble factors can synergize to regulate the intracellular ionic environment. While both basic fibroblast growth factors (bFGF) and adhesion to fibronectin can independently activate the Na^+/H^+ antiporter and raise intracellular pH (pH_i) in endothelial cells, growth factor stimulation of adherent cells is more efficient in the process (Ingber *et al.*, 1990).

Similarly, in fibroblasts, Protein Kinase C (PKC)-dependent activation of the antiporter (and elevation of pH_i) by Platelet Derived Growth Factor (PDGF) requires cell adhesion to ECM. PDGF-stimulated Ca^{2+} mobilization, another ion transient required for cell cycle progression in murine fibroblasts, does not occur in cells in suspension but readily occurs in cells adherent to fibronectin (Turker *et al.*, 1990). The mechanism underlying this regulation is now well known. In adherent cells, PDGF stimulates tyrosine phosphorylation and activation of phospholipase C (PLCγ), which hydrolyzes phosphatidylinositol 4,5-bisphosphate [PI(4,5)P_2] into DAG and inositol triphosphate (IP_3), which in turn activate PKC and increase Ca_i^{2+}. In nonadherent cells, the activation of PLCγ by PDGF still occurs, but there is a dramatic decrease in the level of its substrate, PI(4,5)P_2, and therefore no appreciable generation of diacylglycerol (DAG) and IP_3 can occur (McNamee *et al.*, 1993). Presumably, the adhesion-dependent synthesis of PI(4,5)P_2 is largely caused by the activation of phosphatidylinositol-4-5-kinase (PI4-5K) activity by Rac and Rho, two plasma membrane molecules regulating cell–ECM interaction.

In addition to the examples discussed in detail above, several alternative models for cooperation between ECM receptors and other receptors have emerged. Another clear situation whereby ECM can collaborate with soluble factors is where interaction of an ECM molecule with an adhesion receptor directly activates a growth factor receptor without the need for that receptor's soluble ligand. This seems to be true when $\beta1$ integrins directly activate a PDGFβ receptor (Howe *et al.*, 1998). A second model entails the ligand-mediated activation of growth factor receptors that have been recruited to ECM-dependent adhesion sites. The increased concentration of receptor tyrosine kinases increases the efficiency of receptor activation, as reported in case of the Epithelial Growth Factor receptor, PDGF receptor, and insulin receptor (Vuori and Ruoslahti, 1994). A third model suggests that the adhesion stuctures act as a molecular "scaffold" for the downstream component of signaling cascades, thus allowing more efficient propagation of the signal. For example, within focal adhesions, integrins physically bridge the ECM to the network of cytoplasmic actin microfilaments, a situation that seems particularly well suited for providing an appropriate molecular scaffold for signaling components. This type of event has been reported in fibroblasts for activation of the MAPK cascade.

Another highly controversial question about ECM–cell interactions is that the extracellular matrix molecule composition is heterogeneous in different tissues and, in the same tissue, at different stages of development. The functional significance of this apparent redundancy of ECM component variation is that, at a given time and place, the ECM has the potential to provide specific environmental information to cells. For example, in case of mammary epithelial cells, for a correct signaling induced by prolactin and insulin, the adhesion of cells to the basement membrane components is necessary, while their interaction with ECM proteins, such as collagen I, inhibits the intracellular signal cascades induced by these hormones (Edwards *et al.*, 1998; Lee and Streuli, 1999).

Post-translational modifications also affect the ways in which ECM components interact with each other and with cells. The degree of glycosylation of fibronectin (Jones *et al.*, 1986) and laminin (Dean *et al.*, 1990) and the amount of calcium bound by thrombospondin (Lawler *et al.*, 1988) have all been shown to modulate cell adhesion. Self-aggregation of laminin–nidogen complexes is dependent on calcium ions (Paulsson *et al.*, 1988) while fibronectin becomes incorporated into ECM through transglutaminase-catalyzed cross-linking (Barry and Mosher, 1988). Self-assembly or cross-linking to other matrix components might affect cell adhesive activity by increasing the local concentration of cell-binding sites or, conversely, obscuring the sites. Noncovalent interactions between matrix molecules can affect the activity of adhesive glycoproteins such as fibronectin: such observations have led to the categorization of thrombospondin, tenascin, osteonectin, and, in some circumstances, laminin, as "anti-adhesive" matrix glycoproteins (Sage and Bornstein, 1991; Calof and Lander, 1991). In addition, soluble proteoglycans can inhibit cell adhesion to collagen and fibronectin (Ruoslahti, 1989).

23.3. Growth Factors — Extracellular Matrix Interactions

The second way by which the ECM may affect cell function is through harboring growth factors or growth factor-binding protein (Zhu *et al.*, 1999).

In this case ECM plays an active role in the mobilization of growth molecules rather than passively sequestering such factors. The interactions between growth factors and extracellular matrix regulate cell behavior in many ways. For instance, the direct binding of growth factors to the ECM can affect the local concentrations as well as the biological activity of the growth factors. On the other hand, the transcription, translation, and postranslational modification of ECM macromolecules have been shown to be regulated by various growth factors.

The binding of growth factors to the ECM is regulated by the glycosaminoglycan side chains. The presence of basic aminoacid clusters within regions of α-helical structure of growth factors seems to mediate the binding to the negatively charged heparin sulfate side chains of proteoglycans.

The biological consequences of the matrix-bound growth factors are related to their controlled release. The extracellular matrix is able to limit the diffusion of soluble factors, and thus provides a local store of biologically active molecules that persists after growth factor production has ceased. In case of Fibroblast Growth Factor (FGF), its binding to ECM induces a decrease in its degradation compared to free FGF. On the contrary, TGF-β and PDGF bound to ECM are inactive and can be released by the proteolysis of the matrix (Dallas *et al.*, 1995).

The regulation of specific gene expression is again regulated by growth factor–ECM interaction, as in case of tumor necrosis factor (TNF) production that is increased by neutrophil adhesion to fibronectin.

Several ECM molecules display intrinsic growth factor activity. Some ECM proteins contain repeated epidermal growth factor (EGF)-like sequences and, of these, laminin, tenascin, and thrombospondin-I have been reported to possess mitogenic activity.

All of these observations support the idea that growth factors and ECM proteins collaborate in creating distinct cellular environments or "niches" that regulate proliferation and differentiation, a concept originally formulated for stem cells in self-renewing tissues (Schofield, 1978). Further evidence has come from a number of experimental models of differentiation. In bone marrow, differentiation of progenitor stem cells along separate lineages is directed by growth factors, several of which are presented in a functionally active form by matrix components secreted by fibroblasts of the bone marrow stroma (Gordon, 1988).

23.4. Extracellular Matrix/Biomaterial Interaction

On the basis of the depicted network between cells and extracellular matrix, it appears that the implantation of an artificial prosthesis in the body can interfere with the normal function of the tissue site of implantation just inducing remodeling of the ECM. This remodeling may be caused: (1) by the inflammatory and fibrotic response determined by the tissue injury due to the surgical implantation and/or to the poor biocompatibility of the biomaterial, and (2) by the stresses (or mechanical forces) applied to the tissue by an implant with different viscoelastic properties in comparison with the surrounding biological environment.

23.4.1. Regulation of Tissue Fibrosis, as an Integrated Cellular Response to Biomaterial

Encapsulation of an implanted biomaterial with fibrosis is a highly evolved response of the majority of animal tissue. In humans, the components of the process have been greatly clarified, leading to a coherent view of how wound healing occurs in response to a device implantation. Typically, the biomaterial is present for months to years before significant scar accumulates, although the time course may be accelerated by factors related to the selected prosthesis. Thus, efforts to understand fibrosis focus primarily on events that lead to the early accumulation of scar in hopes of identifying new implantable materials able to avoid or slow its progression.

As the tissue becomes fibrotic, there are both quantitative changes in the composition of the ECM with a 3–5-fold increase in the total content of collagens and noncollagenous components. Since fibroblasts are the key fibrogenic cells, in the next section we shall discuss mainly their behavior in the presence of an exogenous artificial material.

23.4.2. Fibroblast Cell Activation—a Highly Orchestrated Reaction to Biomaterial Implantation

Following biomaterial implantation, fibroblasts undergo a response known as "activation," which is the transition of quiescent cells into proliferative and fibrogenic cellular elements. Fibroblast cell activation is a pleiotropic yet tightly programmed response occurring in a reproducible sequence of events. Early events have been termed "initiation"; it encompasses rapid changes in gene expression and phenotype, and renders the cells responsive to cytokines and other local stimuli. Initiation results from paracrine stimulation related to the rapid effect of tissue injury on the homeostasis of neighboring cells, such as macrophages, and from early changes in ECM composition. Full activation incorporates those cellular events that amplify the "initiation" phenotype through enhanced cytokine expression and responsiveness. This component of activation results from autocrine and paracrine stimulation, as well as from accelerated ECM remodeling (Romer *et al.*, 1996). Stimuli initiating fibroblast activation, for the most part, derive from macrophages in addition to rapid, subtle changes in ECM composition.

Macrophages are well established as critical effector cells in the response to injury, whether this response leads to resolution and re-establishment of normal tissue architecture and function or to the eventual development of fibrosis (Riches, 1996). A considerable body of work suggests that macrophages are recruited to sites of implantation and mediate ECM remodeling by locally inducing or producing factors that affect both tissue resorption, and fibroblast cell proliferation and extracellular matrix accumulation. Although increased production of macrophage-derived growth factors has been documented in many forms of tissue fibrosis (Bitterman *et al.*, 1983; Martinet *et al.*, 1987), the exact mechanisms of resident cell activation by macrophages are not completely understood. In fact, macrophages may be responsible for influencing phenotypic characteristics in fibroblasts other than (or in addition to) those directly resulting in increased interstitial matrix production and proliferation.

Indeed, activated macrophages are spatially and temporally associated with the induction of matrix-degrading metalloproteinase activity in resident fibroblasts and elaborate mediators sufficient for this induction. The metalloproteinase enzymes, or matrixins, broad spectrum proteases able to initiate the ECM degradation events that occur during tissue remodeling, are thought to play an important role in the initiation of the fibroblasts.

Although end-stage fibrotic pathology results from the excessive proliferation and extracellular matrix production of activated resident fibroblasts, these cells must first be induced to migrate to a developing lesion. Normal fibroblasts are embedded in a fibrillar collagen-rich matrix and enclosed by a basement membrane. After biomaterial implantation, fibroblast invasion into granulation tissue surrounding the implant is an early event, regardless of whether the result is restoration of normal tissue architecture or fibrosis. This recruitment is likely mediated by numerous molecules including growth factor, chemotactic cytokines, and matrix components. However, release from the fibrillar collagen-rich matrix surrounding these cells would seem to be absolutely necessary for cell migration to initiate. In this respect, expression of matrix-degrading proteases by fibroblasts granulomatous lesions may be required for their migration within developing lesions.

Both inflammatory and resident cell-derived metalloproteinases are thought to contribute to these processes (Martin, 1997). There are three mammalian interstitial collagenases (collagenase-1, -2, and -3) capable of initiating the degradation of interstitial collagens, each the product of a separate matrix metalloproteinase (MMP) gene. Collagenase-2 (MMP-8) is specifically produced and secreted by neutrophils, while collagenase-1 (MMP-1) and collagenase-3 (MMP-13) seem to be expressed by many different cell types including inflammatory cells, epithelial cells, and fibroblasts. Although increased total collagenase activities have been reported in tissue response a long time after biomaterial implantation, (Shapiro, 1998), it is likely that early localized increases in this enzyme activity are necessary for the initial phases of fibroblast resident cell activation and recruitment (Werb, 1997).

The perpetuation of fibroblast cell activation involves key phenotypic responses mediated by increased cytokine effects and strong remodeling of ECM.

Enhanced cytokine responses occur through multiple mechanisms. Among these, increased expression of cell membrane receptors and enhanced signaling are especially important. Continued ECM remodeling during this phase underlies virtually all cellular responses characterizing progressive tissue injury. The complex matrix network is progressively replaced by one rich in fibril-forming collagen; this fundamental shift in ECM composition affects the behavior of the fibroblast cells, accelerating their activation.

Discrete phenotype responses of fibroblasts can be identified as their activation in response to the biomaterial is perpetuated. These include: (1) proliferation, (2) fibrinogenesis, and (3) cytokine release.

Increased numbers of fibroblasts around the implant arise in part from local proliferation in response to polypeptide growth factors, most of which signal through receptor tyrosine kinases. FGF and PDGF are the best characterized and most potent among these proliferative factors in tissue fibrosis. Injury is associated with both increased autocrine and paracrine PDGF and FGF, and up-regulation of their receptors. Again, as described before, the proliferative response to both growth factors requires all interactions via integrins with the supporting ECM structures.

TGF $\beta 1$ is the dominant stimulus to ECM production by fibroblasts and it is increased in experimental and human tissue fibrosis. There are many sources of this cytokine; however, autocrine expression is most important. TGF $\beta 1$ activity is also enhanced in fibrotic tissue through proteolysis of latent TGF $\beta 1$ present in the ECM in the active cytokine by a urokinase-type plasminogen activator. Up-regulation of collagen synthesis during activation is among the most striking molecular responses of fibroblast to biomaterial and is mediated by both transcriptional and post-transcriptional mechanisms, not all of which can be ascribed to TGF $\beta 1$.

Transcriptional activation of the type I collagen has been extensively characterized; in addition, the half-life of collagen α(I) 1 mRNA increases 20-fold in activated compared with quiescent cells. Increased production and/or activity of cytokines are critical for perpetuation of fibroblast activation. Almost all features of fibroblast activation can be attributed to autocrine cytokines, although ECM is an important reservoir of bound growth factors. Finally, through the up-regulation of tissue inhibitors of metalloproteinases, fully activated fibroblasts can also inhibit the activity of interstitial collagenases, which additionally favors the accumulation of scar.

On the basis of the picture described, what is likely to emerge is an even more coherent paradigm for how complex cellular events are integrated to achieve a distinct biologic end point, the encapsulation of implanted biomaterial by scar. This raises an intriguing question. What happens to activated fibroblasts during resolution of the reaction against the prosthesis? Recently, answers have begun to emerge about either the reversion of activated fibroblasts to quiescent cells or the clearance of activated elements. A key unresolved issue is whether an activated fibroblast can revert to a quiescent state. One stimulus that may control this response is interleukin 10 (IL-10). This cytokine down-regulates inflammation and increases interstitial collagenase activity while it provides a fibrogenic negative signal to limit scar accumulation. In addition, the reconstitution of a normal ECM in the rest of the tissue site of implantation can affect negatively the fibroblast activation.

Finally, one potential fate of activated fibroblast is apoptosis, as fibroblast apoptosis has been documented during the recovery phase of experimentally induced tissue injury.

23.4.3. Mechano/Transduction by Biomaterials and ECM Remodeling

As a consequence of the studies concerning the biocompatibility of the biomaterials, new devices have been synthesized to have appropriate chemical, physical, interfacial, and biomimetic characteristics, which permit one to avoid the adverse tissue reactions.

Although the choice of a material for a specific application is mainly based on its physicochemical and biocompatible properties, the traditional mechanical properties such as impact strength, elasticity, and permeability are essential for specific application. Indeed, the choice of the biomaterial has to be primarily governed by the end use of the device, but the material selection must be done on the basis of an extensive biological characterization of the tissue site of implantation. In other words, biomaterial design requirements are highly dependent on the specific clinical application with the key to materials selection being an understanding of the functional and mechanical characteristics of the ECM present in that specific tissue.

Cells of a tissue have the remarkable ability to receive mechanical stress input from their environment and to respond by improving the capacity of the tissue to accommodate that stress field. For example, stretching a vascular wall causes its cells to produce extracellular matrix to better sustain those same tensional forces (Choquet *et al.*, 1997).

The central question in tissue restoration after biomaterial implantation is: "what causes a cell to remodel the ECM of a tissue surrounding an implant"?

The answer is that cells, such as fibroblasts, adhere to the material surface at multiple sites, thereby sensing the forces to which the device is subjected and consequently producing an ECM that can sustain those forces. Several studies have described this phenomenon using the terms "cellular tensegrity" and "mechanotransduction." For example, by attaching to a bioelastic matrix at each end of a cytoskeletal fiber, the mechanical input of stretching the elastic matrix is borne in part by the cell's cytoskeletal components. The cell response is the activation of genes to produce an extracellular matrix sufficient to sustain the dynamic range and temporal aspects of the applied forces.

The cell sets an internal stress field (the distribution of intracellular forces at mechanical equilibrium) that results from the combination of the forces exerted on the adhesive contacts and the forces generated within the cytoskeleton. These intracellular stress fields influence a number of functions such as apoptosis (Chen *et al.*, 1997), migration (Pelham and Wang, 1997), signal transduction (Shyy and Chien, 1997), nuclear shape (Maniotis *et al.*, 1997), and ECM remodeling (Zhong *et al.*, 1998). The stress fields are not static, because the adhesive contacts continuously remodel (Davies *et al.*, 1994). The stress fields change as the cell receives external mechanical stimuli and, in response, dynamically reorganizes its linkages to integrins, the ECM, and its cytoskeleton. The forces applied to the adhesive contacts therefore modify the internal stress field of a cell and can influence many of its signaling pathways. The internal stress field is also dependent upon cell–cell contacts: cells in contact with other cells are no longer transmitting forces only between their interior and the ECM; cells in contact with other cells are also transmitting forces to their neighbors. These interactions between groups of cells combine with the varied spatial organization of the ECM to define the resting stress field within developing or healing tissues and organs. These resting stress fields are important in defining the shape of developing tissue and may be relevant to the efficiency of its physiological function.

The internal forces that cells generate appear to depend upon the stiffness of the ECM; for example, fibroblasts grown on stabilized collagen gels generate stresses within the gels while fibroblasts cultured on freely floating gels do not. Additionally, only fibroblasts grown on stabilized gels form stress fibers or assemble fibronectin into fibrils (Halliday and Tomasek, 1995). The stiffness of the substrate also affects cell spreading and motility. Cells grown on flexible substrates show reduced spreading and increased rates of motility or lamellipodial activity when compared with cells grown on rigid substrates (Pelham and Wang, 1997). Additionally, the focal adhesions of the cells plated on flexible substrates are irregularly shaped, are highly dynamic, and have a reduced amount of phosphotyrosine when compared to the focal adhesions of cells plated on rigid substrates (Pelham and Wang, 1997). In addition to responding to substrate stiffness with changes in spreading and motility, cells also respond to stiffness by increasing the amount of force they apply against more constrained ECM. In experiments in which beads coated with RGD (a synthetic peptide that is a known fibronectin ligand) were magnetically twisted on a cell surface to apply a tangential force, it was observed that the stiffness of the cells increased with the amount of deformation (Wang *et al.*, 1993).

In this approach, the biomaterial would be able to mirror the tissue site of implantation. For example, it must be elastic when the tissue to be restored is elastic, and able to handle mechanical inputs in a manner similar to natural tissue. The prosthesis not only should match the mechanical properties of the tissue to be restored, but it should contain sites to which the normal cells of the tissue can attach. By multiple adhesions of the cells to the biomaterials, the mechanical stresses sustained by the functional artificial device would be appropriately transmitted to that cell, which can discern the magnitude of the force, its dynamic range, and the time course of any changes. This mechanical sensing by the cell would result in the remodeling of the ECM in a way similar to the natural tissue only in case of devices well integrated in the tissue from a mechanical and biocompatible point of view.

23.5. Future Perspectives

Tissue-engineering approaches typically employ exogenous three-dimensional extracellular matrices (ECMs) to engineer new natural tissues from isolated cells. The exogenous ECMs are designed to bring the desired cell types into contact in an appropriate three-dimensional environment, and also provide mechanical support until the newly formed tissues are structurally stabilized and specific signals to guide the gene expression of cells forming the tissue (Putnam and Mooney, 1996).

One approach to designing exogenous ECMs for tissue engineering is to mimic the functions of the ECM molecules found naturally found in tissues (Fouser *et al.*, 1991). These native ECMs act as a scaffolding to bring cells together in a tissue, to control the tissue structure, and to regulate the cell phenotype (e.g., tissue-specific gene expression) (Alberts *et al.*, 1994).

All synthetic ECMs used to engineer tissues have three primary roles. First, the synthetic ECMs facilitate the localization and delivery of cells to specific sites in the body. Second, they define and maintain a three-dimensional space for the formation of new tissues with appropriate structure. Third, they guide the development of new tissue with appropriate function.

The synthetic ECM should provide temporary mechanical support sufficient to withstand *in vivo* forces and maintain a potential space for tissue development. This mechanical support by the synthetic ECM should be maintained until the engineered tissue has sufficient mechanical integrity to support itself. The cells composing the engineered tissue must express appropriate genes to maintain the tissue-specific function of the engineered tissue. The function of seeded cell is strongly dependent on the specific cell-surface receptors (e.g., integrins) used by cells to interact with the material, on interactions with surrounding cells (Parson-Wingerter and Saltzman, 1993) and on the presence of soluble growth factors (Deuel, 1997). These factors can be controlled by incorporating or integrating a variety of signals, such as cell-adhesion peptides (Hubbell, 1995) and growth factors (Mooney *et al.*, 1996), into the synthetic ECM or subjecting it to mechanical stimuli (Banes, 1993).

The exogenous ECMs for tissue engineering can be fabricated from two classes of biomaterial: naturally derived materials and synthetic materials. Naturally occurring materials, such as collagen, have the potential advantage of specific cell interactions. In addition, naturally derived materials offer limited versatility in designing an exogenous ECM with specific properties (e.g., mechanical strength). Synthetic materials, by contrast, can be manufactured reproducibly on a large scale, and can also be processed into an exogenous ECM in which the macrostructure, mechanical properties, and degradation time can be readily controlled and manipulated. Exogenous ECMs fabricated from biodegradable polymers will eventually erode in the body, avoiding a chronic foreign-body response.

The greatest disadvantage of synthetic materials is, however, the lack of cell-recognition signals. Toward this end, efforts are being made to incorporate cell-adhesion peptides biomaterials, which normally exhibit little cellular interaction. Mechanical signals conveyed to cells via their adhesion to a matrix also clearly regulate the development of various tissues and the gene expression of many cell types in culture. In order to engineer functional structural tissues, the correct mechanical stimuli may be provided during the process of tissue development via an appropriate synthetic ECM. For example, tendons engineered without mechanical stimuli do not have mechanical strength as great as native tendon, although they appear to be histologically identical.

The concept of combining synthetic materials with cell-recognition sites of naturally derived materials is very attractive. These hybrid materials could possess the favorable properties of synthetic materials, including widely varying mechanical and degradative properties, reproducible large-scale production and good processability, as well as the specific biological activites of naturally derived materials. This last property may be needed to engineer complex tissues with multiple cell types organized in specific patterns. Several cell-adhesion ligands with highly specific recognition could potentially be dispayed spatially in a desirable pattern to induce specific cell-organization schemes. This appoach has been investigated to promote endothelial cell adhesion to engineered blood vessels.

In conclusion, engineering tissues may provide an alternative to current therapies used to treat the loss or failure of tissue function. The development of synthetic ECMs is a critical component of this field and research in this area is based on the understanding of native ECM molecules. The matrices developed for tissue engineering may, in turn, provide a novel experimental system to eluidate the mechanisms by which native ECMs regulate tissue development.

References

Alberts, B., Bray, D., Lewis, J., Raff, M., Roberts, K., Waston, J.D. 1994, in: *Molecular Biology of the Cell*, pp. 971–995, Garland Publishing, New York.

Banes, A.J. 1993, in: *Physical Forces and Mammalian Cell* (J.A. Frango, ed.), pp. 81–123, Academic Press, New York.

Barry, E.L., Mosher, D.F. 1988. Factor XIII cross-linking of fibronectin at cellular matrix assembly sites, *J. Biol. Chem.* **263**, 10464–10469.

Bitterman, P.B., Rennard, S.I., Adelberg, S., Crystal, R.G. 1983. Role of fibronectin as a growth factor for fibroblasts, *J. Cell. Biol.* **97**, 1925–1932.

Calof, A.L., Lander, A.D. 1991. Relationship between neuronal migration and cell-substratum adhesion: laminin and merosin promote olfactory neuronal migration but are anti-adhesive, *J. Cell. Biol.* **115**, 779–794.

Chen, C., Mrksich, M., Huang, S., Whitesides, G., Ingber, D. 1997. Geometric control of cell life and death, *Science* **276**, 1425–1428.

Choquet, D., Felsenfeld, D., Sheetz, M. 1997. Extracellular matrix rigidity causes strengthening of integrin-cytoskeleton linkages, *Cell* **88**, 39–48.

Dallas, S.L., Miyazono, K., Skerry, T.M., Mundy, G.R., Bonewald, L.F. 1995. Dual role for the latent transforming growth-factor-β-binding-protein in storage of latent TGF-β in the extracellular-matrix and as a structural matrix protein, *J. Cell Biol.* **131**, 539–549.

Davies, P., Robotewskyj, A., Griem, M. 1994. Quantitative studies of endothelial cell adhesion: directional remodeling of focal adhesion sites in response to flow forces, *J. Clin. Invest.* **93**, 2031–2038.

Dean, III, J.W., Chanrasekaran, S., Tanzer, M.L. 1990. A biological role of the carbohydrate moieties of laminin, *J. Clin. Chem.* **265**, 12553–12562.

Deuel, T.F. 1997, in: *Principles of Tissue Engineering* (R.P. Lanza, R. Langer, W.L. Chick, eds.) pp. 133–149, Academic Press, New York.

Edwards, G.M., Wilford, F.H., Liu, X.W., Hennighausen, L., Djiane, J., Streuli, C.H. 1998. Regulation of mammary differentiation by extracellular matrix involves protein-tyrosine phosphatates, *J. Biol. Chem.* **273**, 9495–9500.

Felsenfeld, D., Choquet, D., Sheetz, M. 1996. Ligand binding regulates the directed movement of b1 integrins on fibroblasts, *Nature* **383**, 438–440.

Fouser, L. Iruela-Arispe, L., Bornstein, P., Sage, E.H. 1991. Transcriptional activity of the alpha 1(I)-collagen promoter is correlated with the formation of capillary-like structures by endothelial cells in vitro, *J. Biol. Chem.* **266**, 18345–18351.

Gordon, M.Y. 1988. Extracellular matrix of the marrow microenvironment, *Br. J. Haemat.* **70**, 1–4.

Halliday, N., Tomasek, J. 1995. Mechanical properties of the extracellular matrix influence fibrobectin assembly in vitro, *Exp. Cell Res.* **217**, 107–117.

Howe, A., Apin, A.E., Alahari, S.K., Juliano, R.L. 1998. Integrin signaling and cell growth control, *Curr. Opin. Biol.* **10**, 220–231.

Hubbell, J.A. 1995. Biomaterials in tissue engineering, *Biotechnology* **13**, 565–576.

Ingber, D.E., Prusty, D., Frangioni, J.V., Cragoe, E.J., Lechene, C., Schwartz, M.A. 1990. Control of intracellular pH and growth by fibronectin in capillary endothelial cells, *J. Cell Biol.* **110**, 1803–1811.

Jones, G.E., Arumugham, R.G., Tanzer, M.L. 1986. Fibronectin glycosylation modulates fibroblast adhesion and spreading, *J. Cell. Biol.* **103**, 1663–1670.

Jones, J.I., Gockerman, A., Busby, W.H., Camachohubner, C., Clemmons, D.R. 1993. Extracelluar-matrix contains insulin-like growth-factor binding protein-5-potentiation of the effects of IGF-I, *J. Cell Biol.* **121**, 679–687.

Lawler, J., Weinstein, R., Hynes, R.O. 1988. Cell attachment to thrombospondin: the role of ARG-GLY-ASP, calcium, and integrin receptors, *J. Cell. Biol.* **107**, 2351–2361.

Lee, Y.J., Streuli, C.H. 1999. Extracellular matrix selectively modulates the response of mammary epithelial cells to different soluble signaling ligands, *J. Biol. Chem.* **274**, 22401–22408.

Maniotis, A., Chen, C., Ingber, D. 1997. Demonstration of mechanical connections between integrins, cytoskeletal filaments, and nucleoplasm that stabilize nuclear structure, *Proc. Natl. Acad. Sci. USA* **94**, 849–854.

Martin, P. 1997. Wound healing-aiming for perfect skin regeneration, *Science* **276**, 75–81.

Martinet, Y., Rom, W.N., Grotendorst, G.R., Martin, G.R., Crystal, R.G. 1987. Exaggerated spontaneous release of platelet-derived growth factor by alveolar macrophages from patients with idiopathic pulmonary fibrosis, *N. Engl. J. Med.* **317**, 202–209.

McNamee, H.P., Ingber, D.E., Schwartz, M.A. 1993. Adhesion to fibronectin stimulates inositol lipid synthesis and enhances PDGF-induced inositol lipid break-down, *J. Cell Biol.* **121**, 673–678.

Mooney, D.J., Baldwin, D.F., Suh, N.P., Vacanti, J.P., Langer, R. 1996. Novel approach to fabricate porous sponges of poly(D,L-lactic-co-glycolic acid) without the use of organic solvents, *Biomaterials* **17**, 1417–1422.

Parsons-Wingerter, P.A., Saltzman, W.M. 1993. Growth versus function in the three-dimensional culture of single and aggregated hepatocytes within collagen gels, *Biotechnol. Prog.* **9**, 600–607.

Paulsson, M., Saladin, K., Landwehr, R. 1988. Binding of Ca^{2+} influences susceptibility of laminin to proteolytic digestion and interactions between domain-specific laminin fragments, *Eur. J. Biochem.* **177**, 477–481.

Pelham, R.J., Wang, Y.-L. 1997. Cell locomotion and focal adhesions are regulated by substrate flexibility, *Proc. Natl. Acad. Sci. USA* **94**, 13661–13665.

Putnam, A.J., Mooney, D.J. 1996. Tissue engineering using synthetic extracellular matrices, *Nat. Med.* **2**, 824–826.

Riches, D.W., Chan, E.D., Winston, B.W. 1996. TNF-alpha-induced regulation and signalling in macrophages, *Immunobiology* **195**, 477–490.

Romer, J., Bugge, T.H., Pyke, C., Lund, L.R., Fick, M.J., Degen, J.L., Dano, K. 1996 Impaired wound healing in mice with a disrupted plasminogen gene, *Nat. Med.* **2**, 287–292.

Ruoslahti, E. 1989. Proteoglycans in cell regulation, *J. Biol. Chem.* **264**, 13369–13372.

Sage, E.H., Bornstein, P. 1991. Extracellular proteins that modulate cell-matrix interactions, *J. Biol. Chem.* **266**, 14831–14834.

Schofield, R. 1978. The relationship between the spleen-colony forming cell and the haematopoietic stem cell, *Blood Cells* **4**, 7–25.

Schwartz, M.A., Baron, V. 1999. Interactions between mitogenic stimuli, or, a thousand and one connections, *Curr. Opin. Biol.* **11**, 197–202.

Schwartz, M.A., Lechene, C. 1992. Adhesion is required for protein Kinase C-dependent activation of the Na^+/H^+ antiporter by platelet-derived growth factor, *Proc. Natl. Acad. Sci. USA* **89**, 6138–6141.

Shapiro, S.D. 1998. Matrix metalloproteinase degradation of extracellular matrix: biological consequences, *Curr. Opin. Cell. Biol.* **10**, 602–608.

Shyy, J.Y., Chien, S. 1997. Role of integrins in cellular responses to mechanical stress and adhesion, *Curr. Opin. Cell Biol.* **9**, 707–713.

Stoker, M., O'Neill, C., Berryman, S., Waxman, V. 1968. Anchorage and growth regulation in normal and virus-transformed cells, *Int. J. Cancer* **3**, 683–693.

Turker, R.W., Meade-Cobun, K., Ferris, D. 1990. Cell shape and increased free cytosolic calcium $[Ca^{2+}]i$ induced by growth factors, *Cell Calcium* **11**, 201–209.

Vuori, K., Ruoslahti, E. 1994. Association of insulin receptor substrate-1 with integrins, *Science* **266**, 1576–1578.

Wang, N., Butler, J., Ingber, D. 1993. Mechanotransduction across the cell surface and through the cytoskeleton, *Science* **260**, 1124–1127.

Werb, Z. 1997. ECM and cell surface proteolysis: regulating cellular ecology, *Cell* **3**, 439–442.

Zhong, C., Chrzanowska-Wodnicka, M., Brown, J., Shaub, A., Belkin, A., Burridge, K. 1998. Rho-mediated contractility exposes a cryptic site in fibronectin and induces fibronectin matrix assembly, *J. Cell Biol.* **141**, 539–551.

Zhu, Y., Oganesian, A., Keene, D.R., Sandell, L.J. 1999. [Type IIa] procollagen containing the cysteine-rich amino propeptide is deposited in the extracellular matrix of prechondrogenic tissue and binds to TGF-b 1 and BMP-2, *J. Cell Biol.* **131**, 539–549.

24

Protein Adsorption and Cellular/Tissue Interactions

Agnese Magnani, Gianfranco Peluso, Sabrina Margarucci, and Krishnan K. Chittur

24.1. Introduction

It is now well accepted that an understanding of protein adsorption to surfaces is required in order to understand how cells and tissues interact with surfaces. We need information about not only how much of a given protein is on a surface but its structure. We will start by a broad overview about what proteins are, and discuss their properties in solution and their critical role in influencing the properties of implanted biomaterials. We will then cover the principles of protein adsorption to surfaces and discuss briefly techniques used to probe proteins on surfaces. The relationship between proteins on surfaces and interactions of cells with surfaces will then be discussed.

The approach used in this section will hopefully be useful for advanced undergraduates with previous background in biochemistry and physical chemistry. The topics will be dealt with in very general terms and information about the state of the art should be obtained from current literature.

Agnese Magnani • Dipartimento di Scienze e Tecnologie Chimiche e dei Biosistemi, Università degli Studi di Siena, Via A. Moro, 2, 53100 Siena, Italy. • **Gianfranco Peluso and Sabrina Margarucci** • Istituto di Biochimica delle Proteine ed Enzimologia, Consiglio Nazionale delle Richerche, Via Toiano 6, 0072 Arco Felice, Napoli, Italy. • **Krishnan K. Chittur** • Chemical and Materials Engineering Department, University of Alabama Huntsville, 301 Sparkman Drive, Huntsville, 35899 Alabama, United States.

Integrated Biomaterials Science, edited by R. Barbucci. Kluwer Academic/Plenum Publishers, New York, 2002.

24.2. Protein Adsorption

24.2.1. What Are Proteins?

Proteins are biological polymers made from building blocks of 20 amino acids. Their unique properties are derived from the sequence in which the amino acids are arranged. The properties of proteins in solution and while adsorbed to surfaces, however, are directly related to this primary sequence. Proteins in solution have definite three-dimensional structures stabilized in some cases by disulfide bonds between different parts of the same linear polymer or by hydrogen bonding interactions. This three-dimensional arrangement of the linear chain of amino acids is determined in some complex way on the primary sequence; the exact rules for protein folding from a linear sequence into a 3-D structure are still largely unknown.

In aqueous environments, the most hydrophobic amino acids (e.g., isoleucine, phenylalanine, valine, leucine, tryptophan, methionine, alanine) will be buried inside the complex 3-D structure while charged and polar amino acids will be on the outside, in contact with water (e.g., arginine, lysine, aspartic acid, glutamine, glutamic acid, histidine, serine, threonine). Some of the amino acid side chains have ionizable groups such as amines or hydroxyls or carboxylic acid groups. The p*K*a values of these ionizable side chains will determine the charge that these groups and (consequently) the protein will carry at different pH values. At the physiological pH of 7.4, a protein may have several amino acid side chains positively charged and several that are negatively charged. The development of a quantitative molecular understanding of protein adsorption to surfaces will require detailed modeling of how these charged groups interact with charged and uncharged groups on a synthetic surface.

The 3-D structure can be understood in terms of a collection of secondary structures such as the α-helix, β-sheet, and random coils. Thus a protein in solution consists of a number of secondary structures arranged together in some unique 3-D arrangement. It is this 3-D structure and the availability of specific amino acid sequences on the outside of the protein that determine its *in vivo* properties.

24.2.2. Protein Structure in Solution and on Surfaces

A number of techniques are available for analyzing protein structure in solution. The current accepted best way for obtaining information on the actual 3-D structure of proteins is X-ray crystallography. Circular dichroism and infrared absorption techniques can provide information about solution protein secondary structure. Proteins can (and do) change their structure upon adsorption to surfaces and a study of protein structure on surfaces can be challenging. It is not possible, for example, to use X-ray diffraction techniques to probe adsorbed protein structure. The technique called circular dichroism relies on the differential absorption of the right and the left circularly polarized light as it travels through the protein sample. This differential absorption is easily detectable for proteins in solution and is a very sensitive technique to monitor the presence or absence of α-helices. Application of circular dichroism to adsorbed proteins requires a significant amplification of the differential absorption by using very large surface area special substrates. Fourier transform infrared spectroscopy can provide information about the secondary structure of proteins adsorbed to surfaces (Magnani and Barbucci, 1993; Barbucci and Magnani, 1993). A discussion of the strengths and limitations of the FTIR technique has been recently published (Chittur, 1998a, b).

The study of proteins on surfaces involves a determination of how the surface changes the distribution of secondary structures like the α-helix and β-sheet in the protein. In addition, we would like to know the spatial orientation of the protein on the surface, since the orientation will determine if the binding site of the protein with cells is available or hidden due to the surface. Infrared spectroscopy and atomic force microscopy can be used to probe protein conformation and orientation on surfaces, though these remain fairly difficult to measure (Chittur, 1998a, b).

Antibody binding techniques can also be used to examine issues related to protein orientation and structure on surfaces. Antibodies are proteins that are generated by the immune system in response to an immune challenge. Techniques to generate antibodies that can bind to different portions of a given protein molecule are now well developed and have been adequately described in textbooks and handbooks. These antibodies are usually targed with a fluorescent label and can therefore be used to probe for the presence of the antigen protein (or a specific part of the antigen protein) on a surface. ELISA (enzyme linked immunosorbent assay) relies on this initial step of protein–antibody binding to detect and quantify proteins on surfaces.

24.2.3. Measurement of Proteins on Surfaces

Labeling proteins with radioactive labels such as 125 iodine remains the most widely used technique for measurement of protein adsorption to surfaces (Slack and Horbett, 1988; Slack and Horbett, 1989; Bale *et al.*, 1988; Wojciechowski *et al.*, 1986). It is difficult, however, to measure real-time kinetics of protein adsorption to surfaces with this technique (Cornelius *et al.*, 1992). The technique relies on covalently attaching the radiolabel to the protein of interest followed by gel filtration or other techniques to separate the labeled protein from free radioactive label and appropriate calibration experiments. Techniques to separate the free radiolabel from the labeled protein are, however, not perfect and a small amount of free radioactive label will remain in the test solution. It is important to account for this unknown amount of free radiolabel while calculating the amount of adsorbed protein from radioactivity measurements.

The radioactive labeling method provides no information on protein structure, however. This is a very sensitive and reliable technique for obtaining quantitative information about proteins adsorbed to surfaces, but offers no information about protein conformation. In addition, waste disposal has become quite complicated and expensive.

Fourier transform infrared spectroscopy with attenuated total internal reflection techniques can be used in combination with radiolabeling techniques to monitor protein adsorption to surfaces in real time (Fink *et al.*, 1987; Pitt *et al.*, 1987). Total internal reflection fluorescence has also been used to provide real-time adsorption information for proteins on surfaces (Hlady *et al.*, 1986; Rockhold *et al.*, 1983).

The Atomic Force Microscope (AFM) can measure the forces of interaction between a probe and features on a surface. This in turn allows an unparalleled view of proteins on surfaces including the ability to image single protein molecules at a time. In a typical configuration, a gold-coated silicon cantilever with a known force constant supports a silicon nitride tip. A piezoelectric scanner is used to raster the sample with this tip. There are three independently controlled piezos, one each for the x, y and z-axis (with z being the distance between the tip and the surface). A laser beam is reflected from the top of the cantilever to a four-quadrant photodetector. As the scanner rasters the sample, the cantilever will be deflected up or down depending on the surface features encountered by the tip. This motion of the cantilever is accurately tracked by the laser beam. The AFM can be operated in a constant-height or a constant-force mode. In the constant-force mode, the computer in the AFM will adjust the z-piezo such that the distance between the silicon nitride tip and the surface is maintained constant based on the information obtained from the photodetector. When the cantilever is deflected up because the tip encounters a raised surface feature, this will change the intensities of the laser beam detected by the two halves of the photodetector. The AFM computer will immediately adjust the voltage to the z-piezo so that these two signal intensities are again back to what they should be. The voltage required to adjust the z-piezo provides the information for the calculation of height of the surface features. Since the cantilever obeys Hooke's Law, from a knowledge of the spring constant, and known deflections, forces between the tip and the surface can be measured quite accurately. The operation of the AFM in what is called the Lateral Force Mode can be explained similarly. The twisting of the cantilever due to changes in the way the tip interacts with the surface will result in differences in the intensities of the laser beam as detected by the left and right halves of the four-quadrant photodetector. This difference can be translated into the actual lateral forces experienced by the cantilever if the physical properties of the cantilever are accurately known. Illustrations describing the operating principles of the AFM (and related techniques) have been published in several journal articles and books (Wilbur *et al.*, 1995; Sarid and Ellings, 1991; Haggerty *et al.*, 1991).

The necessity of maintaining a close contact between a hard probe tip such as silicon nitride and a surface for imaging is a source of continuing problems for the scientist imaging soft materials such as proteins (Andrade *et al.*, 1992). This can be overcome to some extent by using Tapping Mode TM-AFM. In TM-AFM the tip is vibrated at a specific frequency and brought into close contact with the sample surface. If the tip interacts with a surface feature, the amplitude of vibration is changed. The piezoelectric crystals are automatically adjusted by the AFM computer to recover the original amplitudes. The tip can thus be rastered over a surface to generate topographic information. While AFM operated in the Tapping Mode does not destroy proteins and other soft molecules, the image resolutions are not as good as those obtained while using contact AFM.

Images obtained by the AFM in the contact mode reflect features of the surface and the tip itself. Since the tip has finite dimensions, imaging small molecules or surface features of dimensions similar to that of the tip are *contaminated* by the tip itself (Eppel *et al.*, 1993). Techniques to account for the shape of the tip and improve the resolution of the images so obtained have been described in the literature. The idea is to image an object of known dimensions with the tip, create the shape of the tip, and use that to improve the resolution of the final image. The procedure for calculating and using tip shapes has been described as deconvolution (Markiewicz and Goh, 1994, 1995) and using the language of mathematical morphology (Wilson *et al.*, 1995; Villarubia, 1994, 1996).

Atomic Force Microscopy and related techniques offer an unparalleled view of individual protein molecules or small collections of such molecules adsorbed to surfaces (Sarid and Ellings, 1991; Haggerty *et al.*, 1991; Siedlecki *et al.*, 1994; Eppel *et al.*, 1995; Feng and Andrade, 1993). AFM has also been used recently to follow the adsorption and desorption of proteins directly at the solid–liquid interface (Stipp, 1996).

24.2.4. Protein Adsorption to Surfaces: Principles

Following the initial observations of rapid protein adsorption to implanted surfaces, studies have shown that the adsorption process is dynamic. The composition of the adsorbed protein layer depends not only on surface chemistry, morphology, and energy, but also time. Leo Vroman was the first to describe, for example, how fibrinogen adsorbed to a surface from plasma can be displaced at later times by other proteins such as high molecular weight kininogen. In order for a protein to adsorb to a surface, it must first be transported to near the surface; this can happen by molecular diffusion or convection (transport due to thermal gradients are highly unlikely under physiological conditions and so we can safely ignore them). The rate at which the protein then adsorbs to the surface will depend on a number of factors including the nature and distribution of charged groups on the surface, and the magnitude of the van der Waals and hydrophobic interactions between the protein and the surface. The rigorous modeling of protein adsorption to surfaces must be based on all these molecular forces.

In developing an understanding of protein adsorption to surfaces, investigators use two types of measurements: (a) the adsorption isotherm and (b) the adsorption kinetics. Even though protein adsorption is not reversible (like small molecules: for example, gases on adsorbents), investigators have and continue to model the adsorption process in terms of the Langmuir isotherm. An adsorption isotherm is, however, very limited in its ability to convey the dynamics of the adsorption process. During the initial stages of protein–surface contact, the adsorption process may be partially reversible, but as the surface gets covered with protein, almost none of the adsorbed protein molecules can be removed by solvent alone.

Proteins in solution can, however, exchange with adsorbed proteins, albeit at a much smaller rate than the rate of adsorption.

Adsorption kinetics (plot of surface concentration of protein with time) provides perhaps the best information that allows us to understand protein adsorption and its relationship to cellular events. In a mixture of proteins, the protein at the highest concentration and with the highest diffusivity has the best chance of adsorbing to the surface. If this protein binds to the surface at a rate that depletes all available surface sites before any other protein approaches the surface, then the surface will be dominated by this protein. If however, this protein binds to surface sites only loosely, it can be easily replaced by other proteins that may be present at much lower concentrations but may bind to the surface with much higher affinity. A simple reaction diffusion mechanism can therefore be used to explain the dynamics of protein adsorption to surfaces. A complete description of this mechanism and simulations reproducing some of the Vroman effect type of observations made in the literature has been published (Lu *et al.*, 1994; Nadarajah *et al.*, 1995). The significant differences in the affinities of plasma proteins for surfaces and differences in their solution concentration explain why the composition of the proteins on adsorbed surfaces is very different from their relative concentrations in the solution.

We will now illustrate a few principles of protein adsorption to surfaces using idealized kinetic plots. Consider three proteins A, B, and C such that protein A adsorbs to the surface faster than protein B, which in turn adsorbs faster than C. Assuming monolayer adsorption and similar solution densities for the three proteins, an idealized plot of the surface concentration of these proteins as a function of time can be shown as follows in Figure 24.1. Protein A reaches its equilibrium concentration on the surface much faster than proteins B and C.

Notice in this figure that the slope of the curve at equilibrium is zero, i.e., protein adsorption is assumed to stop after a certain time for all three proteins. In examining literature data, however, it is striking that in many cases, the surface concentration of protein does not appear to level to a equilibrium value—the curve never reaches a slope of zero. In a few cases, calculations have shown that indeed, in many cases, the calculated amount

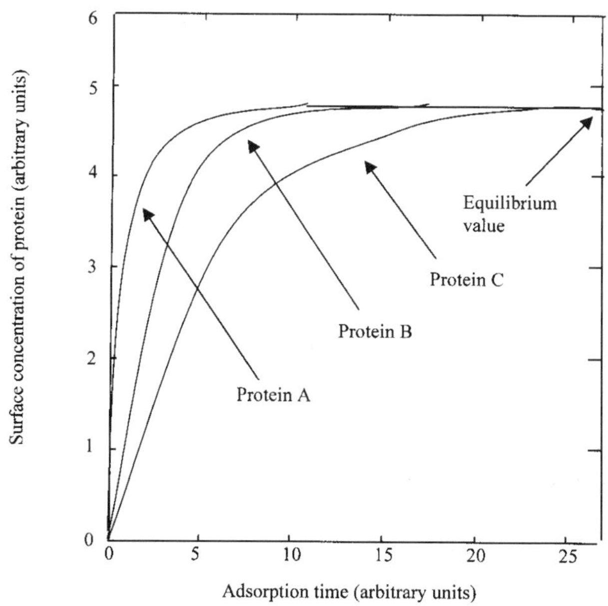

Figure 24.1. Kinetic plot of the adsorption of three different proteins (A, B, and C) to a surface as a function of time.

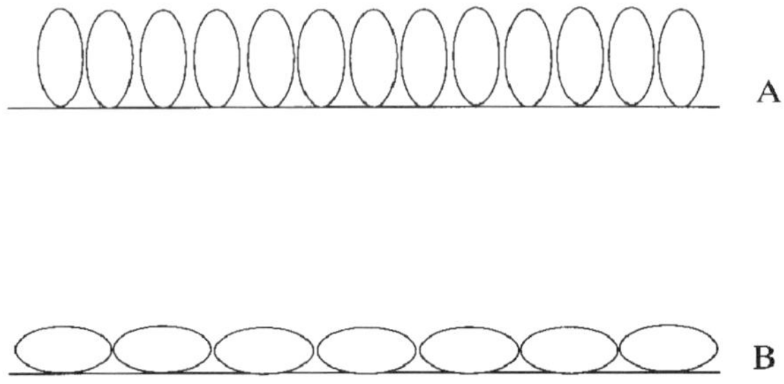

Figure 24.2. Different packing ways of a protein on a surface: (A) end-on way; (B) side-on way.

of protein on a surface is much more than what can be accounted for by a single monolayer. The monolayer assumption derives from the fact that there are only a limited number of sites of adsorption on any given surface and competition for these sites limits the proteins that can be detected on the surface.

In reality, this equilibrium surface adsorbed value varies for different proteins, reflecting differences in the way proteins are packed on the surface. As an example, consider the next Figure 24.2. The density of the surface adsorbed protein will depend on how the protein is packed: the end-on arrangement will, for example, provide a much denser protein layer on the surface than a side-on arrangement.

In spite of a wealth of protein adsorption literature data that include adsorption kinetics with different combinations of surfaces, solution conditions (pH, ionic strength, etc.), and protein types, general rules which will allow us to predict protein adsorption for any general protein–surface combination are not available. A number of empirical approaches have been tried, including multivariate approaches using the "Tatra" plot (Andrade *et al.*, 1992). This approach includes the use of a number of experimentally measurable quantities for both the surface, the protein in solution, and the adsorbed protein to obtain some statistical correlations for the prediction of protein adsorption. Multivariate models based on the partial least-squares algorithm have also been developed to establish a correlation between the surface properties of common polymeric materials and the amount and retention of fibrinogen adsorbed from complex mixtures (Perez-Luna *et al.*, 1994). Statistical approaches like these can be used to extract important variables that are related to a particular dependent variable of interest, such as cell adhesion, bioseparability, biofouling, etc., but are not of general utility. If it was so, we would have developed a general framework through which we could predict the consequence of *any* general protein–surface contact. A general framework for understanding protein adsorption to surfaces will require that we quantify all the important forces between proteins and surfaces and develop techniques to average such interactions over a large collection of proteins.

24.2.5. Importance of Protein Adsorption

The injury caused by the implantation of any artificial material is followed almost instantly by the adsorption of a protein layer on the surface. This observation made more than 40 years ago triggered a number of investigations into the nature of this adsorbed protein layer and its relationship to cellular interactions with the implanted surface. We now know that surface chemistry (the presence of specific functional groups), surface energetics, and surface morphology all influence protein adsorption to surfaces. In addition to mechanical design requirements, biomaterials scientists must design materials that will have the appropriate surface properties so that the implanted device will be *biocompatible.* A *biocompatible* material or device is one that is designed with specific properties and that works *in vivo* precisely in the manner in which it is designed. Biomaterials scientists now have a number of techniques to design materials with precise mechanical and surface properties but have yet to identify which of these properties will lead to the desired *in vivo* functionality.

Platelets are an excellent example to illustrate the role of proteins and surfaces in biomaterial–host interactions. Platelets do not normally bind to soluble fibrinogen unless they are activated by some agonist like ADP (adenosine diphosphate), but they will bind to adsorbed fibrinogen. This is in part due to the concentration and localization of fibrinogen on the surface that has the effect of accentuating the platelet–receptor protein interaction (Horbett, 1996).

A number of studies have clearly shown that often information on the amounts of a particular protein at the interface are insufficient to explain cellular interactions; information about protein structure is essential. For example, surfaces with different chemical compositions which had the same amounts of adsorbed fibronectin (a cell adhesion protein) had different effects on the differentiation responses of fibroblasts and neuronal cells (Sukenik *et al.*, 1989, 1990).

The researchers concluded that these differences were due to differences in fibronectin conformation resulting from different surface chemistries. Using FTIR/ATR, we could detect distinct differences in the conformation of adsorbed fibronectin on these surfaces (Cheng *et al.*, 1994).

The long-term success of prosthetic vascular grafts has been limited to grafts with diameter of 4 mm or larger; with smaller grafts the luminal surface tends to activate components of the coagulation system and leads to implant occlusion. There is therefore a significant interest in the development of novel thromboresistant materials which can be used to make small-diameter vascular grafts. Flow can affect the rate at which proteins and cells are brought to surfaces, but can also affect the rate at which cellular elements including platelets secrete components from their cytoplasm to the immediate surroundings. Investigators are interested in kinetics of thrombus formation, the size and distribution of aggregates on the surface, and the likelihood these aggregates will be removed from the surface. All of these will depend on the nature of the surface and the proteins adsorbed to these surfaces.

In vivo the normal, intact endothelium is perfectly thromboresistant and thus serves as the model against which all synthetic materials and surface modification strategies are compared. There have been numerous attempts at preparing surfaces with a confluent monolayer of endothelial cells for flowing blood contacting situations. These studies have, however, had only limited success owing to the difficulty of growing and maintaining an intact and functional endothelial cell layer on surfaces over long periods of time. The ability of endothelial cells to grow on substrates depends not only on the initial concentration of cell-adhesive molecules such as fibronectin, but the ability of cells to modify and recondition the protein-modified substrate (Detrait *et al.*, 1999). The choice of material used to grow endothelial cells is critical, since the properties of fibronectin depend on the nature of the substrate. Fibronectin is maintained in its native conformation better on hydrophilic surfaces than on hydrophobic surfaces (Grinnel and Feld, 1981, 1982). A recent study has shown that introducing an integrand independent mechanism for binding endothelial cells to surfaces can increase the strength of attachment of the cells and help in cell spreading (Bhat *et al.*, 1998).

24.3. Cells/Tissue Interactions

24.3.1. The Wound Healing Process

Severe tissue injury causes blood vessel distruption with concomitant extravasation of blood constituents. Blood coagulation and platelet aggregation generate a fibrin-rich clot that plugs injured vessels and fills any discontinuity in the wounded tissue. While the blood clot within the vessel lumen re-establishes hemostasis, the clot within the wound space provides a provisional matrix for cell migration. Platelets also have a dual function, since they not only facilitate the formation of a hemostatic plug but also secrete multiple mediators, including growth factors (ten Dijke *et al.*, 1989). In fact the coagulation pathways, as well as the activated complement pathways, and injured or activated parenchymal cell all generate numerous vasoactive mediators and chemotactic factors, which together recruit inflammatory leukocytes to the wounded site. Infiltrating neutrophils clean the wounded area of foreign particles, including bacteria. If excessive microorganisms or indigestible particles have lodged in the wound site, neutrophils will probably cause further tissue damage as they attempt to clear these contaminants through the release of enzymes and toxic oxygen products. When particle clearance has been completed, the generation of granulocyte chemoattractants usually ceases. Effete neutrophils in the wound are either extruded with the eschar or phagocytosed by macrophages or fibroblasts. Peripheral blood monocytes continue to infiltrate the wound site, however, in response to specific monocyte chemoattractants. Once in tissue, monocytes progressively become activated macrophages. Macrophages, like platelets, release growth factors that initiate granulation tissue formation. However, unlike platelets which release stored proteins and peptides but produce little if any of these molecules, macrophages have the ability to continually synthesize and secrete growth factors and cytokines.

On the basis of the above-described summary, the process of wound healing can be divided into three main overlapping stages: inflammation, formation of granulation tissue, and matrix formation and remodeling.

24.3.1.1. Inflammation

Tissue injury results in the release of blood components into the wound site. Contact of the blood plasma with tissue protein and the basement membrane activates the clotting cascade. The clot traps plasma protein and blood cells into a fibrin gel, thereby inducing hemostasis and providing a matrix for the influx of inflammatory cells. Thrombin, formed during the clotting cascade, stimulates release of α-granules from aggregated platelets. These α-granules contain locally acting growth factors such as TGF-β, PDGF, and FGF. The combination, concentration, and timing of growth factor release and activation at the site of injury regulate the complex process of wound healing by controlling cell proliferation, chemotaxis, and activation of a variety of cellular responses.

Platelet aggregation and blood clot formation cease as the stimuli for initiation dissipate. This cessation involves (i) the generation of protein C (which degrades coagulation factors V and VII) (Kisiel *et al.*, 1977), (ii) the release of plasminogen activator (which initiates clot lysis) (Moncada *et al.*, 1976), and (iii) the production of prostaglandins from smooth muscle cells (which inhibit platelet aggregation and PDGF production, thereby providing a feedback control mechanism). The production of growth inhibitors at various steps in the wound healing process may therefore be essential for restraining cell growth in the presence of mitogenic factors.

Neutrophils, attracted by a variety of chemotactic factors, work mainly to remove contaminating bacteria from the injury site. However, they are not essential to wound healing as neutropenia does not interfere with the healing process (Simpson and Ross, 1972). Macrophages, like neutrophiles, remove pathogenic, organism, and tissue debris, including effete neutrophilis. The influx of monocytes and their conversion to macrophages is critical for the initiation of tissue repair. Both cell types are most numerous in the wound site between 3 and 5 days following injury. Macrophages release a variety of biologically active substances, including further amounts of TGF-β and PDGF, which facilitate the recruitment of additional inflammatory cells, augment macrophage-mediated tissue debridement, and initiate granulation tissue formation. TGF-β has been shown to be three orders of magnitude more potent than PDGF as a chemoattractant for both monocytes and fibroblast (Wahl *et al.*, 1987; Postlewaite *et al.*, 1987). TGF-β can also stimulate endothelial cell PDGF production. In addition, TGF-β, PDGF, and TGF-α have been reported to stimulate their own production, thus providing a way to amplify and sustain their respective physiological effects (Van Obberghen-Schilling *et al.*, 1988; Paulsson *et al.*, 1987; Coffey *et al.*, 1987).

After an injury site has been sterilized during inflammation, the secreted products of the activated macrophages may become damaging to healthy cells and tissue. At this stage of wound healing, the suppression of macrophage activities may be critical for protecting the surrounding healthy tissue, and for the transition between inflammation and granulation tissue formation. In this regard, therefore, it is interesting to note that TFG-βs have also been reported to deactivate superoxide production from macrophages (Tsunawaki *et al.*, 1988).

At this point, a speculative scheme can be proposed whereby a stereotyped sequence of inflammatory events results in the resolution of inflammation. For example, injury to endothelial and epithelial cell "barriers" is associated with leakage of fluid and protein. Therefore, reconstitution of normal microvascular permeability occurs by the reforming of cell junctions and the regeneration of cell sheets. Monocytes mature into macrophages to remove cellular debris such as necrotic polymorphonuclear cells. Thus, neutrophil secretion is restricted and aged cell undergoes apoptosis, which determines the macrophage removal of the intact senescent cell without stimulating macrophage release of proinflammatory mediators. There are several steps in this scheme that could go away and lead to circumstances favoring the development of persistent inflammation. For example, if the macrophage fails to develop the appropriate receptors for removing apoptotic cells, neutrophils would eventually become necrotic and disgorge their damaging contents, in the damaged tissues.

24.3.1.2. Granulation Tissue Formation

Granulation tissue consists of a dense population of fibroblasts, macrophages, and neovasculature embedded in a loose matrix of collagen, fibronectin, and hyaluronic acid. TGF-β has a major role in granulation tissue formation. It increases the expression of genes associated with extracellular matrix formation (ECM), such as fibronectin, the fibronectin receptor, various types of collagen, and protease inhibitors. TGF-β has been shown to enhance the contraction of a collagen matrix by fibroblast (Montesano and Orci, 1988), suggesting its possible involvement in connective tissue contraction. In response to growth factors such as PDGF and TGF-β the fibroblasts proliferate, migrate into the wound site, and then undergo a series of phenotypic changes to become myofibroblasts, which have characteristics similar to smooth muscle cells. The myofibroblasts align themselves along the radial axis of the newly deposited extracellular matrix within the wound. The myofibroblasts then form interactions with other cells and extracellular matrix to generate a contractive force that aids in wound closure.

Endothelial cells in the wound proliferate and form new blood vessels (angiogenesis) to supply the injured site with nutrients and oxygen. This nutrient supply is essential for synthesis, deposition, and organization of the extracellular matrix. Basic FGF is a potent mitogen for vascular endothelial cells, derived from either large vessels or capillaries (Gospodarowicz *et al.*, 1985). FGF also stimulates endothelial cells to produce a urokinase-type plasminogen activator, a protease implicated in neovascularization. In addition, bFGF regulates the synthesis and deposition of various extracellular matrix components (Gospodarowicz *et al.*, 1986). Heparin sulfate, a structural component of the ECM, may function to stabilize FGFs, since it protects both bFGF and aFGF from acid or heat inactivation and potentiates their mitogenic activity (Gospodarowicz and Cheng, 1986). It has been suggested that when FGFs are released they become an integral part of the ECM. The hydrolysis of ECM by heparitinase, an inducible enzyme produced by activated platelets and macrophages (Savion *et al.*, 1984; Yahalom *et al.*, 1984), could subsequently lead to solubilization of biologically active heparin sulfate–FGF complexes. Although TGF-βs are not mitogenic for endothelial cells, they are potent angiogenic agents *in vivo*. This is probably due to their ability to chemoattract macrophages and to stimulate macrophages to secrete angiogenic peptides (Roberts *et al.*, 1986) and to their direct affect on capillary formation (Merwin *et al.*, 1991).

24.3.1.3. Re-Epithelialization

Within hours of injury, re-epithelialization begins to restore the integrity of the damaged surface. Re-epithelialization begins with the migration of epithelial cells from the free edges of the tissue across the wound. Within 24 hours, epithelial cells at the original edge of the wound begin proliferating, thereby generating more cells for migration. EGF and other members of the EGF family are chemotactic and mitogenic for epithelial cells (Laato, 1988). Once re-epithelialization is complete, the epithelial cells revert to their nonmigrating phenotype and become attached to the basement membrane through hemidesmosomes.

24.3.1.4. Matrix Formation and Remodeling

The third phase of wound healing is the gradual dissolution of granulation tissue with devascularization and the loss of cells, fibronectin, and type III collagen. The granulation tissue is replaced with connective tissue consisting of a framework of collagen and elastin fibers providing tissue strength and elastin properties, respectively. This framework then becomes saturated with proteoglycans and glycoproteins. Remodeling involves the synthesis of new collagen and the degradation of old collagen. The production of collagen and proteinase inhibitors is stimulated by TGF-β (Sporn *et al.*, 1987), while the production of collagenes by fibroblasts is stimulated by PDGF (Bauer *et al.*, 1985). The final outcome of matrix formation and remodeling is the scar tissue.

24.3.2. *In Vivo* Models

24.3.2.1. Subcutaneous Implants

Several animal models have been developed to gauge the efficacy of growth factors in wound healing. A porous subcutaneous chamber is often used as an *in vivo* model for the healing of deep wounds.

Chambers of stainless steel wire mesh or polyvinyl alcohol sponges are inserted into the backs of rats. The animal encapsulates the chamber with connective tissue, defining a dead space in which growth factors can be injected. The chambers are removed after one to two weeks and the infiltrated granulation tissue is examined by biochemical and histological techniques. While PDGF, FGF, EGF, and TGF-β have all been demonstrated to stimulate granulation tissue formation using this model system, TGF-β appears to be the most effective (Sprugel *et al.*, 1988; Cromack *et al.*, 1987). To examine the intrinsic role of growth factors in wound healing, the presence of endogenous growth factors in wound chamber models has also been determined. Macrophages isolated from wound chambers were found to express elevated mRNA leves for TGF-α, TGF-β, PDGF, and IGF-1 (Rappolee *et al.*, 1988). The concentration of TGF-β was found to peak during the phase of wound healing associated with maximal fibroblast proliferation and collagen synthesis (Cromack *et al.*, 1987).

24.3.2.2. Impaired Healing Model

The efficacy of any wound healing factor is more easily demonstrated in animals with impaired wound healing. Defective wound repair can be induced by chemotherapy, steroids, or streptozotocin. When the effects of EGF, PDGF, TGF-β and insulin on wound healing were compared in adriamycin treated rats, TGF-β, was found to be the most effective growth factor (Lawrence *et al.*, 1986). PDGF and EGF alone had no effect. A combination of EGF, PDGF, and TGF-β resulted in an almost complete reversal of adriamycin inhibition of wound healing. EGF was shown to prevent methyl prednisolone induced inhibition of wound healing in a wound chamber model (Laato, 1988). PDGF restored wound healing in streptozotocin-induced diabetic rats, while insulin had no effect. A combination of PDGF and insulin, however, stimulated a more rapid increase in collagen deposition than PDGF alone (Grotendorst *et al.*, 1985). These animal models indicate that the repair process in the various forms of defective healing requires different growth factors and combinations of growth factors for optimal healing.

24.3.2.3. Angiogenesis Model

Growth factors stimulation of new blood vessel formation *in vivo* can be determined in assays using the avascular rabbit cornea, the hamster cheek pouch, and the chick chorioallantoic membrane. All three assays are scored by blood vessel growth toward the angiogenic factor but are difficult to quantitate. Concordant with the *in vitro* observations, FGFs are potent angiogenic factors in all three assays (Gospodarowicz *et al.*, 1986). As discussed previously, TGF-β is a strong growth inhibitor of capillary endothelial cells *in vitro*, but a potent angiogenic factor *in vivo* (Roberts *et al.*, 1986). Thus, extrapolations between *in vitro* and *in vivo* cannot always be made.

24.3.2.4. Biological Effects of TGF-β

TGF-*β* has been widely viewed as a growth-stimulatory factor for mesenchymal cells and growth inhibitor for epithelial cells. This notion is based largely on the proliferative effects of TGF-*β* in cell culture, the localization of TGF-*β* during embryogenesis to regions of mesenchymal reorganization, and the enhancing effects of TGF-*β* in wound healing and bone formation studies (Barnard *et al.*, 1990). Challenging this view, however, are the observations that TGF-*β*1 is largely growth inhibitory *in vivo*. Silberstein and Daniel (1987) demonstrated reversible inhibition of mammary gland epithelial cell growth by TGF-*β*1 administered in a slow-release pellet. Subsequently, Russell *et al.* (1988) found that intravenously administered TGF-*β*1 and TGF-*β*2 inhibited the early phase of liver regeneration following partial hepatectomy; however, even with continuous administration of TGF-*β*, the regenerative process still proceeded but in a delayed fashion. Finally, *in vivo* administration of TGF-*β* can inhibit lymphoid and myeloid cell proliferation (Goey *et al.*, 1989). Thus, it is perplexing how TGF-*β* can act as a potent growth inhibitor while functioning to enhance connective tissue formation in normal and wound-healing circumstances.

Recent studies using the chicken chorioallantoic membrane have provided some insights into the mechanisms by which TGF-*β* may act *in vivo* (Yang and Moses, 1990). Focal administration of TGF-*β*1 to the chorioallantoic membrane resulted in gross angiogenesis and the rapid formation of a hypercellular lesion involving increased cell density of fibroblasts, epithelial cells, and endothelial cells. Cellular accumulation occurred in the face of marked proliferative inhibition of all cell types, including fibroblastic, epithelial cells, and endothelial cells. Therefore, the accumulation of fibroblasts and epithelial cells was almost certainly due to enhanced cell migration through chemotaxis. Endothelial cell accumulation in the form of capillary sprouts may involve a more complex process. There was evidence of increased cell proliferation at the periphery of the lesion, where exogenous TGF-*β*1 concentrations would be expected to be low or nonexistent.

The results from the chorioallantoic membrane studies are consistent with certain *in vitro* findings. The chemotactic effects of TGF-*β*1 for dermal fibroblasts have been shown to occur at concentrations much lower than those required for growth inhibition or extracellular matrix induction (<10 pg/ml; Postlewaite *et al.*, 1987). At higher concentrations TGF-*β*1 is no longer chemotactic. Thus, it is probable that the diffusion of TGF-*β*1 into the chorioallantoic membrane stimulated the chemotaxis of cells toward its source of delivery and highest concentration. It is speculated that once cells have reached the zone of higher TGF-β1 concentrations, both cell migration and proliferation become inhibited, so that cells may devote their energy to perform differentiated functions. For endothelial cells, the differentiated functions may take the form of capillary tube formation and basement membrane deposition, while differentiated functions for fibroblasts would be extracellular matrix deposition. A possible mechanistic explanation for the increased proliferation peripherally is that TGF-β, while inhibitory for proliferation at higher concentrations, could be an indirect mitogen at lower concentrations.

24.3.2.5. TGF-β as an Indirect Mitogen

TGF-β has been shown to induce both the platelet-derived growth factor (PDGF) A chain gene c-sis (coding for PDGF B chain). More recently, Battegay *et al.* (1990) demonstrated not only TGF-β induction of PDGF-AA synthesis in aortic smooth muscle cells, but also inhibition of TGF-β induced DNA synthesis using neutralizing antibodies to PDGF-AA. This demonstrates that mitogenesis induced by TGF-β is indirect, being mediated by PDGF-AA autocrine stimulation. It was further shown that the TGF-β stimulatory effect occurred only at lower concentrations, while higher concentrations of TGF-β resulted in inhibition of smooth muscle cell proliferation. The inhibitory effect at higher concentrations was correlated with inhibitory expression of the PDGF receptor α subunit, which is required for biological responses to PDGF-AA. These findings provide molecular mechanisms by which TGF-β1 may stimulate and inhibit proliferation in the same cell type.

Both TGF-β stimulation of proliferation at low concentrations and inhibition of proliferation at higher concentrations may be mediated indirectly through other growth factors, such as PDGFs and their cognate receptors. For endothelial cells, indirect mitogenesis involving factors other than PDGFs would be expected. It should also be noted that the effects of TGF-β on PDGF receptor expression cannot explain the growth-inhibitory effects of TGF-β on epithelial cells and probably lymphoid and myeloid cells, because these cell types usually lack PDGF receptors and are unresponsive to PDGFs.

References

Andrade, J.D., Hlady, V., Wei, A.P., Ho, C.H., Lea, A.S., Jeon, S.I., Lin, Y.S., Stroup, E. 1992. Proteins at interfaces: principles, multivariate aspects, protein resistant surfaces, and direct imaging and manipulation of adsorbed proteins, *Clin. Mater.* **11**, 67–72.

Bale, M.D., Mosher, D.F., Wolfarht, L., Sutton, R. C. 1988. Competitive adsorption of fibronectin, fibrinogen, immunoglobulin, albumin and bulk plasma proteins on polystyrene latex, *J. Colloid Interface Sci.* **125**, 516–522.

Barbucci, R., Magnani, A. 1993. Conformation of human plasma proteins at polymer surfaces, the effectiveness of surface heparinization, *Biomaterials* **15**(12), 955–962.

Barnard, J.A., Lyons, R.M., Moses, H.L. 1990. The cell biology of transforming growth factor beta, *Biochim. Biophys. Acta* **1032**(1), 79–81.

Battegay, E.J., Raines, E.W., Seifert, R.A., Bowen-Pope, D.F., Ross, R. 1990. TGF-beta induces bimodal proliferation of connective tissue cells via complex ontrol of an autocrine PDGF loop, *Cell* **63**, 515–524.

Bauer, E.A., Cooper, T.W., Huang, J.S., Altman, J., Deuel, T.F. 1985. Stimulation on *in vitro* human skin collagenase expression by platelet-derived growth factor, *Proc. Natl. Acad. Sci. USA* **82**, 4132.

Bhat, V.D., Truskey, G.A., Reichert, W.M. 1998. Using avidin-mediated binding to enhance initial endothelial cell attachment and spreading, *J. Biomed. Mater. Res.* **40**, 57–65.

Cheng, S.S., Chittur, K.K., Sukenik, C.N., Culp, L.A., Lewandowska K. 1994. The conformation of fibronectin on self-assembled monolayers with different surface composition, An FT-IR/ATR study, *J. Colloid Interface Sci.* **162**, 135–142.

Chittur, K.K. 1998a. Ftir/atr for protein adsorption to biomaterial surfaces, *Biomaterials* **19**, 257–269.

Chittur, K.K. 1998b. Proteins on surfaces, Methodologies for surface preparation and engineering protein function, in: *Biopolymers at Interfaces* (M. Malmsten, ed.), Chapter 6, pp. 143–179, Elsevier Surfactant Series, Elsevier, New York.

Coffey, R.J., Derynck, R. Wilcox, J.N., Bringman, T.X., Goustin, S.A., Moses, H.L., Pittelkow, M.R. 1987. Production and auto-induction of transforming growth factors-β in human keratinocytes, *Nature* **328**, 817–820.

Cornelius, R.M., Wojciechowski, P.W., Brash, J. L. 1992. Measurement of protein adsorption-kinetics by an in situ, real-time, solution depletion technique, *J. Colloid Interface Sci.* **150**(1), 121–133.

Cromack, D.T., Sporn, M.B., Roberts, A.B., Merino, M.J., Dart, L.L., Norton, J.A. 1987. Transforming growth factor-beta levels in rat wound chambers, *J. Surg. Res.* **42**, 622–628.

Detrait, E., Lhoest, J.B., Bertrand, P., van den Bosch de Aguilar, Ph. 1999. Fibronectin pluronic coadsorption on a polystyrene surface with increasing hydrophobicity, Relationship to cell adhesion, *J. Biomed. Mater. Res.* **45**, 404–413.

ten Dijke, P., Iwata, K. K. 1989. Growth factors for wound healing, Biotechnology **7**, 793–798.

Eppell, S.J., Zypman, F.R., Marchant, R.E. 1993. Probing the resolution limits and tip interactions of atomic force microscopy in the study of globular proteins, *Langmuir* **9**, 228–288.

Eppell, S.J., Simmons, S.R., Albrecht, R.M., Marchant, R.E. 1995. Cell-surface receptors and proteins on platelet membranes imaged by scanning force microscopy using immuno-gold contrast enhancement, *Biophys. J.* **68**(2), 671–680.

Feng, L., Andrade, J.D. 1993. Surface atomic and domain-structures of biomedical carbons observed by scanning tunneling microscopy (STM), *J. Biomed. Mater. Res.* **27**(2), 177–182.

Fink, D.J., Hutson, T.B., Chittur, K.K., Leininger, R.I., Gendreau, R.M. 1987. Quantitative surface studies of protein adsorption by infrared spectroscopy. II Quantitation of adsorbed and bulk proteins, *Anal. Biochem.* **167**, 147–153.

Goey, H., Keller, J.R., Back, T., Long, D.L., Ruscetti, F.W., Wiltrout, R.H. 1989. Inhibition of early murine hemopoietic progenitor cell proliferation after in vivo locoregional administration of transforming growth factor-beta 1, *J. Immunol.* **143**(3), 877–880.

Gospodarowicz, D., Cheng, J. 1986. Heparin protects basic and acidic FGF from inactivation, *J. Cell Physiol.* **128**, 475–484.

Gospodarowicz, E., Massoglia, S., Cheng, J., Lui, G-M., Bohlen, P. 1985. Isolation of bovine pituitary fibroblast growth factor purified by fast protein liquid chromatography (FPLC). Partial chemical and biological characterization, *J. Cell Physiol.* **122**, 323–393.

Gospodarowicz, D., Neufeld, G., Schweigerer, L. 1986. Molecular and biological characterization of fibroblast growth factor, an angiogenic factor which also controls the proliferation and differentiation of mesoderm and neuroectoderm derived cells, *Cell Differ.* **19**, 1–17.

Grinnell, F., Feld, M.K. 1981. Adsorption characteristics of plasma fibronectin in relationship to biological activity, *J. Biomed. Mater. Res.* **15**, 363–381.

Grinnell, F., Feld, M.K. 1982. Fibronectin adsorption on hydrophilic and hydrophobic surfaces detected by antibody binding and analyzed during cell adhesion in serum containing medium, *J. Biol. Chem.* **257**, 4888–4893.

Grotendorst, G.R., Martin, G.R., Pencet, D., Soddck, J., Harvey, A.K. 1985. Stimulation of granulation tissue formation by platelet-derived growth factor in normal and diabetic rats, *J. Clin. Invest.* **76**, 2323–2329.

Haggerty, L., Watson, B.A., Barteau, M.A., Lenhoff. A.M. 1991. Ordered arrays of proteins on graphite observed by scanning tunneling microscopy, *J. Vac. Sci. Technol. B* **9**(2), 1219–1222.

Hlady, V., Reinecke, D.R., Andrade, J.D. 1986. Fluorescence of adsorbed protein layers. I. Quantitation of total internal reflection fluorescence, *J. Colloid Interface Sci.* **111**, 555–569.

Horbett, T.A. 1996. Proteins, Structure, properties and adsorption to surfaces, in: *Biomaterials Science: An Introduction to Materials in Medicine* (B.D. Ratner, A.S. Hoffman, F.J. Schoen, J.E. Lemons, eds.), Chapter 3, pp. 133–141, Academic Press, New York.

Kisiel, W., Canfield, W.M., Ericsson, L.H., Davie, E.W. 1977. Anticoagulant properties of bovine plasma protein C following activation by trombin, *Biochemistry* **16**, 5824–5831.

Laato, M. 1988. The effects of epidermal growth factor on granulation tissue formation in the rat, *Acta Chir. Scand., Suppl.* **546**, 1–44.

Lawrence, W.T., Sporn, M.B., Gorschboth, C., Norton, J.A., Grotendorst, G.R. 1986. The reversal of an adriamicin induced healing impairment with chemoattractans and growth factors, *Ann. Surg.* **203**, 142–147.

Lu, C.F., Nadarajah, A., Chittur, K. K. 1994. A comprehensive model for protein adsorption to surfaces, *J. Colloid Interface Sci.* **168**, 152–161.

Magnani, A., Barbucci, R. 1993. Fourier transform attenuated total reflection infrared spectroscopy (ATR/FTIR): application to proteins adsorption studies, in: *Test Procedures for the Blood Compatibility of Biomaterials* (S. Dawids, ed.), pp. 171–184, Kluwer Academic, Amsterdam.

Markiewicz, P., Goh, M.C. 1994. Atomic force microscopy probe tip visualization and improvement of images using a simple deconvolution procedure, *Langmuir* **10**, 5–7.

Markiewicz, P., Goh, M. C. 1995. Atomic force microscope tip deconvolution using calibration arrays, *Rev. Sci. Instrum.* **66**(5), 3186–3190.

Merwin, J.R., Newman, W., Beale, L.D., Tucker, A., Madri, J. 1991. Vascular cells respond differentially to transforming growth factors beta 1 and beta 2 in vitro, *Am. J. Pathol.* **138**, 37–56.

Moncada, S., Gryglewski, R., Bunting, S., Vance, J.R. 1976. An enzyme isolated from arteries transforms prostaglandin endoperoxidoses to an unstable substance that inhibits platelet aggregation, *Nature* **263**, 663–665

Montesano, R., Orci, L. 1988. Transforming growth factor β stimulates collagen-matrix contraction by fibroblasts: implications for wound healing, *Proc. Natl. Acad. Sci. USA* **85**, 4894–4897.

Nadarajah, A., Lu, C.F., Chittur, K.K. 1995. Modelling the dynamics of protein adsorption to surfaces, in: *Proteins at Interfaces*, ACS Symposium Series (T.A. Horbett, J.L. Brash, eds.), Chapter 13, pp. 181–194, American Chemical Society, Columbus, OH.

Paulsson, Y., Hammacher, A., Heldin, C-H., Westermark, B. 1987. Possible positive autocrine feedback in the prereplicative phase of human fibrolasts, *Nature* **328**, 715–717.

Perez-Luna, V.H., Horbett, T.A., Ratner, B.D. 1994. Developing correlations between fibrinogen adsorption and surface properties using multivariate statistics, *J. Biomed. Mater. Res.* **28**, 1111–1126.

Pitt, W.G., Spielgelberg, S.H., Cooper, S.L. 1987. Adsorption of fibronectin to polyurethane surfaces: Fourier transform infrared spectroscopic studies, in: *Proteins at Interfaces: Physicochemical and Biochemical Studies*, Vol. 343 (J.L. Brash, T.A. Horbett, eds.), pp. 324–338, American Chemical Society, Washington, D.C.

Postlethwaite, A.E., Keski-Oja, J., Moses, H.L., Kang, A.H. 1987. Stimulation of the chemotactic migration of human fibroblasts by trasforming growth factor beta, *J Exp. Med.* **165**, 251–256.

Rappolee, D.A., Mark, D., Bande, M.J., Werb, Z., 1988. Wound macrophages express TaF-2 and other growth factors in vivo: Analysis by mRNA phenotyping, *Science* **241**, 708–712.

Roberts, A.B., Sporn, M.B., Assoian, R.K., Smith, J.M., Roche, N.S., Wakefield, L.M., Heine, U.I., Liotta, L.A., Flanga, V., Kehrl, J.H., Fauci, A.S. 1986. Transforming growth factor type β, rapid induction of fibrosis and angiogenesis *in vivo* and stimulation of collagen formation in vitro, *Proc. Natl. Acad. Sci. USA* **83**, 4167–4171.

Rockhold, S.A., Quinn, R.D., Van Wagenen, R.A., Andrade, J.D., Reichert, W.M. 1983. Total internal reflection fluorescence (TIRF) as a quantitative probe of protein adsorption, *J. Electroanal. Chem.* **150**, 261–275.

Russell, W.E., Coffey, R.J. Jr., Ouellette, A.J., Moses, H.L. 1988. Type beta transforming growth factor reversibly inhibits the early proliferative response to partial hepatectomy in the rat, *Proc. Natl. Acad. Sci. USA* **85**(14), 5126–5130.

Sarid, D., Ellings, V. 1991. Review of scanning force microscopy, *J. Vac. Sci. Technol. B* **9**, 431–437.

Savion, N., Vlodawshy, I., Fuks, Z. 1984. Interaction of T lymphocytes and macrophages with cultured vascular endothelial cells, *J. Cell Physiol.* **118**, 169–178.

Siedlecki, C.A., Eppell, S.J., Marchant, R.E. 1994. Interactions of human Von-Willebrand factor with a hydrophobic self-assembled monolayer studied by atomic-force microscopy, *J. Biomed. Mater. Res.* **28**(9), 971–980.

Silberstein, G.B., Daniel, C.W. 1989. Reversible inhibition of mammary gland growth by transforming growth factor beta, *Science* **237**(4812), 291–293.

Simpson, D.M., Ross, R. 1972. The neutrophilic leukocyte in wound repair. A study with antineutrophil serum, *J. Clin. Invest.* **51**, 2009–2023.

Slack, S.M., Horbett, T.A. 1988. Physicochemical and biochemical aspects of fibrinogen adsorption from plasma and binary protein solution onto polyethylene and glass, *J. Colloid Interface Sci.*, **124**, 533–551.

Slack, S.M., Horbett, T. A. 1989. Changes in the strength of fibrinogen attachment to solid surfaces, An explanation of the influence of surface chemistry on the Vroman effect, *J. Colloid Interface Sci.* **133**. 148–156.

Sporn, M.B., Roberts, A.B., Wakefield, L.M., Crombrugghe, B. 1987. Some recent advances in the chemistry and biology of transforming growth factor beta, *J. Cell Biol.* **105**, 1039–1045.

Sprugel, K.H., McPherson, J.M., Clowes, A.W., Ross, R. 1988. The effects of different growth factors in subcutaneous wound chambers, *Prog. Clin. Res.* **266**, 77–91.

Stipp, S.L.S. 1996. In situ, real-time observations of the adsorption and self-assembly of macromolecules from aqueous solution onto an untreated, natural surface, *Langmuir* **12**, 1884–1891.

Sukenik, C.N., Lewandowska, K., Balachander, N., Culp, L.A. 1989. Modulation of fibronectin adhesive functions for fibroblasts and neural cells by chemically derivatized substrata, *J. Cell Physiol.* **141**, 334–341.

Sukenik, C.N., Balachander, N., Culp, L. A., Lewandowska, K., Merritt, K. 1990. Modulation of cell adhesion by modification of titanium surfaces with covalently attached self-assembled monolayers, *J. Biomed. Mater. Res.* **24**, 1307–1311.

Tsunawaki, S., Sporn, M., Ding, A., Nathan, C. 1988. Dectivation of macrophages by transforming growth factor-β, *Nature* **334**, 260–262.

Van Obberghen-Schilling, E., Roche, N.S., Flanders, K.C., Sporn, M.B., Roberts, A.B. 1988. Transforming growth factor $\beta 1$ positively regulates its own expression in normal and transformed cells, *J. Biol. Chem.* **263**, 7741–7746.

Villarrubia, J.S. 1994. Morphological estimation of tip geometry for scanned probe microscopy, *Surf. Sci.* **321**, 287–300.

Villarrubia, J.S. 1996. Scanned probe microscope tip characterization without calibrated tip characterizers, *J. Vac. Sci. Technol. B* **14**, 1518–1521.

Wahl, S.M., Hunt, D.A., Wakefield, L.M., McCartney-Francis, N., Wahl L.M., Roberts, A.B., Sporn, M.B. 1987. Transforming growth factor beta (TGF-beta) induces monocyte chemotaxis and growth factor production, *Proc. Natl. Acad. Sci. USA* **84**, 5788–5792.

Wilbur, J.L., Biebuyck, H.A, MacDonald, J.C., Whitesides, G.M. 1995. Scanning force microscopies can image patterned self-assembled monolayers, *Langmuir*, **11**, 825–831.

Wilson, D.L., Kump, K.S., Eppell, S.J., Marchant, R.E. 1995. Morphological restoration of atomic-force microscopy images, *Langmuir* **11**(1), 265–272.

Wojciechowski, P., ten Hove, P., Brash, J.L. 1986. Phenomenology and mechanisms of the transient adsorption of fibrinogen from plasma (Vroman effect), *J. Colloid Interface Sci.* **111**, 455–461.

Yahalom, J., Eldor, A., Fuks, Z. 1984. Degradation of sulfated proteoglycans in the subendothelial basement membrane by human platelet heparitinase, *J. Clin. Invest.* **74**, 1842–1849.

Yang, E.Y., Moses, H.L. 1990. Transforming growth factor beta 1-induced changes in cell migration, proliferation, and angiogenesis in the chicken chorioallantoic membrane, *J. Cell. Biol.* **111**, 731–741.

25

Inflammatory Response to Polymeric Materials

Denis Labarre and Marie-Paule Carreno

25.1. Introduction

The inflammatory response is historically defined as "A tissue reaction that results in rubor, calor, dolor and functio laesa." This nonspecific response is characterized by the activation of the complement system, chemotactic attraction of phagocytes, and an increased vascular permeability. It consists in a series of primarily local events occurring as the normal response expected from the organism of a healthy individual for its self-protection against any foreign attack, allowing the isolation of the foreign body and the elimination of injured cells, and preparing a normal tissue repair.

Thus, the inflammatory response plays a pivotal role in the biocompatibility of a material considered as a foreign body. In addition to the initial injury induced by its introduction into a living system, the persistent presence of the foreign material in contact with a living tissue induces an inflammatory response which can remain local, benign, and short, or can become systemic, persistent, and health-threatening. A material of optimal biocompatibility should not add to the normal inflammatory response, nor prevent the tissue repair.

The inflammatory response is a time-dependent process. It starts by the acute phase, is followed by the chronic phase, and its normal end is tissue repair. Different types of ions, proteins, mediators, and leukocytes are involved during the different phases. The rate, the intensity and the duration of the events occurring at the molecular level in the surroundings of the

---

Denis Labarre • Laboratoire de Biomatériaux et Polymères, UMR CNRS 8612, Université Paris-Sud XI, 92290 Châtenay-Malabry, France. • **Marie-Paule Carreno** • Laboratoire d'Immunopathologie Humaine, INSERM U430, Hôpital Broussais, 75014 Paris, France.

Integrated Biomaterials Science, edited by R. Barbucci. Kluwer Academic/Plenum Publishers, New York, 2002.

material during the different phases depend on many parameters because the inflammatory response is a very cooperative phenomenon. It starts at a low molecular level on the surface of the material by exchanges of water and hydrated ions, fast adsorption or binding of proteins likely followed by conformational changes. Then it develops by amplification loops owing to activation of humoral systems and recruitment of different cell subpopulations capable of producing and secreting mediators allowing information exchanges and various activities. As a result, the inflammatory response depends strongly on the material, but also on the site of interaction between the material and the living tissue.

Introducing the detailed features of inflammation and of the complement system is far beyond the scope of this chapter and will not be presented. Owing to its ability to induce a nonspecific recognition of particulate foreign bodies, the complement system plays a major role in the induction of the inflammatory response. A schematic view of the role played by complement in cooperation with leukocytes in inflammation and phagocytosis can be found in the paper published by Frank and Fries (1991).

The present chapter deals first with the specifications and the types of polymeric biomaterials in contact with living tissues. Then physicochemical characteristics of the materials such as size, surface area, surface morphology, hydrophilicity and hydrophobicity, crystallinity, surface structure, and surface chemistry, which are involved in the inflammatory response, are presented. Some recent results concerning the assessment of the inflammatory response to materials, either in close contact with blood or in contact with other tissues, are reviewed. After a conclusion, a list of the abbreviations used in the chapter is given in the Appendix.

25.2. Polymeric Materials in Contact with Living Tissues

Polymeric materials have been increasingly used in contact with living tissues. More and more are designed to interact with biological systems, i.e., true biomaterials, but classical polymers are still used for obvious economical reasons. The materials are supposed to be selected according to precise specifications required to match the function. Depending on the physical and chemical characteristics which are required, some of them can be found in different uses while some others are only found in very specialized ones.

25.2.1. Specifications

The choice of a polymeric material designed for being used in contact with living tissues usually involves many requirements and some of them can be relevant to the inflammatory response:

- The choice of a material will be determined mainly by its bulk mechanical or other physical properties required to match the function. They are essentially related to the molecular structure of the polymeric material (semicrystalline, glassy, rubbery) and some can be relevant to the inflammatory process.
- The presence of the lowest amount of low molecular weight species and possibly toxic or irritating leachables in the material matrix or on its surface is a prominent requirement. It is the reason why flexible poly(vinyl chloride) (PVC), which contains significant amounts of plasticizers and stabilizing agents, is not used in implanted devices in spite of its low cost and high versatility. The weak biocompatibility of usual flexible PVC-based materials is not linked to high molecular weight PVC. When examining PVC and an aliphatic polyurethane (Tecoflex) containing various amounts of plasticizers, Lindner *et al.* (1994) demonstrated that an increase in plasticizer weight percent correlated positively in Tecoflex with the increase in host inflammatory response up to 14 days of implantation. Comparing PVC and Tecoflex at a similar polymer-to-plasticizer ratio, a similar acute inflammatory response was observed, but the PVC-based membrane elicited a reduced chronic inflammatory response. PVC is still used as main constituent of simple disposable devices designed for some short-term uses such as catheters or blood bags. Concerning at least the reduction of migration of low molecular weight species, it could be improved with surface treatments (Jayakrishnan and Lakshmi, 1998). Migration of such small molecules is also a major concern in the case of gel-filled silicone breast implants. The polymer constituting the envelope, which is silicone rubber, i.e., poly(dimethyl siloxane) (PDMS), is hydrophobic, amorphous, and compliant. Thus it allows a fast diffusion of hydrophobic molecules through its network. The highly diffusible small molecules "bleed" through the surrounding envelope and migrate, inducing many adverse reactions (Busch, 1994; Rhie *et al.*, 1998). Among several coatings, Bocchiotti *et al.* (1993) proposed to coat such implants with a thin film of turbostratic carbon.
- The requirement of sterility at the end of the manufacturing process for any biomedical or pharmaceutical device designed to be in contact with living systems, is mandatory. The aggressive treatments required to sterilize a device can substantially modify the initial bulk and surface characteristics of its polymeric constituents. For instance, cross-linking or chain scission can be induced during steril-

ization by ionizing radiation. Small toxic molecules are introduced in the polymeric matrix and on its surface following sterilization by ethylene oxide. However, if sterilization procedures can substantially modify the physical properties of the material, the biological response is sometimes unrelated. For instance, the effects of three different sterilization procedures, i.e., by beta irradiation, ethylene oxide, and steam, have been evaluated by Zhang *et al.* (1996) on two polymeric materials, a silicone and a polyurethane (PU), by implantation in rats for 10 and 90 days. The numbers of macrophages, giant cells, fibroblasts and other cells present at the surfaces were evaluated. The PU surface showed signs of degradation already after sterilization, especially after ethylene oxide treatment. However, differences in the biological responses were small and independent of the sterilization method but depended more on the material.

- Another relevant requirement is either the biostability, for instance in the case of materials for permanent implanted prostheses, or, on the contrary, a controlled biodegradability, as in the case of materials for deep sutures, or for injected particulate drug carriers or for internal fracture fixation devices. Even in the case of the so-called biostable materials, the polymers will age at different rates depending on the polymer itself and on its local environment. Local constraints will induce crazes, cracks, and fragmentation which can be relevant to the inflammatory processes. In the case of biodegradable polymers, the type of degraded molecules and their rates of production and elimination are of prime importance. This point will be emphasized in another paragraph.

While the choice of a material is mainly determined owing to its bulk properties, the so-called biocompatibility concerning the inflammatory response is mainly determined by the physical and chemical properties of the surface of the material interacting with its local environment. Consequently, it should be remembered that the capacity to induce inflammation concerning a medical device used by a surgical team can be completely different from the capacity of the pure polymer constituting the bulk of the device. This is again typically exemplified by silicone gel-filled breast implants with gel bleeding and talc deposition on the surface (Kasper and Chandler, 1994). As a lot of confusion concerning the biocompatibility of polymers results from the lack of definition of the material which is actually used, pure polymeric materials should be included as controls in the evaluation tests. Indeed, the community of people interested in the use of materials in contact with living tissues needs to discriminate between the effects due to additives or other leachables or contaminants linked to device processing, and the effects related to pure and well-defined polymers.

25.2.2. Polymeric Materials

Part of defined devices or isolated, polymeric materials have a size, a shape, and a surface morphology. They can be homogeneous or heterogeneous in the bulk or on the surface, e.g., coated, used as coating, or separated into phases. They can be classified through different properties such as their physical state, e.g., rubbery, rigid, amorphous, semicrystalline, or their susceptibility to degradation. Some of them are well-defined concerning their chemical composition, while others resulting mainly from surface modifications by processes such as glow discharge are not so precisely defined.

Owing to its long and successful history in human accidental or deliberate implantation, poly(methyl methacrylate) (PMMA) is widely used on or inside the eye, but also as the main constituent of acrylic cements used to anchor articular prostheses.

Polymers such as high-density polyethylene (HDPE) have been used for artificial hip or knee joints. Polypropylene (PP) is well known as a nondegradable suture material. Poly(ethylene terephthalate) (PET) and expanded poly(tetrafluoroethylene) (ePTFE) have been extensively used as vascular substitutes for large arteries and in reconstructive surgery, or the nonporous PTFE sometimes associated to Proplast (Proplast-Teflon) has been used as temporomandibular joints.

Rubbery polymers have many uses under different forms, either as bulk material or as coating, e.g., catheters, shunts and tentative small-diameter vascular prostheses, breast implants, wrist, elbow, or finger implants, joints, etc. Silicone rubber, mainly poly(dimethyl siloxane) (PDMS), has been the most extensively used. Elastomeric poly(ether urethane)s (PEU) and poly(ether urethane urea)s (PEUU) have also been proposed for such uses.

Even if they are not usually used alone as linear polymers, water-soluble or water-swollen polymers retain their capacity to swell in the presence of water when slightly cross-linked or bound on a surface. Apart from slightly cross-linked poly(2-hydroxyethyl methacrylate) (PHEMA) and substituted polyacrylamides (PAAm), which are used alone, for instance, in ocular lenses (Wichterle and Lim, 1960) or as microspheres for therapeutic embolization (Jayakrishnan *et al.*, 1990; Beaujeux *et al.*, 1996; Laurent *et al.*, 1996), most of the water-soluble polymers and hydrogels, such as poly(ethylene oxide) (PEO), poly(acrylic acid) (PAAc), poly(vinyl pyrrolidone) (PVP), and poly(vinyl alkohol) (PVA), are only used as surface modifiers to endow a substrate with hydrophilic surface properties.

In addition to the water-swollen polymers, several other polymers have been studied as coatings, e.g., silicone, fluorinated polymers, PET, and PEU. Some are surface-grafted by processes such as glow discharge and the resulting polymers are not as precisely defined as classical polymers.

Biodegradable and bioerodible polymers are designed for temporary uses and to be eliminated when they are no longer useful. They are used as tissue adhesive, e.g., poly(alkyl cyanoacrylate)s (PACA), or for sutures in deep wound closure, e.g., poly(glycolic acid) also named polyglycolide (PGA), poly(lactic acid)s also named polylactides (PLA) varying from 100% L PLA (PLLA) to racemic PLA (PLA50), poly(ε caprolactone) (PCL), copolymers of lactic and glycolic acids (PLGA), or copolymers of lactic acid and ε caprolactone. They are increasingly used in reconstructive surgery as plates, screws, films, patches, pins, etc. They can also be used as constituents of nanoparticles designed for drug delivery through parenteral administration or of microparticles for drug delivery through different routes or for short-term embolization purposes.

Finally, the effects resulting from chemical modifications of polymers on various biological systems have been studied with polymers which can be modified rather easily, such as polystyrene (PS), and applied to polymers, such as PEU and PEUU containing phenyl rings.

25.3. Characteristics of the Materials Involved in the Inflammatory Response

Providing that our own cells are normal, they do not induce an autologous inflammatory response, owing to their surface biochemistry. Concerning materials, the question whether the inflammatory response depends on both their physical and chemical characteristics stimulates controversial answers. For instance, Boss *et al.* (1995) conclude from their study on polyethylene that the manner in which the host handles the biomaterials is determined primarily by the physical state of the biomaterials (rather than their chemical composition).

The aim of this section is trying to identify some characteristics of polymeric materials which are involved in the inflammatory response, by examining the influences of their surface features. The surface features can be either purely physical, such as surface area, smoothness, or shape, or physicochemical, such as hydrophilicity, hydrophobicity, lipophobicity, ionic charge, crystallinity, phase separation, of surface mobility, or purely chemical, such as type of linked functional groups or surface contamination.

25.3.1. Size, Surface Area, and Surface Morphology

The inflammatory response is primarily a surface-related phenomenon. Thus it should be exquisitely sensitive to physical surface features such as size and surface area, smoothness and shape, and local curvature radius. This sensitivity can be evidenced with particles used either as models, or as drug carriers, or recovered as wear fragments, for instance in intra-articular prostheses. Concerning nonporous particles, the surface-to-volume ratio (S/V) of particles increases when their average size decreases and this ratio is directly related to the specific surface area by the specific gravity of the material. If the material is porous, the S/V ratio is still increased. It is clear that, concerning biological reactions to materials, comparison between materials should be done on a surface area basis. Taking into account the internal open porosity of the material in these reactions has to be carefully scrutinized.

The S/V ratio and the size are of prime importance for at least two reasons. The first one is that the higher the ratio, i.e., the smaller the size, the higher the surface area at constant volume or weight of material. The second one is that micronic and submicronic particles can be phagocytized and processed by "professional" phagocytes such as macrophages, while larger materials are equally able to induce locally an inflammatory response but cannot be phagocytized. Hence even if the material is the same, the consequences on the fate of the material and on the biological response can be very different depending, for instance, on the elimination rate of the particles. Gelb *et al.* (1994) have evaluated in a subcutaneous rat air-pouch model the *in vivo* effects of the size, morphology, and surface area of poly(methyl methacrylate) (PMMA) particles on the acute inflammatory response and have shown the influence of these parameters.

At least hydrated ions, proteins, and cells are involved and cooperate in the inflammatory response. The size of proteins is in the nanometer range while the size of cells is in the micrometer range. As a result, the smoothness of a material surface is a relative concept, depending on the contacted species.

When the surface of a material is in contact with a living tissue, the first species arriving at the interface are the most diffusible. Coming along with water and ion exchanges, adsorption of proteins is kinetically the initial step in the induction of the inflammatory response. Researchers working in the field of protein separation by chromatographic techniques have demonstrated extensively that proteins can be adsorbed as any macromolecule on almost all kinds of material surfaces. Adsorption characteristics such as the number of adsorption sites, the affinity, and the reversibility with the time of residence depend on the protein–surface pair. As proteins are not rigid, conformational changes are likely to occur to adapt the protein to its new interfacial environment. In addition, if the material is porous, proteins can be retained in the pores, providing that they are larger than the exclusion volume of the proteins.

If the adsorption of individual proteins does need neither a large space nor special steric requirements, the case is already different for some enzymatic sites which need an assembly of proteins and other species to be efficient. Enzymatic sites such as the alternative C3-convertase, which is composed of C3bBb, magnesium ions, and stabilized by protein P, or even more a C5-convertase site which requires additional linked C3b, need a sufficient space. In addition, they should meet steric requirements which could not always be fulfilled, for instance, on the surface of small nanoparticles or liposomes. Harashima *et al.* (1994) have shown that the extent of opsonization and subsequent hepatic uptake of liposomes decreased with the decrease in size of liposomes (from 800 to 200 nm in diameter) and no enhancement of uptake was observed at 200 nm when compared to unopsonized liposomes. However, nanoparticles smaller than 200 nm can be taken up by the Mononuclear Phagocytic System (MPS) (Bazile *et al.*, 1995) and can efficiently activate the complement system (Vittaz *et al.*, 1996).

Cells do not "see" the same material surface as proteins for at least two reasons. The first one is that they are far larger, and the second is that cells usually interact with an already opsonized (i.e., covered with proteins) material surface. But owing to their "large" size, cells are sensitive to materials with sharp angles or short curvature radius and to textured surfaces (Bern *et al.*, 1992; Brohim *et al.*, 1992; Kasper, 1994). Marois *et al.* (1992) have investigated some effects of porous structures of polyurethanes and ePTFE on blood T cell subsets. Another example is given by Lam *et al.* (1995), who studied the influence of surface morphology and wettability on both degradable (PLLA) and nondegradable (PTFE) polymer films and concluded that porosity enhanced the inflammatory response only when the wettability of the material permitted cellular ingrowth. More recently, James *et al.* (1997) evaluated in rats the inflammatory response to a silicone elastomer and compared it with porous and nonporous cellulose acetate filters, in order to show a possible link to carcinogenicity. However, as the surface area of porous materials is increased when compared to that one of nonporous materials, the effects induced by both types of surfaces and not due to such an increase should be evaluated on a surface area basis.

25.3.2. Physicochemical Parameters

When examining a large number of papers devoted to the inflammatory response to materials surfaces, it can be seen that the response depends more on combinations rather than on isolated physicochemical parameters, because it involves very discriminating processes.

25.3.2.1. Hydrophilicity, Hydrophobicity, Lipophobicity, and Critical Surface Tension

Hydrophilicity, hydrophobicity, and lipophobicity of materials are properties which are likely involved in their biocompatibility, but the link between such physical properties and a complex biological response is not obvious. Because such properties are qualitative, a first question is whether they could be easily quantified by a single parameter which could be, for instance, the critical surface tension (CST). CST has been proposed as a key parameter concerning the biocompatibility of polymers.

The CST of a material is supposed to reflect its complete wettability. After determining contact angles (θ) at the interface between the material, different liquids, and their vapors, the CST value of the material is calculated according to classical equations, by extrapolating at $\cos\theta = 1$, i.e., $\theta = 0$.

According to the published data, polytetrafluoroethylene (PTFE) is very hydrophobic and even lipophobic (CST = 19 dynes/cm). The CSTs of poly(dimethyl siloxane) (PDMS) (24 dynes/cm) and poly(vinylidene fluoride) (PVDF) (25 dynes/cm) are almost similar and both materials are supposed to be more hydrophobic than polyethylene (PE) (31 dynes/cm). The CST of poly(2-hydroxyethyl methacrylate) (PHEMA) (37 dynes/cm) is lower than those of poly(methyl methacrylate) (PMMA) (39 dynes/cm) and poly(ethylene terephthalate) (PET) (43 dynes/cm).

The data concerning PHEMA are rather confusing, because this material has been developed as the main constituent of hydrated contact lenses. It can take about one-third of its weight of water and it has been shown that its surface wettability depends on the "history" of the material, mainly on its local environment. When PHEMA is dried, its surface is indeed rather hydrophobic, as reflected by its low CST value. When placed in contact with an aqueous solution, its surface undergoes a very slow rearrangement. But this phenomenon takes a long time at room temperature because the glass transition temperature of PHEMA is above room temperature (T_g is given in the range 328–359 K).

It results that the critical surface tension of a material such as PHEMA is not sufficient to quantify its hydrophilic/hydrophobic properties. If CST cannot reflect properly such properties which are still rather simple, its intrinsic value as a key parameter to correlate with a response as complex as the inflammatory response is highly questionable.

However, there is experimental evidence that the adsorption of proteins on hydrophobic surfaces induces changes of conformation of the adsorbed species, leading to a fast decrease in the reversibility of the adsorption versus time and to modifications of the surface epitopes of the adsorbed protein when compared to those of the soluble native one. This is the reason why surfaces such as polystyrene (PS) (Nilsson *et al.*, 1993a, b) and polypropylene (PP) or silicone (Gobel *et al.*, 1987) can activate the complement system by a mechanism which does not need any covalent binding of nascent C3b on the surface.

Concerning hydrophilic material surfaces, it is to be expected that they can induce complement activation if their hydrophilic character is linked to the presence of nucleophilic chemical groups able to bind nascent C3b (see below concerning the effects linked to surface chemistry). But the presence of such groups is not a necessary requirement to induce complement activation because, as shown above, the contact with a hydrophobic surface can be sufficient to trigger such a response by conformational changes following C3 adsorption on the surface.

25.3.2.2. Crystallinity of Surfaces and Surface Structure

In order to decrease the sharp transition at the interface between a hydrated living tissue and a hydrophobic material, a very popular strategy has been to modify the surface for increasing its hydrophilicity without introducing polymers endowed with a known complement activating capacity. Many water-soluble or very hydrophilic polymers have been tested for this purpose. As the chemical groups which induce hydrophilicity can be very different, the induced effects which are more linked to surface chemistry are examined in a further paragraph.

If we focus on the physicochemical aspects, it was already shown that crystalline, i.e., ordered, polymers such as Nylons induced complement activation through its classical pathway (Herzlinger *et al.*, 1981). It has also been shown that thermal treatments of polymer surfaces resulting in surface crystallization can strongly influence the activation of complement protein C1, probably because of the increased organization of the surface which makes possible an increased recognition by C1 (Niinobe *et al.*, 1988). As a result, the surface modification by hydrophilic polymers devoid of nucleophilic groups and remaining in an amorphous state could be necessary if recognition by C3 and C1 is expected to be avoided.

It could be the case for poly(ethylene oxide) (PEO) modified surfaces. The binding of PEO on surfaces has been proposed for a long time by Merrill and Salzman (1983). However, the results have been sometimes disappointing. Chaikof *et al.* (1992) have found an increased C3 activation in the presence of surfaces bearing low molecular weight (2,000) PEO and a decreased activation in the presence of surfaces bearing higher molecular weight (20,000) PEO. Thus, increasing the surface hydrophilicity by binding of such polymers is not sufficient per se but more the density of PEO and the structure of the hydrophilic surface.

Jeon *et al.* (1991) and Jeon and Andrade (1991) have modeled the interactions between a protein and a surface bearing PEO chains terminally attached by one end to a hydrophobic solid substrate. Their calculations lead to the conclusions that a surface bearing terminally attached PEO with a high surface density and a sufficient chain length should exhibit optimal protein resistance, with the attainment of high surface density being more important than long chain length.

Such models have been experimentally tested with nanoparticulate systems made from polylactides (PLA) and block copolymers of PLA-PEO. Such copolymers composed of one block of PLA 30,000 covalently linked to one block of PEO 2,000 (PLA_{30}-PEO_2) can readily self-organize when placed into aqueous solutions, even without added surfactant, into sterically stabilized nanoparticles with a mean diameter of about 100 nm. The kinetics of complement activation by such particles of PLA-PEO (Vittaz *et al.*, 1996) and their uptake by the MPS (Gref *et al.*, 1994; Bazile *et al.*, 1995) are very slow. Their effects on plasma coagulation proteins are negligible, in contrast to the effects observed in the presence of control PLA particles (Sahli *et al.*, 1997). Fernandez-Urrusuno *et al.* (1995) have shown that after intravenous injection of different kinds of nanoparticles into rats, the production of α1-acid glycoprotein, an acute phase protein, is reduced in the presence of long-circulating nanoparticles made from biblock copolymers PLA-PEO, when compared with particles made from the homopolymer PLA, or polystyrene (PS), or surfactant-coated PS nanoparticles.

The average surface density of PEO on the particles can be decreased by a controlled and limited hydrolysis of some PEO chains, without destabilizing the colloidal suspension and changing the average diameter of the particles. When the average surface density of PEO on the particles is below a given threshold, a fast complement activation has been observed (Vittaz *et al.*, 1996). In another system, nanoparticles were prepared from mixtures of PLA_{20}-PEO_5 copolymers with PLA_{50} and their uptake by phagocytic cells was measured (Gref *et al.*, 1998). Reduction of the uptake was found above a given threshold concerning the proportion of PEO in the mixture. In both cases, the thresholds corresponded to a calculated average distance of about 2.2 nm between two adjacent PEO chains. The latter authors have also shown that a minimal level of adsorption was found for different plasma proteins on PLA-PEO surfaces with PEO chains of molecular weight above 2,000. On increasing the PEO molecular weight to above 5,000, only small changes in plasma protein adsorption were obtained.

The influence of the configuration of PEO on the surface was also examined. Polymerization of isobutylcyanoacrylate (IBCA) was initiated in the presence of either α,ω-dihydroxy-PEO, or α-methoxy, ω-hydroxy-PEO, or α,ω-dimethoxy-PEO. Nanoparticles were formed in both the first cases and not in the latter. Their capacity to activate complement was tested. Both of them activated complement to a lesser extent than control PIBCA nanoparticles. When compared on a surface area basis, the best results were obtained with nanoparticles made from α,ω-dihydroxy-PEO, i.e., PIBCA-PEO-PIBCA, which is supposed to form loops on the surface, i.e., side-on configuration, when compared with nanoparticles made from α-methoxy, ω-hydroxy-PEO, i.e., PIBCA-PEO, which is supposed to form a brush, i.e., end-on configuration, on the surface (Peracchia *et al.*, 1997).

Despite the fact that PEO has been the most studied polymer for this purpose, such steric repulsive effects are not limited to this polymer and dextran has also been tested. Österberg *et al.* (1995) studied the fibrinogen-rejecting ability of surface-bound dextran in end-on and side-on configurations and compared them with end-on PEO. End-on PEO and side-on dextran were more effective than end-on dextran for reducing fibrinogen adsorption on modified aminated polystyrene plates or tubes.

These results support those of Peracchia *et al.* concerning a more protective effect for a side-on configuration. But they seem to be conflicting with those obtained by Carreno *et al.* (1988) and Passirani *et al.* (1998a) on the respective abilities of Sephadex® (cross-linked dextran) and of dextran terminally-linked to the surface of PMMA nanoparticles (Nanodex) to activate complement. In Sephadex, the dextran chains which are cross-linked are likely in a side-on configuration on the surface, while they are likely in an end-on configuration on the surface of Nanodex. When present in Nanodex, dextran was as a poor activator of complement as soluble dextran when compared on a weight basis, and more than twenty times less activator than crushed Sephadex when compared on a surface area basis.

However, the data of Österberg *et al.* are related to fibrinogen, which is not known to possess a binding capacity to surface-bound nucleophilic groups. In the experiments of Peracchia *et al.*, side-on PEO does not present nucleophilic groups to reactive proteins such as nascent C3b, while side-on dextran presents a large number of nucleophilic groups, as is the case in the experiments of Carreno *et al.* Some differences in the complement activating capacities of dextran derivatives could also result from the fact that the curvature radius of Sephadex particles is larger than that of Nanodex, because the average diameter of crushed Sephadex was about two orders of magnitude larger than that of Nanodex. Thus, it could be interesting to compare side-on bound dextran in nanoparticles with Sephadex and

Nanodex concerning their respective abilities to activate complement before drawing a last conclusion concerning the most efficient configuration of bound dextran for decreasing complement activation. Nanodex particles have also been shown to circulate more than 48 hours *in vivo* when injected into mice (compared to less than 1 hour for control PMMA particles), probably owing to a slow recognition by MPS (Passirani *et al.*, 1998b).

From the models of Jeon *et al.* and from the different experimental data obtained with nanoparticles and liposomes, it is clear that the rate and the extent of opsonization by plasmatic proteins, and especially complement and coagulation proteins, can be strongly reduced on surfaces bearing either amorphous PEO chains terminally linked to the surface by one or two ends, or dextran chains linked by one end, with sufficiently high surface density and length. Such a property is already used in clinical studies with long-circulating liposomes bearing on their surface PEO chains anchored into the lipid bilayer and carrying anti-cancer drugs (Allen *et al.*, 1998; Goren *et al.*, 1998).

Such efficient surface modifications should not be limited to PEO and dextran. Other water-soluble macromolecules could also be good candidates, providing that they are bound in an efficient configuration. However, despite the fact that the rate of opsonization and/or complement activation can be reduced owing to a "right" outside structure of PEO, these reactions are not inhibited but only slowed down. Possible long-term effects on the inflammatory response are not known yet. In addition, all these kinds of submicronic particles are self-organized systems and it should be much more difficult from a technical point of view to obtain larger objects regularly covered with a sufficient surface density of PEO or other very hydrated polymers.

25.3.2.3. Surface Chemistry

The prominent role of surface chemistry in the inflammatory response is illustrated by what is known concerning the natural surface of cells. Normal mammalian cells are protected from complement-mediated self-destruction by regulatory membrane proteins, including complement receptor type 1 (CR1), membrane cofactor protein (MCP), and decay-accelerating factor (DAF). On normal cells, such regulatory proteins prevent the amplification processes following a random and low level deposition of nascent C3b or C3b-like-C3 on their surface from blood plasma. Besides such proteins, it has been shown that membrane-associated sialic acid regulates the competition between human factor B and factor H for cell-bound C3b on sheep erythrocytes. Thus, a deficiency of sialic acid diminishes the number of high affinity sites for H and turns a nonactivating into an activating surface on which B can efficiently bind and amplify the initial nonspecific low activation (Kazatchkine *et al.*, 1979a).

The capacity to use different features of the complement system to invade the human host without being destroyed by lysis has been developed for ages by pathogens (Cooper, 1991). Some of them are able to escape complement activation by mimicking some complement regulatory functions. Such a strategy has been developed concerning long-circulating liposomes bearing ganglioside M1 (Allen and Chonn, 1987).

Other compounds are able to modulate the action of complement. For instance, heparin, the well-known anticoagulant, has also been shown to inhibit complement activation at different stages (Ecker and Gross, 1929; Loos *et al.*, 1976; Weiler *et al.*, 1978; Kazatchkine *et al.*, 1981). Binding of heparin to zymosan, which is a powerful particulate complement activator, turns it into a nonactivating surface (Kazatchkine *et al.*, 1979b). Thus, binding of heparin or heparin-like molecules to surfaces has been suggested to be a way of improving blood compatibility of polymeric surfaces by increasing the local activity of inhibitory proteins controlling coagulation and complement activation (Labarre, 1990). However, the way how heparin is bound on the surface is likely important concerning the activity of the resulting modified surface (Mollnes *et al.*, 1995).

Heparin is a mixture of polysaccharides, and it has been shown that despite the fact that the presence of sulfate groups is necessary to obtain both anticoagulant and anticomplement activities, the sites involved in the inhibitory activities are independent (Maillet *et al.*, 1988). As a polysaccharide, heparin is susceptible to degrade, and modification of surfaces by introducing sulfate or sulfonate groups is thus an attractive alternative to heparinization to avoid a possible degradation, and to decrease the inflammatory reactions. Several authors have described different methods for introducing such groups on polymer surfaces. The results are sometimes paradoxical, as illustrated by those of Bitter-Suermann *et al.* (1981), Montdargent *et al.* (1991), Toufik *et al.* (1995), Keogh *et al.* (1996), and a lot of work is still necessary to understand the molecular phenomena occurring at such interfaces.

Concerning the effects of other chemical groups borne by polymeric surfaces on complement activation, it has been shown previously that contact with hydrophobic surfaces such as polystyrene (PS) or polypropylene, in which phenyl rings and methyl groups are respectively borne by a vinylic backbone, could be sufficient to induce complement activation. Decreasing the hydrophobicity of a surface by introducing some hydrophilic groups can further increase this activation if such groups are endowed with nucleophilic characteristics. For instance, Montdargent *et al.* (1991) have modified PS surfaces by grafting an increasing number of hydroxymethyl

(CH_2OH) groups. The modified surfaces remained low complement activators when up to an average of 70% of the phenyl rings were modified, but became strong activators when about 90% (PS-$CH_2OH_{0.9}$) of the rings were modified. Copolymers of hydroxyethyl methacrylate (HEMA) and ethyl methacrylate were also able to activate complement and the activation increased with the percentage of HEMA in the copolymers (Payne and Horbett, 1987). It has been known for more than twenty years now that cellulosic membranes are strong activators of complement (Craddock *et al.*, 1977a).

Thus, the activating capacity of polymeric surfaces bearing hydroxyl groups is well documented, but the relationship between the degree of substitution of a polymeric surface in hydroxyl (OH) groups and its capacity to behave like a strong or a low activator of complement is not well understood. For instance, concerning polymers bearing only OH groups, cross-linked dextran (Sephadex®) and cross-linked poly[N-acryloyl-2-amino-2-(hydroxymethyl)-1,3-propanediol] (Trisacryl®) bear three OH groups per repeating unit of respective molecular weight = 162 and 175, while PS-$CH_2OH_{0.9}$ bears less than one OH group per repeating unit of molecular weight = 135. When their complement activating capacity is compared on a surface area basis, it decreases in the order Sephadex > PS-$CH_2OH_{0.9}$ > Trisacryl, while their density in OH groups decreases in the order Sephadex > Trisacryl ≫ PS-$CH_2OH_{0.9}$ (Labarre and Passirani, 1996).

This means that the presence of OH groups on a polymeric surface increases its complement activating capacity but the capacity is not directly related to their density. In addition, decreasing the density of OH groups on a polysaccharidic surface by substituting them by acetyl, benzyl, carboxymethyl, carboxymethylbenzylamide, or diethylaminoethyl groups (Chenoweth, 1984; Bosch *et al.*, 1987; Carreno *et al.*, 1988; Toufik and Labarre, 1995; Toufik *et al.*, 1995; Bowry and Rintelen, 1998) reduces the activating capacity of the surface, depending on the substituting groups. But the relationship between the reduction and the degree of substitution is usually not linear.

25.4. Assessing the Inflammatory Response to Materials

The inflammatory response to materials has been studied in a very large number of systems. Fundamental studies have usually been performed *in vitro* with proteins, blood fractions, and cells or cell lines. Concerning *in vivo* testing, normal or deficient mice and rats, guinea pigs, rabbits, sheep, goats, horses, pigs, and baboons have been used as animal models. Materials have been implanted in many places, i.e., in different muscles, in the peritoneal cavity, subcutaneously either in direct contact with the tissues, or in a cage system, or in an air pouch system, in the wall of urinary bladder, in a bone or in the knee, in the medullar cavity, or in the vitreal cavity, or in nerve regeneration chambers. They have been tested in direct contact with circulating blood, as aortic, aorto-iliac, femoral, or coronary vascular prostheses, as catheters, as coating for stent grafts, or as constituents of cardiopulmonary bypass or of hemodialyzer circuits. As nano- or microparticles, they have also been injected intravenously or inhaled into the lungs. Ultimate information can be found from clinical studies on materials routinely used in humans.

The inflammatory response to materials implanted in tissues has been usually evaluated as a function of time by several methods either qualitatively or quantitatively, using light, scanning, and transmission electron microscopies to examine histologic slices, and magnetic resonance imaging *in vivo*. The surface area of the inflammatory reaction, or the thickness and organization of the capsule around the implant, the type of tissue, e.g., fibrous or granulomatous, have been evaluated. The number of cells present in an exsudate and their type, e.g., polymorphonuclear (PMN), monocytes/macrophages, foreign-body giant cells (FBGC), B lymphocytes and T-helpers or T-suppressors lymphocytes, fibroblasts, have been measured by methods such as immunocytofluorometry. Monoclonal antibodies have been used to recognize specifically some epitopes on cells present on material surfaces after contact with a living tissue or blood. Measurements of concentration of complement activation products such as C3a, C4a, C5a, C3bi, C5b-9, Bb, or consumption of complement activity (CH50, C4, B,...) in the fluid phase, or production of inflammatory mediators such as the interleukines (IL-1α or β, IL-6), tumor necrosis factor (TNFα), prostaglandins, and derivatives such as PGE2 or leukotriene B4, have been performed. Finally, clinical signs such as fever or nausea have been noted.

25.4.1. Materials in Close Contact with Blood

When materials are placed in close contact with blood, the rate of the events occurring at the interface is very fast because the different species present either in solution, i.e., divalent ions, proteins, and/or their fragments, or the cells in suspension can diffuse very easily. The most apparent feature is usually the development of thrombotic events on the surface of large blood-contacting items. But, even if coagulation is controlled by use of heparin and/or anti-aggregating agents, the inflammatory response is triggered during the contact.

In vivo, the fate of the material depends primarily on the relative sizes of the item and of the encountered phagocytic cells. Inflammation is induced by large blood-contacting devices. As the device is too large to be phagocytized, the activated leukocytes are "at work" on the surface of the device. Inflammation is also induced by injected micronic or submicronic particles. Even if the particles are small enough to cross over the pulmonary capillaries, they are usually phagocytized, distributed, and processed in the organs of the Mononuclear Phagocyte System (MPS), mainly the Kupffer cells of the liver (Borchard and Kreuter, 1996). Because of this very efficient phagocytosis, the possible thrombotic events are usually hidden, providing that the MPS is not saturated.

In vitro, native blood cannot be stored because coagulation is triggered as soon as blood is in contact with the subendothelium injured by the needle used for withdrawing the blood. For the same reason, blood coagulation is also triggered in *ex vivo* bleeding tests, even if there is no effect linked to storage. It results that *in vitro* tests are performed with modified blood and blood fractions, either heparinized, or with serum which is depleted at least in fibrinogen, or with citrated plasma in which divalent ions are chelated, or with isolated leukocytes, or with macrophagic cell lines. Thus, it is not surprising that evaluating the inflammatory response to materials in contact with blood, either by *in vitro* or by *in vivo* methods, can lead to apparent discrepancies.

Polymeric materials have been used in contact with blood for many years with very variable results depending mainly on the local conditions of flow and on the composition of the surface. Their use as constituents of hemodialyzers membranes is probably the most successful one since Kolff (1990) developed this device, and a lot of information is available from this application.

25.4.1.1. Biocompatibility in Hemodialysis

Anaphylatoxins play a key role in mediating the inflammatory response in host defense mechanisms to pathogens as to artificial devices (Craddock *et al.*, 1977b). Cellulosic membranes activate the alternative and classical pathways of complement generating increased plasma levels of the anaphylatoxins C3a and C5a within the first 15 minutes of hemodialysis (Woffindin *et al.*, 1992; Pertosa *et al.*, 1993; Innes *et al.*, 1994). It has been recently described how rapid activation of the complement system by cuprophane membranes is mediated by the classical pathway C3-convertase C4bC2a, suggesting an important role of natural antipolysaccharide antibodies in this activation (Lhotta *et al.*, 1998).

Quantitation of complement activation with polyacrylonitrile-based (PAN) membranes is complicated due to its high capacity to adsorb anaphylatoxins. At this time, the protein layers during contact of blood with hemodialysis membranes play an important role. Cornelius and Brash (1993) demonstrated that C3 is adsorbed on cellulose acetate, cuprophane, poly(methyl methacrylate) (PMMA), and PAN dialysis membranes, and factor D is also adsorbed on PAN (Pascual and Schifferli, 1993) and PMMA (Pascual *et al.*, 1993b). C3 adsorption on dialysis membrane is influenced by the surface hydrophobicity (Lin *et al.*, 1992).

The temporal relationship that has been observed between complement activation, enhanced expression of CD11b/CD18 (Mac-1, CR3) on granulocytes, and leukocyte margination has led to the suggestion that complement activation is primarily responsible for the acute neutropenia occurring during the early phase of bioincompatible hemodialysis (Craddock *et al.*, 1977a). Leukocyte adhesion processes to endothelial cells are activated *in vivo* during hemodialysis procedure and participate to inflammatory response. CD11b/CD18 expression on monocytes and neutrophils in the venous line at the end of dialysis procedure was significantly higher during cuprophane dialysis as compared to Hemophan and polysulfone membranes. Transient nature of adhesive interactions occurring during cell margination is mainly dependent on expression of selectins, such as CD15s, and integrins, such as CD11b/CD18, which are shed by activated cells (Berger *et al.*, 1984). Hemodialysis is associated with an increase of CD62P/CD15s interactions which mediate platelet-leukocyte co-aggregation. A significant correlation was found between the expression of CD15s molecule and neutrophil counts during hemodialysis on low complement activating membranes.

As assessed by CD61 expression on leukocytes, platelets bound significantly on leukocytes during hemodialysis: a significant correlation was found during hemodialysis between the expression of CD11b molecules and the expression of CD61 + on monocytes during hemodialysis. The role of enhanced expression of CD11b/CD18 in the pulmonary sequestration of granulocytes during hemodialysis has, however, been challenged (Hakim and Lowrie, 1982; Combe *et al.*, 1994). Thus, the nadir of granulocytopenia occurs at 15 minutes of dialysis with complement-activating membranes, while the maximal decrease in PaO_2 is observed at 60 minutes of hemodialysis (De Backer *et al.*, 1983). In addition, hemodialysis-associated neutrophil and platelet co-aggregation, upregulation of the platelet-associated CD61 antigen with increased hydrogen peroxide production by granulocytes (Bonomini *et al.*, 1997), were shown to be independent of complement activation (Jacobs *et al.*, 1989).

It is now well documented that several of the acute and chronic inflammatory changes are also associated with extracorporeal circulation, such as an increased cytokine production in patients with end-stage renal failure undergoing chronic hemodialysis (McGregor, 1977; Cheung *et al.*, 1991; Combe *et al.*, 1994). The magnitude of changes is dependent on individual factors and on the nature of the hemodialysis membrane (Cheung *et al.*, 1991; Dinarello, 1992; Schoels *et al.*, 1993; Lin *et al.*, 1996). An early increase in CD11b/CD18 expression on monocytes from dialyzed patients was accompanied by an increase in plasma interleukin-1β later during hemodialysis (Thylen *et al.*, 1992). Several studies support the hypothesis that monocytes produce pro-inflammatory cytokines upon activation by soluble molecules generated through complement activation (Haeffner-Cavaillon *et al.*, 1987) and/or by bacterial derived fragments that may enter in the blood compartment from the dialysate (Kaspar and Gerhrke, 1994). IL-1 and TNFα are closely associated with chronic and acute inflammatory processes in hemodialytic patients. It has been shown that C5a may play a role for induction of IL-1beta-mRNA during hemodialysis procedure (Schindler *et al.*, 1993).

In addition to the production of IL-1 and TNFα, hemodialysis using complement-activating membranes is associated with enhanced concentrations of their natural inhibitors IL-1ra, TNFRII, and IL-10 (Descamps-Latscha *et al.*, 1995; Brunet *et al.*, 1998). IL-1α and TNFα trigger the production of a- and b-chemokines that exert a crucial function of amplifying the immune-mediated inflammatory reaction (Schröder *et al.*, 1990) and several studies have detected enhanced expression of chemokines messengers (IL-8 and MCP-1) in monocytes from hemodialyzed patients (Pertosa *et al.*, 1993).

Patients with chronic renal failure present functional disregulation of the immune response leading to altered immune response to viral and bacterial infections (Moran *et al.*, 1990; Gerez *et al.*, 1991; Hayakawa *et al.*, 1994; Stachowski *et al.*, 1994). Patients on long-term hemodialysis manifested prolonged survival of skin allografts, a high incidence of malignant tumors, anergy in cutaneous delayed hypersensitivity tests, and defective responses to T cell-dependent antigens such as influenza and hepatitis B vaccines (Descamps-Latscha and Herbelin, 1993). Previous work reported that 40% of end-stage renal disease patients failed to respond to Hepatitis B virus (HBV) vaccination, a phenomenon that remains a key problem in the spread of HBV infection among the patients. Although acquired abnormalities of the immune response may obviously contribute to increased morbidity in chronically dialyzed patients, the respective roles of uremia and biocompatibility of the dialysis procedure remain unclear at that time.

Several observations suggest that the primary defect in the attenuated T lymphocyte responses to Hepatitis B antigens observed with cells of hemodialyzed patients may result from a disregulation of the co-stimulatory processes during antigen presentation and recognition as well as from a decreased IL-2 receptor density (Kurz *et al.*, 1986).

25.4.1.2. *In Vivo* Evaluations of Vascular Prostheses and Stent Grafts

Despite the fact that the investigators were usually more interested in the thrombotic events occurring on such devices in contact with blood, some effects on inflammation have also been examined.

Searching for a possible link between inflammation and infection in the presence of vascular prostheses, Olofsson *et al.* (1995) compared explanted infected and uninfected aortic vascular prostheses and concluded that acute and chronic inflammation observed in the presence of such prostheses were not predictive of infection.

The effects of aortic reconstruction and collagen impregnation of Dacron prostheses on the complement system have been examined by De Mol Van Otterloo *et al.* (1992). This study was conducted on 41 patients, who received either a collagen-impregnated or a nonimpregnated prosthesis. Activation of the complement system initiated by both pathways was found in both cases with no statistical difference between the groups of prostheses and a statistical difference with control patients. A close study was performed by Swartbol *et al.* (1996) to determine the inflammatory response in patients receiving aortobifemoral bypass made of either ePTFE or collagen-impregnated knitted Dacron. The authors found that aortobifemoral surgery induced complement activation and release of interleukin-6 but not TNFα. Utoh *et al.* (1997) evaluated the postoperative inflammatory reactions to gelatin- and collagen-sealed knitted Dacron prostheses used for repairing abdominal aortic aneurism and found a higher inflammatory response during the second week following implantation with the gelatin-sealed prosthesis, but not later. Chakfe *et al.* (1996) compared albumin-preimpregnated and preclotted Dacron prostheses in surgery of the abdominal aorta and concluded that the glutaraldehyde cross-linked albumin did not induce any systemic inflammatory reaction.

The recent development of stent grafts has induced evaluations of the inflammatory response to such polymer-coated devices. De Scheerder *et al.* (1995) investigated the response to poly(organo) phosphazene- and amphiphilic polyurethane- (PU) coated, stainless steel stents in porcine peripheral arteries. They found a similar response for the uncoated and the PU-coated stents and a severe reaction to the poly(organo) phosphazene-coated one. In their study on stents made of Dacron-covered nitinol, Hayoz *et al.* (1997) found nonspecific inflammatory reactions in some patients and an *in vitro* activation of neutrophils by the intact stent graft itself, but no activation by both Dacron and nitinol. In another study on Dacron-covered and heparin-coated Dacron-covered stent grafts implanted in sheep, Schurmann *et al.* (1997) found a severe inflammatory response to the heparinized material, a moderate response to the Dacron-covered stent, and almost no response to noncovered ones.

25.4.1.3. *In Vitro* Evaluations of Modified Materials

The main advantage of the *in vitro* evaluations is that they are more focused on some features of the very complex inflammatory response. Conversely, some interactions occurring *in vivo* are obviously hidden. Fundamental studies on the effects of modifications of material surfaces are performed by *in vitro* methods and the activation of the complement system is usually tested. This can be done by checking the decrease in different activities or the increase in the concentration of different markers of the activation in the supernatant fluid phase, but these methods are indirect and can lead to difficulties in interpretation. For instance, native complement components can be adsorbed on some surfaces without being activated (Cheung, 1990), and markers such as C3a and C5a can be adsorbed to a great extent on surfaces (Montdargent *et al.*, 1992).

In order to give a reliable picture of the complement activating properties of material surfaces, Mollnes *et al.* (1995) have developed a novel method for evaluating the biocompatibility of artificial surfaces based on monoclonal antibodies that can specifically identify complement activation products in the fluid phase as well as adsorbed to the surface. Owing to this method, they were able to show significant differences between some fluid-phase and bound complement components on materials. For instance, they found a low fluid-phase formation of C3b and terminal complex, and large amounts of both components on Tecoflex. In contrast, the reverse was found in the presence of silicone tubing. In addition, they have shown that activation of complement was more pronounced for poly(vinyl chloride) than for polyethylene tubings. After surface modifications either by sequential adsorption of polyethylenimine and dextran sulfate or by polyethylenimine followed by covalent end-point immobilization of heparin, the complement activation was reduced both in the fluid phase and on the surfaces. In contrast, surfaces exposing only polyethylenimine caused extensive complement activation.

However, as such very discriminating methods are not widespread yet, the results presented below have been obtained mainly by indirect methods.

Polystyrene (PS) and various derivatives have been extensively studied as a model polymeric surface. PS in the form of microtitre plates activates complement via the alternative pathway by adsorption of C3 in an active conformation (Nilsson *et al.*, 1993a). PS as a reference material, but also ePTFE, a polyurethane, and woven Dacron, have been evaluated concerning the capacity of these materials to induce superoxide release by neutrophils. Kaplan *et al.* (1994) concluded that contact-induced neutrophil activation differed from that described for cells in suspension and showed different mechanisms depending on the presence of serum and on the type of material.

Chemical substitution of PS in the range 0.1–0.7 hydroxymethyl (CH_2OH) groups per phenyl ring endowed PS with a constant complement-activating capacity in serum when evaluated on a constant surface area basis, while substitution with 0.9 CH_2OH groups increased dramatically the activating capacity (Montdargent *et al.*, 1991). Fifty/fifty substitution by CH_2OH and sulfonate groups led to nonactivating surfaces by combined interactions of the surfaces with proteins D and H (Montdargent *et al.*, 1993; Pascual *et al.*, 1993a).

Gemmell (1997) has evaluated various PS microspheres, including aminated and carboxylated ones, and compared them to cross-linked agarose, concerning complement components after incubation with serum. After fluorescently tagging the components by use of monoclonal antibodies against SC5b-9, C3bi, C3d, C4d, Bb, and C1q, this author quantified the components by flow cytometry analysis of the beads and found appreciable amounts of C3bi and SC5b-9 on the surfaces.

After surface modification of PS by radiofrequency plasmas containing methane, hexamethylene-disiloxane and hydroxyethyl methacrylate, the modified surfaces activated the classical pathway, while surfaces modified by 1,2-diaminocyclohexane, acrylic acid, and poly(ethylene glycol) activated the alternative pathway (Golander *et al.*, 1992). Fluorinated, siliconized, nitrogenated, and oxygenated surface-modified PS were examined concerning the adhesion mechanisms of blood monocytes in the presence of C3-depleted or C3-replenished serum. The results suggest adhesive interactions between adsorbed iC3b and the leukocyte integrin CD11b/CD18, with a possible additional action of fibrinogen (McNally and Anderson, 1994).

After end-point attachment of heparin on PS, C3 deposition occurred at reduced level and the net effect was an overall reduction of C3 binding due to obliteration of the alternative pathway (Nilsson *et al.*, 1993b). Such an effect was not found by Gong *et al.* (1996), who studied heparinized polyethylene tubings in a closed loop model and assessed the generation of C3a, C3bi, and terminal complex. The modest effect which was found was attributed to the presence of a large blood–gas interface. Such an effect of air bubbles had already been documented by Ward *et al.* (1984).

Angiographic catheters made out of four different polymers, i.e., polyamide (PA), polyethylene (PE), polyurethane (PU), and PTFE, were compared *in vitro* with silicone-coated latex urinary catheters, with respect to their ability to activate complement. All the polymers tested activated the complement system, but differences were found between the polymers. Activation was most prominent with exposure to PA and least marked with PU (Kuroki *et al.*, 1995).

25.4.2. Materials in Contact with Other Tissues

Polymeric materials are used for different purposes in contact with living tissues in which extensive contact with blood is not the main issue. The net result is that the rate of the inflammatory response is not as fast. Some of the most recent developments are presented in this part.

25.4.2.1. Intraocular Implants

Different materials have been tested in the eye as candidates for intraocular lenses (IOL), ocular drainage implants, or drug delivery systems. The reference material is poly(methyl methacrylate) (PMMA), which has been clinically used for years with rather satisfactory results after Ridley observed the good tolerance of PMMA debris by the eyes of wounded airmen of World War II. Several authors have compared other materials, e.g., silicone (Skorpik *et al.*, 1993; Wenzel *et al.*, 1993) and/or Acrysof or hydrogel (Amon and Menapace, 1992; Hollick *et al.*, 1998), with it. The inflammatory reaction was mild and similar for silicone and PMMA. Acrysof and the hydrogel were the best materials.

Heparin-surface-modified PMMA has also been compared to PMMA in multicenter studies. End-point heparin attachment on PMMA reduced the generation of C3a and fluid phase terminal complex (Pekna *et al.*, 1993). Heparin surface modification reduced the inflammatory response and cellular deposit on the material surface in rabbits and humans (Borgioli *et al.*, 1992; Amon *et al.*, 1996; Kivalo, 1997).

Fifty:fifty poly(DL-lactic-co-glycolic acid) (PLGA) has been evaluated as discs inserted subconjunctivally for a potential depot drug delivery system (Gould *et al.*, 1994) and as microspheres for intravitreous sustained drug delivery (Giordano *et al.*, 1995). The inflammatory reaction was mild in both cases.

25.4.2.2. Materials for Sutures

Materials used for sutures have a high surface-to-volume ratio and this could result in increased effects on inflammation and wound healing. The results obtained by Niessen *et al.* (1997) exemplify such increased effects. Despite the fact that the exact mechanism was not known, these authors have shown that a monofilamentous synthetic absorbable suture material (Monocryl) gave smaller, less reactive scars than a multifilamentous suture material (Vicryl-rapide).

Both biodegradable (or erodible) and stable suture materials have been implanted in different sites of various animal species including humans, and usually compared together. Despite the fact that Prolene (stable) and Vicryl (biodegradable) are probably the most cited suture materials, no actual reference suture material has been systematically included in the different studies and this fact does not allow an easy comparison between materials.

Bakkum *et al.* (1995) have tested in peritoneal defects of a standard side wall-uterine horn adhesion model in rats, three materials, i.e., Prolene, Vicryl, Catgut, with different diameters and knot configurations concerning a possible correlation between the inflammatory reaction and postsurgical adhesion formation. Both the inflammatory reaction and the adhesion percentage showed significant differences within and in between suture characteristics after 14 days; e.g., most variables of the inflammatory response were observed to increase from Prolene to Vicryl to catgut, but no significant correlation between inflammation and adhesion was found.

Beardslay *et al.* (1995) have evaluated a new synthetic fluorescent pigmented polypropylene suture material in rat gluteal muscles and compared it to polypropylene and coated polyamide. Similar reactions were found at day 30 or less after implantation, but differed after. The tissue reactions induced after 30 days by the new suture material were similar to those of polypropylene and significantly less than those induced by coated polyamide.

In 15 patients, who underwent root resections of the upper incisors on both sides, Giray *et al.* (1997) found that the scar formation and the local inflammation were more marked during the healing period on the side sutured with silk than on the side treated with n-butyl-2-cyanoacrylate.

Hanke *et al.* (1994) have compared catgut, polypropylene, and polyglactin 910 in urinary bladder incisions in rabbits and found that the latter was superior to any other suture material as regards the reaction to foreign bodies and inclination to incrustation. However, Soler *et al.* (1993) found a lower biological tolerance with a composite mesh made of Dacron and polyglactin 910 than with a Dacron mesh.

Setzen and Williams (1997) compared the tissue response to a nonabsorbable monofilament suture made of expanded polytetrafluoroethylene (ePTFE), with the response to ten other commercially available absorbable and nonabsorbable monofilamented and multifilamented sutures. In general, sutures made of ePTFE produced a minimal tissue response.

25.4.2.3. Articular Prostheses and Bone Fracture Fixation

Polymeric materials are used in articular prostheses for different purposes: PMMA has been widely used for cemented prostheses, Proplast-Teflon for temporomandibular joints, silicone for wrist, elbow, or finger implants, ultrahigh molecular weight polyethylene (UMWPE) for hip or knee joints, and homopolymers or copolymers of lactic and glycolic acids (PLGA) as pins and screws in arthroscopic fixation.

Boss *et al.* (1993) evaluated the early and late phase reactions on specimens of cemented arthroplasties. On the tenth postoperative day, they observed only a mild and focal inflammatory response, where present. Many years after implantation, a thin and quiescent fibrous interfacial membrane alternating with bone and osteoid, i.e., segmental osseointegration, or a cartilaginous layer abutting on the cement, were revealed.

However, such mild reactions are observed when the cement is unfractionated. Jasty *et al.* (1992) suggest that loosening of total joint prostheses is in part related to the fragmentation of the acrylic cement mantle surrounding the prosthesis, and the biological consequences to the particulate acrylic. They tested particulate-form PMMA in different immunocompetent and immunodeficient strains of mice and observed a foreign-body reaction produced and sustained by nonimmune phagocytosis without contribution by the immune system. The same team (Jiranek *et al.*, 1995) concluded that the foreign-body response to particulate orthopedic biomaterials was macrophage-initiated and maintained that lymphocytes were not essential to this response, although they might modulate it. The aseptic loosening of hip prostheses could actually be due to the presence of particulate debris, because membranes recovered from cementless and cemented prostheses, containing either metal or cement debris, released similar concentrations of gelatinase, collagenase, prostaglandin E2, and interleukin-1 when cultured into conditioned media. Such bioactive products could induce bone resorption (Kim *et al.*, 1993). The findings of Wooley *et al.* (1996) suggest also that the development of a cellular response to particulate debris may be significant in the pathogenesis of aseptic loosening. However, the paper by Van Der Vis *et al.* (1997) seems to disagree. Despite the fact that bone formation was inhibited by polyethylene particles when injected into the knees and the intramedullary femoral cavities of rats, the authors concluded that wear particles per se do not initiate bone resorption.

Proplast-Teflon has been used for temporomandibular joint reconstruction. Exuberant foreign-body reactions, significant osseous changes, and pain have been reported (Chuong *et al.*, 1993; Henry and Wolford, 1993), probably linked to Proplast.

Silicone elastomer implants have a relatively low rate of complications, but inflammatory reactions to debris are reported (Karlsson *et al.*, 1992; Hirakawa *et al.*, 1996). These authors emphasize the role played by particles formed in silicone wrist, elbow, or finger implants.

Biodegradable pins and screws of polyglycolide (PGA), polylactides (PLA), and their copolymers have been used in the treatment of fractures and osteotomies, and nonspecific foreign-body reactions which could not be attributed to infection have been reported. Tegnander *et al.* (1994) have found production of C5adesArg in the presence of PLA. Bostman and co-workers have studied in rabbits and patients the inflammatory effects linked to absorbable internal fixation devices made of PGA and PLA, including poly(L-lactide) (PLLA) (Bostman, 1992; Bostman *et al.*, 1992; Paivarinta *et al.*, 1993; Bostman *et al.*, 1995). The intensity of the inflammatory response decreased from PGA to PLLA. The degradation of PLLA, producing lactic acid at a low rate, is far slower than the degradation of PGA, producing glycolic acid at a high rate. These two phenomena are probably related.

25.4.2.4. *In Vivo* Evaluations of New or Modified Materials

The inflammatory response to polymeric material surfaces, modified or not, has been extensively evaluated in animal models. However, it is rather difficult to have a clear view from the published results because most of them lack reference materials. This is not the case for the paper by Kao *et al.* (1994), who have tried to quantify formation of foreign-body giant cells (FBGC) on implanted polymer surfaces as a function of time. These authors have measured the density of adherent macrophages present initially that participate in FBGC formation (d0) and the rate constant for cell fusion (k) and used both parameters to calculate the time-dependent FBGC density (dfc), up to 5 weeks of implantation. They have tested three poly(ether urethanes) (PEU) varying in weight percentage of hard segment, one poly(ether urethane urea) (PEUU), and compared them to two reference materials: low density polyethylene and silica-free poly(dimethyl siloxane). It was concluded that increase in PEU hard segment weight percentage, surface hardness, and hydrophobicity increased total protein adsorption, d0 and dfc. Such a model shows possibilities of quantifying macrophage adhesion and FBGC formation, and their modulations by various polymer properties.

Rats and mice are the most used animal models. The prevailing site of implantation is subcutaneous, either direct, or in a cage, or in an air pouch. It has been sometimes compared to intraperitoneal implantation and the duration of implantation is variable. The following papers are presented according to the materials.

Owing to its mechanical properties, poly(dimethyl siloxane) (PDMS) is a very useful material, but its inertness has been a matter of controversy. It has been evaluated by different authors and compared to other materials. Krause *et al.* (1993) tested in a rat air pouch model the production of intracellular hydrogen peroxide by inflammatory cells adherent to the surface of PDMS and compared it to ePTFE. It was found that after two days, cells adherent to ePTFE produced almost 3.5 times more hydrogen peroxide than did cells adherent to PDMS, after which the production decreased.

Petillo *et al.* (1994) proposed a technique using subcutaneous cages into rats in conjunction with cytofluorimetric analysis of exsudate leukocytes to evaluate the monocyte/macrophage activation in response to PDMS, two PEUUs, a polyetherimide (PEI), and a poly(etheretherketone) (PEEK). For all tested materials, the maximum numbers of exsudate cells and of Ia-positive macrophages were found on day 7, although the entity of the cell increase was associated with the material. Only in the case of PDMS did the percentage of Ia-positive macrophages remain the same as compared with control empty cage macrophages.

Lansdown *et al.* (1995) implanted subcutaneously in rats samples of Dacron and Silastic tubings used as catheters for peritoneal dialysis. Dacron induced a modest to severe granulomatous reaction with giant cell formation persisting for at least 30 days, which subsided, while Silastic induced a mild reaction that regressed by day 10. The authors concluded that adverse reactions noted in clinical patients may not be attributable to the materials used.

However, Naidu *et al.* (1996) claimed that silicone elastomer particles are acutely inflammatory after injection of particles of Silastic, PMMA, and monosodium urate smaller than 10 microns into a rat subcutaneous air pouch lined with synovial membrane-like cells. After retrieval of exsudate at variable times, the authors measured white blood cell count, tumor necrosis factor, and PGE2.

More recently, Fabre *et al.* (1998) quantified by flow cytometry in exsudates the inflammatory response to cylindrical tubes composed of poly(vinyl chloride) (PVC), PDMS, and a polyurethane (PU) implanted subcutaneously in the dorsal region of rats over a 3-week period. At day 2, PVC induced a predominantly neutrophilic reaction, while PU and PDMS induced a reaction characterized by the presence of a mixture of monocytes and neutrophils. Then the reaction decreased and the number of cell events became too low at day 23 to distinguish the subpopulations.

As already noted in previous paragraphs, various PU and related polymers have been tested and often compared to PDMS. Huang *et al.* (1992) have evaluated the cellular reaction to a poly(ester urethane) vascular prosthesis, Vascugraft, and compared it with Impra, Goretex, and Mitrathane. The tissue reaction surrounding the Vascugraft revealed a mild inflammatory reaction, similar to the one observed with PTFE grafts, and the Mitrathane prosthesis exhibited a moderate inflammatory response, characterized by a level of activation on fibroblasts higher than other grafts.

Sulfonate-grafted poly(ether urethane)s with different degrees of substitution were implanted intramuscularly into rats and evaluated concerning their capacity to modify and stimulate the inflammatory response (Hunt *et al.*, 1996). The authors concluded that surface charge can influence the early-phase acute inflammatory response to an implanted material. Mathur *et al.* (1997) have compared polyether polyurethanes and polycarbonate polyurethanes and found similar responses in the exsudate analysis of the acute and chronic inflammatory responses.

More classical polymers such as poly(ethylene terephthalate) (PET) have been coated with proteins or plasmatic fractions and implanted intraperitoneally for short periods into normal or deficient mice (Tang and Eaton, 1993). These authors claimed that spontaneous adsorption of fibrinogen appeared to initiate the inflammatory response to the implanted polymer, suggesting a nexus between clotting and inflammation in response to biomaterials.

PET has also been surface-modified with poly(ethylene oxide) (PEO) and implanted in the peritoneal cavity of mice by Desai and Hubbell (1992). The control PET showed an initial inflammatory reaction followed by an extensive fibrotic response, while the PEO-modified surface showed only a mild inflammatory response and no fibrotic encapsulation, but a cellular monolayer was formed.

A PET fabric was surface-modified by either Fluoropassiv fluoropolymer (PET/FC) or an RGD-containing peptide (PET/RGD) and implanted subcutaneously in rats (Chinn *et al.*, 1998). Minimal acute and chronic inflammation was associated with the fabrics and fibroblast proliferation was less into PET/FC than into PET and PET/RGD. Cellular exsudate extracted from cages containing the samples showed at one week a higher total leukocyte count for PET/RGD than for the others. Then this parameter decreased for all the samples.

Peptides, namely RGD, RGE, and poly-L-lysine, were also used to coat the surface of ultrahigh molecular weight polyethylene (UHMWPE). The samples were implanted into rats either intraperitoneally or subcutaneously and lactate dehydrogenase (LDH) activity was measured in blood (Johnson *et al.*, 1997). LDH activity was elevated at weeks 1 and 2 for rats implanted with materials when compared to control animals, while from weeks 3–12 it was similar in all groups. At the end of week 12, the implants placed subcutaneously had a less extensive fibrous and vascular tissue formation than those implanted intraperitoneally. At both sites, the RGD- and poly-L-lysine-coated samples had thicker fibrous capsule formation than the RGE-coated samples.

Stimulation of macrophages subpopulations with UHMWPE has been evaluated by Rhodes *et al.* (1997) in the exsudates resulting from subcutaneous implantation in rats. Granulocytes, monocytes, immature and mature macrophages, and T-lymphocytes, but no B-lymphocytes, were found in the exsudates. Different subpopulations identified by their granularity and positivity to specific antibodies were present. The results suggest a possible mechanism by which monocytes were attracted to the site of the implanted material.

Owing to their increasing uses, the biodegradable polymers have been tested in subcutaneous or intraperitoneal implantations. Van Sliedregt *et al.* (1992) concluded that the inflammatory response to polylactide particles injected into the peritoneal cavity of mice was not related to molecular weight. Kinoshita *et al.* (1993) have compared PLLA in different forms to polypropylene when implanted subcutaneously into the back of dogs and concluded that tissue reactions associated with biodegradation of the PLLA mesh were mild. Lam *et al.* (1995) concluded that PLLA films provoked a more intense inflammatory response than nonbiodegradable PTFE films. Recently, Den Dunnen *et al.* (1997) evaluated the degradation and foreign-body reaction of poly(DL-lactide-ε-caprolactone) bars and concluded that the latter was very mild. Bergsma *et al.* (1995) have tested the response to predegraded and as-polymerized poly(L-lactide) (PLLA) cylinders in a cage implant system and did not find significant differences between the samples. A possible explanation for the absence of differences could be that the predegraded particles were sieved before implantation, thus eliminating all small particles that could provoke an increased cellular reaction.

25.5. Conclusion

The inflammatory response is the normal tissue response following a wound, allowing nonspecific self-protection against foreign bodies, the elimination of injured cells, and a normal tissue repair. It is thus a major concern as soon as a polymeric material is placed in contact with any living tissue, inducing the response either by direct contact or through indirect effects.

When a material is implanted, the rate and intensity of the response depend on the site of implantation. For instance, the kinetics of the response is very fast when a material is placed in direct contact with blood, because of the fast diffusion of the species involved in the inflammatory response. Determination of the biocompatibility of a material is thus site-specific.

Concerning the implanted material, the presence in the bulk and on the surface of diffusible small molecules which are soluble either in aqueous or in lipidic media induces usually a strong response. Such molecules can be present owing to different causes. They can be deliberately added to the material or the device for various purposes, e.g., plasticizers, stabilizing agents, silicone oils, pastes, etc. They can be fortuitously introduced on the surface during the processing of the material to make a device, through external lubricants for extrusion, or molding agents. They can be produced by degradative processes, such as aggressive sterilization treatments or a too fast degradation of biodegradable polymers. The small molecules resulting from these different causes are endowed with a variable toxicity and may induce cell death, resulting in necrosis and at least indirect inflammation. Thus the evaluation of the inflammatory response to ready-to-use materials should be performed by comparison with reference pure polymers, and on aqueous and lipidic extracts after contact with the materials.

As the inflammatory process is primarily surface-related, the presence of particles can also induce an increased inflammatory response. Small particles have a high surface-to-volume ratio and an open porosity can still increase this parameter. Such particles can be phagocytized and processed by professional phagocytes and activate production and secretion of inflammatory mediators. The presence of sharp-angled particles can still modulate the reactions. Particles can be produced by degradative processes, e.g., wear debris and degradable materials, or can be introduced during processing, e.g., talc found on retrieved breast prostheses. Thus the inflammatory response to a material should be evaluated at least on a surface area basis, especially when designing a device susceptible to produce particles, and the introduction of particles on the surface should be avoided by using appropriate processes.

The physicochemical features of a material surface are able to modulate the inflammatory response. Intrinsically, rigid hydrophobic surfaces induce irreversible protein adsorptions and changes of conformation resulting, for instance, in complement activation. Increasing the proportion of hard segments into polyurethanes increases the inflammation. Intrinsically, flexible hydrophobic materials can even absorb lipidic species and their surface can undergo rearrangments. Owing to the presence of surface order, crystalline surfaces can induce recognition by proteins such as C1 and activate complement through its classical pathway, even independently of the presence of immunoglobulins. Concerning hydrophilic surfaces, it has been shown that the hydrophilic character of a surface is not per se sufficient to avoid an inflammatory response. For instance, to obtain an efficient repelling (i.e., steric) effect toward proteins, and to delay complement and leukocyte activations, the binding of PEO on a surface needs to be performed with both a sufficient average density and a sufficient length. Terminally attached PEO can be efficient by binding either by one end, i.e., end-on, or by both ends, i.e., side-on. Other hydrophilic polymers can be efficient too. End-on dextran can decrease complement activation and decrease fibrinogen adsorption. Side-on dextran is more efficient to decrease fibrinogen adsorption but induces complement activation.

Concerning the surface chemistry, its prominent role in the modulation of the inflammatory response by natural surfaces has to be remembered. For instance, decreasing the surface concentration of sialic acid on sheep erythrocytes turns a complement nonactivating surface into an activating one. Conversely, the binding of heparin onto the surface of zymosan, a particular polysaccharide, turns a complement-activating surface into a nonactivating one. Providing that heparin is attached by one end, such a modification has proved its efficiency on PMMA intraocular lenses implanted in humans.

However, everything is not yet clear concerning the effects of different chemical groups present on a surface. This is typically the case for sulfate or sulfonate groups supposed to mimic heparin on surfaces, and apparently discrepant results have been reported. Increasing the concentration of the hydrophilic and nucleophilic hydroxyl group on hydrophobic substrates results both in increasing hydrophilicity and complement activation. But the relationship between the increased concentration of OH groups and the increased complement activation is not direct. Decreasing the concentration of this group on polysaccharidic surfaces by substitution can decrease complement activation, but again the relationship is not direct and depends strongly on the type of the groups used for substitution, in addition to their concentration.

The inflammatory response to materials has been assessed in a very large number of *in vivo* and *in vitro* systems, and in the presence of different tissues. A clear effect of the direct contact of the material with blood is to increase the rate of the events involved in the response. A material can be tested *in vivo* either in the form of a device made of it, or as-received, or predegraded, etc., in a given site of an animal model. Usually, the concentration of some proteins and protein fragments, the presence of different types and subtypes of cells and tissues, the production and secretion of different mediators, are evaluated as a function of time.

When a material is in contact with blood *in vivo*, its fate depends primarily on its size, because particles smaller than capillaries could be able to circulate. The inflammatory response which is triggered results in that case in a fast phagocytosis by the encountered resident macrophages. Concerning large items in contact with blood, the cooperation between proteins and cells takes place rapidly on the surface.

The most experience that is available concerning human uses of polymeric materials is probably in the case of the hemodialysis membranes. At short term, the capacity of such membranes to activate complement and adsorb some proteins or protein fragments is well documented. Neutrophils can be activated through complement activation or directly. Different cytokines and their inhibitors are produced and modulate the inflammatory response in hemodialyzed patients. At long term, patients with chronic renal failure present functional disregulation of the immune response to antigens.

Concerning the inflammation induced in the presence of implanted vascular prostheses, it has been shown that complement activation is linked to surgery and that the inflammatory reaction is not predictive of infection. The use of some coatings such as cross-linked albumin or collagen to avoid preclotting of the prosthesis does not increase the reaction.

The fast development of stent grafts has given an impulse to the evaluation of the inflammatory response to such devices. The recent results show that the least reactive stent grafts are the metallic ones, and this is a challenge for polymers.

The *in vitro* evaluations are very useful for testing new or modified materials, because such evaluations are usually simpler and can focus on some features of the very complex *in vivo* response. Conversely, they can be shortsighted and the response even artefactual because, for instance, the tests routinely used to evaluate the inflammatory response to natural foreign bodies in hospitalized patients are not really adapted to the evaluation of materials. In addition, some materials are able to disturb completely the test system itself, for instance by chelation of divalent ions or adsorption of proteins and protein fragments. It can be expected that the novel method for evaluation of complement activating properties of material surfaces developed by Mollnes *et al.* (1995) could give a more reliable picture by identifying complement activation products both in the fluid phase and on the surface of the material.

Polymeric materials are used for different purposes in contact with living tissues in which extensive contact with blood is not the main issue. The net result is that the rate of the inflammatory response is not as fast.

In recent years, devices such as surface-modified and especially heparin-modified intraocular lenses have been compared with similar devices made of PMMA, which is the reference material for this purpose, even in large multicenter evaluations on patients. Different materials for suture, monofilament or multifilament, either biodegradable or not, have been evaluated in contact with different soft tissues in different species including humans. Polymeric materials either biodegradable or not, used in articular prostheses and bone fracture fixation, have been examined, with special emphasis on the production of wear debris and on the rate of production of degradation products.

The inflammatory response to polymeric material surfaces, modified or not, has been extensively evaluated in animal models as a function of time. Rats and mice, either normal or deficient, are the most used animal models. The prevailing site of implantation is subcutaneous, either direct, or in a cage, or in an air pouch. The subcutaneous implantation has sometimes been compared to intraperitoneal implantation. However, it is rather difficult to have a synthetic view of the published results because many of them lack reference materials.

The ultimate conclusion of this chapter could be that the minimal requirement in the assessment of the inflammatory response to materials *in vivo* is a systematic comparison with a few control reference materials in order to allow, in a first step, a better survey of the abundant literature, before trying to understand and quantify the observed effects.

APPENDIX: Abbreviations Used in this Chapter

Bb	the largest fragment obtained by cleavage of protein B by protein D
C1, C2, C3, C4, C5, C9	respectively the first, second, third, fourth, fifth, and ninth protein of the complement system
C3a, C4a, C5a	small fragments obtained by cleavage of C3, C4, and C5 by respective convertases and endowed with an activity of anaphylatoxin
C3adesArg, C5adesArg	C3a and C5a in which the terminal arginine has been cleaved
C3b	the largest fragment obtained by cleavage of C3 by C3-convertases
C3bi	inactive C3b obtained by cleavage of the α chain of C3b by inhibitor protein I
C3bBb	the alternative pathway C3-convertase
C3b-like-C3	hypothetical and circulating active form of C3 in the conformation of C3b
C4b2a	the classical pathway C3-convertase
C5b-9	the terminal lytic complex of complement
CH50	haemolytic technique to assess complement activity
CR1	complement receptor type 1
CR3	complement receptor type 3
CST	critical surface tension
DAF	decay-accelerating factor
ePTFE	expanded poly(tetrafluoroethylene)

FBGC	foreign-body giant cells
HBV	hepatitis B virus
HDPE	high-density polyethylene
IBCA	isobutylcyanoacrylate
IL	interleukine
MCP	membrane cofactor protein
MPS	mononuclear phagocytic system
PA	polyamides (Nylons)
PAAc	poly(acrylic acid)
PAAm	polyacrylamides
PACA	poly(alkyl cyanoacrylate)s
PAN	polyacrylonitrile. PAN hemodialysis membranes are usually made of copolymers of poly(acrylonitrile-co-methallyl sulfonate)
PCL	poly(ε caprolactone)
PDMS	poly(dimethyl siloxane)
PE	polyethylene
PEO	poly(ethylene oxide)
PET	poly(ethylene terephthalate)
PEU	poly(ether urethane)s
PEUU	poly(ether urethane urea)s
PGA	polyglycolide or poly(glycolic acid)
PGE2	prostaglandin E2
PHEMA	poly(2-hydroxyethyl methacrylate)
PLA	polylactides or poly(lactic acid)s including 100% L PLA (PLLA) and racemic PLA (PLA50)
PLA-PEO	block copolymers of polylactides and poly(ethylene oxide)
PLGA	copolymers of lactic and glycolic acids
PMMA	poly(methyl methacrylate)
PMN	polymorphonuclear (leukocytes)
PP	polypropylene
PS	polystyrene
PTFE	poly(tetrafluoroethylene)
PU	polyurethanes
PVA	poly(vinyl alkohol)
PVC	poly(vinyl chloride)
PVDF	poly(vinylidene fluoride)
PVP	poly(vinyl pyrrolidone)
S/V	surface-to-volume ratio
Tg	glass transition temperature
TNFα	tumor necrosis factor α
UHMWPE	ultrahigh molecular weight polyethylene

References

Allen, T.M., Chonn A. 1987. Large unilamellar liposomes with low uptake into the reticuloendothelial system, *FEBS Lett.* **223**, 42–46.

Allen, T.M., Lopes de Menezes, D., Hansen, C.B., Moase, E. H. 1998. Stealth™ liposomes for the targeting of drugs in cancer therapy, in: *Targeting of Drugs 6: Strategies for Stealth Therapeutic Systems* (G. Gregoriadis, B. McCormack, eds), pp. 61–75, Plenum Press, New York.

Amon, M., Menapace, R. 1992. Beurteilung der biologischen Verträglichkeit von PMMA-, heparinmodifizierten PMMA- und Hydrogel-Intraokularlinsen mit Hilfe der Spiegelmikroskopie, *Klin. Monatsbl. Augenheilkd.* **200**, 95–100.

Amon, M., Menapace, R., Radax, U., Freyler, H. 1996. In vivo study of cell reactions on poly(methyl methacrylate) intraocular lenses with different surface properties, *J. Cataract Surg.* **22**, 825–829.

Bakkum, E.A., Dalmeijer, R.A., Verdel, M.J., Hermans, J., van Blitterswijk, C.A., Trimbos, J. B. 1995. Quantitative analysis of the inflammatory reaction surrounding sutures commonly used in operative procedures and the relation to postsurgical adhesion formation, *Biomaterials* **16**, 1283–1289.

Bazile, D., Prud'homme, C., Bassoullet, M.T., Marlard, M., Spenlehauer, G., and Veillard, M. 1995. Stealth Me.PEG-PLA nanoparticles avoid uptake by the mononuclear phagocytes system, *J. Pharm. Sci.* **84**, 493–498.

Beardslay, S.L., Smeak, D.D., Weisbrode, S.E. 1995. Histologic evaluation of tissue reactivity and absorption in response to a new synthetic fluorescent pigmented polypropylene suture material in rats, *Am. J. Vet. Res.* **56**, 1248–1252.

Beaujeux, R., Laurent, A., Wassef, M., Rufenacht, D., Boschetti, E., Merland, J.J. 1996. Trisacryl-gelatin microspheres for therapeutic embolization. Part 1: Development and in vitro evaluation, *Am. J. Neuroradiology* **17**, 533–540.

Berger, M., O'Schea, J., Cross, A.S., Folks, T.M., Chused, T.M., Brown, E.J., Frank, M.M. 1984. Human neutrophils increase expression of C3bi as well as C3b receptors upon activation, *J. Clin. Invest.* **74**, 1566–1571.

Bergsma, J.E., Rozema, F.R., Bos, R.R., Boering, G., de Bruijn, W. C., Pennings, A.J. 1995. Biocompatibility study of as-polymerized poly(L-lactide) in rats using a cage implant system, *J. Biomed. Mater. Res.* **29**, 173–179.

Bern, S., Burd, A., May, J.W. Jr. 1992. The biophysical and histologic properties of capsules formed by smooth and textured silicone implants in the rabbit, *Plast. Reconstr. Surg.* **89**, 1037–1044.

Bitter-Suermann, D., Burger, R., Hadding, U. 1981. Activation of the alternative pathway of complement: efficient fluid-phase amplification by blockade of the regulatory complement protein β1H through sulfated polyanions, *Eur. J. Immunol.* **11**, 291–295.

Bocchiotti, G., Verna, G., Fracalvieri, M., Fanton, E., Datta, G., Robotti, E. 1993. Carbofilm-covered prostheses in plastic surgery: preliminary observations, *Plast. Reconstr. Surg.* **91**, 80–90.

Bonomini, M., Stuad, S., Carreno, M.P., Settefrati, N., Santarelli, P., Haeffner-Cavaillon, N., Albertazzi, A. 1997. Neutrophil reactive oxygen species production during hemodialysis, role of activated platelet adhesion to neutrophils through P-Selectin, *Nephron* **75**, 402–411.

Borchard, G., Kreuter, J. 1996. The role of serum complement on the organ distribution of intravenously administered poly(methyl methacrylate) nanoparticles, effects of pre-coating with plasma and with serum complement, *Pharm. Res.* **13**, 1055–1058.

Borgioli, M., Coster, D.J., Fan, R.F., Henderson, J., Jacobi, K.W., Kirkby, G.R., Lai, Y.K., Menezo, J.L., Montard, M., Strobel, J. 1992. Effect of heparin surface modification of poly(methyl methacrylate) intraocular lenses on signs of postoperative inflammation after extracapsular cataract extraction. One-year results of a double-masked multicenter study, *Ophthalmology* **99**, 1248–1255.

Bosch, T., Schmidt, B., Spencer, P.C., Samtleben, W., Pelger, M., Baurmeister, U., Gurland, H. J. 1987. Ex vivo biocompatibility evaluation of a new modified cellulose membrane, *Artif. Organs* **11**, 144–148.

Boss, J.H., Shajrawi, I., Dekel, S., Mendes, D.G. 1993. The bone-cement interface: histological observations on the interface of cemented arthroplasties within the immediate and late phases, *J. Biomater. Sci. Polym. Ed.* **5**, 221–230.

Boss, J.H., Shajrawi, I., Aunullah, J., Mendes, D.G. 1995. The relativity of biocompatibility. A critique of the concept of biocompatibility, *Isr. J. Med. Sci.* **31**, 203–209.

Bostman, O.M. 1992. Intense granulomatous inflammatory lesions associated with absorbable internal fixation devices made of polyglycolide in ankle fractures, *Clin. Orthop.* **278**, 193–199.

Bostman, O., Paivarinta, U., Partio, E., Vasenius, J., Manninen, M., Rokkanen, P. 1992. Degradation and tissue replacement of a absorbable polyglycolide screw in the fixation of rabbit femoral osteotomies, *J. Bone Jt. Surg. Am.* **74**, 1021–1031.

Bostman, O.M., Pihlajamaki, H.K., Partio, E., Rokkanen, P.U. 1995. Clinical biocompatibility and degradation of polylevolactide screws in the ankle, *Clin. Orthop.* **320**, 101–109.

Bowry, S., Rintelen, T.H. 1998. A cellulosic hemodialysis membrane with minimized complement activation, *ASAIO J.* **44**, M579–M583.

Brohim, R.M., Foresman, P.A., Hildebrandt, P.K., Rodeheaver, G.T. 1992. Early tissue reaction to textured breast implant surfaces, *Ann. Plast. Surg.* **28**, 354–362.

Brunet, P., Capo, C., Dellacasagrande, J., Thirion, X., Mege, J.L., Berland., Y. 1998. IL-10 secretion by peripheral blood mononuclear cells in haemodialysis patients, *Nephrol. Dial. Transplant.* **13**, 1745–1752.

Busch, H. 1994. Silicone toxicology, *Semin. Arthritis Rheum.* **24**, 11–17.

Carreno, M.P., Labarre, D., Jozefowicz, M., Kazatchkine, M.D. 1988. The ability of Sephadex to activate human complement is suppressed in specifically substituted functional Sephadex derivatives, *Mol. Immunol.* **25**, 165–171.

Chaikof, E.L., Merrill, E.W., Callow, A.D., Connolly, R.J., Verdon, S.L., Ramberg, K. 1992. PEO enhancement of platelet deposition, fibrinogen deposition and complement C3 activation, *J. Biomed. Mater. Res.* **26**, 1163–1168.

Chakfe, N., Kretz, J.G., Petit, H., Epailly, E., Nicolini, P., Levy, F., Pasquali, J.L., Eisenmann, B. 1996. Albumin-impregnated polyester vascular prosthesis for abdominal aortic surgery: an improvement?, *Eur. J. Vasc. Endovasc. Surg.* **12**, 346–353.

Chenoweth, D.E. 1984. Complement activation during hemodialysis: clinical observations, proposed mechanisms and theoretical implications, *Artif. Organs* **8**, 281–287.

Cheung, A.K. 1990. Adsorption of unactivated complement proteins by hemodialysis membranes, *Am. J. Kidney Dis.* **14**, 472–477.

Cheung, A.K., Hohnholt, M., Gilson, J. 1991. Adherence of neutrophils to hemodialysis membranes: role of complement receptors, *Kidney Int.* **40**, 1123–1128.

Chinn, J.A., Sauter, J.A., Phillips, R.E. Jr., Kao, W.J., Anderson, J.M., Hanson, S.R., Ashton, T. R. 1998. Blood and tissue compatibility of modified polyester: thrombosis, inflammation and healing, *J. Biomed. Mater. Res.* **39**, 130–140.

Chuong, R., Piper, M.A., Boland, T.J. 1993. Recurrent giant cell reaction to residual Proplast in the temporomandibular joint, *Oral Surg. Oral Med. Oral Pathol.* **76**, 16–19.

Combe, C., Pourtein, M., De Precigout, V., Baquey, A., Morel, D., Potaux, L., Vincendeau, P., Bezian, J.H., Aparicio, M. 1994. Granulocyte activation and adhesion molecules during hemodialysis with cuprophane and a high-flux biocompatible membrane, *Am. J. Kidney Dis.* **24**, 437–442.

Cooper, N.R. 1991. Complement evasion strategies of microorganisms, *Immunology Today* **12**, 327–331.

Cornelius, R.M., Brash, J.L. 1993. Identification of proteins absorbed to hemodialysis membranes from heparinized plasma, *J. Biomater. Sci. Polymer Ed.* **4**, 291–304.

Craddock, P.R., Fehr, J., Dalmasso, A.P., Brigham, K.L., Jacob, H.S. 1977a. Hemodialysis leukopenia: pulmonary vascular leukostasis resulting from complement activation by dialyser cellophane membranes, *J. Clin. Invest.* **59**, 879–888.

Craddock, P.R., Hammerschmidt, D., White, J.G., Dalmasso, A.P., Jacob, H.S. 1977b. Complement (C5a)-induced granulocyte aggregation in vitro, *J. Clin. Invest.* **60**, 260–264.

De Backer, W.A., Verpooten, G.A., Borgonjon, D.J., Vermeire, P.A., Lins, R.R., De Broe, M.E. 1983. Hypoxemia during hemodialysis: effects of different membranes and dialyzates compositions, *Kidney Int.* **23**, 738–743.

De Mol Van Otterloo, J.C., Van Bockel, J.H., Ponfoort, E.D., Brommer, E.J., Hermans, J., Daha, M.R. 1992. The effects of aortic reconstruction and collagen impregnation of Dacron prostheses on the complement system, *J. Vasc. Surg.* **16**, 774–783.

Den Dunnen, W.F., Robinson, P.H., van Wessel, R., Pennings, A.J., van Leeuwen, M.B., Schakenraad, J.M. 1997. Long-term evaluation of degradation and foreign-body reaction of subcutaneously implanted poly(DL-lactide-epsilon-caprolactone), *J. Biomed. Mater. Res.* **36**, 337–346.

Desai, N.P., Hubbell, J.A. 1992. Tissue response to intraperitoneal implants of polyethylene oxide-modified polyethylene terephthalate, *Biomaterials* **13**, 505–510.

Descamps-Latscha, B., Herbelin, A. 1993. Long-term dialysis and cellular immunity: a critical survey, *Kidney Int.* **43**, 135–142.

Descamps-Latscha, B., Herbelin, A., Nguyen, A.T., Roux-Lombard, P., Zingraff, J., Moynot, A., Verger, C., Dahmane, D., de Groote, D., Jungers, P., Dayer, J.M. 1995. Balance between IL-1beta, TNF-alpha and their specific inhibitors in chronic renal failure and maintenance dialysis. Relationship with activation markers of T cells, B cell, and monocytes, *J. Immunol.* **154**, 882–893.

De Scheerder, I.K., Wilczek, K.L., Verbeken, E.V., Vandorpe, J., Lan, P.N., Schacht, E., Piessens, J., De Geest, H. 1995. Biocompatibility of biodegradable and nonbiodegradable polymer-coated stents implanted in porcine peripheral arteries, *Cardiovasc. Intervent. Radiol.* **18**, 227–232.

Dinarello, C.A. 1992. Interleukin-1 and tumor necrosis factor and their naturally occurring antagonists during hemodialysis, *Kidney Int.* **42**, S68–S74.

Ecker, E.E., Gross, P. 1929. Anticomplementary power of heparin, *J. Infect. Dis.* **44**, 250–253.

Fabre, T., Bertrand-Barat, J., Freyburger, G., Rivel, J., Dupuy, B., Durandeau, A., Baquey, C. 1998. Quantification of the inflammatory response in exsudates to three polymers implanted in vivo, *J. Biomed. Mater. Res.* **39**, 637–641.

Fernandez-Urrusuno, R., Fattal, E., Porquet, D., Feger, J., Couvreur, P. 1995. Influence of surface properties on the inflammatory response to polymeric nanoparticles, *Pharm. Res.* **12**, 1385–1387.

Frank, M.M., Fries, L.F. 1991. The role of complement in inflammation and phagocytosis, *Immunology Today* **12**, 322–326.

Gelb, H., Schumacher, H.R., Cuckler, J., Ducheyne, P., Baker, D.G. 1994. In vivo inflammatory response to polymethylmethacrylate particulate debris: effect of size, morphology and surface area, *J. Orthop. Res.* **12**, 83–92.

Gemmell, C.H. 1997. A flow cytometric immunoassay to quantify adsorption of complement activation products (iC3b, C3d, SC5b-9) on artificial surfaces, *J. Biomed. Mater. Res.* **37**, 474–480.

Gerez, L., Madar, L., Shkolnik, T., Kristal, B., Arad., G., Reshef., A., Steinberger., A., Ketzinel., M., Sayar., D., Shassha., S., Kaempfer, R. 1991. Regulation of interleukin-2 and interferon-gamma gene expression in renal failure. *Kidney Int.* **40**, 266–272.

Giordano, G.G., Chevez–Barrios, P., Refojo, M.F., Garcia, C.A. 1995. Biodegradation and tissue reaction to intravitreous biodegradable poly(DL-lactic-co-glycolic)acid microspheres, *Curr. Eye Res.* **14**, 761–768.

Giray, C.B., Atasever, A., Durgun, B., Araz, K. 1997. Clinical and electron microscope comparison of silk sutures and n-butyl-2-cyanoacrylate in human mucosa, *Aust. Dent. J.* **42**, 255–258.

Gobel, R.J., Janatova, J., Googe, J.M., Apple D.J. 1987. Activation of complement in human serum by some synthetic polymers used for intraocular lenses, *Biomaterials* **8**, 285–288.

Golander, C.G., Lassen, B., Nilsson-Ekdahl, K., Nilsson, U.R. 1992. RF-plasma-modified polystyrene surfaces for studying complement activation, *J. Biomater. Sci. Polym. Ed.* **4**, 25–30.

Gong, J., Larsson, R., Ekdahl, K.N., Mollnes, T.F., Nilsson, U., Nilsson, B. 1996. Tubing loops as a model for cardiopulmonary bypass circuits, both the biomaterial and the blood-gas interfaces induce complement activation in an in vitro model, *J. Clin. Immunol.* **16**, 222–229.

Goren, D., Zalipsky, S., Horowitz, A.T., Gabizon, A. 1998. Stealth™ liposomes as carriers of doxorubicin, in: *Targeting of Drugs 6: Strategies for Stealth Therapeutic Systems* (G. Gregoriadis, B. McCormack, eds), pp. 77–85, Plenum Press, New York.

Gould, L., Trope, G., Cheng, Y.L., Heathcote, J.G., Sheardown, H., Rootman, D., Liu, G.S., Menon, I.A. 1994. Fifty:fifty poly(DL glycolic acid-lactic acid) copolymer as a drug delivery system for 5-fluorouracil: a histopathological evaluation, *Can. J. Ophthalmol.* **29**, 168–171.

Gref, R., Minamitake, Y., Peracchia, M.T., Trubetskoy, V., Torchilin, V., Langer, R. 1994. Biodegradable long-circulating polymeric nanospheres, *Science* **263**, 1600–1603.

Gref, R., Quellec, P., Alonso, M.J., Tobio, M., Lück, M., Müller, R.H., Dellacherie, E. 1998. PEG-coated nanospheres, surface optimization and therapeutic applications, in: *Targeting of Drugs 6: Strategies for Stealth Therapeutic Systems* (G. Gregoriadis, B. McCormack, eds), pp. 275–286, Plenum Press, New York.

Haeffner-Cavaillon, N., Cavaillon, J.M., Laude, M., Kazatchkine, M.D. 1987. C3a(C3adesArg) induces production and release of interleukin-1 by cultured human monocytes, *J. Immunol.* **139**, 794–799.

Hakim, R.M., Lowrie, E.G. 1982. Hemodialysis-associated neutropenia and hypoxemia: the effect of dialyser membrane materials, *Nephron* **32**, 32–39.

Hanke, P.R., Timm, P., Falk, G., Kramer, W. 1994. Behavior of different suture materials in the urinary bladder of the rabbit with special reference to wound healing, epithelization and crystallization, *Urol. Int.* **52**, 26–33.

Harashima, H., Sakata, K., Funato, K., Kiwada, H. 1994. Enhanced hepatic uptake of liposomes through complement activation depending on the size of liposomes, *Pharm. Res.* **11**, 402–406.

Hayakawa, M., Hatano, T., Sunabe, T., Higa., I., Osawa., A. 1994. Cytokine production and cytotoxicity of lymphocytes in patients on maintenance short or long term haemodialysis, *Nephrol. Dial. Transplant.* **9**, 144–152.

Hayoz, D. Do, D.D., Mahler, F., Triller, J., Spertini, F. 1997. Acute inflammatory reaction associated with endoluminal bypass grafts, *J. Endovasc. Surg.* **4**, 354–360.

Henry, C.H., Wolford, L.M. 1993. Treatment outcomes for temporomandibular joint reconstruction after Proplast-Teflon implant failure, *J. Oral Maxillofac. Surg.* **51**, 352–360.

Herzlinger, G.A., Bing, D.H., Stein, R., Cumming, R.D. 1981. Quantitative measurement of C3 activation at polymer surfaces, *Blood* **57**, 764–770.

Hirakawa, K., Bauer, T.W., Culver, J.E., Wilde, A.H. 1996. Isolation and quantitation of debris particles around failed silicone orthopedic implants, *J. Hand Surg.* [*Am.*] **21**, 819–827.

Hollick, E.J., Spalton, D.J., Ursell, P.G., Pande, M.V. 1998. Biocompatibility of poly(methyl methacrylate), silicone and Acrysof intraocular lenses, randomized comparison of the cellular reaction on the anterior lens surface, *J. Cataract Refract. Surg.* **24**, 361–366.

Huang, B., Marois, Y., Roy, R., Julien, M., Guidoin, R. 1992. Cellular reaction to the Vascugraft polyesterurethane vascular prosthesis, *in vivo* studies in rats, *Biomaterials* **13**, 209–216.

Hunt, J.A., Flanagan, B.F., McLaughlin, P.J., Strickland, I., Williams, D.F. 1996. Effect of biomaterial surface charge on the inflammatory response, evaluation of cellular infiltration and TNF alpha production, *J. Biomed. Mater. Res.* **31**, 139–144.

Innes, A., Farrel, A.M., Burden, R.P., Morgan, A.G., Powell, R.J. 1994. Complement activation by cellulosic dialysis membranes, *J. Clin. Pathol.* **47**, 155–158.

Jacobs, A.A. Jr., Ward, R.A., Wellhaussen, S.R., McLeish, K.R. 1989. Polymorphonuclear leukocyte function during hemodialysis: relationship to complement activation, *Nephron* **52**, 119–124.

James, S.J., Pogribna, M., Miller, B.J., Bolon, B., Muskhelishvili, L. 1997. Characterization of cellular response to silicone implants in rats: implications for foreign-body carcinogenesis, *Biomaterials* **18**, 667–675.

Jasty, M., Jiranek, W., Harris, W.H. 1992. Acrylic fragmentation in total hip replacements and its biological consequences, *Clin. Orthop.* **285**, 116–128.

Jayakrishnan, A., Lakshmi, S. 1998. Immobile plasticizer in flexible PVC, *Nature* **396**, 638

Jayakrishnan, A., Thanoo, B.C., Rathinam, K., Mohanty, M. 1990. Preparation and bioevaluation of radiopaque hydrogel microspheres based on PHEMA/iothalamic acid and PHEMA/iopanic acid as particulate emboli, *J. Biomed. Mater. Res.* **24**, 993–1004.

Jeon, S.I., Andrade, J.D. 1991. Protein-surface interactions in the presence of polyethylene oxide II. Effect of protein size, *J. Colloid Interface Sci.* **142**, 159–166.

Jeon, S.I., Lee, J.H., Andrade, J.D., de Gennes, P.G. 1991. Protein-surface interactions in the presence of polyethylene oxide I. Simplified theory, *J. Colloid Interface Sci.* **142**, 149–158.

Jiranek, W., Jasty, M., Wang, J.T., Bragdon, C., Wolfe, H., Goldberg, M., Harris, W.H. 1995. Tissue response to particulate polymethylmethacrylate in mice with various immune deficiencies, *J. Bone Jt. Surg. Am.* **77**, 1650–1661.

Johnson, R., Harrison, D., Tucci, M., Tsao, A., Lemos, M., Puckett, A., Hughes, J.L., Benghuzzi, H. 1997. Fibrous capsule formation in response to ultrahigh molecular weight polyethylene treated with peptides that influence adhesion, *Biomed. Sci. Instrum.* **34**, 47–52.

Kao, W.J., Zhao, Q.H., Hiltner, A., Anderson, J.M. 1994. Theoretical analysis of *in vivo* macrophage adhesion and foreign body giant cell formation on polydimethylsiloxane, low density polyethylene and polyurethanes, *J. Biomed. Mater. Res.* **28**, 73–79.

Kaplan, S.S., Basford, R.E., Jeong, M.H., Simmons, R.L. 1994. Mechanisms of biomaterial-induced superoxide release by neutrophils, *J. Biomed. Mater. Res.* **28**, 377–386.

Karlsson, M.K., Necking, L.E., Redlund-Johnell, I. 1992. Foreign body reaction after modified silicone rubber arthroplasty of the first carpometacarpal joint, *Scand. J. Plast. Reconstr. Surg. Hand Surg.* **26**, 101–103.

Kaspar, R.L., Gerhrke, L. 1994. Peripheral blood mononuclear cells stimulated with C5a or lipopolysaccharide to synthesize equivalent levels of IL-1beta mRNA show unequal IL-1 beta protein accumulation but similar polyribosome profiles, *J. Immunol.* **153**, 277–283.

Kasper, C.S. 1994. Histologic features of breast capsules reflect surface configuration and composition of silicone bag implants, *Am. J. Clin. Pathol.* **102**, 655–659.

Kasper, C.S., Chandler, P.J. Jr. 1994. Talc deposition in skin and tissues surrounding silicone gel-containing prosthetic devices, *Arch. Dermatol.* **130**, 48–53.

Kazatchkine, M.D., Fearon, D.T., Austen, K.F. 1979a. Human alternative complement pathway: membrane-associated sialic acid regulates the competition between B and β1H for cell-bound C3b, *J. Immunol.* **122**, 75–81.

Kazatchkine, M.D., Fearon, D.T., Silbert, J.E., Austen, K.F. 1979b. Surface-associated heparin inhibits zymosan-induced activation of the human alternative complement pathway by augmenting the regulatory action of the control proteins on particle-bound C3b, *J. Exp. Med.* **150**, 1202–1215.

Kazatchkine, M.D., Fearon, D.T., Metcalfe, D.D., Rosenberg, R.D., Austen, K.F. 1981. Structural determinants of the capacity of heparin to inhibit the formation of the human amplification convertase, *J. Clin. Invest.* **67**, 223–228.

Keogh, J.R., Wolf, M.F., Overend, M.E., Tang, L., Eaton, J.W. 1996. Biocompatibility of sulphonated polyurethane surfaces, *Biomaterials* **17**, 1987–1994.

Kim, K.J., Rubash, H.E., Wilson, S.C., D'Antonio, J.A., McClain, E.J. 1993. A histologic and biochemical comparison of the interface tissues in cementless and cemented hip prostheses, *Clin. Orthop.* **287**, 142–152.

Kinoshita, Y., Kirigakubo, M., Kobayashi, M., Tabata, T., Shimura, K., Ikada, Y. 1993. Study on the efficacy of biodegradable poly(L-lactide) mesh for supported transplanted particulate cancellous bone and marrow: experiment involving subcutaneous implantation in dogs, *Biomaterials* **14**, 729–736.

Kivalo, M. 1997. The effect of heparin-surface-modification on scar-tissue formation around a subconjunctival poly(methyl methacrylate) implant in the rabbit, *Acta Ophthalmol. Scand.* **75**, 189–193.

Kolff, W.G. 1990. The invention of the artificial kidney, *Int. J. Artif. Organs* **13**, 337–343.

Krause, T.J., Robertson, F.M., Greco, R.S. 1993. Measurement of intracellular hydrogen peroxide induced by biomaterials implanted in a rodent air pouch, *J. Biomed. Mater. Res.* **27**, 65–69.

Kuroki, K., Roy, S., Laerum, F., Mollnes, T.E., Solheim, B.G., Videm, V. 1995. Complement activation by angiographic catheters in vitro, *J. Vasc. Interv. Radiol.* **6**, 819–826.

Kurz, P., Kohler, H., Meuer, S., Hutteroch, T., Meyerzum-Buschenfelde., K. 1986. Impaired cellular immune responses in chronic renal failure: evidence for a T-cell defect, *Kidney Int.* **29**, 1209–1214.

Labarre, D. 1990. Heparin-like polymer surfaces, Control of coagulation and complement activation by insoluble functionalized polymers, *Int. J. Artif. Organs* **13**, 651–657.

Labarre, D., Passirani, C. 1996. Complement activation by polymer surfaces bearing hydroxyl groups, First International Symposium on Polymer Therapeutics, London.

Lam, K.H., Schakenraad, J.M., Groen, H., Esselbrugge, H., Dijkstra, P.J., Feijen, J., Nieuwenhuis, P. 1995. The influence of surface morphology and wettability on the inflammatory response against poly(L-lactic acid): a semi-quantitative study with monoclonal antibodies, *J. Biomed. Mater. Res.* **29**, 929–942.

Lansdown, A.B., Sirivongs, D., Vuttivirojana, A. 1995. Experimental evaluation of local reactions due to Dacron used in Tenekhoff catheters for peritoneal dialysis, *ASAIO J.* **41**, 202–204.

Laurent, A., Beaujeux, R., Wassef, M., Casasco, A., Gobin, Y.P., Aymard, A., Rufenacht, D., Boschetti, E., Merland, J.J. 1996. Trisacryl-gelatin microspheres for therapeutic embolization. Part 2: Clinical evaluation in tumors and arteriovenous malformations, *Am. J. Neuroradiology* **17**, 541–548.

Lhotta, K., Wurzner, R., Kronenberg, F., Oppermann, M., Konig, P. 1998. Rapid activation of the complement system by cuprophane depends on complement component C4, *Kidney Int.* **53**, 1044–1051.

Lin, Y.F., Chang, D.M., Shaio, M.F., Lu, K.C., Chyr, S.H., Li, B.L., Sheih, S.D. 1996. Cytokine production during hemodialysis: effects of dialytic membrane and complement activation, *Am. J. Nephrol.* **16**, 293–302.

Lin, Y.S., Hlady, V., Janatova, J. 1992. Adsorption of complement proteins on surfaces with a hydrophobicity gradient, *Biomaterials* **13**, 497–504.

Lindner, E., Cosofret, V.V., Ufer, S., Buck, R.P., Kao, W.J., Neuman, M.R., Anderson, J.M. 1994. Ion-selective membranes with low plasticizer content: electroanalytical characterization and biocompatibility studies, *J. Biomed. Mater. Res.* **28**, 591–601.

Loos, M., Volanakis, J.E., Stroud, R.M. 1976. Mode of interaction of different polyanions with the first (C1), the second (C2) and the fourth (C4) component of complement. III: Inhibition of C4 and C2 binding sites on C1S by polyanions, *Immunochemistry* **13**, 789–791.

Maillet, F., Petitou, M., Choay, J., Kazatchkine, M.D. 1988. Structure-function relationships in the inhibitory effect of heparin on complement activation: independency of the anti-coagulant and anti-complementary sites on the heparin molecule, *Mol. Immunol.* **25**, 917–923.

Marois, Y., Roy, R., Marois, M., Guidoin, R.G., von Maltzahn, W.W., Kowligi, R., Eberhart, R.C. 1992. T lymphocyte modification with the UTA microporous polyurethane vascular prosthesis: in vivo studies in rats, *Clin. Invest. Med.* **15**, 141–149.

Mathur, A.B., Collier, T.O., Kao, W.J., Wiggins, M., Schubert, M.A., Hiltner, A., Anderson, J.M. 1997. In vivo biocompatibility and biostability of modified polyurethanes, *J. Biomed. Mater. Res.* **36**, 246–257.

McGregor, R.R. 1977. Granulocyte adherence changes induced by hemodialysis, endotoxin, epinephrin, and glucocorticoids, *Ann. Intern. Med.* **36**, 35–41.

McNally, A.K., Anderson J.M. 1994. Complement C3 participation in monocyte adhesion to different surfaces, *Proc. Natl. Acad. Sci. USA* **91**, 10119–10123.

Merrill, E.W., Salzman, E.W. 1983. Polyethylene oxide as a biomaterial, *ASAIO J.* **6**, 60–64.

Mollnes, T.E., Riesenfeld, J., Garred, P., Nordström, E., Høgåsen, K., Fosse, E., Götze, O., Harboe, M. 1995. A new model for evaluation of biocompatibility: combined determination of neoepitopes in blood and on artificial surfaces demonstrates reduced complement activation by immobilization of heparin, *Artif. Organs* **19**, 909–917.

Montdargent, B., Labarre, D., Jozefowicz, M. 1991. Interactions of functionalized polystyrene derivatives with the complement system in human serum, *J. Biomater. Sci. Polym. Ed.* **2**, 25–35.

Montdargent, B., Toufik, J., Carreno, M.P., Labarre, D., Jozefowicz, M. 1992. Complement activation and adsorption of protein fragments by functionalized polymer surfaces in human serum, *Biomaterials* **13**, 571–576.

Montdargent, B., Maillet, F., Carreno, M.P., Jozefowicz, M., Kazatchkine, M., Labarre, D. 1993. Regulation by sulphonate groups of complement activation induced by hydroxymethyl groups on polystyrene surfaces, *Biomaterials* **14**, 203–208.

Moran J., Blumenstein, M., Gurland, H. 1990. Immunodeficiencies in chronic renal failure, *Contrib. Nephrol.* **86**, 91–110.

Naidu, S.H., Beredjiklian, P., Adler, L., Bora, F.W. Jr., Bker, D.G. 1996. In vivo inflammatory response to silicone elastomer particulate debris, *J. Hand Surg.* [*Am.*] **21**, 496–500.

Niessen, F.B., Spauwen, P.H., Kon, M. 1997. The role of suture material in hypertrophic scar formation: Monocryl vs.Vicryl-rapide, *Ann. Plast. Surg.* **39**, 254–260.

Niinobe, M., Matsuda, T., Iwata, H. 1988. Molecular mechanism of complement activation on polymer surfaces: contact activation of reconstituted first component (C1) of classical pathway, in: *Advances in Biomaterials*, Volume 8 (C. de Putter, G.I. de Groot, J.C. Lee, eds), pp. 181–186, Elsevier, Amsterdam.

Nilsson, U.R., Strom, K.E., Elwing, H., Nilsson, B. 1993a. Conformational epitope of C3 reflecting its mode of binding to an artificial polymer surface, *Mol. Immunol.* **30**, 211–219.

Nilsson, U.R., Larm, O., Nilsson, B., Strom, K.E., Elwing, H., Nilsson-Eckdahl, K. 1993b. Modification of the complement binding properties of polystyrene: effects of end-point heparin attachment, *Scand. J. Immunol.* **37**, 349–354.

Olofsson, P., Rabahie, G.N., Matsumoto, K., Ehrenfeld, W.K., Ferrell, L.D., Goldstone, J., Reilly, L.M., Stoney, R.J. 1995. Histopathological characteristics of explanted human prosthetic arterial grafts: implications for the prevention and management of graft infection, *Eur. J. Vasc. Endovasc. Surg.* **9**, 143–151.

Österberg, E., Bergstrm, K., Holmberg, K., Schuman, T.P., Riggs, J.A., Burns, N.L., Van Alstine, J.M., Harris, J.M. 1995. Protein-rejecting ability of surface-bound dextran in end-on and side-on configurations: comparison to PEG, *J. Biomed. Mater. Res.* **29**, 741–747.

Paivarinta, U., Bostman, O., Majola, A., Toivonen, T., Tormala, P., Rokkanen, P. 1993. Intraosseous cellular response to biodegradable fracture fixation screws made of polyglycolide or polylactide, *Arch. Orthop. Trauma Surg.* **112**, 71–74.

Pascual, M., Schifferli, J.A. 1993. Adsorption of complement factor D by polyacrylonitrile dialysis membranes, *Kidney Int.* **43**, 903–911.

Pascual, M., Plastre, O., Montdargent, B., Labarre, D., Schifferli, J.A. 1993a. Specific interactions of polystyrene biomaterials with factor D of human complement, *Biomaterials* **14**, 665–670.

Pascual, M., Schifferli, J.A., Pannatier, J.G., Wauters, J.P. 1993b. Removal of complement factor D by adsorption on polymethylmethacrylate dialysis membranes, *Nephrol. Dial. Transplant.* **8**, 1305–1306.

Passirani, C., Barratt, G., Devissaguet, J.P., Labarre, D. 1998a. Interactions of nanoparticles bearing heparin or dextran covalently bound to poly(methyl methacrylate) with the complement system, *Life Sci.* **62**, 775–785.

Passirani, C., Barratt, G., Devissaguet, J.P., Labarre, D. 1998b. Long-circulating nanoparticles bearing heparin or dextran covalently bound to poly(methyl methacrylate), *Pharm. Res.* **15**, 1046–1050.

Payne, M.S., Horbett, T.A. 1987. Complement activation by hydroxyethylmethacrylate-ethylmethacrylate copolymers, *J. Biomed. Mater. Res.* **21**, 843–859.

Pekna, M., Larsson, R., Formgren, B., Nilsson, U.R., Nilsson, B. 1993. Complement activation by polymethyl methacrylate minimized by end-point heparin attachment, *Biomaterials* **14**, 189–192.

Peracchia, M.T., Vauthier, C., Passirani, C., Couvreur, P., Labarre, D. 1997. Complement consumption by poly(ethylene glycol) in different conformations chemically coupled to poly(isobutyl 2-cyanoacrylate) nanoparticles, *Life Sci.* **61**, 749–761.

Pertosa, G., Tarantino, E.A., Gesualdo, L., Montaniro, V., Schena, F.P. 1993. C5b-9 generation and cytokine production in hemodialyzed patients, *Kidney Int.* **43**, S221–S225.

Petillo, O., Peluso, G., Ambrosio, L., Nicolais, L., Kao, W.J., Anderson, J.M. 1994. In vivo induction of macrophage Ia antigen (MHC class II) expression by biomedical polymers in the cage implant system, *J. Biomed. Mater. Res.* **28**, 635–646.

Rhie, J.W., Han, S.B., Byeon, J.H., Ahn, S.T., Kim, H.M. 1998. Efficient *in vitro* model for immunotoxicologic assessment of mammary silicone implants, *Plast. Reconstr. Surg.* **102**, 73–77.

Rhodes, N.P., Hunt, J.A., Williams, D.F. 1997. Macrophage subpopulation differentiation by stimulation with biomaterials, *J. Biomed. Mater. Res.* **37**, 481–488.

Sahli, H., Tapon-Bretaudiere, J., Fischer, A.M., Sternberg, C., Spenlehauer, G., Verrecchia, T., Labarre, D. 1997. Interactions of poly(lactic acid) and poly(lactic acid-co-ethylene oxide) nanoparticles with the plasma factors of the coagulation system, *Biomaterials* **18**, 281–288.

Schindler, R., Linnenweber, S., Schulze, M., Oppermann, M., Dinarello, C.A., Shaldon, S., Koch, K.M. 1993. Gene expression of interleukin-1 beta during hemodialysis, *Kidney Int.* **43**, 712–721.

Schoels, M., Jahn, B., Hug, F., Deppish, R., Ritz, E., Hänsch, G.M. 1993. Stimulation of mononuclear cells by contact with cuprophan membranes: further increase of beta2-microglobulin synthesis by activated late complement components, *J. Kidney Dis.* **21**, 394–399.

Schröder, J.M., Sticherling, M., Henneicke., H.H., Preissner, W.C., Christophers, E. 1990. IL-1 alpha or TNF-alpha stimulate release of three NAP/IL-8-related neutrophil chemotactic proteins in human dermal fibroblast, *J. Immunol.* **144**, 2223–2229.

Schurmann, K., Vorwerk, D., Bucker, A., Neuerburg, J., Klosterhalfen, B., Muller, G., Uppenkamp, R., Gunther, R.W. 1997. Perigraft inflammation due to Dacron-covered stent–grafts in sheep iliac arteries: correlation of MR imaging and histopathological findings, *Radiology* **204**, 757–763.

Setzen, G., Williams, E.F. 1997. Tissue response to suture materials implanted subcutaneously in a rabbit model, *Plast. Reconstr. Surg.* **100**, 1788–1795.

Skorpik, C., Menapace, R., Scholz, U., Scheidel, W., Grasl, M. 1993. Erfahrungen mit Disklinsen aus Siliconmaterial, *Klin. Monatsbl. Augenheilkd.* **202**, 8–13.

Soler, M., Verhaeghe, P., Essomba, A., Sevestre, H., Stoppa, R. 1993. Le traitement des éventrations post-opératoires par prothèse composée (polyester-polyglactin 910). Etude clinique et expérimentale, *Ann. Chir.* **47**, 598–608.

Stachowski, J., Pollock, M., Barth, C., Maciejewwski, J., Baldamus, C. 1994. Non-responsiveness to hepatitis B vaccination in haemodialysis patients: association with impaired TCR/CD3 antigen receptor expression regulating co-stimulatory processes in antigen presentation and recognition, *Nephrol. Dial. Transplant.* **9**, 144–152.

Swartbol, P., Parsson, H., Truedsson, L., Sjoholm, A., Norgren, L. 1996. Aortobifemoral surgery induces complement activation and release of interleukin-6 but not tumour necrosis factor-alpha, *Cardiovasc. Surg.* **4**, 483–491.

Tang, L., Eaton, J.W. 1993. Fibrin(ogen) mediates acute inflammatory responses to biomaterials, *J. Exp. Med.* **178**, 2147–2156.

Tegnander, A., Engebretsen, L., Bergh, K., Eide, E., Holen, K.J., Iversen, O.J. 1994. Activation of the complement system and adverse effects of biodegradable pins of polylactic acid (Biofix) in osteochondritis dissecans, *Acta Orthop. Scand.* **65**, 472–475.

Thylen P., Lundahl, J., Fernvik, E., Hed, J., Svenson, S.B., Jacobson, S.H. 1992. Mobilization of an intracellular glycoprotein (Mac-1) on monocytes and granulocytes during hemodialysis, *Am. J. Nephrol.* **12**, 393–400.

Toufik, J., Labarre, D. 1995. Relationship between reduction of complement activation by polysaccharide surfaces bearing diethylaminoethyl groups and their degree of substitution, *Biomaterials* **16**, 1081–1088.

Toufik, J., Carreno, M.P., Jozefowicz, M., Labarre, D. 1995. Activation of the complement system by polysaccharidic surfaces bearing carboxymethyl, carboxymethyl-benzylamide and carboxymethylbenzylamide sulphonate groups, *Biomaterials* **16**, 993–1002.

Utoh, J., Goto, H., Hirata, T., Hara, M., Kitamura, N. 1997. Postoperative inflammatory reactions to sealed Dacron prostheses, a comparison of Gelseal and Hemashield, *J. Cardiovasc. Surg. (Torino)* **38**, 287–290.

Van Der Vis, H.M., Marti, R.K., Tigehelaar, W., Schuller, H.M., Van Noorden, C.J. 1997. Benign cellular responses in rats to different wear particles in intra-articular and intramedullary environments, *J. Bone Jt. Surg. Br.* **79**, 837–843.

Van Sliedregt, A., Knook, M., Hesseling, S.C., Koerten, H.K., de Groot, K., van Blitterswijk, C.A. 1992. Cellular reaction on the intraperitoneal injection of four types of polylactide particulates, *Biomaterials* **13**, 819–824.

Vittaz, M., Bazile, D., Spenlehauer, G., Verrecchia, T., Veillard, M., Puisieux, F., Labarre, D., 1996. Effect of PEO surface density on long-circulating nanoparticles which are low complement activators, *Biomaterials* **17**, 1575–1581.

Ward, C.A., Koheil, A., Johnson, W.R., Madras, P.N. 1984. Reduction in complement activation from biomaterials by removal of air nuclei from the surface roughness, *J. Biomed. Mater. Res.* **18**, 255–269.

Weiler, J.M., Yurt, R.W., Fearon, D.T., Austen, K.F. 1978. Modulation of the formation of the amplification convertase of complement C3bBb, by native and commercial heparin, *J. Exp. Med.* **147**, 409–421.

Wenzel, M., Kammann, J., Allmers, R. 1993. Zur Bioverträglichkeit von Intraokularlinsen aus Silicon, *Klin. Monatsbl. Augenheilkd.* **203**, 408–412.

Wichterle, O., Lim, D. 1960. Hydrophilic gels for biological use, *Nature (London)* **185**, 117–118.

Woffindin, C., Hoenich, N.A., Mattews, J.N. 1992. Cellulose-based haemodialysis membranes: biocompatibility and functional performance compared, *Nephrol. Dial. Transplant.* **7**, 340–345.

Wooley, P.H., Nasser, S., Fitzgerald, R.H. Jr. 1996. The immune response to implant materials in humans, *Clin. Orthop.* **326**, 63–70.

Zhang, Y.Z., Bjursten, L.M., Freij-Larsson, C., Kober, M., Wesslen, B. 1996. Tissue response to commercial silicone and polyurethane elastomers after different sterilization procedures, *Biomaterials* **17**, 2265–2272.

26

Inflammatory Response to Metals and Ceramics

Arturo Pizzoferrato, Elisabetta Cenni, Gabriela Ciapetti, Donatella Granchi, Lucia Savarino, and Susanna Stea

26.1. Introduction

The implantation of a prosthetic material produces tissue damage and a defense reaction, namely inflammation. The inflammatory reaction is phylogenetically and ontogenetically the oldest defense mechanism.

The acute inflammation that follows implantation lasts a short time and leaves no signs provided there are no side effects to prolong it. But the material of the prosthesis itself could cause such an effect: this may then lead to chronic inflammation, which may either heal, continue over time, or cause biological damage. If the cause of inflammation is able to interact with the immune system, a cell-mediated or humoral immune response is induced.

This chapter analyses the pathophysiology of the aforementioned phenomena with regard to metal and ceramic prosthetic materials.

26.2. Material Degradation and Inflammation

Materials which come in contact with the biological environment must fulfil a number of requirements; moreover, the inflammatory reaction elicited must be as limited as possible.

Arturo Pizzoferrato, Elisabetta Cenni, Gabriela Ciapetti, Donatella Granchi, Lucia Savarino, and Susanna Stea • Laboratorio di Fisiopatologia degli Impianti Ortopedici, Istituti Ortopedici Rizzoli, Via di Barbiano 1/10, 40136 Bologna, Italy.

Integrated Biomaterials Science, edited by R. Barbucci. Kluwer Academic/Plenum Publishers, New York, 2002.

The chemical composition, additives, manufacturing processes, and decontamination/sterilization of the materials can influence their stability. In addition, all materials contain either minor components or impurities which may be released in the biological environment, so inducing a tissue response even if the main component is stable.

Conversely, the stability of biomaterials is influenced by the biological events that occur at the interface with tissues.

Advanced stages of degradation of a material, i.e., a consistent decrease in its mechanical properties and/or mass, often result in a change of the material properties, as well as in a change of the biological response (Standard ISO/TR 10993-9, 1994).

Products of degradation and/or released constituents may be eliminated (bioresorption) from the body by normal metabolic pathways, without causing acute or chronic damage to any component of the physiological system, or accumulated within the body, leading to adverse local or systemic effects.

It is relatively simple to find materials which satisfy the functional requirements (e.g., strength, fatigue resistance, stiffness, transparency, electrical conductivity). More difficult is to find materials maintaining their performance for a long period of time (more than 20 years in some instances) without degrading or inducing undesired effects, such as inflammation, in the host tissues.

Therefore the characteristics of the materials contacting biological fluids and tissues have to be defined and their long-term stability, as well as the degradation kinetics of resorbable materials, have to be verified: the physicochemical properties of the material, the surface chemistry, and the morphology, all modulate the inflammatory response.

26.2.1. Metals and Alloys

Metals and alloys have a large range of application, especially in orthopedics and dentistry, including devices for partial and total joint replacement, devices for fracture fixation, surgical instruments, external splints, dental implants and amalgams, heart valves, pace-maker cases, conductive leads. The high modulus, strength, and corrosion resistance coupled with the ductility of metals make them suitable for bearing loads, without leading to significant deformations and permanent dimensional changes. Metals and alloys for implants must have minimal tendency to corrode electrochemically; alternatively, this tendency is suppressed by the formation of a protective oxide film on the surface.

A large number of alloys such as stainless steel AISI 316L, cobalt–chrome alloys, and titanium alloys have been widely used for oral and orthopedic implants; they may be designed for short-term function or for the life of the patient, as in total joint replacement. Most of the metal-alloy implants may corrode in a biological milieu and there is no doubt that their degradation plays a role in prosthesis loosening, even if mechanisms are not well known (Dobbs and Minski, 1980; Shahgaldi *et al.*, 1995; Merritt and Brown, 1996).

Notwithstanding the strength and hardness of metal alloys, degradation may occur resulting from electrochemical dissolution, wear, or a synergistic combination of the two mechanisms.

Corrosion, and consequently ion release, represents the main *in vivo* degradation mechanism for such materials since corrosion products represent lower energy states: salts, especially if containing chloride ions, and extracellular proteins are some of the agents of this process.

In vivo corrosion is associated both with the effects of corrosion on the material and with the effect of corrosion products on the tissue. The synergistic interaction between biological, chemical, and electrochemical factors and mechanical stress can lead to the oxidation of specific metal atoms. As a result, metal ions released from the surface of the material into the surrounding tissues and fluids may cause local and systemic responses.

Electrochemical phenomena include generalized and localized corrosion (crevice and pitting corrosion); usually in a metallic alloy several oxidation processes occur at the same time leading to several corrosion mechanisms, such as stress corrosion cracking, corrosion fatigue, and fretting (Lycott and Hughes, 1984). Metal ion release can be further increased by chemical and electrochemical variables and mechanical stresses.

Concerns have been raised regarding the potential hazards posed by metal ions released by corrosion of orthopedic implants, especially metals that are known carcinogens in other situations, such as hexavalent chromium, cobalt, and nickel (Merritt and Brown, 1996). There are several issues to be considered in assessing these hazards, including the corrosion rate, specific chemical species released, the intrinsic toxicity of the products, and their distribution and fate within the body (Jacobs *et. al.*, 1995, 1996), as well as the possible synergistic or antagonistic interactions among the corrosion product components (Timbrell, 1991).

Metal ions may be released at different sites and/or levels, depending on the type and solubility of the reaction products: they are either stored within tissues, or transported to distant organs, or excreted through urine, feces, skin, hair, and nails (Merritt *et al.*, 1980). In some cases local inflammatory responses or systemic diseases can be induced or enhanced. It is reasonably assumed that the local and systemic effects of metal ions are due to a dose-dependent mechanism: they act as essential trace elements, but become toxic if too much. The threshold between the toxic and the physiological dose is often not clear-cut, and an essential element becomes toxic due to a minimal increase in concentration.

Particulate wear debris from material surfaces, mainly from abrasive or three-body wear, may also be a source of metal ions: thus metal ion release is associated with both corrosion of bulk material surfaces and degradation of particulate debris.

A number of studies investigated the biological response to metal particles and how metal particles corrode *in vivo*, often playing an important role in the pathological processes of prosthetic loosening: at the implant site, where the concentration of ions is high and particulates are released, inflammatory and toxic reactions can take place. Wear debris from metal implants induce foreign-body reactions driven by histiocytes and giant cells: these cells have been strongly involved with progressive osteolysis and aseptic loosening of the implant (Goldring *et al.*, 1986; Jiranek *et al.*, 1993). The type of material, the size of the particles, and the total surface area influence the reactions to wear debris (Hirakawa *et al.*, 1996).

Moreover, corrosion products could be responsible for the induction of bone resorbing agents, such as interleukin 1α, interleukin 1β, interleukin 6, and tumor necrosis factor, by macrophages, fibroblasts, and endothelial cells (Jiranek *et al.*, 1993; Yang and Merritt, 1994). As these biological mediators regulate bone remodeling and have the ability to initiate an inflammatory response and bone resorption (Sun *et al.*, 1997), an imbalance in their production may contribute to the process of bone osteolysis and eventually induce prosthesis failure (Thompson and Puleo, 1995; Nichols and Puleo, 1997; Ishiguro *et al.*, 1997).

Also, the immune system can be involved when the corrosion products are drained to the lymph nodes. Conflicting results have been obtained on the mechanism of interaction between metal ions and the immune system: in the bloodstream the ions are diluted and are no longer toxic, but may act as a sensitizer and trigger a specific immune reaction (Lalor and Revell, 1993; Case *et al.*, 1994; Granchi *et al.*, 1995; Lee *et al.*, 1997; Savarino *et al.*, 1999).

26.2.2. Ceramics

Ceramics are largely used in the biomedical field and are classified according to their physiological reactivity. At one end of the range are the inert, or better the nearly inert ceramics, i.e., oxide ceramics such as alumina. At the other end are found some calcium phosphate ceramics, which are degraded and resorbed upon implantation.

Between these extremes are the ceramics of controlled reactivity applied in orthopedics and dentistry because of their biocompatibility and adequate binding with tissues (Klein *et al.*, 1983a).

Inert ceramics are the most biologically accepted of all materials because of their chemical stability; they are much less likely to produce any adverse effects, compared with metals and polymers.

Their intrinsic properties include rigidity, high compressive strength, fatigue resistance, hardness, and corrosion resistance; therefore they are applied mainly in orthopedics as bearing surface of joint prostheses, as well as in dental and maxillofacial surgery (Harms and Mausle, 1979). High-density alumina is the bioinert material most widely used because of its durability and corrosion resistance. Nevertheless, even alumina dissolves somewhat in extracellular fluids, because aluminum forms complexes in aqueous solutions with hydroxyl, fluoride, and phosphate ions. Moreover, some wear can occur that could give rise to an inflammatory response. The tissue reaction of the alumina wear debris has been extensively studied: it has been shown that the effects of wear are generally limited, without any particular cellular reaction, possibly due to the very small size of particles. Only when the ceramic particles are associated with debris from other materials can an intense foreign-body reaction occur (Lerouge *et al.*, 1996; Kubo *et al.*, 1999).

Ceramics of controlled reactivity and *degradable ceramics* include resorbable calcium phosphate materials, sintered apatites, i.e., hydroxyapatite (HA), tricalcium phosphate (TCP), bioactive glasses (BG), and glass ceramics, as well as calcium-phosphates from natural sources, i.e., human bones, banked freeze-dried bones or sintered bones, processed and/or sintered bovine bone. The chemical, physical, and mechanical properties of these materials have been summarized in previous reviews (de Groot, 1983; Van Raemdonck *et al.*, 1984; Ducheyne and Lemons, 1988).

The behavior of such ceramics can be largely influenced by physicochemical properties such as crystallinity, granulometry, and porosity (Daculsi and Passuti, 1990; Bohne *et al.*, 1993; Malard *et al.*, 1999); however, their biocompatibility and bioactive properties, i.e., the ability to elicit or modulate biological activity, have already been demonstrated (Cheung and Haak, 1989; Williams *et al.*, 1993).

For bone replacement materials bioactivity is directly related to bone bonding through the formation of an apatite layer on the ceramic material. Then a variety of events occurs at the bioactive ceramic–tissue interface, such as dissolution from the ceramic, ion exchange and structural rearrangement at the ceramic–tissue interface, solution-mediated effects on cellular activity, deposition of either the mineral phase or the organic phase, with or without integration into the ceramic surface, chemotaxis of cells toward the ceramic surface, cell attachment, proliferation and differentiation, and eventually extracellular matrix formation (Daculsi *et al.*, 1990; Neo *et al.*, 1993; Ducheyne and Qiu, 1999)

Calcium phosphate ceramics are used as bone substitutes in orthopedics, as well as in ear, nose, and throat and oral surgery (de Groot, 1983) although their mechanical properties make this difficult. They have little compressive strength, depending mainly on the porosity, the pore size, the chemical composition, and the grain size (Le Huec *et al.*, 1995). These materials are fragile, brittle, and cannot be shaped during surgical operations. Consequently, they are not designed for load-bearing applications, where local stress and associated wear would be elicited, but are reported to be successful in promoting bone formation when used to repair bone or periodontal defects, and as coatings on load-bearing orthopedic or dental devices for tissue ingrowth. In such applications, the nature of the interface between coating and substrate will significantly affect the material stability, while the properties of the coating material such as crystallinity and chemistry will determine the coating stability.

Among the materials for coating, HA powder has been widely used in orthopedics and in dental surgery, as a source material for plasma-sprayed, bone-like coatings deposited onto metal substrates because of its ability to bond chemically to bone (Jarcho,1981; Tofe *et al.*, 1994).

Thus, artificial components and prostheses with superior mechanical properties, such as dental implants or hip joints, can be implanted within bone and hard tissue when coated with HA (de Groot *et al.*, 1998): push-out tests show that the bond between implant and surrounding bone may approach the shear strength of bone.

Excellent clinical results were reported for hydroxyapatite (HA)-coated implants. Nevertheless, the clinical use of hydroxyapatite (HA) coating is controversial, as far as the long-term performance of the coating and the effects of resorption are concerned, because, after being subject to the elevated temperatures ($>1000\,^{\circ}C$) associated with the plasma spraying process, the coated HA is chemically modified; a noncrystalline or amorphous phase fraction is introduced that, in combination with other Ca-phosphate phases, strongly affects the resorption characteristics of the coating in the human body and therefore its lifespan (Radin and Ducheyne, 1994; LeGeros *et al.*, 1994). The degradation of coatings causes chemical and physical changes which affect their properties and performance. Such changes may lead to crack initiation and propagation, fracture, debonding, chemical transformation and, in some cases, dissolution of the material, wear debris production, and tissue reaction.

Early stage inflammatory reactions toward HA and third-body wear following hip replacement surgery have been identified in recent studies: the early inflammatory response is characterized by local osteoporosis, favorable bonding between the implant and the cortical bone, eosinophilic deposition, nonspecific local inflammation, and bone marrow depletion. Multinuclear cells have been identified in the inflammation area (Korkusuz and Uluoglu, 1999).

With the advent of mass production of coated devices, reliable measures have to be implemented to assure their chemical integrity and the reproducibility of the spraying process.

26.3. Acute Inflammatory Response

Following the implantation of a device in the body the tissue is acutely damaged: this provides a series of stimuli for inflammation, which substantially consists in the migration of serum proteins and cells to the injured areas.

The inflammatory response to the implantation of biomaterials follows a pattern shared by most inflammatory reactions in the body, irrespective of the stimulus. Specific responses may be elicited at a later stage, due to the persistence of the implant or the release of foreign substances. Three phases can be distinguished for the sake of clarity:

(a) the exudative phase, which involves intense signaling and migration of inflammatory cells;

(b) the proliferative phase, marked by active cell division and granulation tissue formation;

(c) the repair phase, characterized by new connective tissue and/or tissue organization.

At the beginning of the process vasoactive and chemotactic agents (bradykinin, prostaglandins, etc.) are produced by the resident cells: the vasodilation with increased blood supply and the generation of new chemotactic factors by blood cells promote, respectively, the exudation of plasma fluid and the adhesion of cells to the endothelium. For the increased capillary permeability caused by retraction of the endothelial cells, first macromolecules, then leukocytes move from bloodstream to the inflammatory site. Some plasma proteins are known to adhere to the biomaterial surface thereby modulating the cell/biomaterial interactions. In the earliest stages of inflammation, neutrophils are prevalent, but later monocytes and lymphocytes migrate toward the injured site.

In the inflamed area the recruited cells are activated and differing activities are performed, including secretion of cytokines, prostaglandins, and lysosomal enzymes, phagocytosis of debris, necrosis of irreversibly damaged cells, production of reactive oxygen species, and so on. The nature of the initial stimulus and/or its persistence dictates the evolution of this firing situation toward resolution or self-perpetuating reaction (chronic response).

The inflammatory response to biomaterials is often studied following implantation in the soft tissues, with subsequent formation of a fibrous capsule, but quantitative studies on cell types and numbers around the implant are rare (Freyria *et al.*, 1991). The composition of the inflammatory exudate surrounding an implanted biomaterial can be determined *in vivo* using the cage implant system in animals without their sacrifice (Marchant *et al.*, 1983).

The type of death of cells irreversibly damaged by biomaterials, i.e., the distinction between necrosis and apoptosis, has become relevant in the network of reaction to implants.

Apoptosis or "programmed cell death" plays an important role in the physiological turnover of cells for the maintenance of tissue organization. In contrast with apoptosis, necrosis is a mechanism of cell death usually determined by high concentrations of the toxic agent.

In vivo the apoptotic death is limited to the involved cells and the complete elimination of such cells by phagocytes prevents an inflammatory response, while the necrosis is accompanied by cell lysis, release of proteolytic enzymes, and other products: inflammation and injury to tissues may follow (Tomei and Cope, 1991). The induction of either necrosis or apoptosis of cells by biomaterials has been recently investigated.

26.3.1. Mediators of the Inflammatory Reaction

The development of the inflammatory reaction is controlled by a number of active substances:

- products of the plasma enzymatic systems—coagulation, kinin and fibrinolytic pathways, complement—are fast-acting mediators which modulate the immediate response;
- lipid mediators—prostaglandins and leukotrienes—cause the accumulation and activation of cells;
- vasoactive mediators released from mast cells, basophils, and platelets;
- cytokines released by leukocytes.

These substances have been identified in the human periprosthetic tissues, and their role in the reaction to implant has been confirmed by *in vitro* studies.

The inflammatory cells interact with the layer of adsorbed proteins onto the material surface, with the composition of this layer depending on the properties of the material. This contact leads to the activation of one or more of the protease cascades, such as coagulation, fibrinolysis, the complement system, and the kallikrein-kinin system, and to the adhesion and activation of platelets and neutrophils.

The type of particle ingested by phagocytes may influence the release of mediators: a number of substances, including PGE2, IL-1, IL-6, and TNF, have been demonstrated to mediate the resorption of bone around the implant. Materials with moderate toxicity but high wear rate have been shown to participate in bone resorption, as they cause a release of inflammatory mediators greater than that induced by a more toxic alloy, which leads cells to death.

26.3.1.1. Complement

The complement system is part of the nonspecific immune response: when this system is activated, a number of proteases are sequentially activated to lead to a stable complex with cytolytic activity. Moreover, the anaphylatoxins C3a and C5a are produced following the activation of complement. These cause increased vascular permeability, smooth muscle contraction, and release of histamine and other inflammatory mediators from basophils and mast cells. C5a is a potent chemotactic agent and activator of polymorphonuclear leukocytes, too: granulocytes and monocytes are induced to adhere to the endothelium and, after migration into tissues, to release their enzymes.

Complement activation onto the biomaterial surface may influence biocompatibility. Usually biomaterials activate the complement through the alternative pathway, even though the involvement of the classic pathway cannot be excluded (Jahns *et al.*, 1993). Following transportation of the activated factors along the bloodstream, systemic effects are reported.

The evaluation of complement activation is included in Standard ISO 10993-4: the assay of the classical, the alternative and the common pathways are recommended, as well as the membrane attack complex.

The C4a and C4d fragments are markers of the classical pathway. Bb, C3a and iC3b (inactivated-C3b) are markers of the alternative pathway, while C5a is a marker of the common pathway.

The membrane attack complex is generated by the assembly of C5 through C9 as a consequence of the complement activation by either the classical or the alternative pathway. Complexes formed in the absence of a target membrane bind to a regulatory serum protein, the S protein. The S protein binds to C5b-9 complexes, forming the soluble, nonlytic SC5b-9 complex.

a. Complement and Metals. Cobalt, silver, and nickel powder may activate complement; but complement activation was not detected in serum incubated with chromium powder (Remes and Williams, 1991a). Other authors demonstrated increased deposition of C3c and iC3b onto chromium surfaces after incubation in plasma or in serum. C3 convertases (C4d or Bb fractions) were not observed. A low or transient complement activation via the classical pathway was indicated on ethanol-washed chromium, since deposition of C1q was observed only after short incubation times (Walivaara *et al.*, 1996).

After contact of blood with titanium oxide (TiO_2), the complement was adsorbed initially onto titanium surface, then the amount of deposited complement decreased with time, and the amount of adsorbed high molecular weight kininogen increased (Kanagaraja *et al.*, 1996).

The effects of titanium dioxide on C3 adsorption from diluted human plasma was found to depend on the Ti crystal structure and on the exposure time (McAlarney *et al.*, 1996).

b. Complement and Ceramics. Complement activation may be involved in the mechanism by which some ceramic implants are resorbed. Macrophages have receptors for C3b and these receptors cause cells to adhere to other cells or to particles bearing C3b on their surface, facilitating phagocytosis. C3b may also stimulate frustrated phagocytosis by cells, a process which would result in degradative enzymes and high-energy oxygen species being secreted over the implant surface. Both phagocytosis and frustrated phagocytosis may lead to resorption of the ceramic implant. In addition, C3 deposition mediates the recruitment of mononuclear osteoclast precursors to the exposed mineralized bone surface (Mangham *et al.*, 1993).

It was demonstrated that at increasing serum concentrations of both calcium hydrogen phosphate and coral (calcium carbonate) powder, the quantity of C3 activation increased (Remes and Williams, 1991b).

Other authors found that sintered tricalcium phosphate (β-whitlockite) does not activate complement, while HA powders after sintering induce conversion of C3 (Klein *et al.*, 1983b).

26.3.1.2. Prostaglandins

Prostaglandins derive from arachidonic acid through the cyclo-oxygenase pathway. The arachidonic acid is converted by the microsomal enzyme cyclo-oxygenase into cyclic endoperoxide PGG_2, which in turn is transformed into PGH_2 by hydroperoxidase PGHS. There are two separate PGHS enzymes: constitutive PGHS (PGHS-1) and inducible PGHS

(PGHS-2). Following conversion by a number of isomerases and synthetases, prostacyclin, thromboxane, PGD_2, PGE_2, and $PGF_{2\alpha}$ are produced.

PGE_2 (produced by macrophages, monocytes, neutrophils, and osteoblasts) is pyrogenic, enhances vascular permeability and sensitivity to pain, and stimulates leukocyte cAMP. In addition, it is likely to mediate bone resorption induced by cytokines, contributing to hip prosthesis loosening. PGE_2 can also have an anabolic effect on bone (stimulating the collagen synthesis and preosteoblast replication), probably through IGF-1 or TGFβ. $PGF_{2\alpha}$ (produced by macrophages, monocytes, osteoblasts, and platelets) can stimulate bone resorption, but its effect is partially mediated by an increase in endogenous PGE_2 production. Thromboxane A_2 (produced by monocytes, macrophages, and platelets) induces platelet aggregation and blood vessel constriction. Prostacyclin is a potent vasodilator and inhibits platelet aggregation. PGD_2 is produced by mast cells, while PGI_2 is produced by endothelial cells and osteoblasts.

Prostaglandin synthesis is increased by IL-1, TNF, bradykinin, thrombin, TGFβ, TGFα, EGF, PDGF, FGF; it is inhibited by IFNγ, and IL-4. Conversely, the production and activity of cytokines are induced by prostaglandins (Ibbotson *et al.*, 1985).

a. PGE_2 and Metals. The release of PGE_2, mainly by macrophages after particle ingestion, has to be considered due to its activity in resorbing bone. Internalization of particles, necessary for cytokine secretion, is not required for the release of PGE_2: the synthesis of PGE_2 is induced by simple particle–cell membrane interaction, without phagocytosis. This phenomenon of "frustrated phagocytosis" is frequently observed during interaction of cells with other nonphagocytosable particles (Shanbhag *et al.*, 1995). PGE_2 is secreted by osteoblasts and fibroblasts, too, and some bone-resorbing cytokines, including IL-1, IL-6, and TNF, are released, as well.

Chemical composition, size, concentration, and aging of particles are key factors for the release of PGE_2 from macrophages. It was found that Co^{2+} and Cr^{3+} ions increased the release of PGE_2 from leukocytes, while Ti^{3+} ions were associated with a decrease in the release of PGE_2 (Liu *et al.*, 1999). In another study, the macrophages exposed to commercially pure Ti (1–3 μm) released TNF, while PGE_2 was produced by osteoblasts exposed to the macrophage-conditioned medium (Gonzales *et al.*, 1996).

The discrepancy in results may be due to the different source of macrophages used in the different studies: human monocytes, murine peritoneal macrophages, and immortalized cell lines may well respond differently to Ti.

Concerning the size of particles, Ti alloy particles ranging over 0.1–10 μm stimulated the release of PGE_2 from cultured human monocytes/macrophages (Maloney *et al.*, 1996). The effect of size and concentration of Ti particles was studied by Glant *et al.* (1993). Particulates in the non-phagocytosable size range had very little or no effect on PGE_2 production by peritoneal macrophages, while Ti particulates $<1\,\mu$m in size stimulate peritoneal macrophages to secrete PGE_2. The maximum response to 1–3 μm Ti particles is observed at a concentration of 0.1% (approximately 10–15 Ti particulates per cell).

The aging of particles may influence the response, too: aged particles of CoCr and AISI 316L stainless steel, from implant retrieval, were less toxic than freshly produced particles, but stimulate the release of more IL-6 and PGE_2 from monocytes (Haynes *et al.*, 2000).

It has been found, using immortalized cell lines *in vitro*, that the inflammatory response of macrophages to CoCr, including PGE_2 secretion, is amplified by the presence of osteoblasts: if this is the case *in vivo*, bone resorption would be increased (Horowitz *et al.*, 1998). Macrophage-secreted PGE_2 stimulates the production of IL-6, with an increased osteolytic reaction, as was shown with TiAlV particles (Haynes *et al.*, 1996).

b. PGE_2 and Ceramics. A drawback with HA or HA/TCP coatings on implant devices is their tendency to fragment and generate particulate wear debris. Following the release of particles in the implant bed, an adverse tissue reaction is triggered, similar to that associated with fragmented PMMA or polyethylene, which have been implicated in peri-implant granuloma formation and aseptic loosening after total joint replacement. Human bone marrow mononuclear cells exposed to HA particles release PGE_2, indicating that HA or HA/TCP have significant proinflammatory effect when transformed from an intact surface coating to a particulate form (Kim *et al.*, 1993).

The HA/TCP particles derived from different sintering temperatures exhibit different effects on cultured human monocyte/macrophages. The HA/TCP particles dried at 110 °C were the most biologically active, stimulating significant release of PGE_2. Other particles, sintered at either 900 or 1200 °C, did not stimulate PGE_2 production. HA/TCP particles from plasma-spray coatings also failed to release proinflammatory products (Harada *et al.*, 1996).

26.3.1.3. Cytokines

Cytokines are soluble glycoproteins or peptides which act nonenzymatically in picomolar to nanomolar concentrations through specific receptors to provide intercellular signals.

Cytokines are synthesized, stored, and released by various cell types. They act mostly on neighboring cells in the microenvironment where they have been released. They are characterized as local hormones and their secretion is brought about by autocrine or paracrine mechanisms. During paracrine secretion some cytokines may escape cell binding and may spill over into the general circulation.

The central role of cytokines is to control the direction, amplitude, and duration of immune responses and to control the modeling of tissues, developmentally programmed, constitutive, or unscheduled. Unscheduled remodeling is that which accompanies inflammation, infection, wounding, and repair. Individual cytokines can have pleiotropic, overlapping, and sometimes contradictory functions depending on their concentration, the type of target cells, and the presence of other cytokines and mediators. It is supposed that all cytokines form the specific system or network of communication signals between cells of the immune system, and between the immune system and other organs. Their activities, particularly secretion and receptor expression, are strictly regulated. Additional regulatory mechanisms are provided by the concomitant action of different cytokines and the presence in biological fluids of specific inhibitory proteins, soluble cytokine-binding factors, and specific autoantibodies. The cytokine system is a very potent force in homeostasis when activation of the network is local and cytokines act vicinally in surface-bound or diffusible form, but when their production is sustained and/or systemic there is no doubt that cytokines contribute to the signs, symptoms, and pathology of inflammatory, infectious, autoimmune, and malignant diseases.

IL-1, IL-6, TNFα, IL-11, IFNγ, and some members of the chemokine superfamily, produced by activated macrophages, are proinflammatory cytokines, i.e., they up-regulate the inflammatory reactions. The anti-inflammatory cytokines IL-4, IL-10, and IL-13 belong to the T cell-derived group and down-regulate inflammation through suppression of the production of proinflammatory cytokines. This inhibitory effect may be exerted even when the production of proinflammatory cytokines is induced by wear particles. In fact, it has been shown *in vitro* that IL-10 inhibits the secretion of TNFα and IL-6 by titanium-stimulated monocytes (Pollice *et al.*, 1998).

Around prosthetic implants, mononuclear phagocytes may be activated by wear particles to release cytokines. TNFα has been shown to inhibit osteoblast proliferation and differentiation. In addition, IL-1β and TNFα released by particle-activated mononuclear phagocytes stimulate the release of IL-6, TNFα, and PGE_2 from human osteoblastic cells. In this way mononuclear phagocytes reduce the number of bone-forming cells; osteoblasts may amplify bone loss by releasing bone-resorbing mediators in response to particle-activated mononuclear phagocytes (Haynes *et al.*, 1997).

a. Cytokines and Metals. The release of cytokines from macrophages is influenced by the chemical composition, size, and concentration of wear particles, in the same way as occurs for PGE_2. According to some authors, the effect of metals is not direct but as a result of bacterial endotoxin adsorbed onto the material surface. Therefore, the differences found among metals with regard to the stimulation of cytokine secretion would be due to the fact that surface material chemistry and microstructure affect the concentration and configuration of adsorbed molecules (Ragab *et al.*, 1999; Daniels *et al.*, 2000).

Co^{2+} increased the release of TNFα and IL-6 from leukocytes. Cr^{3+} ions did not increase the release of TNFα but increased the secretion of IL-6. Ti^{3+} ions were associated with a decrease in the release of TNFα and a minimal change in IL-6 (Liu *et al.*, 1999).

Human monocytes were challenged *in vitro* with metal particles of 0.5–3 μm diameter, similar to the size of metal wear debris found near failed implants. Stainless steel particles greatly stimulated IL-1β release at concentrations of 2.5×10^6 particles/ml and above. CoCr and TiAlV particles stimulated IL-1β release at 4×10^7 particles/ml. There was no significant difference between cast and forged CoCr particles. TNFα release was stimulated by stainless steel, TiAlV, forged, and cast CoCr, at 4×10^7 particles/ml. TiAlV particles stimulated IL-6 release at 4×10^7 particles/ml, but CoCr and stainless steel particles failed to stimulate IL-6 release (Haynes *et al.*, 1998).

Results are therefore contradictory among the various authors, above all with regard to chromium. Also, using the murine-macrophage cell line J774A.1 it was found that CoCr particles only at high concentration stimulated cell activity (Prabhu *et al.*, 1998). Chromium may therefore have a stimulating and inhibiting effect on the secretion of cytokines, depending on the experimental conditions.

Other authors demonstrated that 0.7×10^8 titanium particles challenged *in vitro* with 10^6 macrophage-like cells induced IL-1β release 7-fold higher than that of the negative control, 3-fold IL-8 release, 170-fold TNFα release (Rader *et al.*, 1999a). Titanium alloy is able to promote the expression of monocyte chemoattractant protein-1 (MCP-1) and monocyte inflammatory protein-1α (MIP-1α) from human macrophages *in vitro* in a dose- and time-dependent manner (Nakashima *et al.*, 1999a).

Stainless steel filters for the preparation of leukocyte depleted blood products were also found to induce receptors of interleukin-1, which inhibits the inflammatory reaction (Yamaji *et al.*, 1997).

The mechanism by which metal ions may stimulate cytokine release has been suggested, at least for titanium. Titanium ions probably activate adenylcyclase inducing the production of cAMP. This in turn activates protein kinase A inducing the expression of the specific mRNA for cytokines. Furthermore, Ti ions may also stimulate phospholipase A of the cell membrane with the activation of the arachidonic acid metabolic pathway and the production of PGE_2 and PGE_1, which in turn stimulate adenylcyclase (Blaine *et al.*, 1997).

Another mechanism was suggested by Nakashima *et al.*, at least with regard to IL-6 and TNFα. They showed that the phagocytosis of Ti particles by macrophages is not necessary to induce the production of cytokines in culture. Titanium alloy particles interact with the macrophage cell-surface Mac-1 receptors (CD11b/CD18). This process is influenced by the opsonization of metal particles with complement or their fragments. Mac-1 receptors, in fact, also bind with the fragment CR3bi. Binding between the metal particle and the receptor, through phosphorylation of selected proteins, induced the tyrosine and serine/threonine kinase activity that ultimately resulted in the translocation of the specific transcription factors Nuclear Factor-kB and Nuclear Factor-IL-6 from the cytoplasm to the nucleus. The transcription factors modulated specific mRNA expression (Nakashima *et al.*, 1999b).

Probably, multiple signaling pathways are involved in the mechanism by which metal particles stimulate cell functions. The stimulation of cytokine release can be observed only during the first day of contact between peritoneal macrophages and titanium, at least with regard to IL-6, and then basal levels are restored (Giudiceandrea *et al.*, 1998).

The presence of blood serum that binds to the titanium particles increases the cytokine release from macrophages in the first 12 hours, at least *in vitro*. After 24 hours this phenomenon can be observed only with high concentrations of metal particles (Maloney *et al.*, 1998).

b. Cytokines and Ceramics. Ceramic materials induce less cytokine release from macrophages than metals do. In fact, it has been shown that, compared to the negative control, the release of TNFα is 4-fold greater with alumina, 5-fold greater with zirconium dioxide, and 25-fold greater with cobalt (Rader *et al.*, 1999b). Even hydroxyapatite does not induce an increase in the synthesis of IL-1α by murine splenic B lymphocytes when they are cultured directly on the surface of this biomaterial (Takebe *et al.*, 1998).

26.3.1.4. Other Mediators

a. The Kinin-Forming System. The kinins, bradykinin and lysylbradykinin, are basic peptides responsible for pain induction and vasodilation; they increase vascular permeability, cause the contraction of smooth muscle, and stimulate NO production by endothelium and arachidonic acid metabolism. Kinins are liberated in plasma from precursor molecules, high and low molecular weight kininogen (HMWK and LMWK, respectively), and T-kininogen, by the action of various proteases, such as kallikrein.

Hageman factor, kallikrein, and HMWK are adsorbed onto foreign surfaces, such as metals. Research into the plasma protein adsorption on titanium has shown an initial adsorption of fibrinogen, which was then replaced by HMWK. On vanadium and silver, high adsorption of both fibrinogen and HMWK was observed. Only small amounts of factor XII, prekallikrein, and HMWK bound to chromium surfaces after incubation in plasma (Vroman *et al.*, 1985; Elwing *et al.*, 1991; Walivaara *et al.*, 1996).

b. Histamine. Histamine is derived from the aminoacid histidine by the action of the histidine-decarboxylase. It is a normal constituent of many tissues and is stored in a form of an inactive macromolecular complex. In humans, histamine is stored in mast cells and basophil granules, largely complexed to mucopolysaccharides (glycosaminoglycans). Histamine has a number of functions including primary, local dilation of small vessels; widespread arteriolar dilatation; local increased vascular permeability by contracting endothelial cells; the contraction of nonvascular smooth muscle; chemotaxis for eosinophils; and blockage of T lymphocyte function.

A number of different cells have receptors for histamine. These can be of three types: H1, H2, and H3. The H1 receptors mediate acute vascular effects together with smooth muscle constriction in the bronchi and the stimulation of eosinophil chemotaxis. In contrast, the H2 receptors mediate a number of anti-inflammatory effects, including the inhibition of eosinophil chemotaxis, but cause vasodilatation. The H3 receptor is mainly involved in the control of histamine release by different cells.

c. Eicosanoids. Eicosanoids are prostaglandins and leukotrienes: they are synthesized and released in response to an appropriate stimulus. They are derived from a polyunsaturated essential fatty acid, arachidonic acid, which is easily released from phosphatidylcholine and phosphatidylinositol, which are on the cell membrane, after hydrolysis by phospholipase A_2 and C, respectively. Arachidonic acid is metabolized by two major routes, the cyclo-oxygenase and lipoxygenase pathways. The cyclo-oxygenase pathway produces prostaglandins, prostacyclin, and thromboxanes; the lipoxygenase pathway produces in one branch leukotrienes, and in the second branch lipoxins.

d. Leukotrienes. The second metabolic pathway of arachidonic acid leads to the formation of leukotrienes. Lipoxygenase enzymes add oxygen to the arachidonic acid giving rise to intermediate hydroperoxides.

Leukotrienes have been identified in neutrophils, eosinophils, basophils, macrophages, and mast cells. The three peptidoleukotrienes LTC_4, LTD_4, and LTE_4, originally called Slow Reacting Substance of Anaphylaxis (SRS-A), cause vasoconstriction and increase vascular permeability during inflammation. LTB_4 is chemokinetic and chemotactic for neutrophils and stimulates the aggregation of PMN and the release of lysosomal enzymes.

e. PAF. Platelets produce a group of acetyl-alkylglycerol ether analogs of phosphatidylcholine, called platelet-activating factor (PAF). Like eicosanoids, PAF is not stored inside the cell but synthesized after cell activation: the hydrolysis of membrane phospholipids, by the phospholipase enzyme A_2, leads to the production of arachidonic acid and a substance, lyso-PAF, which is both the forerunner and the metabolite of PAF. Most of the PAF produced in the inflammatory cells remains associated with the cell itself. PAF that causes platelet aggregation is a potent phagocyte chemoattractant and provides stimuli for the release of lysosomal enzymes and reactive oxygen products by neutrophils, eosinophils, and macrophages. In addition, PAF increases the stickiness of endothelial cells for leukocytes, so promoting the outcome of plasma fluids.

26.3.2. Leukocyte Exudation

26.3.2.1. Interactions between Blood Cells and the Endothelium

The endothelium is involved in the main events of acute inflammatory response:

- Vasodilation with increased blood supply to the inflamed tissue.
- Increased capillary permeability caused by retraction of the endothelial cells, in response to soluble mediators. Large molecules may escape from the capillaries, and thus soluble mediators are allowed to reach the site of inflammation.
- Leukocytes, i.e., neutrophils first, and monocytes and lymphocytes later, migrate out of the capillaries into the surrounding tissues.

In order to move out, leukocytes express proteins on their membrane (such as LFA-1, Mac 1/CR3, and LECAM-1), adhering to ligands on endothelial cells.

Biomaterials able to change specific receptors would alter the adhesion of leukocytes to the vascular wall.

LFA-1 and Mac-1/CR3 belong to the β_2 integrin subfamily. LFA-1, recognized by the monoclonal antibodies belonging to the cluster differentiation CD11a/CD18, is expressed on lymphocytes, neutrophils, and monocytes, and mediates their adhesion to the endothelium through the ligands ICAM-1, ICAM-2, and ICAM-3.

Mac-1, recognized by CD11b/CD18, is expressed on neutrophils, monocytes, natural killer cells, and macrophages. Its main function is to mediate the adherence of both monocytes and neutrophils to vascular endothelium for subsequent extravasation through the ligands ICAM-1, fibrinogen, factor X, and iC3b (Arnaout, 1990).

LECAM-1 belongs to the selectin family and is recognized by CD62L. It is expressed on all leukocytes but one subpopulation of memory lymphocytes. It plays a crucial role in the early phase of the leukocyte extravasation during the inflammatory process (Kansas, 1992). The ligands of LECAM-1 are glycoconjugates expressed on the endothelium surface (Mebius and Watson, 1993).

Endothelial cells express a wide spectrum of surface molecules: some are constitutively found while others are increased or induced *de novo* after activation of cells. Main receptors on endothelial cells are ICAM 1 and 2 (Intercellular Adhesion Molecule-1 or 2), ELAM-1 (Endothelial Leukocyte Adhesion Molecule-1), and VCAM-1 (Vascular Cell Adhesion Molecule-1).

ELAM-1 is a glycoprotein of the selectin family: its *de novo* synthesis is induced by endotoxin, interleukin 1 (IL-1), and Tumor Necrosis Factor (TNF). ICAM-1 (CD54) is an adhesive protein of the immunoglobulin superfamily. It increases remarkably in the presence of endotoxin or IL-1.

VCAM-1 belongs to the immunoglobulin superfamily as well. The expression of this adhesion on the endothelial cell membrane increases significantly after exposure to endotoxin, IL-1, and TNF. VCAM-1 favors the adhesion and transendothelial migration of lymphocytes and monocytes. The proinflammatory mediators induce a signal transduction from the cell membrane to the nucleus, involving different protein kinases and transcription factors. The effect of metal ions on the endothelial adhesion molecules has been studied by many authors (Klein *et al.*, 1994). Very low concentrations of metal ions (Ni, Co, Zn), with no influence on cell morphology, elicited a significant dose-dependent expression of ELAM-1 and ICAM-1. Therefore, extremely low concentrations of metal ions could play a significant role in inflammatory processes around metallic prosthetic devices.

Endothelial adhesions play a relevant role also in the pathogenesis of contact hypersensitivity induced by metals. Two common contact sensitizers, $NiCl_2$ and $CoCl_2$, were shown to induce the expression of ELAM-1, ICAM-1, and VCAM-1, on human umbilical vein endothelial cells, and the expression of ELAM-1 and ICAM-1, but not VCAM-1, on microvascular endothelium from foreskin. The induction depends on *de novo* mRNA and protein synthesis (Goebeler *et al.*, 1993). Nickel and cobalt ions induce NF-κB binding activity that subsequently modulates transcription of adhesion molecule genes, and also transcription factor AP-1 activity (Goebeler *et al.*, 1995; Wagner *et al.*, 1998).

In patients with aseptic loosening of orthopedic prostheses, the presence of E-selectin, VCAM-1, ICAM-1, and the receptors LFA-1 and CR3 was demonstrated at the bone–implant interface obtained during revision arthroplasty. E-selectin was upregulated and correlated strongly with the presence of metal wear debris. VCAM-1 was more frequently observed in the lining cells on the implant side. ICAM-1 was strongly expressed by aggregates of macrophages and multinucleated giant cells on the implant side. These macrophage aggregates coexpressed both ICAM-1 and CR3 (al-Saffar *et al.*, 1995a). The expression of proinflammatory molecules on the endothelial cell surface may be induced by titanium. In the soft tissue adjacent to the surface of titanium miniplates used in the treatment of mandibular fractures, hypertrophic endothelial cells were observed, expressing HLA-DR, CD54, and CD62P antigens (Katou *et al.*, 1996).

26.3.3. Cells of the Inflammatory Acute Reaction

26.3.3.1. Neutrophils

Neutrophils (PMNs) represent about 60% of the circulating leukocytes. They are derived from immature cells in the bone marrow, which come to maturation by formation of specific enzyme-containing granules and development of phagocytic and migrating properties. The circulating PMN is an end-stage cell with a half-life of about 8 hours: the multilobed nucleus and the cytoplasm rich in granules make it easily recognizable. Membrane-associated receptors of PMNs include receptors for IgG subclasses, complement fragments, chemotactic peptides, and lipids. The neutrophils which usually live adherent to the endothelium respond to chemotactic factors crossing the membrane to gather at the injured site. Using a battery of enzymes and an oxygen metabolite-generating system, PMNs are able to kill bacteria, viruses, and mammalian cells. Moreover, they are able to produce arachidonic acid metabolites, such as leukotriene B4 (LTB4): together with neutrophil-secreted platelet activating factor (PF4) it is involved in PMN recruitment with self-perpetuation of inflammation.

PMNs die within the tissue and the cell debris are removed by macrophages. It has been ascertained that PMNs are induced to degranulation with release of their enzymes and to ROS production by a number of biomaterials (Kaplan and Simmons, 1995). In our lab, PMNs from healthy people were challenged *in vitro* with chromium, cobalt, nickel, molybdenum, titanium, aluminum, and vanadium, prepared as aqueous extracts in phosphate buffered saline (PBS): Mo, Al, and V have been found to increase ROS generation by PMNs, while signals not different from unstimulated PMNs were recorded for Cr, Co, Ni, and Ti (Ciapetti *et al.*, 1998). When PMNs of patients with implant loosening were analyzed, it was found that ROS generation was different depending on the implant: patients with stainless steel devices responded to chromium with a ROS release higher than that recorded for controls, while patients with CrCoMo hip prostheses released less ROS than controls when challenged with Cr and Co (Ciapetti *et al.*, 1997). The hypothesis that leukocytes from patients with implants are "sensitized" and react to metal components differently from controls, deserves further investigation.

26.3.3.2. Monocytes/Macrophages

After maturation in the blood marrow and circulation in the blood stream, monocytes are destined to migrate into the tissues where they transform into macrophages and exert their biological activities. The random migration of monocytes through vessel membrane becomes directional when chemotactic factors are produced at the inflammation site.

Unlike PMNs, macrophages are much longer-lived cells which reside in tissues interfacing with implants for extended periods of time (months). A key element in the tissue response to implants is the degree and extent of macrophage activation. Macrophage is the central cell type involved in inflammation and immune response: its behavior after contact with biomaterials is therefore extremely important in regulating the host response. Upon functional activation, all the macrophage activities, including adhesion and spreading, phagocytosis, receptor expression, lysosomal content, oxygen species generation, and cytokine secretion, are increased. These properties make the macrophages more efficient in bacteria and cell killing, while through IL1, TNF, and chemotactic products they recruit PMNs, sustain inflammation, and possibly are self-activating. A unique feature of macrophages is their ability to fuse together, forming giant cells: these are responsible for ingestion and degradation of large particles. Wear particles are commonly found within macrophages and giant cells in the fibrous membrane between loose prosthetic components and the host bone undergoing resorption. It has been shown that monocytes/macrophages can be stimulated by metals *in vitro* to release more active oxygen species (Mu *et al.*, 2000). Macrophages have been recently shown to play a key role in the initiation of osteolysis via cytokine production after particle phagocytosis (Horowitz *et al.*, 1998; Trindade *et al.*, 1999).

26.3.3.3. Mast Cells

These are resident cells in mucosae and connective tissue whose predominant feature is the high content in histamine stored as an inactive macromolecular complex. A variety of stimuli trigger their degranulation with discharge of histamine, prostaglandin D2, leukotrienes, acid hydrolases, and chemotactic factors: this makes the mast cell actively participating to the inflammatory reaction. According to a recent study, mast cells and their products, mainly histamine, are important in recruitment of inflammatory cells to biomaterial implants (Tang *et al.*, 1998).

26.3.4. Chemotaxis

Chemotaxis is the ability of cells to migrate in response to the presence of a concentration gradient of a chemotactic factor (Pizzoferrato *et al.*, 1986). This function mainly applies to phagocytes, and is different from the mechanism of "contact guidance," which describes the movement of cells (mainly epithelial cells and fibroblasts) along specific structures (e.g., collagen fibrils). Different from chemotaxis is the process of chemokinesis, i.e., the random movement of cells triggered by chemokinetic substances in the milieu. The process of "polarization" of cells, that is the cell with the characteristic morphology with a "leading front" and an elongated "tail," precedes both the mechanisms of movement.

During inflammation, migration of phagocytic cells is mediated by a number of molecules. *N*-formylmethionyl-leucyl-phenylalanine (FMLP), complement fraction C5a, transforming growth factor β (TGF-β), leukotriene B4 (LTB4), tumor necrosis factor-α (TNFα), 12-hydroxyeicosatetranoic acid (12-HETE) are all molecules with chemotactic activity for blood monocytes. Moreover, different types of cells are stimulated by different inducers, including interleukins, bacterial lipopolysaccharides (LPS), phorbol-myristate acetate (PMA), mitogens, to secrete multiple chemotactic cytokines, designated chemokines. Monocyte chemotactic proteins, like monocyte-chemotactic protein-1, -2, and -3 (MCP-1, MCP-2, and MCP-3), belong to the C-C subfamily (i.e., with two adjacent residues of cysteine), while in the C-X-C subfamily (with two cysteines separated by an amino acid) are collected the chemotactic proteins for PMNs, e.g., interleukin 8 (IL8) and granulocyte-chemotactic protein-2 (GCP-2) (Wuyts *et al.*, 1994).

Chemotaxis may be measured either *in vivo* or *in vitro*. The first method developed for the evaluation of cellular chemotaxis *in vivo* was the Rebuck skin window (Gangarosa *et al.*, 1955): after abrading a patch of skin, a glass coverslip coated with the sample to be tested was applied on the abraded area. The coverslip was then removed and analyzed for cell type and number after a defined duration of time. Other authors used the injection of samples to be tested in animal tissues such as the pleural cavity, eye, knee, or lung, to characterize the cell accumulation thereafter (Tang and Eaton, 1993).

Different assays have been developed to measure cell chemotaxis *in vitro*, including the migration through filters (Boyden, 1962), the time lapse cinematography (Ramsey, 1972), the cell orientation assay (Zigmond and Hirsch, 1973), and the migration under an agarose layer (Nelson *et al.*, 1975), with the filter-based Boyden chamber method still being the most widely used.

The leukocyte migration inhibition assays have been the most popular technique for *in vitro* investigation of cell mediated immune response to biomaterials (Merritt and Brown, 1985).

The mechanism of chemotaxis related to a biomaterial/device has been poorly investigated. After two pioneering papers concerning mainly MMA effect on chemotaxis *in vitro* (Beard *et al.*, 1976; Petty, 1978), a study on the chemotaxis of leukocytes from patients with THJ replacement suggested a relationship between decreased chemotactic ability and incidence of bacterial infection (Endler *et al.*, 1982).

An *in vitro* study of chemotaxis of macrophages after *in vivo* challenge with powdered biomaterials was performed by our group. Alumina, though endocytosed by macrophages, did not alter their chemotactic properties, while chromium was found to reduce the migration of such cells (Pizzoferrato *et al.*, 1984, 1986).

Neutrophils (PMNs) have been often used as they are recognized as the main cells reacting to implanted devices in the early inflammatory reaction, but many studies concern the PMNs/polymers interactions (Kaplan *et al.*, 1990; Papatheofanis and Barmada, 1991; Campoccia *et al.*, 1993; Tang *et al.*, 1998).

A considerable effort in studying chemotaxis and chemokinesis of cells with biomaterials was made by D.F. Williams and his group. First, a correlation between *in vitro* chemokinesis/chemotaxis and *in vivo* extent of the tissue reaction to metals was attempted: a strong chemotactic activity *in vitro* would mean a narrow area of inflammatory cells around the *in vivo* implant. Aluminum and copper fit in well with this hypothesis, with aluminum inducing an intense migration *in vitro* and a minimal inflammatory area *in vivo*, while copper was found to migrate less but to cause an intense local response. Nickel had an intermediate behavior (MacNamara *et al.*, 1984). Nickel and copper were further studied for their chemokinetic properties *in vitro* and were found to stimulate a proportion of the neutrophil population to take up an oriented morphology and to move (Hunt *et al.*, 1992).

Different results were obtained in our lab, where AISI 316L stainless steel, Ti, Ni, Co, Cr, Mo, and Cu were extracted according to the ASTM guidelines for materials, and examined for their ability to change neutrophil spherical shape. All these metals were found to modify the morphology of a limited portion of cells, ranging from 4.6 to 12.7%: the reason for the discordance is likely to be the different ion concentrations in the metal solution used in the tests, which cause a different cell response (Ciapetti *et al.*, 1992). This is confirmed by a study on metal ions used for dental restorations: zinc, copper, and nickel induced PMN polarization and enhanced the migration of PMNs in the concentration range of 0.5–1.0 mM, while chromium and iron were unable to cause such enhancement. The conclusion was that zinc, copper, and nickel ions attract leukocyte by chemotaxis and may therefore modulate the inflammatory response of host tissue around such metals (Hujanen *et al.*, 1995).

Also, ceramics were found to induce complement activation and neutrophil polarization *in vitro*. The ceramic powders tricalcium phosphate, coral, and calcium hydrogen phosphate were shown to activate complement when added to human serum. Moreover, it was also suggested that there may be a relationship between the neutrophil polarization response to serum incubated with ceramic powders and C3 activation (Remes and Williams, 1991a).

The chemotaxis of monocytes in response to nearly pure alumina, alumina-titania, synthetic hydroxyapatite, and natural hydroxyapatite was recently measured using the under-agarose migration assay (Bosetti *et al.*, 1999). All the ceramics lowered cell migration when the size of particles was less than 50 micrometers, while both HAs at greater size promoted migration. Using other data from this study it was concluded that natural apatite is better tolerated than synthetic apatite, which in turn is better tolerated than alumina.

In conclusion, there is little doubt that cells are recruited to biomaterial implant site by chemotactic stimuli, but the nature of such substances are still largely unknown. According to a recent study, two chemokines—macrophage inflammatory protein 1(α and monocyte chemoattractant protein 1—are required for phagocyte chemotaxis toward biomaterial surface (Tang *et al.*, 1998).

26.3.5. Phagocytosis

It is known that the extent of an inflammatory response to an implant is a function of the exposed surface. As a consequence, even "bioinert" materials can evoke an intense inflammatory reaction when in the form of particulates. In our lab, it was found that the aluminum oxide particles injected in the peritoneal cavity recruited a number of inflammatory cells higher than in controls and increased their chemotactic activity (Pizzoferrato *et al.*, 1987).

Particles within tissues surrounding the implant are generated by wear and micromovements. Monocytes/macrophages and tissue histiocytes are the cells in charge of clearing the implant area *in vivo*. Several activities of phagocytic cells are stimulated by the ingestion of particles, depending on the nature, number, and size of particles. Also, extracellular particles may elicit cell reactions. Therefore, the cell/particle interaction influences the tissue response at the interface with the implant.

Wear debris is now considered to be the main factor responsible for aseptic loosening of orthopedic devices (Lohmann *et al.*, 2000).

26.3.5.1. Metals

Among metals, titanium shows excellent biocompatibility but not good wear resistance as CoCr alloy and stainless steel: this is the reason for the number of studies on Ti particles.

Shanbhag and co-workers tested titania particles on P388D1 macrophages and found that at low dose Ti stimulated IL 1 release and bone resorption, while fibroblast proliferation was not increased. When given with a higher surface area, the same particles inhibited DNA synthesis (Shanbhag *et al.*, 1994). The authors did recommend the use of the "surface area ratio" (SAR), which is a ratio of the total surface of the given particles to the surface area of cells, when measuring the effect of particles onto cells *in vitro*. This was confirmed by the same authors using blood monocytes: phagocytosable Ti and TiAlV particles induced the release of various cellular mediators, with TiAlV being the most competent to elicit the synthesis and release of inflammatory mediators (Shanbhag *et al.*, 1995). An inverse relationship between toxicity and release of mediators *in vitro* was found by other authors: using rat peritoneal macrophages, exposed to either CoCr alloy or TiAlV particles, they demonstrated that TiAlV particles, which were less cytotoxic, induced significantly more release of PGE_2, IL-1, IL-6, and TNF than did the CoCr particles, which were more cytotoxic (Haynes *et al.*, 1993). TiAlNb particles have less marked effects than TiAlV because of its enhanced corrosion resistance (Rogers *et al.*, 1997). When mononuclear cells from interfacial membranes of patients with TJR are stimulated *in vitro* with chromium or titanium particles, high levels of inflammatory interleukins and prostaglandin E2 were produced. These substances are then inducers of local osteolysis and aseptic loosening (Lee *et al.*, 1997).

That metal particles could be dangerous to tissues through different mechanisms was suggested by Kane *et al.* (1994), who found titanium particles promoting first collagenase production by macrophages and then strong adsorption of it onto the surface: the enzyme may be responsible for local bone resorption.

Instead, using the "bone harvest chamber" implanted in rabbits, titanium particles small enough to be phagocytosed by macrophages were shown not to hamper bone ingrowth (Goodman *et al.*, 1995). The same authors injected low (10^{-6}–10^{-7}) and high (10^{-8}–10^{-9}) doses of phagocytosable (< 10 micron) particles of Ti-6Al-4V, and HDPE for comparison, in the rabbit bone and found that after 16 weeks a histiocytic reaction without extensive fibrosis, necrosis, or granuloma had been evoked (Goodman *et al.*, 1996a). The conclusion is that an ongoing generation of such particles over a more extended period might be necessary to interfere with the process of bone remodeling: this is likely to occur *in vivo*. Ti was also tested *in vitro* on bone-resorbing cells: after phagocytosis Ti-containing osteoclasts were fully functional, hormone-responsive, and bone-resorbing (Wang *et al.*, 1997b). When applied *in vitro* to osteoblast-like stromal cells, phagocytosed titanium and chromium–cobalt, as well PMMA and UHMWPE, did not abrogate their ability to undergo osteoclast differentiation (Sabokbar *et al.*, 1998).

In conclusion, the metal debris ranging over 0.1–10 micron are ingested by phagocytes, while larger particles are engulfed by giant cells. The fibroblasts, monocytes/macrophages, and giant cells may be activated by intracellular wear particles (0.1–5 microns), with production of cytokines and prostaglandins (mainly E_2) which, in turn, activate osteoclasts to resorb bone.

26.3.5.2. Ceramics

Ceramics are usually coupled to ceramic or UHMWPE: despite their good wear properties some fine particles or grains are generated *in vivo*. The particles are not totally inert: different activities of cells responding to ceramic particles have been reported. In a study *in vitro* on calcium hydroxide and hydroxyapatite particle effect on fibroblasts, [$Ca(OH)_2$] was found to alter cell morphology, DNA and protein synthesis, ALP activity, in accordance with necrosis observed after *in vivo* implantation; hydroxyapatite less than 10 micron was ingested and did not damage cells, even if proliferation was affected (Alliot-Licht *et al.*, 1994). That granuloma formation or inflammation was not induced by HA particles, and that bone ingrowth was not adversely affected, were confirmed by an *in vivo* study using the "bone harvest chamber" (Wang *et al.*, 1994).

After ingestion, some particles interact with macrophages: in the presence of HA microcrystals they showed less acid phosphatase and lactate dehydrogenase activities and higher intracellular calcium content than macrophages cultured in the presence of calcined HA and alumina (Fukuchi *et al.*, 1995). In a recent study *in vitro*, the acidic environment of macrophagic organelles was reproduced and HA particles were monitored for their dissolution: both calcium and phosphate ions were found in the medium, with different time course, so confirming the possibility that HA is digested inside macrophage-like acid environment. Caution was recommended in interpreting such results, due to so many factors (size, number, time) playing a role (Bloebaum *et al.*, 1998). Phagocytosis of small particles (<15 micron) of HA and SiC did not alter monocyte viability, even if morphological changes and IL 1β release were elicited, in contrast with diamond particles which were found to be inert (Nordsletten *et al.*, 1996). Functional integrity up to 24 h, with respect to morphology and respiratory burst, was found for human neutrophils following phagocytosis of HA (Dowsett *et al.*, 1997).

Human osteoblasts from spongy bone were cultured onto alumina and HA disks: they showed good spreading and outgrowth, with no metabolic impairment of cells. After 10 days of cultivation the only difference was a better proliferation on alumina vs HA (Labat *et al.*, 1995).

That the good compatibility of HA, and its "osteoconductivity," is linked to proper collagen formation was shown *in vivo* (Lindholm *et al.*, 1996) and *in vitro* (Rovira *et al.*, 1996). When BCP, alone or combined with other materials, is implanted to fill bone defects, macrophages and giant cells are involved in phagocytosis of particles: cell-mediated degradation of the material was observed up to 78 weeks in the rabbit femurs (Dupraz *et al.*, 1998). To summarize, most ceramic particles, generated from ceramic/ceramic and ceramic/UHMWPE couplings, are usually sized 0.2–5 micron and are easily ingested by macrophages and histiocytes. Once ingested, such particles seem not to alter the specific functions of phagocytosing cells.

26.4. Chronic Inflammation

As previously illustrated, a "physiological" wound healing reaction due to surgery itself will occur following biomaterial implantation in the body. The wound healing process lasts about 7–10 days after implantation, with the properties of the material determining what happens next. If the material is totally inert and not subjected to biodegradation, once the initial acute inflammatory response has subsided, it becomes encapsulated by fibrous tissue, to stay so interminably. Therefore this material is considered to be biocompatible. If the material is degradable, an extra dimension is added to host reaction: the breakdown process may re-activate the inflammatory process or even never let it end. The signs of inflammation accompanying that reaction may be aggravated due to the release of toxic substances.

A number of factors will determine the evolution of the inflammatory response. Roughly these factors are distinguished in two groups: (1) the physical properties and (2) the chemical properties of the biomaterial.

Among the physical properties, the surface roughness or microtopography, the wettability, and the size of wear particles are crucial, while the intrinsic toxicity and the release of toxic substances are main aspects linked to material composition. High wettability will promote tissue adherence; low wettability will result in the opposite.

Concerning the surface of the implant, both geometrical configuration and surface irregularities are involved in determining the inflammatory response. Cylindrical configuration evokes a zone of fibrosis more limited than that seen around sharp-edged implants: using the same material, angular implants show collagen fibers oriented parallel to the surface but a persisting chronic inflammation at angularities, too.

Rough irregular implants induce foreign-body giant cell response, which is a sign of frustrated phagocytosis, and indefinite persistence of chronic inflammation cells (Goodman *et al.*, 1990).

Chronic inflammation is characterized by mononuclear cells, mainly monocytes and macrophages, but also lymphocytes, plasmacells, fibroblasts, as well as by proliferation of capillary buds and increase in connective tissue. Macrophages arrive at the site of an inflammatory response more slowly than granulocytes, but their persistence and their stronger ability to phagocytose promote the reorganization of the tissue and lead to final repair. Moreover, macrophages are more resistant to the acidic conditions resulting from degranulation process of neutrophils, so functioning as the ultimate scavenger cells (Figure 26.1).

Giant cells are formed at the site of chronic inflammation from the fusion of macrophages. Their phagocytic ability is less developed than that of macrophages, but their role is mainly the ingestion of particles too large to be phagocytosed by a single cell. This is particularly seen in the presence of plastic wear (polyethylene in joint prostheses) (Figure 26.2) or when a rough surface is implanted (artificial ligament or multifilament sutures); on the contrary, it is rather unusual around ceramic and metal implants.

Lymphocytes are characteristically present at sites of chronic inflammation, even if their role and the presence of plasma cells, too, is not completely understood (Figure 26.3).

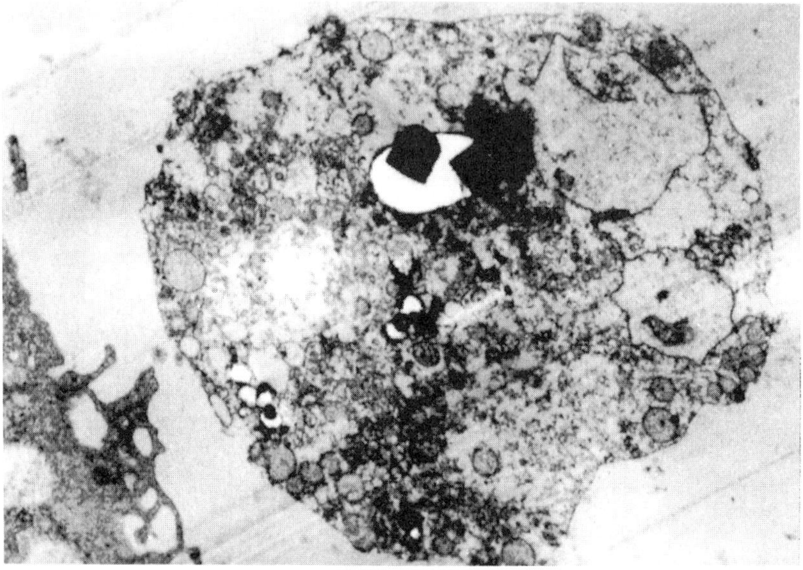

Figure 26.1. Macrophage ingesting ceramic particles. View in transmission electron microscopy

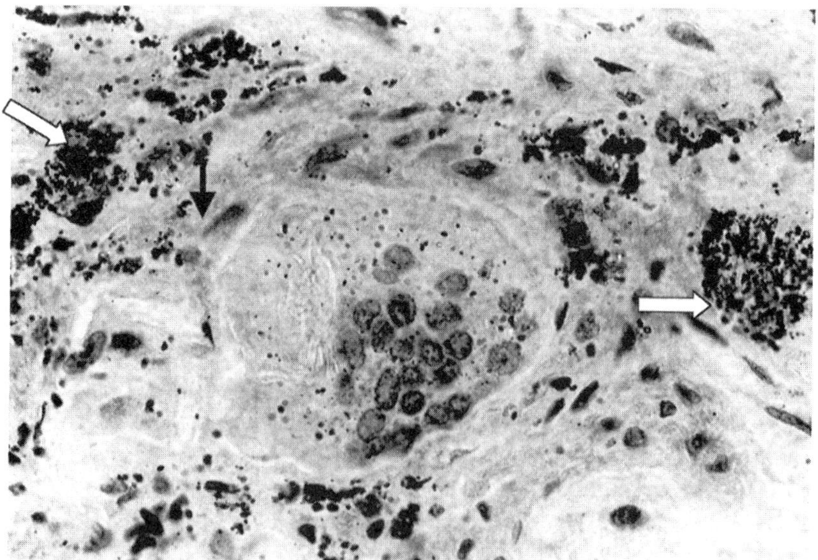

Figure 26.2. A giant cell in reaction tissue. Black arrow shows a big plastic wear particle ingested by the cell. White arrows point to metallic wear. Particles are black in transmitted light (Hematoxylin–Eosin, 100 ×).

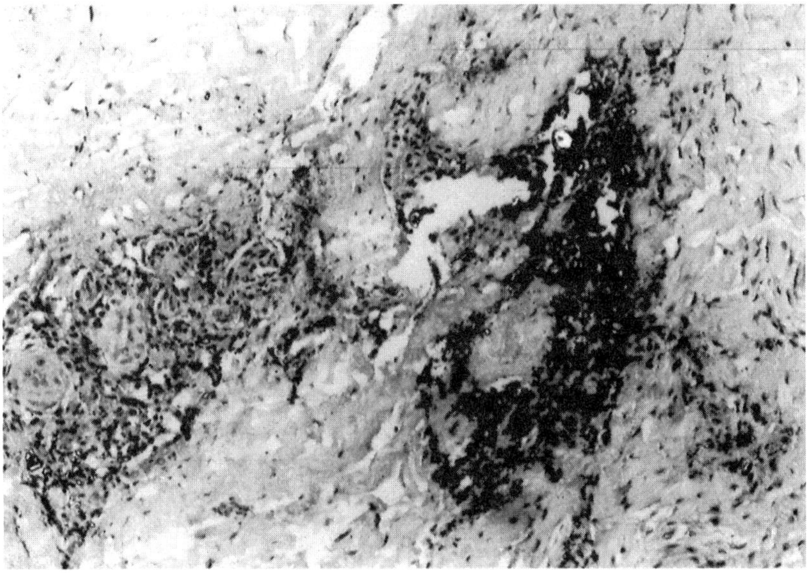

Figure 26.3. Ceramic particles in the neocapsule. On the left-hand side of the picture, some lymphocytes are present in the perivascular area (Hematoxylin–Eosin, 25 ×).

When acute inflammation subsides, granulation tissue forms at the site of the implant. It is a specialized tissue with the precise task of repairing the injury, to be replaced in the near future. It consists in capillaries, collagen secreting fibroblasts, contractile fibroblasts (myofibroblasts), and chronic inflammatory cells.

Within such tissue, a rapid blood flow provides the metabolic environment which allows the fibroblasts to proliferate and to secrete reparative collagen, while myofibroblasts give considerable force for contraction to the granulation site.

The extent and duration of granulation tissue around prosthetic implants are related to the size and the surface characteristics: extensive areas of granulation tissue are seen around implants with large and rough surfaces.

When joint prostheses are implanted and wear particles are produced, the histological pictures observed in the tissues are often related to the type, and sometimes the size, of the particulate material (Kubo *et al.*, 1999).

Using immunocytochemistry, it has been shown that periprosthetic CD68+ wear-debris-laden macrophages are the most prominent cell type which is positive for inducible nitric oxide synthase (iNOS), nitrotyrosine, and cyclo-oxygenase-2 (COX-2) and contribute to the periprosthetic bone resorption. If nitric oxide and peroxynitrite generation is high, macrophages may die with the release of phagocytosed wear debris into the extracellular matrix. A detrimental cycle of events is then established with further phagocytosis by newly-recruited inflammatory cells and subsequent NO, peroxynitrite, and prostanoid synthesis. Since both NO and PGE2 have been implicated in the induction and maintenance of chronic inflammation with final loss of bone, these substances may participate in the aseptic loosening of joint prostheses (Hukkanen *et al.*, 1997).

Other chemical mediators have been claimed to be involved in periprosthetic bone loss, as described elsewhere in this chapter.

When analyzing the specimens retrieved from loosened joint prostheses, particles derived from the surfaces undergoing wear are a constant finding, even if with a different extent (Savio *et al.*, 1994). Metal particles appear black when observed by transmitted light microscopy, with an irregular form and a small size (1–5 μm) for the most part, so they are easily ingested by mononuclear histiocytes (Winter, 1974; Williams, 1982; Pazzaglia *et al.*, 1988). Particles less than 10 microns are phagocytosed by macrophages, while larger particles, which are rarely found in metal implants, can be found within foreign-body giant cells (Agins *et al.*, 1988) (Figures 26.4 and 26.5).

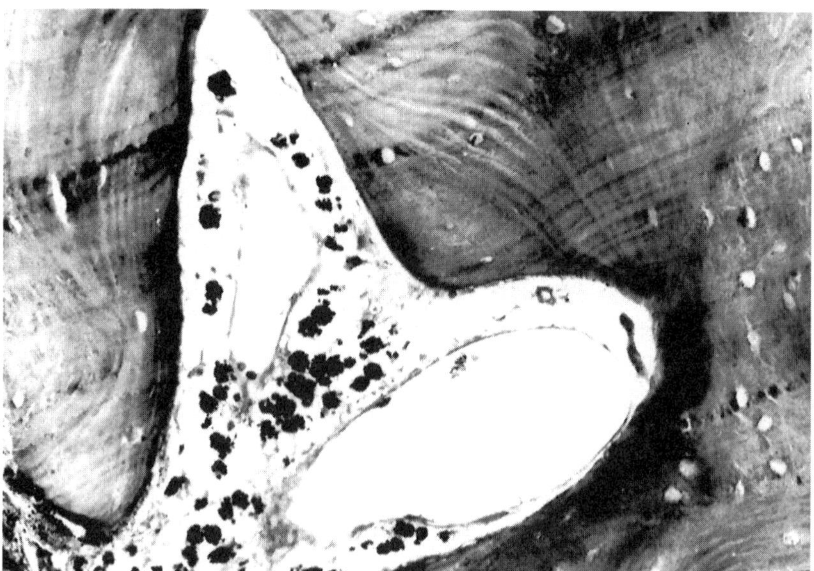

Figure 26.4. Black metal particles in the bone marrow (Hematoxylin–Eosin, 40 ×).

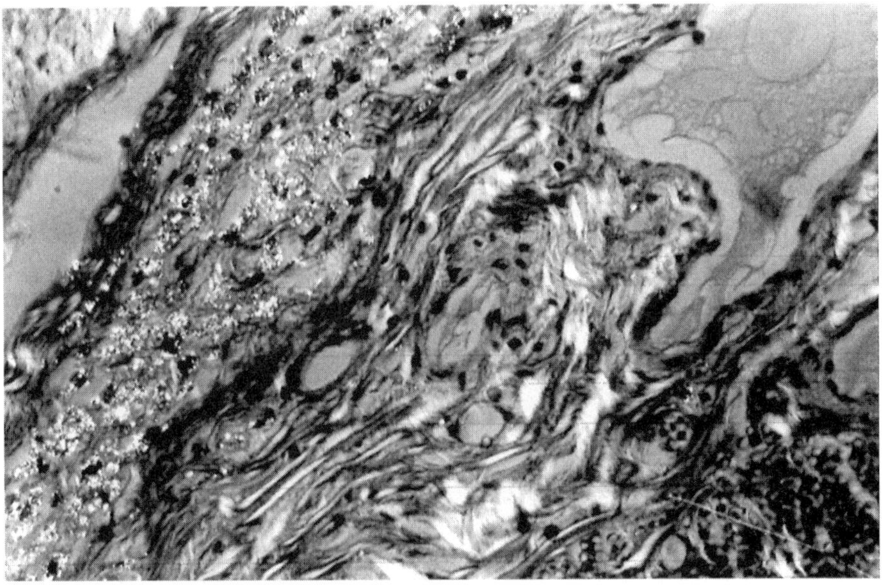

Figure 26.5. A big quantity of metallic particles is evident in the upper-left corner of the image. Particles appear as bright spots as the slice is observed in polarized light (Van Gieson, 40 × polarized light).

Ceramic particles are less common, as ceramic wear is very limited in joint prosthesis. When present in the tissue, a mild inflammatory response is seen (Figure 26.6). Ceramic debris may originate in larger amounts from coating of metallic implants: also, in this case no strong adverse reaction is seen. The scarce toxicity of ceramic materials can be proved also *in vitro*: the effect of tricalcium phosphate (TCP), hydroxyapatite (HA), and aluminum-calcium-phosphorous oxide (ALCAP) on the adherence and viability of human monocyte and monocyte-derived macrophages was tested *in vitro*. Monocytes and macrophages were found to be living on the surface of these ceramics for several days, despite the changes in the material surface (Ross *et al.*, 1996).

Frustrated phagocytosis does not involve engulfment of the material, but rather the extracellular release of leukocyte products such as enzymes and reactive oxygen species in an attempt to degrade the material.

Cytokines. It has already been said that cytokines regulate the duration and extent of the inflammatory process.

Most of the research has been performed on orthopedic implants, with particular attention to loosening of the hip prosthesis. The loosening is the

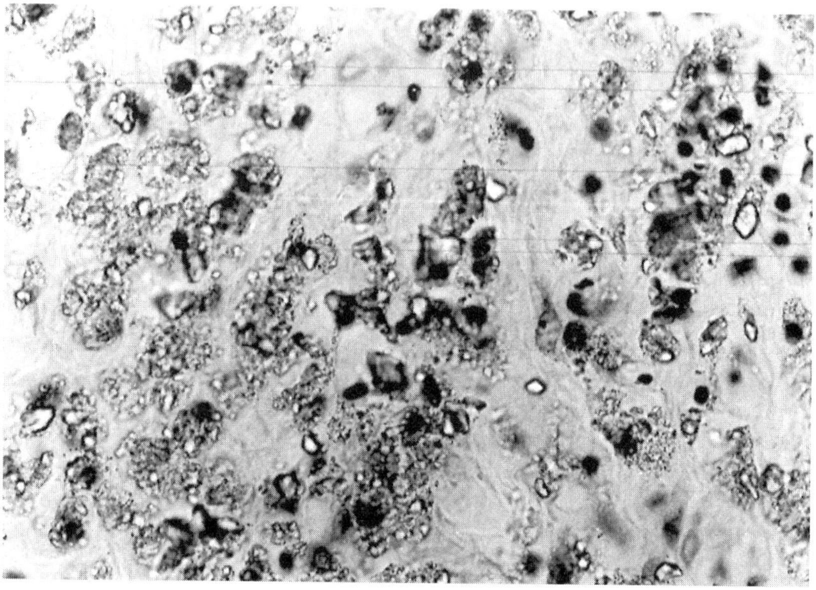

Figure 26.6. Ceramic particles in the soft tissue collected from the newly formed joint capsule of a hip prosthesis. Wear debris are phagocytosed by histiocytes or localized in the extracellular spaces (Hematoxylin–Eosin, 40× polarized light).

result of mechanical, chemical, and biological factors: following their interaction a chronic inflammatory process, which contributes to resorption of periprosthetic bone, is established. The correlation between the severity of osteolysis around the prosthesis and the presence of proinflammatory cytokines at the bone/loosened prosthesis interface was demonstrated by many authors. The cytokine release is probably due to wear particles, which stimulate monocytes and macrophages to secrete these factors. This hypothesis is supported by many studies on tissue samples and *in vitro* cultured cells. A remarkable activity of proinflammatory cytokines and CSFs has been highlighted following *in vitro* culture of the tissues surrounding the failed prostheses. By *in situ* hybridization of the membranes, high levels of IL-1b mRNA in macrophages were also demonstrated (Chiba *et al.*, 1994). Moreover, *in vitro* experiments showed that both cobalt–chromium and titanium–aluminum–vanadium particles promote the release of inflammatory cytokines involved in the osteolytic process (al-Saffar *et al.*, 1995b). The chromium corrosion products were shown to be potent macrophage/monocyte activators and to mediate osteolysis and aseptic loosening (Jiranek *et al.*, 1993; Merkel *et al.*, 1999).

A study on 39 patients with loosening of the hip joint prosthesis who underwent revision surgery was performed in our lab. Bioptic samples were retrieved from the bone/implant interface close to the stem or the head, and IL1 α, IL1 b, IL 6, and TNF α were detected by immunohistochemistry. The amount of cytokine was found not to depend on the time-to-failure of the implant and was not correlated to the pain score; as expected, the levels tend to be lower in subjects being treated with nonsteroidal anti-inflammatory drugs. The proportion of positive cells varied greatly according to the site of collection, but in general the amount of cytokine was higher in patients carrying a polyethylene acetabular component; moreover, they were associated to plastic wear particles, even though a direct correlation between the extent of wear and the amount of cytokines was not found. A significant negative correlation between metal wear and IL6 was seen (Stea *et al.*, 1999). Metal debris were rarely observed, so that no correlation was found with the positive cells: the ability of metal ions released from the implant to induce the cytokine release in the peri-implant tissues was not excluded. To support this hypothesis it was observed that the exposure to chromium extract slightly increased the release of proinflammatory cytokines, such as TNFa and IL-6, from peripheral blood mononuclear cells (PBMC) (Granchi *et al.*, 1998a).

This finding confirms the idea that a sustained chromium release from the implant induce PBMC to produce bone-resorbing cytokines, which in the long term could be responsible for irreversible tissue damage. Moreover, we observed that GM-CSF was increased in the serum of patients with aseptic loosening of hip prosthesis (Granchi *et al.*, 1998b). Our experience confirms the ability of the orthopedic devices to promote the release of cytokines. That happens not only for the inflammatory action of wear particles, but it is probably due to the chemical features of the material, which influence the cytokine release directly.

26.5. Toxicity of Biomaterials and Inflammation

The inflammatory potential of a biomaterial is related to its toxicity. When a biomaterial is investigated for biocompatibility, its cytotoxic activity is a crucial point to be assessed; moreover, it has to be ascertained whether cell death is due to necrosis or apoptosis, as the biological significance of these two events is very different.

That apoptosis has a role in cell/material interaction has been suggested quite recently. Some hemodialysis membranes with increased levels of protein phosphorylation in mononuclear cells, which means expression of activation surface molecules and cell death for apoptosis, were classified as "nonbiocompatible" (Carracedo *et al.*, 1998). Recent data suggest that metal ions released from dental alloys or other biomaterials, such as Pt^{4+}, Co^{2+}, Ga^{3+}, and Ni^{2+}, induced apoptosis in the mast cell line HMC-1 and the myeloid cell line HL-60, while in human fibroblast L929 all cytotoxic metal ions produced cell necrosis (Schedle *et al.*, 1995, 1998).

We found that the cytotoxic effects of the extracts of chromium, nickel, and cobalt on isolated mononuclear cells depends on the type of metal, on the extract concentration, and on the time of contact between cells and extract (Granchi *et al.*, 1998c).

Cell death by apoptosis may be important in implants which release metal ions by corrosion or wear: the phenomen may have been underestimated up to now, as it is a "clean" way of cell death, leading to limited damage in the surrounding tissues (Stea *et al.*, 2000). Apoptotic cells were identified *in situ* in 54 tissue biopsies from loosened hip joint prostheses. A high proportion of apoptotic cells was found in the tissue sections where metal particles were present (24% apoptotic cells), if compared to areas where no wear (6%), or plastic wear (2.8%), or ceramic wear (1.5%) was observed. Apoptosis was neither related to the presence of bone cement, nor to the time-to-failure of the implant.

In recent years a number of methods has been developed to distinguish between necrosis and apoptosis. Assays currently used to measure apoptosis include detection of morphological changes, DNA fragmentation, flow cytometric analysis, and detection of genes for apoptosis.

Cells undergoing apoptosis show structural changes which can be observed by electron microscopy. Briefly, the morphological features of apoptosis include the loss of specialized membrane structures, such as microvilli and desmosomes, followed by the rapid blebbing of plasma membrane, that is a membrane-invested extension of cytosol. This is followed by rapid, irreversible condensation of cytoplasm, with an increase in cell density, compaction of cytoplasmic organelles, and condensation of the nuclear chromatin to form dense structures underlying the nuclear membrane.

The DNA fragmentation is a landmark of the cellular apoptosis due to the activation of nucleases that degrade the highly ordered chromatin structure of DNA into internucleosomal fragments (50 to 300 kilobases) and subsequently into smaller DNA pieces of about 200 base pairs in length. These DNA fragments can be extracted from apoptotic cells and result in the appearance of "DNA laddering" when the DNA is analyzed by agarose gel electrophoresis; the DNA of nonapoptotic cells, which remain largely intact, does not display this "laddering," while the denaturated DNA of necrotic cells show a large smear near the deposition area.

Flow cytometry can be applied to differentiate the two modes of cell death, and several methods have been described for cells undergoing DNA fragmentation (Darzynkievicz *et al.*, 1992).

The large number of DNA fragments in apoptotic cells results in a multitude of 3′-hydroxyl termini of DNA ends: apoptotic cells can be identified by labeling the DNA breaks with fluorescent-tagged deoxyuridine triphosphate nucleotides (f-dUTP). The enzyme terminal deoxynucleotidyl transferase (TdT) catalyzes a template independent addition of F-dUTP to the 3′-hydroxyl DNA ends of double- or single-stranded DNA.

Another method for detection of apoptosis on a per-cell basis by flow cytometry has been described (Vermes *et al.*, 1995). In normal blood cells the plasma membrane exhibits significant phospholipid asymmetry, with phosphatidylcholine and sphingomyelin predominantly on the external leaflet, and most of the membrane phosphatidylethanolamine and phosphatidylserine on the inner leaflet. In the early stages of apoptosis the phosphatidylserine translocates from the inner part of the plasma membrane to the outer layer, to be exposed at the external surface of the cell: the recognition and the phagocytosis of apoptotic cells by macrophages seems to be promoted by this event. It was shown that the anticoagulant annexin V preferentially binds to negatively charged phospholipids like phosphatidylserine. Thus, fluorescein isothiocyanate (FITC)-labeled Annexin V can be used for the quantification of apoptosis. Since phosphatidylserine is exposed also by necrotic cells also following the loss of membrane integrity, a DNA stain, such as the exclusion dye propidium iodide, is applied simultaneously. The apoptotic cells became Annexin V-positive as soon as the nucleus has condensated, but before the cell had become permeable to propidium iodide.

The coordinated structural changes of the apoptotic process represent the final effect of an intricate network of events. All living cells contain various molecules that participate in these events, but in a form which requires activation. The process of programmed cell death is the result of an interaction between initiating stimuli, such as toxic substances, and "factors" which determine the susceptibility of the cells to start the cascade of events responsible for the structural changes. These "factors" are specific genes which coordinate and regulate apoptosis, as well as cell growth and differentiation. Bcl-2 is a potent suppressor of apoptosis, while ICE, c-myc, and p53 can induce apoptosis.

Because most substances become cytotoxic, depending on their concentration, some authors suggest that the threshold for the onset of cell death can be determined by the expression levels of genes which promote or suppress apoptosis: these are measured by PCR on the RNA of cells exposed to toxic substances (Hickmann and Boyle, 1996). Monoclonal antibodies, conjugated with either fluorochromes or enzymes, are now available, and the presence of the gene products can be revealed by flow-cytometric and histochemical techniques.

26.6. Specific Immune Response

If the cause of inflammation persists and interacts with the immune system, that is to say it has immunogenic characteristics, a humoral or cell-mediated *specific immune response* is induced. The immune system is made up of a set of cells and molecules, whose fundamental task is to defend the organism against the aggression of something foreign. This occurs through the ability to recognize and differentiate autologous from heterologous substances with an antigenic action, and the ability to react in a specific way toward a "non-self" target. The specific immune response starts when the antigen is exposed on the surface of an "antigen presenting cell" together with a class II HLA molecule. By this molecule, the T helper lymphocytes CD4+ through the T Cell Receptor (TCR) recognize the antigen. At the same time the macrophage discerns IL-1, which acts on T helper lymphocytes, aiding the production of IL-2 and increasing the number of receptors for IL-2 on the B lymphocytes and CD8+ cytotoxic T lymphocytes. By IL-2, the CD4+ T lymphocytes induce the clonal expansion of CD8+ cytotoxic lymphocytes that recognize the antigen on the target cell, presented by a class I HLA molecule, and carry out their cytolytic function. The helper T lymphocytes also induce the proliferation and the differentiation of plasma cells to B lymphocytes through mediators such as IL-2, IL-5, IL-4, and IL-6.

In recent years many studies have been published showing how some materials can interact with the immune system (Rodgers *et al.*, 1997). The current opinion of many experts is that the mechanisms of such interaction should be explored by standardized experimental models in order to be adopted even in the preclinical assessment of a device. Furthermore, some devices that have been used for years produce undesirable effects that can be attributed to an immune response. In both cases, i.e., preclinical testing or intolerance to the device, the strategy is the same. A recent document on immunotoxicity testing has been developed (FDA-CDRH, 1999). According to the document, immunotoxicity is any adverse effect on the structure or function of the immune system, or on other systems as a result of immune system dysfunction. Immunotoxicity testing has to be carried out on all materials, even those with immunotoxic effects, which have not been completely studied. The document follows the ISO classification scheme based on type and duration of contact with the body and it provides a guide to potential immunotoxic effects that might be associated with medical device materials, with regard to the scientific and medical literature on the matter.

Once a material has been found to be potentially immunotoxic, it is important to know what kind of response is induced. This could be immunostimulation, immunosuppression, hypersensitivity, or autoimmunity. Finally, taking into account the pathophysiology of the immune response, the most appropriate test can be used for immunotoxicity (Table 26.1).

According to the literature, metal implants are thought to be able to induce all the above-mentioned immunotoxic effects, regardless of the duration and type of contact. On the contrary, ceramic implants are not able to elicit a specific immune response, but chronic inflammation alone.

26.6.1. Immunogenicity of Metals and Ceramics

A material is immunogenic if it has certain physicochemical characteristics, incuding (i) high molecular weight, (ii) notable internal chemical complexity, (iii) solubility or solubilizable by phagocytes, (iv) extraneity to the species in which it is introduced. Immunogenic molecules have a more or less high number of antigens that can be recognized by specific structures of the immune response, such as membrane receptors of T lymphocytes and soluble antibodies. Generally speaking, a biomaterial, despite being considered as something biologically inert, can induce a tissue reaction in the host, and an immune response as well. The material *per se* is not an antigen, but it has been shown that the proteins that are adsorbed on the surface of a material can change their structure to become "non-self" (Stern *et al.*, 1972). Small molecules released from the material can act as haptens, binding to a protein carrier, or as adjuvants, that is either forming an insoluble complex with the antigen thereby extending its presence in the body or increasing its size so that phagocytes become more active (Merritt, 1986).

a. Metals. The potential immunogenicity of metals has been widely studied and demonstrated (Merritt and Brown, 1996; Remes and Williams, 1992; Yang and Merritt, 1996). The sensitizing metals are haptens, which are not able to act as antigens by themselves. There is evidence that a combination of the metals with circulating or tissue proteins gives rise to new antigens. An alternative hypothesis is that these metals interfere with

Table 26.1. Tests for the Evaluation of the Immunotoxicity

Immune response	Functional assays	Soluble mediators	Phenotyping	Histology
Humoral response	Antibody response to antigen + adjuvant Lymphocyte proliferation Antibody-dependent cell-mediated cytotoxicity Passive cutaneous anaphylaxis Direct anaphylaxis	Complement fractions Immune complexes	Cell surface markers Intracellular markers	Histomorphology Cell surface markers Intracellular markers *In situ* hybridization
Cellular response T lymphocytes	Guinea pig maximization test Lymphocyte proliferation (LTT) Mixed lymphocyte reaction	Cytokine patterns indicative of T cell subsets (Th1 and Th2)	Cell surface markers Intracellular markers	Histomorphology Cell surface markers Intracellular markers *In situ* hybridization
Natural killer	Biochemical activation (MTT) Tumor cytotoxicity		Cell surface markers	Cell surface markers

the antigen recognition phase of the immune response. Sensitivity to nickel, cobalt, and chromium is commonly found among the general population. The identification of these sensitivities is generally got by the detection of cell-mediated immunity, but also metal-specific antibodies were found in patients with total joint replacements (Yang and Merritt, 1994)

b. Ceramics. Most studies about tissue reaction induced by ceramics have shown that these materials can induce a chronic inflammatory response. Cases of allergic dermatitis caused by professional contact with ceramics have been described, but there is little information about the immunogenicity of ceramics used as biomaterials. Tricalcium phosphate ceramics were found to be able to elicit tuberculin-type delayed skin reactions in guinea pigs (Sasaoka *et al.*, 1989), as well as a significant footpad swelling in C57BL mice (Nagase, 1985). The antigenicity of alumina and hydroxyapatite has not been demonstrated.

26.6.2. Interaction between Biomaterials and the Immune System

The interaction between biomaterial and the immune system may lead to *immunostimulation*: this does not necessarily mean disease, but self-maintenance of the inflammatory process may be promoted. The immunostimulation may be defined as "unintended or inappropriate antigen-specific or nonspecific activation of the immune system," which includes the unintended immunogenicity of biomaterials (e.g., antibody and/or cellular immune response to a foreign protein) or the enhancement of the immune response to an antigen by a material with which it is mixed *ex vivo* or *in situ*.

The inhibition of the specific immune response (i.e., antibody and T cell responses) that is immunosuppression may be just as generic; one potential consequence is more frequent and serious infections resulting from reduced host defense. Biomaterials can deprime the immune response. In that case the risk of infection is notably higher. Besides nonspecific immune response inhibition, depressive effects on the production of antibodies (Wang *et al.*, 1997a) and on cell-mediated immune response are also known. Some studies suggest that the presence of metal ions, mainly chromium, released from prosthesis components could be associated with a decrease in lymphocyte subpopulations in patients with joint prosthesis loosening (Savarino *et al.*, 1999; Granchi *et al.*, 1995). Moreover, some metals, such as chromium, seem to inhibit the IL-2-dependent response of mononuclear cells so that they are not able to trigger an efficient cell-mediated immune response (Granchi *et al.*, 1998a). Other authors demonstrated a toxic effect of the metals against the immune system. In a postmortem study of hip prosthesis carriers, the necrosis of lymph nodes and changes in T lymphocytes, due to metal dissemination from implant, were observed (Case *et al.*, 1994). The stimulation of PBMC by phytohaemoagglutinin is largely affected by chromium extract: both cell viability and DNA synthesis were diminished, and cytokine release was inhibited as well (Granchi *et al.*, 1998a; Wang *et al.*, 1996).

Pathologic immune reactions consist of *hypersensitivity* and *autoimmunity*. Hypersensitivity is defined as an increased reactivity to an antigen to which a person (or animal) has been previously exposed, with an adverse rather than protective effect. The complex mechanisms that determine the adaptation of the immune system to each new antigenic emergency are prone to errors, resulting in altered immunoregulation disease or hypersensitivity. Four types of immunoreaction causing anatomoclinical damage have been described.

Type I Immediate or Anaphylactic Hypersensitivity. More commonly defined as allergic diseases, they are mediated by IgE. The basic requirements for an allergic disease are specificity and passive transferability. It has been shown how subcutaneous inoculation of the serum of a subject sensitive to an antigen followed by the antigen itself can induce an erythematous reaction. The Fc portion of the IgE binds to the receptors on basophils and mast cells: a series of biochemical mediators, inducing the clinical manifestations of an allergic reaction, such as skin rash, urticaria, and edema, are released into the microenvironment. The immediate hypersensitive reaction to biomaterials can be recognized by the positivity to the subcutaneous inoculation of the antigen, or the identification of specific serum immunoglobulins.

Type I hypersensitivity reactions were not observed for metals and ceramics, while they were demonstrated for other materials (Alenius *et al.*, 1993; Heese *et al.*, 1997; Rodgers *et al.*, 1997).

Type II or Antibody-Dependent Cytotoxic Hypersensitivity. These are reactions triggered by the interaction between an antibody (IgM or IgG) and an antigen on a cell membrane. The damage is caused by the activation of the complement system, either by recruiting phagocytes by the Fc of the Igs and C3b, or by the antibody-dependent cell-mediated cytotoxicity (ADCC). In the latter case killer cells bind to the Fc fragment-receptor on target cells and bring about their death by releasing lytic substances. Actually, because the effect or mechanisms of antibody-dependent cytotoxic hypersensitivity are not easily demonstrated, its role is still purely speculative and may be attributed to the materials that release wear particles that can adhere to the cell membrane.

Type III or Hypersensitivity Mediated by Immunocomplexes. The immunocomplexes (IC) that normally form in the antibody–antigen reaction are destined to be phagocytosed. Their persistence in the circulation and in tissues is the prerequisite for a type III reaction. This depends on several factors, such as the size of the complexes, their electrical charge, and the characteristics of the antigen. The mechanism by which tissues are damaged is common to all IC diseases and is represented by the triggering of the inflammation events. Immunoglobulins sterically modified in their interaction with the antigen acquire some properties they do not have as free molecules, i.e., bind and activate the complement and interact with all the cells carrying the receptor for the Fc fragment of the Igs, as mononucleated phagocytes and platelets. Depending on the way the ICs are formed, two groups of diseases can be distinguished, i.e., ICs formed *in situ* and circulating ICs. The experimental models are represented respectively by the reaction of Arthus and by acute and chronic serum disease. From a theoretical point of view, a biomaterial that has weak antigenic properties and is slowly degraded should induce a type III reaction, but even in this case it is difficult to demonstrate the effector mechanisms.

Type IV or Delayed Cell Hypersensitivity. Unlike the previous reactions, these are not mediated by antibodies, but by T lymphocytes, and especially CD4+ T lymphocytes which, after stimulation of the antigen, proliferate and cause tissue damage. Some lymphocytes attract and activate macrophages (which take on the morphology of epithelioid or giant cells) for cytotoxic activity, while others are directly cytotoxic. The final result is the formation of a granuloma. Due to the nature of the biomaterial itself, its application, tissue reaction, and slow degradation, type IV hypersensitive reactions are more often associated with the implantation of a device. Metal implants are most often responsible for type IV hypersensitivity. That has been proven and discussed in many studies on orthopedic implants (Deutman *et al.*, 1977; Carlsson *et al.*, 1980; Cancilleri *et al.*, 1992; Amstutz and Grigoris, 1996; Granchi *et al.*, 1999) and dental implants (Greppi *et al.*, 1989; Kim and Johnson, 1999; Jia *et al.*, 1999). The metals act as haptens and bind to the proteins in peri-implant tissue, producing the sensitizing antigen. This is captured and processed by the macrophages that carry it to the T lymphocytes within the satellite lymph nodes. T lymphocytes become activated, proliferate, and cause tissue damage by two mechanisms: cytokine production and cytotoxic lymphocyte activation. The sensitization process may last 1–2 weeks; the subsequent and continuous contact with the antigen, which is released by degradation at the implant site, leads to the onset of the hypersensitive reaction. That is accompanied by an inflammatory response, which in turn causes more and more marked tissue damage until it is necessary to remove the prosthesis (Gruber, 1991; Jiranek *et al.*, 1993; Lalor and Revell, 1993).

Another pathologic event linked to immune reaction is the *autoimmune response* to the body's own constituents. It is indicated by the presence of auto-antibodies or T lymphocytes reactive with host tissue or cell antigens, and may result in autoimmune disease with chronic, debilitating, and sometimes life-threatening tissue and organ injury. Theoretically, a biomaterial can act as an adjuvant which may induce an autoimmune response; for example, the coupling with a foreign protein may induce IgG or IgM antibodies that cross-react with a human protein and cause tissue damage by activating the complement system.

Reliable tests for auto-antibodies (e.g., ELISA) and auto-reactive T cells (e.g., lymphocyte proliferation) are available, and several animal models have been developed to study certain human autoimmune diseases (Rose, 1997). However, auto-antibodies and auto-reactive T lymphocytes may only be indicators of an autoimmune response. Even if an autoimmune response can be demonstrated in preclinical testing, convincing evidence that a biomaterial causes autoimmune disease in animals is difficult to obtain, and no evidence has been found for metal and ceramic implants.

26.6.3. Methods for Testing the Immune Specific Response

Histology of tissue biopsies from several peri-implant sites is used for characterization of the cells at the tissue–implant interface and may be useful in the case of *humoral* or *cell-mediated response.* Neutrophils, eosinophils, lymphocytes, plasma cells, lymphoid follicles, and mono- and multinuclear histiocytes are recognized according to their morphology .

Around orthopedic prostheses wear particle are observed and the extent of wear is correlated to cellular events (Pizzoferrato *et al.*, 1991). Furthermore, immunotoxicity is also connected to the condition of the lymph nodes near the prosthesis. These may be modified by the toxic effect of the material (presence of wear particles, lymph node necrosis, apoptosis) or by immunostimulant effects (increase in the lymph node volume, or increase in lymph node follicles).

Lymphocyte subsets are not morphologically distinguished: lymphocytes are differentiated according to some characteristics of the membrane and/or intracytoplasmic antigens. Immunohistochemistry on tissues provides further information about the type of cell involved in peri-implant reaction (Lalor and Revell, 1993). T lymphocytes are CD3 and CD2 positive cells, while B lymphocytes are identified by the presence of CD19 antigens: lymphocytes CD4 (helper inducer, CD4+CD29+, and suppressor inducer CD4+CD45RA+) and CD8 (cytotoxic suppressor). Furthermore, lymphocytes expressing activation antigens, including the receptor for interleukin (CD25), the receptor for transferrin (CD71), the expression of the HLA-DR of the major histocompatibility complex on T cells, and the "early activation antigen" (CD69) are identified (Biselli *et al.*, 1992). NK cells are recognized using CD16, CD56, and CD57 antigens.

Some cytokines are identified in tissues by immunohistochemistry, with TNF-α, IL-6, IL-1, and chemokines found in aspecific reactions, while IL-2 indicates a specific immune reaction. Sometimes immunohistochemical testing alone cannot determine whether the presence of a cytokine is a consequence of the activity of the cells at the interface, or if they have a different origin: this can be solved by *in situ* hybridization of the mRNA (Jiranek *et al.*, 1993; Goodman *et al.*, 1996b).

a. Humoral Response. Specific humoral response involves the production of antibodies against the molecules released by the material. An ADCC is established or circulating immunocomplexes are formed. Furthermore, even the levels of some complement fragments, such as C3a, C5a, TCC, Bb, iC3b, C4d, and SC5b-9, are modified in humoral response. Specific antibodies can be found in the plasma of patients who developed a humoral hypersensitive reaction against a material. Type I hypersensitivity is indicated by specific IgE, passive transferability, or by the direct reaction to the antigen. B lymphocytes are quantified and plasma cells are recognized for their intracytoplasmatic immunoglobulins. If the specific humoral immunity is inhibited by the material, a state of immunodepression is established, with reduction of the host's resistance to opportunistic infections, viruses, and tumors. The state of immunodepression is ascertained measuring the amount of known antibodies, such as isohemoagglutinin, anti-streptococcus antibodies, anti-staphylococcus antibodies, or antibodies against vaccine antigens.

b. Cell-Mediated Response. In specific immune response T and B lymphocytes are involved; they are identified by phenotype characteristics (Granchi *et al.*, 1995). This type of test is useful for people with prostheses because there are quantitative variations in the distribution of lymphocyte subsets. T and B lymphocytes are identified by the presence of the antigens described in the paragraph about tissue response. The state of lymphocyte activation can be determined by functional testing.

The biochemical activation of cells may be explored also by the MTT test or the formazan salt reduction test (3-(4,5 dimethyltiazol-2-yl)-2,5 diphenyl tetrazolium bromide) (Ciapetti *et al.*, 1993). The salt is reduced by the active mitochondrial enzymes of the cell: this is therefore an indirect but accurate measure of the viability and/or activation of the cells.

The Lymphocyte Transformation Test (LTT) measures the ability of lymphocytes to respond *in vitro* to an exogenous stimulus. Using plant lectins the lymphocytes turn into blasts, which are usually bigger than "resting" lymphocytes because they have duplicated their DNA content. Tests to determine that transformation has taken place are based on this biochemical event. A precursor of DNA, that can be radioactive (tritiated thymidine) or fluorescent, is taken up during the S phase (synthesis of DNA) of the cell cycle. Alternatively, a substance that intercalates in the double chain which is formed and thus acts as an index of the total quantity of DNA (Blaheta *et al.*, 1991) can be used.

The most informative method for studying the function of natural killer cells is to measure their cytotoxic activity against tumor cells, such as the K562 cell line. The cytotoxic activity of NK cells is analyzed by assessing the incorporation of propidium iodide or the release of ^{51}Cr in target cells (Vitale *et al.*, 1989).

Specific immune response occurs through an IL2-dependent mechanism: upon evaluation of this cytokine or its soluble receptor it can be said if lymphocytes are activated through a specific recognition system. Using other molecules, the Th1 lymphocytes involved in cell-mediated reactions are distinguished from Th2, which are, respectively, involved in the type I hypersensitivity reaction and immune response against parasites (Romagnani, 1992.). Th1 lymphocytes differ from Th2 lymphocytes inasmuch as they produce high levels of TNF-α, IFN-γ, and IL2, but not IL4 or IL5. Other cytokines, i.e., IL6, IL10, IL3 and GMCSF, are produced by Th1 to a lesser extent than Th2. Our studies on cytokine release in mononuclear cells of patients with Co–Cr hip prostheses demonstrated that when PBMCs were challenged with metal extract, the release of both TNF-α and GM-CSF was higher than in normal donors, while IL6 was lower. Metal concentrations in serum from patients were significantly higher and correlated with TNF-α release in PBMCs stimulated with both metal extracts. The prevalence of cells that produce TNF-α and IL-6 differently recall the pattern of release which differentiates Th1 from Th2 lymphocytes. The Th1 cells are responsible for the cell-mediated hypersensitivity reaction and their increase would justify the sensitization to the metals (Granchi *et al.*, 1999). The expression of the activation antigen (CD69 or "early activation" antigen) on CD3/T-lymphocytes cultured with metal ions was assessed by flow cytometry. The chromium-induced activation index was significantly higher in patients with implant loosening than in healthy donors and in preimplants. Moreover, a "high activation index" (=2) was observed only for the chromium-stimulated PBMCs of the patients with prostheses, especially those with implant loosening. The cobalt extract was able to inhibit CD69 expression in healthy subjects, while in patients with prosthesis loosening the toxic effect of the extract was less evident, as demonstrated by the activation index significantly higher than in healthy individuals.

The high sensitizing ability of chromium could be due to its persistence in the tissue. Indeed, chromium is eliminated more slowly than nickel and cobalt: these are rapidly transported away from the implant site and excreted with the urine (Merritt and Brown, 1996).

In vivo tests can be used for the preclinical assessment of specific cell-mediated response to a material: the closed patch sensitization test (topical application) and the maximization sensitization test (intradermal and topical application) are commonly used (EN 30993—Part 10). Both assays, which are sensitization tests on guinea pigs, assess the potential of the material to produce skin sensitization. They entail three consecutive phases: the preliminary phase is intended to determine the optimal concentrations of the test material to be used; the induction phase is the first contact with the potentially sensitizing material; and the last phase, or challenge, is performed some weeks after the induction and shows the ability of materials to sensitize the animals by inducing a skin reaction.

If a biomaterial is suspected to produce a delayed hypersensitive reaction in humans, the patch test should be recommended. It is a skin provocation test, because the allergen is directly in contact with the organ (skin) that presents the symptoms. The allergen is a chemical substance that acts as a hapten and reacts with the sensitized skin T lymphocytes. The most common method used is the closed patch test: the substance applied onto the skin is covered with a plaster, which is removed after 48 h. The reaction is positive when papules or blisters appear. A negative reaction is examined again at 72–96 h.

The effectiveness of *in vitro* testing to detect hypersensitivity to metals has been widely demonstrated. Lymphocytes from patients with total joint replacement have a high proliferative response and cytokine release when they were cultured with metal salts (Bjurholm *et al.*, 1990) and particles of cobalt–chromium alloy and polymethylmethacrylate (Wooley *et al.*, 1996, 1997; Toumbis *et al.*, 1997).

The *in vitro* finding of sensitized lymphocytes does not necessarily call for *in vivo* evidence of hypersensitivity, and these data in patients with orthopedic implants often disagree (Rooker and Wilkinson, 1980; Carlsson and Moller, 1989). It is reasonably assumed that the activation of specific lymphocytes evolves in different ways. In a few cases a strong hypersensitive reaction with skin symptoms, which disappeared after removal of the implant, was described (Rostoker *et al.*, 1987), but for the most part sensitized lymphocytes were detected *in vitro* without a corresponding positive reaction to the patch test. This disagreement between laboratory results and clinical findings could be explained with the tissue-specific homing of T-cells, which enhances the efficiency of the immune system by targeting immune surveillance and effector response to tissue similar to those where the antigen initially entered the body, and conversely may act to reduce opportunities for autoimmune cross-reaction with unrelated tissue (Picker *et al*., 1993). It is well known that T lymphocytes involved in the local skin immunity express the "cutaneous lymphocytes antigen" (CLA), which represents a skin homing receptor for T cells. On the contrary, T cells migrating to different sites of inflammation, such as synovium and joints, do not express this antigen: this movement is probably regulated by other organ-specific homing mechanisms (Pitzalis *et al*., 1996).

In conclusion, the acute inflammatory reaction is part of the normal defence reaction against the foreign material: under this assumption cells and fluid are recruited at the implant site soon after implantation. The physiological progression toward tissue repair and sometimes sequestration of the device by a fibrous capsule represents the conclusion of the surgical insertion.

If the surface of the material changes following interaction with tissues or particulates are generated, the response may evolve toward chronic inflammatory reaction. Granulomatous reactions need more time to heal and the persistence of inflammation may evolve up to osteolysis phenomena and loosening of the implant. Interaction of biomaterials with immune cells may trigger reactions with final modulation of some immune responses.

Research in orthopedics should tend to better understanding of the local reactions between cells and materials, as well as to development of surfaces eliciting positive biological response.

References

Agins, H.J., Alcock, N.W., Bansal, M., Salvati, E.A., Wilson, P.D., Pellicci, P.M., Bullough, P. G. 1988. Metallic wear in failed titanium alloy total hip replacements. A histological and quantitative analysis, *J. Bone Jt. Surg.* **70**, 347–356.

al-Saffar, N., Mah, J.T., Kadoya, Y., Revell, P.A. 1995a. Neovascularisation and the induction of cell adhesion molecules in response to degradation products from orthopaedic implants, *Ann. Rheum. Dis.* **54**, 201–208.

al-Saffar, N., Revell, P.A., Khwaja, H.A. Bonfield, W. 1995b. Assessment of the role of cytokines in bone resorption in patients with total joint replacement, *J. Mat. Sci. Mater. Med.* **6**, 762–767.

Alenius, H., Palosuo, T., Kelly, K., Kurup, V., Reunala, T., Makinen-Kiljunen, S., Turjanmaa, K., Fink, J. 1993. IgE reactivity to 14 KD and 27 KD natural rubber proteins in latex allergic children with spina bifida and other congenital anomalies, *Int. Arch. Allerg. Immunol.* **102**, 61–66.

Alliot-Licht, B., Jean, A., Gregoire, M. 1994. Comparative effect of calcium hydroxide and hydroxyapatite on the cellular activity of human pulp fibroblasts in vitro, *Arch. Oral Biol.* **39**, 481–489.

Amstutz, H.C., Grigoris, P. 1996. Metal on metal bearings in hip arthroplasty, *Clin. Orthop.* **329**, S11–34.

Arnaout, M.A. 1990. Structure and function of the leukocyte adhesion molecules CD11/CD18, *Blood* **75**, 1037–1050.

Beard, R.B., Carim, H., De Rosa, J.F., Dubin, S., Koerner, R., Miller, A.S. 1976. Biocompatibility of electrodes for implantable power sources, in: *Biocompatibility of Implant Materials* (D.F. Williams, ed.), Chap. 16, Sector Publishing, London.

Biselli, R., Matricardi, P.M., D'Amelio, R., Fattorossi, A. 1992. Multiparametric flow cytometric analysis of the kinetics of surface molecule expression after polyclonal activation of human peripheral blood T lymphocytes, *Scand. J. Immunol.* **35**, 439–447.

Bjurholm, A., al-Tawil, N.A., Marcusson, J.A., Netz, P. 1990. The lymphocyte response to nickel salt in patients with orthopedic implants, *Acta Orthop. Scand.* **61**, 248–250.

Blaheta, R.A., Franz, M., Auth, M.K.H., Wenish, H.J.C., Markus, B.H. 1991. A rapid non-radioactive fluorescence assay for the measurement of both cell number and proliferation, *J. Immunol. Meth.*, **142**, 199–206.

Blaine, T.A., Pollice, P.F., Rosier, R.N., Reynolds, P.R., Puzas, J.E., O'Keefe, R.J. 1997. Modulation of the production of cytokines in titanium-stimulated human peripheral blood monocytes by pharmacological agents. The role of cAMP-mediated signaling mechanisms, *J. Bone Jt. Surg., Am. Vol.* **79**, 1519–1528.

Bloebaum, R.D., Lundeen, G.A., Bachus, K.N., Ison, I., Hofmann, A.A. 1998. Dissolution of particulate hydroxyapatite in a macrophage organelle model, *J. Biomed Mater. Res.* **40**, 104–114.

Bohne, W., Pouezat, J.A., Peru, L., Daculsi, G. 1993. Heating of calcium phosphate crystals: morphological consequences and biological implications, *Cells Mater.* **3**, 377–382.

Bosetti, M., Ottani, V., Kozel, D., Raspanti, M., De Pasquale, V., Ruggeri, A., Cannas, M. 1999. Structural and functional macrophages alterations by ceramics of different composition, *Biomaterials* **20**, 363–370.

Boyden, S. 1962. The chemotactic effect of mixtures antibody and antigen on polymorphonuclear leucocytes, *J. Exp. Med.* **115**, 453–458.

Campoccia, D., Hunt, J.A., Doherty, P.J., Zhong, S.P., Callegaro, L., Benedetti, L., Williams, D.F. 1993. Human neutrophil chemokinesis and polarization induced by hyaluronic acid derivatives, *Biomaterials* **14**, 1135–1139.

Cancilleri, F., De Giorgis, P., Verdoia, C., Parrini, L., Lodi, A., Crosti, C. 1992. Allergy to components of total hip arthroplasty before and after surgery, *Ital. J. Orthop. Traumatol.* **18**, 407–410.

Carlsson, A., Moller, H. 1989. Implantation of orthopaedic devices in patients with metal allergy, *Acta Derm. Venereol.* **69**, 62–66.

Carlsson, A., Magnusson, B., Moller, H. 1980. Metal sensitivity in patients with metal-to-plastic total hip arthroplasties, *Acta Orthop. Scand.* **51**, 57–62.

Carracedo, J., Ramirez, R., Martin Malo, A., Rodriguez, M., Aljama, P. 1998. Nonbiocompatible hemodialysis membranes induce apoptosis in mononuclear cells: the role of G-protein, *J. Am. Soc. Nephrol.* **9**, 46–53.

Case, C.P., Langlamer, V.G., James, C., Palmer, M.R., Kemp, A.J., Heap, P.F., Solomon, L. 1994. Widespread dissemination of metal debris from implant, *J. Bone Jt. Surg. Br. Vol.* **76**, 701–712.

Cheung, H.S., Haak, M.H. 1989. Growth of osteoblasts on porous calcium phosphate ceramics: an *in vitro* model for biocompatibility study, *Biomaterials* **10**, 63–67.

Chiba, J., Rubash, H.E., Kim, K.J., Iwaki, Y. 1994. The characterization of cytokines in the interface tissue obtained from failed cementless total hip arthroplasty with and without femoral osteolysis, *Clin. Orthop.* **300**, 304–312.

Ciapetti, G., Roda, P., Landi, L., Facchini, A., Pizzoferrato, A. 1992. In vitro methods to evaluate metal-cell interactions, *Int. J. Artif. Organs* **15**, 62–66.

Ciapetti, G., Cenni , E., Pratelli, L., Pizzoferrato, A. 1993. In vitro evaluation of cell/biomaterial interaction by MTT assay, *Biomaterials* **14**(5), 359–364.

Ciapetti, G., Granchi, D., Verri, E., Savarino, L., Savioli, F., Dallari, D., Gualtieri, G., Pizzoferrato, A. 1997. Effect of metal ions on leucocytes from patients with metal implants, 13th European Conference on Biomaterials, Goteborg (Sweden), 4–7 September 1997, Abstract P127.

Ciapetti, G., Granchi, D., Verri, E., Savarino, L., Cenni, E., Savioli, F., Pizzoferrato, A. 1998. Fluorescent microplate assay for respiratory burst of PMNs challenged in vitro with orthopedic metals, *J. Biomed. Mater. Res.* **41**, 455–460.

Daculsi, G., Passuti, N. 1990a. Effect of the macroporosity for osseous substitution of calcium phosphate ceramics, *Biomaterials* **11**, 86–87.

Daculsi, G., LeGeros, R.Z., Heughebaert, J.C., Barbieux, I. 1990. Formation of carbonate-apatite crystals after implantation of calcium phosphate ceramics, *Calcif. Tissue Int.* **46**, 20–27.

Daniels, A.U., Barnes, F.H., Charlebois, S.J., Smith, R.A. 2000. Macrophage cytokine response to particles and lypopolysaccharide in vitro, *J. Biomed. Mater. Res.* **49**, 469–478.

Darzynkievicz, Z., Bruno, S., Del Bino, G., Gorczyca, W., Hotz, M.A., Lassota, P., Traganos, F. 1992. Features of apoptotic cells measured by flow cytometry, *Cytometry* **13**, 795–808.

de Groot, K. 1983. Ceramics of calcium phosphates, preparation and properties, in: *Bioceramics of Calcium-Phosphate* (de Groot K, ed.), pp. 99–114, CRC Press, Boca Raton.

de Groot, K., Wolke, J.G.C., Jansen, J.A. 1998. Calcium phosphate coatings for medical implants, *J. Eng. Med.* **212**, 137–148.

Deutman, R., Mulder, T.J., Brian, R., Nater J.P. 1977. Metal sensitivity before and after total hip arthroplasty, *J. Bone Jt. Surg. Am. Vol.* **59**, 862–865.

Dobbs, H.S., Minski, M.J. 1980. Metal ion release after total hip replacement, *Biomaterials* **1**, 193–198.

Dowsett, S.A., Hyvonen, P.M., Kowolik, M.J. 1997. Functional integrity of human neutrophils following 24 hour incubation with hydroxyapatite and fluoride, *J. Biolumin. Chemilumin.* **12**, 215–221.

Ducheyne, P., Lemons, J.E. (eds.), 1988. *Bioceramics: Materials Characteristics versus In Vivo Behavior*, NY Academic Science, New York.

Ducheyne, P., Qiu, Q. 1999. Bioactive ceramics: the effect of surface reactivity on bone formation and bone cell function, *Biomaterials* **20**, 2287–2303.

Dupraz, A., Delecrin, J., Moreau, A., Pilet, P., Passuti, N. 1998. Long-term bone response to particulate injectable ceramic, *J. Biomed. Mater. Res.* **42**, 368–375.

Elwing, H., Tengvall, P., Askendal, A., Lundstrom, I. 1991. "Lens-on-surface": a versatile method for the investigation of plasma protein exchange reactions on solid surfaces, *J. Biomater. Sci. Polym. Ed.* **3**, 7–15.

Endler, M., Endler, T.A., Zielinski, C. 1982. Influence of hip arthroplasty upon chemotactic behaviour of leucocytes, *Acta Orthop. Scand.* **53**, 795–799.

Freyria, A.M., Chignier, E., Guidollet, J., Luisot, P. 1991. Peritoneal macrophage response: an in vivo model for the study of synthetic materials, *Biomaterials* **12**, 111–118.

Fukuchi, N., Akao, M., Sato, A. 1995. Effect of hydroxyapatite microcrystals on macrophage activity, *Biomed. Mater. Eng.* **5**, 219–231.

Gangarosa, E.J., Inglefield, J.T., Thomas, C.G.A., Morgan, H.R. 1955. Studies on hypersensitivity of human tissues in vitro, *J. Exp. Med.* **101**, 425–433.

Giudiceandrea, F., Iacona, A., Cervelli, G., Grimaldi, M., Maggiulli, G., Cococcetta, N., Cervelli, V. 1998. Mechanisms of bone resorption: analysis of proinflammatory cytokines in peritoneal macrophages from titanium implant — an experimental design, *J. Craniofac. Surg.* **9**, 254–259.

Glant T.T., Jacobs, J.J., Molnar, G., Shanbhag, A.S., Valyon, M., Galante, J.O. 1993. Bone resorption activity of particulate–stimulated macrophages, *J. Bone Miner. Res.* **8**, 1071–1079.

Goebeler, M., Meinardus-Hager, G., Roth, J., Goerdt, S. and Sorg, C., 1993, Nickel chloride and cobalt chloride, two common contact sensitizers, directly induce expression of intercellular adhesion molecule-1 (ICAM-1), vascular cell adhesion molecule-1 (VCAM-1), and endothelial leukocyte adhesion molecule (ELAM-1) by endothelial cells, *J. Invest. Dermatol.* **100**, 759–765.

Goebeler, M., Roth, J., Brocker, E.B., Sorg, C., Schulze-Osthoff, K. 1995. Activation of nuclear factor-kappa B and gene expression in human endothelial cells by the common haptens nickel and cobalt, *J. Immunol.* **155**, 2459–2467.

Goldring, S.R., Jasty, M., Roelke, M.S., Rourke, C.M., Bringhurst, F.R., Harris, W.H. 1986 Formation of a synovial-like membrane at the bone-cement interface: its role in bone resorption and implant loosening after total hip replacement, *Arthritis Rheumatol.* **29**, 836–842.

Gonzales, J.B., Purdon, M.A., Horowitz, S.M. 1996. In vitro studies on the role of titanium in aseptic loosening, *Clin. Orthop.* **330**, 244–250.

Goodman, S.B., Fornasier, V.L., Lee, J., Kei, J. 1990. The effects of bulk versus particulate titanium and cobalt chrome alloy implanted into the rabbit tibia, *J. Biomed. Mater. Res.* **24**, 1539–1549.

Goodman, S.B., Aspenberg, P., Spang, Y., Doshi, A., Regula, D., Lidgren L. 1995. Effects of particulate high-density polyethylene and titanium alloy on tissue ingrowth into bone harvest chamber in rabbits, *J. Appl. Biomater.* **6**, 27–33.

Goodman, S.B., Davidson, J.A., Song, Y., Martial, N., Fornasier, V.L. 1996a. Histomorphological reaction of bone to different concentrations of phagocytosable particles of high-density polyethylene and Ti-6Al-4V alloy in vivo, *Biomaterials*, **17**, 1943–1947.

Goodman, S.B., Knoblich, G., O'Connor, M., Song, Y., Huie, P., Sibley, R. 1996b. Heterogeneity in cellular and cytokine profiles from multiple samples of tissue surrounding revised hip prostheses, *J. Biomed. Mater. Res.* **31**, 421–428.

Granchi, D., Ciapetti, G., Stea, S., Cavedagna, D., Bettini, N., Bianco, T., Fontanesi, G., Pizzoferrato, A. 1995. Evaluation of several immunological parameters in patients with aseptic loosening of hip arthroplasty, *Chir. Organi Mov.* **80**, 399–408.

Granchi, D., Verri, E., Ciapetti, G., Savarino, L., Cenni, E., Gori, A., Pizzoferrato, A. 1998a. Effects of chromium extract on cytokine release by mononuclear cells, *Biomaterials* **19**, 283–291.

Granchi, D., Verri, E., Ciapetti, G., Stea, S., Savarino, L., Sudanese, A., Mieti, M., Rotini, R., Dallari, D., Zinghi, G., Montanaro, L. 1998b. Bone resorbing cytokines in serum of patients with aseptic loosening of hip prosthesis, *J. Bone Jt. Surg.* **80**, 912–917.

Granchi, D., Cenni, E., Ciapetti, G., Savarino, L., Stea, S., Gamberini, S., Gori, A., Pizzoferrato, A. 1998c. Cell death induced by metal ions, necrosis or apoptosis? *J. Mater. Sci., Mater. Med.* **9**, 31–37.

Granchi, D., Ciapetti, G., Stea, S., Savarino, L., Filippini, F., Sudanese, A., Zinghi, G., Montanaro L. 1999. Cytokine release in mononuclear cells of patients with Co–Cr hip prosthesis, *Biomaterials* **20**, 1079–1086.

Greppi, A.L., Smith, D.C., Woodside, D.G. 1989. Nickel hypersensitivity reactions in orthodontic patients. A literature review, *Univ. Tor. Dent. J.* **3**, 11–14.

Gruber, H.E. 1991. Bone and the immune system, *Proc. Soc. Exp. Biol. Med.* **197**, 219–225.

Harada, Y., Wang, J.T., Doppalapudi, V.A., Willis, A.A., Jasty, M., Harris, W.H., Nagase, M., Goldring, S.R. 1996. Differential effects of different forms of hydroxyapatite and hydroxyapatite/tricalcium phosphate particulates on human monocyte/macrophages *in vitro*, *J. Biomed. Mater. Res.* **31**, 19–26.

Harms, J., Mausle, E. 1979. Tissue reaction to ceramic implant material, *J. Biomed. Mater. Res.* **13**(1), 67–87.

Haynes, D.R., Rogers, S.D., Hay, S., Pearcy, M.J., Howie, D.W. 1993. The difference in toxicity and release of bone-resorbing mediators induced by titanium and cobalt-chromium-alloy wear particles, *J. Bone Jt. Surg., Am. Vol.* **75**, 825–834.

Haynes, D.R., Rogers, S.D., Howie, D.W., Pearcy, M.J., Vernon-Roberts, B. 1996. Drug inhibition of the macrophage response to metal wear particles in vitro, *Clin. Orthop.* **323**, 316–326.

Haynes D.R., Hay, S.J., Rogers, S.D., Ohta, S., Howie, D.W., Graves, S.E. 1997. Regulation of bone cells by particle-activated mononuclear phagocytes, *J. Bone Jt. Surg., Br. Vol.* **79**, 988–994.

Haynes, D.R., Boyle, S.J., Rogers, S.D., Howie, D.W., Vernon-Roberts, B. 1998. Variation in cytokines induced by particles from different prosthetic materials, *Clin. Orthop.* **352**, 223–230.

Haynes, D.R., Crotti, T.N., Haywood, M.R. 2000. Corrosion of and changes in biological effects of cobalt chrome alloy and 316L stainless steel prosthetic particles with age, *J. Biomed. Mater. Res.* **49**, 167–175.

Heese, A., Peters, K.P., Koch, H. 1997. Type I allergies to latex and the aeroallergenic problem, Eur. *J. Surg. Suppl.* **579**, 19–22.

Hickmann, J.A., Boyle, C.C. 1996. Apoptosis and cytotoxins, *Br. Med. Bull.*, **52**, 632–643.

Hirakawa, K., Bauer, T.W., Stulberg, B.N., Wilde, A.H. 1996. Comparison and quantitation of wear debris of failed total hip and knee arthroplasty, *J. Biomed. Mater. Res.* **31**, 257–263.

Horowitz, S.M., Luchetti, W.T., Gonzales, J.B., Ritchie, C.K. 1998. The effects of cobalt chromium upon macrophages, *J. Biomed. Mater. Res.* **41**, 468–473.

Hujanen E.S., Seppa S.T., Virtanen K. 1995. Polymorphonuclear leukocyte chemotaxis induced by zinc, copper and nickel in vitro, *Biochim. Biophys. Acta* **1245**, 145–152.

Hukkanen, M., Corbett, S.A., Batten, J., Konttinen, Y.T., McCarthy, I.D., Maclouf, J., Santavirta, S., Hughes, S.P., Polak, J.M. 1997. Aseptic loosening of total hip replacement. Macrophage expression of inducible nitric oxide synthase and cyclo-oxygenase-2, together with peroxynitrite formation, as a possible mechanism for early prosthesis failure, *J. Bone Jt. Surg., Br. Vol.* **79**, 467–474.

Hunt, J.A., Remes, A., Williams, D.F. 1992. Stimulation of neutrophil movement by metal ions, *J. Biomed. Mater. Res.* **26**, 819–828.

Ibbotson, K.J., Twardzic, D.R., D'Souza, S.M., Hargreaves, W.A., Todaro, G.K., Mundy, G.R. 1985. Stimulation of bone resorption *in vitro* by systemic transforming growth factor-alpha, *Science* **228**, 1007–1011.

Ishiguro, N., Kojima, T., Ito, T., Saga, S., Anma, H., Kurokouchi, K., Iwahori, Y., Iwase, T., Iwata, H. 1997. Macrophage activation and migration in interface tissue around loosening total hip arthroplasty components, *J. Biomed. Mater. Res.* **35**, 399–406.

Jacobs, J., Urban, R.M., Gilbert, J.L., Skipor, A.K., Black, J., Jasty, M., Galante, J.O. 1995. Local and distant products from modularity, *Clin. Orthop.* **319**, 94–105.

Jacobs, J., Skipor, A., Doorn, P., Campbell, P., Schmalzried, T., Black, J., Amstutz, H. 1996. Cobalt and chromium concentrations in patients with metal on metal total hip replacements, *Clin. Orthop.* **3295**, S256–S263.

Jahns, G., Haeffner-Cavaillon, N., Nyddegger, U.E., Kazatchkine, M.D. 1993. Complement activation and cytokine production as consequences of immunological bioincompatibility of extracorporeal circuits, *Clin. Mater.* **14**, 303–336.

Jarcho, M., 1981, Calcium phosphate ceramics as hard tissue prosthetics, *Clin. Orthop. Relat. Res.* **157**, 259–278.

Jia, W., Beatty, M.W., Reinhardt, R.A., Petro, T.M., Cohen, D.M. 1999. Nickel release from orthodontic arch wires and cellular immune response to various nickel concentrations, *J. Biomed. Mater. Res.* **48**, 488–495.

Jiranek, W.J., Machado, M., Jasty, M., Jesevar, D., Wolfe, H.J., Goldring, S.R., Goldberg M.J., Harris, W.H. 1993. Production of cytokines around loosened cemented acetabular components. Analysis with immunohistochemical techniques and in situ hybridization, *J. Bone Jt. Surg., Am. Vol.* **75**, 863–879.

Kanagaraja, S., Lundstrom, I., Nygren, H., Tengvall, P. 1996. Platelet binding and protein adsorption to titanium and gold after short time exposure to heparinized plasma and whole blood, *Biomaterials* **17**, 2225–2235.

Kane, DeHeer, D.H., Owens, S.R., Beebe, J.D., Swanson, A.B. 1994. Adsorption of collagenase to particulate titanium: a possible mechanism for collagenase localization in periprosthetic tissue, *J. Appl. Biomater.* **5**, 353–360.

Kansas, G.S., 1992, Structure and function of L-selectin, *APMIS* **100**, 287–293.

Kaplan, S.S., Basford, R.E., Kormos, R.L., Hardesty, R.L., Simmons, R.L., Mora, E.M., Cardona, M., Griffith, B.L. 1990. Biomaterial associated impairment of local neutrophil function, *ASAIO Trans.* **36**, M172–175.

Kaplan, S.S., Simmons, R.L. 1995. Neutrophil biomaterial interactions: implications for host defense and inflammation, in: *Encyclopedic Handbook of Biomaterials and Bioengineering*, Part A: *Materials*, Vol. 1 (D.L. Wise, D.J. Trantolo, D.E. Altobelli, M.J. Yaszemski, J.D. Gresser, E.R. Schwartz, eds.), pp. 457–491, Marcel Dekker, Inc., New York.

Katou, F., Andoh, N., Motegi, K., Nagura, H. 1996. Immuno-inflammatory responses in the tissues adjacent to titanium miniplates used in the treatment of mandibular fractures, *J. Craniomaxillofac. Surg.* **24**, 155–162.

Kim, H., Johnson, J.W. 1999. Corrosion of stainless steel, nickel-titanium, coated nickel-titanium, and titanium orthodontic wires, *Angle Orthod.* **69**, 39–44.

Kim, K.J., Sato, K., Kotake, S., Katoh, Y., Itoh, T. 1993. Biochemical and histochemical analysis of bone marrow cells activated by HA particles, in: *Bioceramics*, Vol. 6 (P. Ducheyne, D. Christiansen, eds.), pp. 365–369, Butterworth-Heinemann Ltd., Philadelphia.

Klein, C.L., Nieder, P., Wagner, M., Kohler, H., Bittinger, F., Kirkpatrick, C.J., Lewis, J.C. 1994. The role of metal corrosion in inflammatory processes: induction of adhesion molecules by heavy metal ions, *J. Mater. Sci., Mater. Med.* **5**, 798–807.

Klein, C.P., Driessen, A.A., de Groot, K. 1983a. Biodegradation behaviour of various calcium phosphate materials in bone tissue, *J. Biomed. Mater. Res.* **17**, 769–784.

Klein, C.P., de Groot, K., van Kamp, G. 1983b. Activation of complement C3 by different calcium phosphate powders, *Biomaterials* **4**, 181–184.

Korkusuz, F., Uluoglu, O. 1999. Non-specific inflammation and bone marrow depletion due to intramedullary porous hydroxyapatite application, *Bull. Hosp. Jt. Dis.* **58**, 86–91.

Kubo, T., Sawada, K., Hirakawa, K., Shimizu, C., Takamatsu, T., Hirasawa, Y. 1999. Histiocyte reaction in rabbit femurs to UHMWPE, metal, and ceramic particles in different sizes, *J. Biomed. Mater. Res.* **45**, 363–369.

Labat, B., Chamson, A., Frey, C. 1995. Effects of γ-alumina and hydroxyapatite coatings on the growth and metabolism of human osteoblasts, *J. Biomed. Mater. Res.* **29**, 1397–1401.

Lalor, P.A., Revell, P.A. 1993. T-lymphocytes and Titanium Aluminium Vanadium (TiAlVa) alloy: evidence for immunological events associated with debris deposition, *Clin. Mater.*, **12**, 57–62.

Le Huec, J.C., Schaeverbeke, T., Clement, D., Faber, J., Le Rebeller, A. 1995. Influence of porosity on the mechanical resistance of hydroxy-apatite ceramics under compressive stress, *Biomaterials* **16**, 113–118.

Lee, S.H., Brennan, F.R., Jacobs, J.J., Urban, R.M., Ragasa, D.R., Glant, T.T. 1997. Human monocyte/macrophage response to cobalt-chromium corrosion products and titanium particles in patients with total joint replacements, *J. Orthop. Res.* **15**, 40–49.

LeGeros, R.Z., Zheng, R., Kijkowska, R., Fan, D., LeGeros, J.P. 1994. Variations in composition and crystallinity of "hydroxyapatite (HA)" preparations, in: *Characterization and Performance of Calcium Phosphate Coatings for Implants* (E. Horowitz, J.E. Parr, eds.), pp. 45–53, ASTM STP 1196, American Society for Testing and Materials, Philadelphia.

Lerouge, S., Huk, O., Yahia, L.H., Witvoet, J., Sedel, L. 1996. Characterization of *in vivo* wear debris from ceramic-ceramic total hip arthroplasties, *J. Biomed. Mater. Res.* **32**, 627–633.

Lindholm, T.C., Gao, T.J., Lindholm, T.S. 1996. Time-related deviations of fibronectin and type I, II and III collagen on the interface between a hydroxyapatite disc and the rim of a calvarial trephine defect in rabbits, *Biomaterials* **17**, 1515–1520.

Liu, H.C., Chang, W.H., Lin, F.H., Lu, K.H., Tsuang, Y.H., Sun, J.S. 1999. Cytokine and prostaglandin E_2 release from leukocytes in response to metal ions derived from different prosthetic materials: an in vitro study, *Artif. Organs* **23**, 1099–1106.

Lohmann, C.H., Schwartz, Z., Zoster, G., Jahn, U., Buchhorn, G.H., MacDougall, M.J., Casasola, D., Liu, Y., Sylvia, V.L., Dean, D.D., Boyan, B.D. 2000. Phagocytosis and wear debris by osteoblasts affects differentiation and local factor production in a manner dependent on particle composition, *Biomaterials*, **21**, 551–561.

Lycott, R.W., Hughes, A.N. 1984. Corrosion, in: *Metal and Ceramic Biomaterials*, Vol. 2 (P. Ducheyne, G.W. Hastings, eds.) pp. 91–118, CRC Press, Boca Raton.

MacNamara, A., Crowley, H.K., Williams, D.F. 1984. Metal-cell incubation products: chemotactic potential, in: *Biomaterials and Biomechanics 1983, "Advances in Biomaterials 5"* (P. Ducheyne, G. Van der Perre, A.E. Aubert, eds.), pp. 307–312, Elsevier Science Publishers B.V., Amsterdam.

Malard, O., Bouler, J.M., Guicheux, J., Heymann, D., Pilet, P., Coquard, C., Daculsi, G. 1999. Influence of biphasic calcium phosphate granulometry on bone ingrowth, ceramic resorption, and inflammatory reactions: preliminary in vitro and in vivo study, *J. Biomed. Mater. Res.* **46**, 103–111.

Maloney, W.J., James, R.E., Smith, R.L. 1996. Human macrophages response to retrieved titanium alloy particles in vitro, *Clin. Orthop.* **322**, 268–278.

Maloney, W.J., Sun, D.H., Nakashima, Y., James, R., Smith, R.L. 1998. Effects of serum protein opsonization on cytokine release by titanium-alloy particles, *J. Biomed. Mater. Res.* **41**, 371–376.

Mangham, D.C., Scoones, D.J., Drayson, M.T. 1993. Complement and the recruitment of mononuclear osteoclasts, *J. Clin. Pathol.* **46**, 517–521.

Marchant, R., Hiltner, A., Hamlin, C., Rabinovitch, A., Slobodkin, R., Anderson, J.M. 1983. In vivo biocompatibility studies: I. The cage implant system and a biodegradable hydrogel, *J. Biomed. Mater. Res.* **17**, 301–325.

McAlarney, M.E., Oshiro, M.A., McAlarney, C.V. 1996. Effects of titanium dioxide passive film crystal structure, thickness, and crystallinity on C3 adsorption, *Int. J. Oral Maxillofac. Implants* **11**, 73–80.

Mebius, R.E., Watson, S.R. 1993. L- and E-selectin can recognize the same naturally occurring ligands on high endothelial venules, *J. Immunol.* **151**, 3252–3360.

Merkel, K.D., Erdmann, J.M., McHugh, K.P., Abu-Amer, Y., Ross, F.P., Teitelbaum, S.L. 1999. Tumor necrosis factor-alpha mediates orthopedic implant osteolysis, *Am. J. Pathol.* **154**, 203–210.

Merritt, K. 1986. Hypersensitivity induction, in *Handbook of Biomaterials Evaluation* (A.F. Von Recuum, ed.), pp. 179–187, Macmillan Publishing Company, New York.

Merritt, K., Brown, S.A. 1985. Biological effects of corrosion products from metal, in: *Corrosion and Degradation of Implant Materials* (A.C. Fraker, C.D. Griffith, eds.), pp. 195–207, *Second Symposium, ASTM STP 859*, American Society for Testing and Materials, Philadelphia.

Merritt, K., Brown, S.A. 1996. Distribution of cobalt chromium wear and corrosion products and biological reaction, *Clin. Orthop.* **329**, S233–S243.

Merritt, K., Mayor, M.B., Brown, S.A. 1980. Evaluation of sensitivity to metallic implants, in: *Evaluation of Biomaterials* (G. D. Winter, J.L. Leray, K. de Groot, eds.), pp. 315–324, J.Wiley & Sons, New York.

Mu, Y., Kobayashi, T., Sumita, M., Yamamoto, A., Hanawa, T. 2000, Metal ion release from titanium with active oxygen species generated by rat macrophages in vitro, *J. Biomed. Mater. Res.* **49**, 238–243.

Nagase, M. 1985. Antigenicity of alumina ceramic and calcium phosphate ceramics-genetic control of the immune response, *Nippon Seikeigeka Gakkai Zasshi* **59**, 183–191.

Nakashima, Y., Sun, D.H., Trindade, M.C., Chun, L.E., Song, Y., Goodman, S.B., Schurman, D.J., Maloney, W.J., Smith, R.L. 1999a. Induction of macrophage C-C chemokine expression by titanium alloy and bone cement particles, *J. Bone Jt. Surg., Br. Vol.* **81**, 155–162.

Nakashima, Y., Sun, D.H., Trindade, M.C., Maloney, W.J., Goodman, S.B., Schurman, D.J., Smith, R.L. 1999b. Signaling pathways for tumor necrosis factor-alpha and interleukin-6 expression in human macrophages exposed to titanium-alloy particulate debris in vitro, *J. Bone Jt. Surg., Am. Vol.* **81**, 603–615.

Nelson, R.D., Quie, P.G., Simmons, R.L. 1975. Chemotaxis under agarose, a new and simple method for measuring chemotaxis and spontaneous migration of human polymorphonuclear leukocytes and monocytes, *J. Immunol.* **115**, 1650–1656.

Neo, M., Nakamura, T., Ohtsuki, C., Kokubo, T., Yamamuro, T. 1993. Apatite formation on three kinds of bioactive materials at an early stage in vivo: a comparative study by transmission electron microscopy, *J. Biomed. Mater. Res.* **27**, 999–1006.

Nichols, K.G., Puleo, D.A. 1997. Effect of metal ions on the formation and function of osteoclastic cells in vitro, *J. Biomed. Mater. Res.* **35**, 265–271.

Nordsletten, L., Hogasen, A.K.M., Konttinen, Y.T., Santavirta, S., Aspenberg, P., Aasen, A.O. 1996. Human monocytes stimulation by particles of hydroxyapatite, silicon carbide and diamond: in vitro studies of new prosthesis coatings, *Biomaterials* **17**, 1521–1527.

Papatheofanis, F.J., Barmada, R. 1991. Polymorphonuclear leukocyte degranulation with exposure to polymethylmethacrylate nanoparticles, *J. Biomed. Mater. Res.* **25**, 761–771.

Pazzaglia, U.E., Ghisellini, F., Barbieri, D., Ceciliani, L. 1988. Failure of the stem in total hip replacement. A study of aetiology and mechanism of failure in 13 cases, *Arch. Orthop. Trauma Surg.* **107**, 195–202.

Petty, W. 1978. The effect of methylmethacrylate on chemotaxis of polymorphonuclear leucocytes, *J. Bone Jt. Surg.* **60**, 492–497.

Picker, L.J., Treer, J.R., Ferguson-Darnell, B., Collins, P.A., Bergstresser, P.R., Terstappen L.W.M.M. 1993. Control of lymphocyte recirculation in man. II. Differential regulation of the cutaneous lymphocyte associated antigen, a tissue-selective homing receptor for skin homing T-cell, *J. Immunol.* **150**, 1122–1136.

Pitzalis, C., Cauli, A., Pipitone, N., Smith, C., Barker, J., Marchesoni, A., Yanni, G., Panayi, G.S. 1996. Cutaneous lymphocytes antigen-positive T lymphocytes preferentially migrate to the skin but not the joint in psoriatic arthritis, *Arthritis Rheum.* **39**, 137–145.

Pizzoferrato, A., Vespucci, A., Tarabusi, C., Ciapetti, G., Stea, S. 1984. Chemotactic response of macrophages from biomaterial injected mice, in: *Biomaterials and Biomechanics 1983, Advances in Biomaterials 5* (P. Ducheyne, G. Van der Perre, A.E. Aubert, eds.), pp. 301–306, Elsevier Science Publishers B.V., Amsterdam.

Pizzoferrato, A. Vespucci, S., Ciapetti, G., Stea, S. 1986. Chemotactic behavior of macrophages under biomaterial influence, in: *Techniques of Biocompatibility Testing*, Vol. II (D.F. Williams, ed.), pp. 110–121, CRC Press, Inc., Boca Raton.

Pizzoferrato, A., Vespucci, A., Ciapetti, G., Stea, S., Tarabusi, C. 1987. The effect of injections of powdered biomaterials on mouse peritoneal cell populations, *J. Biomed. Mater. Res.* **21**, 419–428.

Pizzoferrato, A., Ciapetti, G., Stea, S., Toni, A. 1991. Cellular events in the mechanisms of prosthesis loosening, *Clin Mater.* **7**, 51–81.

Pollice, P.F., Hsu, J., Hicks, D.G., Bukata, S., Rosier, R.N., Reynolds, P.R., Puzas, J.E., O'Keefe, R.J. 1998. Interleukin-10 inhibits cytokine synthesis in monocytes stimulated by titanium particles: evidence of an anti-inflammatory regulatory pathway, *J. Orthop. Res.* **16**, 697–704.

Prabhu, A., Shelburne, C.E., Gibbons, D.F. 1998. Cellular proliferation and cytokine responses of murine macrophage cell line J774A.1 to polymethylmethacrylate and cobalt-chrome alloy particles, *J. Biomed. Mater. Res.* **42**, 655–663.

Rader, C.P., Sterner, T., Jakob, F., Schutze, N., Eulert, J. 1999a. Cytokine response of human macrophage-like cells after contact with polyethylene and pure titanium particles, *J. Arthroplasty* **14**, 840–848.

Rader, C.P., Baumann, B., Sterner, T., Rolf, O., Hendrich, C., Schultze, N., Jakob, F. 1999b. TNFα secretion by human macrophage-like cells in response to wear particles and its modification by drugs, *Biomed. Tech. (Berl.)* **44**, 135–141.

Radin, S. and Ducheyne, P. 1994. Changes in characteristics arising from processing and the effect on in-vitro stability of calcium phosphate ceramics, in: *Characterization and Performance of Calcium Phosphate Coatings for Implants*, (E. Horowitz, J.E. Parr, eds.) pp. 111–123, ASTM STP 1196, American Society for Testing and Materials, Philadelphia.

Ragab, A.A., Van De Motter, R., Lavish, S.A., Goldberg, V.M., Ninomiya, J.T., Carlin, C.R., Greenfield, E.M. 1999. Measurement and removal of adherent endotoxin from titanium particles and implant surfaces, *J. Orthop. Res.* **17**, 803–809.

Ramsey, W.S. 1972. Analysis of individual leucocyte behaviour during chemotaxis, *Exp. Cell Res.* **70**, 129–139.

Remes, A., Williams, D.F. 1991a. Neutrophil polarization and immunoelectrophoresis assay in the study of complement activation by biomaterials, *Biomaterials* **12**, 607–613.

Remes, A., Williams, D.F. 1991b. Relationship between chemotaxis and complement activation by ceramic biomaterials, *Biomaterials*, **12**, 661–667.

Remes, A., Williams, D.F. 1992. Immune response in biocompatibility, *Biomaterials* **13**, 731–743.

Rodgers, K., Klykken, P., Jacobs, J., Frondoza, C., Tomazic, V., Zelikoff, J. 1997. Immunotoxicity of medical devices, *Fund. Appl. Tox.* **36**, 1–14.

Rogers, S.D., Howie, D.W., Graves, S.E., Pearcy, M.J., Haynes, D.R. 1997. In vitro human monocytes response to wear particles of titanium alloy containing vanadium or niobium, *J. Bone Jt. Surg., Br. Vol.* **79**, 311–315.

Romagnani, S. 1992. Induction of Th1 and Th2 response, a key role for the 'natural' immune response? *Immunol. Today* **13**, 379–381.

Rooker, G.D., Wilkinson, J.D. 1980. Metal sensitivity in patients undergoing hip replacement. A prospective study, *J. Bone Jt. Surg., Br. Vol.* **62**, 502–505.

Rose, N.R. 1997. Immunologic diagnosis of autoimmune disease, in: *Handbook of Human Immunology*, (M.S. Lefell, A.D. Donnenberg, N.R. Rose, eds.), pp. 111–123, CRC Press, Boca Raton.

Ross, L., Benghuzzi, H., Tucci, M., Callender, M., Cason, Z., Spence, L. 1996. The effect of HA, TCP and ALCAP bioceramic capsules on the viability of human monocyte and monocyte derived macrophages, *Biomed. Sci. Instrum.* **32**, 71–79.

Rostoker, G., Robin, J., Binet, O., Blamoutier, J., Paupe, J., Leissana Leibowitch, M., Beduelle, J., Sonneck, J.M., Garrel, J.B., Millet P. 1987. Dermatitis due to orthopedic implants. A review of the literature and report of three cases, *J. Bone Jt. Surg., Am. Vol.* **9**, 1408–1412.

Rovira, A., Amedee, J., Bareille, R., Rabaud, M. 1996. Colonization of a calcium phosphate/elastin-solubilized peptide-collagen composite material by human osteoblasts, *Biomaterials* **17**, 1535–1540.

Sabokbar, A., Pandey, R., Quinn, J.M., Athanasou, N.A. 1998. Osteoclastic differentiation by mononuclear phagocytes containing biomaterial particles, *Arch. Orthop. Trauma Surg.* **117**, 136–140.

Sasaoka, K, Seto, K, Tsugita, M., Tsuru, S. 1989. An immunological study of tricalcium phosphate supplied by three different manufacturers, *J. Clin. Lab. Immunol.* **30**, 197–202.

Savarino, L., Granchi, D., Ciapetti, G., Stea, S., Donati, M.E., Zinghi, G., Fontanesi, G., Rotini, R., Montanaro, L. 1999. Effects of metal ions on white blood cells of patients with failed total joint arthroplasties, *J. Biomed. Mater. Res.* **47**, 543–550.

Savio, J.A., Overcamp, L.M., Black, J. 1994. Size and shape of biomaterial wear debris, *Clin. Mater.* **15**, 101–147.

Schedle, A., Samorapoompichit, P., Rausch-Fan, X.H., Franz, A., Füreder, W., Sperr, W.R., Sperr, W., Ellinger, A., Slavicek, R., Boltz-Nitulescu, G., Valent, P. 1995. Response of L929 fibroblast, human gingival fibroblasts and human tissue mast cells to various metal cations, *J. Dent. Res.* **74**, 1513–1515.

Schedle, A., Samorapoompichit, P., Füreder, W., Rausch-Fan, X.H., Franz, A., Sperr, W.R., Sperr, W., Slavicek, R., Simak, S., Klepekto, W., Ellinger, A., Ghannadan, M., Baghestanian, M., Valent, P. 1998. Metal ion-induced toxic histamine release from human basophils and mast cells, *J. Biomed. Mater. Res.* **39**, 560–567.

Shahgaldi, B.F., Heatley F.W., Dewar A., Corrin, B. 1995. In vivo corrosion of cobalt–chromium and titanium wear particles. *J. Bone Jt. Surg., Br. Vol.* **77**, 962–966.

Shanbhag, A., Jacobs, J.J., Black, J., Galante, J.O., Glant, T.T. 1994. Macrophage/particle interactions: effect of size, composition and surface area, *J. Biomed. Mater. Res.* **28**, 81–90.

Shanbhag, A., Jacobs, J.J., Black, J., Galante, J.O., Glant, T.T. 1995. Human monocyte response to particulate biomaterials generated in vivo and in vitro, *J. Orthop. Res.* **13**, 792–801.

Standard ISO 10993–4, 1992. Biological evaluation of medical devices — Part 4: Selection of tests for interaction with blood, International Organization for Standardization.

Standard ISO/TR 10993–9, 1994. Biological evaluation of medical devices. Part 9: Degradation of materials related to biological testing, International Organization for Standardization.

Standard EN/ISO 10993–10, 1995. Biological evaluation of medical devices. Part 10: Tests of irritation and sensitization, International Organization for Standardization, pp. 1–43.

Stea, S., Visentin, M., Granchi, D., Melchiorri, C., Soldati, S., Sudanese, A., Toni, A., Montanaro, L., Pizzoferrato, A. 1999. Wear debris and cytokine production in the interface membrane of loosened prostheses, *J. Biomat. Sci., Polym. Ed.* **10**, 236–247.

Stea, S., Visentin, M., Granchi, D., Cenni, E., Ciapetti, G., Sudanese, A., Toni, A. 2000, Apoptosis in peri-implant tissue, *Biomaterials* **21**, 1393–1398.

Stern, I.J., Kapsalis, A.A., DeLuca, B.L., Pieczynski, W. 1972. Immunogenic effects of foreign materials on plasma proteins, *Nature* **238**, 151–152.

Sun, Z.L., Wataha, J.C., Hanks, C.T. 1997. Effects of metal ions on osteoblast-like cell metabolism, *J. Biomed. Mater. Res.* **34**, 29–37.

Takebe, J., Itoh, S., Ariake, T., Shioji, H., Shioyama, T., Ishibashi, K., Ishizawa, H. 1998. The effect on immunocytes of anodic oxide titanium after hydrothermal treatment, *J. Biomed. Mater. Res.* **42**, 272–277.

Tang, L., Eaton, J.W. 1993. Fibrin(ogen) mediates acute inflammatory responses to biomaterials, *J. Exp. Med.* **178**, 2147–2156.

Tang, L., Jennings, T.A., Eaton, J.W. 1998. Mast cell mediate acute inflammatory responses to implanted biomaterials, *Proc. Natl. Acad. Sci. USA* **95**, 8841–8846.

Thompson, G.J., Puleo, D.A. 1995. Effects of sublethal metal ion concentrations on osteogenic cells derived from bone marrow stromal cells, *J. Appl. Biomater.* **6**, 249–258.

Timbrell, J.A. 1991. *Principles of Biochemical Toxicology*, Taylor & Francis, London.

Tofe, A.J., Brewster, G.A., Bowerman, M.A., Myers, R.N., Hurson, S.M. 1994. Hydroxylapatite powders for implant coatings, in: *Characterization and Performance of Calcium Phosphate Coatings for Implants* (E. Horowitz, J.E. Parr, eds.), pp. 9–15, ASTM STP 1196, American Society for Testing and Materials, Philadelphia.

Tomei, L.D., Cope, F.O. (eds.), 1991. *Apoptosis: The Molecular Basis of Cell Death*, Current Communications on Cell and Molecular Biology, Vol. 3, Cold Spring Arbor, NY.

Toumbis, C.A., Kronick, J.L., Wooley, P.H., Nasser S. 1997. Total joint arthroplasty and the immune response, *Semin. Arthritis Rheum.* **27**, 44–47.

Trindade, M.C., Nakashima, Y., Lind, M., Sun, D.H., Goodman, S.B., Maloney, W.J., Schurman, D.J., Smith R.L. 1999. Interleukin-4 inhibits granulocyte-macrophage colony-stimulating factor, interleukin-6, and tumor necrosis factor-alpha expression by human monocytes in response to polymethyl methacrylate particle challenge in vitro, *J. Orthop. Res.* **17**, 797–802.

U.S. Department of Health and Human Services, Food and Drug Administration—Center for Devices and Radiological Health, Guidance for industry and FDA reviewers, Immunotoxicity Testing Guidance, Document issued on May 6, 1999, Pages 1–16.

Van Raemdonck, W., Ducheyne, P., De Meester, P. 1984. Calcium-phosphate ceramics, in: *Metal and Ceramic Biomaterials*, Vol. II, *Strength and Surface* (P. Ducheyne, G.W. Hastings, eds.), pp. 143–166, CRC Press, Boca Raton.

Vermes, I., Haanen, C., Steffen-Nakken, H., Reutelingsperger, C. 1995, A novel assay for apoptosis. Flow cytometric detection of phosphatidylserine expression on early apoptotic cells using fluorescein labelled Annexin V, *J. Immunol. Methods* **184**, 39–51.

Vitale, M., Neri, L.M., Comani, S., Falcieri, E., Rizzoli, R., Rana, R., Papa, S. 1989. Natural killer function in flow cytometry. II. Evaluation of NK lytic activity by means of target cell morphological changes detected by right angle light scatter, *J. Immunol. Methods* **121**, 115–120.

Vroman, L., Adams, A.L., Brakman, M. 1985. Lack of exchange among plasma proteins in narrow spaces on glass, demonstrated with metal oxide coatings, *Haemostasis* **15**, 300–303.

Wagner, M., Klein, C.L., van Kooten, T.G., Kirkpatrick, C.J. 1998. Mechanisms of cell activation by heavy metal ions, *J. Biomed. Mater. Res.* **42**, 443–452.

Walivaara, B., Askendal, A., Krozer, A., Lundstrom, I., Tengvall, P. 1996. Blood protein interactions with chromium surfaces, *J. Biomater. Sci., Polym. Ed.* **81**, 49–62.

Wang, J.S., Goodman, S., Aspenberg, P. 1994. Bone formation in the presence of phagocytosable hydroxyapatite particles, *Clin Orthop.* **304**, 272–279.

Wang, J.Y., Tsukayama, D.T., Wicklund, B.H., Gustilo, R.B. 1996. Inhibition of T and B cell proliferation by titanium, cobalt, and chromium: role of IL-2 and IL-6, *J. Biomed. Mater. Res.* **32**, 655–661.

Wang, J.Y., Wicklund, B.H., Gustilo, R.B., Tsukayama D.T. 1997a. Prosthetic metals impair murine immune response and cytokine release in vivo and in vitro, *J. Orthop. Res.* **15**, 688–699.

Wang, W., Ferguson, D.J., Quinn, J.M., Simpson, A.H., Athanasou, N.A. 1997b. Biomaterial particle phagocytosis by bone-resorbing osteoclasts, *J. Bone Jt. Surg., Br. Vol.* **79**, 849–856.

Williams, D.F. 1982. Tissue reaction to metallic corrosion products and wear particles in clinical orthopaedics, in: *Biocompatibility of Orthopaedic Implants*, Vol. I (D.F. Williams, ed.), CRC Press, Inc., Boca Raton.

Williams, D.F., Black, J., Doherty, P.J. 1993. Second consensus conference on definitions in biomaterials, in: *Biomaterial–Tissue Interfaces: Advances in Biomaterials*, Vol. 107 (P.J. Doherty, D.F. Williams, eds.), pp. 525–533, Elsevier Applied Science, London.

Winter, G.D. 1974. Tissue reactions to metallic wear and corrosion products in human patients, *J. Biomed. Mater. Res.* **5**, 11–26.

Wooley, P.H., Nasser, S., Fitzgerald, R.H. Jr. 1996. The immune response to implant materials in humans, *Clin. Orthop.* **326**, 63–70.

Wooley, P.H., Petersen, S., Song, Z., Nasser, S. 1997. Cellular immune response to orthopedic implant materials following cemented total joint replacement, *J. Orthop. Res.* **15**, 874–880.

Wuyts, P., Proost, W., Put, J., Lenaerts, P., Paemen, L., Van Damme, J. 1994. Leukocyte recruitment by monocyte chemotactic proteins (MCPs) secreted by human phagocytes, *J. Immunol. Methods* **174**, 237–247.

Yamaji, K., Yamane, S., Niimi, Y., Sueoka, A., Nose, Y. 1997. Strategy of leukocyte filtration for immunomodulation: development of stainless steel leukocyte filter, *Ther. Apher.* 1, 63–66.

Yang, J., Merritt, K. 1994. Detection of antibodies against corrosion products in patients after Co-Cr total joint replacements, *J. Biomed. Mater. Res.* **28**, 1249–1258.

Yang, J., Merritt, K. 1996. Production of monoclonal antibodies to study corrosion products of CoCr biomaterials, *J. Biomed. Mater. Res.* **31**, 71–80.

Zigmond, S.H., Hirsch, J.G. 1973. Leukocyte locomotion and chemotaxis. New method for evaluation, and demonstration of a cell-derived chemotactic factor, *J. Exp. Med.* **137**, 387–410.

27

Biocompatibility and Biological Tests

Antonietta M. Gatti and Jonathan C. Knowles

27.1. Definition

It is widely known that before a material can be declared clinically usable, it must undergo biological tests to prove its biocompatibility. Until the 1970s, this term was related to the biological inertness of the material, since an inert material does not interact physically with the biological tissues it comes into contact with and develops no reaction capable of compromising the life of the implant and the health of the biological environment (NIH Consensus, 1988).

One must think that a foreign material put in the human body always causes a reaction, but, if the material is "inert," the reaction consists only of the formation of a fibrous capsule that segregates the material from the biological environment.

With the improvement in materials technology and instrumentation, particular materials have appeared on the scientific horizon that can degrade in the biological tissues and whose degradation products can interact "positively" with the living cells and their metabolism, thus bringing about favorable biological reactions for the implant life and its functionality. The utilization of these active materials induced the biomaterials community to reconsider the definition of biocompatibility.

During the Consensus Conference in Liverpool in 1991 (II Consensus, 1991), that property was defined as "the ability of a material to perform with an appropriate host response in a specific application."

Antonietta M. Gatti • INFM, Laboratorio dei Biomateriali, Dipartimento di Discipline Chirurgiche e delle Emergenze, Universita di Modena e Reggio Emilia, Via del Pozzo 71, 41100 Modena, Italy. **Jonathan C. Knowles** • Department of Biomaterials-Eastman Dental Institute, University College London, London, 256 Gray's Inn Road, London WC1X 8LD, UK.

Integrated Biomaterials Science, edited by R. Barbucci. Kluwer Academic/Plenum Publishers, New York, 2002.

This means that also reabsorbable or active materials can be regarded as biocompatible and offer an appropriate behavior within the human body. The definition is necessary, because nobody knows what characteristics a material has to possess to be biologically safe.

This chapter summarizes and analyzes the *in vitro* and *in vivo* tests stated by the European Community and those not yet standardized, that a material and a prosthesis must undergo before being released for clinical implantation, to be accepted by and work in the human body. However, before that it is necessary to illustrate the philosophy that rules this matter.

The block diagram of Figure 27.1 shows the theoretical path we ought to follow before developing a medical device meant for human use. First, we must know the biological problems we are called to solve and the function

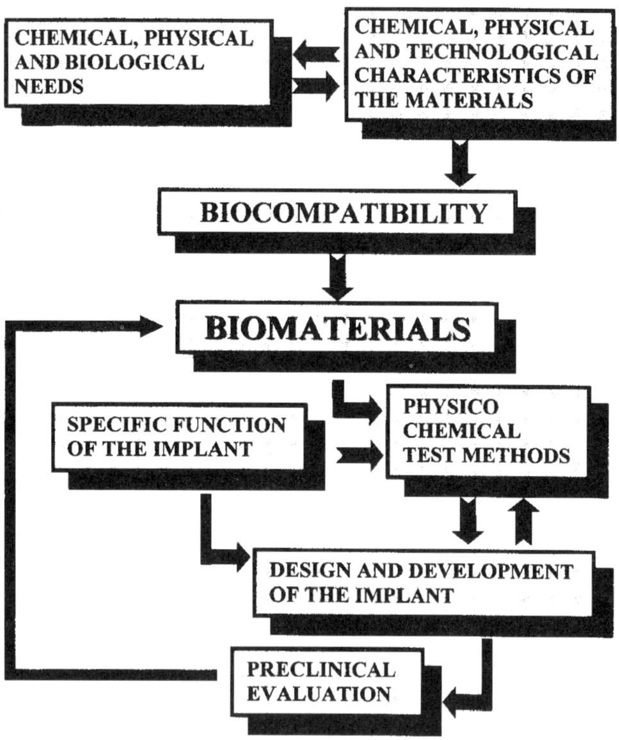

Figure 27.1. Block diagram of the philosophy of biocompatibility tests for biomaterials and medical devices.

a prosthesis is to substitute. Knowledge of the parameters regulating this function, and especially of the values or the range of values that they assume, gives elements to choose the materials suitable for the particular biological needs.

The material selection occurs within the list of the proper ones developed by engineers or chemists. By consulting the physicochemical handbooks it is possible to check the chemical and physical characteristics of the materials commercially available, that better fit the range of values of the biological parameters within which we are to act. For every material it is also possible and advisable to consult the technical sheet published by the producer, a document that contains more details, including the technology to obtain and/or to work it. These technical data are particularly important when the materials in question are polymers.

If, for instance, we take the case of a hip joint replacement, we have to consider the anatomy of the site (the acetabulum size or the range of possible sizes, the length and diameter of the femoral channel where a stem is to be placed), the biomechanics of the hip joint particularly during the ambulation, and the physiology of bone. These studies provide us with a set of data that must be taken into consideration in the selection of the suitable materials.

In fact, leafing through some handbooks, it is possible to list a set of materials with mechanical properties such as the capability to bear the ambulatory loads, a prerequisite characteristic in the case of our example.

Biomaterials generally may be divided into three main classes: metals, ceramics, and polymers. If we are to choose a material for the hip joint mentioned in our example, we compare materials coming from different classes. It is easy to see that metals offer the more favorable mechanical characteristics, though, for instance, ceramics are better, hardness-wise; but in many instances their brittleness prevents the possibility to use them for our purpose.

In the case of the replacement of a vascular segment where the prosthesis is not called to support load, a soft material is necessary, so polymers are often preferred. A biomedical material is selected as a function of a specific medical application. Once a material is chosen for its physical characteristics, its biocompatibility must be checked.

27.2. Biocompatibility Tests and Their Rules

The biocompatibility of a material must take into account all its different interactions with the different biological surroundings. For that purpose many biological tests exist as described in Table 27.1. That is part of a standard of the European Community (ISO/EN 30993-1, 18) concerning the biological testing of dental and medical devices.

Only after having passed some of the tests listed can one material be considered as a "biomaterial" and a subclass of materials called biomaterials can be delimited. The biological tests regard three principal groups of devices:

(a) surface devices,
(b) external communicating devices,
(c) internal devices.

Every group is divided into subgroups dealing with specific devices that establish different kinds of contacts with specific biological tissues or cells, i.e., blood, and soft and hard tissues. In Table 27.1 another parameter appears, and that is the time of contact of the material with the biological environment: less than 24 hours, more than 24 hours but less than 30 days, more than 30 days.

All these variables try to define how high the risk is related to that particular prosthesis. The higher the risk, the more numerous are the biological tests that the material must undergo.

The materials the researcher would use in the construction of medical devices are not required to undergo all the tests, but just those related to the type (external, external/internal, internal) and duration of the contact between device and tissue(s).

27.3. Biological Tests

27.3.1. Cytotoxicity

The simplest biological test considers the *in vitro* interaction of the material with the simplest organism: the cell. If the sample is toxic, the cell dies. There are three main ways of testing cytotoxicity:

1. Exposing the cells to extracts from the biomaterial in question.
2. Indirect contact via, for example, a diffusion layer such as agar.
3. Direct contact with the biomaterial surface (ISO/EN 30993-5).

Direct contact is obtained by immersing the biomaterial in an extractant, that is often a culture medium either with or without serum supplement. Following incubation at 37 °C for at least 24 hours, the extractant liquid is filtered off and then diluted (neat, 50%, 10%, and 1%, for example) and the cells exposed to these dilutions in triplicate for different periods of

Table 27.1. Types of Medical Devices versus the Biological Tests (from ISO/EN30993-1)

		Biocompatibility tests											
	Contact duration (days)	Cytotoxicity	Sensitization	Intracutaneous reactivity	Systematic toxicity (acute)	Subchronic toxicity	Genotoxicity	Implantation	Haemocompatibility	Chronic toxicity	Carcinogenicity	Reproductive/developmental	Degradation
Surface devices													
Skin	<1	√	√	√									
	1–30	√	√	√									
	>30	√	√	√									
Mucous membrane	<1	√	√	√									
	1–30	√	√	√									
	>30	√	√	√		√	√						
Breached surface	<1	√	√	√									
	1–30	√	√	√									
	>30	√	√	√		√	√						
External communicating devices													
Blood path indirect	<1	√	√	√					√				
	1–30	√	√	√					√				
	>30	√	√		√	√	√		√	√	√		
Tissue/bone/dentin	<1	√	√	√									
	1–30	√	√				√	√					
	>30	√	√	√	√	√	√		√	√	√		
Circulating blood	<1	√	√	√									
	1–30	√	√				√	√					
	>30	√	√				√	√		√	√		
Implant devices													
Bone/tissue	<1	√	√	√									
	1–30	√	√				√	√					
	>30	√	√				√	√		√	√		
Blood	<1	√	√	√	√		√	√					
	1–30	√	√	√	√		√	√	√				
	>30	√	√	√	√	√	√	√	√	√	√		

time, for example 24 h, 48 h, and 72 h, with near-confluent monolayers of the selected cell line. It may be achieved either by inoculating the cells directly onto the material surface or by placing the test material directly onto a near-confluent monolayer. The former method has problems in that it can be difficult to obtain reproducible numbers of cells on the piece of test material as they can easily wash off when the well is flooded with more medium, unless the sample fits very closely into the culture well. A way round this is to inoculate with a small drop which does not flood over the side of the test sample and incubate this for a short while to allow the cells to adhere to the sample surface. After that, the well may then be filled with more medium and the cells should remain adherent to the test material, unless it is highly toxic and the cells may round up.

Since the *in vitro* tests are simple and less expensive, many, more suitable and meaningful methods have been designed. The following tests are not considered in the European normative, but represent innovative assessments of the biocompatibility.

27.3.1.1. New Diagnostic Methods for Assessment of Biocompatibility: Flow Cytometry (FCM)

Flow cytometry (Watson, 1991; Lopes *et al.*, 1998) is a technique that measures specific parameters for individual particles in a suspension and those parameters include light scatter, optical density, and fluorescence emission. Each measurement is extremely fast and this allows data collection for an extremely large number of particles. As a basic parameter, the light scattering in a forward and side direction gives information on the cell dimensions and overall volume. These measurements, if the values are well defined, may be used to actually sort cells if a mixed population of cells is run through the flow cytometer. This has major advantages over conventional assays used. For a mixed population of cells, where a particular marker is being measured (for example, markers for bone formation) by back analysis, the individual population of cells expressing the marker or markers may be found.

The staining methods used in flow cytometry are quite different from conventional stains for surface-adherent cells. The cells first need to be suspended in an aqueous medium to allow a passage through the flow cytometer, the stain must be specific and must adhere well to its site of attachment without diffusing into the surrounding aqueous medium, the cells must be easily excited by the specific wavelength of the incident light, and, if cell sorting is a requirement, must be nontoxic.

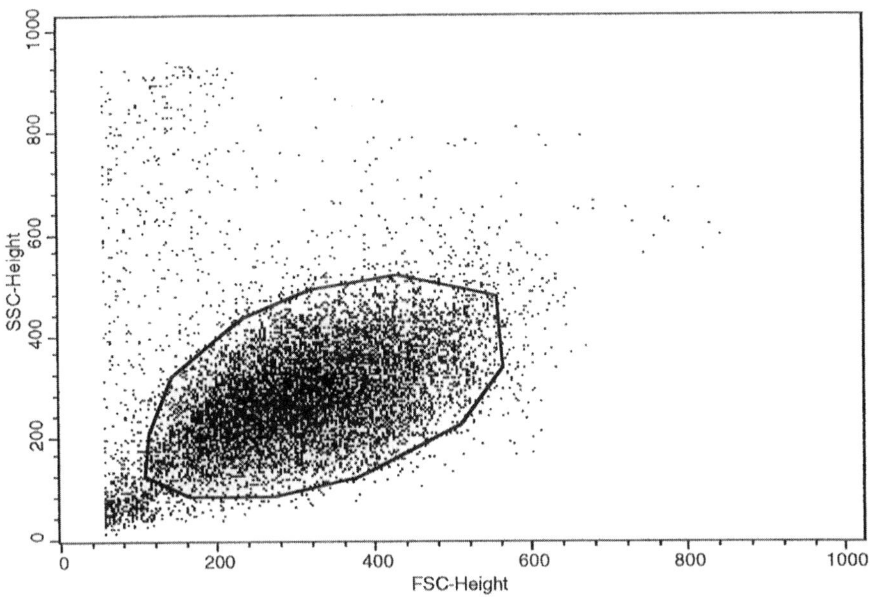

Figure 27.2. Representative flow cytometry dot-plot profile for 1,000 cells, grown on hydroxyapatite for 10,000 individual cells grown on hydroxyapatite for 6 days, showing the forward and side scatter distribution of the cells.

a. Immunofluorescent Staining of Antigens. In order to use flow cytometry to measure stained antigens, the cells must first be resuspended by trypsinization and then permeabilized with, for example, saponin. Primary antibodies are then applied, followed by fluorescein isothiocyanate (FITC)-conjugated secondary antibodies. Thus when running the flow cytometry experiment, the green fluorescence of the FITC may be detected. Figure 27.2 shows the FCM dot plot of 10,000 cells grown on hydroxyapatite for 6 days, showing the forward scatter and side scatter distribution of the cells. Also included on the diagram is a gate, indicated by the solid line. The application of this gate allows in this case the cellular debris to be screened out, but also highlights how in a mixed primary cell culture the individual populations may be analyzed.

b. DNA Staining with Propidium Iodide (PI). Propidium iodide intercalates in the nucleic acid helix, with a resultant increase in fluorescence of about 20-fold. Once the PI has been applied, it may be simultaneously detected as a red fluorescence at the same time as the green fluorescence for

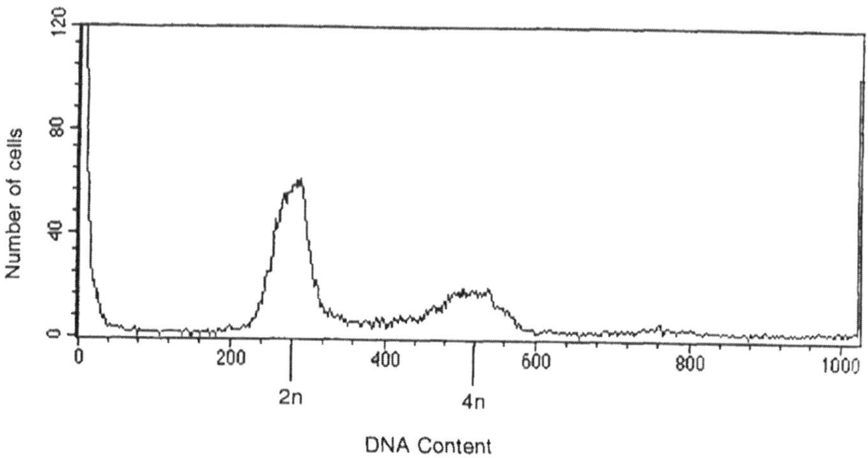

Figure 27.3. Histogram for MG63 cells cultured on sintered hydroxyapatite discs. A representative histogram of the DNA content of cells grown on hydroxyapatite and stained with propidium iodide.

the FITC. This shows not only how basic cell shape may be measured from the forward and side scatter data, but also how other measurements may also be made simultaneously. Figure 27.3 shows a typical histogram for MG63 cells, cultured on sintered hydroxyapatite discs. The graph shows three major features: the main peak, corresponding to the G0/G1 phase (resting phase), the minor peak due to G2 + M levels of DNA (post-DNA synthesis), and the intervening trough due to the S phase (DNA synthesis phase). Comparative analysis of these peaks allows determination of whether materials are inhibiting cells moving into any of their growth phases.

27.3.1.2. Molecular Biological Techniques

Numerous powerful techniques developed to give a fundamental understanding of the biological process in different cell types are now being applied to biomaterials and the understanding of the cellular processes occurring on implantation, and this may in future lead to ways of controlling these reactions at the genetic level. These techniques have given us valuable information about the processes associated with inflammatory processes and the molecules, which mediate immune processes.

The synthesis of any new protein or glycoprotein must have an associated messenger RNA (mRNA) present within the cell. These mRNA molecules are formed when the genetic information within the cell nucleus is transcripted. This also represents the genetic information at any time point in use to make protein. Thus the analysis of the mRNA is a way of checking which protein (or proteins) is being synthesized. In the majority of cases, detection of a specific mRNA points to the active synthesis of the corresponding protein.

The measurement of mRNA is not limited just to *in vitro* cell culture techniques, but may be applied to *in vivo* experiments. This offers the possibility of comparative *in vitro* and *in vivo* experiments, which may offer the possibility of correlating what is seen in cell culture with implant biopsy tests and this may give considerable insight into the host response. Again, future experiments may be envisaged, which may help to resolve the differences seen between *in vivo* animal and human implant studies and may allow a selection of more suitable animal models, dependent on the device under test (Ziats *et al.*, 1988).

The isolation of RNA is routinely carried out either by established techniques or readily available kits. While the total levels of mRNA in the RNA isolated are low, further purification is usually unnecessary due to the analysis methods available for examining specific mRNA expression.

27.3.1.3. Reverse Transcription Polymerase Chain Reaction (RT-PCR)

RT-PCR is the most commonly used technique for detection of mRNA. This technique has been used widely for the examination of surface proteins, for example, and is so extensively used because of its efficiency, relatively low cost, high specificity, and speed of use. The technique is valuable as only a very small number of cells is required, thus allowing 96-well plates to be used, which can also lead to good statistical results as 8 to 10 wells may be used for each point as opposed to the more usual triplicate. Further advantages are gained in that this single small sample may be used to analyze for multiple transcript expression.

The experiment proceeds by first making a cDNA copy of the mRNA by reverse transcriptase. The cDNA copy is then amplified up using DNA polymerase, which is thermostable, and two sequence specific oligonucleotide primers. A number of very specific heating stages are now undertaken to first separate the DNA strands (at 94 °C), then cooling to allow the primers to bind (55 °C), and then activation of the copying process by the DNA polymerase. Each cycle doubles the DNA content and thus by cycling many times (between 30 and 50 cycles) a product of 200NNN600 base pairs is obtained for further analysis.

While this at first looks simple, it should be borne in mind that the key element to this process and also its advantage is the specificity of the oligonucleotides used in the priming. The most obvious starting point for implementing these techniques is to make use of those already documented in the literature. Other resources may be drawn upon for the more experienced, such as use of databases for DNA sequences, for which primers can be made.

27.3.2. Genotoxicity

Historically, biomaterials have always been viewed as inert. However, this view is false, as even the most chemically stable materials undergo some degradation, albeit at very low levels. Recent years have seen dramatic advances in more chemically and biologically active biomaterials (ISO/EN 30993-3, 1993; OECD 481), which may degrade and may also be combined with active inorganic or organic species. This can give a very complex pattern of local and systemic interactions: With recent advances in detection techniques, the evaluation of biomaterials and their influence on cell cycle must be critically evaluated. The methods for quantitative assessment of genotoxicity are not well developed. Furthermore, latency effects are also poorly understood, thus complicating the issue. A mutagenic material is one which increases the rate of mutation of either individual genes and/or chromosomal mutations. A number of well-known tests are available, such as the Ames test for *in vitro* gene mutation or the micronucleus test for *in vivo* chromosomal damage (Ames *et al.*, 1975; UNI 9582/6, 1991). Mutagens may be classified into two types, those that damage DNA directly and those that damage DNA indirectly, with an intermediate conversion step.

The test verifies the mutagenic potential of the extract of the material on mammalian or nonmammalian cell culture, with a positive mutagenic material as a control.

27.3.3. Carcinogenicity

The carcinogenic potential of a material can be evaluated through implantation on rodents using a noncarcinogenic material such as polyethylene as a control, whose lack of carcinogenic potential is well-documented (ISO/EN 30993-3, 1993). These tests need very extended time periods, as long as 1 year, and sometimes they need to be exhaustive. Sometimes they are only indicative, due to ignorance of some aspects of biocompatibility or the complexity of some biological parameters.

If the carcinogenicity test is negative, we may not be sure that the material, once implanted, will not induce a carcinogenic response. For instance, for years many silicone breast prostheses were implanted in women. Silicones had been preventively tested for the biological evaluation

(James *et al.*, 1997), but in 1992 FDA alerted the users about the possible carcinogenicity of such materials and important manufacturers were forced to discontinue production.

Hindsight tells us now that those further tests would have been necessary in order to put safer prostheses on the market.

27.3.4. Reproductive Toxicity

The reproductive toxicity tests are described in the same standard of carcinogenicity and mutagenicity, being different aspects of the same adverse response to a material (ISO/EN 30993-3, 1993). These tests are indicated for intrauterine devices, energy-depositing devices, and resorbable or leachable materials or devices. Recently, some *in vitro* tests were designed to detect the potential toxicity of a material or device during the reproductive cycle of the cells. New experiments use transgenic animals, namely animals with their cellular genetic patrimony changed by the DNA manipulation, for example, by introducing human DNA segments.

In the future more importance is likely to be given to the *in vitro* tests with cells containing manipulated DNA and the significance of the results will increase due to the DNA manipulation and hence a closer affinity with human DNA.

27.3.5. Irritation and Sensitization

These tests try to estimate the potential for contact sensitization of materials or extracts (ISO/EN 30993-10, 1993). Amounts of leachables can induce allergic or irritative reaction. A classic example is the allergic reaction to nickel-containing metal alloys in contact with the skin, in women wearing non-noble jewels.

These tests are also performed via a patch test. Guinea pigs are treated with a patch embedded with an extract of the material and an untreated patch as a control. Skin irritation zones are checked after stated times. The sensitization test is divided into two phases: induction and challenge. The results compare zones of the dorsal skin of guinea pigs treated with the material extracts and a proven allergic compound (Freund compound).

27.3.6. Local Effect after Implantation

A series of implantation tests is described in order to assess the local effect of the implantation of the material or its extracts in living tissue, from macroscopic and microscopic points of view. Since the test is designed to assess the biological interface developed by the material or device, it is not

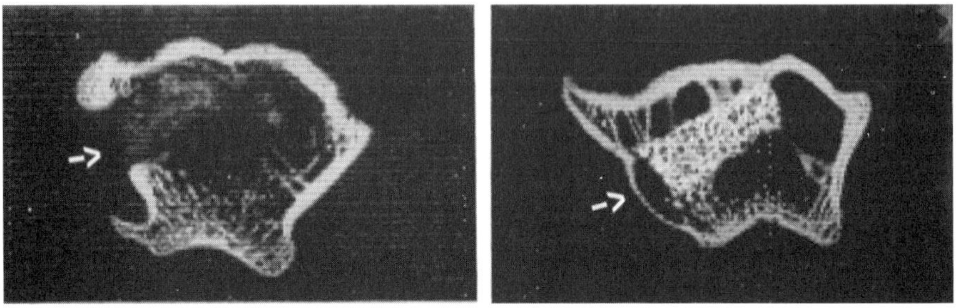

Figure 27.4. Two X-ray images of implants in rabbit's femural diaphyses: at left, a composite material (collagen/hydroxyapatite granules); at right, a cylinder of tricalcium phosphate (TCP).

necessary to implant the biomechanically correct device, as *in vivo* (ISO/EN 30993-6, 1993; ASTM F361).

The implantation can be undertaken in mice through incisions from the sacrum toward the neck, producing a subcutaneous pocket where the material can be inserted. The tunnel can be created intraperitoneally, subcutaneously, or intramuscularly. For orthopedic materials the insertion can be made in rabbit femoral diaphyses. The biological reaction around the material can indicate its biocompatibility.

Figure 27.4 shows two X-ray images of implants in rabbit's femoral diaphyses, a composite material (collagen/hydroxyapatite granules) (left), and a porous cylinder of tricalcium phosphate (right).

The bone reaction is different in the two sites after 40 days. The composite material seems to slow the new bone growth; in fact at higher magnification (Figure 27.5), under a scanning electron microscope in a backscattered mode, it is possible to see the bone wall, few bone trabeculae, densely crossed by blood vessels, and the material. On the other hand, in the picture on the right, the cylinder is well integrated in newly-formed trabeculae (Figure 27.6). At higher magnification the new bone ingrowth into the pores is seen. The close contact of the material with bone is evidence of the full stability and functioning of the prosthesis during the work.

Figure 27.7 shows a scanning electron image in a backscattered mode of a titanium dental implant surrounded by new bone grown that follows the surface morphology. At higher magnification it is possible to appreciate the interface between bone and titanium.

27.3.7. Systemic Toxicity

These tests are intended to evaluate the possible toxicity in a living body caused by leachables from a device at sites distant from the implant

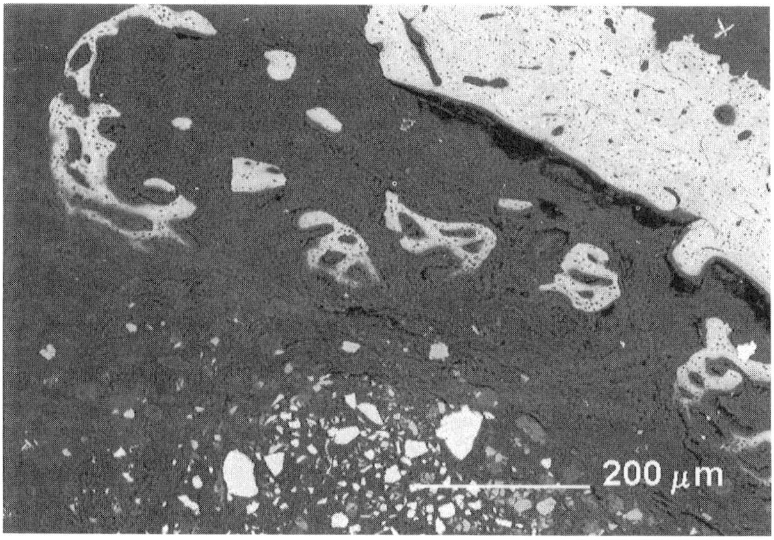

Figure 27.5. Scanning electron microscopic image, in backscattered mode, of the bone wall with few new bone trabeculae, densely irrorated, and the granules of hydroxyapatite.

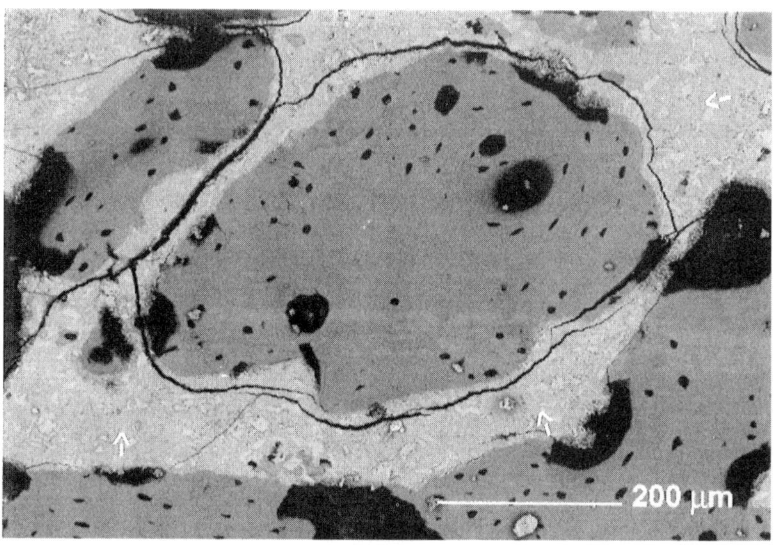

Figure 27.6. Scanning electronic microscopic image of some pores of the TCP cylinder (white arrows) completely rehabited by newly formed bone trabeculae.

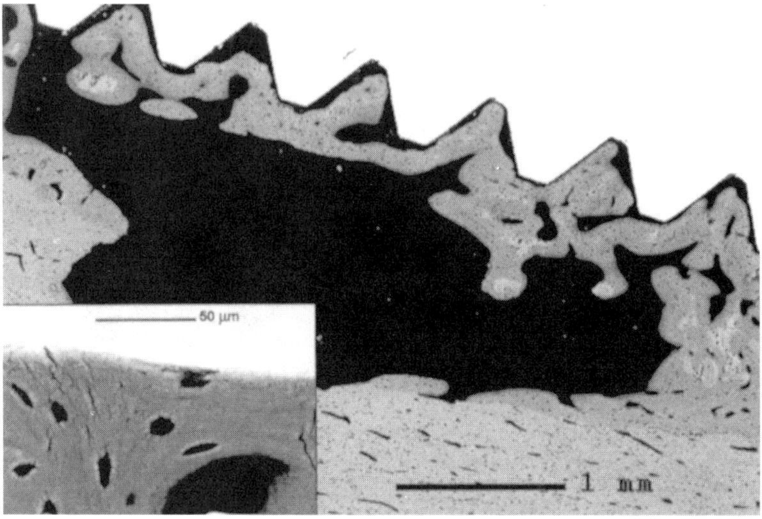

Figure 27.7. Scanning electron image (in backscattered mode) of a dental titanium implant (white) after implantation in sheep's jaw surrounded by new bone trabeculae.

site. It is obvious that a material can be biocompatible in its massive form, but the leached components or the products that the released components form with the host's organic ones might not be so (ISO/EN 30993-11, 1993). The evaluation takes into account many aspects, such as:

- acute toxicity for oral application (US FDA, 1982),
- subacute for intraperitoneal application (OECD 411),
- subchronic toxicity for oral, dermal, intravenous application, and for inhalation (OECD 413),
- pyrogenicity in order to check the increase of temperature due to the inoculation of extracts of the material for oral, dermal intravenous applications; this test also checks the behavior of pyrogenic substances of endotoxin and nonendotoxin origin (USP XXII 151 and 85),
- chronic toxicity and carcinogenicity.

Anatomopathologic evaluations of the principal organs, such as liver, kidney, and lungs, must be carried out at the time of sacrifice of the implanted animals. Also, this test can be not meaningful; in fact the toxicity of leachables depends not only on their chemistry, but also on their quantity released in unit time (release rate). Probably for every compound there is a threshold value, above which the toxicity becomes evident.

27.3.8. Hemocompatibility

Assessing the hemocompatibility of a material is not simple, because blood is a very complex tissue from chemical, biological, and biomechanical points of view. The main consideration is that when blood interacts with a material, it changes its properties as a function of the presence of the implant. When it is extracted for a simulation, its properties are a function of the method of extraction and of the surface chemistry of the new container. So the designed tests are not reliable and reproducible and do not predict the clinical performance of the device or material. The standardized tests try to evaluate the hemolytic properties of a candidate material to blood implantation (ISO/EN 30993-4, 1993).

Hemolysis can be caused by many factors:

- *Mechanical forces:* For instance, an increase in osmotic pressure in the red cell membrane can cause the cell membrane rupture. The rupture can be caused also by rheological factors, such as the increase of shear forces in high-velocity blood flow. This can occur, for instance, by the presence of implanted mechanical cardiac valves.
- *Biochemical factors:* For instance, a deficiency of nutritional factors or metabolic energy (ATP) can result in the loss of the discoid shape and microvesiculation of hemoglobin. Chemical, bacterial endotoxins, pH, and metabolic changes induced by temperature can bring about the rupture of the red-cell membrane.

The *in vitro* test can give an idea of the interaction, but it is not to be regarded as exhaustive. In animals, the evaluation of the free hemoglobin can give an idea of the hemolytic properties of the device, but it is impossible to know whether they depend on mechanical, chemical, or biochemical factors.

27.3.9. Degradation

These tests (ISO/EN 30993-13, -14, -15, 1993) are relatively new. Some are not yet standardized and only a draft exists. They are designed for the resorbable materials that are now starting to be used routinely as implants. The degradable implant is usually designed to function as a temporary implant. It performs its function until the tissue has been reconstructed; during or after that the material degrades and is reabsorbed via chemical and/or cellular pathways, thus saving secondary surgery for implant removal.

The degradation components must, of course, be biocompatible, but may not interfere with cell metabolism. The rate of release should also be such as not to dramatically affect the local pH or osmotic pressure, etc., and the release rate should be within the buffering capacity of the cells.

The tests clearly try to reproduce the degradative processes for metals, ceramics, polymers, and leachables as closely as possible to those found in the biological system. Metals and alloys degrade via corrosion. Corrosion can be chemical or electrochemical, but in both cases new compounds are formed, often soluble, that may not be biocompatible.

Ceramics, and in particular the porous ones, degrade and can release debris, to which the human body may react via a foreign-body reaction. In this case cells can react against the chemistry of the material, but also against the physical size of the debris. Particles sized 10 to 100 microns can induce a microphagic reaction. The macrophages try to digest these debris but do not succeed. A similar process can also be seen with polymers, such as polyethylene, which is used to make the acetabular cup in hip joint prostheses and, when it wears, the higher the amount of debris, the greater the inflammatory response.

The chemical degradation is the most difficult process to simulate. Of course, if the plastics are boiled, many components (chemical stabilizers, antioxidants, catalyzers, polymerization retardants or accelerants, plasticizers, fillers, dies, etc.) are extracted and are not always biocompatible.

However, in the human body the temperature does not exceed 40 °C, so the simulated test does not reproduce the *in vivo* conditions. This area of research is of interest as a number of devices for both short- and long-term implantation are becoming available.

At present, researchers are trying to develop materials that degrade releasing not only biocompatible components, but also elements or compounds that interact positively with the biological environment stimulating some processes or functions: these are called bioactive materials.

Active glasses such as Bioglass® and apatite-wollastonite glass are examples (Hench and Ethridge, 1982; Gatti and Zaffe, 1992). These vitreous materials degrade when in contact with body fluids and release ions such as sodium, calcium, and phosphorus, which stimulate the bony growth but also develop a chemical bond with the bone.

Figure 27.8 shows a scanning electron microscopic image (in backscattered mode) of granules of bioactive glass granules implanted in sheep's jaw bone defects and their X-ray dot maps for calcium, silicon, sodium, and potassium developed with an energy dispersive system. The sectioned granules appear not homogeneous after degradation and, in backscattered mode, we can distinguish three zones, differing in their electron density. Already after 30 days implantation in sheep, the external layer is composed only of calcium and phosphorus, the intermediate one of silicon, and the internal core has the original composition. Note the calcium phosphate crystal grown on the surface of the glass.

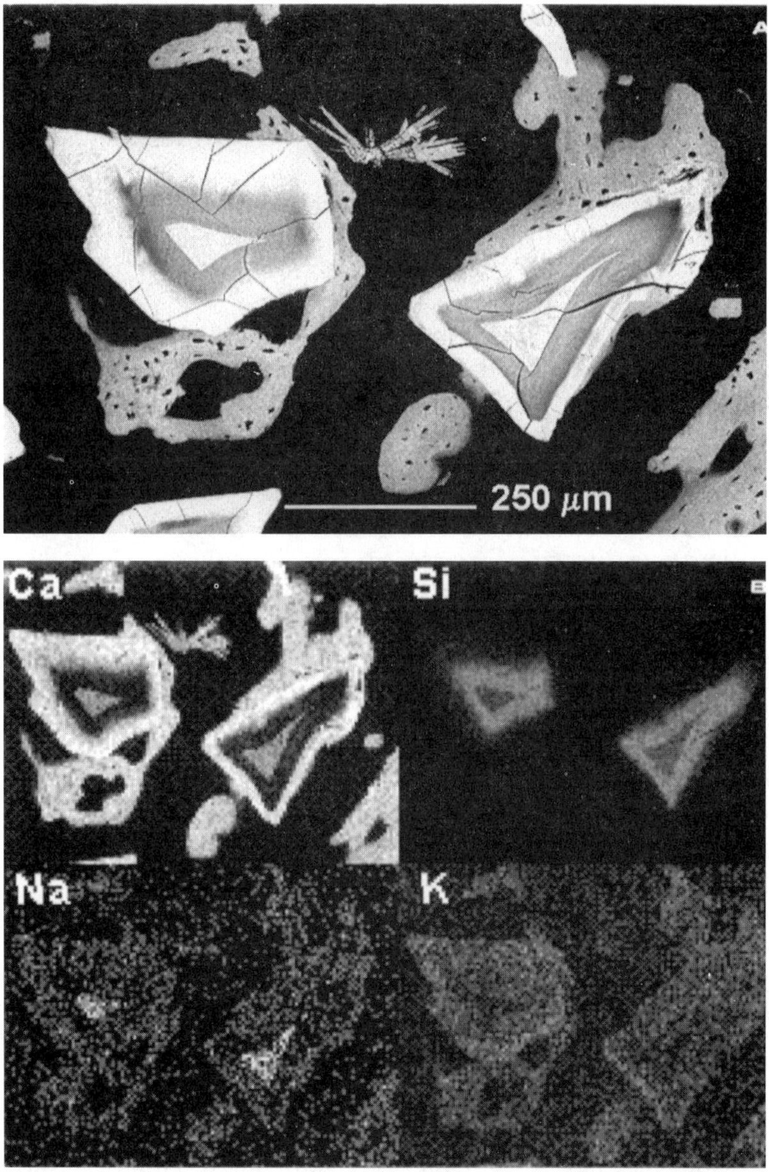

Figure 27.8. (A) Scanning electron image (in backscattered mode) of bioactive glass granules implanted in sheep's jaw bone defects and (B) their X-ray dot maps for calcium, silicon, sodium, and potassium. Note the new bone and the calcium phosphate crystal grown on the surface of the degraded glass.

Bioactive materials are very innovative, but require a detailed understanding of the kinetics of degradation; in fact the rate of the released compounds must be optimized. If the release rate changes, becoming faster or slower, the material may become inefficient (nonbioactive) or nonbiocompatible.

27.4. Biofunctionality Tests

If the materials selected to construct a prosthesis have been shown to be "biomaterials," the device is not necessarily biocompatible or may not be so for all its life. The *in vivo* performance of the device can be different from that expected or calculated from a theoretical point of view. For instance, the shaped material can degenerate under the biological attack. So it is necessary, before *in vivo* implantation, to perform suitable physical and chemical tests considering the physiological conditions in which the "designed" device is required to work. It is therefore necessary to carry out so-called simulation tests. Machines are needed where the physiological conditions, when known, are reproduced and where the prosthesis can work for a certain period. The parameters of the simulator can be varied in order to check how the prosthesis behaves in different, also extreme, situations. These tests can be called tests of "biofunctionality," as they are designed to check the bioperformance of the prosthesis during its functioning.

For instance, considering the specific case of a hip-joint prosthesis, the tribological behavior of the selected matching materials must be tried through suitable tests to evaluate their friction coefficient and their wear. The instruments can be pin-on-disc, ring-on-disc, block and journal, or journal and bush (Gatti and Trentani, 1976; Gatti, 1980). The results of the study show the behavior of the wear developed between two materials, and suggest the material(s) to choose in order to obtain the least possible wear. To obtain results as close as possible to the real working conditions, researchers constructed specific simulators for hip-joint prostheses to test the spherical matching.

Machines, mimicking circulating blood to test cardiac valves, were designed to verify, for instance, the fatigue that the prosthesis undergoes.

The primary consideration in the construction of a simulator is: how many parameters have to be reproduced to obtain meaningful results? The more numerous the parameters, the more complicated the machine will turn out to be and the more complete the interpretation of the results will be.

The second set of questions includes: Are all the physiological data known to build the machine? When a parameter varies between a minimum and a maximum, which value or range of values should the machine reproduce?

Simple answers to these questions do not exist. Usually researchers consider each parameter individually, and develop machines that realize the best compromise among the parameters reproduced and the significance of the results obtained.

Table 27.2 shows some of the main problems of biomaterials while in working conditions, related to each of the three classes of materials generally used in manufacturing prostheses or implantable medical devices.

Metals can corrode and the prosthesis, losing its morphology, compromises its functionality. The same lack of performance is reached for problems of wear, while high friction can lead to stoppage of the relative motion between two surfaces. Metals can be magnetic or paramagnetic; so prostheses immersed in the blood flow, as a vena cava filter, can be displaced if the patient undergoes a nuclear magnetic resonance test. Such a displacement can even lead to the death of the patient.

Ceramics must be checked as to degradation, wear, and friction since they are used to construct hip-joint components and cardiac valves. Polymers are the most intriguing materials: In fact it is possible to tailor them as the necessity demands, but they are weak and can adsorb and desorb, releasing first the components not chemically bound to the polymeric structure such as catalyzers, filler, etc. The chemical instability is an aspect of their weakness. But the greatest problem with these materials is that they are made essentially of C, H, and O, the same elements as the human body. So the degradation *releases ions or compounds* chemically recognizable by the cells that can interact, not always positively, with the metabolic processes. Since the released amounts are small and not always detectable by instrumentation in a simulation degradative test, these materials, even now, have a higher level of risk for human health.

After tests in simulators, the prosthesis must be implanted *in vivo* in animals to achieve a further degree of safety for the product. The preclinical trials serve to check the behavior of the prosthesis with its final design. After all these tests the prostheses have a reasonable level of security for the patient. Sometimes in the human body the implants can develop unpredictable behaviors that can compromise the life of the device itself. An example: while an artificial heart was undergoing clinical validation in Italy, the researchers involved in the project noticed that, if some bacteria adhered to the internal surface of the implanted biocompatible prosthesis or the external tubing carrying blood, they changed their stereoscopic morphology, thus keeping the antibiotics from acting on them. In that case, the biocompatibility of the material is so good as to allow undesired bacteria to live. In such a case, a selective behavior of the material in terms of "nonadhesivity" is desirable.

Knowledge of these interactions can induce the bioengineers, on one hand, to select (Figure 27.1) other biomaterials for the prosthetic construction or to change the design, and, on the other hand, to develop new biofunctionality tests to check other phenomena.

ACKNOWLEDGMENTS

The authors thank Dr. Monari, Ms. Piaggi, and Ms. Salvatori for their technical assistance.

References

Ames, J., McCann, J., Yamasaki, E. 1975. Methods for detecting carcinogens and mutagens with salmonella/mammalian microsome mutagenicity tests, *Mutat. Res.*, **31**, 347–374.

ASTM F361, Practice for assessment of compatibility of metallic materials for surgical implants with respect to effect of materials on tissue, in: *ASTM, Médical Devices and Services, 1990, Vol. 13*.

Gatti, A.M. 1980. Simulation: Problems relating to mechanical tests on hip joint replacements, *Inst. Mech. Eng.* **9** (1), 17–21.

Gatti, A.M., Trentani, C. 1976. Puntualizzazioner dei tests di simualzione per protesi d'anca, *Chir. Organi. Mov.* **63**(6) 543–550.

Gatti, A.M., Zaffe, D. 1992. Bioactive glasses and chemical bond, in: *Biomaterials: Hard Tissue Repair and Replacement* (D. Munster, ed.), pp. 97–106, Elsevier Science, Amsterdam.

Hench, L.L., Ethridge, E.C. 1982. *Biomaterials: An Interfacial Approach*, Academic Press, New York.

II Consensus Conference on Definitions in Biomaterials. 1991. In: *Biomaterial–Tissue Interface: Advances in Biomaterials* (E. Doherty, D.F. Williams, L. Williams, eds.), pp. 525–533, Elsevier Science, Amsterdam.

ISO/ EN 30993-1. 1993. Biological evaluation of medical and dental materials and devices: Part 1–16.

ISO/EN 30993-10. 1993. Biological evaluation of medical and dental materials and devices: Part 10, Irritation and sensitization.

ISO/EN 30993-11. 1993. Biological evaluation of medical and dental materials and devices: Part 11, Test for systemic toxicity.

ISO/EN 30993-13. 1993. Biological evaluation of medical and dental materials and devices: Part 13, Identification and quantification of degradation products from polymers.

ISO/EN 30993-14. 1993. Biological evaluation of medical and dental materials and devices: Part 14, Identification and quantification of degradation products from ceramic materials.

ISO/EN 30993-15. 1993. Biological evaluation of medical and dental materials and devices: Part 15, Identification and quantification of degradation products from metallic materials.

ISO/EN 30993-3. 1993. Biological evaluation of medical and dental materials and devices: Part 3, Test for genotoxicity, carcinogencity, and reproductive toxicity.

ISO/EN 30993-4. 1993. Biological evaluation of medical and dental materials and devices: Part 4, Selection of tests for interactions with blood.

ISO/EN 30993-5. 1993. Biological evaluation of medical and dental materials and devices: Part 5, Cytotoxicity.

ISO/EN 30993-6. 1993. Biological evaluation of medical and dental materials and devices: Part 6, Test for local effects after implantation.

James, S.J., Progribna, M., Miller, B.J., Bolon, B., Muskhelishvili, L. 1997. Characterization of cellular response to silicone implants in rats: implications for foreign-body carcinogenesis, *Biomaterials* **18** (9), 667–675.

Lopes, M.A., Knowles, J.C., Kuru, L., Santos, J.D., Olsen, I. 1998. Flow citometry for assessing biocompatibility, *J. Biomed, Mater. Res.* **41**(4), 649–656.

NIH Consensus Development Conference in *Clinical Applications of Biomaterials.* 1988., In: *Implant Materials in Biofunction: Advances in Biomaterials* (C. De Putter *et al.*, eds.), Vol. VIII, pp. 11–16, Elsevier Science, Amsterdam.

OECD Guideline for testing of chemicals n.411. 1981. *Subchronic dermal toxicity: 90-day study.*

OECD Guideline for testing of chemicals n.413. 1981. *Subchronic inhalation toxicity: 90-day study.*

OECD Guidelines for testing of chemicals n.481. 1986. *Genetic toxicology: Saccaromyces cerevisiae, mitotic recombination assay.*

UNI U 42.05.031.6, 9582/6. 1991. *Biocompatibilit di materiali e dispositivi per uso medico: Mutagenicità (prova di Ames)*, 1–12.

US FDA. 1982. Bureau of Foods: *Toxicological principles for the safety assessment of direct food additives*, appendix II, 19.

USP XXII, NF XVII (151), (1981). *Pyrogen test*, p. 1515.

USP XXII, NF XVII (85), (1983). *Bacterial endotoxin tests*, p. 1493 ff.

Watson, J.V. 1991. *Introduction to Flow Cytometry*, Cambridge University Press, Cambridge.

Ziats, N.P., Miller, K.M., Anderson, J.M. 1988. In vitro and in vivo interactions of cells with biomaterials, *Biomaterials* **9**(1), 5–13.

28

Infection and Sterilization

Roberto Giardino and Nicolò Nicoli Aldini

28.1. Infection

Like every other type of foreign body, biomaterials can enhance infections after implantation into the organism. In 1957, Elek and Conen demonstrated that the number of bacteria (*Staphylococcus pyogenes*) required to produce local infections was inferior in the presence of nonresorbable suture material (braided silk). Afterward, infections related to the use of prostheses or medical devices gained wide attention (Norman and Yoshikawa, 1994), biomaterials being increasingly used in the field of medicine. In a series of 1703 breast implants, Gabriel *et al.* (1997) observed an infection rate equal to 1.3%, which corresponded to 7.1% of all complications. A total of 177 McKee-Farrar and Charnley total hip arthroplasties collected by Jacobsson *et al.* (1996) required revision for sepsis in 2.8% of the cases. Sepsis was also classified as one of the most dangerous complications related to the permanence of a central venous catheter for prolonged time intervals (Corticelli *et al.*, 1990)

The recurrence of sepsis after reintervention in the presence of an infected graft is another challenging problem, observed in 35% of the infected vascular prosthetic grafts reoperated on by Taylor (Taylor *et al.*, 1996).

Various characteristics have been proven to affect susceptibility to infections when a material is implanted into the organism, such as size and shape of the implant, stability of the device, surface characteristics, and chemical composition of the material.

Among factors related to the increasing number of infections, the following should be carefully evaluated: local damage to tissues, impairment

---

Roberto Giardino and Nicolò Nicoli Aldini • Experimental Surgery Department, Codivilla-Putti I.O.R. Research Institute, Via di Barbiano 1/10, 40136 Bologna, Italy.

Integrated Biomaterials Science, edited by R. Barbucci. Kluwer Academic/Plenum Publishers, New York, 2002.

of the neutrophil granulocyte function, protection of bacteria by the material, and bacterial adherence to the foreign-body surface.

28.1.1. Tissue Reactivity to the Implant

The reactivity of tissues to the implant gives rise to an inflammatory stimulus, and acute inflammation results in local damage to tissues. Such damage is directly proportional to the grade of the inflammatory stimulus. Tissue destruction creates environmental conditions that are favorable for bacterial survival and multiplication. In particular, Gristina *et al.* (1989a,b) suggested that collagen and hydroxyapatite crystal exposure occurs when bone is traumatized, and this may provide an optimal environment for bacterial growth. Organic debris represents a source of nutrient materials for bacteria, also in traumatized soft tissues. Endothelial cells are characterized by an outer polysaccharide capsule: when it is traumatized, fibronectin receptor sites are exposed and susceptible to bacterial adherence and colonization. Vascular graft infections can be explained through this mechanism. Platelet vegetation, fibronectin, and fibrin on artificial heart valves may allow for bacterial adherence to tissues and subsequent development of bacterial endocarditis. The role played by fibronectin on the surface of implanted metallic devices as a determinant of bacterial colonization is also emphasized in the studies of Delmi *et al.* (1994).

28.1.2. The Neutrophil Impairment

The contact between the material and neutrophil granulocytes results in an impairment of the bactericidal properties of these cells. According to Klock and Baynton (1976), the chemotactic response seems not to be affected. The reason may be the release of toxic lysosomal enzymes and oxygen free radicals, with subsequent cell damage. These cells may also be unable to exert the bactericidal activity, being devoid of the lysosomal enzymes.

28.1.3. The Protection of the Microorganisms

Also, the physical properties of the material may play a role in the protection of the microorganisms. For instance, pores provide a recess where bacteria can be isolated and protected from host defenses. This is a reason for the onset of early infections; in fact, when pores are colonized by host tissues, bacteria penetration is not possible. Disruption of the material produced by mechanical agents, corrosion or wear, creates environmental conditions that facilitate bacterial colonization. Manufacturing defects of the

Table 28.1. *Staphylococcus epidermidis* Adhesiveness to Different Central Venous Catheters (*In Vitro* Evaluation—Turbidimetric Method)[a]

Material	No guide	Guide
Teflon	2.7 ± 0.1	3.3 ± 0.2
Polyethylene	2.5 ± 0.2	4.0 ± 0.1
Polyvinylchloride	2.9 ± 0.2	
Polyurethane 1	2.4 ± 0.2	2.4 ± 0.2
Polyurethane 2	1.7 ± 0.3	1.7 ± 0.2

[a] Values are expressed in turbidimetric units.

device, as well as damages during implantation, may create a place of elective bacterial colonization.

In a study on Central Venous Catheters, Buscaroli *et al.* (1990b, 1991) correlated the susceptibility of these devices to infections, type of material, as well as structure and surface characteristics. The materials tested were teflon, polyethylene, polyvinylchloride, and polyurethane. Two sets of samples were prepared; in the first group, no maneuvers were performed on the catheter, while in the second one a guide was inserted into the lumen and was then removed following a sterile procedure according to the Seldinger technique. Afterward, the distal parts of the catheters were placed in culture with *Staphylococcus epidermidis* (64 TU—Turbidimetric Unit) for 72 hours at 37°. After careful washing with saline solution to remove nonadherent bacteria, the parts were re-incubated in a sterile culture medium for 72 hours at 37°. Bacterial growth in the medium was then evaluated with the turbidimetric method. The catheter sample underwent scanning electron microscopy (SEM) to detect the presence of defects of the wall. Results are summarized in Table 28.1 and demonstrate that the type of material seems to be scarcely related to bacterial adhesive properties; on the other hand, the passage of the guide increases the bacterial adhesive action to teflon and polyethylene catheters but not to polyurethane catheters. This procedure and the subsequent damage to the inner surface of the wall due to the guide seem to be favorable for the growth of microorganisms. Microfractures on the inner surface, as well as manufacturing defects, were confirmed by SEM observation.

28.1.4. Bacterial Adherence

The bacterial adhesive action to the biomaterial surface is also important (Darouiche *et al.*, 1997). *Staphylococcus epidermidis* produces a glycocalyx that allows its adherence and growth on the surface of the prosthesis. A slime capsule may be produced by the many microorganisms infecting the implants. "Slime" is an exopolysaccharide produced by bacteria that plays an important role in biomaterial-centered infections. In addition to surface adherence, it is also a medium for nutritional exchanges and protects the microorganism against phagocytosis and antibodies. There is evidence that slime-producing stains of bacteria are more likely to cause infections than other bacteria.

Concerning bacterial adherence, two phases can be considered: an initial, nonspecific attachment, related to characteristics of the microorganism, fluid interface, and substratum, and a second specific, irreversible adherence, involving interactions among the specific proteins known as adhesins and the receptors (Gristina *et al.*, 1989a,b).

A short time after adherence, if favorable conditions occur, a spread of bacterial colonies on the biomaterial surface is observed. Extracellular polysaccharides are produced and form a biofilm matrix. This matrix seems to be involved not only in bacterial adherence, but also in virulence (Merrit *et al.*, 1996), and it also enhances resistance to host defenses and protects against the penetration of antibiotics. As emphasized by Gristina *et al.* (1989a,b), the microzone is an environmental condition, in which host defense factors are blunted by protective bacterial polymers.

The contact between the material and bacteria may occur through one of three pathways: direct contamination, contiguous spread, and hematogenous spread.

In the early phases of adherence, surface electrical charges of the bacterium and surface energy of the material are involved (Morra and Cassinelli, 1997); subsequently, there is an interaction between fimbrial adhesions and substratum receptors.

At implantation, the surface of a biomaterial is an easy and competitive target for both tissue cells and bacteria. Gristina named this phenomenon "the race for the surface." If cell colonization occurs first, it is an obstacle to bacterial invasion, as in the case of metals. Many polymers have a surface free energy that is antiadhesive for tissue cells. Therefore, bacterial colonization may precede tissue ingrowth, and susceptibility to infections may be enhanced. From this perspective, a strategy to prevent infections can be the improvement of the biomaterial surface adhesive action to tissue cells, in order to enhance rapid colonization by host tissues.

Aricola *et al.* (1990) evaluated the bacterial adhesive properties of *Staphylococcus epidermidis* in relation to different types of suture materials. The assessment of the adhesive action grade was performed by means of the turbidimetric method, according to the procedure described for the Central Venous Catheters. The materials submitted to the test and the results are

Table 28.2. *Staphylococcus epidermidis* Adhesiveness to Different Types of Suture Materials (*In Vitro* Evaluation—Turbidimetric Method)[a]

Silk	NR	B	38 TU
Catgut	R		35 TU
Polyglycolic acid	R	B	28 TU
Polyglactin 910	R	B	30 TU
Poliglyconate	R	M	30 TU
Polypropylene	NR	B	26 TU
Nylon	NR	M	24 TU
Polyester	NR	B	27 TU

[a] NR = nonresorbable, R = resorbable, B = braided, TU = turbidimetric units.

summarized in Table 28.2. The adhesive property turned out to be higher in resorbable than in nonresorbable threads, and natural filaments were more prone to the adhesive action than synthetic ones.

Methylmethacrylate is a substrate where bacterial growth can easily occur, and it may also inhibit host defenses. In a series of total knee replacements, Gristina reported a significantly higher rate of infections in those patients where methylmethacrylate was used with respect to uncemented prostheses. Animals studies confirmed a lower rate of infections when metals were implanted without methylmethacrylate.

Bacteria can participate in metal corrosion. It is demonstrated that strains of *Pseudomonas aeruginosa*, *Escherichia coli*, and *Staphylcoccus aureus* possess enzymes that can break down metals. Their maximal virulence depends on the availability of metallic ions, and subsequently, metallic corrosion products may increase the virulence on the biomaterial surface.

28.1.4.1. Bacteria

Staphylococcus epidermidis is the microorganism more frequently isolated in polymeric biomaterial-centered infections. *Staphylococcus aureus* is associated with metals (Green and Ripley, 1984) and is the major pathogen in bone, joint, and soft tissue infections related to biometallic implants (Table 28.3): it can be found also in association with *S. epidermidis* and gram-negative microorganisms. *In vitro* studies (Merrit and Turner, 1985) demonstrated a preferential adherence of *S. epidermidis* to the surface of polymers. *Staphylococcus epidermidis* should be present also in metal-related

Table 28.3. Biomaterials and Infections: More Frequently Involved Types of Microorganism Related to the Materials and the Devices

Microorganism	Device/material
Staphylococcus epidermidis	Vitallium
	High-density polyethylene
	Methacrylate
	Vascular catheters
	Vascular grafts
	Heart valves
Staphylococcus aureus	Metallic internal fixation devices

polymicrobial infections, but in association with other organisms: in this case, the pathogenic action of the microorganisms is enhanced.

Dougherty (1986) emphasized the role of *S. epidermidis* as a cause of infection in vascular prosthetic grafts and hip prostheses. According to the same author, this microorganism was involved in 60% of the aortofemoral graft infections and in 67% of the prosthetic valve endocarditis infections.

In a survey of 139 silicone implants removed from symptomatic patients, Ahn *et al.* (1996) found positive cultures in 47% of the cases. Involved microorganisms were *Propionibacterium acnes* (57.5%), *S. epidermidis* (41%), and *E. coli* (1.5%). These authors noted that culture positivity was not significantly associated with systemic symptoms.

Experimental investigations on bacterial colonization of biomaterials were conducted by Gristina *et al.* (1989a,b). The microorganisms were *S. epidermidis* and *S. aureus*, and tests were performed on vitallium, nickel–cobalt chromium alloys, stainless steel, and polymethylmethacrylate (Leake *et al.*, 1982). Results demonstrated that the initial attachment time for *S. aureus* was significantly longer for all of the materials. *Staphyloccus epidermidis* showed a preference for polymers rather than metals, while the behavior of *S. aureus* was the opposite. In experimental conditions (rabbits) and after local inoculation of *S. aureus*, Arens *et al.* (1996) registered a rate of infections significantly higher for steel implants than for titanium implants. Wassall *et al.* (1997) observed that a silver coating on orthopedic external fixation pins reduced the adhesive action of *E. coli*, *P. aeruginosa*, and two strains of *S. aureus*, when compared to stainless steel controls. An experimental evaluation of the effects of the commonly used implant materials on the infection rate was performed by Petty *et al.* (1985) in a canine model. The tested materials were stainless steel, cobalt chromium alloys, high-density polyethylene, *in vivo* pre-polymerized and polymerized polymethylmethacrylate. In control cases, no implants were applied. These authors noted that all of the implants were significantly associated with *S. aureus* infections in comparison with controls. The incidence of *E. coli* and *S. epidermidis* infections in *in vivo* polymerized polymethylmethacrylate was higher than in the other implants.

The resistance of the biomaterial surface to infections can be maintained by sterilization and antibiotic impregnation or by improving colonization by host tissue cells.

With regard to the origin, many infections are likely to be related to the endogenous flora of the patient. Focuses of infections in the organism may also be involved. Antibiotic administration after stomatologic or urological procedures is suggested in patients with hip prosthesis to prevent hematogenous dissemination of bacteria (Shaw and Greer, 1994). The role of bacteriemia in the onset of prosthetic infections is, however, controversial. Experimentally, Moore (1987) observed that the intravenous infusion in dogs of 10^7 *S. aureus* during vascular grafting surgery or in the early postoperative period led to the infection of all the grafts. Late infusion (3 to 12 months) was followed by a rate of infections ranging from 30% to 57%. Once pseudointimal healing had occurred, no infections were registered.

Environmental contamination, as well as contamination from medical devices such as venous or cardiac catheters, endotracheal tubes, and bladder catheters, should be considered, too. Air-borne implant contamination can be reduced by using laminar flow in the operating theater. This seems to be demonstrated for total joint arthroplasty (Ritter, 1984; Fitzgerald and Peterson, 1984).

Another possible factor of infection is the positioning of the prosthesis in a traumatic—and therefore likely to be contaminated—area. In such a clinical situation, the appropriate use of prophylactic antibiotics, adequate wound debridement, and timely soft tissue coverage is recommended (McClinton and Helgemo, 1997). The scarce vascularization of the tissues, such as in bone or joint capsule, may be a first cause for the lack of protective factors in the implant site. The surface of a prosthesis is usually a wide area to which bacteria can adhere, and therefore a relatively small number of microorganisms can cause infection. On the other hand, vascular and heart valve prostheses, which are in direct contact with blood, are more protected, and a larger amount of germs is required to cause infection.

Finally, an important role in the onset of implant infections is played by the patient's condition or diseases. Systemic illnesses, such as diabetes or immunodeficiencies, nutritional depletion, intercurrent infections, chronic use of drugs such as steroids, and previous surgical procedures in the same area are related to a high susceptibility to sepsis when a prosthetic device is positioned.

The prevention of infections related to biomaterial implantation is not only the result of appropriate sterilization procedures, which will be discussed in the following section, but depends also on the introduction of several pre-, intra-, and postoperative measures. Cleaning and disinfection of the skin within the operative field should be performed accurately; antiseptic products like iodine tincture, iodophor, and clorexidine are recommended. The operative field should be accurately surrounded by sterile drapes. Only people directly involved in surgical procedures should have access to the operation room. The role of antibiotic prophylaxis is still under debate. Graft material-bonding antibiotics and antibiotic impregnation of bone cement are employed. In an experimental model on rabbits, Bradley *et al.* (1997) evaluated the effectiveness of cross-linked albumin coatings applied on pure titanium implants, in the prevention of infections exposed to *S. epidermidis*: he registered a significantly lower rate of infections in coated (27%) versus uncoated (62%) implants.

In conclusion, the adherence of bacteria to the material surface and its colonization are the core of biomaterial-related infections. Host defenses and use of antibiotics have poor or no efficacy against sepsis, and the only effective procedure is the removal of the device.

28.2. Sterilization

Any device that is to be implanted in the organism must comply with sterile conditions. Therefore, the sterilization process is of primary importance, but the method is often limited by the characteristics of the material.

The commonest sterilization procedures are the following:

1. Steam and dry heat.
2. Ethylene oxide (EtO) and other chemical agents.
3. Gamma irradiation.
4. Electron (E-beam) radiation.

In a survey of the trends characterizing the methods of sterilization for medical devices, Pearson (1966) reported the following percentages: steam 52.5%, dry heat 10.0%, EtO 54.2%, gamma irradiation 11.7%, E-beam irradiation 2.5%, and other methods 2.5%. The principal advantages and disadvantages of each method are outlined in Table 28.4.

Table 28.4. Advantages and Disadvantages of the Principal Sterilization Methods

Steam and dry heat

Advantages	Disadvantages
Easy and safe Low costs No environmental contamination	Thermic damage of the device Not suitable for many materials

Ethylene oxide and other chemical agents

Advantages	Disadvantages
Suitable for many materials Well-experienced procedure	Not effective in sealed cavities Inflammable and explosive Requires decontamination Quarantine periods of 7–14 days Many process variables (pressure, temperature, humidity, EtO concentration, time)

Gamma irradiation

Advantages	Disadvantages
Complete product penetration Immediate release of the material No residuals Environmental safety Unique variable of the process (time)	Degradation of some plastic products Brittleness of some materials

Electron (E-beam) radiation

Advantages	Disadvantages
Rapid dose-rate Based on the electricity	Complex dosimetry Limited product penetration Heating of the material Equipment maintenance

28.2.1. Steam and Dry Heat

Steam is the most classical sterilization procedure, but the involvement of a high-temperature process severely restricts its use (Link and Buttner, 1992). In fact, many biomaterials cannot be exposed to high temperature or humidity without a modification of their physicochemical properties. It is more effective than dry heat (see above), because steam thermal conductivity is higher and its condensation and penetration into materials enhance its effects. The procedure should be performed in autoclaves, where high-pressure boiling of water is obtained. Time/temperature rates are inversely proportional. According to the Medical Research Council, the standards for steam sterilization are 15 min at 121°C, 10 min at 126°C, or 3 min at 134°C.

The dry heat procedure is carried out in Pasteur's stoves, where a flow of warm air is obtained by means of a forced ventilation system. There is a direct relationship between temperature and exposure time to reach sterilization: at 120°C, 6 hours are required; at 160°C, 120 minutes; and at 180°C, 30 minutes. The materials suitable for this method are only steel, titanium, alloys, and, in general, metallic devices.

28.2.2. Ethylene Oxide and Other Chemical Agents

Chemical sterilization is obtained with various types of products, among which the most important is ethylene oxide (Dorman Smith, 1991; Barker, 1995). Ethylene oxide (EtO) is a colorless, highly reactive, explosive and inflammable gas (Ernst and Doyle, 1968). Its killing power on bacteria, spores, mycetes, and viruses is well demonstrated. Bactericidal properties are related to the penetration of the gas into the microorganism, the reaction with cell proteins, and the block of vital functions. To obtain an effective sterilization with EtO, some parameters have to be determined, such as gas concentration, exposure time, temperature, humidity, and pressure. EtO concentration is the most important factor and should be about 700–800 mg/l. Time varies from 1.5 to 12 hours. The range of temperatures is 37°–87°C and an increase in this parameter shortens the sterilization time. The procedure is performed in autoclaves. At the end of sterilization, the material contains a significant amount of gas and should therefore be degassed before its use. This operation is carried out in the same autoclave with sterile air or nitrogen circulation. The main advantages of EtO sterilization are that it can treat those materials or devices that can be damaged by high temperatures (steam or dry heat). Disadvantages are toxicity, prolonged sterilization times, and need for postventilation. The residues of EtO or its by-products, such as ethylene glycol or ethylene chloride, are dangerous for the organism. Inadequate ventilation can cause irritation to the tissues. Ventilation time varies with the composition and features of the material. At room temperature 7 days may be necessary, at 50° with forced ventilation 12 hours, and at 60°, 8 hours. Polyvinylchloride is the material that requires the longest period of time; nonporous materials, such as glass or metals, require shorter time intervals.

To improve safety, many attempts were made (Berth and Wolftbrandt, 1992) to obtain nonexplosive mixtures using diluents for EtO, such as chlorofluorocarbon (Freon 12). Following the EC rules on abolition of this gas, alternative diluents were investigated, such as carbon dioxide, nitrogen, and hydrofluorocarbon.

Another chemical sterilizing product is formaldehyde, which is a colorless gas, highly irritant to eyes and mucosae. It has a well-demonstrated microbicidal effect, with a wide range of action on Gram+ and Gram− bacteria, spores, mycetes, and viruses. However, its effect may be impaired by the organic residues present on the surface of the material, which therefore has to be carefully cleaned before starting the procedure.

Sterilization is carried out in autoclaves, where the gas obtained through evaporation of an aqueous solution of formaldehyde circulates. The effectiveness of this process is related to the concentration of formaldehyde, exposure time, pressure, and temperature. In standard conditions, the bactericidal power is obtained with a concentration of 1500 mg/l. In a steam atmosphere and at a temperature of 65°C, concentration drops to 65 mg/l. Also, exposure time varies with temperature: 2 hours at 80°C, 4 hours at 55°C.

The advantages of this procedure are mainly represented by the possibility of sterilizing materials that cannot be exposed to high temperatures; the product is not explosive or inflammable and involves low cost. The limit to its use is the product toxicity.

28.2.3. Irradiation

Today, irradiation sterilization is a widely employed procedure (Brinston, 1991). Since the discovery of radioactivity, the feasibility of its use in this field had been considered, but it came into general use in the late 1950s. The gamma rays used for this purpose are photons of electromagnetic radiations with an energy range of 1–10 MeV (Henon, 1992). Interactions between radiations and material involve three types of consequences:

a. *Physical events*: Interactions between atoms and radiations produce unstable molecules (primary products).
b. *Physicochemical events*: Primary products react with each other and produce highly reactive ions and radicals.
c. *Chemical events*: There are interactions and reactions among the unstable reactive groups.

The resulting damage to the material is proportional to the energy absorbed.

The commonest source of radiation is ^{60}Co. Radiations are produced during the spontaneous transformation of the isotope into nonradioactive nickel. The dose is the quantity of energy deposited per mass unit, and is expressed in Grays (Gy). The dose most commonly used is 25 kGy. The sterilizing effect is based on the alterations induced on the DNA chains of the microorganisms, with the block of the cell metabolism or reproduction. These changes are dimerization of DNA bases, scission, and cross-linking of the sugar phosphate backbone of molecules.

Different types of microorganisms give different responses to radiation (Tallentire, 1980). Many of the potential effects of radiation on the microbial cells are reversible, and this reversibility correlates with the microorganism ability to repair the damage induced by radiation. In bacterial cells, this ability is related to the presence of enzymes that remove the lethal dimers produced by radiation. Among the external factors that may protect or sensitize microorganisms against radiation, oxygen and water play a fundamental role. It is demonstrated that microorganisms irradiated under anaerobic conditions are less sensitive than those irradiated in aerobic conditions. On the contrary, the presence of water reduces the sensitizing effects of oxygen (Halls, 1992).

The most important consideration about gamma irradiation is that exposure modifies the physical properties of some polymers, thus changing the pattern of their chains which can be more cross-linked or broken (Tables 28.5 and 28.6). So, if the polymer is resorbable, the degradation properties will be modified with important effects on the *in vivo* behavior of the device. Changes in mechanical properties were observed in polyacetals and polyamides; polycarbonates and polypropylene became brittle; changes in physical appearance were registered for some polymers, such as polyvinylchloride, polypropylene, or polycarbonate.

Table 28.5. Gamma Irradiation: Selection of Materials

No restrictions	Cautions	To be avoided
Styrene	Polymethylmethacrylate and its copolymers	Acetals
Polyethylene	Polyvinylchloride	Polytetrafluoroethylene
Polycarbonates	Polypropylene	Cyanoacrylates
Polyethylene terephthalate	Polylactides	Nylon and polypropylene (films)
Urethanes		Chitosan
Cellulose		
Elastomers (silicone)		
Polyamides		

Table 28.6. Gamma Irradiations: Effects on Some Materials

Material	Effects
Polyacetals	Embrittlement, yellowing
Polytetrafluoroethylene	Embrittlement
Cyanoacrylates	Loss of tensile properties
Nylon and propylene films	More sensitivity to radiation and oxidation changes
Polypropylene	Loss of elongation, embrittlement, continues to degrade after irradiation
Polymethylmethacrylate	Modest loss of physical effects. Temporary color shift
Polyvinylchloride	Anticipate color shift. Odor

The construction of an implant for gamma-ray sterilization is very expensive and is therefore justified only if many devices are to be treated. If a huge quantity of materials is to be processed, this procedure offers the following advantages: safety, ease, reliability, and cost.

28.2.4. Electron (E-Beam) Radiation

Electron beam sterilization is a procedure generating great interest at present (Doué, 1992), E. beam accelerators are used in industry for different purposes, such as cross-linkage of cables and tubes, hardening of surface coatings, and vulcanization of elastomers. High-energy industrial accelerators that deliver electron beams with an energy greater than 5 MeV can also be used for sterilization of medicosurgical devices (Ross and Saart, 1991). They are adequately modified and equipped with platforms to load and unload products, separate bays for treated and untreated materials, and a cell containing the sterilization unit. This unit is equipped with a linear accelerator, with power ranging from 1.7 to 20 kW. At high electron-beam dose rates, treatment time decreases: at 25 KGy sterilization can take 5 minutes.

The depth (Barnard, 1991) to which electrons from a 10-MeV beam can penetrate for product sterilization is 40–80 cm, assuming the density of the materials is 0.1–0.2 g/cm^3; this depth of insertion is appropriate for sterilization of medical devices.

One advantage of high-dose sterilization is that exposure time to radiation is shortened. Therefore, the peroxidation damage caused by the diffusion of the atmospheric oxygen in the material is reduced. As mentioned above, there are medical polymers whose properties can be modified by radiation. It is demonstrated that a high dose of radiation causes less damage (Ishigaki *et al.*, 1989).

E-beam radiation on materials produces free ions and radicals by breaking the chemical bonds. Polymerization, cross-linkage, and scission are some of the reactions induced in plastics. The rate of these changes depends on the radiation dose, dose rate, environment (temperature, humidity, presence or absence of oxygen), and type of monomer.

The main advantages of E-beam sterilization are speed, precision, and flexibility. The high cost of the equipment restricts its use to those companies who have a large quantity of materials to sterilize.

The choice of the most appropriate method of sterilization is of great importance, because a biocompatible device may become unacceptable to the organism through an inappropriate procedure. For this reason, a device should be evaluated for its toxicity even when previous tests have demonstrated that all its components are biologically compatible.

White *et al.* (1996). observed that mechanical properties were significantly affected by sterilization methods; for instance, EtO caused less microstructural damage than gamma radiation to ultrahigh molecular weight polyethylene components of arthroprostheses, thus resulting in higher toughness and percent elongation. Moreover, a loss of fracture toughness and a decrease in tearing after gamma irradiation were also confirmed for this polymer by others (Pascaud *et al.*, 1997). Besong *et al.* (1998) demonstrated that sterilization by gamma irradiation in air of ultrahigh molecular weight polyethylene components for joint replacement caused chain scission and started a long-term oxidative process that degraded chemical and mechanical properties of the polymer. Furthermore, gamma irradiation and thermal annealing were proven to increase creep resistance of hydroxyapatite-reinforced polyethylene composites (Suwanprateeb *et al.*, 1998).

Paganetto *et al.* (1991) demonstrated that EtO sterilization and a 1.25 Mrad gamma irradiation dose had the same degradation effect on 700,000 MW poly-L-lactic acid samples.

In addition, the effects of the manufacturing features should be taken into account and added to those of the sterilization procedures. De Lollis (1991) and Giannini *et al.* (1994) observed that the compression-molding process of the poly-L-lactic acid used to obtain internal fixation devices made the molecular weight of the original polymer drop from 410,000 D to 240,000 D. Sterilization of these devices was performed by both EtO and gamma irradiation (2.5 Mrad). A further decrease in molecular weight was then registered and was more significant with gamma irradiation (138,000 D) than EtO (200,000 D). Also, the elastic module was affected, but without significant differences between the two procedures.

Chitosan is a polysaccharide obtained from chitin and has many potential fields of application as a biomaterial (Rao and Sharma, 1997). The effects of the different methods of sterilization on this biopolymer were investigated by Rao and Sharma (1995). Gamma irradiation showed a modification in mechanical properties, with a reduction in mechanical strength due to the scission of the proteic chains; the main problem with this treatment was related to the gas left as a residue in the material. Steam autoclaving and glutaraldehyde treatment appear to be adequate methods of sterilization. Lim *et al.* (1998) emphasized that irradiation in air might improve the tensile strength of chitosan films, while irradiation in anoxia did not affect film properties significantly. These authors concluded by saying that both the polymer structure and the conditions of irradiation were major determinants of radiation-induced reactions.

Muller *et al.* (1998) compared the impact of the method of sterilization (steam and EtO) on polysulfone membranes for dialysis, and concluded by asserting that the use of steam instead of EtO improved biocompatibility of these devices.

In conclusion, when selecting a method of sterilization, the following factors have to be taken into account: susceptibility to heat and water vapor; thermolability, absorption and desorption of volatile gases; and radiation sensitivity.

The influence of sterilization on the surface properties of the material should also be evaluated, and it was observed after EtO treatment that some residues of EtO remain in the polymeric matrix and can diffuse on the surface with adverse biological consequences, especially when in direct contact with blood.

When none of the previously mentioned methods can be employed, as a last resort an aqueous chemical disinfectant can be used, followed by accurate washing with sterile saline solution or distilled water.

To conclude, the choice of the method of sterilization is mainly influenced by technical criteria, and polymers react differently to different sterilization procedures. For these reasons, all of the principal sterilization techniques (gamma irradiation, EtO, and E-beam irradiation) play an important role and should be selected according to the material characteristics and properties.

References

Ahn, C.Y., Ko, C.Y., Wagar, E.A., Wong, R.S., Shaw, W.W. 1996. Microbial evaluation: 139 implants removed from symptomatic patients, *Plast. Reconstr. Surg.* **98**(7), 1225–1229.

Arciola, C.R., Buscaroli, S., Rocca, M., Farinetti, A., Fini, M., Manfrini, M., Giardino, R. 1990. Studio in vivo dell'adesivit dello *Staphylococcus epidermidis* sui fili di sutura, *Giorn. Chir.* **11**(3), 141–143.

Arens, S., Schlegel, U., Printzen, G., Ziegler, W.J., Perren, S.M., Hansis, M. 1996. Influence of materials for fixation implants on local infection. An experimental study of steel versus titanium DCP in rabbits, *J. Bone Jt. Surg. Br. Vol.* **78**(4), 647–651.

Barker, J. 1995. Ethylene oxide sterilization update, *Med. Dev. Technol.* **6**, 23–24.

Barnard, J. W. 1991. E-Beam processing in the medical device industry, *Med. Dev. Technol.* **2**(5), 34–41.

Berth, L., Wolffbrandt, K. 1992. Improving the ethylene oxide sterilization, *Med. Dev. Technol.* **3**(5), 38–44.

Besong, A.A., Tipper, J.L., Ingham, E., Stone, M.H., Wroblewsky, B.M., Fisher, J. 1998. Quantitative comparison of wear debris from UHMWPE that has and has not been sterilized by gamma irradiation, *J. Bone Jt. Surg. Br. Vol.* **80**(2), 340–344.

Bradley, J., Powers, D., Friedman, R.J. 1997. The prevention of prosthetic infections using a cross-linked albumin coating in a rabbit model, *J. Bone Jt. Surg. Br. Vol.* **79**(5), 816–819.

Brinston, R. 1991. Gaining the competitive edge with Gamma Sterilization, *Med. Dev. Technol.* **2**(5), 28–33.

Buscaroli, S., Arciola, R.C., Ciapetti, G., Fini, M., Rocca, M., Stea, S., Giardino, R. 1990a. In vitro study on the relationship between polymer structure and surgical infections, Proceedings of II World Week of Professional Updating in Surgery and in Surgical and Oncological Disciplines, Milan.

Buscaroli, S., Fini, M., Rocca, M., Maraldi, N.M., Squarzoni, S., Coprticelli, A.S., Rossi, R., Leprotti, S., Giardino, R. 1990b. Cateteri venosi centrali. struttura ed adesività batterica, Atti del VI Congresso Nazionale SIATeC, Bologna.

Buscaroli, S., Fini, M., Leprotti, S., Rocca, M., Squarzoni, S., Maraldi, N.M., Arciola, C.R., Giardino, R. 1991. Central Venous Catheters: technological or acquired defects and bacterial adhesion, Proceedings of 4th European Symposium on Biomaterials, Siena.

Corticelli, A.S., Buscaroli, S., Fini, M., Giardino, R., Maraldi, N.M., Paladini, R., Rocca, M., Rossi, R., Squarzoni, S. 1990. Cateteri venosi centrali e rischio di infezioni: studio clinico e sperimentale, Atti del VI Congresso Nazionale SIATeC, Bologna.

Darouiche, R.O., Landon, G.C., Patti, J.M., Nguyen, L.L., Fernau, R.C., Mcdevitt, D., Greene, C., Foster, T., Klima, M. 1997. Role of staphylococcus aureus surface adhesion in orthopedic device infections. Are results model-dependent?, *J. Med. Microbiol.* **46**(1), 75–79.

Delmi, M., Vaudaux, P., Lew, D.P., Vasey, H. 1994. Role of fibronectin in staphylococcal adhesion to metallic surfaces used as models of orthopedic devices, *J. Orthop. Res.* **12**(3), 432–438.

De Lollis, A. 1991. Mezzi di sintesi in acido polilattico, Atti del simposio sui Biomateriali polimerici, Bologna, pp. 168–178.

Dorman Smith V. 1991. Considerations when using ethylene oxide for the sterilization of medical devices, *Med. Dev. Technol.* **2**(5), 42–45.

Doué, B. 1992. Electron Beam Accelerators. A technology adapted for the sterilization of medical devices, *Med. Dev. Technol.* **3**(5), 48–53.

Dougherty, S.H. 1986. Implant infections, in: *Handbook of Biomaterial Evaluation* (*A. van Recum, ed.*), pp. 276–289, McMillan Publishing Co., London.

Ernst, R.R., Doyle, J.E. 1968. Sterilization with gaseous Ethylene Oxide: a review of physical and chemical factors, *Biotechnol. Bioeng.* **10**(1),

Fitzgerald, R.H., Peterson, L.F.A. 1984. Wound colonization and deep wound sepsis, in: *Infections in Joint Replacement Surgery* (N.S. Etekjiar, ed.), pp. 151–165, Mosby, St Louis.

Gabriel, S.E., Woods, J.E., O Fallon, W.M., Beard, C.M., Kurland, L.T., Melton, L.J. 1997. Complications leading to surgery after breast implantation, *N. Engl. J. Med.* **366**(10), 677–682.

Giannini, S., Grimaldi, M., Ceccarelli, F., Bertelli, R. 1994. The manufacturing details and mechanical aspects of the PLLA implants, in: *Biodegradable Implants in Fracture Fixation.* (Leung Kwok-sui, Hung Leung-kim, Leung Ping-chung, eds.), pp. 59–66, Word Scientific Publishing, Singapore.

Giardino, R., Maraldi, N.M., Squarzoni, S., Corticelli, A.S., Buscaroli, S., Rocca, M., Fini, M. 1990a. Central Venous Catheters and bacterial adhesion: in vitro and in vivo evaluation, Proceedings of the 92° Congrés Francais de Chirurgie, Paris, October 1–4.

Giardino, R., Maraldi, N.M., Squarzoni, S., Sabatelli, P., Corticelli, A.S., Rossi, R., Fini, M., Buscaroli, S., Rocca, M. 1990b. Central venous catheters: an ultrastructural study, *Int. J. Artif. Organs* **13**, 586.

Green, S.A., Ripley, M.J. 1984. Chronic osteomyelitis in pin tracks, *J. Bone Jt. Surg., Am. Vol.* **66**(7), 1092–1098.

Gristina, A., Barth, E., Webb, L. 1989a. Microbial adhesion and the pathogenesis of biomaterial centered infections, in: *Orthopaedic Infections: Diagnosis and Treatment* (R. Gustilo, R. Gruninger, D. Tsukayama, eds.), W.B. Saunders, Philadelphia.

Gristina, A., Barth, E., Webb, L. 1989b. Microbes, metals and other non-biological substrata in man, in: *Orthopedic Infections: Diagnosis and Treatment*, (R. Gustilo, R. Gruninger, D. Tsukayama, eds.), W.B. Saunders, Philadelphia.

Halls, N. 1992. The microbiology of irradiation sterilization, *Med. Dev. Technol.* **3**(6), 36–45.

Henon, Y. 1992. Gamma Processing: The state of the art, *Med. Dev. Technol.* **3**(5), 30–37.

Ishigaki, I., Yoshii, F., Makunchi, K., Tamura, N. 1989. Radiation effects on polymeric materials, Proceedings of the International Kilmer Memorial Conference on the Sterilization of Medical Products, Moscow, Sept. 1989.

Jacobsson, S.A., Djerf, K., Wahlstrom, O. 1996. Twenty Year results of Mc Kee-Farrar versus Charnley prosthesis, *Clin. Orthop.* **329**(S), 60–69.

Klock, J.C., Baynton, D.F. 1976. Degranulation and abnormal bactericidal function of granulocytes procured by reversible adhesion to nylon wool. *Blood* **48**, 149.

Leake, E.S., Gristina, A.G., Wright, M.J. 1982. Use of chemotaxis chambers for studying in vitro bacterial colonization of biomaterials, *J. Clin. Microbiol.* **15**(2), 320–323.

Lim, L.Y., Khor, E., Koo, O. 1998. Gamma irradiation of chitosan, *J. Biomed. Mater. Res.* **43**(3), 282–290.

Link, A., Buttner, K. 1992. Steam sterilization: a suitable alternative, *Med. Dev. Technol.* **3**(5), 45–47.

McClinton, M.A., Helgemo, S.L. 1997. Infection in the presence of skeletal fixation in the upper extremity, *Hand Clin.* **14**(4), 745–760.

Merrit, K., Turner, G.E. 1985. Adherence of bacteria to biomaterials, Abstract, 11 Annual Meeting of the Society for Biomaterials, San Diego.

Merrit, K., Gaind, A., Anderson, J.M. 1996. Detection of bacterial adherence on biomedical polymers, *J. Biomed. Mater. Res.* **39**(3), 415–422.

Moore, W.S. 1977. Experimental studies relating to sepsis in prosthetic vascular grafting in: *Infections of Prosthetic Hearth Valves and Vascular Grafts* (R.L. Duma, ed.), pp. 267–285, University Park Press, Baltimore.

Morra, M., Cassinelli, C. 1997. Bacterial adhesion to polymer surfaces: a critical review of surface thermodynamic approaches, *J. Biomater. Sci. Polym. Ed.* **9**(1), 55–74.

Muller, T.F., Seitz, M., Eckle, I., Lange, H., Kolb, G. 1998. Biocompatibility differences with respect to the dialyzer sterilization method, *Nephron* **78**(2), 139–142.

Norman, D.C., Yoshikawa, T.T. 1994. Infections of the bone, joint and bursa, *Clin. Geriatr. Med.* **19**(4), 703–718.

Paganetto, G., Mazzullo, S., De Lollis, A., Buscaroli, S., Rocca, M., Fini, M., Giardino, R. 1991. Poly-L-lactic acid: biointeraction and processing variable relationships, *Biomateriali* **2**, 179–183.

Pascaud, R.S., Evans, W.T., McCullagh, P.J., Fitspatrick, D.P. 1997. Influence of gamma irradiation sterilization and temperature on the fracture toughness of ultra-molecular-weight-polyethylene, *Biomaterials* **18**(10), 727–735.

Pearson, L.S. 1996. Sterilization survey, *Med. Dev. Technol.* **7**, 58–64.

Petty, W., Spanier, S., Shuster, J.J., Silverhome, C. 1985. The influence of skeletal implants on incidence of infections. Experiments in a canine model, *J Bone Jt. Surg, Am. Vol.* **67**(8), 1236–1284.

Rao, S.B., Sharma, C.P. 1995. Sterilization of chitosan: implications, *J. Biomater. Appl.* **10**, 136–143.

Rao, S.B., Sharma, C.P. 1997. Use of Chitosan as a biomaterial: study on its safety and hemostatic potential, *J. Biomed. Mater. Res.* **34**, 21–28.

Ritter, M.A. 1984. Ecology of the operating room, in: *Infections in Joint Replacement Surgery* N.S. Eftekhar, ed.), pp. 131–148, Mosby, St Louis.

Ross, A., Sadat, T. 1991. Industrial applications of high energy electrons for sterilization, *Med. Dev. Technol.* **2**(8), 20–26.

Shaw, J.A., Greer, R.B. 1994. Complications of total hip replacement, in: *Complications Orthopaedic Surgery* (C.H. Epps, ed.), Lippincott Company, Philadelphia.

Suwanprateeb, J., Tanner, K.E., Turner, S., Bonfield, W. 1998. Influence of sterilization by gamma irradiation or thermal annealing on creep of hydroxyapatite-reinforced polyethylene composites, *J. Biomed. Mater. Res.* **39**(1), 16–22.

Tallentire, A. 1980. The spectrum of microbial radiation sensitivity, *Radiat. Phys. Chem.* **15**, 83.

Taylor, S.M., Weatherford, D.A., Langan, E.M., Lokey, J.S. 1996. Outcomes in the management of vascular prosthetic graft infections confined to the groin. A reappraisal, *Ann. Vasc. Surg.* **10**(2), 117–122.

Wassall, M.A., Santin, M., Isalberti, C., Cannas, M., Denyer, S.P. 1997. Adhesion of bacteria to stainless steel and silver coated orthopedic external fixation pins, *J. Biomed. Mater. Res.* **5**(36), 325–330.

White, S.E., Paxson, R.D., Tanner, M.G., Whiteside, L.A. 1996. Effects of sterilization on wear in total knee arthroplasty, *Clin. Orthop.* **331**, 164–171.

29

Drug Delivery Systems

Francesco M. Veronese and Paolo Caliceti

29.1. Introduction

Drugs, in the majority of cases, are toxic at high doses however, they must be present in the circulation for a time sufficient to reach therapeutically useful results. This is commonly achieved by repeated drug administrations, which give rise to peak and valley drug concentration. Such a method of administration has two disadvantages: on the one hand the low compliance by the patient and, on the other, the risk of reaching toxic levels. This chance is very severe in particular for new biotechnological drugs such as peptides, proteins, or oligonucleotides that usually are very active and often have a very narrow therapeutic window.

A solution to these problems comes now from the drug controlled release technology, meaning with this word also programmable or pulse release from insoluble matrices. The chemical modification of the drug by soluble polymers to increase the residence time in blood, as well as to convey more favorable properties such as the reduction of antigenicity or increased stability toward enzymes, is also considered part of the technology. In any of these cases not only desirable and constant drug levels are reached, but also a release that may last for a long time, up to one year. To reach this goal the drug is usually entrapped when the matrix is produced or shaped, and only in rare cases is it absorbed into the matrix from a concentrated drug solution.

The technology described above does not apply only to systemic drug treatment, i.e., distribution through the whole body via the blood, but also sometimes to localization in a particular area, as occurs, for instance, in wound treatment and in medication of inflamed epidermis as well as of eyes,

---

Francesco M. Veronese and Paolo Caliceti • Department of Pharmaceutical Sciences, University of Padova, Via F. Marzolo, 5, 35131 Padova, Italy.

Integrated Biomaterials Science, edited by R. Barbucci. Kluwer Academic/Plenum Publishers, New York, 2002.

ears, or vagina. Often these results may be obtained by special devices as those based on adhesion.

It must be also remembered that the controlled release technology is not limited to therapeutic treatments but may be exploited in the most varied and unexpected cases, as, for instance, in household products release, in agriculture, for antifouling products release in boat painting, in animal feeding, in antiparasites for animals, in plant aerial seeding, just to cite the most well-known cases. All of these products require special designs, but less care is needed in regard to the homogeneity of the components and purity than for products devised for human use. The advantage is that the spectrum of usable polymers for the device preparation is higher, with more probability of success and low cost.

A final, but no less important way to deliver drugs is to conjugate them to soluble polymers with chemical bonds that are either cleavable into the body to release the starting drug or stable to leave drug–polymer conjugates free to circulate as a new therapeutic product. In this latter case the binding must be studied in order to maintain the drug active moiety free for receptor binding.

The advantage of such a conjugation is a prolonged circulating time by the reduction in kidney filtration due to the increased size of the drug–polymer complex. Furthermore, an increased stability to proteolysis and reduced immunogenicity is achieved.

29.2. Controlled or Programmable Drug Release versus Slow or Sustained Release

Slow or sustained drug release means control of the drug pharmacokinetics by the use of long known techniques, namely compresses, tablets, suspensions, emulsions, and enteric formulations. More sophisticated and chemically based systems are also considered in this category, such as the preparation of drug complexes. With any of these methods the release of a drug is retarded, but the disadvantage of being not easily reproducible *in vivo* does exist, since they depend on environmental conditions and are also related to interindividual variations. Further limits of the methods are the difficulty in reducing the peak concentration levels in blood and reaching a long-time release.

These disadvantages may be overcome by a more sophisticated use of polymer to achieve what is called controlled release. The controlled drug delivery systems can be classified in three main categories: controlled, targeted, and prolonged or sustained delivery.

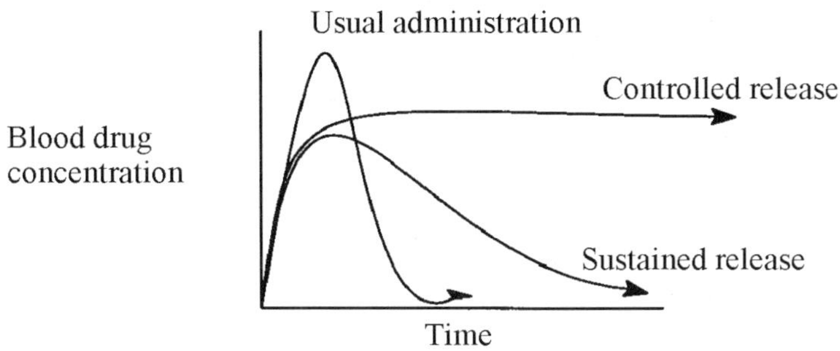

Figure 29.1. Blood drug concentration following different routes of administration.

Controlled release systems are designed in order to release proper drug amounts continuously or under specific physiological, chemical, or physical stimulation. Several sophisticated stimuli responsive devices have been developed, though most of them are only experimental tools.

Targeted delivery is better defined as a strategy to get the drug to the site of action. This can be realized by exploitation of pro-drugs, drug–carrier conjugates, and *in situ* administration using suitable dosage formulations.

Prolonged or sustained drug delivery systems act by maintaining constant therapeutic levels in the body for a long time. These systems are often considered, with some exceptions, as the advanced development of traditional dosage forms. The variety of sustained drug delivery systems recently developed makes this group the biggest one. This class of advanced drug delivery systems comprises in fact many implantable, long circulating devices, or devices for external use.

In the best known controlled release technology, the polymer acts as a cage containing the drug, which can escape at a rate that depends upon the pore size of the cage itself: a proper turning of the pore size and cage characteristics maintains the release of the drug for the desired time and rate (Figure 29.1).

In those cases in which so-called "intelligent polymers" are used, the pore size of the release matrix may be varied on demand and a modification of the release rate is achieved yielding the desired drug/blood concentration profile. This is an active area of research that, in the most sophisticated applications, mimics in some way the feedback regulation of biological phenomena. As far as one can understand, this study may give significant results only through serious collaboration among pharmacists, polymer chemists, and biologists.

29.3. Biodegradable and Nonbiodegradable Polymers

The specific need for controlled release applications dictates on each occasion the choice of polymer. Usually, the demand is minor if the device is designed for external use or for oral administration, while it is much more stringent if it must be given intravenously or subcutaneously or for application into a delicate and not easily accessible cavity like the airways. For external use, the polymer may be nonbiodegradable, such as those having a carbon–carbon or silica–oxygen backbone, while in the second group of applications a biodegradable polymer is in great demand.

Polymer biodegradability may be related to backbone cleavage by water alone or by the action of proteolytic enzymes, the shortening of the chains usually being accompanied by increased solubility. Typical examples of the first class are the hydrolysis of ester or anhydride bonds, while an example of the second class is the hydrolysis of amide bonds.

Biodegradation may also be related to hydrolysis taking place in backbone side chains, provided that this yields to solubilization of the entire polymer (Table 29.1).

In the majority of cases, the chemical reactions at the basis of biodegradation are known processes and, like all chemical reactions, they may be controlled at a rate by the proper choice of close substituent end groups. A typical example is the solubilization of cyanoacrylates as compared to acrylates. By suitable exploitation of chemistry one may therefore tailor the release rate of the drug entrapped in the polymer and the duration of the polymer itself inside the body.

The polymers that will be described in more detail below do not represent an exhaustive list, but are the most interesting or promising to date. They do not correspond to those employed, since the commercial

Table 29.1. Typical Biodegradable and Nonbiodegradable Polymers Used in Controlled Release Technology

Nondegradable	Degradable
Polysiloxanes	Polylactides and polyglycolides
Polyacrylates	Polycyanoacrylates
Polyurethanes	Polyorthoesters
Polyethylenes	Polyphosphazenes
	Polyanhydrides
	Polysaccharides
	Polycarbonates
	Poly-ε-caprolactones

exploitation of polymers is often dictated not only by the superiority of properties, but by marketing and patenting situations as well.

29.4. Polymers for Controlled Release Applications

Some of the most important biodegradable and nonbiodegradable polymers used in drug release technology are reported in this section (Chasin and Langer, 1990; Dumitru, 1994; Park *et al.*, 1993). The former are preferred for internal application although some nonbiodegradable ones, such as polysiloxanes, are largely used both inside the body as well as in delicate body cavities.

29.4.1. Polysiloxanes

Polysiloxanes may be considered the first class of polymers employed in controlled drug release. They are also known as silicones, a historic name that originated from the old idea that they were ketones in structure. Their use in drug release came from the observation by Folkman and Lony while studying polysiloxane heart valves. These authors found that a lipid soluble dye like Sudan was adsorbed and could then diffuse in silicon elastomer membranes, unlike water-soluble dyes like methylene blue. A study with dyes and drugs of different structures demonstrated that this property is common to many substances and depends upon their hydrophilic/hydrophobic ratio; furthermore, penetration into the polymer matrix is due to hydrophobic interaction.

From the structure reported below, which is at the basis of the most common products, one may understand the reason for the chemical inertness of polysiloxanes. They may be degraded, in fact, by a few chemicals such as ozone or nitrogen oxides. For this reason, heat or chemical means are much used methods of sterilization.

Their special oligomeric properties are explained by the chemical structure (**I**). The Si–O length of 1.64 exhibits high rotation for lower

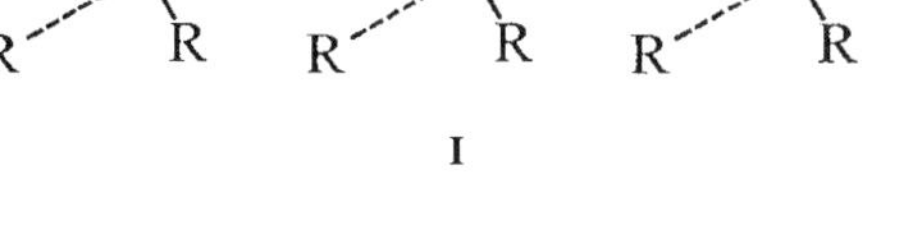

I

intramolecular steric hindrance as compared to all the polymers based on carbon backbone in which the C–C distance is 1.53 Å. The very low torsion barrier for the rotation along the skeleton bonds is the reason for the high flexibility and low Tg.

Polysiloxanes may be present in various structures and with a variety of substitutions that are reflected in their properties. For example, the linear polymer with —CH_3 as Si substituent (II) presents a Tg of $-125\,^{\circ}C$, but if a benzene ring is present in the chain the Tg may be $-48\,^{\circ}C$ or $-18\,^{\circ}C$ depending upon the *meta* or *para* position in the benzene substitution.

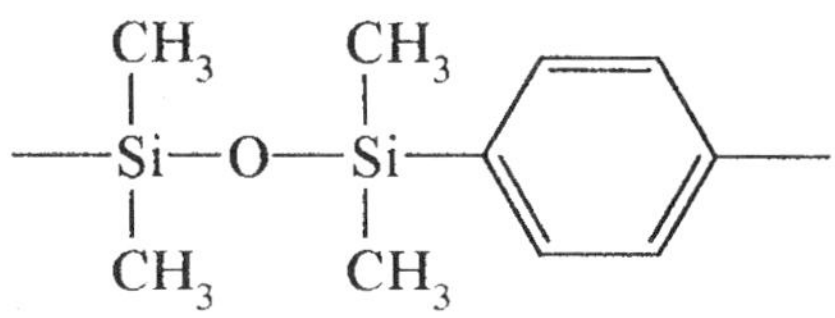

II

More complex structures are also present in a polymer, as in the case of sesquisiloxanes (**III**) which exhibit a high melting for the decreased flexibility of the structure.

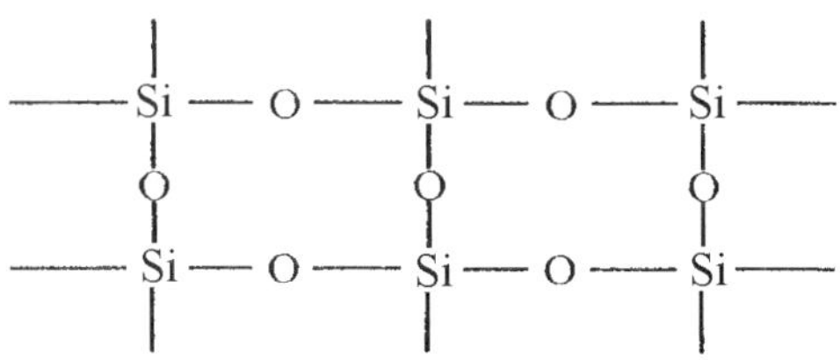

III

Other properties are changed with proper Si substitution. Of interest among these is the gas permeability, which is very high when trimethylsylil groups are present in carbon chain polymers. Chloride, nitrogen, alkyl, or aryl groups also convey to polysiloxanes not only gas permeability but also selectivity.

The synthesis of polysiloxanes starts from cyclic structure (**IV**), which

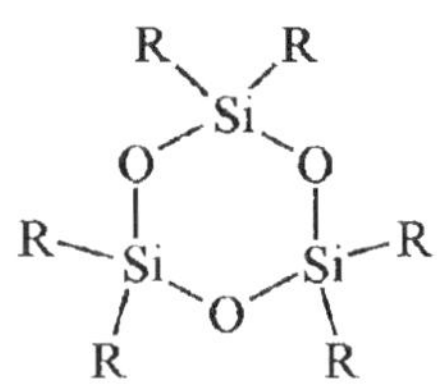

IV

may undergo anionic or cationic polymerization. Copolymers may be obtained as well.

Further polymerization of linear polysiloxanes is obtained by cross-linking through different mechanisms:

- vinylic addition in case of polymers bearing a vinyl group in the substituents;
- alkoxy condensation based on addition of the terminal hydroxyl group of a chain to Si of a tetraalkyloxysilane with concomitant displacement of the alkyl groups;
- acetoxy condensation through the addition of the terminal hydroxyl group of a chain to Si of methyltriacetoxysilane, with convenient displacement of acetate.

Drugs may be added to these cross-linked mixtures, in addition to solid compounds such as SiO_2 or carbon, to convey new physical properties to the polymer.

The great biocompatibility of these polymers, accompanied by absence of toxicity or irritability and high stability both *in vitro* and *in vivo*, make them suitable for several applications.

In drug release: The major application started in the 1960s, in steroid release for contraception, where the drug-loaded polymers were prepared in quite different shapes and a constant drug release was obtained lasting for over one year.

In artificial skins: This application was studied, but good results were obtained only following protein grafting to the surface to yield hydrophilicity to the hydrophobic silicon polymers.

In contact lenses: In this case too the hydrophobicity is the major problem, and many approaches are described in order to take advantage of the magnificent optical properties of this polymer, namely very high transparency even in the presence of additives and good gas permeability.

29.4.2. Polyphosphazenes

This is a second, important class of inorganic polymers with a great range of applications thanks to their very large range of properties. Polyphosphazenes differ from silicones because many terms are biodegradable for hydrolytic chain cleavage.

The repeated unit is reported below (**V**), with n being equal to or above 15,000 while R is an alkylic or arylic substituent.

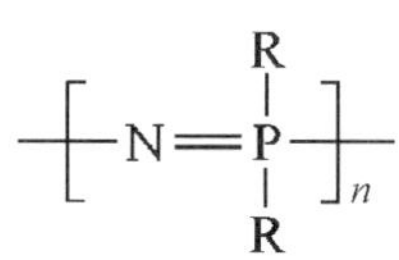

V

The nature of R is more important in dictating the polymer property than the value of n: the structure of R determines whether the polyphosphazenes are hydrophilic or hydrophobic, water insoluble or soluble. As an example, if they bear fluoroalkoxy side groups then they present a contact angle in the range of 107°, similar to that of teflon, while it drops to 101° in case of an unsubstituted benzene ring and to 0° when the ring is partially sulfonated. Important substituents are the amino acid esters with or without other amino bearing groups such as imidazole or other hydrophilic substituents that confer biodegradability on the polymer. In this case the rate of degradation depends upon the type of amino acid and the presence and amount of imidazole. In many polyphosphazenes a high degree of biocompatibility was found.

The synthesis of polyphosphazenes generally starts from phosphate pentachloride and ammonia to yield hexachlorophosphazene (**VI**).

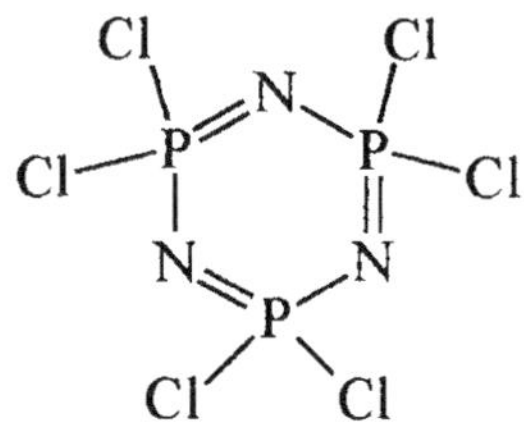

VI

Chloride may be substituted by the required derivative at this step, or after polymerization to polydichlorophosphazene achieved by heat.

The chloride was also substituted by amino group bearing drugs and the conjugate was used as such in drug release as classical prodrugs after their insolubilization to degradable matrix. More commonly, however, the drugs are physically entrapped in insoluble polyphosphazenes matrices by one of the common procedures to yield microspheres, slides, or rods.

From polyphosphazene matrices the drug release is not always based on diffusion process, but on a combination of diffusion and erosion, so the overall rate of release depends upon the relative rate of drug diffusibility and polyphosphazene erosion. This polyphosphazene behavior allows high molecular weight drugs to be released such as peptides and proteins.

Until now we are unaware of drugs that have reached a state of commercialization following polyphosphazene entrapment, although some are at an advanced state of clinical trials.

29.4.3. Lactic/Glycolic Acid Polymers

These polyester-based polymers may be regarded as the most interesting and, so far, most exploited polymers in drug delivery as well as biomaterials. The starting monomers, glycolic and lactic acid, are natural compounds, the second being present also in the citric acid cycle that may be used as such in the polymerization to yield polyesters by heat catalyzed removal of water. However, this simple procedure gives low molecular weight products, not above 10,000 D, while high molecular weight products are obtained with polymerization, usually catalyzed by trialkylaluminum (but cadmium, tin, and lead derivatives are also used) of the cyclic glycolic or lactic acid dimers. These compounds, called lactides or glycolides, may in turn be obtained by heat in the presence of proper metal oxides as catalysts.

Since the lactide may be present in three structures, different forms of polymers may be obtained (**VII**).

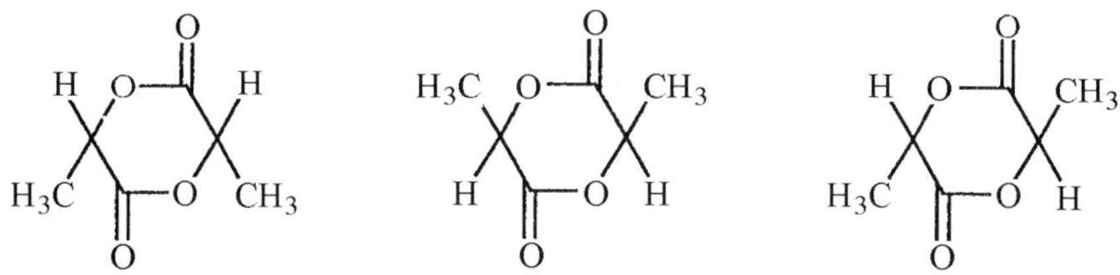

L (-) lactide D (-) lactide meso-lactide

VII

By common use, polymers obtained from linear forms are called polylactic or polyglycolic, while those obtained from cyclic forms are called polylactide or polyglycolide, respectively. Copolymers are obtained as well.

As expected, the various polymeric forms are reflected in different properties of the matrices and drug release behavior that is based on drug diffusion inside the matrices, but also on its erosion. It was clearly demonstrated that the ester cleavage rate is in turn related to polymer composition, molecular weight, crystallinity etc.

A few polymer properties and applications are reported in Table 29.2.

Table 29.2. Correlation between Polymer Composition, Degradation Rate, and Drug Release Suitability

Polymers	Tg (°C)	Degradation time	Released drugs
Poly-L-lactide	60–67	Months–years	Vaccines
Polyglycolide	36	Months	Growth promoters
Poly-D,L-lactide	57–59	Months–weeks	Contraceptive
Poly-D,L-lactide-glycolide	40–60	Months–weeks	LHRH
Poly-L-lactic acid		Few weeks	Antibiotic for local activity
Poly-glycolic acid		Days	FSH

If polymer erosion and dissolution is higher than drug diffusion, a constant drug release takes place with diffusion as the rate-determining step, but if the polymer does not degrade during the drug release the rate would slowly decline, because the diffusion path length increases as the drug is depleted from the polymer. Such a declining release is avoided by selecting a polyester that hydrolyzes, breaking the matrices into smaller pieces.

The polymer may be shaped in different forms, but for drug release rods or microspheres are most commonly used. The first were mainly used for animal administration, for instance to release estrogen for cattle synchronization. Microspheres are preferred for human use for easy administration when their diameter is small enough that they can pass through the syringe needle.

A further advantage due to polymer degradation is the possibility of releasing high molecular weight drugs such as polypeptides and proteins, which would not leave the matrix by diffusion only. Of great interest was the release of luteinizing hormone releasing hormone (LHRH), the first polypeptide released from microspheres that reached a state of broad commercialization, as well as the release at higher molecular weight vaccines.

There is a problem with sterilization of drug-loaded matrices. It can only be carried out by radiation processing, since steam sterilization would degrade the labile ester bond while dry heating would soften the matrix or change the polymer structure, since the Tg of the polymer is easily reached in this process.

29.4.4. Poly-ε-Caprolactones

These polymers were considered of great interest to release substances of low value, since they may be obtained with easy chemistry from cheap starting products. In fact they were first used for the preparation of biodegradable containers to release seeds in aerial planting of conifers.

The ε-caprolactone monomer is easily obtained by cyclohexanone oxidation with peracetic acid, as reported (**VIII**), while polymerization is carried out by an anionic, cationic, or coordinated mechanism.

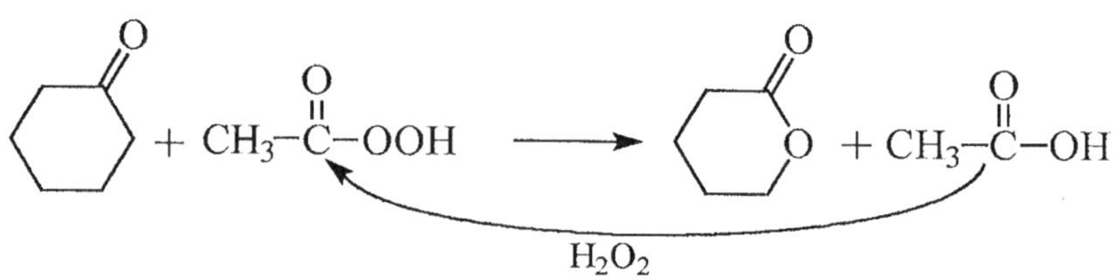

VIII

Polymerization carried out according to the first mechanism is slow and, for concurrent intramolecular transesterification with chain cleavage, low molecular weight polymers are obtained. Polymerization carried out according to the second mechanism is difficult to control due to the instability of the terminal cationic group. High molecular weight products may be obtained by coordination polymerization using Zn^{2+}, Sn^{2+}, and Al^{3+} or Ti derivatives as catalysts. Since in this case the transesterification process is very low compared to the growing chain, a high mass and narrow molecular weight distribution are reached. Radical polymerization is also possible, but this is a more expensive and tedious procedure.

Polycaprolactones are semicrystalline with a mp of 59–64 °C, depending upon the molecular weight. This is an important parameter in controlled release, because it is reflected in the permeability of drugs and degradability of the polymer. Thus crystalline polymers, which occur at low molecular weight, are less degradable for low accessibility of water. Furthermore, there is a little permeability of drugs due to the tortuosity of the crystalline form.

The Tg of polymers is very low, below −60 °C, but it may be higher with consequent increased biodegradability in copolymers: for instance, it is +20 °C in the presence of 80% polylactide. Biodegradation may be modified also in blends, for which cellulose propionate, cellulose acetate butirrate, or polylactic acid is commonly used.

It is noteworthy that the diffusibility in the polymer (D) observed in many drugs is lower by three orders of magnitude than that observed in silicon resins, while the solubility in the polymer (CS) is much higher, and therefore the drug flux (J) is similar for the two polymers.

Films, tubes, or microspheres of polycaprolactones were prepared, the method of preparation being important to determine the release properties. In many cases the release follows the Higuchi equation for spheres. A similar profile is observed in blends of microspheres in which the relative concentration of the two components is reflected in the release rate. Typical examples are blends with cellulose propionate, where the chlorpromazine release after one hour is 15, 28, 50, or 100% when polycaprolactone is present at 100, 75, 50, 25, or 0% concentration, respectively.

Reserve systems were also prepared to obtain, as expected, a constant release profile; the most important example is the release of levonorgestrel for fertility control. A zero-order drug release is obtained for over one year, the commercial product being called Capronor®. In this case, as often occurs, the *in vivo* release is somehow lower than that observed *in vitro* due to different sink situations.

The caprolactone degradation presents a characteristic behavior: two slopes in the molecular weight vs. time profile, the first having a higher rate due to an autocatalytic cleavage of the ester bonds while the second exhibits a lower rate related to the formation of crystalline polymer due to the formation of shorter chains in the polymer degradation.

29.4.5. Polyanhydrides

The starting monomers for these degradable polymers are aliphatic or aromatic bicarboxylic acids that are characterized, in both cases, by hydrophobic character. Mostly used are *p*-carboxyphenoxy-propane (**IX**), -ethane, -octane or -valeric acid, often copolymerized with sebacic acid (**X**) or with vinyl groups bearing bicarboxylic acids.

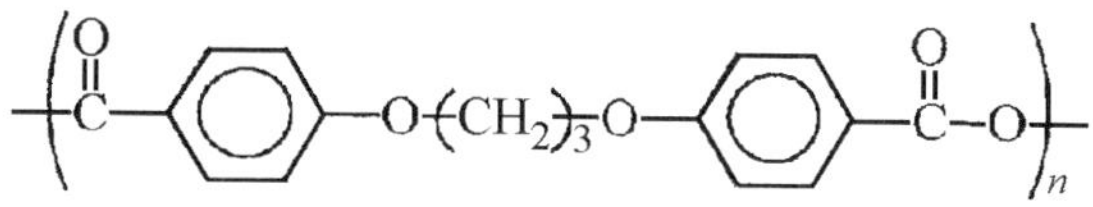

IX

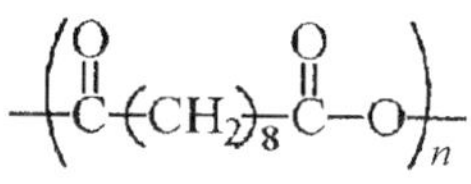

X

The polymerization of the bicarboxylic monomers may be achieved by fusion, dehydration, or dehydrochlorination: the first procedure may give good results but is not easy to carry out, while the second yields good quality polymers but is very expensive. On the other hand, the last polymerization procedure is the most convenient for the quality of polymers, and meanwhile it is cheap enough regarding the low cost of the starting acid chloride monomers.

The hydrophobicity of these polyanhydrides is reflected by a very low penetration of water in the matrices, so protecting the entrapped drugs from hydrolytic degradation while the polymer is eroded at the surface only for the hydrolysis of the anhydride bond exposed at the surface.

This characteristic is of great advantage in the release of labile drugs, because many biotechnological products are, on the one hand, labile to water and, on the other, due to their high hindrance, they do not diffuse easily through the polymer network. A typical example of the potential of this polymer is the release of insulin, a polypeptide of over 50 amino acids, which is released from a copolymer with sebacic acid in about one week with a rate of insulin release that is superimposable on the copolymer degradation. The coincidence of the two processes demonstrates that the release takes place by erosion of the matrix.

Polymer degradation in water is greatly dependent upon the polymer composition; for instance, the presence of sebacic acid in the *p*-carboxyphenoxypropane–sebacic acid copolymer increases the polymer hydrolysis up to 100 times. The degradation is also increased by decreasing the aliphatic chain between the two carboxyphenoxy groups. Polyanhydrides are resistant in the dry state or in organic solvents, but exhibit a water degradation that depends upon the composition; for example, the aliphatic polyanhydrides are less stable than the aliphatic-aromatic ones. They may reacts with some drugs; the chemistry explains, for instance, that they easily react with drugs bearing amino groups.

An important example of the therapeutic application of polyanhydrides is the release of the chemotherapic agent carmustine in brain and the local release of gentamycine to treat osteomyelitis.

29.4.6. Polyalkyl Acrylates

Two polyacrylate structures are useful in drug release: polyalkyl acrylate and polyalkyl cyanoacrylate prepared from acrylate (**XI**) and cyanoacrylate (**XII**) monomers, respectively. The second, characterized by biodegradation followed by solubilization, has being used for many years as tissue glue in surgery.

Unlike the polymers previously reported, these are not shaped in the desired form starting from already polymerized material, but microspheres or microcapsules are directly obtained during the polymerization step.

$$CH_2{=}CH{-}COOR \qquad\qquad \begin{array}{l} CH_2{=}C{-}COOR \\ \qquad\ \ | \\ \qquad\ CN \end{array}$$

XI **XII**

Polymethyl methacrylate nanoparticles are preferentially prepared by emulsion-free polymerization in aqueous media initiated by peroxodisulfate or gamma rays. The properties and size of particles may be changed by affecting the monomer concentration, addition of casein to decrease the flocculation during the polymerization, and temperature or initiator concentration.

Polyalkyl cyanoacrylate nanoparticles, on the other hand, are obtained by an anionic polymerization mechanism. The initiator is usually the OH- of water in an acidic medium of pH 2–3, since the hydroxyl ion concentration present in alkaline, and also in neutral medium, is too high to allow discrete particle formation.

The polymerization carried out in the presence of a drug and of emulsifiers yields very small particles, in the range of 30–300 nm, a size very

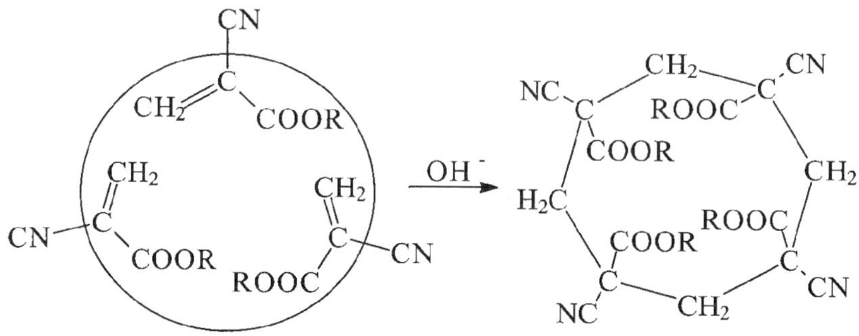

Figure 29.2. Capsule formation by interfacial polymerization.

close to that of the pores of the filters used for sterile filtration. This small particle size dictates their characteristic distribution in a body: a free circulation in blood and localization in some organs only, namely lungs and bone marrow. A useful captation by some tumors was also observed for the enhanced endocytotic activity of these tissues.

The nanocapsules (Figure 29.2) are instead formed by creating oil-in-water emulsion with the oily phase containing ethanol in addition to the dissolved cyanoacrylate. The ethanol, with its high water solubility, diffuses into the aqueous phase leaving only the oil, which forms very small nanodroplets. The monomer in turn diffuses out from the oily phase to reach the water, where it polymerizes according to the above-reported base-catalyzed mechanism.

The incorporation of drugs into the acrylate nanospheres may be explained on the basis of a Langmuirian-type or partitioning-type isotherm. Nanospheres can entrap a significant amount of drugs for their large surface area. Drugs may be either adsorbed during the polymerization process or bound at the surface of preformed capsules. The entrapment capacity depends upon several factors, such as the nature of monomer, the p*K*a of the drug, the concentration in the polymerization media, and the relative hydrophobicity of the drug and monomer. In nanocapsules instead, the adsorption is mainly related to drug solubility into the oily compartment since, in this case, the drugs are present in the internal space, although adsorption at the surface is not excluded.

29.4.7. Polyacrylate Hydrogels

Hydrogels are hydrophilic matrices of great interest for parenteral and external use. The main characteristic of these systems is their high water absorption capacity which, on the one hand, confers on them good biocompatibility and, on the other, can modulate the drug release kinetic. Water absorption and the other physicochemical, mechanical, biological, and pharmaceutical properties depend strictly on the chemical composition of the polymer. The possibility of using copolymers of different qualitative and quantitative composition therefore makes these systems highly versatile and of great interest in pharmaceutical technology. The proper choice of copolymer composition can in fact achieve a huge variety of physically and chemically inert or stimuli-responsive hydrogels. Recently, a number of sophisticated devices based on thermal or pH responsive hydrogels have been successfully investigated for drug release. The most interesting hydrogel-forming polymers are those obtained by gamma-ray induced polymerization of glass-forming monomers at low temperature (Scheme 29.1). Most used among these monomers is 2-hydroxyethyl acrylate (**XIII**), but the methacrylate (**XIV**) derivative and vinyl pyrrolidone (**XV**) are often used also, while ethylen glycole dimetacrylate (**XVI**) is the cross-linking agent most often employed.

$$CH_2{=}CH{-}COOC_2H_4{-}OH$$

XIII

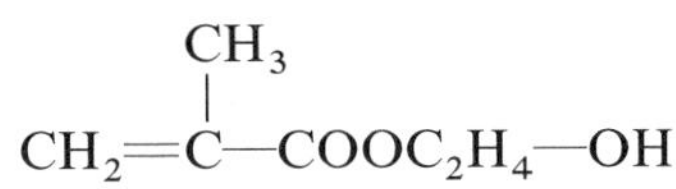

XIV

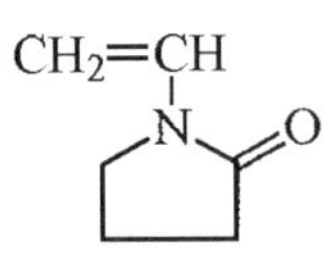

XV

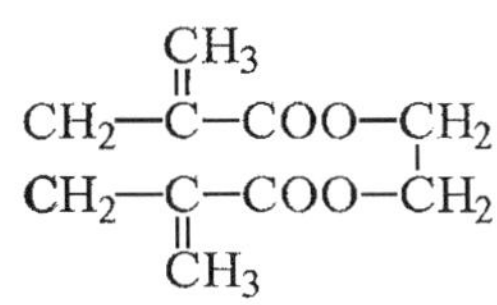

XVI

These hydrogels are obtained by freezing at very low temperature, usually with dry ice, a mixture of monomer or monomers, cross-linking agent, and drug, all dissolved in water or buffer. If the monomer has a sufficiently low Tg it does not crystallize but remains in a fluid state, while water crystallizes finely dispersed in the monomer. The irradiation at this temperature gives rise to a polymeric mass that, once thawed, has a hydrogel appearance with a sponge-like structure when examined by scanning electron microscopy. Note that congealing prevents drug precipitation and denaturing during the polymerization reaction.

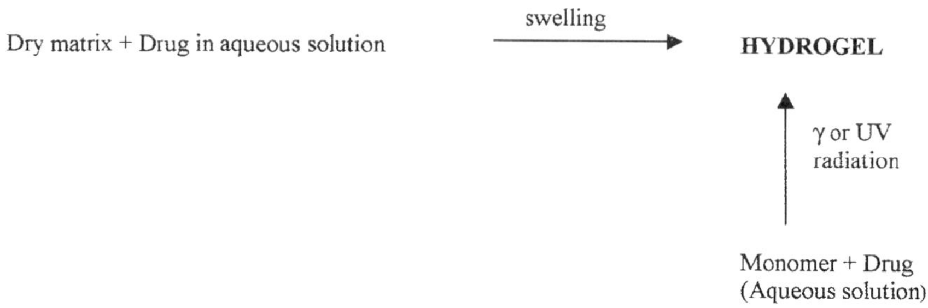

Scheme 29.1

The concentration of monomer in the starting water solution may vary over a large range, between approximately 20 and 80, while the cross-linking agent always possesses low concentration, usually a few percent. The polymerization gives rise to a very soft or hard gel, depending upon the monomer and cross-linking concentrations. As expected from a dense and cross-linked hydrogel, a drug is released following diffusion-controlled kinetics at a rate that mostly depends on the properties and solubility of the drug.

One potential use of these polymers is the easy immobilization of enzymes, which generally maintain their native active conformation during the low-temperature radiation-induced polymerization. However, enzyme leakage is also observed from these matrices and the degree depends upon the enzyme structure, although it is always unpredictable.

Another method for preparing hydrogels is preformed matrix swelling in the presence of drug aqueous solution (Scheme 29.1). This procedure presents the advantage of drug loading under nondenaturating conditions. Nevertheless, a limited drug load is often yielded.

29.4.8. Other Polymers for Controlled Release

Nylon: This polymer is used in the preparation of microcapsules employed in several technological applications apart from drug release. These include the entrapment to keep separate during storage substances otherwise nonmiscible, or to maintain separated fragrances with different properties.

Cellulose acetate: Relatively large particles are prepared with cellulose acetate by a coacervation process to entrap chemotherapeutic drugs. These large drug-loaded particles are localized in the required areas by directed injection in the arterea creating a so-called chemoembolization with simultaneous release of the drug.

Jaluronic acid: As such this natural polymer, similarly to many other polysaccharides, is not suitable for controlled drug release due to its high water solubility, which makes any formulation too unstable. The drawback was solved by chemical derivatization with hydrophobic acids, usually aliphatic ones, that temporarily insolubilizes jaluronic acid (**XVII**). It was found that the chain length is critical to reach a required erosion rate accompanied by drug release which, however, never exceeds few days.

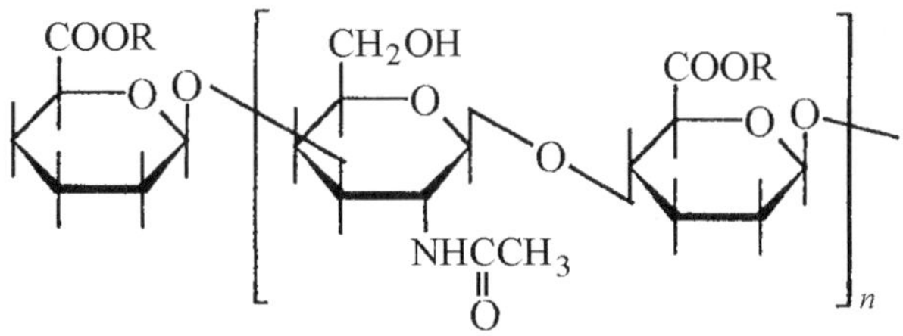

XVII

A proper choice of acid yields products devoid of toxicity or immunogenicity and with good biocompatibility, all properties that also make them suitable for the preparation of biomaterials, as in the case of artificial skin. A further possibility of jaluronic acid in drug release is the conjugation of the drug itself to the hydroxy or carboxy groups of the polysaccharide. A significantly lower release rate takes place in this case due to physical erosion of the polymer matrix by solubilization, and also to the chemical cleavage of the drug–polysaccharide bond.

Polyacroleine: The vinyl bond of acroleine is polymerized by the usual methods to yield an insoluble product, which may be used as such for controlled release or, in turn, may be derivatized with amino containing drugs to yield reversible Shiff base. In this case the drug release takes place by concurrent erosion and hydrolytic mechanisms, as described above for jaluronic acid esters.

29.5. Novel Drug Delivery System Preparations

Several different procedures are available for the preparation of polymeric drug delivery systems. The choice of preparation method depends upon the physicochemical properties of the system components and the required architectural and geometrical characteristics of the device to be prepared (Guiot and Couvrier, 1986; Park *et al.*, 1993; Robinson, 1978; Tyle, 1990).

29.5.1. Monolithic Matrices

Implantable polymeric matrices are in the majority of cases monolithic devices with suitable geometry and high biocompatibility that are inserted subcutaneously or, more rarely, intraperitoneously or intramuscularly.

The simplest method to prepare monolithic matrices with defined geometrical shape and dimension is casting in a mold of a properly concentrated organic solution of the polymer containing the drug, followed by slow solvent evaporation (Scheme 29.2). All polymers soluble in organic solvents are potential candidates for this preparation method. Evaporation must be carried out under controlled conditions in order to avoid drug deposition and the formation of bubbles or chinks; high polymer concentration, possibly over 30%, is recommended at this step. Furthermore, the solvent must be completely eliminated in order to avoid toxicity. The inherent insolubility or low solubility of the polymer in the physiological liquids must guarantee the maintenance of the physical structure of the matrix, otherwise cross-linking agents must be added.

Another method of monolithic matrix preparation is the *in situ* γ-ray or chemically induced polymerization of a monomer/drug mixture (Scheme 29.2). The γ-ray induced polymerization has already been discussed in this chapter for the preparation of hydrogels. With respect to this technique, polymerization by chemical initiators avoids exposure of the drug to potentially denaturing radiation but the chemicals employed are often toxic, so their complete removal is required. Elimination of the initiator residues is, however, not a straightforward task, since it should be carried out by repeated extraction with the risk that this procedure could significantly affect the properties and performance of the formulation.

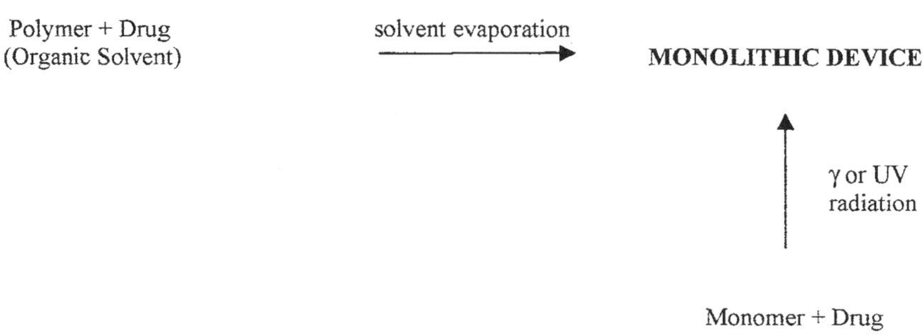

Scheme 29.2

29.5.2. Microspheres and Nanospheres

Microspheres and nanospheres are pharmaceutical dosage forms for the parenteral route of administration that can be obtained by a number of different manufacturing processes.

Emulsion/solvent extraction and emulsion/solvent evaporation techniques have been widely used with a number of polymers soluble in organic solvents (Scheme 29.3). These methods are based on the formation of an emulsion obtained by injecting an organic solution of the polymer containing the drug, the "internal phase," in the "continuous phase," usually a water buffer, under controlled stirring, temperature, and pressure. The microspheres or nanospheres are formed by solvent evaporation under vacuum or by slow solvent diffusion from the microdroplets to the external phase. This last procedure is time-consuming and, in addition, may induce drug crystallization. Alternatively, the solvent of the internal phase is rapidly extracted by strong dilution of the external phase. The success of the preparation is dictated by the proper choice of the operative conditions: the physicochemical natural of the solvents, polymer concentration in the internal phase, injection rate, internal-volume/external-volume ratio, stirring speed, pressure, temperature, physicochemical properties, and amount of surfactants and other additives.

A similar approach for the preparation of microspheres and nanospheres is by double emulsion and solvent elimination (Scheme 29.4). The difference, with respect to the single emulsion method reported above, is that a drug solution is previously emulsified in the polymer solution (1st emulsion) and the obtained dispersion is further emulsified in the external phase (2nd emulsion). This procedure is often followed when the drug is not soluble in the polymer organic solution.

Spray drying is a very efficient method for microparticle preparation and can be employed with both synthetic and natural polymers (proteins and polysaccharides). In this technique a polymer solution containing the drug is injected into a dry chamber under vacuum in order to allow for instantaneous solvent evaporation. The complete solvent elimination is the major advantage of this method, while possible drug degradation represents a serious drawback. Also, with this technique the operative conditions must

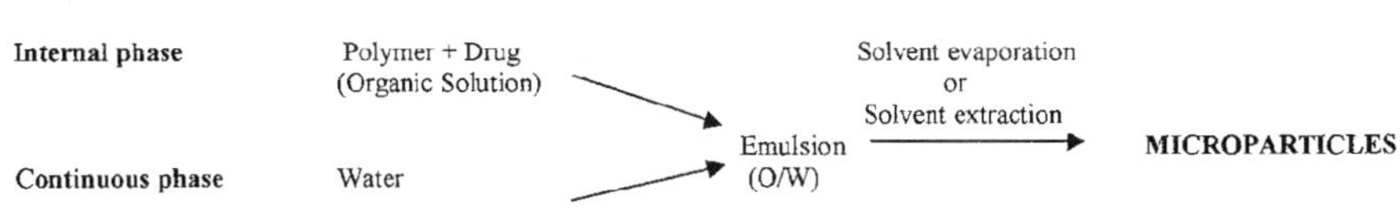

Scheme 29.3

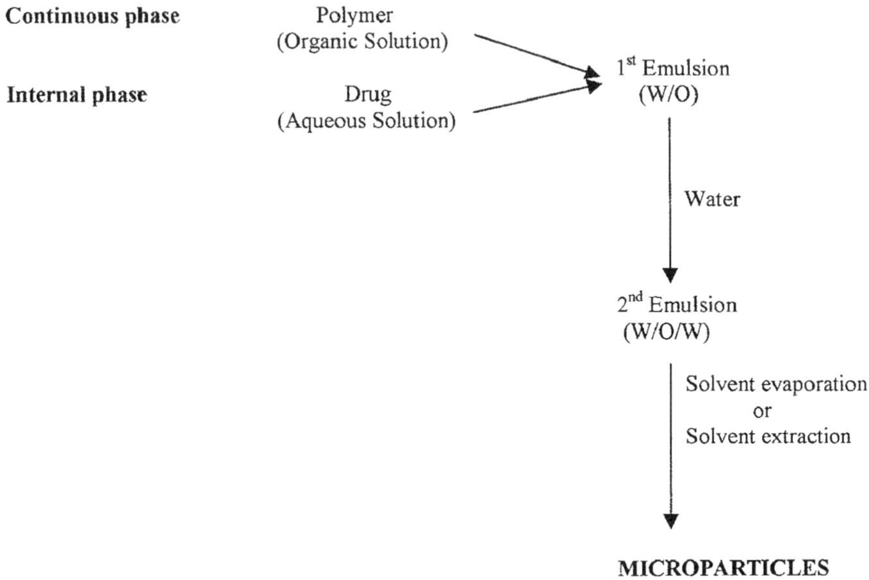

Scheme 29.4

be determined accurately in order to obtain the desired product. Other similar procedures are spray-congealing and freeze drying.

Acrylic- and cyanoacrylic microspheres and nanospheres can be fairly easily obtained by inducing polymerization of the monomer dispersed in a proper solvent as reported in the previous section.

29.5.3. Microcapsules and Nanocapsules

Microparticles and nanoparticles constituted by a core containing the drug and an external polymeric film controlling the drug release are better defined as microcapsules and nanocapsules.

These reservoir dosage formulations can be obtained through the modification of one of the above-reported methods or by coacervation or interfacial polymerization. In the coacervation procedure, the drug is suspended or emulsified in a colloidal dispersion of the polymer and the physicochemical conditions of the mixture are changed so that the polymer initially concentrates on the drug particle surface (coacervate formation) and then precipitates around it. In *simple coacervation*, the coacervate is obtained by changing the ionic force, pH, temperature, or by addition of a miscible nonsolvent for the polymer, since modification of the physicochemical properties of the mixture can reduce polymer solavation and induce its precipitation. In *complex coacervation*, a second polymer, usually with a charge opposite to that of the first one, is added to the mixture in order to allow for the formation of an insoluble polymer–polymer complex around the drug particles. The microcapsules obtained by simple or complex coacervation are hardened by desiccation or by cross-linking agent addition. Coacervation is used with many synthetic and natural polymers, namely polyesters and proteins; a typical example of complex coacervation is gelatin–arabic gum complex formation.

Interfacial polymerization is one of the less versatile methods to obtain microcapsules. The method is based on the preparation of an emulsion (generally W/O) where the dispersed phase contains the drug and a monomer, while a second reactive monomer is subsequently added to the external phase. The two monomers react at the emulsion interface to give a synthetic polymeric film. This procedure is followed when preparing nylon microcapsules using sebacic acid as monomer in the internal organic phase and hexamethylendiamine in the aqueous continuous phase.

More sophisticated reservoir systems are intraocular, intrauterine, and transdermal devices or osmotic pumps.

29.6. Internally or Externally Controlled Drug Delivery Systems

The possibility of control from either outside or inside the body is the ambitious goal of second-generation drug release systems (Heller 1993; Gurny et al. 1993; Langer 1998). Many attempts have been carried out so far, always very original and sometimes also successful, following different approaches. The release in fact was controlled by temperature variation or pH changes or triggered by ultrasound, electrical impulse, or magnetic fields as well as by the actions of enzymes in turn controlled by substrate concentration.

29.6.1. Device Erosion Controlled by pH

a. Methylvinylether–Maleic Anhydride Copolymer. With this copolymer esters may be easily obtained by reaction of the anhydride groups with aliphatic alcohol of various chain lengths, leading to an insoluble polyanionic product (**XVIII**). The solubility of the product is related to the pH of the solution and also to the chain length of the alcohol.

It was in fact demonstrated that a nearly linear correlation does occur between matrix dissolution and size of alcoholic group in half ester of methylvinylether–maleic acid copolymer. On the other hand, it was also observed that once the alcohol is fixed, the solubility depends linearly on the degree of esterification.

On this basis one may design a polymer that, at a required pH, attains the needed number of ionized carboxylic groups to begin the solubilization with simultaneous release of the entrapped drug. The possibility of self-regulation of this matrix was demonstrated by a system that entraps a drug together with the enzyme urease into the properly designed copolymer. In this case drug release occurs in response to incoming urea, because this substance is hydrolyzed by the enzyme to ammonia with concomitant increase in pH. In other words, urea stimulates release of the entrapped drug once a proper pH-sensitive polymer is used.

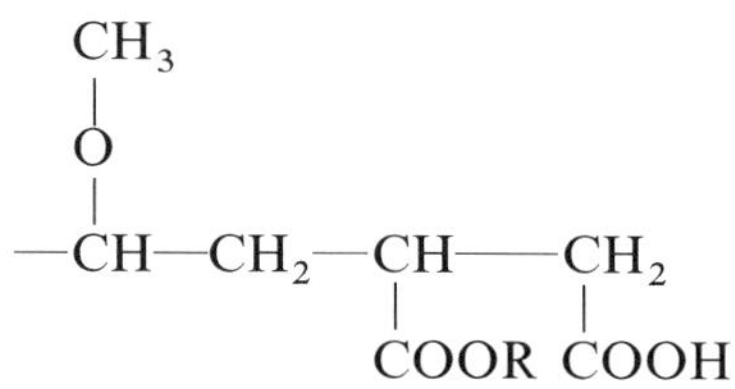

XVIII

b. Poly(orthoesters). These polymers are characterized by increased erosion rate as the pH is decreased, where the polymer is hydrolyzed giving rise to simple aliphatic acids and diols both devoid of toxicity. In this respect they present an erosion behavior that is the opposite of that exhibited by the previously described polymer, since the former is eroded by solubilization on increasing pH while poly(orthoesters) are eroded by ester cleavage toward acidity.

This behavior of poly(orthoesters) makes them suitable for the release of insulin from a matrix where it is entrapped together with the enzyme glucose oxides. When glucose is increased in blood, as occurs in diabetics, for diffusion it reaches a higher level in the matrix, and here it is oxidized to gluconic acid by glucose oxidize with a concomitant rise in local H^+ concentration. This situation is reflected in increased polymer erosion and increased release of insulin.

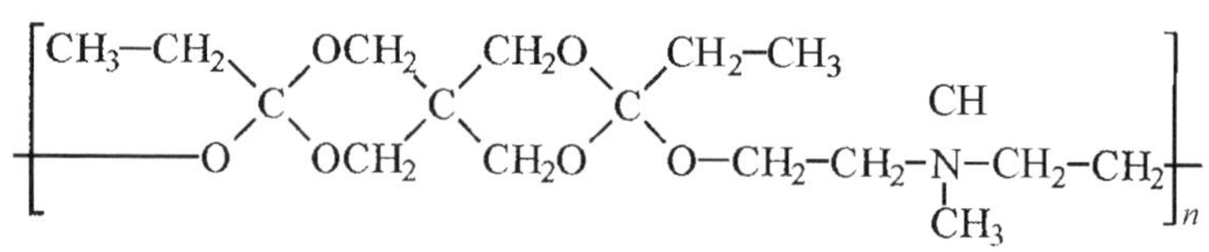

XIX

It was found, however, that with the described polymer the sensibility of the system was not enough to release the required insulin amount with the relatively low pH variation in the microenvironment and therefore a new, more successful poly(orthoester) was later synthesized that incorporates amino groups into the polymeric structure (**XIX**). A pulsatile insulin release was achieved in this case, although it was found to work only for a limited number of glucose shots.

29.6.2. Self-Modulated Devices

a. Poly(acrylic) Polymers. The potential of these polymers to permanently entrap enzymes without activity loss (see above) was exploited to create a pulsatile insulin release system taking advantage, also in this case, of the catalytic properties of glucose oxidase. It was in fact found that glucose oxidase can be immobilized at high yield in these polymers by radiation-induced polymerization at low temperature. Several release matrices were studied, the one with the best results being composed of a copolymer prepared with 2-hydroxyethyl acrylate, 4-trimethylsilyl styrene, and the basic moiety *N,N*-diethylaminoethyl methacrylate (**XX**). In this case, the protons of gluconic acid released by glucose oxidase in the presence of glucose protonates the polymer-bound amino groups, giving positive charge repulsion and hydration with final chain swelling and release of insulin.

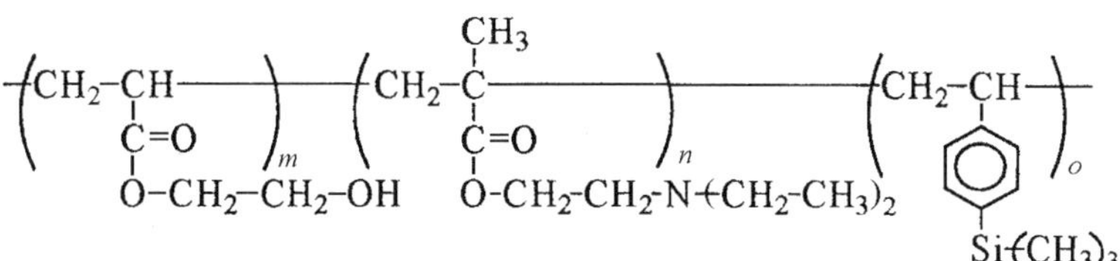

XX

This system, as opposed to those previously described, is not based on erosion, and may last for a longer time without need of replacement. Furthermore, it is characterized by reversible swelling and shrinking on concentration of the substrate present in its surrounding.

b. Self-Regulated Microporous Membranes. To the surface of microporous membranes, such as those based on poly(vinylidene fluoride), having pore size of 0.2 μm, carboxylic and amine groups were bound by air plasma treatment followed by polyacrylamide grafting and proper chemical reactions. It was demonstrated that at neutral pH the COOH groups are dissociated and solvated, thus closing the pores that in such a state prevent

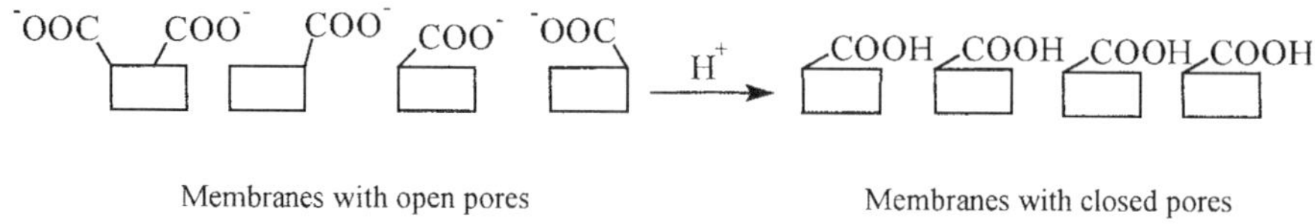

Figure 29.3. Microporous membrane with pH-controlled pore opening.

the insulin from leaking out the membrane. On the other hand, in the presence of glucose, gluconic acid is liberated and this lowers the pH causing the chain of acrylic acid to collapse with concomitant opening of the pores that allows insulin to leak (Figure 29.3).

c. Boronic Acid Derivatives. An original-type gel that swells in the presence of diols containing products such as glucose was devised. It is based on the ability of borate moiety to form reversible complexes with diols.

This property was exploited preparing an *N*-vinylpyrrolidone polymer with phenylboronic acid as pendant group (**XXI**). When mixed with poly(vinyl alcohol) a tight hydrogel is formed, for the cooperative binding between borate on one polymer and diols in PVA.

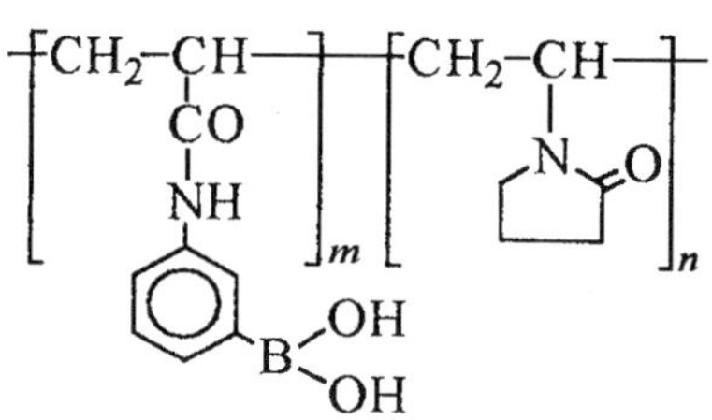

XXI

If, in this hydrogel, a drug such as insulin is entrapped, an incoming diol containing a substrate, such as glucose, causes some bonds between the two polymers to be broken for a competitive effect, with consequent swelling of the gel, and the entrapped insulin is released.

d. Antibody Regulated Release. An antibody-controlled system for an addict's treatment was studied for a reversible release of naltroxone, a morphine antagonist, only in the presence of morphine. The system is placed inside a proper membrane, as a dialysis membrane, permeable to small molecules only. Naltroxone is entrapped in a polymer that undergoes

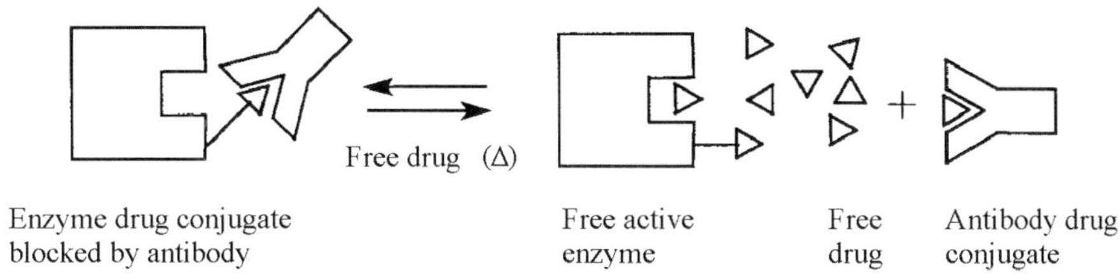

Figure 29.4. Antibody controlled system for an addict's treatment.

surface erosion in the presence of water and this polymer, in turn, is covered by a lipid layer that prevents the entrance of water. The bag also contains the enzyme lipase with a morphine analogue covalently linked close to the lipase active site together with an antibody specific toward morphine.

In the absence of morphine the antibody is bound to the lipase linked morphine, blocking the active site and thus preventing its enzymatic activity. When morphine is present in the addict's blood it enters the dialysis bag, displacing the linked morphine from the antibody and in this way leaving lipase free to act. Under the action of lipase the lipid layer is modified, water may enter with consequent erosion of the polymer containing naltroxone, which is now free to diffuse out (Figure 29.4).

29.6.3. Externally Triggered Devices

a. Ultrasonic Modulated Devices. In some polymers ultrasound has the effect of increasing the release rate of entrapped drugs, such as in the case of ethylene–vinylacetate copolymer in the release of high molecular weight molecules like bovine serum albumin or insulin. In the first case an irradiation of 75 kHz with 16 volt intensity was used. Ultrasound was found to increase also the erosion rate of other polymers, as demonstrated in the case of poly(anhydrides) or poly(orthoesters). The mechanism of these effects is not very clear, although most likely the acoustic cavitation generated by ultrasound seems to be the major cause of the activity.

b. Magnetically Modulated Devices. The effect of magnetic field in increasing the release rate of drugs from magnetic beads containing devices was demonstrated in different experimental models. Ethylene–vinyl acetate copolymer or alginate gels were used among others, while the magnetic beads were either dispersed into the matrix or sandwiched between drug-containing polymer films. Entrapped polypeptides were released at a rate up to 50-fold higher upon exposure to a magnetic field than in the ground state.

This dramatic effect seems related to squeezing of the polypeptides from the polymer pores due to the their alternating expansion and contraction induced by the oscillating magnetic field. For a satisfactory result the magnetic field strength, the polymer matrix structure, the polymer elasticity, and the magnetic bead size seem to be important. For instance, a correlation was found between magnetic field elasticity as measured by Young's modulus and the magnetic field effect.

c. Electrically Modulated Erosion of Devices. When mixed together, poly(ethyloxazoline) and poly(methacrylic) form an insoluble complex due to hydrogen bonding if they are in a solution below pH 5.0 that, however dissolves above pH 5.4. It was found that if this system is placed in a salty solution and an electric current applied, the matrix surface facing the cathode begins to dissolve as a consequence of the hydroxyl ions formed at the cathode and act on the polymer as an increase in pH. On this basis, a device was prepared for diabetics treatment that was able to release insulin many times, by simply turning on and off an externally applied current (Figure 29.5).

d. Temperature-Triggered Polymers. This polymer release method is based on the unusual property, characteristic of several polymers and their copolymers, of shrinking and become insoluble at high temperature and swelling below what is called the lower critical solution temperature (LCST). The most common polymer is poly(*N*-isopropylacrylamide) (**XXII**), which, present as a hydrogel above the LCST of 31°C, becomes soluble below this temperature. It was also found that the use of copolymers may even improve the mechanical properties of thermally reversible hydrogels, such as the case of *N*-isopropylacrylamide, *n*-butyl methacrylate, and ethylene glycol dimethacrylate copolymer.

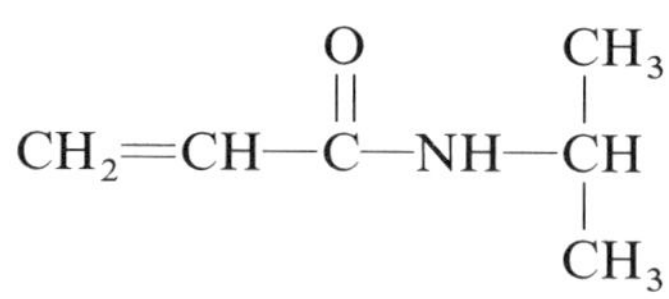

XXII

Proper blends may also give rise to useful thermosensitive hydrogels, of interest, for instance, in the mixture of two copolymers obtained by separate polymerization of *N*-polyacryloylpyrrolidone with ethylene dimethacrylate, on the one hand, and polyoxyethylene with 1,2,3-propanetryl

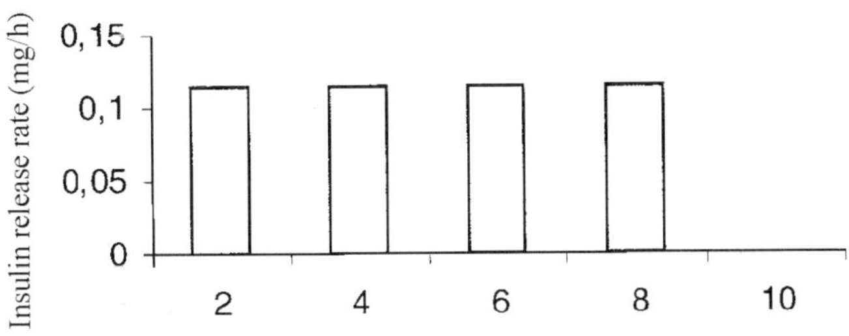

Insulin release from a 160 mg device following on and off application of a 5 mA current in 0.9%

Figure 29.5. Electrically regulated system for insulin release.

tris(3-isocyanate-4-methylcarbamilate) on the other. These copolymers give rise to two interpenetrating but not covalently linked chains. Other copolymers were studied, among those of interest being the hydrogel prepared from *N*-isopropylacrylamide and *n*-butyl methacrylate which presents an on–off shrinking and swelling with concomitant drug release.

e. Injectable Thermosensitive Polymers. These involve quite different and interesting applications of thermosensible polymers that may respond to the important and desirable request of creating *in situ*, in the body, an insoluble releasing matrix. In one very successful case the system is based on the use of a buffered solution of poly(ethylene oxide)–poly(lactic acid) block copolymer, soluble at 45°C, which dissolved the drug. The aqueous solution is injected with a regular syringe into the body, where it forms a hydrogel with the entrapped drug since the body temperature is below the LCST of the polymer.

29.7. Transdermal Therapeutic Delivery Systems

In recent years transdermal delivery has been largely studied to provide an alternative route to the administration of several therapeutics. In this respect many new transdermal therapeutic systems (TTSs) have been developed either for local or systemic drug delivery (Chien, 1987; Robinson, 1978). These new formulations are aimed at obtaining prolonged and constant drug delivery, allowing for drug targeting, reducing dose and side effects, improving patient compliance, and finally enhancing the therapeutic performance of many molecules.

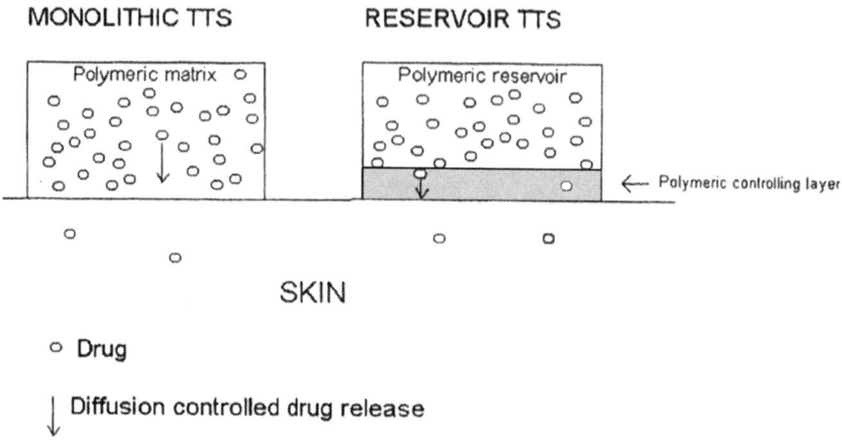

Figure 29.6. Monolithic and reservoir transdermal therapeutic systems.

The rationale of these innovative dosage forms is to control the drug delivery rate by a proper device applied on the skin while the skin itself acts as a sink. The release rate from the device is therefore the means to dictate the drug bioavailability (Figure 29.6).

From a technological point of view, the most successful TTSs are fabricated by a combination of different polymeric matrices that represent the structural and functional elements of the device. A good knowledge of the physicochemical, mechanical, and biological properties of the polymers used to prepare of these devices is therefore a fundamental step in obtaining a suitable system. General requisites for polymers used for the realization of TTSs are physical and chemical stability, physical and chemical compatibility with the drug or the other additives, and absence of toxicity.

The polymeric transdermal delivery systems can be classified into two main categories on the basis of their architecture: monolithic and reservoir devices.

29.7.1. Monolithic Devices

Monolithic devices are basically constituted by a single polymeric matrix that contains the drug molecularly dispersed or suspended in a fine state and controls its release. The physicochemical properties of the polymer and the physical structure of the matrix are the key elements dictating the drug release rate. The release occurs by diffusion mechanisms, following the second Fink's law, and therefore the drug must be partially soluble in the polymeric network.

The maintenance of the device at the application site of the skin is a relevant issue for proper efficacy of a TTS. The device must in fact be easily applied by mild pressure, must adhere uniformly to the skin, remain at the site of application during the therapy duration, and be completely and easily removed without any lesion to the skin.

If the polymer used to prepare monolithic TTSs possesses *per se* adhesive properties, the "patch" can be applied directly on the skin. On the other hand, if the monolithic matrix is devoid of an adhesive nature, a suitable polymeric layer is stratified on the matrix at the side in contact with the skin in order to allow for adhesion of the system. In this latter case, the adhesive layer must not affect the drug release. Silicones and acrylates are among the polymers most used for the preparation of adhesive layers.

Structural elements of monolithic TTSs are the backing layer and the protective liner. The backing layer is a polymeric film stratified on the device at the side exposed to the atmosphere. It should preserve the physical and chemical stability of the drug and the materials comprising the device, but must not be occlusive. Among the most common polymers used for these purposes are polyvinylchloride, high-density or low-density polyethylene, polypropylene, ethylene vinyl acetate, polyesters, and nylon. The protective liner is a removable film that protects the adhesive side of the device before applying the TTS.

Several such monolithic TTSs are already on the market, the best known being Nitrodisc®, Nitro-Dur®, and Frandol Tape® designed for long-term release of nitroglycerine or isosorbide dinitrate, and are already used successfully in angina treatment.

29.7.2. Reservoir Devices

Reservoir TTSs are complex systems obtained by assembling two or more polymeric layers. The layers provide for different functions and must therefore be prepared with polymers possessing different physicochemical, mechanical, and biological properties. An inert matrix containing the drug in a molecularly dispersed or aggregated state constitutes the reservoir layer. This element is constructed in order that the polymer properties or the physical structure of the polymeric network are physically and chemically compatible with the drug and do not affect the drug release. On the other hand, biocompatibility of this matrix is a minor requisite since this TTS component is not applied directly to the skin. Polymeric reservoirs can be prepared using carboxypolymethylene, polyacrylamide, celluloses, silicone elastomers, rayons, and polyurethanes.

Drug release from reservoir TTSs is controlled by a polymeric layer stratified on the side of the reservoir matrix that interfaces the device and the skin. The release rate is modulated by the physicochemical properties of the polymers or by using membranes with different microstructure. The most common rate-controlling membranes are prepared with ethylene-vinyl acetate, polypropylene, polycarbonates, polyvinylchloride, silicones, and cellulose acetate/nitrate. Some polymers used to prepare the rate control layer also possess adhesive properties that guarantee maintenance of the device at the site of application. Alternatively, a further adhesive layer, devoid of release rate-controlling properties, can be applied, as reported for the monolithic systems.

The backing layer and the protective liner are additional elements comprising the reservoir TTS, as already reported for the monolithic devices.

Several reservoir TTSs have already been developed and used extensively for the release of hormones, cardiovascular drugs, analgesics, antihistaminics, central nervous drugs, anti-inflammatories, etc. Transderm-Nitro® for nitroglycerine, Transderm-Scop® for scopolamine, Estraderm® for estradiol, and Catapress-TTSR for isosorbide dinitrate release are among these.

29.7.3. Skin Permeability Enhancers

Although very successful, TTS technology is still an open and controversial area of research due to the potential toxicological risk and the difficulty in reaching and controlling the skin permeability since many factors dictate their performance and safety.

Skin impermeability is one of the main problems affecting the efficacy of transdermal administration. The skin is a complex tissue constituted by various layers with different structure and physiology of fundamental importance in protection from infectious organisms and pollutant penetration as well as from dehydration. Nevertheless, this barrier represents the main obstacle to drug penetration, thus limiting transdermal delivery. From a theoretical standpoint alone, drugs with an inherent high capability of penetration are good candidates for transdermal delivery, so that a transdermal device can efficiently control their systemic delivery. On the other hand, low diffusion through the skin layers can reflect on the lack of release rate control by the device, insufficient drug absorption, low bioavailability, lack of therapeutic efficacy, and, finally, local toxicity. Moreover, low or irregular permeation in some skin layer can result in drug accumulation which, on the one hand, may represent a further element of toxicity and, on the other, makes difficult eventual therapy interruption. In order to reduce skin resistance to drug permeation, physical and chemical techniques have been studied. One of the most effective methods is the use of skin permeation

Table 29.3. Permeation Enhancers and Suggested Mechanisms of Action

Dimethylsulfoxide, Dimethylformamide, *N*-methyl-2-pyrrolidone	Lipid, lipoprotein and nucleoprotein extraction; protein binding water displacement
Propylene glycol	Alpha keratin solvation and occupation of hydrogen-binding sites
Azone	Probably acts by partitioning and destructuring the lipid bilayer
Coleic acid	Similar action of azone but the lipid structure does not appear so drastically disrupted
Sodium lauryl sulfate	Destruction of corneum stratum integrity by uncoiling and extracting the alpha-keratin helix, opening up the protein-controlled polar pathway
Decylmethylsulfoxide	Destruction of corneum stratum integrity by modification of intercellular lipids and cellular keratin. FDA approved
Ethanol and other alcohols	Polar lipid extraction
SEPA®, unsaturated cyclic ureas, salicilates, alkylazacycloalkanones, etc.	Enhancers with miscellaneous mechanisms

chemical enhancers. These chemicals are usually associated with the drug in the TTS and provide a disorganization of the skin structure, allowing for better diffusion of the therapeutic. The main requisites that these chemical enhancers must possess are drug compatibility, rapid induction and reversibility of action, and nonlocal or systemic toxicity. Several molecules with skin permeation enhancer properties are presently available, though their often unclear mechanism of action and potential toxicity greatly limit their use, especially in a long-term treatment. The enhancers may possess quite different molecular structures that, with their physicochemical nature, interact more easily with proteins or lipids present in the skin with a destructuring effect. The compounds most used are reported in Table 29.3.

In a quite different approach iontophoresis, sonophoresis, electroporation, and thermal treatment are some of the physical methods have also been successfully employed in many experimental trials to promote drug permeation. These methods have the advantage of avoiding the use of chemical enhancers that can induce toxic effects, but their application often needs sophisticated devices which must be accurately calibrated.

The great importance of skin permeation enhancers in transdermal delivery is attested by the active research that is presently being carried out on developing new physical and chemical methods to enhance skin permeability. Recent advances in this field allow us to foresee transdermal administration also in case of drugs with low physicochemical properties, such as high molecular weight molecules and peptides.

Another relevant issue in transdermal delivery is the presence of a number of deactivating enzymes in the epidermal layer. The enzymatic activity in this layer is very similar to the liver, and for this reason it represents a further limit to the exploitation of transdermal devices. In order to overcome this problem, enzyme inhibitors associated with the drugs in the device seem a promising solution.

Finally, it is noteworthy that the TTS, designed for intimate and prolonged contact with the skin, can provoke some adverse reactions, such as irritation and inflammatory responses which can give rise to toxic phenomena and infections. In order to avoid these side effects, only well-established biocompatible materials must be used for the preparation of these systems and biocompatibility tests must be carried out not only on polymers, but also on the final devices.

Apart from technological and biological considerations pertaining to TTS preparation, particular attention must be paid to the pharmacological properties of a candidate drug for transdermal delivery. Two main problems face the choice of drug: difficulty of high TTS loading and difficulty of therapy interruption in case of toxicity. This implies that only drugs with high pharmacological potency and high therapeutic index can be considered for transdermal delivery. Moreover, TTSs are often erroneously developed for drugs with poor pharmacokinetic properties, though in many cases the maintenance of constant high levels of a drug is a trivial solution since it is not reflected in enhanced efficacy. Many drugs in fact display their therapeutic activity on the basis of the biological rhythms of the organism or of the pathology evolution. Hormones, for example, are usually active by intermittent administration, while prolonged release of trinitrates is considered devoid of utility since the incidence of angina and stroke is higher in the morning and this drug can be rapidly administered by sublingual dosage forms. Drug pharmacodynamics, and not only pharmacokinetics, must therefore be carefully taken into consideration.

29.8. Mechanisms of Drug Release

Polymeric systems for prolonged drug delivery are designed in order that the polymeric matrix controls the drug release and thus becomes the rate-determining step of drug delivery. Therefore, the *in vitro* drug release analysis of these systems is carried out considering only the transport of the drug from the matrix, while the other events that can influence the release, such as dissolution in the releasing medium, must be minimized. This is why sink conditions (below 30% of the saturation concentration of the drug in the releasing medium) must be maintained throughout the time of release. It is, however, important to note that, despite the relevance of *in vitro* analysis in the development of drug delivery systems, this release does not always reflect the *in vivo* behavior, since in this latter case many anatomical, physiological, and pathological factors can concur in determining the release profile.

The mechanism, as well as the kinetics and rate of drug release from a polymeric delivery system depend upon the physicochemical properties of the drug, the materials, and the device construction (Park *et al.*, 1993; Robinson, 1978; Tyle, 1990). Furthermore, since drug release occurs with different mechanisms for undegradable and unswellable, and swellable and biodegradable matrices, all these situations will be discussed separately.

29.8.1. Undegradable and Unswellable Devices

Drug release from monolithic undegradable and unswellable matrices is dictated by diffusion mechanisms defined by the well-known second Fick's law, which describes the diffusion process in a nonequilibrium situation:

$$\delta c/\delta t = \delta^2 c/\delta x \tag{29.1}$$

This equation can be applied to polymeric compact or porous systems with different geometry, containing the drug molecularly dispersed or suspended in the network. However, the second Fick's equation has often been improperly used in drug release analysis, and for this reason many other simpler equations have been found useful for application to the pharmaceutical field. Higuchi and Peppas, in particular, elaborated the second Fick's law in order to obtain equations that could be easily applied to polymeric matrices with different characteristics.

Higuchi considered the release of a drug suspended in a fine state from a compact and porous matrix that in both cases takes place by a two-step process: (1) dissolution in the matrix and (2) diffusion. Assuming that the rate-determining step of the drug release from a compact nonporous system is diffusion through the matrix network, the equation that describes the drug release is

$$Q = \sqrt{[Dt(2A - C_s)C_s]} \tag{29.2}$$

where Q is the amount of drug released after time t per unit exposed area, D is the diffusion coefficient of the drug in the polymeric network, A is the total drug amount in the matrix per unit volume, and C_s is the drug solubility in the matrix.

On the other hand, if the rate-limiting step is the diffusion process in the buffer permeating the microchannels of a porous matrix the diffusion coefficient D in the Higuchi equation must be replaced by $D\varepsilon/\tau$, where D is the diffusion coefficient of the drug in the permeating fluid, ε is the matrix porosity, and τ is the microchannel tortuosity.

In Higuchi's equations we observe a linear correlation between the released drug and $\sqrt{t}$.

Peppas elaborated a general semiempirical equation which could be applied, with some limitation, to several different devices that release the drug by different mechanisms.

First, the release of a drug molecularly dispersed in a monolithic nonporous matrix is considered. In this case the drug dissolved in the polymer matrix diffuses through the polymeric network. In the short-time analysis, the second Fick's law for a diffusional process from a thin film can be approximated as follows:

$$M_t/M_\infty = 4[Dt/\pi l^2]^{1/2} \tag{29.3}$$

where M_t is the amount of drug released at time t, M_∞ is the amount of drug released after infinite time (corresponding to the drug loaded in the matrix), and l is half the film thickness.

For a cylinder, the release is described by

$$M_t/M_\infty = 4[Dt/\pi a^2]^{1/2} \tag{29.4}$$

where a is the radius, while from a sphere the release is given by

$$M_t/M_\infty = 6[Dt/a^2]^{1/2} \tag{29.5}$$

where a is the radius.

As already reported for Higuchi's elaboration, all these equations indicate a linear correlation between the released drug and $\sqrt{t}$, but their validity range lies between 0 and 60% of the total released drug in the case a thin layer, 0 and 15% in the case of a cylinder, and 0 and 20% in the case of a sphere.

Equations (29.2)–(29.5) can be summarized in equation (29.6):

$$M_t = Kt^{1/2} \tag{29.6}$$

where K represents the properties of the systems.

Equation (29.6) can also be written in a more general form:

$$M_t = Kt^n \tag{29.7}$$

which represents Peppas's semiempirical equation.

This last equation indicates that a Fickian diffusive process takes place when a linear correlation between the released drug and $\sqrt{t}$ ($n = 0.5$) is obtained in the short-time analysis.

In order to overcome the limitation of the analysis during the very short time of release from cylinders and spheres, dimensional parameters have been taken into consideration in the definition of the n. A range of validity between 0 and 60% of the released drug can be obtained for cylinders when $n = 0.45$, and for spheres when $n = 0.43$.

29.8.2. Swellable and Undegradable Matrices

Drug release from swellable and undegradable matrices is a much more complex process than that discussed for unswellable and undegradable monolithic systems. However, only matrices that swell more than 25% of their original volume, such as hydrogels, can be considered swellable systems. In this case, the drug is released by dissolution and diffusion in the penetrating medium. The penetration rate, and in turn the matrix relaxation, can control the release rate and, under particular conditions, zero-order release can be achieved.

The influence of matrix relaxation and the diffusion process on drug release can be estimated by the Deborah number De:

$$\mathrm{De} = \lambda/\theta \tag{29.8}$$

where De is the ratio of a characteristic relaxation time (λ) to a characteristic diffusion time (θ).

Equation (29.8) indicates that $\mathrm{De} \ll 1$ is obtained when the relaxation is much faster than the diffusion, and in this case drug release is controlled by diffusion in the fluid filling the swollen matrix. This condition usually occurs with swellable systems well above the glass transition temperature (Tg) that swell rapidly and reach equilibrium before drug release takes place.

$\mathrm{De} \gg 1$ indicates that the matrix is characterized by a very long relaxation and drug release is controlled by diffusion in an unchanged matrix. The drug diffuses in fact from an unswollen region, such as from a matrix in the glassy state (well below the Tg).

In the cases of $\mathrm{De} \ll 1$ and $\mathrm{De} \gg 1$, the drug is released by diffusion through a system with constant boundary conditions. The relaxation process does not interact with drug release, so the same speculations reported above for Fickian diffusion release from undegradable and unswellable devices can be applied. This process is also defined as Case I transport.

When the characteristic relaxation time and diffusion time are comparable, De $\cong 1$ is obtained. In this case, the relaxation interacts with the diffusion process and drug release takes place under nonconstant boundary conditions. This anomalous non-Fickian transport is observed when the drug is released during a change of the matrix from a glassy to a rubber state.

A third case of drug release from swellable and undegradable matrices is observed when the glassy fraction of a swelling system relaxes with observable rate, but much more slowly than the diffusion of the drug in the rubbery fraction of the matrix. In this process, defined as Case II transport, the release kinetic is controlled by the relaxation of the glassy fraction of the matrix. For a thin film, for example, the drug release can be described by

$$M_t = (4k_0 A/l)t \tag{29.9}$$

where M_t is the amount of drug released at time t, A is the surface area, l is the film height, and k_0 is the case II relaxation constant. Equation (29.9) can also be referred to as the general Peppas semiempirical equation (29.7) where $n = 1$, and therefore the analysis of drug release from swellable and undegradable matrices can be examined with this equation.

In swellable systems, Case I transport, or Fickian diffusion (De $\ll 1$ or De $\gg 1$), is defined for $n = 0.5$, 0.45, and 0.43 for thin films, cylinders, and spheres, respectively; anomalous non-Fickian diffusion (De $\cong 1$) is defined for $0.5 < n < 1$, $0.45 < n < 0.89$, and $0.43 < n < 0.85$, while case II transport is defined for $n = 1$, $n = 0.89$, and $n = 0.85$.

29.8.3. Reservoir Systems

Reservoir systems are usually designed so that the drug is contained in an oversaturation concentration in the core of the system and release is controlled by diffusion through a surrounding undegradable membrane. Release is defined by the first Fick's law, which describes the flux of a substance through the membrane at a steady state:

$$J_{\mathrm{d}} = -D dc/dx \tag{29.10}$$

The first Fick's equation can be elaborated for matrices with different geometrical shape.

Assuming that the drug has the same solubility in the system core and in the external medium, the release for a sandwich or slab reservoir is described by

$$M_t = s_d k_d (C_1 - C_2) t / l \tag{29.11}$$

where M_t is the released amount of drug at time t, s_d is the releasing surface area, l is the thickness of the polymeric membrane, k_d is the membrane/medium distribution coefficient, C_1 is the drug concentration in the core, and C_2 is the drug concentration in the external medium.

Similar equations have been derived for devices with different geometrical shape, such as spheres and cylinders. In these cases the geometrical parameters describing the dimension and shape of the devices are present in the equation describing the release.

In all cases a constant drug release takes place until the saturation constant in the core is maintained, and a zero-order kinetic is observed.

29.8.4. Biodegradable Matrices

In the case of biodegradable matrices the drug release can be controlled by diffusion or by degradation of the matrix. If diffusion is much more rapid than matrix degradation, this last event does not influence the drug release and the matrix behaves as an undegradable system. In this case, the analysis can be carried out as above for undegradable and unswellable systems. On the other hand, when diffusion is a slow process compared to degradation of the matrix, this last process governs the release.

Hopfenberg noted an equation that can be applied in release from surface-degrading devices when a drug is uniformly dispersed in the matrix. Since in these systems release is affected by the change in surface area during the analysis, the geometrical shape and dimensional parameters of the device must be considered.

For a slab, the release is described by

$$M_t / M_\infty = k_0 t / C_0 a \tag{29.12}$$

where C_0 is the initial drug concentration in the matrix, k_0 is the degradation rate constant, and a is the half-thickness. Since the exposed surface is supposed to be constant during release, a zero-order kinetic is obtained.

Similarly to what was observed for the other systems, the geometrical parameters describing the dimension and shape of the device must be introduced in the equation.

Analyses of drug release from matrices that undergo bulk degradation (homogeneous degradation) are much more complex than surface-degrading systems. In this case, the matrix lost with time and permeability through the polymer will increase, accelerating drug release, as in the case of polyester systems. A mathematical and complex analysis of these systems has been carried out by Baker.

In this section we have analyzed separately the different mechanisms and kinetics of drug release from matrices with different physicochemical properties. It is, however, worth noting that the drug is usually released by more than one mechanism. Matrix degradation and diffusion in the undegraded fraction, or matrix swelling and diffusion in the unrelaxed network can, for example, occur simultaneously in drug release.

29.9. Overviews of Problems Involving Long-Term Contact between Tissues and Drug Delivery Systems

Similarly to devices designed for replacing body tissues, drug delivery systems will have to sustain prolonged contact with body regions: tissues, organs, and fluids (Dumitru, 1994; Silver and Doillon, 1989). For this reason, the impact that these devices and all of their components may have on the biological structures as well as their capability to induce biological alterations is of primary concern. Biological compatibility and nontoxicity are therefore prerequisites for any candidate material for *in vivo* application.

In the case of drug delivery systems biocompatibility depends on several factors: route of administration, site of localization, time of application, chemical composition, degradation products, physical structure, and fate of the constituent material and of the whole device.

In the case of polymers, the most extensively used materials for fabrication of sustained delivery systems, the biological compatibility, and potential toxicity depend strictly on the chemical and physical properties of the monomers and the final polymers, i.e., the type of monomers, polymer composition and architecture, molecular weight, dispersivity, process of preparation, degradation products, additives, etc. A satisfactory chemical characterization of the polymers is required and represents the first step in the study, but the physical structure and microstructure of the final device are further parameters that deeply affect the biocompatibility and safety of the system. For these reasons a complex battery of *in vitro* and *in vivo* tests, on both the raw material and the final device, must be carried out.

Toxicological tests are usually carried out by incubation of the raw materials and their extracts or degradation products with cells of different lines, and by evaluation of cellular death, inhibition or abnormal cell growth, and replication. Functional and morphological damage to cells, tissues, and organs can also be evaluated by *in vivo* investigations. In these studies both local and systemic toxicity must be estimated.

In case of long-acting dosage formulations designed for prolonged circulation in blood, special tests are needed due to the fragility of the circulation system. The main problems that can be generated by these materials are deactivation of blood clotting, interference with platelet adhesion and aggregation, blood coagulation, blood flow obstruction by deposition of blood cells and molecules, and electrolyte depletion. *In vitro* tests for hemocompatibility evaluation involve incubation of the materials and systems with blood at various operative conditions, and estimation of clotting time, clot weight, number of adherent platelets, thrombin time, prothrombin time, partial thromboplastin time, platelet factor release, and platelet counts.

Platelet adhesion and morphology and blood protein adhesion (i.e., albumin and fibrinogen) can also be evaluated using platelet or protein-enriched solutions. Blood cell compatibility instead can be tested by measurement of cell attachment, replication, and protein synthesis in cell culture.

However, despite the fact that *in vitro* studies can give interesting information, *in vivo* tests carried out by implantation of the materials in a highly perfused body region are also usually required for the hemocompatibility determination of the materials. Hemocompatibility evaluation is required also for implantable devices that are designed for prolonged intimate contact with soft vascularized biological tissues.

Subcutaneous and intramuscular implants usually generate irritation and, in some cases, acute and chronic inflammation. These events depend strictly upon the site of implantation together with the physical structure of the device, the material, and its degradation products. The relevance of the hydrophilic or hydrophobic nature of the materials on tissue biocompatibility has been extensively discussed and it is still a controversial problem; actually, many hydrophilic and hydrophobic matrices display good biocompatibility. Smoothness of the matrix surface in contact with biological tissues and structural flexibility of the system are instead of primary importance in preventing tissue damage and inflammation. Acute inflammatory response is characterized by the presence of inflammatory cells around or inside the implant and the presence of multinucleated giant cells. The persistence of inflammatory cells, the growth of fibroblasts, and the formation of highly vascularized and collagen enriched fibrotic tissue indicate a chronic inflammatory state. Histological analysis after *in vivo* implantation is necessary to establish the inflammatory degree and safety of the system. In these studies, evaluations of cell death, area of tissue necrosis containing dead macrophages, released enzymes (alkaline phosphatase), and phagocytic activity are carried out.

Drug delivery systems for external use, on the other hand, involve much less investigation, although the impact that these devices can have on biological tissues must not be underestimated. Particular attention must be paid to devices designed for prolonged contact with external mucosae, such as intraocular and bioadhesive systems for oral or gastrointestinal delivery. Irritation is the most common phenomenon that these systems can induce, and is often erroneously considered a minor inconvenience since irritation can represent the first signal of an incoming inflammatory response and, for this reason, must not be underevaluated. Damage to the mucosae can also significantly affect organ functionality, because mucosae are highly vascularized tissues and their structural alteration can reduce the protective function toward penetration of infectious microorganisms or pollutants. Overdosing due to rapid drug absorption can also be a consequence of tissue lesion.

As already reported, skin irritation is one of the most common drawbacks of transdermal delivery systems. A mild redness indicating erythema formation can be due to the polymer adhering to the skin or to the additives. More severe inflammatory disorders, such as ester and oedema formation, are generally due to low molecular weight derivatives deriving from the polymer and device preparation processes: monomers, polymer fragments, catalysts, plasticizers, stabilizers, etc. These chemicals can, in fact, penetrate the skin and act as sensitizers or induce systemic toxicity as the residual monomer of polyvinyl chloride or polyacrylates. For this reason only medical grade materials must be used to prepare a TTS. Irritation and skin lesions can also be due to the physical abrasive structure of the device or to the stickiness of the adhesive layer. For all the above reasons *in vivo* tests are strictly recommended for the final TTS in order to establish skin compatibility.

References

Chasin, M., Langer, R. (eds.). 1990. *Biodegradable Polymers as Drug Delivery Systems, Drugs and the Pharmaceutical Sciences*, Volume 45, Marcel Dekker, Inc., New York.

Chien, Y.W. (ed.). 1987. *Transdermal Controlled Systemic Medications, Drugs and the Pharmaceutical Sciences*, Volume 31, Marcel Dekker, Inc., New York.

Dumitru, S. (ed.). 1994. *Polymeric Biomaterials*, Marcel Dekker, Inc., New York.

Guiot, P., Couvrier, P. (eds.). 1986. *Polymeric Nanoparticles and Microspheres*, CRC Press, Inc, Boca Raton.

Gurny, R., Jungiger, H.E., Peppas, N.A. (eds.). 1993. *Pulsatile Drug Delivery—Current Applications and Future Trends*, Volume 33, Wissenchatliche Verlagsgesellschaft mbH Stuttgart, Stuttgart.

Heller, J. 1993. Modulated release from drug delivery devices, *Crit. Rev. Ther. Drug Carrier Syst.* **10**(3), 253–305.

Langer, R. 1998. *Drug delivery and targeting*, Nature **392**, 6–10.

Park, K., Shalaby, W.S.W., Park, H. (eds.). 1993. *Biodegradable Hydrogels for Drug Delivery*, Technomic Publishing Co., Inc., Lancaster.

Robinson, J.R. (ed.). 1978. *Sustained and Controlled Release Drug Delivery Systems, Drugs and the Pharmaceutical Sciences*, Volume 6, Marcel Dekker, Inc., New York.

Silver, F., Doillon, C. (eds.). 1989. *Biocompatibility—Interactions of Biological and Implantable Materials, Polymers*, Volume 1, VCH Publishers, Inc., New York.

Tyle, P. (ed.). 1990. *Specialized Drug Delivery Systems—Manufacturing and Production Technology, Drugs and the Pharmaceutical Sciences*, Volume 41, Marcel Dekker, Inc., New York.

30

Gene Delivery as a New Therapeutic Approach

Libero Vitiello and Francesco M. Veronese

30.1. Introduction

Thanks to the increasingly fast pace of the human genome's characterization, the use of nucleic acids as therapeutic agents has become a very promising area of investigation in modern medicine. In fact, even though gene therapy was initially envisaged only for the treatment of genetic disorders, it has now become clear that also many acquired diseases, such as cancer, viral infections, vascular diseases, and neurodegenerative disorders, could be treated by the delivery of the appropriate genetic material.

The curative relevance of gene therapy is based on the greater specificity, potency, and versatility of action that specifically designed nucleic acids can have, compared to the traditional pharmaceutical or biopharmaceutical agents. For example, one of the most attractive features of gene-based therapy is that it holds the potential for a permanent correction of an otherwise chronic metabolic dysfunction, thereby eliminating the need for life-long drug administration. The therapeutic capacity of protein-encoding nucleic acids is not necessarily limited to the tissue(s) in which they are delivered. Therapeutic nucleic acids can exert their effect not only locally but also systemically, by exploiting the recipient cells as bioreactors to produce and release the desired therapeutic product. This latter approach can be carried out either totally *in vivo*, e.g., by injecting naked DNA into the muscle tissue, or *ex vivo*, by implanting in the patient

---

Libero Vitiello • Department of Biology, University of Padova, Via U. Bassi 58/B, 35121 Padova, Italy. **Francesco M. Veronese** • Department of Pharmaceutical Sciences, University of Padova, F. 35131 Padova, Italy.

Integrated Biomaterials Science, edited by R. Barbucci. Kluwer Academic/Plenum Publishers, New York, 2002.

small capsules of biocompatible materials containing genetically modified cells that produce the desired therapeutic product (Rizzuto *et al.*, 1999; Chang, 1997).

30.2. Different Kinds of Therapeutic Nucleic Acids

Therapeutic nucleic acids are not necessarily just coding sequences. In fact, in the last decade there have been many experimental gene-transfer approaches that employed other forms of DNA and RNA, or even hybrid molecules. For instance, DNA oligonucleotides can be used to prevent the transcription of specific genes in the treatment of tumors or viral infection and quite often the oligos contain sulfur instead of phosphorus in their backbone, in order to increase their half-life in the cytoplasm. For the same reason, increased resistance to DNAse, a new kind of oligonucleotides, in which the bases are linked by an aminoethyl–pseudopeptide bond, has recently been developed (Nielsen, 2000). Another possible application of oligonucleotides is to induce specific exon-skipping processes, in order to bypass a specific mutation present in the patient. RNA has also been widely experimented as a therapeutic nucleic acid, in the form of antisense molecules that interfere with the translation (or the maturation) of genes involved in the pathologic processes (Gibson, 1996). Another very promising application of RNA is in the form of ribozymes, i.e., particular single stranded RNA molecules that can specifically recognize and cleave mRNA, usually of viral or tumoral origin (Earnshaw and Gait, 1997). Finally, hybrid DNA/RNA molecules—"chimeraplasts"—have recently been designed to correct point mutations by site-specific recombination (Kren *et al.*, 1999).

Regardless of the kind of nucleic acid, any *in vivo* gene-based therapeutic approach has to face the challenge of delivering a sufficient amount of DNA or RNA in an active form to the right target, without inducing significant adverse effects in the patient. In other words, the delivery system must allow the genetic material to overcome a number of anatomic and metabolic barriers such as the RES, the serum with its opsonins and nucleases, the complement, and, most important, the crossing of the plasma membrane and nuclear envelope. The intrinsic features of nucleic acids—negatively charged, hydrophilic, often of high molecular weight, easily subjected to both chemical and enzymatic degradation—make their formulation difficult with the traditional techniques of drug delivery. The research toward the ideal gene-delivery vector has therefore followed two paths: the use of recombinant viruses and the development of artificial vectors.

30.3. Viral Vectors

In these systems the viral genome is altered in order to disable the pathogenic pathways and at the same time create the extra space needed to accommodate the exogenous DNA that has to be transduced. So far, many kinds of viral vectors have been developed, mainly from adenovirus and adeno associated virus, herpes virus, and several rctroviruses. All of them can be quite efficient in their gene-transfer activity (each for a given set of target tissues), given that they exploit a pathway of infection that has specifically evolved to deliver and express foreign genes in the host body.

Despite their efficiency, the use of viral vectors is still hampered by problems related to their immunogenicity and/or toxicity, as well as by the fact that many of them can accommodate only a limited amount of DNA. Last but not least, their production and purification from replication competent helper viruses (often necessary) is quite laborious and costly, especially with GMP standards.

30.4. Synthetic Vectors

Since the second half of the 1980s, there has been an extensive number of reports focusing on the design of DNA artificial delivery systems. In general, the approaches that have been proposed are based either on the use of cationic polymers (like, for instance, poly-L-lysine), or on the use of cationic lipids, or a combination of the two. Recently, the nomenclature of DNA-delivering complexes prepared in different ways has been standardized as polyplexes, lipoplexes, and lipopolyplexes, respectively (Felgner *et al.*, 1997) (Table 30.1). In all cases, the mechanism(s) of action of synthetic vectors are still not well characterized. At this time, it is generally accepted that complexes are internalized by cells mainly, if not exclusively, through an endocytic process and are targeted for degradation into the lysosomal compartment. In order to exert its effect, the therapeutic DNA must then escape from the endosomes into the cytoplasm and enter the nucleus (Figure 30.1). However, the molecular details of the single steps can vary among the different formulations and are presently the object of intense research.

An excellent and comprehensive description of synthetic vectors can be found in a recent book edited by Huang *et al.* (1999).

30.4.1. Polyplexes

Cationic polymers have a natural tendency to interact with the negatively charged DNA and are known to be able to condense plasmid

Table 30.1. Standardized Nomenclature of DNA-Delivering Complexes

Vector	Composition	Possible modifications	Main properties
Polyplexes	DNA plus cationic polymers (e.g., poly-L-lysine, PEI, synthetic peptides).	Targeting moieties like transferrin and galactosamine can be linked to the cationic polymer. Endosomal-releasing agents like adenovirus capsides can also be included.	Condensation of plasmid DNA with poly-cations generates toroidal particles of less than 100 nm in diameter. Polyplexes have been used both *in vitro* and *in vivo*, but some formulations are not serum-resistant.
Lipoplexes	DNA plus cationic lipids, formulated either as liposomes (unilamellar or multilamellar) or micelles. The liposomes can also contain a neutral lipid (usually DOPE or cholesterol) that plays an important role in destabilizing the membrane of the endosomes.	Targeting moieties can be included in the formulation, either separately or linked to PEG molecules that protrude from the lipid bilayer of the liposomes. The presence of PEG within the liposome bilayer also stabilizes the formulation and and prolongs its half-life *in vivo*.	The actual structure of lipoplexes varies according to the kind of lipid(s), method of preparation, and DNA/lipid ratio. In all cases, except for the encapsulated systems, the DNA is not enclosed within single vesicles. Rather, X-ray diffraction studies suggested a columnar, multilamellar structure. The size of the particles varies from 0.1 to 1 μm. Many formulations are serum-resistant and can be successfully used *in vivo*.
Lipopolyplexes	DNA is first precondensed with a poly-cationic polymer or protein (e.g., polylysine, protamine, histones) and then added to a cationic lipid component.	Same as lipoplexes; certain precondensing agents (e.g., synthetic peptides) can also contain *nls* signals.	Same as lipoplexes; DNA precondensation usually reduces the average size of the particles.

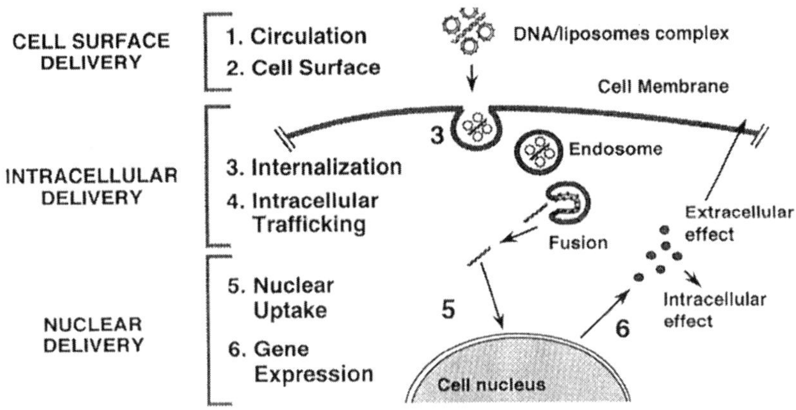

Figure 30.1. Schematic representation of the processes involved in lipid-mediated gene transfer by means of lipoplexes. Note that the structure of the DNA/liposome complexes depicted in the picture is not meant to represent the actual shape of lipoplexes (image kindly provided by INEX Pharmaceuticals, Inc).

molecules into a more compact, toroidal particle with a diameter of less than 100 nm. The first formulations used for gene transfer were based on poly-L-lysine, often conjugated to targeting molecules like transferrin or endosomal-release agents like adenovirus capside proteins (Wagner *et al.*, 1992). Such ternary systems (DNA/polylysine/targeting moiety) exhibited quite high levels of transfection *in vitro*, but mostly lost their efficiency in the presence of serum.

More recently, a different kind of cationic polymer, polyethylenimine, has yielded quite impressive results in terms of DNA delivery, both *in vitro* and *in vivo*. This kind of polymer is capable of delivering the DNA *per se*, that is, without the aid of any targeting or endosomal-releasing factor. In this regard, it has been proposed that its high buffering capability is responsible for the release of the transfected DNA from the endosomes, thanks to the so-called "proton-sponge" effect. In such a model, polyethylenimine would buffer the protons pumped into the endosomes for their acidification, thereby leading to the accumulation of water and, eventually, to the rupture of the vesicle (Boussif *et al.*, 1995).

30.4.2. Lipoplexes

Anionic liposomes have been used sporadically as DNA-delivery agents since the late 1970s, but it was only in 1987, with the publication of the first paper reporting the use of cationic liposomes as a transfection agent, that the idea of lipid-based vectors really took off (Felgner *et al.*, 1987). The vast majority of lipid formulations available today are indeed based on some kind of cationic lipid, either alone or in combination with a neutral colipid (DOPE or cholesterol). The lipidic moieties of the lipoplexes are usually preformulated either as LUV (large unilamellar vesicles), MLV (multilamellar vesicles), or micelles, and the DNA, in aqueous solution, is added just before use. In all cases, the result is a supramolecular aggregate, whose specific structure varies depending greatly on the specific cationic lipid and method of preparation. Several authors have attempted to describe the shape of lipoplexes by using electron microscopy, but the results have always been quite inconsistent among the various reports. The only cases in which the structure of the complexes was more clearly defined were those in which MLVs were actually prepared from a film of dried lipid and resuspended in an aqueous solution containing the DNA. With this method of preparation, a fraction of DNA, usually not much higher than 50%, is actually entrapped between the layers of the MLVs.

More recently, however, a new generation of lipoplexes, termed "encapsulated systems," has been designed, in which few plasmid DNA molecules are actually entrapped into a single lipid bilayer. These systems present several advantages over the conventional lipoplexes. For one, they are much smaller, less than 100 nm, and having a well-defined and homogeneous structure it is much easier to include in their formulation extra molecules on their external surface, like, for instance, targeting peptides. A particular kind of encapsulated system called single plasmid lipid particles (SPLP), carry PEG polymers on their external surface. The presence of PEG increases their stability in serum and also offers a suitable "dock" for conjugating additional functional moieties (Wheeler *et al.*, 1999).

PEG polymers can also be added to the cationic liposomes used to prepare standard lipoplexes, to improve their *in vivo* performance. As for SPLP, the presence of PEG provides the double benefit of increasing the stability of the suspensions, thereby allowing one to reach higher DNA concentrations per ml, as well as increasing the half-life of the complexes in the bloodstream, probably by inhibiting the opsonin coating of the particles. The protective hydrophilic shield created by PEG, however, has a relevant side effect: in the absence of specific targeting moieties it greatly decreases the endocytic uptake of the complexes. For this reason, the choice of the aliphatic "anchor" that links the PEG to the bilayer is of paramount relevance. A longer side chain will slow down the release of the PEG from the liposomes and will therefore provide a prolonged circulation time for the particles, but at the cost of low transfection efficiency. On the other hand, a shorter anchor, like, for instance, ceramide-C8, will generate a much shorter half-life but greater transfection efficiency.

30.4.3. Lipopolyplexes

The combination of the two formulations described above, polyplexes and lipoplexes, leads to lipopolyplexes, formulations in which the DNA is first precondensed with a cationic polymer (or a highly charged protein) and is then added to a suspension of cationic liposomes. Several compounds have been used so far in the precondensing step, the most common being polylysine, protamine, purified histones, and synthetic peptides. The precondensing step in general leads to a decrease in the size of the particles, which is known to be beneficial for *in vivo* applications, but there are also other advantages. For instance, it has been reported that polylysine precondensation increases the resistance of the complexes to the inhibitory action of serum (Vitiello *et al.*, 1996). Also, the use of histones or artificial peptides containing one or more *nls* (*n*uclear *l*ocalization *s*ignal) has been shown to increase the efficiency of the complexes. The idea behind this approach was obviously to improve the transfer of the DNA from the cytoplasm to the nucleus, a process that is known to be the main bottleneck for lipid-mediated transfection. However, given the fact that *nls* sequences are positively charged themselves, it was hard to determine which of the two factors—precondensation of the DNA and specific nuclear targeting—was contributing to the enhanced transfection efficiency. In this regard, a recent report has elegantly demonstrated that in order to obtain an actual nuclear localization effect one has to covalently link *nls* peptides to the plasmid DNA in a 1:1 (one peptide per plasmid) ratio (Zanta *et al.*, 1999).

30.5. Clinical Applications of Gene Transfer

The first gene therapy protocol involving a human patient dates back to 1990, when a child suffering from ADA deficiency was treated by transducing *ex vivo* its T lymphocytes with a modified retrovirus containing a functioning copy of the adenosine deaminase gene. Since then, almost 3500 patients have been enrolled worldwide in more than 500 different trials that used both viral and nonviral vectors. Among them, the viral vectors are the vast majority, almost 75%, while lipid-based vectors and naked DNA account for the 13% and 9%, respectively.* It is also interesting to note that the focus of researchers soon shifted from inherited diseases to cancer, whose treatment has been the object of most (~63%) of the trials carried out so far.

*http://www.wiley.co.uk/wileychi/genmed/clinical/

Despite such massive efforts, virtually all the trials, both terminated and ongoing, were either phase I or II and therefore no gene-based established cure exists as of now. This said, encouraging results have been reported by several groups; in particular, significant improvements of the clinical condition of patients affected by ADA deficiency, X-linked SCID, and familial hypercholesterolaemia were obtained following *ex vivo* transduction with retroviral vectors.* As for cancer protocols, partial remission of metastatic lesions was reported after intratumoral injection of lipid-based vectors.*

In conclusion, gene therapy is a field in its infancy, but there is little doubt that in the future it will become one of the most powerful therapeutic tools available to medical science.

References

Boussif, O., Lezoualc'h, F., Zanta, M.A., Mergny, M.D., Scherman, D., Demeneix, B., Behr, J.P. 1995. A versatile vector for gene and oligonucleotide transfer into cells in culture and in vivo: polyethylenimine, *Proc. Natl. Acad. Sci. USA* **92**, 7297–7301.

Chang, P.L. 1997. Microcapsules as bio-organs for somatic gene therapy, *Ann. NY Acad. Sci.* **831**, 461–473.

Earnshaw, D.J., Gait, M.J. 1997. Progress toward the structure and therapeutic use of the hairpin ribozyme, *Antisense Nucleic Acid Drug Dev.* **7**, 403–411.

Felgner, P.L., Barenholz, Y., Behr, J.P., Cheng, S.H., Cullis, P., Huang, L., Jessee, J.A., Seymour, L., Szoka, F., Thierry, A.R., Wagner, E., Wu, G. 1997. Nomenclature for synthetic gene delivery systems [editorial], *Hum. Gene Ther.* **8**, 511–512.

Felgner, P.L., Gadek, T.R., Holm, M., Roman, R., Chan, H.W., Wenz, M., Northrop, J.P., Ringold, G.M., Danielsen, M. 1987. Lipofection: a highly efficient, lipid-mediated DNA-transfection procedure.

Gibson, I. 1996. Antisense approaches to the gene therapy of cancer—"Recnac," *Cancer Metastasis Rev.* **15**, 287–299.

Huang, L., Hung, M.C., Wagner, E. (eds). 1999. *Nonviral Vectors for Gene Therapy*, Academic Press, San Diego.

Kren, B.T., Metz, R., Kumar, R., Steer, C.J. 1999. Gene repair using chimeric RNA/DNA oligonucleotides, *Semin. Liver Dis.* **19**, 93–104.

Nielsen, P.E. 2000. Peptide nucleic acids: on the road to new gene therapeutic drugs, *Pharmacol. Toxicol.* **86**, 3–7.

Rizzuto, G., Cappelletti, M., Maione, D., Savino, R., Lazzaro, D., Costa, P., Mathiesen, I., Cortese, R., Ciliberto, G., Laufer, R., La Monica, N., Fattori, E. 1999. Efficient and regulated erythropoietin production by naked DNA injection and muscle electroporation, *Proc. Natl. Acad. Sci. USA* **96**, 6417–6422.

Vitiello, L., Chonn, A., Wasserman, J.D., Duff, C., Worton, R.G. 1996. Condensation of plasmid DNA with polylysine improves liposome-mediated gene transfer into established and primary muscle cells, *Gene Ther.* **3**, 396–404.

*http://www.wiley.co.uk/wileychi/genmed/clinical/

Wagner, E., Zatloukal, K., Cotton, M., Kirlappos, H., Mechtler, K., Curiel, D.T., Birnstiel, M.L. 1992. Coupling of adenovirus to transferrin-polylysine/DNA complexes greatly enhances receptor-mediated gene delivery and expression of transfected genes, *Proc. Natl. Acad. Sci. USA* **89**, 6099–6103.

Wheeler, J.J., Palmer, L., Ossanlou, M., MacLachlan, I., Graham, R.W., Zhang, Y.P., Hope, M.J., Scherrer, P., Cullis, P.R. 1999. Stabilized plasmid-lipid particles: construction and characterization, *Gene Ther.* **6**, 271–281.

Zanta, M.A., Belguise Valladier, P., Behr, J.P. 1999. Gene delivery: a single nuclear localization signal peptide is sufficient to carry DNA to the cell nucleus, *Proc. Natl. Acad. Sci. USA* **96**, 91–96.

31

Tissue Engineering

Giovanni Abatangelo, Paola Brun, Marco Radice, Roberta Cortivo, and Marcus K.H. Auth

31.1. Introduction

Several definitions have been proposed to characterize and classify the research areas and main goals of tissue engineering. Some authors, going back to one of the earliest religious documents, the book of *Genesis*, noticed that the first example of tissue engineering was represented by the creation of Eve. A rib of the first donor of mankind, Adam, was used to reconstruct his Paradise-mate. From more recent history, there is evidence that ancient people, like Etruscans and Romans, used to prepare some artificial tissue substitutes, such as teeth, to replace damaged ones.

Apart from these interesting historical considerations, at the present time tissue engineering represents a very new frontier of modern science arising from the integration of knowledge about biology, chemistry, engineering, materials science, and medical disciplines. A formal definition of tissue engineering has been formulated in the following terms: "the application of the principles and methods of engineering and life sciences toward the fundamental understanding of structure–function relationships in normal and pathological mammalian tissues and the development of biological substitutes that restore, maintain, or improve tissue function" (Skalak and Fox, 1988).

It becomes clear that the main goal of tissue engineering is the reconstruction of living tissues to be used for the replacement of damaged

---

Giovanni Abatangelo, Paola Brun, Roberta Cortivo, and Marco Radice • Institute of Histology and Embryology, Faculty of Medicine, University of Padova, Viale G. Columbo, 3, 35121 Padova, Italy. **Marcus K.H. Auth** • Universitätskinderklinik, Abteilung Allgemeine Kinderheilkunde mit Schwerpunkt, Neuropädiatrie, Klinikum der Universitäts-Gesamthochschule, Essen, Germany.

Integrated Biomaterials Science, edited by R. Barbucci. Kluwer Academic/Plenum Publishers, New York, 2002.

or lost tissues/organs of living organisms. To achieve such an aim it is necessary to combine the use of cells together with natural or synthetic scaffolds in or onto which cells must develop, organize, and behave as if they are in their native tissue. Therefore, cells must receive signals from the environment to carry out in an ordered way proliferation and differentiation programs finalized to tissue/organ formation. With regard to these biological processes cells need a continuous flow of signals from the surrounding extracellular milieu that allow for specific genetic program fulfillment. In this respect, it is tempting to generalize that in all tissues cells live in contact with matrices or scaffolds. Since the early developmental phases, embryonic cells produce their own extracellular scaffolds, by secreting many types of substances into the surrounding space, according to a well-defined program of differentiation (Karin, 1992; Lin and Bissell, 1993; Adams and Watt, 1993; Damsky *et al.*, 1993; Vaino and Müller, 1997; Streuli *et al.*, 1993). The different spatial organization of these secreted molecules gives rise to a great variety of natural scaffolds in which cells continue to proliferate and to organize themselves in order to build tissues and to accomplish all their natural functions. The understanding of cell differentiation and functions means the understanding of cell/cell and cell/extracellular matrix communication mechanisms. In this respect, if one looks at the complexity of tissue extracellular matrix (ECM) components, one will not be surprised at the same great variety and complexity of existing interactions between cells and ECM, part of which have been recently characterized, thanks to the tremendous progress in cell and molecular biology. Unlike extracellular matrix that represents the result of a millenary natural evolution, artificial biomaterials do not have such a complex structure and chemical composition. In consequence of this, the information content of man-made devices is very low and the quantity of signals they can transmit to the cells is scarce. Bearing these basic considerations in mind our efforts in trying *in vitro* tissue reconstruction must be driven toward the exact knowledge of cell function on one hand, and, on the other hand, toward the knowledge of interactions and signals that cells must receive from the environment to behave as in natural tissues. We know that ECM plays an instructive role for cellular activities and that cells possess on their surface receptors to respond to extracellular signals. As soon as ligand–receptor interaction is established, the biochemical machinery involved in the control of gene expression starts.

To understand the mechanisms by which ECM can regulate cell behavior, it is essential to take into account tissue extracellular matrix composition, cell surface receptors that recognize the signals, and the transduction system used by cells to transmit information from cell surface to the intracellular transcriptional apparatuses. The understanding of these fundamental processes can help researchers in the choice of appropriate natural or artificial biomaterials on or into which to seed either undifferentiated or specialized cells.

Apart from the biochemical interactions between ECM and cells, another interesting aspect of the environmental influence on development, maintenance and tissue remodeling is represented by the mechanical stimuli that can affect cell behavior. The importance of mechanical forces is particularly evident in tissues such as bone, cartilage, blood vessels, tendons, and muscles, where the physical stimuli, such as mechanical loading, deformation, pressure, and fluid flow, are transduced into electrical or biochemical messages. This process has been defined as mechanotransduction and represents a new interesting area of multidisciplinary research applied to tissue engineering (see Gooch *et al.*, 1998).

To complete this provisional list of the main regulatory mechanisms involved in tissue/organ development and differentiation, growth factors (GF) and cell–cell interactions must be taken into account. Growth factors interact either directly with cell receptors as free substances or after binding to the extracellular matrix molecules. In the latter case, the ECM may function as a local reservoir of GF that can be available for cells even if growth factor production has ceased. In addition, the ECM-bound growth factors are degraded more slowly than in free form (Klagsbrun, 1990) or, in some cases, are inactive (Yamaguchi *et al.*, 1990; Raines *et al.*, 1992). Lastly, some ECM protein share similar sequences with growth factors and therefore possess intrinsic growth factor activity (Engel, 1989; Argraves *et al.*, 1990; Maslen *et al.*, 1991; Ferns *et al.*, 1992). From these observations it is clear that growth factors and ECM components can create a particular environment that influences biological activities of cells, mainly proliferation and differentiation. Cell–cell interactions are also important in regulating cell expression, as demonstrated by several differentiating processes, such as *in vitro* culture systems of rat mammary epithelial cells and human keratinocytes. When mammary rat epithelial cells are cultured on plastic in secondary culture, they form a monolayer and are unable to produce the "late" milk protein WAP (whey acidic protein). The production of this class of milk protein involves a complex mechanism of cell/cell and cell/ECM contacts. In fact, when dissociated cells are cultured on basement membrane extracts (Lin and Bissell, 1993), WAP is not expressed by single or two-cell clusters, while the formation of multicellular structure with closed lumen is required. The regulation of keratinocyte function represents another example of how cell/cell contacts in association with cell/ECM interactions are important to avoid keratinocyte terminal differentiation. Basal epidermal cells in contact either each other or with the basal lamina do not express involucrin, a marker of later stages of differentiation, while in suspension culture these cells lose their contacts and express involucrin, the major precursor of the cornified envelope (Green, 1977; Adams and Watt, 1989).

The knowledge of the main existing relationships among cells, extracellular environment, growth factors, and hormones, physical stimuli, may help in the strategy for the development of scaffolds designed for tissue engineering. Ideally, a scaffold capable of inducing tissue reconstruction should provide a temporary guide for cells growing in it and create an environment that allows cells, under appropriate culture conditions, to accomplish their differentiation programs, that is tissue building, as the artificial framework disappears.

Lastly, in this introductory note it is worth remarking that tissue engineering has received in the last two decades a great impetus from increasing dramatic clinical needs of organ and tissue transplants. It is well known that many tissue defects arising from trauma and diseases or from congenital abnormalities can be repaired only by transferring healthy tissues obtained from donors to the injured sites. Moreover, organ failure represents the major cause of illness and death. Heart, kidney, lung, liver, and pancreas are the organs that can be surgically substituted by a transplant of new organs available from donors. Unfortunately, while the demand for organs to be transplanted is continuously increasing, there are many problems arising from these life-saving treatments that make them unavailable for the majority of the waiting list patients. Donor scarcity, technical difficulties, intensive postsurgical care, and the high cost represent serious limiting factors that have encouraged and pushed scientists toward the search for bioartificial organs as well as for creating scaffolds to be implanted into the body either without or with cells.

In the next sections only the basic aspects of cell culture related to the *in vitro* tissue engineering will be considered.

31.2. Cell Culture and *In Vitro* Tissue Development

The fundamentals of tissue engineering, as already mentioned in the Introduction, are essentially based on knowledge of cell/tissue physiology and structure. Tissues exist as three-dimensional structures formed by cells and the surrounding extracellular scaffold (Gumbiner, 1996). Cells can be completely surrounded by ECM, as in the case of chondrocytes, or may face ECM only on one side. Epithelial and endothelial cells belong to this last category. In some stratified epithelia, only the basal layers are in contact with ECM, while in the upper cell layers no ECM can be detected. As already mentioned, cell–cell and cell–ECM contacts play a role in regulating cell phenotype and differentiation. The mechanisms by which these contacts are involved in such a regulatory function remained largely unknown until recently, when a sufficient amount of data on ECM composition, cell-binding molecules, transmembrane receptors, signal transduction mechanisms, growth factors, hormones, and ion channel structures were available. If the goal of tissue engineering is, in an ultimate analysis, the imitation of natural tissues, all this mass of information will help researchers in developing materials, templates, and scaffolds for *in vitro* reconstruction of tissues.

31.2.1. ECM Composition

The extracellular matrix is composed of a great variety of molecules and includes collagen family, elastic fibers, glycosaminoglycans and proteoglycans, and adhesive glycoproteins. The different combination, immobilization, and spatial organization of these secreted substances give rise to different types of scaffolds that characterize the different body tissues and organs.

Collagens. Collagen is the most abundant protein in the vertebrate body which constitutes a heterogeneous class of proteins that shares some similarities, such as triple helical domains and some characteristic amino acid repeat units along the molecular backbone in which glycine is present at every third amino acid (Gly-Xaa-Yaa). Up to now about 20 different collagens have been characterized which exhibit different mechanical and functional properties. Some collagens are specific for a given tissue, such as type II collagen, which is found only in cartilage. Types I, II, and III are the most abundant collagens of the human body that form fibrils responsible for the tensile strength of the tissue. Other collagens, such as types IV, VII, IX, X, and XII are found associated with collagen fibrils or organized in networks as in basal laminae. In addition to mechanical and structural functions, collagens play an important role in determining cell attachment and spreading. In consequence of these properties, collagens influence cell differentiation and movement. With regard to the role collagen can play in tissue engineering techniques, it must be said that in various cell culture systems the coating of the plastic surface of culture plates with collagen or collagen-derived products (gelatin) is essential to promote cell adhesion and proliferation, such as in the case of endothelial cell and hepatocyte cultures. Cell adhesion is specifically mediated by the presence of cell surface receptors that bind either directly to collagen or via interactive glycoproteins (fibronectin, laminin, etc). Moreover, cross-linking of collagens with chemical agents such as formaldehyde or glutaraldehyde allows the formation of thermoset materials that can be molded in various shapes to obtain seminatural scaffolds useful for tissue engineering and cell culture.

Glycosaminoglycans and Proteoglycans. Glycosaminoglycans (GAG) are linear polysaccharides formed by repeating disaccharide units that may contain sulfate groups. The most common GAGs are chondroitins, keratans, and dermatans, which are sulfated, and hyaluronan, which is not. Another class, the heparans, are mainly associated with cells and basement membranes. With the exception of hyaluronan, all GAGs can be associated to a protein backbone and give rise to the so-called proteoglycans. Cartilage aggrecans are well characterized large proteoglycans whose structure consists of a linear polypeptide on which several chondroitinsulfate (CS) and keratansulfate (KS) molecules are covalently attached. These aggrecans are, in turn, assembled in large aggregates by means of specific binding sites of their core protein to hyaluronan. In this case a single molecule of hyaluronan is able to link in a noncovalently way several aggrecan molecules to form huge water-containing dominions. The swelling pressure caused by these aggregates on the collagen network allows cartilage tissue to withstand compression generated during the joint movement. Similarly, in other tissue, such as skin, proteoglycans in associations with other structural molecules form specific complexes responsible for hydration and spatial organization of ECM. Proteoglycans are also present on a cell surface and act there as receptors by binding to collagens, fibronectin, and trombospondin, and to some growth factors.

Among the glycosaminoglycans, hyaluronan represents a unique nonsulfated polysaccharide that can exist in free form, with no covalently bound protein. It is present in all living organisms and plays an important role in many biological processes, such as matrix structure, water balance, lubrication, cell movement, and differentiation. During embryonic development hyaluronan represents the major constituent of the early extracellular matrix, being substituted during the late phases of the development by other structural ECM components.

Due to the above-mentioned biological properties, proteoglycans and glycosaminoglycans are often used, in association with other ECM molecules such as collagen, to create supporting biomaterials to be employed in tissue engineering (Yannas *et al.*, 1980; Murphy *et al.*, 1990; Orgill and Yannas, 1997). Recently, chemical modification (deacetylation, desulfatation, esterification) of some GAG molecules has made possible the production of new classes of biomaterials suitable for cell culture and *in vitro* tissue reconstruction. Hyaluronan has also been modified by esterification of the carboxyl groups along the backbone with aliphatic or aromatic alcohols. This modification lowers the water solubility of the molecule and make possible the manufacture of various devices, such as spun fibers, woven and nonwoven textiles, films, etc. (Giusti and Callegaro, 1994). These biomaterials can be used both for soft tissue augmentation and as scaffolds for cell culture and tissue engineering.

Adhesive Glycoproteins. This class of ECM molecules includes interactive glycoproteins (proteins with sugar chains attached to them) that exist in several variant forms (family of closely related peptides) and possess multiple binding domains capable of binding collagen and proteoglycans, as well as binding to the cell surface. The binding domains possess specific amino acid sequences that interact with cell surface receptors and serve as adhesion recognition signals. Fibronectin, laminin, vitronectin, thrombospondin, tenascin, and some other glycoproteins are members of this class of extracellular matrix molecules.

a. Fibronectin. Fibronectin is formed by two similar peptides linked at one end by a disulfide bond. There are variant forms of fibronectin which arise from alternative splicing in its mRNA precursor. Along the backbone of the molecule are present multiple RGD (Arg-Gly-Asp), RGDS (Arg-Gly-Asp-Ser), LDV (Leu-Asp-Va-), and REDV (Arg-Glu-Asp-Val) sequences that are responsible for cell binding, while other domains represent binding sites for other ECM molecules such as collagens, fibrin, heparan sulfate, etc. Fibronectin plays an important role in cell attachment to the substrate, in cell movement, and differentiation. Due to its broad binding properties fibronectin is widely used in cell culture systems, in order to favor cell adhesion and spreading. Fibronectin acts also as a negative regulatory signal for preventing involucrin expression by keratinocytes, thus avoiding their terminal differentiation.

b. Laminin. Laminin is found mainly associated with basement membranes. It consists of three chains that form a cross-shaped structure. Laminin exists in different forms, all of which are the product of closely related genes. These interactive proteins are characterized by high binding affinity for cell surface as well as for heparin and type IV collagen. Laminin-5 isoform is typically found associated to the basement membrane. RGD sequences are also present along the backbone of the molecule chains together with other specific sequences, such as PDSGR, YIGSR, and IKVAV sequences that are able to recognize and bind to cell-surface receptors. Interestingly, laminins possess some growth factor-like sequences that become available to cells only upon degradation. These domains are EGF-like peptides and can stimulate cell proliferation and differentiation. Given its high cell binding affinity, laminin alone or in combination with other ECM molecules is widely used to coat cell culture dishes and plates in order that cell attachment and spreading can be enhanced.

c. Thrombospondin. Activated platelets and several cells can produce and release the interactive glycoprotein called thrombospondin. This is a trimeric glycoprotein whose backbone is provided with cell-binding domains, among which an RGD sequence is also present. Thrombospondin has binding sites for collagens, and laminin, as well for fibrinogen. This interactive glycoprotein can be found in ECM associated with fibronectin or with heparan sulfate proteoglycan. Depending on cell type, thrombospondin can either facilitate or inhibit cell attachment and spreading.

d. Vitronectin. This adhesive glycoprotein, also known as S-protein, can be found, like fibronectin, in soluble form in blood, and in fibrillar form in the ECM of several tissues. Again, in this molecule RGD sequences are present and recognize and bind to integrin receptors of the cell surface. Vitronectin also binds to collagens, heparin, and plasminogen activator inhibitor. All these binding properties make this molecule a good candidate for tissue remodeling and cell attachment and migration.

To the above-mentioned adhesive glycoproteins that are the most common and well characterized ones, other molecules with similar biological functions must be added. Tenascin, for example, is another important glycoprotein formed by six oligomer structural units that contain several EGF and fibronectin repeats. The von Willebrand factor (vWf) is a large glycoprotein found in the vascular ECM and plays an important role in platelet adhesion and activation. Other glycoproteins of ECM have RGD sequences involved in cell recognition, such as chondronectin, bone sialoprotein, osteospontin, and fibrillin. Given the heterogeneous and complex composition of ECM, it is not surprising that in future other components will be added to this interesting family of interactive glycoproteins.

Elastic Fibers. The elastic fibers are composed by an amorphous protein, elastin, whose structural characteristic is elasticity. Arterial walls, dermis, and lungs are the sites where a large quantity of elastic fibers can be found. With regard to tissue engineering and cell culture systems, up to now elastin has not received much attention and for this reason we encourage the reader to consult the specific literature for more detailed and exhaustive information on this ECM molecule. Only very recently, however, have some repeat peptide units of elastin been obtained by recombinant techniques (McPherson *et al.*, 1992). Cross-linking of these peptides by gamma irradiation give rise to hydrogels which can be used as substrate for tissue reconstruction.

31.2.2. ECM Receptors

Cell adhesion is crucial for tissue formation and integrity. For tissue engineering strategies it is essential to know how cells can interact with ECM and transduce the information received by the extracellular molecules into an intracellular event. As mentioned in previous paragraphs, the identification of cell binding sites within extracellular molecules is a key step toward identifying the mechanisms of cell–ECM interactions. Cell surfaces possess two kind of receptors: nonintegrin and integrin receptors.

a. Nonintegrin Receptors. Proteoglycans, CD36, and some laminin-binding proteins belong to this class of cell surface receptors. The most studied, however, are the cell surface proteoglycans syndecan and CD44. Syndecan is a transmembrane proteoglycan comprising a cytoplasmic domain, a hydrophobic membrane region, and an extracellular domain. The glycosaminoglycan side chains are represented by chondroitin sulfate and heparan sulfate. Syndecan receptors are a family of related proteoglycans which differ mainly in the extracellular domain GAG composition. These cell surface receptors, in addition to binding collagens, fibronectin, and thrombospondin, bind bFGF (Bernfield and Sanderson, 1990). The colocalization to the cell surface of both growth factors and ECM molecules makes syndecan a unique molecule capable of assembling signaling complexes, probably in combination with other receptors. During *in vivo* tissue development, the expression pattern of syndecan follows morphogenetic rather than histological boundaries. For this reason, syndecan expression during the *in vitro* development of tissues may represent for cell biologists a particular marker of differentiation and development.

CD44 is a cell surface glycoprotein which carries N- and O- liked sugars and GAG side chains. Alternative splicing and posttransductional modifications give rise to different tissue specific forms. The binding of CD44 to type I and IV collagens and hyaluronan play a vital role in cell adhesion and movement (Hardingham and Forsang, 1992).

b. Integrins. Integrins represent a large group of a glycoprotein family, the structure of which consists of a heterodimeric noncovalent association of α and β subunits. The family has been classified into two subgroups according to the identity of the β subunit to which different α subunits combine to give rise to several specific receptors (Hynes, 1992). However, the possibility that some α subunits can combine with several β subunits adds a further level of complexity to the binding capacity of these cell surface receptors. Each of the major ECM components can be recognized by one or more integrins, but the significance of this apparent redundancy is not clear at present. The expression of proper receptors during *in vitro* development of tissues may indicate that the environmental conditions in which cell are cultivated is permissive for cell differentiation. An example is represented by cultured human keratinocytes that are able to express $\beta 1$ and $\beta 4$ integrin subunits when in contact with a dermal-like support (Zacchi *et al.*, 1998). Like *in vivo, in vitro* multipotent cells can also be induced to differentiate along different lineage by a variety of agents that are able to induce specific expression of integrins (Watt, 1991). With regard to tissue engineering, it may be possible to induce specific integrin expression by altering the extracellular milieu in order to guide cultured cells toward specific phenotype expression. Finally, differentiation is not only associated with changes in integrin expression, but also with down-regulation mechanisms of receptor function, probably related to changes in receptor conformation.

31.2.3. Signal Transduction

ECM molecules that interact with a cell surface must induce gene activation in order to enable cells to express specific gene products which, in turn, are responsible for cell and tissue specialized functions. Among the various cell receptors, integrins have been indicated as the main candidates able to transduce signals from the external space to the inner cell compartments, down to the nucleus. The interaction of integrins with ECM molecules requires both subunits and the specific α/β pairing in order to have the binding of the ligand. While β subunits seem to have a nonspecific role in ligand binding activity, α subunits on the contrary confer high specificity of signal transduction (Hemler, 1990). Molecular biology studies have demonstrated that the β_1 cytoplasmic domain of integrins plays an important role in cytoskeletal association. As soon as ECM molecules bind to their specific integrin or nonintegrin receptors, a change in the cytoplasmic domain of the receptor occurs, which associates with cytoskeleton at the focal adhesion sites. Consequently, an assembly of the focal contact proteins with other intercellular components, such as phosphorylated proteins, happens. These changes can promote cytoskeleton rearrangement, which may determine at nuclear level differential interaction of chromatin and nuclear matrix. The dynamic association of integrin receptors with the actin cytoskeleton may also induce changes in cell shape, which in turn alter the ability of cells to proliferate or differentiate. A great amount of work, however, has been done in this field and the reader is referred to some reviews (Stoker *et al.*, 1990; Damsky and Werb, 1992). Briefly, downstream of the binding of ECM molecules to integrins the following steps may be included: clustering of the receptors, activation of intracellular protein kinases and subsequent phosphorylation of cytoskeleton and other associated proteins, and transmission of the signals generated by receptor occupancy to the transcriptional machinery in the nucleus. Growth factors and hormones act in concert with ECM, even though the regulation of gene expression by ECM has a mechanism distinct from those known for soluble factors.

If we consider that the ultimate goal of a cell culturist is to provide cells with appropriate environmental scaffolds and supports, then it is reasonable to think that the utilization of ECM molecules and suitable growth factors can facilitate the development of artificial tissues.

31.2.4. Testing Biomaterials and New Strategies for *In Vitro* Tissue Culture

The increased amount of knowledge obtained from cell and molecular biology in the field of cell–substrate interactions have made possible progress in the preparation of both synthetic and natural biomaterials. From historical considerations, it must be said that wound management products research started the era of development of biomaterials. In 1816 the first patent was presented to consider the adoption of linteum-based dressings as wound-covering materials in hospitals in the U.K. Oakum fiber based devices were other dressing materials proposed during the American Civil War (1870). Almost at the same time, cotton wool, a material used only as a packing material for jewels, was made more absorbent by bleaching. This material was the forerunner for today's "gauze and cotton tissue." All these materials belong to the passive dressing group whose function is mainly absorption. Recently other substances, such as cellulose and viscose, have been used either alone or in combination with cotton to improve the absorption of wound fluids. Given the enhanced adhesion properties of these materials when in contact with a wound surface, their use has been discouraged recently. In 1979 the performance parameters of an ideal wound covering material were specified (Turner, 1979) and the search for new interactive materials started. The first advancement toward interactive wound products was represented by the development of wound dressing with high absorption capacity and low adherence. Impregnated dressings, like paraffin gauzes, deodorizing and polymeric dressings, polymeric films and foams, hydrogels, and hydrocolloids were the new interactive materials that matched some of the parameters of an ideal wound dressing, such as fluid absorbency, gas permeability, maintenance of high humidity at the wound site, easy removal without trauma, and protection against secondary infections (for review see Turner, 1997). Following the development of interactive materials the "bioactive" concept arose from experimental evidence that some substance (tissue extracts) could stimulate by topical application the cellular and acellular processes of wound repair. These substances have to be considered "bioactive," since they produce a localized stimulation of the events in tissue repair. Among the various bioactive substances, the ECM components have received particular attention such as glycosaminoglycans (hyaluronan, chondroitin sulfate, dermatan sulfate), collagen and noncollagenic proteins (fibronectin, laminin, etc.), given their ability to influence the wound microenvironment. Also, polymeric materials such as pectins, alginates, and chitosan have been studied since they can act as pro-oxidants. Hydrogels and hydrocolloids have been shown to possess antioxidant activity which may contribute to both the rate of healing and repair of soft tissues in patients whose antioxidant defenses are compromised.

More recently, bioactive materials have been utilized as supporting scaffolds for *in vitro* tissue reconstruction and cell cultures. The first biomaterials were obtained from natural sources, such as ECM components. Advances in polymer chemistry have also made possible the generation of biomedical polymers such as polyethylene, polytetrafluoroethylene, polymethacrylate, polyamides, and polyurethanes. All these synthetic polymers have been used successfully in tissue engineering, even though they are not bioerodible and bioresorbable and, consequently, when implanted they remain as an integral part of the body tissues. The need to obtain temporary resorbable scaffolds has encouraged the search for hydrolyzable polymers of either natural or synthetic origin.

The main polymers of natural origin used for tissue engineering are proteins such as collagens, albumin, fibrin, fibronectin, and glycosaminoglycans, and also polysaccharides, such as hyaluronan, chondroitin sulfate, keratan sulfate, and chitin. Chemical modification of these natural substances or copolymerization give rise to swellable hydrogels which can be used as tissue substitutes as well as cell delivery scaffolds. Association of collagens with glycosaminoglycans (Orgill and Yannas, 1997) has made possible the preparation of dermal-like tissue substitute. Among GAGs, hyaluronan has been chemically modified by the esterification of its carboxyl groups with different kind of alcohols. With such a chemical modification, a water-insoluble polymer is obtained that can be processed to produce several biomaterial devices useful for tissue engineering, such as membranes, gauzes, woven and nonwoven meshes, and tubes. The extent of molecular modification modulates the soluble and viscous nature of hyaluronan in aqueous solutions and it has been found that the higher the percentage of esterification of hyaluronan, the lower its solubility in water (Barbucci *et al.*, 1993). The total benzyl ester of hyaluronan has been successfully used in both the nonwoven and membrane forms as scaffolds for cell cultures and *in vitro* tissue reconstruction (Andreassi *et al.*, 1991; Zacchi *et al.*, 1998; Brun *et al.*, 2000).

Acidic polysaccharides, such as carboxymethylcellulose, carboxymethylchitin, and carboxymethyl starch, have also been chemically modified in order to obtain unique biomaterials (for a review see Sawhney and Drumheller, 1998) that can be used as drug delivery or cell carriers.

In addition to the above-mentioned natural substances, hydrolyzable synthetic polymers were recognized as suitable biomaterial candidates. The family of poly-α-hydroxyacids, mainly polylactic (PLA) and polyglycolic acids (PGA), have been extensively studied and used in tissue engineering as scaffolds for cell cultures and tissue engineering (Widmer and Mikos, 1998). Polymers and copolymers can be obtained with these hydroxyacids.

Polycarbonates as well as polydioxanones, polyphosphazones, and polyanhydrides can also be processed to obtain various biomaterials. Hydrogels constitute another group of synthetic polymers that have an extended history in the medical and pharmaceutical field (Sawhney and Drumheller, 1998).

The above-reported short list of natural and synthetic polymers gives some idea about the large variety and possible value of these substances being used either as medical devices or as scaffolds in tissue engineering research. From a general point of view, it must be said that the main parameter to be taken into account for biological evaluation of polymeric scaffolds is the information content these biomaterials possess. It is well established from experimental evidence that many cell types exhibit good biological activities, such as proliferation, adhesion, and movement, when cultured on ECM proteins rather than on plastic surfaces. This physiological behavior depends on the signal that cells receive from the environment and consequently it turns out that synthetic materials cannot transmit a great amount of signals since their simple chemical components have a low content of information. From this consideration it is reasonable to think that conjugation of bioactive substances to synthetic polymers could improve the biological properties of the resulting biomaterials. Many biomedical polymers possess reactive functional groups that can be utilized to attach natural substances such as structural ECM peptides (collagen, fibronectin, laminin, etc.), growth factors, enzymes, or carbohydrates (Drumheller and Hubbell, 1995). Also functional groups, such as lysine, aspartic acid, and glycine, may be attached to the backbone of some synthetic polymers, to change their characteristics at the molecular level.

In conclusion, the passive or interactive materials whose traditional role was of support, after suitable chemical modification, can be changed into bioactive materials that can exhibit biological interactions within cells. Therefore, these scaffolds can be used as tissue substitutes to replace tissue defects either with or without cells. In the first case they should guide and facilitate the ingrowth of surrounding tissue cells. In the second case the scaffolds are used as substrate for cell culture in order to obtain an *in vitro* reconstructed tissue to be transplanted.

31.2.5. Association of Gene Therapy to Tissue Engineering

The possibility of introducing genes in cells represents a powerful tool to allow a cell to express new functions or enhance existing cellular activities. This technology was developed originally for the treatment of inherited diseases and now its use has been proposed also for the therapy of several acquired diseases such as cancer, infections, and degenerative and autoimmune diseases. Gene transfer technology can be applied successfully to tissue engineering whose main goal is to create substitutes to replace damaged tissues or organs. In this case, the presence of genetically modified cells can aid in the performance of a tissue substitute.

Genes can be transferred to cells either *in vitro* or *in vivo*. In the first case a biopsy of the desired tissue is needed and its cells must be cultured and expanded. Then cells can be genetically modified and returned to the patient. The first experiments to show the feasibility of this *ex vivo* gene therapy utilized bone marrow stem cells obtained from mice, while lymphocytes were used for the first clinical trial in man (Rosemberg, 1992). Other cells have been used for gene transfer, such as keratinocytes, fibroblasts, endothelial cells, chondrocytes, and hepatocytes. In these cases either autologous cells can be used (obtained from the same patient who will be treated) or allogeneic ones (from donors). In some instances cells can be xenogeneic, that is, obtained from different species.

With regard to gene transfer technology, different techniques can be adopted that include recombinant retroviruses and adenoviruses, DNA–liposome complexes, and gene guns with DNA-coated particles (for a review see Morgan and Yarmush, 1998). Depending on the methods adopted it is possible to obtain permanent or temporary genetic modification. In permanent genetic modification the transferred genes are replicated when a cell divides, while in temporary genetic modification genes are not replicated and will persist and be expressed by the cell for a limited time. The choice of technique depends on the therapeutic application that is needed to treat a disease.

As already mentioned gene transfer technology can be associated with tissue engineering. Up to now gene therapy has been combined with tissue engineering of skin, the cardiovascular system, the muscoloskeletal system, and in tissue engineering for diabetes and for nervous tissue.

In vitro reconstructed epidermis is widely used to correct acquired skin defects such as burns, chronic ulcers, and surgical wounds. The possibility of using genetically modified keratinocytes in tissue engineering of epidermis may offer several therapeutic benefits not only for the treatment of skin associated lesions, but also to correct impaired functions of other tissues/organs. Human keratinocytes were genetically modified by transferring genes encoding human growth hormone (hGH) (Morgan *et al.*, 1987) or clotting factor IX (Gerrard *et al.*, 1993). In this way gene therapy associated to tissue engineering may create an ectopic site of functional cells which secrete soluble substance that diffuses into the systemic circulation of grafted animals. Modification of keratinocytes with genes encoding wound healing factors may allow these cells to express a high level of PDGF (Eming *et al.*, 1995) or insulin-like growth factor (IGF) (Eming *et al.*, 1996). The overexpression of these factors by transplanted cells stimulates the local wound healing processes, thus avoiding the administration of large quantities of recombinant growth factors.

Fibroblasts of the dermis can also be manipulated in order to make them express several factors such as transferrin, factor IX, factor VII, and erythropoietin (Morgan and Yarmush, 1998). When implanted in the body they form an ectopic tissue that secretes soluble factors in the systemic circulation.

Endothelial cells have been genetically modified in order to overexpress antithrombotic enzymes such as tissue plasminogen activator (Dichek *et al.*, 1996). Modified cells, seeded onto luminal surfaces of artificial vessels, are able to reduce the thrombogenicity of the prostheses.

It is well known from the literature that cartilage has poor regenerating capacity when damaged in consequence of various diseases such as trauma, osteoarthritis, and rheumatoid arthritis. Cultured chondrocytes represent a new option for the treatment of cartilage defects (Brittberg *et al.*, 1994a). Polymeric matrices made up of hyaluronan derivatives or synthetic polymers (PLA, PGA) can also be utilized as scaffolds for *in vitro* reconstruction of cartilage to be used as tissue substitute. Genetically modified chondrocytes have been shown to enhance the therapeutic efficacy of these transplantable cells. Human chondrocytes were modified by transferring genes encoding interleukin-1 receptor antagonist (IL-1RA) (Baragi *et al.*, 1995) that blocks interleukin-1 induced degradation activity. When seeded onto the surface of osteoarthritic cartilage in organ culture, transformed chondrocytes were able to protect cartilage from IL-1 induced matrix degradation.

Another example of how tissue engineering can be utilized to treat some degenerative diseases is represented by nervous tissue. An example is represented by Parkinson's disease in which there is a deficiency of neurotransmitter dopamine production. In such cases it is possible to use genetically modified fibroblasts in which transferred genes encode tyrosine hydroxylase that converts tyrosine to L-dopa (Suhr and Gage, 1993). When implanted in rats in which an experimental model of Parkinson's disease was induced, a significant improvement was detected.

From the above-reported examples on gene therapy it is reasonable to think that application of this technology to tissue engineering may represent further progress in the performance of tissue/organ substitutes.

31.3. Artificial Skin

The skin is the largest organ of the mammalian body. The function of the skin resides, essentially, in the protection of the organism from the external environment by helping to maintain temperature homeostasis, antimicrobial control, and social communication.

The skin is composed of four different tissues: epidermis, dermis, basement membrane, and subcutis. The epidermis is the tissue in direct contact with the external environment and consists of epithelial cells, known as keratinocytes, forming a 10-layer-thick fragile sheet (around 0.1 mm). The dermis is a thicker tissue made essentially of a loose array of fibroblasts (mesenchymal cells) and vasculature (endothelial cells) forming an approximately 2–5-mm-thick connective tissue sustaining the overlaid epidermis which is separated from the dermis by a 20-nm-thick multilayered membrane (basement membrane). Finally, the subcutis is a 0.4–4-mm-thick tissue almost composed of fat cells (adipocytes) underneath the dermis. Skin is also composed of a series of appendages known as adnexa, such as hair follicles, sweat glands, and sebaceous glands generally embedded in the dermis.

Because the skin serves as a protective barrier against the outside world, any break in it must be rapidly and efficiently amended. The physiological mechanism which coordinates the ordered repair of cutaneous tissues is generally referred to as wound healing and consists in a well-orchestrated series of temporary overlapping actions involving different cell and biochemical types (Martin, 1997).

In general, by taking into account the time of healing, cutaneous lesions can be divided into two large categories, acute and chronic lesions. The former refers to a group of pathologies which has been provoked by a trauma such as burns or accidents, while the latter refers to permanent, and often unsolved, lesions such as ulcers or genetic diseases. In both cases, an impairment of the healing process is at the basis of the poor clinical result which affects the patient for the rest of its life.

From a surgical point of view, pathologies such as those described above still represent a challenge for the clinician who has to deal, in almost all cases, with a problem related to tissue loss. Historically, the treatment of skin loss has traditionally focused on the design of a temporary wound closure (Yannas, 1995). Attempts to cover wounds and severe burns have been reported from historical sources at least as far back as 1500 B.C., and since then, a very large number of temporary wound dressings have been designed. These include membranes or sheets fabricated from natural and synthetic polymers, skin grafts from human cadavers (homografts, or allografts), and skin grafts from animals (heterografts, or xenografts).

Considering acellular coverage, it has to be emphasized that this represents only temporary dressing, since it does not generally integrate with the cutaneous tissues. Thus, either surgical removal or natural rejection occurs within a short term. Several drawbacks have been demonstrated on humans using synthetic polymers, such as wound contamination and delay in natural remodeling. Similarly, when using natural or natural-derived coverage (devitalized homologous or heterologous skin), the immunogenic issue is the major limiting factor in the application of such a device.

Thus, it is now evident that the ideal wound coverage for cutaneous lesions is an autologous graft which provides both full immunocompatibility and permanent functionality, since it is completely integrated over time. Although possible, the technique is not always available to the surgeon, for example in case of large deep burns. In addition, problems such as donor site morbidity and morbility may add unwanted complications to the pathology treated. Therefore, a series of compromises have arisen using a combination of self and nonself devices.

However, things suddenly changed when in 1952 it was demonstrated that keratinocytes obtained from skin specimens treated with trypsin maintained viability (Billingham and Reynolds, 1952). Further research aimed at the culture of human keratinocytes culminated in the work by Rheinwald and Green (1975), who determined the fundamental procedure for keratinocyte growth *in vitro*. Other significant advances followed this first successful experiment, related mostly to triming the best culture conditions (Leigh and Watt, 1994), but most important was the concept to bring cultured human cells from the laboratory bench to the operating room (Gallico *et al.*, 1984, 1989; Limova and Mauro, 1995; Limat *et al.*, 1996). The most recent advances in the tissue engineering of skin equivalents and practical approach for clinical applications will be described in the following paragraphs.

31.3.1. Epidermis

As mentioned above, after the breakthroughs of Rheinwald and Green in the mid 1970s, the technology of cultured epithelial autograft (CEA) is now available at a large number of hospitals worldwide. In addition, cell culture parameters, harvest procedures, and usage indications have been strictly defined (Leigh, 1994) and CEA production is also being performed on an industrial basis.

However, cumulative clinical data on CEA application, mostly for extensive burn management, have revealed several limitations of this technique. First of all, time requirements for the production of CEA are high, as keratinocytes in standard conditions form epithelial sheets at least 3 weeks later after initiation of the culture. Second, take rates of the grafts and number of implantation procedures are often unpredictable. Furthermore, the use of enzymes to detach CEA from a plastic culture dish and contraction of epithelial sheets represent additional problems (Hansbrough *et al.*, 1993). Thus, for the second generation of CEA, it has been acknowledged that a proper delivery vehicle, namely a biomaterial, should have been developed to overcome almost all limitations of CEA grafting (Rennekampff *et al.*, 1996).

The ideal delivery vehicle, as in general for all tissue engineering scaffolds, should possess relevant properties in terms of biocompatibility and tolerability, then should be totally degradable, in order to avoid device removal, and, finally, should guarantee effective epithelial sheet stability once grafted onto the patient. A large number of biomaterials have been tested so far, in both preclinical and clinical experimental conditions (Boyce *et al.*, 1988; Kaiser *et al.*, 1994; Rennekampff *et al.*, 1996). Among those, one of the most promising backing material to culture human autologous keratinocytes is constituted by a hyaluronic-acid-based microperforated membrane. The convincing rationale for the use of hyaluronan-derived products in skin repair is mostly the fact that the molecule plays a key role in the wound healing process (Oksala *et al.*, 1995).

The commercially available product referred to as Laserskin® (FIDIA Advanced Biopolymers, Abano Terme, Italy) is a 20-μm-thick membrane composed of a benzylic derivative of hyaluronan (HYAFF®11). The innovation of such a device is the microperforation, a regular array of holes (80 μm diameter; 80 μm separated) generated by a laser which allows the colonization of both sides of the membrane, giving rise to a mature epithelial sheet composed of several layers of differentiated keratinocytes (Andreassi *et al.*, 1991). Following a series of preliminary experiments *in vivo* (Myers *et al.*, 1997), the microperforated membrane seeded with human keratinocytes has been applied onto patients (Andreassi *et al.*, 1998) and the major advantage in CEA technique is represented by the use of preconfluent cells, thus decreasing the time needed for grafting (Harris, 1998).

31.3.2. Dermis

A subsequent step forward in the designing of the ideal skin equivalent came from basic research and clinical observations, which demonstrated that CEA take is strongly dependent on the wound bed condition, that is the dermal layer (Fusenig, 1994; MacKenzie, 1994; Rennekampff *et al.*, 1996). In particular, several studies have shown that the presence of a dermal layer is of great importance for the regulation of growth and differentiation of cultured keratinocytes; indeed fibroblasts embedded in their extracellular matrix (ECM) constitute a permissive and regulatory layer for those cells. The first experience to stimulate take rates of CEA was constituted by the improvement in the wound bed preparation using meticulous débridement and/or biointeractive dressings. A further approach is the use of an acellular dermal substitute such as cadaver or heterologous dermis made devitalized by means of particular protocols to avoid a strong graft versus host reaction (Wainwright *et al.*, 1996). After these first attempts, given that fibroblasts are the main constituent of the dermis and are normally used to grow keratinocytes, the concept of a coculture was introduced in order to produce *in vitro* a composite skin replacement composed of an epithelial layer overlaid onto a dermal substitute.

The importance of the scaffold for a dermal-like tissue must be stressed. In fact, the design of a dermal-like tissue depends critically on the use of an ideal scaffold which must allow the dermis to develop into a three-dimensional architecture. One of the most important features of the scaffold is its porosity, which has to fit the neovessel ingrowth from the host tissue (angiogenesis) during the wound healing process. In addition, the biomaterial should be fully biocompatible and totally degradable, being substituted by a full functional ECM in the long term. Finally, the material should be resistant to mechanical forces and easy to apply on the wound area.

Biomaterial technology has produced a series of different scaffolds tested for fibroblast culture and synthesis of a neoextracellular matrix, which plays a key role in CEA attachment via the basement membrane (Shahabeddin *et al.*, 1991; Auger *et al.*, 1995; Lamme *et al.*, 1996). In order to obtain a dermal-like tissue, fibroblasts have been cultured into various kind of scaffolds, such as PGL meshes, acemannan polymers, collagen lattices, etc. Recently an allogeneic cultured human skin equivalent has been used for the treatment of venous ulcers (Falanga *et al.*, 1998). This living skin equivalent consists of a dermal equivalent composed of type I bovine collagen that contains living human dermal fibroblasts with an overlying cornified epidermal layer of living human keratinocytes (Wilkins *et al.*, 1994). A different approach to obtain a dermal-like equivalent is based on the assumption that autologous fibroblasts, when cultured into appropriate scaffolds, can proliferate and deposit the main extracellular components, giving rise to a living dermal equivalent. Based on the fact that hyaluronan is a fundamental component of the nonproteic fraction of the ECM, a nonwoven scaffold constituting the benzylester of hyaluronan has been utilized as a temporary scaffold for the reconstruction of a dermal-like tissue. Experiments conducted *in vitro* showed that the material was a suitable three-dimensional scaffold both for human fibroblast and for

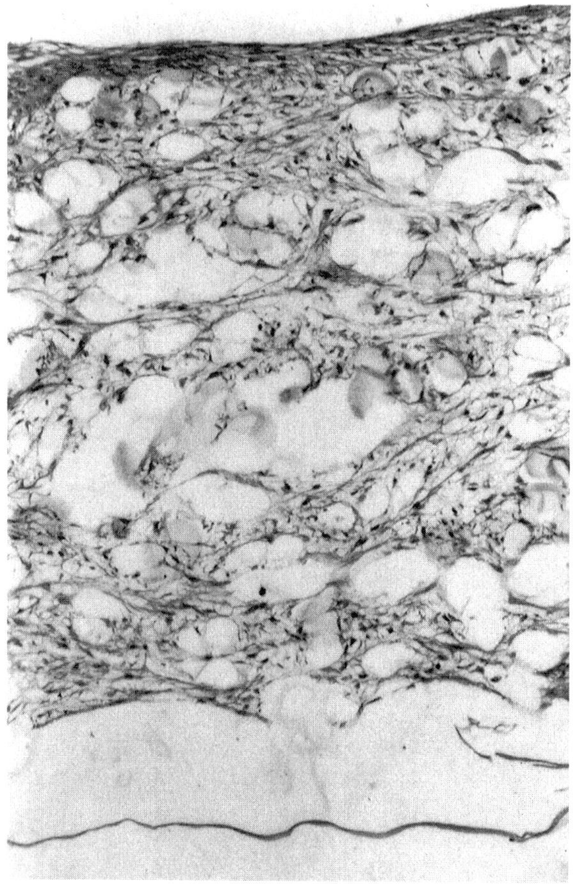

Figure 31.1. Histological analyses on paraffin-embedded specimens of human fibroblasts cultured for 2 weeks on the three-dimensional fiber structure of the nonwoven mesh. Cells appeared randomly dispersed among fibers and a thin fibrillar network secreted by cells was present. Hematoxylin and eosin. Original magnification $\times 200$.

cocultured keratinocytes (Zacchi *et al*, 1998). In particular, it was shown that fibroblasts seeded onto the nonwoven HYAFF® 11 fleeces gave rise to a typical dermal-like tissue with the expression of the main ECM molecules (Figures 31.1 and 31.2). These living dermal equivalents can be used in clinical practice for the treatment of different skin defects, such as full thickness surgical wounds or chronic ulcers (Harris *et al*, 1999; Galassi *et al.*, 2000).

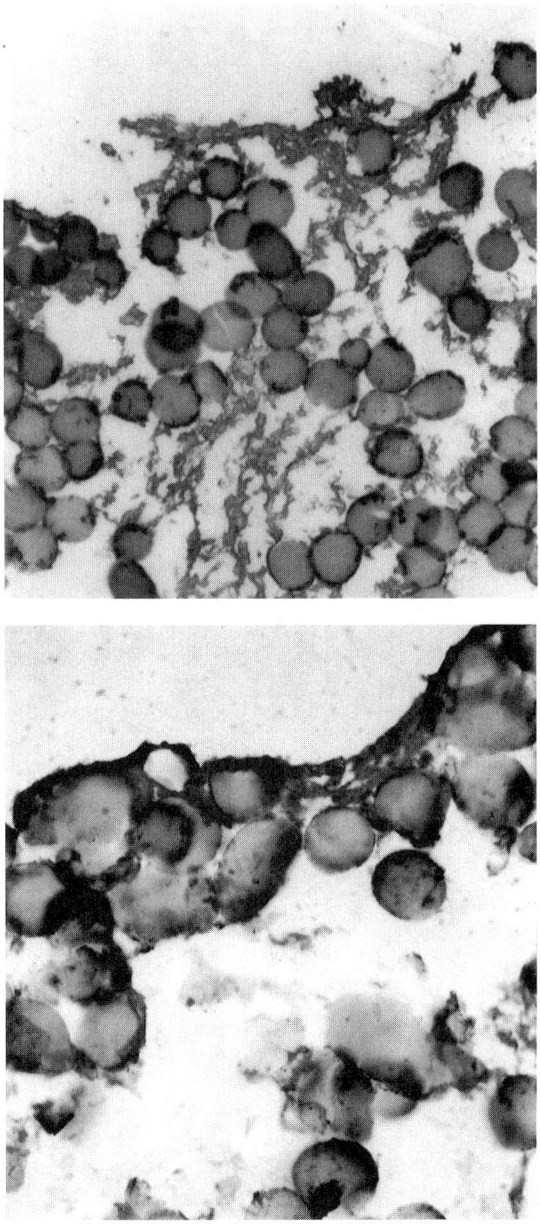

Figure 31.2. Immunolocalization of dermal ECM molecules in the dermal construct. Fibroblasts cultivated for 2 weeks secreted collagen type I (a), fibronectin (b), laminin (c), and PDGF (d). Counterstained with Mayer hematoxylin. Original magnification $\times 200$.

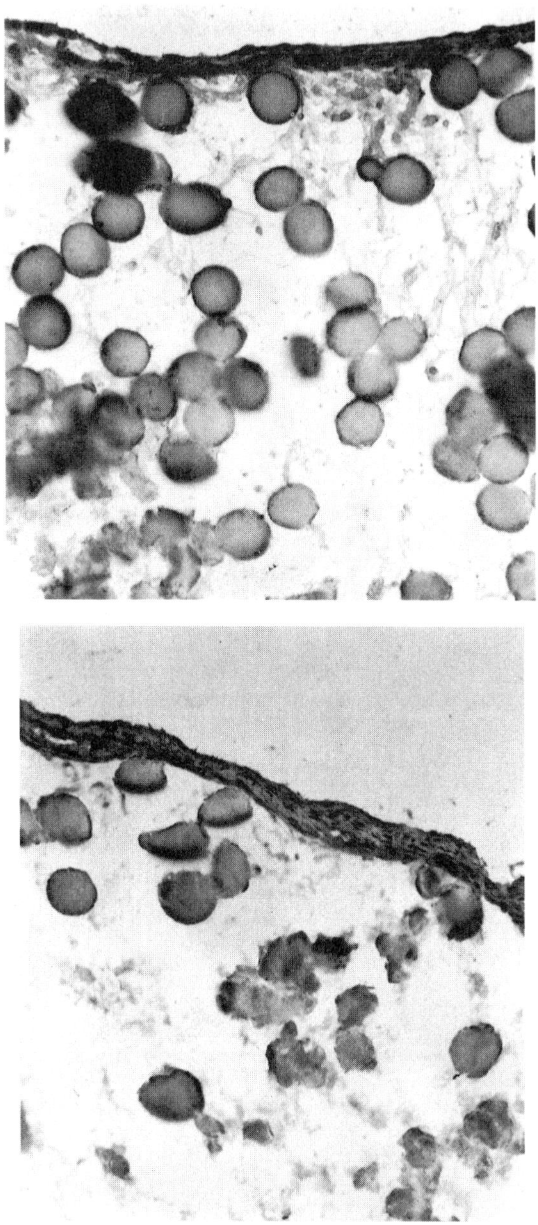

Figure 31.2. *Continued.*

31.3.3. Conclusions

One can conclude that the actual state of art for the creation of a complete cutaneous substitute is far from perfection. The many studies conducted so far reveal that tissue engineering of the skin is only at the beginning of its use in human applications. Burn paticnts were the first targets for such tissue substitutes, then chronic diseases, such as venous ulcers, followed. The more experience that is gained from the surgeon, the more feedback for the basic scientist to improve the product and to broaden clinical indications. For example, it is now clear that for some wounds it is necessary to apply first a dermal substitute and then cover it with an epidermal substitute. In other cases, a single, one-step procedure could be definitive, grafting a dermal–epidermal equivalent.

Nowadays, progress in cell culture and biomedical material technologies have added two important spare parts: epidermis and dermis to the surgeon's toolbox which can be reconstituted in the laboratory from small biopsies of the same recipient. Other parts will follow in a few years, with the final aim to generate a full transplantable replica of the skin with adnexa and vasculature.

31.4. Artificial Cartilage

Cartilage regeneration in adults is usually poor due to its avascularity and the lack of sufficient precursors able to divide and restore the original tissue architecture and function. Vital functioning can be maintained by the replacement of damaged tissue with interventions such as reconstructive plastic surgery using tissue transplantation (i.e., periosteum and perichondrium resurfacing, osteochondral grafts), orthopedic surgery, and/or artificial prosthetic devices. The aim of therapy is to fill the defect and/or stimulate the growth of new cartilaginous tissue. While the repaired tissue should ideally have the mechanical properties, composition, and structure of natural cartilage, the use of either autogenous or allogenous tissue transplantation or alloplastic materials results in inconsistencies in the morphology of the newly healed tissue with mechanical properties that are less than ideal. Moreover, after surgery, problems such as infection or extrusion may occur. Recent studies on the *in vitro* reconstruction of cartilage-like tissue and on transplantation in animal models or in human cells derived from *in vitro* proliferation of biopsy samples have demonstrated that tissue engineering may be most indicated for the repair of articular defects which are not too far advanced.

Current obstacles to the development of cartilage tissue engineered replacements include the low proliferation rate of chondrocytes in culture, their tendency to lose their differentiation assuming a fibroblast-like shape, and the change in collagen phenotype expression when cultivated in flat plastic culture devices, resulting subsequently in their inability to form *in vitro* a three-dimensional organization with cartilaginous characteristics. Some research groups recently have focused on the engineering of cartilage grafts to treat a small variety of joint cartilage pathologies using two different approaches: injection of culture-expanded autologous cells capable of chondrogenesis into the site of the defect, or transplantation of *in vitro*-grown tissue constructs obtained by cultivating biopsied cells onto three-dimensional biocompatible scaffolds. The first approach is founded on the results of recent studies of Brittberg (1994a) which demonstrated how cell therapy enhanced cartilage repair. The second clinical application was pioneered by Vacanti and Upton (1991), who demonstrated the possibility of developing a subcutaneous neocartilage from *in vitro* reconstructed tissue in nude mice. In addition to the use of chondrocytes, an alternative approach to cartilage repair involves the use of progenitor stem cells (Caplan *et al.*, 1997) which have a higher mitotic potential and are immuno-privileged as compared to chondrocytes from older donors.

31.4.1. Properties of Normal and Injured Cartilage

Cartilage is a specialized avascular connective tissue distributed throughout the body which performs many functions due to its ability to resist forces of compression and tension. It originates from the mesenchyme and is composed of chondrocytes, cells which are characterized by a highly specialized extracellular matrix of collagens, proteoglycans, and noncollagenous proteins. These substances maintain water homeostasis within the matrix, thus conferring its unique mechanical properties. Traditionally, three different kinds of cartilage have been described on the basis of the characteristics of this matrix: hyaline cartilage, elastic cartilage, and fibrocartilage. Hyaline cartilage is the most abundant cartilage in the body and is the precursor to bone during development. In the adult, hyaline cartilage is present around the articular surfaces on the bone surface, in the structural framework of the trachea, bronchi, and larynx, in the nose, and at the ends of the ribs. It is composed of cells surrounded by spaces called lacunae and embedded in a matrix made up of collagens (type II, 90–95% type IX and type XI), proteoglycans, and 50–70% water. Typically, hyaline collagen is divided into four zones in which cell size, shape, metabolic activity, and matrix composition all vary, rendering a superficial, transitional, radial, or calcified cartilage.

Cartilage is surrounded by a capsule of connective tissue called the perichondrium which contains a cell layer of chondrocyte precursors. The normal functioning of articular cartilage depends on the maintenance of both the content and structure of the principal extracellular matrix components by a constant turnover of collagen and proteoglycan. Under normal conditions, there is an equilibrium between synthesis and degradation of cartilage ECM molecules but in many clinical conditions, such as trauma, congenital abnormalities, and aging, degradation predominates. The response to a partial-thickness injury is characterized by necrosis, cell proliferation, and matrix synthesis. Full-thickness defects are characterized by damage to the subchondral plate bone with subsequent inflammation and formation of a reparative tissue in which the matrix and cells are more typical of fibrocartilage, a form of cartilage in which the matrix contains thick collagen type I fibers, instead of collagen type II fibers. The inability of cartilage to regenerate a functional tissue poses a serious clinical problem in adults, since chondral lesions eventually develop into a progressive degenerative process that leads to osteoarthritis, a pathology with great social impact which is characterized by moderate chronic inflammation and erosion of articular cartilage. Patients are usually treated with anti-inflammatory pharmacological therapy in conjunction with débridment of the damaged area or abrasion arthroplasty to alleviate short-term symptomatology. When the pathology reaches an advanced stage, articular damage is irrevocable.

31.4.2. Chondrocyte Cultures *In Vitro*

Because of the limited source of cartilage, chondrocytes must be amplified *in vitro* to obtain a sufficient cell number for injection in the area of osteochondral damage (cell therapy) or to form cartilage-like constructs to be transplanted *in vivo*. Experimental evidence demonstrates that these cells cultivated *in vitro* in a two-dimensional microenvironment undergo phenotype modifications. Chondrocytes normally grow and differentiate inside a typical ECM which regulates its cellular activities. Chondrocytes in culture tend to dedifferentiate, assuming an elongated shape and synthesizing a different pattern of collagen molecules. At initial passages (2–4), cultured cells demonstrate varying levels of collagen-type II and collagen type I synthesis, but after long-term culture, a complete switch from type II to type I collagen expression (Benya and Padilla, 1986; Horton *et al.*, 1993; Ramdi *et al.*, 1993) is revealed. Moreover, chondrocytes have a limited capacity to proliferate. The rate of proliferation is generally known to be a function of the age of the cartilage donor, with chondrocytes from younger donors significantly more metabolically active. However, cartilage defects and, consequently, cartilage reconstruction occur more frequently in older adults.

The final step in the development of *in vitro* artificial cartilage is the use of human chondrocytes isolated from a small autologous or allogenic biopsy and amplified by means of *in vitro* culture, to be used directly for transplantation (cell therapy) or after *in vitro* seeding onto an appropriate biodegradable and biocompatible biomaterial. Thus, the optimal *in vitro* culture conditions which allow for the maintenance of chondrocyte phenotype and proliferation need to be identified.

In recent years, researchers have attempted to cultivate cells in various ways, having aimed to maintain the original cell phenotype or to regain their potential to regenerate cartilage. Initial studies involved the use of static Petri dishes in a 37 °C humidified 5% CO_2 incubator, then spinner flasks containing a magnetic stir bar mixed at 50–100 rpm, rotating bioreactors described by Schwarz and colleagues (1992). It was then discovered that differentiation was maintained when cells were placed onto collagen gels (Benya *et al.*, 1977; Horton *et al.*, 1993) or three-dimensional scaffolds, the chondrocytes having regained their phenotypical round shape (Vacanti *et al.*, 1991; Kolettas *et al.*, 1995).

Proliferation rate has been improved by the addition of bioactive molecules in the culture medium. Several studies have analyzed the influence of various growth factors on cartilage synthesis. In two-dimensional cultures, cell number increases, allowing for up to 35 passages, in a medium supplemented with growth factors, namely transforming growth factor β (TGF-β) and basic fibroblast growth factor (bFGF). These factors also help to maintain cell phenotype as there is evidence that TGF-β and bFGF can stimulate cartilage formation and repair (Hunziker and Rosenberg, 1994; Fujisato *et al.*, 1996).

It can be concluded that, to obtain a typical cartilage ECM, chondrocytes have to be seeded onto three-dimensional biomaterials or used for cell therapy after only a few passages. Differentiation of cells may be regained or maintained after several days of proliferation on three-dimensional scaffolds.

31.4.3. *In Vitro* and *In Vivo* Studies: Cell Therapy

Longevity of articular cartilage depends on its extracellular matrix molecules (collagen fibrils, proteoglycans, and glycoproteins). Any tissue capable of replacing damaged articular cartilage must replicate the native structure of the tissue. In the last three decades, much research has attempted to achieve wound healing of full-thickness cartilage defects by the transfer of isolated chondrocytes into articular defects. This therapeutic approach involves the harvesting of autologous chondrocytes obtained arthroscopically from a selected anatomical site which are expanded *in vitro* and subsequently injected under a periosteal flap into the lesion (Brittberg *et al.*, 1994a). The first results of autologous chondrocyte transplantation were promising for partial-thickness defects and those of relatively small size, but were not completely satisfactory. In a small group of treated patients, the central area of the implant was not well fixed to the surrounding tissues; this seemed to be related to a loose attachment to the underlying bone (Messner and Gillquist, 1996). This method was laborious, and led to degenerative changes in the articular cartilage surrounding the defect.

As mentioned previously, Benya and colleagues (1977) demonstrated that dedifferentiation was avoided when cells were cultured in collagen gels. In recent years, collagen has been used by many researchers as a natural delivery vehicle for cells, supplying an appropriate environment for proliferation. Wakitani and colleagues (1989) have implanted chondrocytes delivered in a collagen type I vehicle gel into a full-thickness patellar groove cartilage defect of the rabbit knee. Cells rapidly proliferated, having produced a metachromatic extracellular matrix which filled the entire defect. However, also in this case, the newly formed tissue did not integrate with the host cartilage and thus could not be indicated for the repair of full-thickness defects. A recent study of Kawamura and colleagues (1998) seemed to have partially solved this problem by transplanting a cartilage-like construct obtained from allogenic chondrocytes cultivated for two weeks in a collagen type I gel-biomatrix into a full thickness defect in the rabbit knee. At day 1 after implantation the repair tissue had the morphology of hyaline cartilage, and at 24 weeks host and donor cartilage appeared to have integrated, although not completely. These results suggest that cultivating chondrocytes in a gel-biomatrix may lead to a three-dimensional structure which resembles cartilage tissue, with the physical stability and mechanical properties necessary for the incorporation of the implant into surrounding tissues.

31.4.4. Cartilage-like Tissue Constructs

In the last decade, many studies have demonstrated that the *in vivo* implantation of cartilage-like tissue constructs allowed for the regeneration of the damaged cartilage (Vacanti *et al.*, 1992; Vacanti and Upton, 1994). The reconstruction of an *in vitro* engineered cartilage has been attempted using different kinds of biomaterials with the final aim of obtaining an engineered structure which shares similar properties with the native tissue. In general, autologous or allogenic chondrocytes need to be amplified *in vitro*, seeded onto the biomaterials where they would actively proliferate and synthesize an ECM similar to that in native tissue. The scaffolds need to provide a framework for cell proliferation and ECM deposition which, once transplanted, can offer physical stability and integrity. Moreover, biocompatibility and degradability of biomaterials are essential requisites for their clinical application and depend, as well as the mechanical properties, on scaffold design and *in vitro* culture conditions. For these reasons, the availability of an appropriate biomaterial scaffold is crucial to allow chondrocyte growth and the development of a cartilaginous tissue.

While researchers initially used agarose or collagen gels as vehicles for chondrocytes, this technique evolved more recently into the culture for up to three weeks in a collagen matrix to obtain a cartilage-like construct which has the physical and mechanical properties to regenerate cartilage once implanted *in vivo*. Other studies have been performed using synthetic polymers of polyglactin to obtain cartilage-like constructs to be implanted *in vivo* (Vacanti *et al.*, 1991). Numerous natural or synthetic three-dimensional polymers have been investigated as alternatives to agarose gel, collagen gel, and polyglactin and have been tested for their biocompatibility and biodegradability both *in vitro* and *in vivo*. In recent years, polylactic acid (PLA), fibrous polyglycolic acid (PGA) meshes, and carbon fiber pads have been used as synthetic scaffolds for chondrocytes cultures which were to be subsequently transplanted *in vivo*. Chu and colleagues (1995) expanded rabbit chondrocytes in culture, subsequently seeding the cells onto PLA scaffolds prior to implantation into rabbit femoral condyles. Freed and colleagues (1993) cultivated both bovine and human chondrocytes on PGA scaffolds. The cells which attached to the fibers retained their characteristic spherical *in vivo* morphology and produced cartilage matrix molecules. When chondrocyte-PGA constructs were then grafted subcutaneously in nude mice and intra-articularly in rabbits (Freed *et al.*, 1994), neocartilage containing GAGs and collagen types I and II was formed.

In the absence of cells, PGA scaffolds were shown to promote chondrogenesis, probably by guiding host cells into the defect and providing a framework for cell migration. However, in the longer term, six months after implantation, chondrocyte-seeded scaffolds were shown to be superior in repairing defects than scaffolds alone. Kim and colleagues (1994) used PGA fibers immersed in a poly-L-lactic acid (PLLA) solution to obtain a synthetic scaffold to be seeded with chondrocytes for transplantation. Other authors (Hemmen *et al.*, 1991) have reported the use of carbon fiber pads embedded with chondrocytes. Angele *et al.* (1998) and Haisch *et al.* (1998) experimented with cultivated chondrocytes mixed in fibrin glue and then seeded onto synthetic polymers (i.e., vycril and poly-dioxanon fleeces, polytetrafluorethylene membranes).

Of these various substrates, hyaluronan and its derivatives are very promising scaffolds for cell proliferation and differentiation. Hyaluronan is known to have a fundamental role in embryonic development (Cortivo *et al.*, 1990; Abatangelo *et al.*, 1994; Moriarity *et al.*, 1996) and wound healing in both adult and fetal life stages (Knudson and Knudson, 1990; Moriarty *et al.*, 1996; Oksala *et al.*, 1995). Various preparations of esterified hyaluronan were tested to assess their biocompatibility and biodegradability (Cortivo *et al.*, 1991; Benedetti *et al.*, 1993). The most suitable device for cell culture was identified as the total esterified derivative of hyaluronan called HYAFF®11 used in the form of nonwoven meshes (40-μm-thick fibers) and microperforated membranes (Zacchi *et al.*, 1998). Hyaluronan was previously shown to maintain the chondrogenic potential of chick embryo chondrocytes cultured for subsequent transplantation (Robinson *et al.*, 2000). Chick embryo chondrocytes (Brun *et al.*, 2000) were seeded on HYAFF®11 nonwoven meshes and cells were allowed to grow for up to three weeks and then harvested for immunohistological analyses. Results indicated that avian chondrocytes adhered and proliferated within the biomaterial where they synthesized glycosaminoglycans and type II collagen (Figures 31.3 and 31.4). When transplanted in nude mice (Campoccia *et al.*, 1998), HYAFF®11-chondrocyte constructs seemed to generate a cartilage-like tissue.

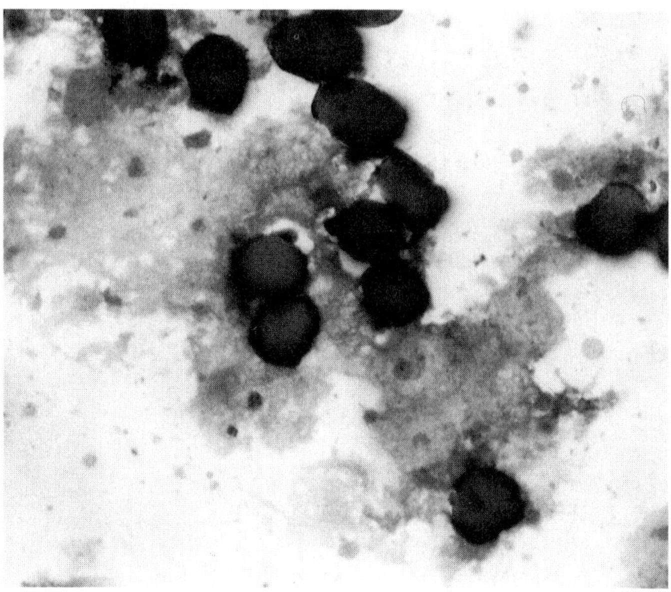

Figure 31.3. Chick embryo chondrocytes grown onto HA-based meshes stained with 1% Toluidine blue after 1 week from seeding. Note the positive methachromatic staining around cell clusters. Original magnification $\times 100$.

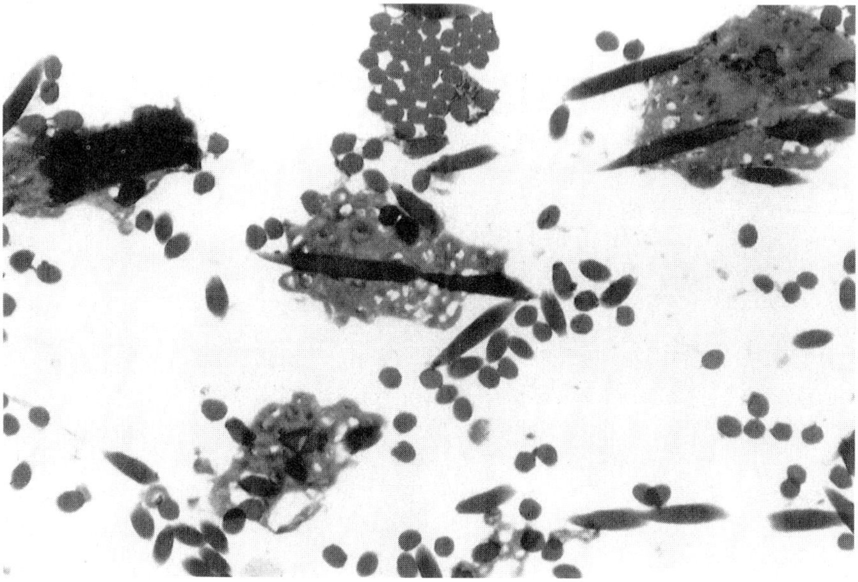

Figure 31.4. Immunolocalization of collagen type II in chick embryo chondrocytes after 3 weeks from seeding into HYAFF nonwoven mesh. Counterstaining with hematoxylin. Original magnification ×400.

When cells are seeded onto any type of biomaterial, high cell density (Puelacher *et al.*, 1994) and the addition of growth factors have been shown to be crucial parameters which improve proliferation and matrix deposition.

In conclusion, in all of these animal studies, the use of three-dimensional biocompatible and biodegradable scaffolds seeded with chondrocytes was demonstrated to promote the repair of cartilage defects or subcutaneous cartilage.

31.4.5. Mesenchymal Stem Cells

Since regeneration in much of adult human tissues is poor, the repair of a damaged tissue often leads to a structure significantly different in physiological properties and ECM compositions from the native tissue (e.g., fibrocartilage versus normal cartilage). The discovery that *in vitro* mesenchymal stem cell cultures have the potential to generate differentiated phenotypes (i.e., myoblasts, chondroblasts, osteoblasts, adipocytes, and fibroblasts) (Young *et al.*, 1995) is now recognized as a potentially powerful tool in tissue engineering which may help resolve this fundamental problem in wound healing. It is well known that these mesenchymal cells differentiate during development and, in progressive stages, form the structural tissues of the body. With the knowledge that wound healing is multiphasic, resembling the stages of embryonic development, the use of multipotent mesenchymal precursors in tissue repair might have real clinical potential.

Among these multipotent cells are the stem cells in the marrow (Caplan, 1991) that are easily sampled by a bone marrow needle aspiration (Lazarus *et al.*, 1995). Bone marrow stroma has been shown to contain precursor cells of the osteogenic lineage, including osteoblasts and chondroblasts, that have the ability to differentiate into cartilage when transplanted *in vivo* (Caplan, 1994; Radice, 2000). Furthermore, the use of various combinations of growth factors in culture have been found to induce a specific phenotype development (Rogers *et al.*, 1995). With the aid of specific histological staining of different ECM molecules and the currently available antibodies against markers that trace a specific cell phenotype, these differentiated cell subpopulations can be identified.

In one report, the development of a precartilaginous phenotype from mesenchymal cells was described morphogenically as aggregations of round cells bound by flattened cells and surrounded by a dense pericellular matrix. Positive metachromatic staining with toluidine blue revealed its glycosaminoglycan content and its expression of collagen type IIA to be precartilaginous in nature (Sandell *et al.*, 1991).

Mesenchymal stem cells may be expanded *in vitro* and either be directly implanted at high concentrations in damaged sites or first cultured in the presence of the appropriate growth factors to reconstruct a tissue similar to the native one in which they will be implanted (Kasugai *et al.*, 1991; Dixon *et al.*, 1996). These cells implanted in sites of osteochondral defects completely repair and restore the physiological function of the tissue. Studies of implanted cells, conducted to demonstrate that the local microenvironment drives the precursors to proceed into the appropriate differentiation steps (Wakitani *et al.*, 1994; Butnariu-Ephrat *et al.*, 1996; Grigoriadis *et al.* 1988), actually revealed an incomplete integration of the injected cells with the surrounding tissues. For this reason, although needle re-infusion of a cell suspension can be an effective and convenient method of grafting, temporary scaffolds of suitable biomaterials should be used to ensure the delivery of these cells into the damaged area and avoid their dispersion into the vascular or lymphatic system. The biomaterials previously described for cartilage reconstruction (PLA, PGA, and natural molecules or hyaluronan-based devices) are also indicated as structural supports of *in vitro* proliferation of mesenchymal cells for *in vivo* transplantation.

Recently, some researchers have seeded the biomaterial, HYAFF®11, with bone marrow stem cells. These cells proliferated actively into the scaffold and secreted a ECM rich in collagen type I and collagen type IIA, molecules that are typical of a prechondrogenic phenotype. Tissue constructs were than implanted in the rabbit knee, where they developed a cartilage tissue that seemed to integrate very well with the surroundings tissues (Radice *et al.*, 2000). These results further demonstrate the great potential of mesenchymal stem cells for the development of cartilaginous implants *in vitro* and *in vivo*.

31.4.6. Conclusions

Since cartilage has no regenerative properties, tissue engineered replacements which provide to the defect site isolated cells, alone or in conjunction with a structural scaffold of biodegradable biomaterials, allow for long-term integrated repair of the tissue and are thus indicated for the surgical treatment of arthritis, trauma, or congenital abnormalities. Chondrocytes and mesenchymal stem cells show great potential in the development of cartilage-like tissue both *in vitro* and *in vivo*. Bioengineered *in vivo* tissue transplantation holds advantages over cell therapy since the presence of an ECM matrix may not only provide a stable support for cells, but also ensures that the transplanted cells remain in the treated site and act as a source for growth factors which stimulate correct cell differentiation.

31.5. Artificial Bone

Bone is a part of the musculoskeletal system and the loss of bony substance may affect not only the specific tissue physiology but also a whole working apparatus which enables human beings to stand and move within the environment. Bone functions may be impaired by a series of pathologic events ranging from congenital inherited diseases (e.g., osteogenesis imperfecta) to acute traumatic accidents. Although bone is one of the tissues capable of self-regeneration/repair, in many situations this event does not occur. Thus, the common diseases of bone, including osteoporosis, segmental bone defects, and periodontal disease, require the use of agents to stimulate bone growth and regeneration.

The first goal in the management of bone loss is the reconstitution of its biomechanical activity. This has generally being accomplished initially by the use of both synthetic implants, reviewed elsewhere (see chapters dealing with hard tissue regeneration and reconstruction and dental materials and implants, and also Park *et al.*, 1995), and bone grafts (Buttermann *et al.*,

1996; Mankin *et al.*, 1996). Metals, nonbiodegradable polymeric materials, and ceramics provide custom-tailored prostheses and readily weight-bearing devices, but are generally not "incorporated" into the host environment and necessitate programmed surgical revision(s) over time. Bone grafting, either autogenous or homogeneic, represents actually the mainstream therapy used for bone repair, but its liability has prompted the development of alternative products.

This section will focus on the development of such innovative products which basically rely, as other tissue engineered constructs, on the intrinsic regenerative/repair potential of the body.

31.5.1. Basic Histology and Physiology of Bone

Bone tissue is composed of three basic elements: the cellular component, and the extracellular matrix further divided into organic and calcified matrix (for more detailed information see also Vaughan, 1981; Mundy, 1996). Cells which populate bone are osteoblast/osteocyte, stem cells (both hematopoietic and mesenchymal), bone marrow stroma (composed of various cell types such as adipocytes, fibroblasts, etc.), nerve, endothelial cell, and osteoclast.

The most important components of a healthy adult bone are, however, osteoblast/osteocyte and osteoclast, since those cells are responsible for the tissue homeostasis by a well-regulated turn-over mechanism which accounts for 2–10% year of bone remodeling. In addition, hematopoietic progenitors, supported by stromal cells, provide the formation and regulation of blood components (see below).

With regard to repair/regeneration in adults, other cells take part of the mechanism. Mesenchymal cells provide appropriate precursors for the neoformation of the bone matrix and reconstitution of the correct cell/matrix ratio. In addition, endothelial cells are essential in sustaining bone tissue formation by providing nutrients and gases and exporting catabolic substances. The invasion of new vasculature after damage is generally known as angiogenesis.

Bone is divided, from a histological point of view, into two broad categories: the trabecular (spongy) bone and the cortical (compact) bone. Differences among them stem from both their origin and three-dimensional configuration.

Trabecular bone comes from endochondral ossification, that is a primitive cartilaginous intermediae made from mesenchymal tissue (chondrocytes). The cartilaginous template eventually degenerates and ossifies to form new bone. Endochodral ossification is found in the embryonic formation of long bones, in fracture repair, in physeal growth of the immature skeleton, and in the incorporation of bone grafts. Trabecular bone occurs in the interior of flat bones, and near the ends of long bones in the region of the joint surface. Cortical bone derives from intramembranous ossification, without the formation of a cartilaginous network, but rather directly from condensed mesenchymal tissue. Cortical bone occurs in the walls of the shafts of long bones and as the outer shell of flat bones, such as the pelvis.

The structure of trabecular bone is characterized by a porous network of interconnected lamellar bone rods and plates (trabeculae). The main biomechanical function of trabecular bone is to resist compression. Cortical bone is dense compared to trabecular bone, and contains closely spaced groups of concentric lamellar bone rings called osteons. Due to its compact structure with small pores, cortical bone can resist compression, tension, and torsion. Given those biomechanical characteristics of bone from different parts of the body, tissue engineering should, in general, take into account differences in designing appropriate bone substitutes.

From a physiological point of view, bone is not limited to "passive" mechanical and protective functions, but it also regulates homeostasis of important elements, such as phosphorus and calcium, by means of continuous deposition/resorption of the ossified tissue and exchange with the bloodstream. Moreover, hematopoiesis, the generation of components of blood, takes place, in the adult, in almost all bone cavities of the red bone marrow. Thus, bone acts as a reservoir of hematopoietic stem cells which allow the body to survive and fight occasional infection or tumor development.

31.5.2. Acellular Approaches for Tissue Engineering of Bone

Theoretically, two strategies can be applied to the engineering of bone, namely the design and fabrication of acellular and cellular substitutes (tissue engineered tissues). This subsection will briefly describe available acellular approaches on the market or still in development, while the next will rather focus on tissue engineered products.

The main concern in designing acellular substitutes for bone repair/regeneration is the effective stimulation of neoformation of bone tissue by host environment. Thus, materials have to fulfil not only osteoconductive but also relevant osteoinductive requisites. Available or candidate substrates for such products are acellular bone graft, and synthetic or semisynthetic materials.

The first category actually represents the "gold" standard for the treatment of bone loss, when enough autologous bone is not available for autografting. Positive aspects are the active biological role of freeze-dried or frozen, sterilized and processed (crushed, molded, etc.) allogeneic bone graft. Indeed, it is well known that acellular bone has hidden osteogenic growth factors (OPs, BMPs) entrapped in the organic extracellular matrix and they will most likely be released during resorption of the graft into the host tissue (Brekke, 1996; Mundy, 1996). Moreover, bone graft possesses other properties such as load bearing and osteoconduction by the three-dimensional porous structure which also encourages vascular ingrowth. Negative aspects of bone grafting are the allogeneic origin with concern in respect of cross-infection and immunological reactions (rejection). Furthermore, bone grafts lack moldability to fit "difficult" lesion sites and sometimes fail to integrate completely with the generation of fragile areas.

Historically, synthetic or semisynthetic materials offered some advantages over natural bone substitutes, such as moldability and unlimited supply. However, difficulties in manufacturing and processing and lack of long-term osteointegration relegate those products only as alternative materials. Significant advancements in material design and manufacturing have, however, brought about a new series of substrates capable of overcoming such problems. Of particular interest are polyester and polyanhydride formulations arranged in three-dimensional configurations such as nonwoven and sponges (Yaszemski *et al.*, 1996; Ashammakhi and Rokkanen, 1997).

The three-dimensional structure is an important feature in improving osteoconduction by the porous network enabling vasculature invasion and bone regeneration. Moreover, those materials are totally biodegradable, thus avoiding the need of re-operation. However, concerns are still pending on long-term degradation products of those materials.

A parallel line of development has taken into consideration the chemical and/or physical modification of natural polymers, such as collagen, hyaluronic acid, and combinations thereof. Advantages of these materials are their active biological role in bone development and homeostasis, being natural components of the organic extracellular matrix. However, three-dimensional configurations essentially lack mechanical properties and lot-to-lot variabilities are known to occur for proteic substrates.

Finally, the discovery and isolation of different osteogenic factors (Urist, 1965) resulted in a further tool to improve the development of acellular bone substitutes. The main problem beside the use of a liquid osteogenic factor resides in its correct delivery. Injectable liquid substances are likely to be rapidly cleared from the application site by surrounding circulatory systems, i.e., bloodstream or lymphatic. Also, in case of large defects, a constant gradient of bone promoting factor should be released in a controlled fashion to maintain stimulating activity for the time needed to completely generate new bone tissue. Thus, a supportive, completely biodegradable matrix should be developed to control the delivery of the drug, possibly providing also mechanical stability of the implant and allowing for neotissue formation. Examples of such delivery vehicles are injectable hydrogels or suspensions composed mainly of collagen occasionally combined with hyaluronic acid, or solid supports such as sponges combined with a specific promoting factor (Cook *et al.*, 1994; Hollinger *et al.*, 1996; Sciadini *et al.*, 1997).

All these new materials and complex systems rely on the body's self-reparative response to various stimuli, however due to the great interindividual variability and underlying basal significant diseases affecting natural repair mechanisms, acellular devices may not be effective in all cases. In addition, delivery of the right dose of growth factor may be hard to trimmer, especially in subjects at risk for excessive cellular proliferation (tumors).

31.5.3. Cellular Approaches for Tissue Engineering of Bone

Cellular devices to engineer bone are actually being used, that is autologous bone graft. However, due to donor site morbidity and surgical problems, this technique cannot be widely applied, especially for large bone resection or complex anatomy of the bone to be substituted (maxillofacial reconstruction). Thus, a complete and readily available source of autologous bone must be developed to treat such difficult lesions.

As already described, a tissue engineered construct is composed at least of two elements: cells supported by a scaffold. In bone regeneration applications, a great deal of preclinical research both *in vitro* and *in vivo* has been done, but clinical trials or case reports are still limited, so far. Tissue engineering of bone starts from cell harvesting and, as far as this aspect is concerned, either adult differentiated (osteoblast/osteocyte and chondrocyte) or progenitor (from marrow stroma, periosteum, perichondrium) cells can be used (Shimomura *et al.*, 1975; Niedzwiedzki *et al.*, 1993; Vacanti *et al.*, 1993; Brittberg *et al.*, 1994; Scammell and Roach, 1996; Breitbart *et al.*, 1998; Nevo *et al.*, 1998). Differentiated osteoblast/osteocyte is not easy to culture and has intrinsic low duplication properties, so that a large amount of bone cannot be replicated *in vitro*. Chondrocyte has been used and demonstrated to form bone tissue, but reproducibility and donor site morbidity may be unacceptable for clinical applications.

Attention was then referred to the use of progenitor bone cells which have been found to reside in different tissues (Young *et al.*, 1995; Warejcka *et al.*, 1996; Prockop, 1997). The basic rationale of using such a cell is that natural repair/regeneration mechanisms of bone rely definitely on the recruitment and commitment of stem elements which recapitulate the embryonic development of this tissue.

Advantages offered by progenitor or stem cells are clearly their high duplication potential and morphogenic plasticity. Also, in this particular case, progenitor mesenchymal cells can easily be harvested, e.g., by a small bone-marrow needle biopsy from iliac crests, and easy to isolate and culture. The major concern in using progenitor elements, however, is differentiation, namely the risk of implanting a stem cell which may not develop eventually into bone but, unexpectedly, into a different tissue such as dermis or adipose tissue.

Various experiments conducted *in vitro* likely suggest that mesenchymal progenitor cells can be easily pushed through the osteoblast/osteocyte differentiation lineage using specific inducers (Kasugai *et al.*, 1991; Dixon *et al.*, 1996; Young *et al.*, 1998). In addition, some evidence has been shown that *in vivo* progenitor mesenchymal cells may be driven to the correct differentiation pathway by the influence of different stimuli exerted by the surrounding microenvironment (Wakitani *et al.*, 1994).

Thus, two different approaches can actually be hypothesized using such a primitive element, either construct *in vitro* a bone substitute to be transplanted back into the patient, or deliver previously expanded progenitors directly *in vivo*, hypothesizing that microenvironment could drive autologous cells through the correct differentiation cascade.

Once the cellular source has been chosen, the supporting material must be developed to fit two general requirements: cellular compatibility and support, and host compatibility and biodegradability. The "ideal" biomaterial which can meet these different needs is not easy to design and, considering bone, problems are increasing due to biomechanical properties of the recipient site. Two categories of scaffold can be used: soft- or hard-based biomaterials. The former group is composed of many candidates, either synthetic, semisynthetic, or natural, while the latter group relies basically on natural (acellular matrices) and ceramic materials. To add more complexity, combination of the above-mentioned materials is, in general, always possible.

Based on clinical experience from implanted resorbable orthopedic implants, few materials have been experimented in regenerating new bone *in vitro*. The most extensively tested synthetic materials are actually PLA and PGA with addition of osteoblast or mesenchymal progenitors (Breitbart *et al.*, 1998).

An alternative to synthetic scaffolds is represented by modified natural molecules such as collagen and hyaluronic acid. Hyaluronic acid seems to be very promising as tissue engineering scaffold, based on previous reports of its osteoinductive capacity (Sasaki and Watanabe, 1995), and its fundamental role in embryonic development (Toole, 1997) and wound healing (Weigel *et al.*, 1988).

Hyaluronic acid is a component of the organic matrix of bone and exerts various important biological functions. In particular, hyaluronic acid plays a key role in cell–cell and cell–matrix interactions (Toole, 1991). In addition, high tolerability, sequence conservation, wide availability from animal sources, and standardized isolation methods make this polysaccharide a good candidate for biomaterial design and fabrication.

Currently, a series of hyaluronan derivatives have been obtained by the physicochemical modification of hyaluronic acid extracted from chicken rooster combs (see also previous sections). Those hyaluronan-based devices have been studied *in vitro* and *in vivo* and various scaffold configurations have been investigated during recent years, in particular microfibers, sponges, and nonwoven fabrics for tissue engineering purposes (Campoccia *et al.*, 1998). Among them, some configurations have already been used as a delivery vehicle for tissue engineered skin (Andreassi *et al.*, 1991; Zacchi *et al.*, 1998) and cartilage (Aigner *et al.*, 1998), and, recently, also in osteochondral regeneration (Barry and Murphy, 2000; Solchaga *et al.*, 2000). In particular, preliminary reports show that hyaluronic based sponges coated with fibronectin are able to support mesenchymal progenitors adhesion and proliferation, and deposition of bone extracellular matrix.

With respect to hard scaffold for tissue engineering, only ceramics have been considered so far based on previous preclinical and clinical evidence. Different formulations of tricalcium phosphate (TCP) and both synthetic and natural (coral) hydroxapatite are commercially available for orthopedic applications. Experimentally, hydroxapatite alone (Iyoda *et al.*, 1993), and a combination of TCP/hydroxapatite in cylinder form have been tested on bone regeneration (Liebergall *et al.*, 1994) with positive results. Another example comes from a combination of porous alumina ceramic seeded with rat marrow cells and implanted in the back of syngeneic rats. Results of implanted engineered construct compared to biomaterial-alone performances demonstrated that only implants with bone marrow cells have inherent osteogenic capacity and that neo-osteogenesis in the biomaterial pores prevents the ingrowth of fibrous tissue (Okumura *et al.*, 1992).

In summary, data originating from these different experiences conducted both *in vitro* and *in vivo* demonstrate that tissue engineering of bone can become an alternative therapeutic tool in the hand of the physician for the treatment of bone loss (Burgess and Hollinger, 1998).

31.5.4. Tissue Engineered Products: Clinical Considerations

The end stage in the development of a tissue engineered bone substitute is the application of this technology to clinical needs. The construction of a bone-like tissue may be useful for two basic reasons:

1. Investigation of the physiology of bone tissue using representative models.
2. Grafting of tissue engineering products on patients.

The first aspect is intimately related to basic and applied research, in that a model which can reproduce a human bone *in vitro* can help in understanding tissue physiology in both health and disease, for example to study hematopoiesis mechanisms (Mantalaris *et al.*, 1998). Furthermore, such a model can be included in the researcher's toolbox, along with "classical" *in vitro* and *in vivo* protocols (cell cultures, animal models), to test a variety of new drugs or medical devices to predict tolerability and efficacy, thus improving the design of clinical trials.

As long as the second aspect is considered, the implantation of an autologous bone-like tissue may represent a great improvement for the field, because of the chronic donor shortage of human spare parts and various drawbacks related to the application of natural and synthetic available orthopedic implants. The application of one particular engineered product in a structural tissue such as bone, however, could not apply to all pathologic conditions that a surgeon may face, given also the fact that the human body is composed of hundreds of different bone segments with rather different biological characteristics. For example, the treatment of a large tissue resection in a load-bearing joint due to osteosarcoma is completely different from the management of a small nonunion fracture in a non-weight-bearing area.

In the first case, a hard and slow-degrading biomaterial should be indicated for such a condition, in order to give enough time for implanted cells to reconstitute an efficient woven bone. Then, when the biomaterial degradation/resorption process begins, a mature lamellar bone could be deposited with the progressive regain of biomechanical characteristics, specific of the lost tissue, by the effect of increasing load due to natural joint movement or rehabilitation protocol. In addition, a massive stimulation of vessel ingrowth must be provided readily after implantation by either a surgical technique (vascular pedicle) or chemical induction (growth factor), to prevent necrosis of the inner part of the implant and rapid osteointegration.

In the second situation, a soft biomaterial seeded with cells can be used, possibly by means of a minimally invasive arthroscopical injection (hydrogel). Then, biomaterial may rapidly degrade leaving delivered cells *in situ*, entrapped in a provisional fibrin matrix due to clot formation, to bridge the gap between the apposing edges of the defect and permit fusion.

Given these two examples, there should be a point in the development of tissue engineering strategies for repairing or regenerating bone, in which all the experts involved, such as biologists, physicists, chemists, engineers, pharmacologists, and physicians, could meet and exchange ideas and knowledge to achieve a common target. Indeed, different critical criteria must be met in order to reach a final engineered bone substitute. For instance, the toxicological profile of the biomaterial and the cell culture method adopted should comprise the source and identification of all components used (sera, growth factors, etc.), as well as the surgical pre-op (cell harvesting), intra-op (product application and fixation), and post-op (rehabilitation and medication) procedures. Once the specific pathology, the best clinical approach, and the tissue engineering strategy have been focused, a product should then be developed and, for a cellular device, both a reproducible biomaterial fabrication and an affordable cell culture technique must be precisely combined.

In addition, further complexity may be added if a scale-up of the cellular tissue engineered product is required so as to transfer the technology to an industrial environment (Mayhew *et al.*, 1998). Since slightly less than half a million bone grafting procedures are estimated to be performed each year in the US alone (data source: Advances, MDI, 1997), it is easy to understand that a single academic laboratory cannot supply even a small part of such a huge number of requests. Thus, additional parameters should be considered in adopting tissue engineered strategies to be applied to very frequent bone pathologies, namely cost, risk/benefit, and other industrial considerations.

Moreover, general rules, guidelines, and standards developed for drugs, biologies, and medical devices could not be applied to a tissue engineered product, which requires a different regulatory approach. Indeed, only recently government authorities, such as FDA (Proposed, 1997), have started to consider these new products.

31.5.5. Summary

In this chapter a short overview of the state-of-the-art in structural bone defect repair and regeneration has been presented. Then, some general concepts and a few examples of tissue engineering of bone, especially related to cellular-based tissue substitutes, have briefly been described.

Finally, different strategies for the clinical treatment of bone diseases have been considered and discussed with regard also to a feasible industrial scenario.

Compared to available methods of treating bone deficiencies, tissue engineering may offer various advantages such as autologous grafting, limited donor site morbidity, relatively good mechanical performance, ease of handling, reduced surgical invasivity, and precise custom-tailored prosthesis. Despite the great amount of preclinical data that have been collected, there is still a lack of clinical trials necessary to evaluate the effective potential of such products on humans. This is primarily because some biomaterials have not completely met certain biomedical criteria such as full biocompatibility, especially in the long term, or because the degradation profile or manufacturing process is still unpredictable. Second, further biological data are needed in order to use promising cells such as mesenchymal progenitors. On the other hand, impressive advancements in molecular biology techniques have opened to biomedical engineers new possible frontiers in the treatment of chronic and heritable diseases by the use of genetically manipulated cells, and push researchers to constantly develop innovative approaches and products.

In conclusion, the need to replace or repair bone when natural mechanisms fail will remain in the future. The eventual solution to this problem would preferably be universal, choosing between prosthetic, drug-based, and acellular or cellular tissue engineering options. However, it seems most likely that a specific combination of these products for each specific pathology should have the capacity to address some of the clinical open problems in the treatment of musculoskeletal tissue diseases.

31.6. Glandular Parenchyma: The Liver

31.6.1. Introduction

Tissue engineering of the liver has become a subject of growing scientific and economic interest in recent years. Advances in organ transplantation have made orthotopic liver transplantation a successful therapy for treatment of acute and chronic liver disease. However, the lack of sufficient donor organs and the sudden dramatic deterioration of patients with acute liver failure make a temporary liver support necessary. The complexity of liver function requires synthesis (e.g., of clotting factors and plasma proteins), metabolism (of endogenous and exogenous substances), and elimination (bile secretion) of specific substances over prolonged periods.

While different approaches have been made with respect to hybrid organ devices, we will here focus on options on a cellular level for liver tissue engineering. To meet the demand of differentiated liver function, synthetic liver functions include production of proinflammatory (fibrinogen, alpha-1-antitrypsin) and noninflammatory (albumin, most of the clotting factors) proteins. Among the various metabolic liver functions ammonia detoxification, gluconeogenesis, phase I (microsomal cytochrome P450 activity) and phase II (conjugation) enzymatic activity, fatty acid metabolism, and bile production and elimination are of major impact.

31.6.2. Anatomy

Liver development results from interactions between the endoderm, which differentiates into parenchymal cords, and the mesoderm, which gives rise to endothelial cells lining the blood sinusoids. Cell–cell interactions remain essential for maintaining and modulating the hepatic functional capacities *in vivo* and *in vitro* (Guguen-Guillouzo, 1983).

31.6.3. Liver Microarchitecture

Liver cells are organized in functional and anatomical units called acini. These are hexagonal structures bordered by six portal triads. A portal triad consists of a branch of the portal vein, hepatic artery, and a bile duct. The hepatocytes are surrounded by two layers of fenestrated endothelium and form cords that stretch from the portal triads to the central vein. In the liver, hepatocytes (HC) are organized into a polarized epithelium. The basolateral surfaces of HC appose the sinusoid, while the apical surfaces appose the bile canaliculi. HC secrete plasma proteins across the basolateral surface to enter circulation, while bilirubin is excreted across the apical surface to enter the biliary tree.

This particular architecture is of great importance for liver function, because it involves interaction of parenchymal and nonparenchymal cells and it requires a gradient of specific hepatocellular function along the perisinusoidal blood stream. Our current understanding is that the subdivision of the acinus separates three zones with different capacity for synthesis, major metabolic pathways, and blood glucose regulation. While periportal hepatocytes take part in gluconeogenesis, urea synthesis, ketogenesis, sulfatations, bile acid secretion, and monooxygenation, the function of pericentral hepatocytes involves glycolysis, fatty acid synthesis, glutamine synthesis, biotransformation, and glucuronidation (Arias *et al.*, 1994). Therefore, any tissue engineering concept must reflect these features if the whole spectrum of hepatic function is to be substituted.

31.6.4. Parenchymal and Nonparenchymal Liver Cells

Five distinct cell types occupy close to 80% of the liver volume, the remaining 20% being filled by extracellular matrix components and extracellular spaces (e.g., the space of Disse). Hepatocytes, the liver parenchymal cells, account for 65% of all liver cells and fulfil most of the liver specific functions.

Sinusoidal cells regulate the hepatic circulation, partly by synthesis and release of cytokines. They comprise sinusoidal endothelial cells, which are responsible for exchange of fluids and contents between the sinusoidal lumen and the space of Disse. This is accomplished by abundance of endothelial cell fenestrae with a mean diameter of 150 nm.

Among the other perisinusoidal cell types, Kupffer cells, the hepatic macrophages, modulate metabolic responses in parenchymal liver cells by release of cytokines or eicosanoids and by phagocytotic activity.

The role of Ito (fat storing) cells, located in the space of Disse, involves uptake and release of vitamin A, synthesis of cytokines, and growth factors. Their main impact, however, seems to be synthesis and secretion of extracellular matrix proteins (collagen types I, III, IV, V, VI, fibronectin, laminin, tenascin, undulin, hyaluronic acid, proteoglycans, heparan sulfate) plus synthesis and secretion of extracellular matrix degrading metalloproteinases.

Finally, intrahepatic bile duct epithelial cells are the only cell type with direct cell contact with hepatocytes, forming a complex, three-dimensional network of interconnecting tubular structures from the canals of Hering to the draining extrahepatic bile ducts. They participate in bile secretion and reabsorption, contributing to bile production and elimination via transport of conjugated bilirubin and amino acids, transport of proteins from plasma or lymph into bile, and transport and metabolism of bile acids. Because their metabolic capacities include phase I and II enzymatic activity, biliary epithelial cells contribute to detoxification of xenobiotics (Arias *et al.*, 1994).

31.6.5. Extracellular Matrix

The extracellular space is crucial for exchange of nutrients and metabolic products, and communication with other cells. The very complex extracellular matrix (ECM) of the liver is composed of at least five distinct types of collagen, seven classes of noncollagenous proteins (e.g., laminin and fibronectin), and a number of proteoglycans and glycosaminoglycans (e.g., perlecan). It is noteworthy that a continuous basement membrane between hepatocytes and endothelial cells does not exist. The liver ECM binds cytokines and growth factors, triggers cellular responses, and modulates cell phenotype and differentiation.

31.6.6. Factors Affecting Liver Cell Function

a. Extracellular Matrix. The understanding that the ECM induces cellular polarity and tissue organization has resulted in the development of a fundamental liver cell culture concept. In order to mimic liver architecture, where hepatocytes are surrounded by two basolateral surfaces facing the ECM, a model was established which enables plating of isolated hepatocytes between two layers of collagen gel (Dunn *et al.*, 1989). In this sandwich configuration, HC cluster into cords, can be maintained for more than 7 weeks in culture, and secrete albumin longer and higher as opposed to HC plated on a single collagen layer. Transcription of the liver-specific genes appears to be responsible for the maintenance of liver-specific functions in the sandwich system (Dunn *et al.*, 1992; Yarmush *et al.*, 1992). In that matrix configuration, an orientated cytoskeleton without stress fibers is provided and the maintained cellular polarity expresses intracellular signals for gene transcription and translation (Ezzell *et al.*, 1993).

Further investigations on the composition of the three-dimensional matrix showed that matrix proteins resembling basement membrane have a similar effect on cultured hepatocytes (Musat *et al.*, 1993). Interestingly, the density of ECM molecules determines the ability to switch HC from differentiation to growth (Mooney *et al.*, 1992). When HC are cultured with a low ECM density, increased levels of albumin, transferrin, and fibrinogen are observed. In contrast, higher ECM coating density results in enhanced cell proliferation, while concomitantly differentiated cell functions are down-regulated. This effect is not limited to a single ECM molecule (laminin, fibronectin, collagen type I or type IV), or the three-dimensional geometry.

One step further, it has been demonstrated that cell shape and function can be engineered by these findings. Using an elastomeric stamp, gold surface imprints with monolayers of alkanethiols were coated with extracellular matrix proteins of defined size and concentration (Singhvi *et al.*, 1994). These experiments indicated that it is the degree to which the cell extends that dictates whether the cell will grow or differentiate. Accordingly, hepatocytes grown on unpatterned surfaces could spread without restriction, and showed highest DNA synthesis, but rapid loss of differentiated function. In contrast, hepatocytes plated on the smallest adhesive islands fully restricting cell extension maintained albumin secretion almost like *in vivo*. The technique may promise to synchronize large population of hepatocytes to increase rates of production of specific proteins, or to stimulate relevant metabolic pathways or secretory pathways.

b. Oxygenation. Conventional cell culture systems are limited in providing adequate oxygen supply to the cell layer, therefore hybrid organ devices have been developed (see the relevant chapters). Here, we report briefly on the significant impact of oxygen sensitivity on cultured hepatocytes.

During the initial phase of culture (plating period) HC are most vulnerable to hypoxia. The oxygen partial pressure can be increased by removing any excessive medium soon after cell attachment, and combining confluent seeding density with a medium depth of 2 mm. On long-term culture, HC seem to have adapted to their new environment (Yarmush *et al.*, 1992).

c. Effect of Growth Factors. The hepatocyte function in culture can be improved by application of hepatotrophic factors. In this respect, the hepatocyte growth factor (HGF) has been shown to exert not only mitogenic stimulus to HC, but also influences the effect of other hepatic genes. For instance, the synthesis of albumin and fibrinogen is enhanced (Gomez-Lechon *et al.*, 1995; Block *et al.*, 1996). Other authors found that HC in monolayer had an unchanged effect of albumin production, but decreased cytochrome P450-activity (MEGX-production) in response to HGF (Hu *et al.*, 1995). However, this was true only for monolayer culture, while HC in collagen gel did not exhibit metabolic effects in response to HGF. Therefore, further studies in three-dimensional culture systems under more physiological conditions are required to assess the effect of various growth factors on the functional capacity of liver cells *in vitro*.

d. Role of Cell Type. If the full spectrum of hepatic functions is to be substituted, transformed liver cell lines will exhibit limitations of various degree (Stange *et al.*, 1995). When comparing normal rat hepatocytes and well-differentiated Hep G2 cells (a cell line clinically used in a bioartificial liver device), rat hepatocytes significantly outperformed Hep G2 cells in all categories of biotransformation, such as urea genesis, glucuronidation, sulfation, and oxidative metabolism (Sussman and Kelly, 1993; Nyberg *et al.*, 1994). Therefore, liver tissue engineering should be based upon primary isolated hepatocytes.

e. Cellular Interactions: Coculture Models. In vitro systems based upon only parenchymal liver cells completely lack the dynamic interactions occurring *in vivo*, where different liver cell types communicate not only by means of cytokines or growth factors, but also by expression of cell–cell contacts, e.g., intercellular junctions, and deposition of extracellular matrix (Lescoat *et al.*, 1987). As we have mentioned before, hepatocytes account for only 65% of the liver cell mass, and their complex synthetic and metabolic function requires a specific cell microenvironment.

This section summarizes the significant advances regarding coculture of hepatocytes with other nonparenchymal liver cell types in respect of tissue engineering.

f. The Role of Hepatocyte Density on HC Function and Proliferation in Different Coculture Models. Primary hepatocytes can be maintained on a feeder layer of different cell types, such as fibroblasts or sinusoidal cells which provide some collagen substrata (Michalopoulos *et al.*, 1979; Wanson *et al.*, 1979); however, the specific functions of HC rapidly decrease under these simplified conditions. When, however, HC at higher density were plated on vascular endothelial or sinusoidal endothelial cells, HC in coculture remained longer than 3 weeks viable, secreted albumin at higher levels and longer in coculture (over 3 weeks) than in controls alone (5 days) (Morin and Normand, 1986), and HC exhibited junctional complexes and bile canaliculi between adjacent cells (James *et al.*, 1992).

Investigating the mitogenic capacity of HC in coculture, Shimaoka *et al.*, 1987) plated HC/nonparenchymal cells (NPC) in a ratio of 1:10, demonstrating a labeling index of HC at 54% in coculture as opposed to 12% when cultured alone. Notably, the NPC fraction was not labeled in coculture. A maximal labeling index was observed at lowest HC density and a progressive index decline with increasing HC density. Notably, HC alone had a lower labeling index at all different densities than in coculture, suggesting a mitogenic effect by coculture with NPC.

However, the proliferative potential of HC of different species is variable alone and in coculture. Comparing the proliferative potential of low-density plated rat and pig hepatocytes in pure primary culture or in coculture with rat liver epithelial cells (RLEC), using a HC/NPC of 0.13:1.1, rat HC showed a much lower basal growth and response to added growth factors than pig hepatocytes (Wegner *et al.*, 1992). Strikingly, coculture with RLEC resulted in a controversial effect on the different HC types: pig HC were further stimulated by coculture with RLEC, while rat HC were almost blocked in growth.

Continuous hepatocyte proliferation in coculture has been achieved in a different coculture system (Roberts *et al.*, 1994). Isolated human hepatocytes were cocultured with rat liver epithelial cells (RLEC) for 6 weeks in the presence of a conditioned medium from previous hepatocyte lines. During that time, clusters of hepatocytes, being surrounded by RLEC, proliferated and gradually replaced the RLEC in the well, yielding continuous subcultures over 2 years. In the absence of conditioned medium, hepatocytes deteriorated and RLEC predominated. In the absence of RLEC, HC in conditioned medium lost the typical hepatocellular morphological features. The continuous cocultures, consisting of 95% human hepatic cells after 2 years, retained differentiated hepatocellular functions, such as albumin and transferrin synthesis and drug-metabolizing enzyme activities. It is therefore concluded that proliferating hepatocytes produce soluble growth factors which promote growth of hepatocytes but not nonparenchymal epithelial cells in coculture. On the other hand, maintenance of differentiated hepatocellular functions is supported by heterotypic cell interactions by nonparenchymal liver cells.

g. The Extracellular Matrix in Cocultures of HC with Nonparenchymal Cells: A Prerequisite or Produced by Cocultured Liver Cells In Vitro? Adhesion to the extracellular matrix plays a critical role in directing the migration, proliferation, and differentiation of cells; and aberrations in such interactions can lead to pathological disorders (Clark and Brugge, 1995). Adhesion-induced changes mediate the cell activities in two crucial aspects: first, adherence to the ECM is critical for stimulation of cell proliferation by growth factors or serum in most cell types. Second, such specific cell surface receptors regulate intracellular signal transduction pathways, mediating adhesion-induced changes in cell physiology by integrin links to intracellular cytoskeletal complexes and actin filaments (Clark and Brugge, 1995).

While we have mentioned before the crucial effect of added ECM on HC polarity *in vitro*, we will now report on the ECM production in various coculture systems. Guguen-Guillouzo described first that HC cocultured with rat liver epithelial cells (RLEC) were covered in a cocoon of organized extracellular fibers, reaching a maximum after 7–8 days of coculture on uncoated plastic dishes (Guguen-Guillouzo *et al.*, 1983). These reticulin positively stained fibers in pure HC cultures and were absent or sparsely present in RLEC at confluence. Hence, secretion and organization was an effect of coculturing HC with RLEC, and could be demonstrated in various amounts and distribution around cords of adult and fetal human HC, or rat HC, which were cocultured with RLEC.

Characterization of the ECM, accumulated around the HC, demonstrated type I and type III collagen and fibronectin (Clement *et al.*, 1994). More important, the extracellular matrix network around adult hepatocytes of rat or human origin contains basement membrane components including laminin, collagen type IV, and heparan sulfate proteoglycan (Clement *et al.*, 1988a,b). Interestingly, HC secrete laminin only in soluble form when cultured alone. In contrast, laminin accumulated around HC cords when they were cocultured with RLEC (Clement *et al.*, 1988b), both cell types being capable of synthesizing and secreting it. Under *in vitro* conditions, HC are able to express the whole set of basement membrane components when put in culture, i.e., collagen IV, laminin, and entactin/nidogen (Rescan *et al.*, 1993).

Strikingly, deposition of perlecan (heparansulfate proteoglycan) occurs in coculture only, following reestablishment of specific cell–cell interactions. Although the main source in coculture appears to be RLEC, HC being a lower producer, perlecan deposition requires cellular cooperation, because RLEC in pure culture do not express perlecan extracellularly. Thus, HC may act as a potent regulator of its aggregation within a basement membrane. In conclusion, cocultures of HC with RLEC produce an extracellular matrix network, which includes key elements for assembly of basement membranes. Cocultures of primary HC with Ito cells or with sinusoidal endothelial cells showed a similar pattern of ECM network formation like HC with RLEC (Goulet *et al.*, 1988; Loreal *et al.*, 1993; Gressner *et al.*, 1995).

Increased tissue-specific gene transcription of HC in coculture was mediated by expression of cell surface receptors regulating cell–cell recognition. A plasma membrane protein was demonstrated at the cell surface of both adult HC and RLEC, named liver regulating protein (LRP) because of its involvement in hepatocyte differentiation (Corlu *et al.*, 1991). Blocking of the LRP receptor by an antibody resulted in cytoskeletal disturbances, loss of ECM deposition (few remaining reticulin fibers in coculture), and disturbance of the functional capacity of HC in culture, while cell–cell aggregations and cell adhesion to ECM were still maintained. The authors demonstrated that liver epithelial cells of different species and HC from different species were able to interact and were maintained in a higher functional stability in coculture. The protein regulates ECM deposition but is distinct from an ECM receptor, suggesting that cell–cell interactions in coculture regulate HC differentiation at a different level than ECM receptors.

Summing up the various study results, primary HC strongly contribute to the formation of the ECM network *in vitro*, thus differing partly from the normal conditions *in vivo*. Illustrating this, the deposition of reticulin fibers is located around HC, but requires coculture with nonparenchymal cells, including liver epithelial cells, Ito cells, or sinusoidal endothelial cells.

Thus, the extracellular matrix network requires cellular interactions and is, at least partly, regulated by a cell membrane protein. Although the models described here were only based upon coculture with two liver cell types, these systems offer a great opportunity for further studies on liver tissue engineering.

h. Dependency of the Cell Type Used for Coculture with HC for the Induction of Liver-Specific Functions. As far as the differentiated HC function is concerned, a major improvement by cocultures is obtained in providing confluent nonparenchymal cell layers around HC clusters within a day of culture. In Guguen-Guillouzo's coculture system, direct cell–cell contacts of hepatocytes and rat liver epithelial cells (RLEC) with confluence were provided within 24 hours (Guguen-Guillouzo *et al.*, 1983). Results showed that cocultured HC could be maintained for more than 2 months on plastic, exhibiting a characteristic morphology with expression of bile-canalicular-like structures. Remarkably, this correlated with maintained albumin secretion in coculture over 6 weeks in the presence or absence of fetal calf serum in the culture medium, compared to loss of albumin secretion after 2 weeks in pure HC controls. Hence, HC viability and differentiated function can be most effectively improved in a coculture system with liver epithelial cells enabling confluence within 24 hours.

With regard to the impact of cell densities in that model, Morin and co-workers (1986) clearly showed that in coculture with HC, a higher density of nonparenchymal cells (they were using sinusoidal cells) yielded higher albumin secretion, accordingly. The best ratio was found to be 7 HC/5 SEC in coculture.

Several groups later investigated if the beneficial effect of coculturing HC was related to junctional communication between homotypic or even the heterotypic cell types used. Mesnil and co-workers (1987) postulated that coculture of HC with liver epithelial cells (RLEC) improved the differentiated function of HC by means of their cell contact but not junctional communication. They were able to show that junctional communication, as demonstrated for the epithelial cells for the whole culture period, and detected among the HC after 2 weeks in culture, did not occur between HC and liver epithelial cells. Their findings indicated that HC colonies without contact to RLEC died within 5 days. In contrast, HC colonies surrounded by RLEC regained their normal morphology and survived, no matter what density RLEC were added. Therefore, a RLEC density enabling fast confluence by filling the spaces between HC was favorable for maintenance of HC function. When cocultured with RLEC, adult rat HC produce also acute-phase proteins in serum-free medium, including haptoglobin, α2-macroglobin, and hemopexin at stable levels over 20 days. In addition, plasma protein fibrinogen, α1-acute-phase-protein, α1-acid-glycoprotein, and α1-antitrypsin are produced under these conditions (Guillouzo *et al.*, 1984).

However, regardless of the cell density used, no gap junction communication was ever detected between HC and RLEC. Goulet *et al.* (1988) examined if junctional communication between HC and nonparenchymal cells of different types was required to promote tissue-specific HC functions. In cocultures, reaching confluence within 48 hours, HC remained morphologically intact, retaining junctional channels, secreted albumin longer than 10 days, and contributed to biomatrix deposition together with different coculture cell types. However, no junctional communication was observed between HC and fibroblasts, sinusoidal or vascular endothelial cells, or liver epithelial cells. In conclusion, improved synthetic functions of HC (e.g., albumin production) do not depend on junctional communication between HC and NPC.

With regard to the metabolic function of HC in cocultures, experiments were performed with different NPC types. In one model, HC were plated with different nonparenchymal cell types. While xenobiotic metabolizing enzyme activities rapidly dropped in HC controls, HC in cocultures were well stabilized over 1 week, suggesting that cell membrane-bound molecules on the coculture cells may help to support the HC function (Utesch *et al.*, 1991). Diener and co-workers (1994) examined in the same coculture system the gap junctional intercellular communication of cultured rat hepatocytes cocultured with nonparenchymal epithelial cells (RLEC). Results showed an increased and stabilized intercellular communication among HC in coculture as compared to pure HC controls. However, a heterotypic gap junctional communication between parenchymal and nonparenchymal liver epithelial cells was not observed in that system.

The only evidence for functional gap junctions between HC and other liver cells *in vitro* has been reported by Rojkind and co-workers (1995), establishing a coculture system of HC with Ito cells. Requiring a close contact between HC and Ito cells, a number of differentiated HC functions, such as secretion of albumin, coeruloplasmin, and fibrinogen, was enhanced. Most significantly, functional gap junctions are expressed between the two cell types in coculture. The capacity of different Ito cell clones to form gap junctions correlated with the survival of the cocultures over two weeks.

In conclusion, for improvement of differentiated HC functions in cocultures direct cell contacts between the two cell types are required. While this usually leads to an expression of gap junctions between either HC or NPC, functional gap junctions between HC and nonparenchymal cells have been described *in vitro* only for Ito cells. The synthetic function of HC is enhanced by coculture with liver epithelial, liver endothelial, and Ito cells. Liver-derived nonparenchymal cells generally support the HC function better than cell types of other origin. Cellular interactions are partly mediated by a cell surface protein, expressed on both parenchymal and nonparenchymal liver cells.

Utesch and co-workers (1991) carefully examined several independent metabolic functions of liver parenchymal cells in cocultures with rat liver nonparenchymal epithelial cells or mouse embryo fibroblasts. Comparing testosterone metabolism in HC monoculture with cocultures, a drastically significant reduction occurred only in monoculture, but was equally well maintained in both coculture systems. In the coculture systems, P-450s were well preserved, independent of the cell line used, but demonstrated that the coculture of liver parenchymal cells with nonparenchymal cells significantly improved the differentiated status of the HC.

Accordingly, the activities of various xenobiotic metabolizing enzymes were also much better stabilized in cocultures of rat HC than in monoculture over 1 week (Utesch and Oesch, 1992). Comparing the effect of two different rat epithelial cell lines in coculture with rat HC, activities of cytosolic epoxide hydrolase, glutathione S-transferase, and alpha-naphthol UDP-glucuronosyl transferase were generally measured higher in cocultures with one epithelial cell line. Interestingly, cocultures of HC with mouse embryo fibroblasts coculd also further enhance the activity of glutathione S-transferase and additionally induce the activity of microsomal epoxide hydrolase. These results suggest that the *in vitro* stabilization of differentiated HC functions depend on the cell type used for coculture.

Finally, the authors investigated how far gap junctional intercellular communication (GJIC) occurring in coculture mediate these effects (Diener *et al.*, 1994). While cocultures of HC with a rat liver epithelial cell line resulted in increased and stabilized intercellular communication of the HC, coculture with a rat liver fibroblast cell line did not support the communication. Although a heterotypic gap junctional communication between parenchymal and nonparenchymal cells was not observed, coculture with liver epithelial cells was responsible for the stabilization of the gap junctions between rat HC.

Therefore, cocultures of HC with nonparenchymal cells also improve the metabolic function of parenchymal liver cells. However, stabilization of differentiated functions depends on the type of cells used for coculture with HC. Liver epithelial cells and liver endothelial cells have been proven to be successful in maintaining metabolic HC functions over longer periods, while most fibroblast cell types were ineffective.

In our experiments, we have investigated the effect of primary HC on intrahepatic biliary epithelial cells (BEC). Using autologous human HC and intrahepatic BEC, the final BEC/HC ratio of approximately 1.25% resembled the distribution in the human liver. By plating these cocultures either on a single layer of rat tail collagen gel (SG) or between a double layer of collagen gel (DG), we were able to grow HC with BEC for more than 7 weeks in culture medium devoid of serum or added exogenous growth factors other than insulin or corticoids. While BEC normally require addition of exogenous growth factors HGF, EGF, and fetal calf serum to induce proliferation, in this coculture system proliferation of BEC was not dependent on these factors (Joplin *et al.*, 1992; Auth *et al.*, 1995a,b; 1996). Strikingly, inside collagen double gel aggregates of BEC reorganized themselves to three-dimensional cyst-like structures within a week of coculture, in the absence of exogenous morphogenic factors such as HGF/SF. From these cystic complexes, BEC grew out to form tubular structures with clearly identifiable lumen, gradually forming a network of corresponding ductular configurations over the next 4–6 weeks in culture. Ultrastructurally, the three-dimensional tubular structures were built by polarized BEC, demonstrating apical microvilli toward the duct lumen, basolateral nuclei, and expression of junctional complexes between adjacent cells. The number and differentiation of three-dimensional cyst-like structures of BEC in coculture could even be enhanced by culture in a conditioned medium of previous cocultures, but not by addition of exogenous growth factors HGF or EGF.

In conclusion, our experiments prove the beneficial effect of primary HC on growth and differentiation of human intrahepatic BEC (Auth, 1999). The mechanisms of cellular interactions are mediated by direct cellular contacts, but also by secretion of soluble factors released by cocultures of HC and BEC. These experiments suggest that epithelial interactions play an important role in liver growth and development. Further experiments with other nonparenchymal liver cells are required to examine whether liver regeneration is feasible *in vitro*.

31.6.7. Perspectives

Experiments with liver parenchymal and nonparenchymal cells from different species have demonstrated that cellular interactions are crucial for differentiated hepatic functions, such as synthesis and metabolism. If appropriate cell types are combined, these cocultured liver cells are capable of producing a liver-specific extracellular matrix. The differentiated liver function also requires the presence of specific hepatotrophic factors. It is currently unclear if hepatic cells produce all necessary factors *in vitro*, or if exogenous supply is essential for maintained function.

To provide the initial scaffold for the various liver cells to re-establish the organotypic three-dimensional architecture, matrix gels have proven to be effective tools. However, these culture systems have limitations in terms of upgrading for high cell densities, and dynamic interactions of several liver cell types. Future developments in biodegradable tubular scaffolds may help in giving rise to complete hepatic tissue engineering.

References

Abatangelo, G., Brun, P., Cortivo, R. 1994. Hyaluronan (Hyaluronic acid): an overview, in: *Novel Biomaterials Based on Hyaluronic Acid and Its Derivatives* (D.F. Williams, ed.), pp. 8–18, Proceedings of a Workshop Held at the Annual Meeting of the European Society for Biomaterials, Pisa, Italy.

Adams, J.C., Watt, F.M. 1989. Fibronectin inhibits the terminal differentiation of human keratinocytes, *Nature* **340**, 307–309.

Adams, J.C., Watt, F.M. 1993. Regulation of the development and differentiation by extracellular matrix, *Development* **117**, 1183–1198.

Advances in biotechnology and tissue engineering in musculoskeletal applications. 1997. MDI report #RP-651147, Irvine.

Aigner, J., Tegeler, J., Hutzler, P., Campoccia, D., Pavesio, A., Hammer, C., Kastenbauer, E., Naumann, A. 1998. Cartilage tissue engineering with novel nonwoven structured biomaterial based on hyaluronic acid benzyl ester, *J. Biomed. Mater. Res.* **42**, 172–181.

Andreassi, L., Casini, L., Trabucchi, E., Diamantini, S., Rastrelli, A., Donati, L., Tenchini, M.L., Malcovati, M. 1991. Human keratinocytes cultured on membranes composed of benzyl ester of hyaluronic acid suitable for grafting, *Wounds* **3**, 116–126.

Andreassi, L., Pianigiani, E., Andreassi, A., Taddeucci, P., Biagioli, M. 1998. A new model of epidermal culture for the surgical treatment of vitiligo, *Int. J. Dermatol.* **37**, 595–598.

Angele, P., Nerlich, A., Kujat, R., Faltermeier, H., Moller, H.D., Weigel, B., Nerlich, M. 1998. Chondrocyte differentiation in fibrin-coating on polytetrafluorethylene membranes, in: *Biological Matrices and Tissue Regeneration* (G.B. Stark, R. Horch, E. Tanczos, eds.), pp. 173–177, Springer-Verlag Berlin, Heidelberg.

Argraves, W.S., Tran, H., Burgess, W.H., Dickerson, K. 1990. Fibulin is an extracellular matrix and plasma glycoprotein with repeated domain structure, *J. Cell Biol.* **111**, 3155–3164.

Arias, I.M., Boyer, J.L., Fausto, N., Jakoby, W.B., Schachter, D.A., Shafritz, D.A. 1994. *The Liver: Biology and Pathobiology*, 3rd edn., Raven Press, New York.

Ashammakhi, N., Rokkanen, P. 1997. Absorbable polyglycolide devices in trauma and bone surgery, *Biomaterials* **18**, 3–9.

Auger, F.A., Lopez Valle, C.A., Guignard, R., Thremblay, N., Noel, B., Goulet, F., Germain, L. 1995. Skin equivalent produced with human collagen, *In Vitro Cell. Dev. Biol. Animal* **31**, 432–439.

Auth, M.K.H., Joplin, R., Fabris, L., Keogh, A., Gallacher, R.E., Neuberger, J.M., McMaster, P., Strain, A.J. 1995a. Structural and functional studies of human hepatocytes and biliary epithelial cells cocultured in collagen gels, *Hepatology* **22**(4), 215–A.

Auth, M.K.H., Joplin, R., Wallace, L., Keogh, A., Wilton, J.A., Strain, A.J. 1995b. Coculture of human biliary epithelial cells and hepatocytes in collagen gels, *FASEB J.* **9**(Pt II) , A-852.

Auth, M.K.H., Sadamoto, T., Okamoto, M., Joplin, R., Neuberger, J.M., Strain, A.J. 1996. Proliferation and formation of polarised luminal ducts by human biliary epithelial cells in vitro, *Hepatology* **24**(4), II, 129-A.

Baragi, V.M., Renkievicz, R.R., Jordan, H., Bonadio, J., Hartman, J.W, Roessler, B.J. 1995. Transplantation of transduced chondrocytes protects articular cartilage from interleukin-1 induced extracellular matrix degradation, *J. Clin. Invest.* **96**, 2454–2460.

Barbucci, R., Magnani, A., Da Costa, M.L., Bauser, H., Hellwig, G., Martuscelli, E., Cimmino, S. 1993. Physico-chemical surface characterization of hyaluronic acid derivatives as a new class of biomaterials, *J. Biomater. Sci. Polym. Ed.* **4**(3), 245–273.

Barry, F.P., and Murphy, J.M. 2000. Chondrogenic differentiation of mesenchymal stem cells on matrices of hyaluronan derivatives, in: *New Frontiers in Medical Sciences: Redefining Hyaluronan* (G. Abatangelo and P.H. Weigel, eds.) pp. 247–253, Elsevier Science.

Benedetti, L., Cortivo, R., Berti, T., Pea, F., Mazzo, M., Moras, M., Abatangelo, G. 1993. Biocompatibility and biodegradation of different hyaluronan derivatives (Hyaff) implanted in rats, *Biomaterials* **14**(15), 1154–1160.

Benya, P.D., Padilla, S.R., Nimni, M.E. 1977. The progeny of rabbit articular chondrocytes synthesize collagen type I and type III and type I trimer, but not type II: verifications by cyanogen bromide peptide analysis, *Biochemistry* **16**, 865–872.

Benya, P.D., Padilla, S.R. 1986. Modulation of the rabbit chondrocyte by retinoic acid terminates type II collagen synthesis without including type I collagen: the modulated phenotype differs from that produced by subculture, *Dev. Biol.* **118**(1): 296–305.

Bernfield, M., Sanderson, R.D. 1990. Syndecan, a developmentally regulated cell surface proteoglycan that binds extracellular matrix and growth factors. *Phil. Trans. R. Soc. Lond.*, Ser. B **327**, 171–186.

Billingham, R.E., Reynolds, J. 1952. Transplantation studies on sheets of pure epidermal epithelium and on epidermal cell suspensions. *Br. J. Plast. Surg.* **5**, 25–36.

Block, G., Locker, J., Bowen, W.C., Peterson B.E., Katyal, S., Strom, S.C., Riley, T., Howard, T.A., Michalopoulos, G.K. 1996. Population expansion, clonal growth, and specific differentiation patterns in primary cultures of hepatocytes induced by HGF/SF, EGF and TGF-α in a chemically defined (HGM) medium, *J. Cell Biol.* **132**(6), 1133–1149.

Boyce, S.T., Christianson, D., Hansbrough, J.F. 1988. Structure of a collagen-GAG skin substitute optimized for cultured human epidermal keratinocytes, *J. Biomed. Mater. Res.*, **22**, 939–957.

Breitbart, A.S., Grande, D.A., Kessler, R., Ryaby, J.T., Fitzsimmons, R.J., Grant, R.T. 1998. Tissue engineered bone repair of calvarial defects using cultured periosteal cells, *Plast. Reconstr. Surg.* **101**, 567–574.

Brekke, J.H. 1996. A rationale for delivery of osteoinductive proteins, *Tissue Eng.* **2**, 97–114.

Brittberg, M., Lindahl, A., Nilsson, A., Ohlsson, C., Isaksson, O., Peterson, L. 1994a. Treatment of deep cartilage defects in the knee with autologous chondrocyte transplantation, *N. Engl. J. Med.* **331**, 889–895.

Brittberg, M., Faxen, E., Peterson, L. 1994b. Carbon fiber scaffolds in the treatment of early knee osteoarthritis, a prospective 4-year follow-up of 37 patients, *Clin. Orthop.* **307**, 155–164.

Brun, P., Abatangelo, G., Radice, M., Zacchi, V., Guidolin, D., Daga-Gordini, D., Cortivo, R. 2000. Chondrocyte aggregation and reorganization into three-dimensional scaffolds, *J. Biomed. Mater. Res.* **46**, 337–346.

Burgess, E.A., Hollinger, J.O. 1998. Options for tissue engineering bone, in: *Frontiers in Tissue Engineering* (C.W. Patrick, Jr., A.G. Mikos, L.V. McIntire, eds.), pp. 383–399, Pergamon, New York.

Butnariu-Ephrat, M., Robinson, D., Mendes, D.G., Halperin, N., Nevo, Z. 1996. Resurfacing of goat articular cartilage by chondrocytes derived from bone marrow, *Clin. Orthop. Relat. Res.* **330**, 234–243.

Buttermann, G.R., Glazer, P.A., Bradford, D.S. 1996. The use of bone allografts in the spine, *Clin. Orthop. Relat. Res.* **324**, 75–85.

Campoccia, D., Doherty, P., Radice, M., Brun, P., Abatangelo, G., Williams, D.F. 1998. Semisynthetic resorbable materials from hyaluronan derivatization, *Biomaterials* **19**, 2101–2127.

Caplan, A.I. 1991. Mesenchymal stem cells, *J. Orthop. Res.* **9**(5), 641–650.

Caplan, A.I. 1994. The mesengenic process, *Bone Rep. Reg.* **21**, 429–435.

Caplan, A.I., Elyaderani, M., Mochizuki, Y., Wakitani, S., Goldberg, V.M. 1997. Principles of cartilage repair and regeneration, *Clin. Orthop. Relat. Res.* **342**, 254–269.

Chu, C.R., Coutts, R.D., Yoshioka, M., Harwood, F.L., Monsov, A.Z., Amiel, D. 1995. Articular cartilage repair using allogenic perichondrocyte-seeded biodegradable porous polylactic acid (PLA): a tissue-engineering study, *J. Biomed. Mater. Res.* **29**, 1147–1154.

Clark, E.A., Brugge, J.S. 1995. Integrins and signal transduction pathways: the road taken, *Science* **268**, 233–239.

Clement, B., Laurent, M., Guguen-Guillouzo, C., Lebeau, G., Guillouzo, A. 1988a. Types I and IV procollagen gene expression in cultured rat hepatocytes, *Collagen Relat. Res.* **8**, 349–359.

Clement, B., Rescan, P.Y., Baffet, G., Loreal, O., Lehry, D., Campion, J.P., Guillouzo, A. 1988b. Hepatocytes may produce laminin in fibrotic liver and in primary culture, *Hepatology* **8**(4), 794–803.

Clement, B., Guguen-Guillouzo, C., Campion, J.P., Launois, B., Nicol, M. 1994. Long-term co-cultures of adult human hepatocytes with rat liver epithelial cells: modulation of albumin secretion and accumulation of extracellular material, *Hepatology* **4**(3), 373–380.

Cook, S.D., Dalton, J.E., Tan, E.H., Whitecloud, T.S., Rueger, D.C. 1994. *In vivo* evaluation of recombinant human osteogenic protein (rhOP-1) implants as a bone graft substitute for spinal fusions, *Spine* **19**, 1655–1663.

Corlu, A., Kneip, B., Lhadi, C., Leray, G., Glaise, D., Baffet, G., Bourel, D., Guguen-Guillouzo, C. 1991. A plasma membrane protein is involved in cell contact-mediated regulation of tissue-specific genes in adult hepatocytes, *J. Cell Biol.* **225**(2), 505–515.

Cortivo, R., De Galateo, A., Castellani, I., Brun, P., Giro, M.G., Abatangelo, G. 1990. Hyaluronic acid promotes chick embryo fibroblast and chondroblast expression, *Cell Biol. Int. Rep.* **14**, 111–122.

Cortivo, R., Brun, P., Rastrelli, A., Abatangelo, G. 1991. In vitro studies on biocompatibility of hyaluronic acid esters, *Biomaterials* **12**, 727–730.

Damsky, C., Sutherland, A., Fisher, S. 1993. Extracellular matrix 5: Adhesive interactions in early mammalian embryogenesis, implantation and placentation, *FASEB J.* **7**, 1320–1329.

Damsky, C.H., Werb, Z. 1992. Signal transduction by integrin receptors for extracellular matrix: cooperative processing of extracellular information, *Curr. Opin. Cell Biol.* **4**, 772–781.

Dichek, D.A., Anderson, J., Kelly, A.B., Hanson, S.R., Harker, L.A. 1996. Enhanced *in vivo* antithrombotic effects of endothelial cells expressing recombinant plasminogen activators transduced with retroviral vectors, *Circulation* **93**, 301–309.

Diener, B., Beer, N., Durk, H., Traiser, M., Utesch, D., Wieser, R.J., Oesch, F. 1994. Gap junctional intercellular communication of cultured rat-liver parenchymal-cells is stabilized by epithelial-cells and their isolated plasma-membranes, *Experientia* **50**(2), 124–126.

Dixon, K.P., Murphy, R.W., Southerland, S.S., Young, H.E., Lucas, P.A. 1996. Recombinant human bone morphogenetic proteins-2 and -4 induce several mesenchymal phenotypes in culture, *Wound Rep. Reg.* **4**, 374–380.

Drumheller, P.D., Hubbell, J.A. 1995. Surface immobilization of adhesion ligands for investigations for cell-substrate interactions, in: *Biomedical Engineering Handbook* (J.D. Bronzino, ed.), pp. 1583–1596, CRC Press, Boca Raton.

Dunn, J.C., Yarmush, M.L., Koebe, H.G., Tompkins, R.G. 1989. Hepatocyte function and extracellular matrix geometry: long-term culture in a sandwich configuration, *FASEB J.* **3**, 174–177.

Dunn, J.C., Tompkins, R.G., Yarmush, M.L. 1992. Hepatocytes in collagen sandwich: evidence for transcriptional and translational regulation, *J. Cell Biol.* **116**(4), 1043–1053.

Eming, S.A., Lee, J., Snow, R.G., Tompkins, R.G., Yarmush, M.L., Morgan, J.R. 1995. Genetically modified human epidermis over-expressing PDGF-A directs the development of a cellular and vascular connective tissue stroma when transplanted to athymic mice, *J. Invest. Dermatol.* **105**, 756–763.

Eming, S.A., Snow, R.G., Yarmush, M.L., Morgan, J.R. 1996. Targeted expression of IGF-1 to human keratinocytes: modification of autocrine control of keratinocyte proliferation, *J. Invest. Dermatol.* **107**, 113–120.

Engel, J. 1989. EGF-like domains in extracellular matrix proteins: localised signals for growth and differentiation, *FEBS Lett.* **251**, 1–7.

Ezzell, R.M., Toner, M., Hendricks, K., Dunn, J.C., Tompkins, R.G., Yarmush, M.L. 1993. Effect of collagen gel configuration on the cytoskeleton in cultured rat hepatocytes, *Exp. Cell Res.* **208**, 442–452.

Falanga, V., Margolis, D., Alvarez, O., Auletta, M., Maggiacomo, F., Altman, M., Jensen, J., Sabolinsky, M., Hardin-Young, J. 1998. Rapid healing of venous ulcers and lack of clinical rejection with allogeneic cultured human skin equivalent, *Arch. Dermatol.* **134**, 293–300.

Ferns, M., Hoch, W., Campanelli, J. T., Rupp, F., Hall, Z.W., Scheller, R.H. 1992. RNA splicing regulates agrin-mediated acetylcholine receptor clustering activity on cultured myotubes, *Neuron* **8**, 1079–1086.

Freed, L.E., Marquuis, L.J., Nohria, A., Emmanual, J., Mikos, A.G., Langer, R. 1993. Neocartilage formation *in vitro* and *in vivo* using cells cultured on synthetic biodegradable polymers, *J. Biomed. Mater. Res.* **27**, 11–23.

Freed, L.E., Grande, D.A., Lingbin, Z., Emmanual, J., Marquis, J.C., Langer, R. 1994. Joint resurfacing using allograft chondrocytes and synthetic biodegradable polymer scaffolds, *J. Biomed. Mater. Res.* **28**, 891–899.

Fujisato, T., Sajiki, T., Liu, Q., Ikada, Y. 1996. Effect of basic fibroblast growth factor on cartilage regeneration in chondrocyte-seeded collagen sponge scaffold, *Biomaterials* **17**, 155–162.

Fusenig, N.E. 1994. Epithelial-mesenchymal interactions regulate keratinocyte growth and differentiation *in vitro*, in: *The Keratinocyte Handbook* (I. Leigh, B. Lane, F.M. Watt, eds.), pp. 71–94, Cambridge University Press, Cambridge.

Galassi, G., Brun, P., Radice, M., Cortivo, R., Zanon, G.F., Genovese, P., Abatangelo, G. 2000. In vitro reconstructed dermis implanted in human wounds: degradation studies of the HA-based supporting scaffold, *Biomaterials* **21**, 2183–2191.

Gallico, G.G., III, O'Connor, N.E., Compton, C.C., Kehinde, O., Green, H. 1984. Permanent coverage of large burn wounds with autologous cultured human epithelium, *New Engl. J. Med.* **311**, 448–451.

Gallico, G.G., III, O'Connor, N.E., Compton, C.C., Remensnyder, J.P., Kehinde, O., Green, H. 1989. Cultured epithelial autografts for giant congenital nevi, *Plast. Reconstr. Surg.* **84** 1–9.

Gerrad, A.J., Hudson, D.J., Brownlee, G.G., Watt, F.M. 1993. Gene therapy for haemophilia B using primary human keratinocytes, *Nature* **3**, 180–183.

Giusti, P., Callegaro, L. 1994. *World patent Application No. WO 94/01468*.

Gomez-Lechon, M.J., Castelli, J., Guillen, I., O'Connor, E., Nakamura, T., Fabra, R., Trullenque, R. 1995. Effect of hepatocyte growth factor on the growth and metabolsim of human hepatocytes in primary culture, *Hepatology* **21**, 1248–1254.

Gooch, K.J., Blunk, T., Vunjak-Novakovic, G., Langer, R., Freed, L., Tennant, C.J. 1998. Mechanical forces and growth factors utilized in tissue engineering, in: *Frontiers in Tissue Engineering* (C.W. Patrick, Jr., A.G. Mikos, L.V. McIntire, eds.), pp. 61–82, Pergamon, New York.

Goulet, F., Normand, C., Morin, O. 1988. Cellular interactions promote tissue-specific function, biomatrix deposition and junctional communication of primary cultured hepatocytes, *Hepatology* **8**(5), 1010–1018.

Green, H. 1977. Terminal differentiation of cultured epidermis cells, *Cell* **11**, 405–416.

Gressner, A.M., Lahme, B., Brenzel, A. 1995. Molecular dissection of the mitogenic effect of hepatocytes on cultured hepato-stellate cells, *Hepatology* **22**, 1507–1518.

Grigoriadis, A.E., Heersche, J.N.M., Aubin, J.E. 1988. Differentiation of muscle, fat, cartilage and bone from progenitor cells present in a bone-derived clonal cell population: effect of dexamethasone, *J. Cell Biol.* **106**, 2139–2151.

Guguen-Guillouzo, C., Clement, B., Baffet, G., Beaumont, C., Morel-Chany, E., Glaise, D., Guillouzo, A. 1983. Maintenance and reversibility of active albumin secretion by adult rat hepatocytes co-cultured with another liver epithelial cell type, *Exp. Cell Res.* **143**, 47–54.

Guguen-Guillouzo, C., Clement, B., Lescoat, G., Glaise, D., Guillouzo, A. 1984. Modulation of human fetal hepatocytes survival and differentiation by interactions with a rat liver epithelial cell line, *Dev. Biol.* **105**, 211–230.

Guillouzo, A., Delers, F., Clement, B., Bernard, N., Engler, R. 1984. Long term production of acute-phase proteins by adult rat hepatocytes co-cultured with another liver cell type in serum-free medium, *Biochem. Biophys. Res. Commun.* **120**(2), 311–317.

Gumbiner, B.M. 1996. Cell adhesion: The molecular basis of tissue architecture and morphogenesis, *Cell* **84**, 345–357.

Haisch, A., Rathert, T., Schultz, O., Janke, V., Burmester, G.R., Sittinger, M. 1998. In vitro engineered cartilage for reconstructive surgery, using biocompatible, resorbable fibrin glue/polymer structures, in: *Frontiers of Tissue Engineering* (C.W. Patrick, A.G. Mikos, L.V. McIntire, eds.), pp. 179–187, Pergamon, New York.

Hansbrough, J.F., Morgan, J., Greenleaf, G. 1993. Advances in wound coverage using cultured cell technology, *Wounds* **5**, 174–194.

Hardingham, T.E., Forsang, A.J. 1992. Proteoglycans: many forms and functions. *FASEB J.* **6**, 861-870.

Harris, P.A. 1998. Pre-confluent keratinocyte grafting: the future for cultured skin replacements? *Burns* **24**, 591–593.

Harris, P.A., di Francesco, F., Barisoni, D., Leigh, I.M., Navsaria, H.A. 1999. Use of hyaluronic acid and cultured autologous keratinocytes and fibroblasts in extensive burns, *Lancet* **353**, 35–36.

Hemler, M.E. 1990. VLA proteins in the integrin family: structures, functions and their role on leukocytes, *Annu. Rev. Immunol.* **8**, 365–400.

Hemmen, B., Archer, C.W., Bentley, G. 1991. Repair of articular cartilage defects by carbon fiber plugs loaded with chondrocytes, *Trans. Orthop. Res. Soc.* **16**, 278.

Hollinger, J.O., Brekke, J.B., Gruskin, E., Lee, D. 1996. Role of bone substitutes, *Clin. Orthop. Relat. Res.* **324**, 55–65.

Horton, W.A., Machado, M.A., Ellard, J., Campbell, D., Puttam, E.A., Aulthause, A.L., Sun, X., Sandell, L.J. 1993. An experimental model of human chondrocyte differentiation, *Prog. Clin. Biol. Res.* **383B**, 533–540.

Hu, M.Y., Cipolle, M., Sielaff, T., Lovdahl, M.J., Mann, H.J., Remmel, R.P., Cerra, F.B. 1995. Effects of hepatocyte growth factor on viability and biotransformation functions of hepatocytes in gel entrapped and monolayer, *Crit. Care Med.* **23**, 1237–1242.

Hunziker, E.B., Rosenberg, L. 1994. Induction of repair in partial thickness articular lesion by timed release of TGF-β, *Trans. Orthop. Res. Soc.* **19**, 236.

Hynes, R.O. 1992. Integrins: versatility, modulation and signalling in cell adhesion, *Cell* **69**, 11–25.

Iyoda, K., Miura, T., Nogami, H. 1993. Repair of bone defect with cultured chondrocytes bound to hydroxyapatite, *Clin. Orthop. Relat. Res.* **288**, 287–293.

James, N.H., Molloy, C., Soames, A.R., French, N.J., Roberts, R.A. 1992. An in vitro model of rodent nongenotoxic hepatocarcinogenesis, *Exp. Cell Res.* **203**, 407–419.

Joplin, R., Hishida, T., Tsubouchi, H., Daikuhara, Y., Ayres, R., Neuberger, J.M., Strain, A.J. 1992. Human biliary epithelial cells proliferate in vitro in response to human hepatocyte growth factor, *J. Clin. Invest.* **90**, 1284–1289.

Kaiser, H.W., Stark, G.B., Kopp, J., Balcerkiewicz, A., Spilker, G., Kreysel, H.W. 1994. Cultured autologous keratinocytes in fibrin glue suspension, exclusively and combined with STS-allograft (preliminary clinical and histological report on a new technique, *Burns* **20**, 23–29.

Karin, M. 1992. Signal transduction from cell surface to nucleus in development and disease, *FASEB J.* **6**, 2581–2590.

Kasugai, S., Todescan, R., Jr., Nagata, T., Yao, K.L., Butler, W.T., Sodek, J. 1991. Expression of bone matrix proteins associated with mineralized tissue formation by adult rat bone marrow cells in vitro: inductive effects of dexamethasone on the osteoblastic phenotype, *J. Cell Physiol.* **147**, 111–120.

Kawamura, S., Wakitani, S., Kimura, T., Maeda, A., Caplan, A.I., Shino, K., Ochi, T. 1998. Articular cartilage repair, *Acta Orthop. Scand.* **69**(1), 56–62.

Kim, W.S., Vacanti, J.P., Cima, L.G., Mooney, D., Upton, J., Puelacher, W.C. 1994. Cartilage engineered in predetermined shapes employing cell transplantation on synthetic biodegradable polymers, *Plast. Reconstr. Surg.* **94**, 233–237.

Klagsbrun, M. 1990. The affinity of FGF for heparin: FGF-heparan sulphate interactions in cells and extracellular matrix, *Curr. Opin. Cell Biol.* **2**, 857–863.

Knudson, C.B., Knudson, W. 1990. Similar epithelial-stromal interactions in the regulation of hyaluronate production during limb morphogenesis and tumor invasion, *Cancer Lett.* **52**, 113–122.

Kolettas, E., Buluwela, L., Bayliss, M.T., Muir, H.I. 1995. Expression of cartilage-specific molecules is retained on long term culture of human chondrocytes, *J. Cell Sci.* **108**, 1991–1999.

Lamme, E.N., De Vries, H.J.C., Van Veen, H., Gabbiani, G., Westerhof, W., Middelkoop, E. 1996. Extracellular matrix characterization during healing of full-thickness wounds treated with a collagen/elastin dermal substitute shows improved skin regeneration in pigs, *J. Histochem. Cytochem.* **44**, 1311–1322.

Lazarus, H.M., Haynesworth, S.E., Gerson, S.L., Rosenthal, N.S., Caplan, A.I. 1995. *Ex vivo* expansion and subsequent infusion of human bone marrow-derived stromal progenitor cells (mesenchymal progenitor cells): implications for therapeutic use, *Bone Marrow Transplant.* **16**, 557–564.

Leigh, I.M. 1994. Keratinocyte autografting, allografting and wound healing, in: *The Keratinocyte Handbook* (I. Leigh, B. Lane, F.M. Watt, eds.), pp. 503–511, Cambridge University Press, Cambridge.

Leigh, I.M., Watt, F.M. 1994. The culture of human epidermal keratinocytes, in: *The Keratinocyte Handbook* (I. Leigh, B. Lane, F.M. Watt, eds.), pp. 43–51, Cambridge University Press, Cambridge.

Lescoat, G., Pasdeloup, N., Kneip, B., Guguen-Guillouzo, G. 1987. Modulation of alpha-fetoprotein, albumin and transferrin gene expression by cellular interactions and dexamethasone in cocultures of fetal rat hepatocytes, *Eur. J. Cell Biol.* **44**(1), 128–134.

Liebergall, M., Young, R.G., Ozawa, H. 1994. The effects of cellular manipulation and TGF-β in a composite bone graft, in: *Bone Formation and Repair* (C.T. Brighton, G. Friedlaender, J.M. Lane, eds.), pp. 367–378, American Academy of Orthopaedic Surgeons, Rosemont.

Limat, A., Mauri, D., Hunziker, T. 1996. Successful treatment of chronic leg ulcers with epidermal equivalents generated from cultured autologous outer root sheath cells, *J. Invest. Dermatol.* **107**, 128–135.

Limova, M., Mauro, T. 1995. Treatment of leg ulcers with cultured epithelial autografts: treatment protocol and five year experience, *Wounds* **7**, 170–180.

Lin, C.Q., Bissell, M.J. 1993. Multi-faceted regulation of cell differentiation by extracellular matrix, *FASEB J.* **7**, 737–743.

Loreal, O., Levavasseur, F., Fromaget, C., Gros, D., Guillouzo, A., Clement, B. 1993. Cooperation of Ito cells and hepatocytes in the deposition of an extracellular matrix in vitro, *Am. J. Pathol.* **143**(2), 538–544.

MacKenzie, I. 1994. Epithelial-mesenchymal interactions in the development and maintenance of epithelial tissues, in: *The Keratinocyte Handbook* (I. Leigh, B. Lane, F.M. Watt, eds.), pp. 243–257, Cambridge University Press, Cambridge.

Mankin, H.J., Gebhardt, M.C., Jennings, L.C., Springfield, D.S., Tomford, W.W. 1996. Long-term results of allograft replacement in the management of bone tumors, *Clin. Orthop. Relat. Res.* **324**, 86–97.

Mantalaris, A., Keng, P., Bourne, P., Chang, A.Y., Wu, J.H. 1998. Engineering a human bone marrow model: a case study on ex vivo erythropoiesis, *Biotechnol. Prog.* **14**, 126–133.

Martin, P. 1997. Wound healing—Aiming for perfect skin regeneration, *Science* **276**, 75–81.

Maslen, C.L., Corson, G.M., Maddox, B.K., Glanville, R.W., Sakai, L.Y. 1991. Partial sequence of a candidate gene for the Marfan syndrome, *Nature* **352**, 334–337.

Mayhew, T.A., Williams, G.R., Senica, M.A., Kuniholm, G., du Moulin, G.C. 1998. Validation of a quality assurance program for autologous cultured chondrocyte implantation, *Tissue Eng.* **4**(3), 325–334.

McPherson, D.T., Morrow, C., Minehan, D.S., Wu, J.G., Hunter, E., Urry, D.W. 1992. Production and purification of a recombinant elastomeric peptide $G(VPGVG)^{19}VPGV$ from *Escherichia Coli*, *Biotech. Prog.* **8**, 347–352.

Mesnil, M., Fraslin, J.M., Piccoli, C., Yamasaki, H., Guguen-Guillouzo, C. 1987. Cell contact but not junctional communication (dye coupling) with biliary epithelial cells is required for hepatocytes to maintain differentiated functions, *Exp. Cell Res.* **173**, 524–533.

Messner, K., Gillquist, J. 1996. Cartilage repair, *Acta Orthop. Scand.* **67**, 523–529.

Michalopoulos, G., Russell, F., Biles, C. 1979. Primary cultures of hepatocytes on human fibroblasts, *In Vitro* **15**(10), 796–806.

Mooney, D., Hansen, L., Vacanti, J., Langer, R., Farmer, S., Ingber, D. 1992. Switching from differentiation to growth in hepatocytes: control by extracellular matrix, *J. Cell Physiol.* **151**, 497–505.

Morgan, J.R., Yarmush, M.L. 1998. Gene therapy in tissue engineering, in: *Frontiers in Tissue Engineering* (C. W. Patrick, Jr., A.G. Mikos, L.V. McIntire, eds.), pp. 278–310, Pergamon, New York.

Morgan, J.R., Barrandon, Y., Green, H., Mulligan, R.C. 1987. Transfer and expression of foreign genes in transplantable human epidermal cells, *Science* **237**, 1476–1479.

Moriarty, K.P., Crombleholme, T.M., Gallivan, E.K., O'Donnell, C. 1996. Hyaluronic acid-dependent pericellular matrices in fetal fibroblasts: implication for scar-free wound repair, *Wound Rep. Reg.* **4**, 346–352.

Morin, O., Normand, C. 1986. Long-term maintenance of hepatocyte functional activity in co-culture: requirements for sinusoidal endothelial cells and dexamethasone, *J. Cell Physiol.* **129**, 103–110.

Mundy, G.R. 1996. Regulation of bone formation by bone morphogenetic proteins and other growth factors, *Clin. Orthop. Relat. Res.* **323**, 24–28.

Murphy, G.F., Orgill, D.P., Yannas, I.V. 1990. Partial dermal regeneration is induced by biodegradable collagen-glycosaminoglycans graft, *Lab. Invest.* **63**, 305–313.

Musat, A.I., Sattler, C.A., Sattler, G.L., Pitot, H.C. 1993. Reestablishment of cell polarity of rat hepatocytes in primary culture, *Hepatology* **18**, 198–205.

Myers, S.R., Grady, J., Soranzo, C., Sanders, R., Green, C., Leigh, I.M., Navsaria, H.A. 1997. A hyaluronic acid membrane delivery system for cultured keratinocytes: clinical "take" rates in the porcine kerato-dermal model, *J. Burn Care Rehabil.* **18**, 214–222.

Nevo, Z., Robinson, D., Horowitz, S., Hasharoni, A., Yayon, A. 1998. The manipulated mesenchymal stem cells in regenerated skeletal tissues, *Cell Transplant.* **7**, 63–70.

Niedzwiedzki, T., Dabrowski, Z., Miszta, H., Pawlikowski, M. 1993. Bone healing after bone marrow stromal cell transplantation to the bone defect, *Biomaterials* **14**, 115–121.

Nyberg, S.L., Remmel, R.P., Mann, H.J., Peshwa, M.V., Hu, W.S., Cerra, F.B. 1994. Primary hepatocytes outperform Hep G2 cells as the source of biotransformation functions in a bioartificial liver, *Ann. Surg.* **220**(1), 59–67.

Oksala, O., Salo, T., Tammi, R., Hakkinen, L., Jalkanen, M., Inki, P., Larjava, H. 1995. Expression of proteoglycans and hyaluronan during wound healing, *J. Histochem. Cytochem.* **43**, 125–135.

Okumura, M., Ohgushi, H., Takakura, Y., van Blitterswijk, C.A., Koerten, H.K. 1992. Analysis of primary bone formation in porous alumina: a fluorescence and scanning electron microscopic study of marrow cell induced osteogenesis, *Biomed. Mater. Eng.* **2**, 191–201.

Orgill, D.P., Yannas, I.V. 1997. Design of an artificial skin. IV. Use of island graft to isolate organ regeneration from scar synthesis and other processes leading to skin wound closure, *J. Biomed. Mater. Res.* **39**, 531–535.

Park, S.-H., Llinás, A., Goel, V.K., Keller, J.C. 1995. Hard tissue replacements, in: *The Biomedical Engineering Handbook* (J.D. Bronzino, ed.), pp. 672–703, CRC Press, Boca Raton.

Prockop, D.J. 1997. Marrow stromal cells as stem cells for non hematopoietic tissues, *Science* **276**, 71–74.

Proposed approach to regulation of cellular and tissue-based products. 1997. The Food and Drug Administration, Docket Number 97N-0068.

Puelacher, W.C., Kim, W., Vacanti, J.P., Schloo, B., Mooney, D., Vacanti, C.A. 1994. Tissue engineered growth of cartilage: The effect of varying the concentration of chondrocytes seeded onto synthetic polymer matrices, *Oral Maxillofac. Surg.* **23**, 49–53.

Radice, M., Brun, P., Cortivo, R., Scapinelli, R., Bataillard, C., Abatangelo, G. 2000. Hyaluronan based biopolymers as delivery vehicles for bone marrow-derived mesenchymal progenitors, *J. Biomed. Mater. Res.* **50**, 101–109.

Raines, E.W., Lane, T.F., Iruela-Arispe, M.L., Ross, R., Sage, E.H. 1992. The extracellular protein SPARC interacts with PDGF-AB and -BB and inhibits the binding of PDGF to its receptor, *Proc. Natl. Acad. Sci. USA* **89**, 1281–1285.

Ramdi, H., Legay, C., Lievremont, M. 1993. Influence of matricidal molecules on growth and differentiation of entrapped chondrocytes, *Exp. Cell Res.* **207**, 449–454.

Rennekampff, H.O., Kiessig, V., Hansbrough, J.F. 1996. Current concepts in the development of cultured skin replacement, *J. Surg. Res.* **62**, 288–295.

Rescan, P.Y., Loreal, O., Hassell, J.R., Yamada, Y., Gillouzo, A., Clement, B. 1993. Distribution and origin of the basement membrane component perlecan in rat liver and primary hepatocyte culture, *Am. J. Pathol.* **142**, 199–208.

Rheinwald, J.G., Green, H. 1975. Serial cultivation of strains of human epidermal keratinocytes: the formation of keratinizing colonies from single cells, *Cell* **6**, 331–343.

Roberts, E.A., Letarte, M., Squire, J., Yang, S. 1994. Characterization of human hepatocyte lines derived form normal liver tissue, *Hepatology* **19**, 1390–1399.

Robinson, D., Halperin, N., Nevo, Z. 1990. Regenerating hyaline cartilage in articular defects of old chickens using implants of embryonal chick chondrocytes embedded in a new natural delivery substance, *Calcif. Tissue Int.* **46**, 246–253.

Rogers, J.J., Young, H.E., Adkinson, L.R., Lucas, P.A., Black, A.C., Jr. 1995. Differentiation factors induces expression of muscle, fat, cartilage and bone in a clone of mouse pluripotent mesenchymal stem cells, *Am. Surg.* **61**, 231–236.

Rojkind, M., Novikoff, P.M., Greenwel, P., Rubin, J., Rojas Valencia, L., de Carvalho, A., Stockert, R., Spray, D., Hertzberg, E.L., Wolkoff, A.W. 1995. Characterization and functional studies on rat liver fat-storing cell line and freshly isolated hepatocyte coculture system, *Am. J. Pathol.* **146**, 1508–1520.

Rosemberg, S.A. 1992. Immunization of cancer patients using autologous cancer cell modified by insertion of gene for tumor necrosis factor, *Human Gene Ther.* **3**, 57–73.

Sandell, L.J., Morris, N., Robbins, J.R., Goldring, M.B. 1991. Alternatively spliced type II procollagen mRNAs define distinct populations of cells during vertebral development: differential expression of the amino-propeptide, *J. Cell Biol.* **114**, 1307–1319.

Sasaki, T., Watanabe, C. 1995. Stimulation of osteoinduction in bone wound healing by high-molecular hyaluronic acid, *Bone* **16**, 9–15.

Sawhney, A.S., Drumheller, P.D. 1998. Polymer synthesis, in: *Frontiers in Tissue Engineering* (C.W. Patrick, Jr., A.G. Mikos, L.V. McIntire, eds.), pp. 85–106, Pergamon, New York.

Scammell, B.E., Roach, H.I. 1996. A new role for the chondrocyte in fracture repair: endochondral ossification includes direct bone formation by former chondrocytes, *J. Bone Miner. Res.* **11**, 737–745.

Schwarz, R.P., Goodwin, T.J., Wolf, D.A. 1992. Cell culture for three-dimensional modeling in rotating-wall vessel: an application of simulated biogravity, *J. Tissue Cult. Method* **14**, 51–57.
Sciadini, M.F., Dawson, J.M., Johnson, K.D. 1997. Evaluation of bovine-derived protein with a natural coral carrier as a bone-graft substitute in a canine segmental defect model, *J. Orthop. Res.* **15**, 844–857.
Shahabeddin, L., Damour, O., Berthod, F., Rousselle, P., Saintigny, G., Collombel, C. 1991. Reconstructed skin from co-cultured human keratinocytes and fibroblasts on a chitosane cross-linked collagen GAG-matrix, *J. Mater. Sci. Mater. Med.* **2**, 222–226.
Shimaoka, S., Nakamura, T., Ichihara, A. 1987. Stimulation of growth of primary cultured adult rat hepatocytes without growth factors by coculture with nonparenchymal cells, *Exp. Cell Res.* **172**, 228–242.
Shimomura, Y., Yoneda, T., Suzuki, F. 1975. Osteogenesis by chondrocytes from growth cartilage of rat rib, *Calcif. Tissue Res.* **19**, 179–187.
Singhvi, R., Kumar, A., Lopez, G.P., Stephanopoulos, G.N., Wang, D.I.C., Whitesides, G.M., Ingber, D.E. 1994. Engineering cell shape and function, *Science* **264**, 696–698.
Skalak, R., Fox, C.F. 1988. *Tissue Engineering*, pp. 55–63, Alan R. Liss, New York.
Solchaga, L.A., Goldberg, V.M., Caplan, A.I. 2000. Hyaluronic acid-based biomaterials in tissue engineered cartilage repair, in: *New Frontiers in Medical Sciences: Redefining of Hyaluronan* (G. Abatangelo and P.H. Weigel, eds.), pp. 233–246.
Stange, J., Mitzner, S., Strauss, M., Fischer, U., Lindemann, S., Peters, E., Holtz, M., Drewelow, B., Schmidt, R. 1995. Primary or established liver cells for a hybrid liver? Comparison of metabolic features, *ASAIO* **41**(3), M310–315.
Stoker, A.W., Streuli, C.H., Martins-Green, M., Bissel, M.J. 1990. Designer microenvironment for the analysis of the cell and tissue function, *Curr. Opin. Cell Biol.* **2**(5), 864–874.
Streuli, C.H., Schmidhauser, C., Kobrin, M., Bissell, M.J., Derynck, R. 1993. Extracellular matrix regulates expression of the TGF-beta 1 gene, *J. Cell Biol.* **120**(1): 253–260.
Suhr, S.T., Gage, F.H. 1993. Gene therapy for neurological disease, *Arch. Neurol.* **50**(11), 1252–1268.
Sussman, N.L., Kelly, J.H. 1993. Improved liver function following treatment with an extracorporeal liver assist device, *Artif. Org.* **17**, 27–30.
Toole, B.P. 1991. Proteoglycans and hyaluronan in morphogenesis and differentiation, in: *Biology of Extracellular Matrix*, 2nd edn. (E.D. Hay, ed.), pp. 305–341, Plenum Press, New York.
Toole, B.P. 1997. Hyaluronan in morphogenesis, *J. Intern. Med.* **242**, 35–40.
Turner, T.D. 1979. Hospital usage of absorbent dressings, *Pharm. J.* **222**, 421–426.
Turner, T.D. 1997. The development of wound management products, in: *Chronic Wound Care* (D. Krasner, D. Kane, eds.), pp. 124–138, Health Management Publications, Inc., Wayne.
Urist, M.R. 1965. Bone formation by autoinduction, *Science* **150**, 893–899.
Utesch, D., Oesch, F. 1992. Dependency of the in vitro stabilization of differentiated functions in liver parenchymal cells on the type of cell line used for co-culture, *In Vitro Cell Dev. Biol.* **28A**, 193–198.
Utesch, D., Molitor, E., Platt, K.L., Oesch, F. 1991. Differential stabilization of cytochrome-p-450 isoenzymes in primary cultures of adult-rat liver parenchymal-cells, *In Vitro Cell Dev. Biol.* **27**(11), 858–863.
Vacanti, C.A., Upton, J. 1994. Tissue-engineered morphogenesis of cartilage and bone by means of cell transplantation using synthetic biodegradable polymer matrices, *Bone Rep. Reg.* **9**, 318–321.
Vacanti, C.A., Langer, R., Schloo, B., Vacanti, J.P. 1991. Synthetic polymers seeded with chondrocytes provide a template for a new cartilage formation, *Plast. Reconstr. Surg.* **88**, 753–759.
Vacanti, C.A., Cimma, L.G., Ratkowski, D. 1992. Tissue engineered growth of new cartilage in the shape of a human ear using synthetic polymers seeded with chondrocytes, *Mater. Res. Soc.* **252**, 367–373.

Vacanti, C.A., Kim, W., Upton, J., Vacanti, M.P., Mooney, D., Schloo, B., Vacanti, J.P. 1993. Tissue-engineered growth of bone and cartilage, *Transplant. Proc.* **25**, 1019–1021.

Vaino, S., Muller, U. 1997. Inductive tissue interactions, cell signaling and the control of kidney organogenesis, *Cell* **90**, 975–978.

Vaughan, J.M. 1981. *The Physiology of Bone*, 3rd edn., Clarendon Press, Oxford.

Wainwright, D., Madden, M., Luterman, A., Hunt, J., Monafo, W., Heinbach, D., Kagan, R., Sittig, K., Dimick, A., Herndon, D. 1996. Clinical evaluation of an acellular allograft dermal matrix in full-thickness burns, *J. Burn Care Rehabil.* **17**, 124–136.

Wakitani, S., Kimura, T., Hirooka, A., Ochi, T., Yuneda, M., Owaki, H., Ono, K., Yasui, N. 1989. Repair of rabbit articular surfaces with allograft chondrocytes embedded in collagen gel, *J. Bone Jt. Surg.* **71**, 74–80.

Wakitani, S., Goto, T., Pineda, S.J., Young, R.G., Mansour, J.M., Caplan, A.I., Goldberg, V.M. 1994. Mesenchymal cell-based repair of large, full-thickness defects of articular cartilage, *J. Bone Jt. Surg.* **76-A**, 579–592.

Wanson, J.C., Mosselmans, R., Brouwer, A., Knook, D.L. 1979. Interaction of adult rat hepatocytes and sinusoidal cells in coculture, *Biol. Cell* **36**, 7–16.

Warejcka, D.J., Harvey, R., Taylor, B.J., Young, H.E., Lucas, P.A. 1996. A population of cells isolated from rat heart capable of differentiating into several mesodermal phenotypes, *J. Surg. Res.* **62**, 233–242.

Watt, F.M. 1991. Cell culture models of differentiation, *FASEB J.* **5**, 287–294.

Wegner, H., Schareck, W., Bayer-Helms, H., Gebhardt, R. 1992. Different proliferative potential of rat and pig hepatocytes in pure primary culture and coculture, *Eur. J. Cell Biol.* **58**, 411–417.

Weigel, P.H., Frost, S.J., McGary, C.T., LeBoeuf, R.D. 1988. The role of hyaluronic acid in inflammation and wound healing, *Int. J. Tissue React.* **10**, 355–365.

Widmer, M.S., Mikos, A.G. 1998. Fabrication of biodegradable polymer scaffolds for tissue engineering, in: *Frontiers in Tissue Engineering* (C.W. Patrick, Jr., A.G. Mikos, L.V. McIntire, eds.), pp. 107–120, Pergamon, New York.

Wilkins, L.M., Watson, S.R., Prosky, S.J., Meunier, S.F., Parenteau, N.L. 1994. Development of a belayered living skin construct for clinical applications, *Biotechnol. Bioeng.* **1994**, 747–756.

Yamaguchi, Y., Mann, D.M., Ruoslathi, E. 1990. Negative regulation of TGF-β by the proteoglycan decorin, *Nature* **346**, 281–284.

Yannas, I.V. 1995. Artificial skin and dermal equivalents, in: *Biomedical Engineering Handbook* (J.D. Bronzino, ed.), pp. 2025–2038, CRC Press, Boca Raton.

Yannas, I.V., Burke, J.F., Gordon, P.L., Huang, C., Rubenstein, R.H. 1980. Design of an artificial skin. II. Control of chemical composition, *J. Biomed. Mater. Res.* **14**, 65–81.

Yarmush, M.L., Toner, M., Dunn, J.C.Y., Rotem, A., Hubel, A., Tompkins, R.G. 1992. Hepatic tissue engineering, *Ann. N.Y. Acad. Sci.* **665**, 238–252.

Yaszemski, M.J., Payne, R.G., Hayes, W.C., Langer, R., Mikos, A.G. 1996. Evolution of bone transplantation: molecular, cellular and tissue strategies to engineer human bone, *Biomaterials* **17**, 175–185.

Young, H.E., Mancini, M.L., Wright, R.P., Smith, J.C., Black, A.C., Jr., Reagan, C.R., Lucas, P.A. 1995. Mesenchymal stem cells reside within the connective tissues of many organs, *Dev. Dyn.* **202**, 137–144.

Young, H.E., Wright, R.P., Mancini, M.L., Lucas, P.A., Reagan, C.R., Black, A.C., Jr. 1998. Bioactive factors affect proliferation and phenotypic expression in progenitor and pluripotent stem cells, *Wound Rep. Reg.* **6**, 65–75.

Zacchi, V., Soranzo, C., Cortivo, R., Radice, M., Brun, P., Abatangelo, G. 1998. *In Vitro* engineering of human skin-like tissue, *J. Biomed. Mater. Res.* **40**, 187–194.

32

Assist Devices

Gerardo Catapano

32.1. Introduction

An assist device could be defined as "*an apparatus used to support or partially replace the function of a failing organ.*" Assist devices are also referred to as "artificial or bioartificial organs," the latter term being used in the case that the device combines living elements (i.e., tissues or cells) with synthetic materials. The therapeutic concept underlying the use of assist devices is that a disease due to a failing organ can be healed by supporting or replacing the lacking function(s) with an artificial (vs. bioartificial) analogous device. Assist devices are designed to resemble the function(s) of the organ they are to replace rather than its anatomical structure. As a result, they bear scarce similarity to the natural organ. Each human organ fulfils multiple functions all important to survival of the organism. Assist devices, instead, can only replace those functions known to be essential and which can be described in quantitative terms. In fact, only these functions can be incorporated in the device design. Owing to the scarce knowledge of the pathophysiology of many diseases, currently available assist devices are still somewhat primitive and scarcely efficient when compared to natural organs (Table 32.1). They do not adapt perfectly to the changing state of the patient (e.g., during therapy itself, or upon changing the diet regime) nor do they allow for body growth. They have also limited operation life, as they come in contact with the aggressive fluids and tissues of the human body owing to wear or decay of their transport and separation properties. In a therapy, these features limit treatment time and schedule and may require repeated substitution of the device (even when implanted). Nonetheless, assist devices have permitted us to extend life expectancy of patients with

---

Gerardo Catapano • Department of Chemical and Materials Engineering, University of Calabria, 87036 Arcavacata di Rende (CS), Italy.

Integrated Biomaterials Science, edited by R. Barbucci. Kluwer Academic/Plenum Publishers, New York, 2002.

Table 32.1. Main Features of the Normal Lung and of a Typical Artificial Device for Gas Exchange (Artificial Lung) (adapted from Cooney, D.O. 1980. *Biomedical Engineering Principles*, Marcel Dekker Inc., New York

Lung	Natural	Artificial
Blood flow in lung (l/min)	5	5
Pressure drop (mm Hg)	12	200
Blood volume in lung (l)	1	4
Blood residence time in lung (s)	0.1–0.3	3–30
Gas exchange area (m^2)	50–100	2–10
Venous-alveolar O_2 gradient (mm Hg)	40–50	650

otherwise fatal diseases. As an example, uremic patients have been reported to survive on hemodialysis for longer than twenty years. Depending upon medical needs and the device operation life, assist devices can be located external to the body yet connected to it (i.e., extracorporeal devices) or implanted inside the body (i.e., intracorporeal devices). They can be connected to the body via the blood circulation (i.e., intravascular devices) or embedded in the tissues (i.e., extravascular devices). Therapeutic use of assist devices is generally temporary, to support the failing organ function till its recovery (e.g., the heart-lung machine) or as a bridge to transplantation of a histocompatible organ (e.g., the artificial kidney, the bioartificial liver). There are a few cases where assist devices permanently replace an organ (e.g., the left ventricular assist device). Treatments based on assist devices can be intermittent and repeated over a long time, where there is no stringent need for continuous support to the organ, or continuous, when the device operation life permits it.

Assist devices are made of synthetic materials, which are mostly commodity plastics developed for industrial applications. The limitations to structural and transport properties of synthetic materials, far from being intrinsic to the material, are to be related to the changes occurring as materials come into contact with body fluids or living tissues. The important role played by phenomena occurring at the fluid (vs. tissue)–material interface in any therapy has eventually made engineers and physicians aware of the fact that:

- Fluid (vs. tissue) constituents instantaneously, at first, and then continuously adsorb on the surface of all materials contacting body fluids or living tissues, thereby altering their transport and separation properties, as well as their surface properties.

- All body fluids and living tissues contacting a material they sense "foreign" undergo a large number of biological reactions (triggered by the immune defence of the organism) affecting the general state of the patient and her/his immune response perhaps even long after the contact with the material has ended.

As a result, only a few of the available industrial plastics have been proven feasible for incorporation in assist devices. Recognition of these effects has also prompted definition of material specifications (as well as tests) that qualify a material which can be used in assist devices with minimal side effects. The set of specifications, and derived properties, is often referred to as "biocompatibility" of a material, a concept that changes very rapidly as new analytical tools are available. In recent years, functional materials have been (and still are being) developed which exhibit *ex vivo* performance and biocompatibility exceeding those of industrial plastics.

Table 32.2 provides a rather comprehensive picture of available assist devices updated to 1995. Many listed devices are dealt with elsewhere in this book. In this chapter, we will focus mainly on the biomaterials used in assist devices for extracorporeal blood processing. In fact, despite the large number of therapies proposed over the years the most important application of assist devices with respect to both the number of units sold in the world per year and the amount of money involved still remains hemodialysis together with its derived treatments. At the beginning of the 1990s, it was estimated that more than 400,000 patients were on the hemodialysis treatment worldwide with about 7 million treatments per year in the United States alone. As a whole, about 55 million membrane modules have been used clinically for extracorporeal blood processing, resulting in sales totalling about US$5,500 million per year. In particular, we will discuss the materials that are used in such devices and how they are processed to deliver the required performance. Last, we will briefly deal with the biocompatibility of these materials.

32.2. Biomaterials Used in Extracorporeal Blood Processing

Devices used for extracorporeal blood processing are often classified in two categories, namely "artificial and bioartificial devices" (vs. organs). Artificial devices essentially perform one function, generally to remove endo-(vs. eso-)genous toxins by means of semipermeable barriers. Sometimes, correction of a disorder requires replacing an increasing number of functions, a higher specificity, or even some regulatory or synthetic function needs to be replaced. In these cases, function replacement is best accom-

Table 32.2. State of the Art in the Development of Assist Devices, Updated to 1995 (adapted from Bronzino, J.D. 1995. *The Biomedical Engineering Handbook*, CRC Press Inc., Boca Raton)

Current status	Artificial devices	Bioartificial devices
Established in clinical practice	Hemodialysis and hemo(dia)filtration	
	Peritoneal dialysis	
	Large-joint prostheses	
	Bone fixation systems	
	Cardiac valves	
	Intra-aortic balloons	
	Large vascular grafts	
	Intraocular lenses	
	Dental implants	
	Skin substitutes	
Accepted with reservation	Breast implants	Bioartificial skin
	Small joint prostheses	
	Plasmapheresis	
	Hemoperfusion	
	ECMO in children	
Limited clinical application	ECMO in adults	
	Ventricular assist devices	
	Artificial pancreas	
	Artificial skin	
	Artificial limbs	
	Artificial tendon	
	Immunoadsorption	
Experimental stage	Artificial blood	Bioartificial liver
	Nerve guidance channels	Bioartificial blood
	Total artificial heart	Bioartificial pancreas
	Intravenous blood oxygenation	Bioartificial devices for delivery of active species
	Artificial esophagus	

plished by incorporating into artificial devices living tissues or cells known to perform the required functions. Such devices are termed bioartificial devices.

32.3. Artificial Devices

Artificial devices are designed to process blood for a variety of therapeutic purposes. They share the common feature that the therapeutic goal is accomplished by separating one or more species from the patient's blood. Blood is generally fed in extracorporeal circulation to a device where membranes act as semipermeable barriers between the blood and a stripping

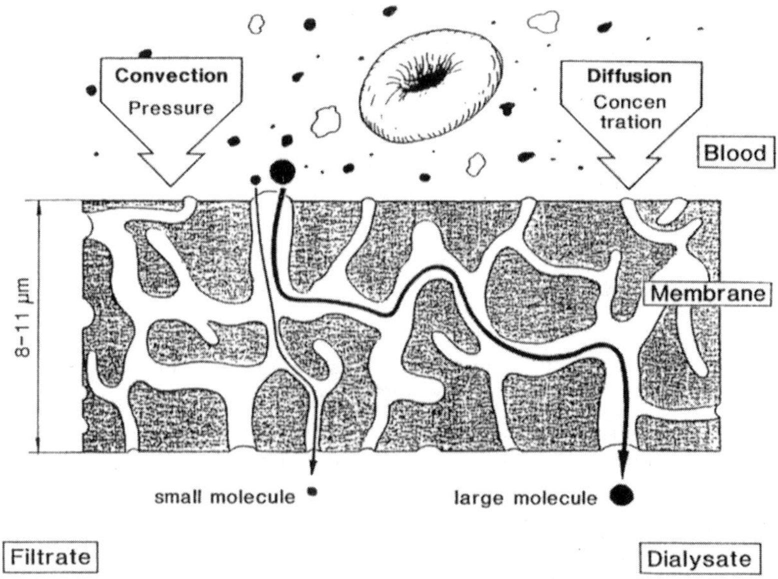

Figure 32.1. General scheme of a membrane-based blood treatment process.

fluid (e.g., a buffered physiological solution for hemodialysis, an oxygen-rich gas stream for blood oxygenation) generally to remove selectively metabolic wastes or exogenous toxins from the blood (Figure 32.1). Mass transfer across a membrane occurs by diffusive and/or convective mechanism and is driven by the applied transmembrane concentration or pressure gradient, respectively. Subsequently, we will refer to the stripping fluid as the dialysate unless otherwise noted.

32.3.1. Membranes and Their Properties

A membrane can be defined as "a phase acting as a barrier that prevents the net motion of mass but permits the regulated and restricted passage of one or more species." Membranes are classified according to many different criteria, e.g.:

- the chemical nature of the polymer (natural vs. synthetic);
- the wall structure (symmetric vs. asymmetric, porous vs. nonporous);
- the separation mechanism (the size of the permeating molecule vs. its solubility in the polymer);

- the driving force for transmembrane transport (solute concentration vs. hydrostatic pressure difference);
- the physicochemical properties (hydrophobic vs. hydrophilic).

Transport across a membrane is indeed promoted by the different chemical potential in the phases at either side of the membrane. Chemical potential may be expressed for ideal solutions as follows:

$$\mu = \mu'(T, P) + R_g T Ln(C) \tag{32.1}$$

(The nomenclature at the end of this chapter defines the symbols.)

Hence, transport of a solute across the membrane can be promoted by the existence of a transmembrane difference of solute concentration, hydrostatic pressure, but even temperature. Such forces are highly interactive. For instance, a transmembrane concentration difference of osmotically active species will establish a transmembrane osmotic pressure difference that counteracts that species transport driven by a hydrostatic pressure difference. However, the rate at which species permeate across a membrane does not depend only upon the existing driving force. Size and geometry of pores in the membrane wall, the pore size distribution, species interaction with the membrane, and the dynamics of fluids on either side of the membrane all contribute to the actual membrane performance. In the following, we will assume that resistance to mass transport from the bulk of the fluid on either side of the membrane to the membrane is negligible. Hence, we will focus on transport parameters intrinsic to the membrane.

For the sake of simplicity, let us refer to a two-component mixture exceedingly rich in a species, the solvent, and poor in another one, the solute. According to the phenomenological approach of irreversible thermodynamics, the net mass (vs. volume) of solvent and solute crossing the membrane per unit time and membrane surface area (i.e., the flux) can be expressed as follows:

$$J_v = L_p(\Delta P - \sigma \Delta \Pi) \tag{32.2}$$

$$J_s = P_M \Delta C + J_v(1 - \sigma) C_{avg} \tag{32.3}$$

Equations (32.2) and (32.3) show that membrane transport and separation properties are described by means of three parameters, namely L_p, the hydraulic permeability, P_M, the diffusive permeability, and σ, Stavermann's reflection coefficient. Stavermann's reflection coefficient measures the solute capacity to permeate the membrane. It ranges from 0 to 1, for solute freely permeating or completely rejected by the membrane, respectively.

The quantity P_M is the reciprocal resistance to solute transport across the membrane in the absence of net solvent flux (i.e., pure diffusive transport). It is easily estimated by measuring the steady-state solute transport across a membrane under a constant transmembrane concentration difference in the absence of solvent flow (i.e., $J_v = 0$). To a first approximation, P_M can be related to solute effective diffusivity in the membrane and membrane wall thickness as follows:

$$P_M = \frac{D_M}{\delta} \tag{32.4}$$

where D_M accounts also for possible solute partitioning between the membrane and the neighboring fluid phase. Fluids on either side of the membrane are also assumed to exhibit the same interactions with the permeating solute.

The quantity L_p is easily estimated by measuring solvent flux across the membrane under increasing transmembrane hydrostatic pressure differences, in the absence of any solute. Pressure drop along the module length on the two sides of the membrane sometime cannot be neglected. Under such circumstances, the transmembrane hydrostatic pressure difference is often obtained by averaging out the hydrostatic pressures at module inlet and outlet as follows:

$$\Delta P \approx \frac{P_{Bi} + P_{Bo}}{2} - \frac{P_{Di} + P_{Do}}{2} \tag{32.5}$$

It has been shown that $L_p \alpha 1/\eta\delta$, thus suggesting that the higher viscosity of plasma will result in a membrane hydraulic permeability lower than those measured with pure water. Figure 32.2 shows the flux–pressure relationship typical of membranes used for different blood treatment processes. The initial slope of each line yields a direct estimate of L_p. We notice that a few mm Hg suffice to promote quite high solvent fluxes across the microporous membranes used in plasmapheresis, while low-flux dialysis membranes offer quite a high resistance to water transport.

The capacity of a solute to permeate a membrane is often established experimentally by estimating how much of it is transported across the membrane under a given transmembrane hydrostatic pressure difference, usually in the absence of a fluid flowing on the membrane side opposite to that of the blood. Membrane sieving capacity is estimated in terms of its sieving coefficient, S, defined as

$$S = \frac{C_p}{C_B} \approx \frac{2C_p}{C_{Bi} + C_{Bo}} \tag{32.6}$$

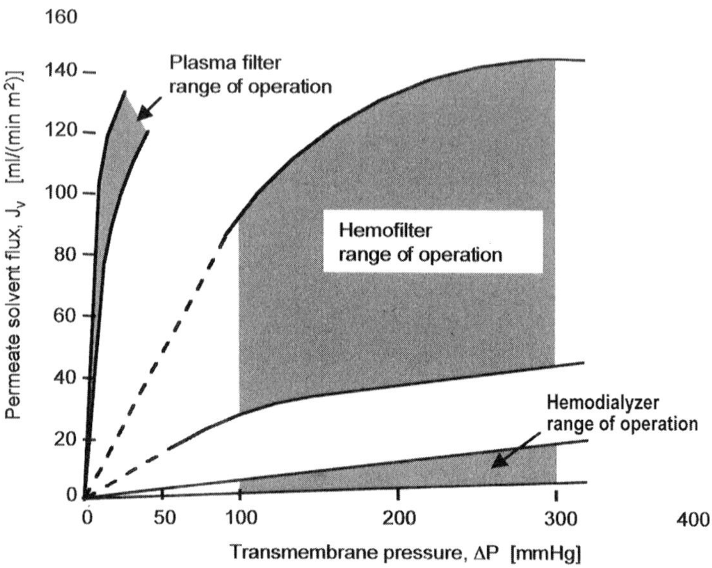

Figure 32.2. Typical relationship between permeate solvent flux and transmembrane hydrostatic pressure for membranes used for different blood treatment processes.

where C_p and C_B are solute concentrations in the permeate and in the fluid on the blood side, respectively. If the solute freely permeates the membrane pores, thus rendering its concentration equal in the bulk plasma water and in the permeate, then $S = 1$. If the membrane is completely impermeable to the solute, then $S = 0$. Membrane capacity to reject a solute is also often expressed in terms of its rejection coefficient, R, where $R = 1 - S$.

In hemodialysis, the rate at which a solute is transported across a membrane is often expressed in terms of clearance (or dialysance) in analogy to the clearance concept in renal physiology. Clearance is defined as the amount of solute removed from the blood per unit time divided by the incoming blood concentration, as follows:

$$\mathrm{CL} = \frac{(C_{\mathrm{Bi}} - C_{\mathrm{Bo}})Q_{\mathrm{Bi}}}{C_{\mathrm{Bi}}} + \frac{Q_{\mathrm{P}} C_{\mathrm{Bo}}}{C_{\mathrm{Bi}}} \tag{32.7}$$

CL represents the solute volumetric rate removal. Caution should be exerted in attributing a given CL only to the membrane properties. In fact, CL is rather determined by both membrane properties and the fluid dynamics of the blood and dialysate compartments in the module.

In blood processing, the most important feature of a membrane is its capacity to reject species with a given molecular weight (MW) (vs. size) and to be freely permeable toward other species. This feature is often expressed by means of a sieving coefficient (vs. clearance) spectrum where membrane sieving is reported for solutes with increasing molecular weight (vs. size). Figure 32.3 shows sieving coefficient spectra typical of membranes used in different blood treatment processes. Pores in the membrane wall generally have not all the same size, nor have they uniform size across the wall thickness. The slope of each curve reflects the actual membrane pore size distribution and suggests how selective the membrane is. Steeper slopes are associated with more selective membranes. Membranes whose sieving spectrum features a smooth slope will not be able to separate solutes with similar MW (vs. size). The sieving coefficient spectrum of a membrane is traditionally determined by evaluating membrane rejection properties with respect to solutes (often proteins) with different MW. Such solutes often have entirely different physicochemical properties. Hence, different interactions with the membrane material and pH-induced shape changes closely relate the spectrum to the specific solutes used in the rejection experiments rather than to the membrane structure only. These difficulties can be overcome by characterizing membrane sieving coefficient toward a homologous series of glucose oligomers. This method makes it possible to use the same technique for

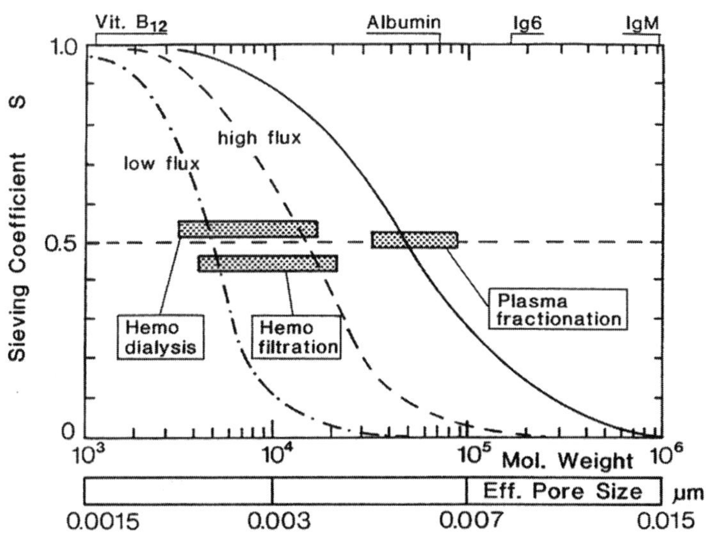

Figure 32.3. Sieving coefficient spectrum typical of membranes used for different blood treatment processes.

assessing solute concentration and noticeably reduces the time required to characterize a membrane. Separation properties of a membrane are also characterized in terms of its molecular weight cut-off (MWCO). By MWCO is generally indicated the MW (vs. size) of a solute toward which the membrane exhibits a set sieving coefficient. Depending on the application, this value ranges from $S = 0.95$ to $S = 0.999$. Thus, theoretically a small number of pores does exist through which much larger molecules than that suggested by the MWCO may cross the membrane. Figure 32.3 shows that membranes feasible for hemodialysis exhibit a much lower MWCO than membranes for plasmapheresis.

32.3.2. Therapeutic Membrane Processes

Even before membranes were used in industrial applications, membrane processes had become established in the clinical practice for the treatment of uremia. In 1943, Kolff and Beck in the Netherlands successfully used an artificial kidney to remove catabolites from the blood of a uremic patient who would have otherwise died. The device was rather primitive (as compared to devices available today) and consisted of a 30-m-long cellophane tube wrapped around a rotating drum immersed in a 100-l dialysate bath. In 1967, the first dialyzer consisting of a cylindrical housing in which hollow fiber membranes were arranged in a "shell-and-tube" configuration was introduced in the clinics. Most of today's membrane modules are still built according to this or a similar configuration (Figure 32.4). Since then, technological development in the preparation of membranes and membrane modules has enabled us to expand the field of application of membrane processes and the number of patients who benefit from membrane-based therapies. Membrane processes are used for the treatment of patients with rather different pathologies from renal failure (hemodialysis, hemo(dia)filtration, etc.), to a variety of hematological and autoimmune disorders (plasmapheresis) or to exchange gas with the blood (as in blood oxygenation).

a. Hemodialysis. In hemodialysis (HD), semipermeable membranes are used in the treatment of patients with chronic or acute renal failure. The therapeutic objective is to remove from the blood urea, uric acid, creatinine, and other wastes of protein metabolism in substitution of the failing kidney. Assist devices aim at simulating the function of the nephron, the functional unit in the kidney in charge of the elimination of waste metabolites and excess fluid. The nephron consists of a passive filtration unit with a sharp sieving spectrum, the glomerulus, followed by a series of active reabsorption units, the tubules. About 120 ml/min filtrate containing waste metabolites

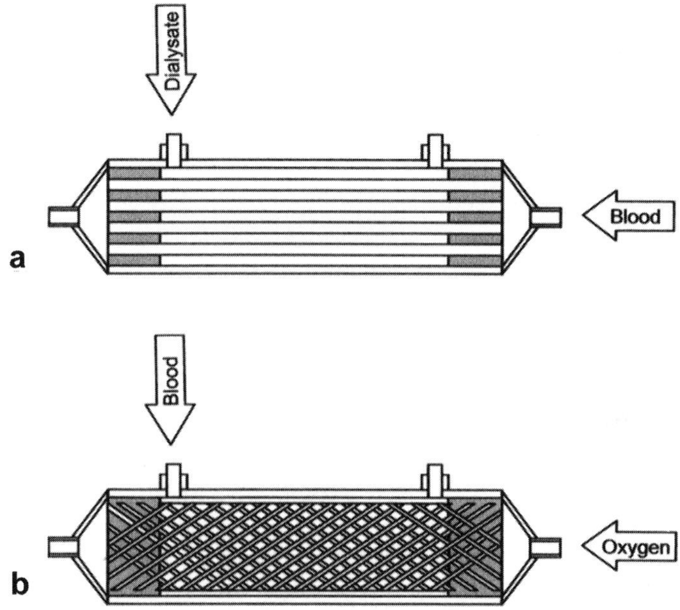

Figure 32.4. Typical configurations of hollow fiber membrane modules: (a) "shell-and-tube"; (b) extraluminal flow.

but also electrolytes is formed in the glomerulus and goes to the tubules. Here, osmotic and selective activated transport phenomena reabsorb fluid, essential nutrients, and electrolytes and concentrate the waste metabolite in the remaining 1 ml/min stream that becomes urine. In hemodialysis, arterial blood generally flows at 200–300 ml/min on one side of a dialysis membrane (0.5–2 m^2 surface area) while a buffered isotonic dialysate solution flows on the other membrane side usually in countercurrent mode. Low MW waste metabolites diffuse across the membrane in response to a transmembrane concentration difference. In order to remove the excess fluid, hemodialyzers are occasionally operated under a small transmembrane pressure (about 0.2 bar). Although effective, the treatment bears but a pale resemblance to the natural nephron. In contrast to the natural function the HD treatment is discontinuous, patients being dialyzed three times per week for about four hours. Species are removed from the blood by diffusion and separation occurs on the basis of molecular size only, making it a rather nonspecific process. As a result, low MW essential nutrients (e.g., amino acids) are removed together with the wastes. The MWCO of dialysis membranes is fairly lower than that of the glomerulus. As a result, dialysis membranes are almost impermeable to solutes with 5,000–12,000 MW which would be cleared by the natural kidney. Accumulation of such species has been recently correlated with some side-effects and morbidity in long-term dialysis patients, as is the case for the occurrence of amyloidosis associated with the accumulation of β_2-microglobulin.

b. Hemo(dia) filtration. In hemofiltration (HF) and hemodiafiltration (HDF), metabolic wastes and excess fluid are removed by filtering the blood against a membrane under a transmembrane hydrostatic pressure difference. In HDF, the permeate is discarded and replaced with a sterile, nonpyrogenic electrolyte solution. HF is used for patients with massive fluid retention and lost fluids are not replaced. Species are transported across the membrane by convection, only. Separation occurs on the basis of the relative size of the permeating species and of pores in the membrane, which acts as a sieve. Figure 32.3 shows that the MWCO of membranes used in HDF and HF is greater than that of HD membranes, yet is substantially lower than that of the glomerulus. Moreover, the broad pore size distribution of HDF and HF membranes and drag effects exerted by plasmatic water on the permeating molecule make these membranes less selective than either the glomerulus or HD membranes, as confirmed by the slanted sieving coefficient spectra. However, the process permits fast removal of toxins that is advantageous in the case of drug detoxification.

c. Plasmapheresis. Therapeutic plasmapheresis (TP, or plasma exchange) is a treatment for the correction of hematological, autoimmune, and metabolic disorders mediated by proteins, antibodies, immune complexes, and high MW toxins which does not aim at simulating any natural function. Table 32.3 shows a list of disorders for which the efficacy of TP has been or is being ascertained. The aim of the therapy is to remove the mediators of the disorder by filtration of the patient's blood against a membrane (0.2–0.5 m^2) under a transmembrane hydrostatic pressure difference. Membranes used in TP feature pores with 0.1–0.8 μm average diameter. Their high MWCO makes it possible to retain in the blood only its cellular components. Fluid, albumin, and coagulation proteins are also removed together with the mediators of the disorder. To maintain the osmotic balance among the different body compartments and blood coagulation properties, the permeate, removed at 10–60 ml/min, is discarded and replaced with a sterile, nonpyrogenic electrolyte solution supplemented with human albumin or fresh frozen plasma. The treatment lasts until 1–2 plasma volumes have been exchanged and may be repeated up to 6–10 times over two weeks. In the treatment of chronic disorders, patients undergo treatment on a daily to monthly schedule depending upon the

Table 32.3. Some Disease States Treated with Plasmapheresis

Nature of disease	Disease
Neurologic	Chronic inflammatory demyelinating polyneuropathy
	Guillan–Barré syndrome
	Myasthenia gravis
Hematologic	Coagulation factor inhibitors
	Cryoglobulinemia
	Hyperviscosity syndrome
	Rh incompatibility
	Sickle cell anemia
	Thrombotic thromocytopenic purpura
Rheumatologic	Rheumatoid arthritis
	Systemic lupus erythematosus
Renal	Goodpasture's syndrome
	Renal allograft rejection
Other	Pemphigus

disorder and patient's response. Limitations to the treatment are mainly related to the cost of plasma replacement solutions and to their possible contamination with viral infections (e.g., AIDS, hepatitis, etc.).

d. Plasma Fractionation. Plasma fractionation (PF) is a therapy complementary to plasmapheresis which was introduced to minimize its cost and risks. In PF, the patient's own plasma removed by TP is filtered across semipermeable membranes which are permeable to low MW proteins and protein-borne toxins but retain blood coagulation factors and immunoglobulins. The toxin-containing plasmatic fraction goes to waste, while the latter fraction is continuously returned to the patient's blood. In PF, patients need no infusion of plasma protein substitutes, which results in reduced cost of therapy and risk of infection.

e. Blood Oxygenation. Assist devices for extracorporeal blood oxygenation (Ox) were first proposed by Kolff in 1965 and Hill in 1968 to replace the lung respiratory function in open heart surgery and in the treatment of the acute respiratory distress syndrome. Devices are designed to saturate venous blood with oxygen and to strip carbon dioxide to maintain the normal blood pH. In the treatment, the blood is drawn from a large systemic vein (e.g., the cava vein) and is pumped at 2–5 l/min to the membrane blood oxygenator. Another pump returns the blood to a branch of the aorta. In blood oxygenators, membranes are essentially used to provide a large surface area (2–10 m^2) to favor contact between the blood and an oxygen-rich gaseous stream while retaining all blood components. To fulfil such a requirement, membranes have to be completely impermeable to liquids but permeable to gases. Thick, homogeneous silicone membranes have been initially used for this purpose. The recent availability of microporous, hydrophobic membranes has permitted us to minimize the resistance to oxygen transport across the membrane and to reduce the membrane surface required to provide the needed oxygen supply. In any case, the gas exchange surface area of artificial devices is much lower than that of the natural lung, as Table 32.1 shows. As a result, blood saturation requires longer blood residence times in the oxygen exchanger and the use of gaseous streams richer in oxygen than air.

32.3.3. Materials in Artificial Devices

Polymeric materials are mostly used in assist devices owing to their advantageous features, such as lightness in weight and easy and versatile processing. In fact, available polymerization and chemical modification techniques offer a broad range of possibilities to prepare objects with the desired properties. The chemical nature of the monomer used is only one of the factors which influence transport and separation properties of polymeric materials, as well as their interactions with body tissues and fluids. Polymeric objects used in assist devices are prepared in a number of steps, each one potentially affecting its properties, namely monomer purification, preparation of the polymeric dope, fabrication of the object, and sterilization. Monomer purification is intended to prevent unwanted toxic species from getting in contact with body tissues and fluids. Monomers are then polymerized (vs. copolymerized) and mixed with other ingredients to fabricate the object. At this stage, a number of additives are used. Catalysts or initiators are added to promote polymerization. Plasticizers and fillers are added to induce the required mechanical and separation properties, respectively, or even modify the material surface properties. Antioxidants are added to prevent chemical alteration of the polymer. Leaching of any of the additives into the body tissues or fluids may be hazardous to the patient undergoing the treatment. The fabrication procedure is critical to the preparation of objects with required transport and separation properties and has definite effects on the morphology of the material surface contacting body fluids, for instance. Sterilization of the polymeric object may also introduce leachable toxic chemicals or even alter its transport and separation properties. The complex preparation of a polymeric object makes it easy to appreciate the problems in maintaining a consistent production of efficient devices which do not harm patients. In the artificial devices briefly discussed above, the blood comes into contact with synthetic materials in the form of cannulae, tubing, bubble traps, blood bags, etc., as it flows in the extracorporeal circuit, and in the form of membranes, potting and housing material, as it flows in the membrane module. Below, we will discuss only polymeric materials and techniques to prepare semipermeable membranes because their blood contacting surface area largely exceeds that of other accessories.

Until a few years ago, membrane polymers were selected based on their capacity to yield membranes with defined structure and performance. Typical criteria were:

- membrane-forming properties of the polymer;
- polymer solubility in commonly used solvents;
- storage stability of the polymeric dope;
- polymer "wettability";
- additives needed and their extractability from the membrane structure;
- stability against oxidation;
- heat stability during extrusion and sterilization.

Additional economic and environmental criteria are to be considered when producing hundreds to millions of kilometers of membranes with constant and reproducible properties:

- polymer availability and cost;
- molecular weight distribution of the polymer, this parameter determining membrane mechanical resistance and handling;
- solvent type and cost;
- type of casting or spinning process;
- nature and amounts of additives required;
- possibility of solvent recovery and environmental impact.

Availability of innovative analytical techniques have made physicians and manufacturers aware of the importance of the biochemical consequences of blood/material interactions and biological safety features (or biocompatibility issues) are being introduced as additional development criteria. Unfortunately, the market volume of most processes is still too small to justify development of polymers custom-made for any given application.

32.3.4. Membrane Preparation Techniques

The separation and transport properties of a membrane are determined by the chemical nature of the polymer and by the structure of the membrane wall. The former influences solute solubility into the polymeric

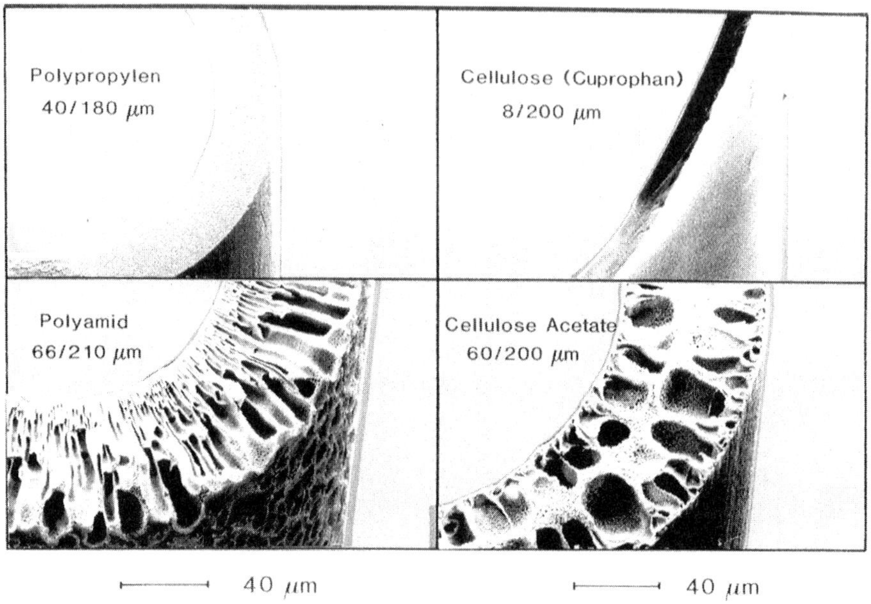

Figure 32.5. Wall structure of membranes made of different polymeric materials and used for different blood treatment processes.

matrix and solute adsorption to the membrane structure (hence, CL and S). The latter influences membrane sieving properties (hence, CL and S) and resistance to mass transport (hence, P_M and L_p). Figure 32.5 shows the typical wall structure of membranes used in blood treatment processes. Membranes are said to be symmetric when their wall is homogeneous or has pores whose size is uniform throughout the wall thickness. Homogeneous membranes for hemodialysis or microporous membranes for plasmapheresis are generally symmetric. Asymmetric membranes feature a thin dense layer (i.e., the skin layer) 0.1–1 μm thick supported by a porous substratum (i.e., the sponge layer) up to about 200 μm thick. The skin layer is the truly selective part of the membrane whose porosity, chemical nature, and thickness determine the actual separation and transport properties of the membrane. The sponge layer serves only to provide mechanical resistance to the skin layer. In terms of function, symmetric membranes basically operate similarly to depth filters while asymmetric membranes operate similarly to surface filters.

Most membranes used in medicine are prepared according to the *phase inversion technique*. Figure 32.6 shows the basic steps for membrane preparation:

- The polymeric dope is prepared by dissolving it in a solvent and by adding plasticizers and/or limited amounts of a nonsolvent for the polymer.
- The dope is sent to the extrusion head (in the case of flat sheet membranes) or to a spinneret consisting of two concentric needles (in the case of hollow fiber or capillary membranes).
- The solvent is extracted and porous membranes are obtained upon polymer precipitation.
- Membranes are thermally treated (i.e., annealed) to enhance their mechanical and separation properties.
- Additives are added to prevent shrinkage and membranes are stored (generally dry).

Both the thermodynamics of the polymeric mixture and the kinetics of solvent extraction determine the actual membrane wall structure and performance. If solvent extraction occurs more rapidly at the surface than in the bulk of the polymeric dope, polymer precipitates locally and forms a skin layer. After formation of the skin layer, solvent continues to be extracted from the underlying dope until it de-mixes in two phases, the one polymer-rich, the other polymer-poor. As the solvent is extracted, the polymer solidifies and coats the polymer-poor zones. As time goes by, the

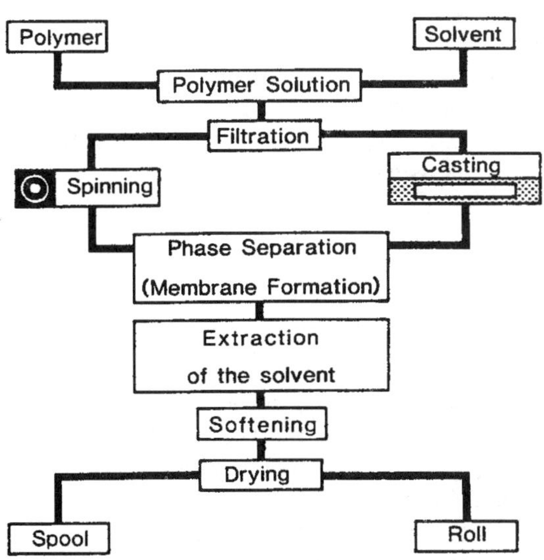

Figure 32.6. Scheme of membrane preparation according to the phase-inversion technique.

polymer-poor zones thicken up till they break the polymer coating and yield an interconnected porous structure (i.e., the sponge layer). Slow, uniform solvent extraction generally yields symmetric membranes.

Different techniques for solvent extraction characterize different phase inversion techniques and yield different membrane wall structure. Those mostly used for the preparation of medical membranes extract the solvent by thermal precipitation and by immersion precipitation. In the thermal precipitation technique, the polymer is dissolved in a solvent at high (vs. low) temperature and is spun in a spinneret or is extruded. In the preparation of hollow fiber membranes, the fiber lumen is generally filled with a gas through the inner concentric needle to prevent its mechanical collapse. Phase separation occurs by suddenly cooling down (vs. heating up) the dope. Membrane formation is generally followed by a thorough extraction of the remaining solvent and other extractables. Symmetric and asymmetric membranes can be prepared according to this technique. Microporous polypropylene (PP) membranes for TP and blood oxygenation are obtained by cooling down the polymeric dope. The same technique can also be used to prepare membranes of polyethylene (PE), polyvinylidenfluoride (PVDF), polyacrylonitrile (PAN), and polysulfone (PS). Polyamide (PA) and cellulosic membranes are precipitated by heat evaporation of the solvent. Most commercial membranes are prepared according to the immersion precipitation technique. Also in this case, the polymer is dissolved in a solvent (vs. a solvent/nonsolvent mixture) and is spun in a spinneret (vs. extruded) to shape the dope. Phase separation occurs by immersing the dope in a coagulation bath containing large amounts of nonsolvent for the polymer. As a result of solvent diffusion out of the dope and nonsolvent diffusion into the dope, the dope separates into a polymer-rich and a polymer-poor phase. Polymer precipitation occurs as its concentration exceeds the solubility limit according to the mechanism previously described. Symmetric and asymmetric membranes made of a number of different polymers (e.g., cuprammonium (Cu), cellulose acetate (CA), PAN, PS) are prepared according to this technique.

32.3.5. Membrane Materials

The first membranes used in hemodialysis were made of cellophane, a type of regenerated cellulose. At the beginning of the 1970s, Cuprohan™ (Cu), another type of regenerated cellulose, was successfully used in hemodialysis and until recently has remained the membrane material most used in medical applications. Membranes were prepared according to the cuprammonium process by dissolving cellulose in an ammoniacal solution of copper hydroxide to form a copper–ammonia–cellulose

Table 32.4. Polymeric Materials Clinically Used for Blood Treatment Processes

Membrane material	Blood treatment process
Regenerated cellulose (Cu, RC)	HD
Cellulose derivatives (CA, CTA, HP, SMC)	HD, HDF, HF
Polyacrylonitrile and copolymers (PAN)	HD, HDF, HF, PF
Polysulfone (PS)	HD, HDF, HF, PF
Polycarbonate (PC)	HD, HDF, HF
Polyamide and blends (PA)	HDF, HF, PF
Polyethylene and copolymers (PE)	HD, HDF, HF, TP, Ox
Polypropylene (PP)	TP, Ox

complex. Extrusion of the dope in an acid bath resulted in the formation of a thick, homogeneous membrane containing cuprammonium radicals apparently enhancing the membrane transport properties. Since then, better understanding of the effect of the thermodynamics of polymer/solvent/nonsolvent ternary mixtures and of the kinetics of solvent extraction on the resulting membrane structure has made it possible to produce semipermeable membranes made of a large number of technological polymers. The materials mostly used for membrane production are summarized in Table 32.4. Polymers made of cellulose or its derivatives are often termed "natural," while those made of monomers not found in nature are termed "synthetic." In the following, preparation and the main features of families of these materials will be briefly discussed.

a. Cellulose and Cellulose Derivatives. Cellulose is a natural semicrystalline polymer consisting of repeating cellobiose molecules. Membranes are generally made by dissolving or melting the natural insoluble cellulose as a cellulose derivative. For instance, soluble cellulose acetate is prepared by esterification with acetic anhydride in the presence of small amounts of perchloric or sulfuric acid. The acetylated cellulose is generally hydrolyzed to the diacetate derivative which can be dissolved in organic solvents (vs. melted) and used to prepare porous membranes, in the presence of plasticizers. The insoluble cellulose form is eventually regenerated by removing the ester moiety by hydrolysis with mild alkali and is referred to as regenerated cellulose (RC). When cellulose is regenerated by saponification of cellulose acetate, the material is referred to as saponified cellulose ester (SCE). Water-soluble cellulose derivatives have also been made by formation of copper–amine complexes (as in the cuprammonium process).

Immediately after preparation cellulose membranes are strongly swollen in water. After every drying/wetting cycle, the membrane gel structure undergoes an irreversible collapse to an extent that depends on temperature, rate of drying, and the amount of plasticizers in the membrane. After equilibration with water, membranes used in HD generally contain 45–50% (w/w) water and can be classified as hydrogels. In such membranes, solutes diffuse through swollen amorphous regions in which pores form dynamically as a result of cellulose polymer chains' constant random motion. The highly crystalline regions in the matrix prevent cellulose from dissolving and provide the membrane with mechanical strength. Cellulose membranes are generally shipped containing 4–50% glycerine by weight of polymer to maintain their hydration state and to ensure high permeability after long-term storage. Membranes made of regenerated cellulose are quite low in cost, effectively remove low MW toxins, and do not promote rapid activation of the coagulation cascade. However, they have only limited capacity to eliminate middle to high MW toxins. Moreover, the hydroxyl groups activate the complement system and the blood cells.

Cellulose derivatives. To improve performance and biocompatibility of cellulose membranes, while retaining the convenient features of cellulose, materials have been recently developed by substituting some hydroxyl groups with other functional moieties. As previously described, cellulose acetate is prepared by esterification of cellulose with acetic anhydride in the presence of acid catalysts. Acetylation can be taken to completion to form cellulose triacetate (CTA) (i.e., degree of substitution DS = 3.0) which can be later randomly hydrolyzed to the diacetate derivative (CA or CDA) (DS = 2.5). Cellulose acetate membranes can be prepared by phase separation for immersion precipitation from organic solvents. Alternatively, a mixture of polymer and plasticizers is melted at high temperature, spun (vs. extruded), and phase separation is induced by cooling in a cold gas stream. These membranes swell in water to a lower extent and expose to blood a more hydrophobic surface than membranes of regenerated cellulose. As a result, they adsorb larger amounts of proteins and more rapidly. The hydroxyl groups in each cellobiose unit may also be etherified with anion-exchanger dimethylaminoethyl (DEAE) or benzyl groups. Membranes made of such cellulose derivatives are commercially available with the tradenames Hemophan™ (HP) and SMC™ (synthetically modified cellulose), respectively. Cellulosic membranes are easily prepared and may exhibit high water fluxes coupled to good separation properties. Their main drawbacks are the scarce resistance to temperature and pH. In fact, the polymer hydrolyzes in acid solutions and is deacetylated in alkaline solutions. They are also extremely susceptible to microbial attack and undergo compaction more easily and to a larger extent than synthetic membranes.

b. Synthetic Polymers. The better comprehension of the mechanisms of membrane formation gathered in the last twenty years made it possible to prepare membranes from synthetic engineering thermoplastics. A variety of hydrophobic materials have been used, such as acrylic (co-)polymers, polysulfone, polyamide, polycarbonate, polyolefines, and blends thereof.

Acrylic polymers. Polyacrylonitrile (PAN) used for medical membranes is a copolymer consisting of a mixture of an acrylic and acrylonitrile monomer (approximately 15:85, mole:mole) and a copolymer such as allylsulfate or methyl acrylate. Membranes are mostly produced by phase separation for immersion precipitation of the polymer from organic solvents into an aqueous coagulation bath. PAN is rather more hydrophobic than cellulosic materials. As a result, it retains only small amounts of water and readily adsorbs globular proteins. The latter feature enhances membrane apparent rejection toward middle molecular proteins (e.g., β_2-microglobulin) and endotoxins. These membranes are dried and stored with glycerine. Details on the preparation of polymethylmethacrylate (PMMA) and polyethylene-co-vinylalcohol (EVAL)/vinylacetate (PVA) membranes manufactured for hemodialysis, hemo(dia)filtration, and plasmapheresis are not available.

Polysulfone. The molecular structure of the polymer features repeating phenolic rings which give this material high rigidity, resistance to tensile stress and compression, as well as high thermal and mechanical stability. Polysulfone (PS) is one of the most hydrophobic materials used in medicine and equilibrates at room temperature with only 0.85–21% water. The polymer is often made more hydrophilic by addition of polyvinylpirrolidone (PVP) to the dope or by chemical insertion of hydrophilic moieties into the polymeric backbone. As with most glassy polymers, it is possible to prepare PS asymmetric membranes in a number of configurations and with a broad range of permeability and sieving spectra (e.g., MWCO from 1,000 to 500,000). Owing to the polymer properties, PS membranes can be heat-sterilized at 121 °C and may be repeatedly exposed to pH from 1 to 13 without significant alteration of membrane properties.

Polyamide. The chemical structure of polyamides features a (-R_1-CONH-R_2-) amidic bond where R may be either an aliphatic or an aromatic group. Good blood biocompatibility has recently been exhibited by membranes made of an aromatic–aliphatic copolyamide. Membranes are prepared by casting a dope made of copolyamide and PVP in dimethylsulfoxide (DMSO) in an aqueous bath. The use of DMSO as a solvent is quite convenient. In fact, in addition to being a good solvent, the polymeric blend is easily removed with water and has been reported to have low biological toxicity. The good miscibility of the copolyamide and PVP reportedly results in the formation of hydrophobic and hydrophilic domains (approx.

100 nm large) during membrane precipitation that seem to determine its good blood biocompatibility.

Polycarbonate. Polycarbonate (PC) membranes have been reported to exhibit quite good biocompatibility. They are easily degraded by alkaline solutions, which limits the possibility to clean, sanitize, and re-use them. Housings of membrane modules are generally made of polycarbonate. The use of PC membranes in a PC housing makes it possible to heat-seal the module ends, thus making potting easy without need of any sealant. However, glycerine added to the membranes to maintain integrity of their pore structure may sometime interfere with the sealing process.

Polyolefins. Polypropylene (PP) and low density polyethylene (PE) have been used for the preparation of microporous membranes for plasmapheresis and blood oxygenation. The maximal pore size ranges from 0.1 to 0.45 μm. Membranes with lower MWCO are not available for processes such as HD, HDF, and HF. Membranes are formed by mixing the polymer with a liquid which acts as a solvent only at high temperature. Then, the dope is spun at high temperature through a spinneret. Polymer precipitation is started by cooling down the spun fiber in a temperature-controlled air gap and is completed by quenching the fiber in a liquid bath. The solvent remaining in the fiber is then removed in an extraction bath, fibers are dried and wound onto spools. Membranes made of olefines are chemically inert but also very hydrophobic. They can be used as such for blood oxygenation. Treatment with surfactants is necessary prior to their use for plasma separation from blood (i.e., TP).

Symmetric and/or asymmetric membranes made of synthetic polymers generally proved useful in filtration processes (e.g., HDF, HF, TP). In hemo(dia)filtration or high flux dialysis, synthetic membranes are generally less restrictive to transport of middle to high MW toxins and activate the complement cascade to a lower extent than cellulosic membranes. However, the cost of these membranes is still high and their performance in terms of permeating water flux and separation properties depend strongly on protein adsorption (i.e., fouling) at the membrane surface or within its pores.

32.3.6. Biocompatibility Issues

Any of the therapeutic treatments considered herein aims at reestablishing the patient's healthy status. The therapeutic objective is at the same time the main limitation to the treatment. In fact, the treatment is expected to remove (vs. administer) given amounts of catabolites or toxins (vs. oxygen) but the treatment itself does not have to do any harm to the patient. The same concept is often expressed by saying that biomaterials used in a treatment (and the treatment as a whole) have to be "biocompatible." As was done before, below we will refer only to membrane-related biocompatibility issues because membranes are often held responsible for any adverse effects of membrane-based therapies. In the past, membranes were considered as passive permselective barriers and biocompatible membrane materials were expected to exhibit the following properties:

1. Material does not have to trigger any thrombogenic, toxic, allergic, or inflammatory reaction.
2. Contact with material does not have to bring damage to blood cells.
3. Neither immunologic nor carcinogenic reactions have to develop after contact with material.

Not a single material available today fulfils all three requirements. It must be accepted that biomaterials are not ideal and cannot be expected to behave similarly to the natural endothelium. When the blood contacts a biomaterial, a series of local reactions takes place involving plasma proteins, blood cells, immune and coagulation factors that activate the immune systems of the host. Accounting for this unavoidable response, biocompatibility could be better defined as "the ability of a material to perform without a clinically significant host response in a specific application," as proposed by the European Society for Biomaterials. Hence, also membranes ought to be considered as barriers actively taking part in reactions with the immune competent blood components. The selection of suitable parameters of the blood response and their correlation with certain characteristics of the biomaterial is the objective of ongoing research. Homeostasis of the human organism following exposure to a stimulus is accomplished by activation of certain pathways closely related by feedback control mechanisms that shut off each process only as the organism returns to a healthy state. Extracorporeal circulation through a membrane module subjects the homeostatic mechanisms to a multiplicity of stimuli to which their response is extraordinarily complex. In fact, the local reactions at the biomaterial surface may have systemic effects on both the blood and the organism as a whole which may, in turn, affect their response to the biomaterial. Things are made even more complex by the fact that clinical consequences often cannot be observed and are frequently a matter of speculation. For these reasons, in this chapter we will briefly discuss only those parameters most commonly used to evaluate the biocompatibility of membrane materials. The interested reader is referred to more advanced textbooks and publications for further information.

32.3.7. Activation of Blood Coagulation (Thrombogenicity)

Still today, thrombus formation at the blood/biomaterial interface is the major problem in the therapeutic use of artificial devices. Blood clots form following thrombin production mostly as a result of the activation of the intrinsic system via a platelet-dependent mechanism. The first step to clot formation is the adsorption of plasma proteins at the biomaterial surface where they undergo conformational rearrangement. Experiments with individual proteins suggest that only adsorbed glycoproteins, such as fibrinogen, are able to interact with platelets and to favor their adhesion at the membrane surface. Adherent platelets undergo morphological changes and spread on the membrane surface. Adhesion is accompanied by the release of serotonin and thromboxan (e.g., TXA_2 and TXB_2) that favor platelet aggregation and, further, substantial release of platelet enzymes, such as platelet factor 4 (PF4) and β-thromboglobulin (β-TG). Release reactions at the membrane surface are followed by the slower but essential activation of the coagulation proteases (e.g., Factor Va and Xa, prothrombin) leading eventually to thrombin generation and the formation of fibrin.

Thrombogenicity of a given membrane material is most commonly evaluated by measuring the extent to which it activates blood coagulation or platelets. A sensitive and rapid assay for the activation of blood coagulation, available in ELISA format, detects inhibition of thrombin by its natural inhibitor antithrombin III with which it forms a complex known as thrombin/antithrombin III (TAT) complex. Although it detects only nonproductive thrombin (i.e., thrombin irreversibly inhibited), the assay is quite useful to detect evolving thrombi. Platelet activation by a given material is generally evaluated by estimating the release of enzymes from the platelet granules. PF4 and β-TG are established markers for the release reactions which take place predominantly during platelet aggregation and represent an advanced stage of platelet activation. Upon platelet activation, arachidonic acid is converted by cyclooxygenase to TXA_2, a potent mediator of platelet aggregation. TXA_2 has a short half-life after which it is transformed into the stable TXB_2 form. Measurements of TXB_2 provide a direct and effective estimate of platelet activation. In fact, unlike β-TG and PF4, TXB_2 is not present in the nonactivated platelets but is generated only upon activation. Figure 32.7 shows that blood contact with PMMA membranes results in a higher TXB_2 generation than that obtained contacting blood with Cu, PAN, or PS membranes. *Ex vivo* investigations consistently show that membranes made of PA, PMMA, and PS elicit a higher PF4 and β-TG release than Cu and PAN membranes. These findings suggest that membranes made of PMMA and other synthetic membranes are more thrombogenic than either those made of cellulosic or PAN. It is interesting to note that clinical investigations do not show any definite trend. The reason might be that membrane material and configuration is only one variable affecting the thrombogenicity of membrane modules. In extracorporeal circulation blood coagulation may be activated by trauma

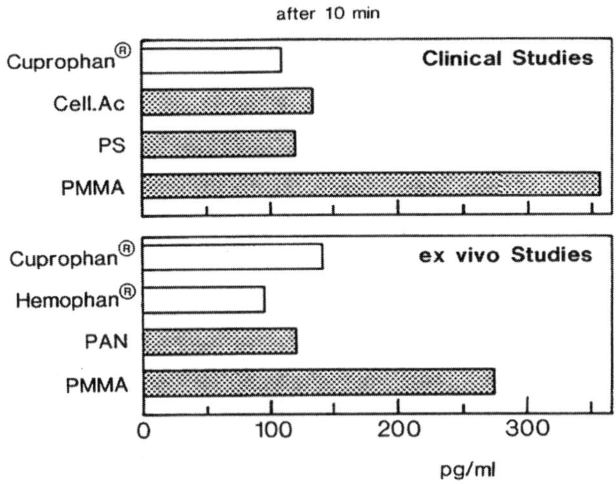

Figure 32.7. TXB_2 generation activated by hemodialysis membranes made of different polymeric materials.

inflicted upon blood constituents by blood pumps, flow disturbances, variations in blood flow, or by contact with air. Dose and MW of the heparin used as anticoagulant during dialysis may also contribute to affect the actual generation of thrombin. Numerous heparin-binding and neutralizing proteins are present in plasma or can be released by activated platelets. Heparin itself is known to activate platelets. An additional factor, particularly in dialysis, is heparin loss through the membrane. This effect is likely to be more significant when low MW heparin (MW = 4000–10,000) is used in combination with high flux membranes.

32.3.8. Complement Activation

The complement system is a nonspecific defence mechanism which is a part of the immune system of the organism. It consists of more than 20 different proteins indicated by the letter "C" followed by a numeral ranging from 1 to 9 and is in charge of protecting the host against bacteria and endotoxins. The complement system may be activated by two pathways: the classical pathway, initiated by immune complexes, and the alternative pathway, which is mainly involved in the activation by biomaterials and is considered in what follows. As the blood contacts the membrane (vs. any biomaterial), some of the C3b molecules in plasma bind to the membrane surface and lead to the increased formation of the enzyme C3-convertase.

Such enzyme cleaves more C3 to form further C3b and C3a, a low MW peptidic fragment. The C3b fragments at the membrane surface form with Factor B the enzymatic complexes known as C3- and C5-convertase. The latter cleaves plasmatic C5 molecules to form the fragments C5a and C5b which are released in the plasma. C5b forms a large molecular complex together with the proteins C6 to C9, called the membrane attack complex (MAC), whose geometry is similar to that of a channel. When it inserts into the cellular membrane of cells or also bacteria, it disrupts their ordered lipid bilayer forming pores that permit leakage of small molecules out of the cell. Further enlargement of the MAC size results in the enlargement of pores and may lead to an early cell death. C3a and C5a are small cationic polypeptides also known as anaphylatoxins, because they promote reactions that lead to anaphylactic shock. Their activity is generally lost or decreased when the polypeptides lose their carboxyl terminal arginine residue and are transformed in their des Arg analogues. C5a is a potent inflammatory mediator and plays a central role in white blood cell activation. C5a and C5a des Arg bind to receptors on neutrophils, monocytes, and macrophages and activate these cells inducing a variety of responses, such as chemotaxis of cells into an inflammatory site, release of degradation enzymes and of oxygen species that mediate cell killing, or the production of other mediators or cytokines, such as interleukin 1 (IL-1).

Activation of the complement system has been reported in all extracorporeal treatments, such as hemodialysis, plasmapheresis, and blood oxygenation. C3b reacts more easily with membranes (vs. biomaterials) presenting surface nucleophilic groups such as the carbohydrates present in the cellular membrane of endotoxins. The presence of hydroxyl groups in the polysaccharidic structure of cellulosic membranes makes them good substrates for C3b, remarkably activating the complement system, as Figure 32.8 shows. Substitution of some hydroxyl groups with either acetyl or DEAE groups results in membranes less complement activating. Figure 32.8 shows that also membranes made of materials without hydroxyl groups activate complement although promoting formation of low (PS, PC) or minimal (PAN) amounts of anaphylatoxins. In these cases, C3b is thought to bind to plasma glycoproteins adsorbed on the surface of the hydrophobic membranes.

Complement activation induced by a membrane is generally assessed by measuring the generation of either C3a, or C5a, or both. Although the pathological consequences of complement activation have yet to be clarified, C5a production is a relevant parameter upon which to judge the biocompatibility of various membranes. However, caution should be exerted in drawing clear-cut conclusions from C5a or C3a generation data from the literature because a number of factors other than membrane interactions with proteins of the complement system may determine a given outcome.

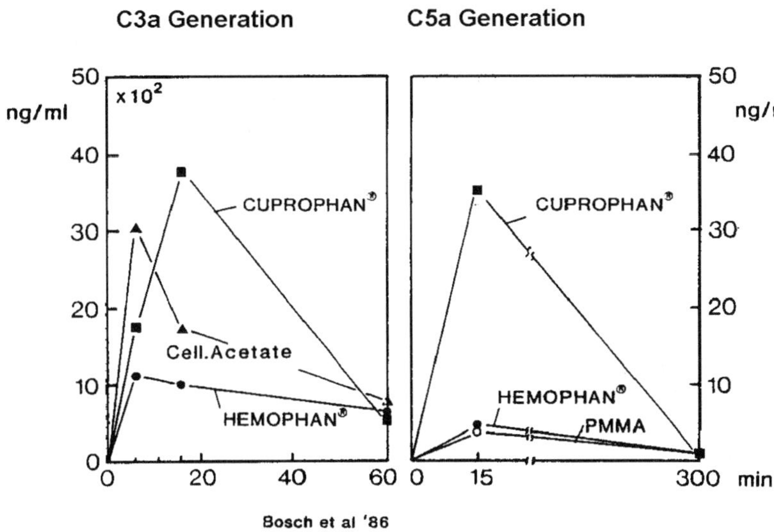

Figure 32.8. Complement activation activated by hemodialysis membranes made of different polymeric materials.

The most relevant among these are membrane interactions with inhibitors of the alternative pathway and anaphylatoxin disappearance by permeation across the membrane wall or adsorption at the membrane wall.

32.3.9. Cell Activation

Modification to physiology or biochemistry of blood cells (e.g., platelets, leukocytes, macrophages) may occur as a result of direct cell contact with the membrane surface or indirectly as a result of the activation of blood coagulation or the complement system. Interactions between blood cells and the humoral components of both defence mechanisms complicate the interpretation of phenomenological evidence.

Experimental evidence shows that extracorporeal blood treatments, particularly hemodialysis and blood oxygenation, upset the regulation of phagocyte (i.e., cells whose primary purpose is to eliminate bacteria from the organism) functions aimed at preventing either inappropriate cell activation resulting in damage to healthy tissue, or an ineffective response to invading bacteria. The most evident clinical effect of synthetic membranes on blood cells was provided by Kaplow and Goffinet in 1968. They reported that during hemodialysis the number of circulating neutrophils and monocytes (i.e., the two principal types of phagocytes) would temporarily decrease within the first hour of dialysis, a phenomenon termed "leukopenia." Cell number begins to decrease immediately after initiation of dialysis, attains a minimum after 10–20 min, goes back to the predialysis level after about 60 min, and rebounds to higher values at the end of the treatment in a pattern generally consistent from patient to patient (Figure 32.9). A similar pattern is observed in other treatments, but for a shift toward longer times. For the sake of comparison, during TP the minimal cell count is attained after about 60 min. Figure 32.9 shows that the minimum number of circulating cells is strongly affected by the membrane material and that cellulose membranes yield the largest transient reduction of cell count. In 1977 Craddock and colleagues demonstrated that the leukopenia is associated with activation of the alternative pathway of the complement system by the membranes used for the treatment. Later, other studies showed that the extent of leukopenia depends on the amounts of active complement components released into the plasma, as Figures 32.8 and 32.9 clearly show. It is today accepted that C5a molecules induce an increased expression of neutrophil adhesion receptors that lead to phagocyte aggregation and their sequestration in the lungs. After a short time, these cells return to blood circulation. The clinical relevance of the membrane-induced leukopenia is still unclear. Firstly, leukopenia interests only a minor fraction of total body neutrophils and monocytes (about 2% and 25%, respectively) which normally circulate in the blood, the rest being sequestered in the capillaries of the lungs, liver, and spleen. Secondly, cell count

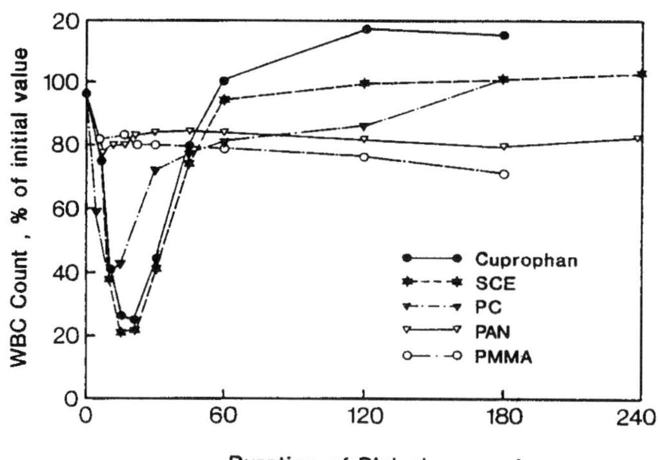

Figure 32.9. Transient leukopenia in uremic patients during hemodialysis with membranes made of different polymeric materials.

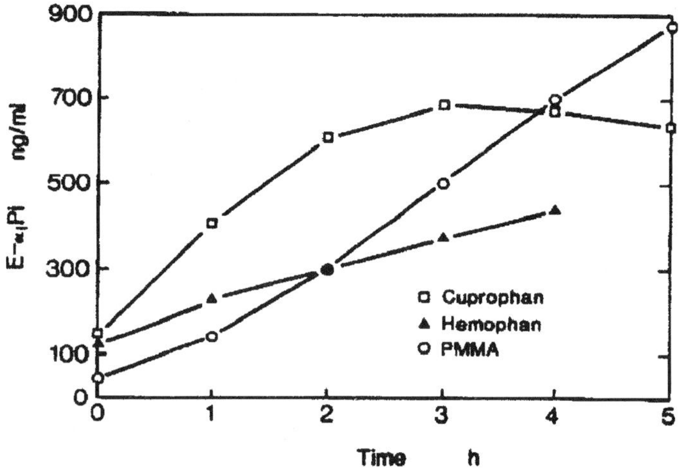

Figure 32.10. Plasma accumulation of granulocyte elastase activated by hemodialysis membranes made of different polymeric materials.

reduction is transient. Phagocyte dysfunction in uremic patients is always associated with the presence of, or the risk of, infection which is quite a problem for hemodialysis patients. However, it has yet to be clarified whether repeated acute stimulation of phagocytes by complement-activating membrane material is directly correlated with a reduction and a chronic down-regulation of phagocyte bactericidal functions.

The direct interaction between polymorphonuclear nucleophiles (PMN), or granulocytes, and membranes of different materials has been known to stimulate the release into the plasma of different amounts of proteases (e.g., elastase and lactoferrin) present in their cytoplasmic granules. Figure 32.10 shows that high amounts of elastase are released upon cell contact with membranes made of PMMA and Cu. PA membranes have been reported to induce release of high amounts of lactoferrin. Experimental evidence suggests that degranulation of the granulocytes does not appear to depend on complement activation because membranes that do not activate complement (e.g., PMMA, PA) also induce release of granulocyte proteases. The clinical relevance of enzyme release has yet to be ascertained.

In summary, there is little doubt that blood contact with membranes activates the immune response of the patients, but its clinical relevance is still uncertain. The extent of activation has been shown to increase as the blood-contacting membrane surface area increases. This suggests that membrane modules delivering a given clearance with smaller membrane surface areas could contribute to minimize complications of the treatment.

32.4. Bioartificial Devices

Physical removal of some toxins from the blood does not yield successful therapeutic outcomes in case that the failing organ is normally in charge of regulating the level of metabolites (e.g., the pancreas), synthesizing metabolites, or removing a large number of differentiated toxins (e.g., the liver). Nor are artificial drug dispensers very effective when a patient needs continuous administration of large doses of low concentrations of biologically active species. In the former case, the ultimate solution is transplantation of a histocompatible donor organ. Scarce availability of donor organs and host rejection of the graft make this therapy available only to a limited number of patients. Transplanted patients are also subjected to life-long immune suppressive therapy which is costly and may have serious complications. Bioartificial devices have been (and are still being) developed that could be effectively used in the treatment of this dysfunction.

Bioartificial devices, or organs, are devices made of synthetic materials which incorporate living cells or tissues known to perform the same function of the failing organ. Cells (vs. tissues) are generally isolated from the same organ of mammals of another species (i.e., xenograft). Immortalized cell lines have been occasionally used to overcome long-term storage problems and the metabolic requirements of primary cells. Figure 32.11 shows some devices that have been proposed over the years either to replace the pancreas (a, c, d) or liver (a–d) function, or to alleviate symptoms of patients with Parkinson's disease or pain in terminal cancer patients (d).

32.4.1. Proposed Bioartificial Devices

a. Bioartificial Liver. The natural liver fulfils more than 1,000 metabolic functions critical to the homeostasis of our organism. Acute liver failure (ALF) is a syndrome resulting from infection, drug intoxication, or as a part of a multiple organ failure that disrupts the liver capacity to accomplish its vital tasks. ALF patients rapidly develop ascites, oedemas, and bleeding followed by hepatic encephalopathy, coma, and eventually death in a matter of weeks, sometimes days. The elective treatment of ALF is liver transplantation, when a donor organ is available in a short time. However, the liver has the potential of regeneration after suffering tissue damage. The artificial devices proposed for liver assist until availability of a histocompatible liver have not resulted in significant improvement of the mortality rate, which remains high at about 80%. Bioartificial devices in which living hepatocytes (i.e., parenchymal liver cells) are incorporated have been recently proposed for liver support. In fact, isolated hepatocytes are capable of supporting nearly all vital hepatic functions and may supply bioactive species promoting regeneration of the natural liver tissue. Such devices are generally termed "bioartificial livers" (BALs). The aim of a BAL is the temporary replacement of the failing liver functions until the tissue damage is self-repaired or to bridge the patient to liver transplantation, if the liver cannot regenerate. To fulfil these requirements a BAL has to replace essential liver functions, such as the elimination of toxic wastes and exogenous toxins, the synthesis of plasma proteins and coagulation factors, storage of essential nutrients, as well as the synthesis of liver regeneration factors, when needed. Both implantable and extracorporeal BALs have been proposed over the last decade. Only a few have been, or currently are, under clinical investigation to assess safety of the treatment. Below, reference will be made only to these devices by the term BAL. The BALs are located external to the patients and are connected to the blood circulation via extracorporeal circuitry closely resembling those used for hemodialysis. Most BALs are fed with plasma which is continuously removed from the blood by plasmapheresis membrane modules: plasma leaving the BAL is mixed to the blood before it returns to the patient. Porcine primary hepatocytes or C3a cells, an immortalized line derived from liver tumor cells, are cultured either outside hollow fiber membranes arranged in a housing in a "shell-and-tube" configuration, in adhesion on the membrane surface or attached to beads, (Figure 32.11a) or in nonwoven fabrics or around hollow fiber membranes arranged in a three-dimensional network (Figure 32.11b). In the former configuration, plasma flows in the membrane lumen and nutrients and toxins (vs. liver-specific products) diffuse to (vs. away from) the cells. In the latter, plasma directly bathes the cells. In BALs incorporating primary hepatocytes, the flowing plasma is enriched in oxygen via blood oxygenation membranes located either upstream from the BAL or incorporated into the BAL itself (Figure 32.11b). Devices are generally operated as arterovenous shunts. Most BALs *in vitro* exhibited some of the essential detoxification and synthetic liver-specific functions. The BAL incorporating C3a cells successfully regained dog models of ALF to conscience and could support them in a healthy status for months. Unfortunately, clinical scale devices were not as successful in the treatment of ALF patients. BALs using hepatocytes showed prolonged survival of pig models of ALF with respect to the untreated animals. Some of them have also successfully bridged patients in hepatic coma to liver transplantation, although for short times only.

b. Bioartificial Pancreas. The treatment aims at regulating within a physiological range the glycemia of patients suffering from insulin-dependent diabetes mellitus. The syndrome is traditionally treated with diet and

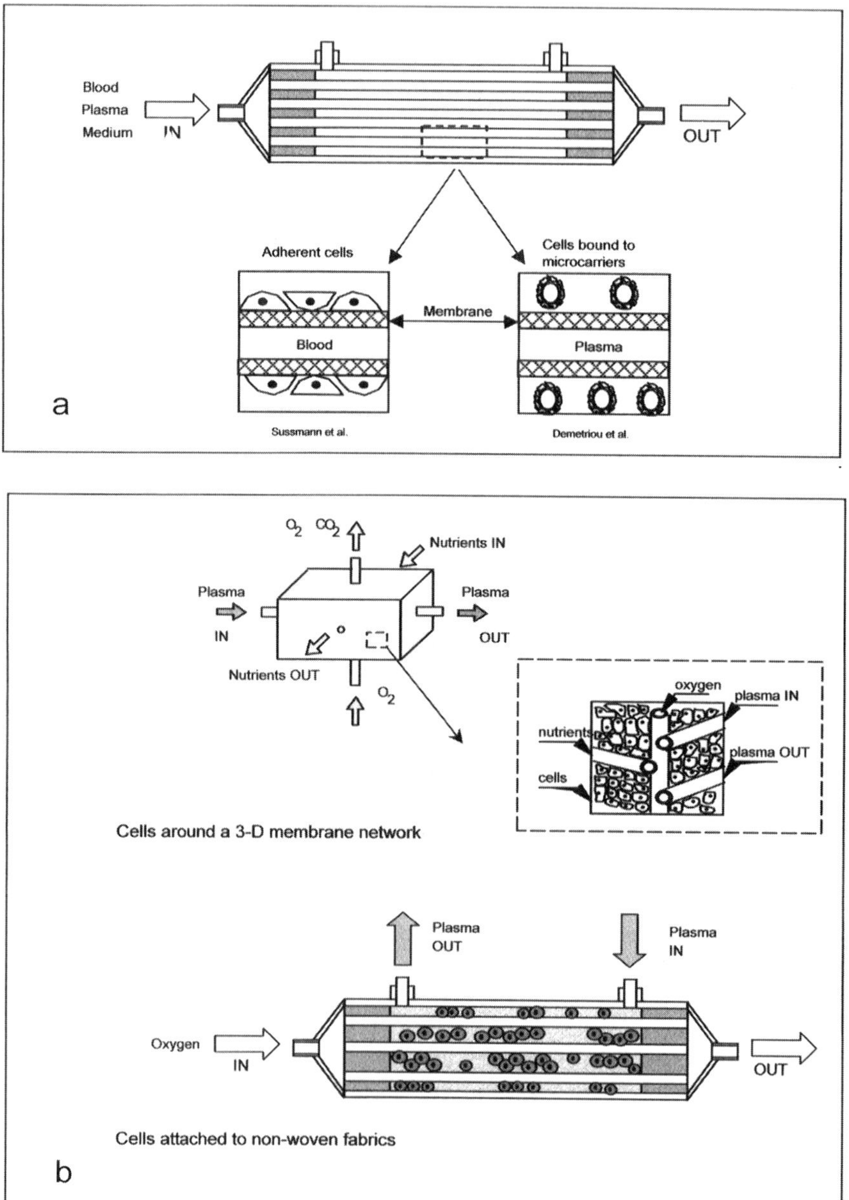

Figure 32.11. Configuration of some proposed bioartificial devices.

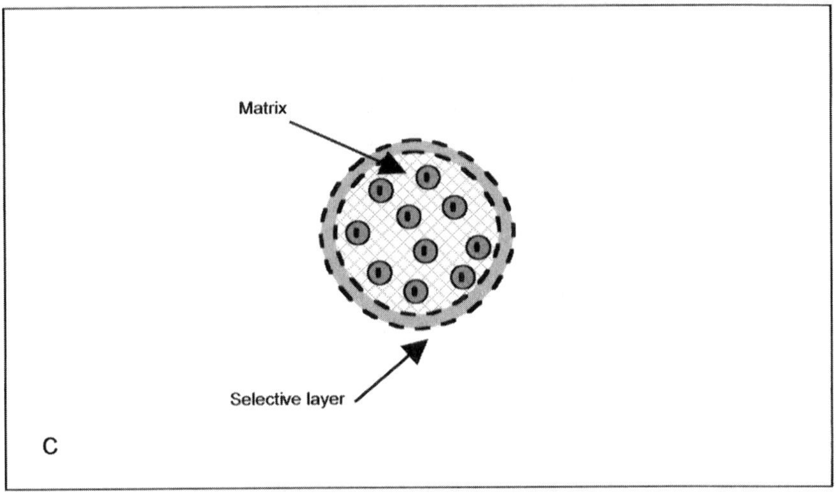

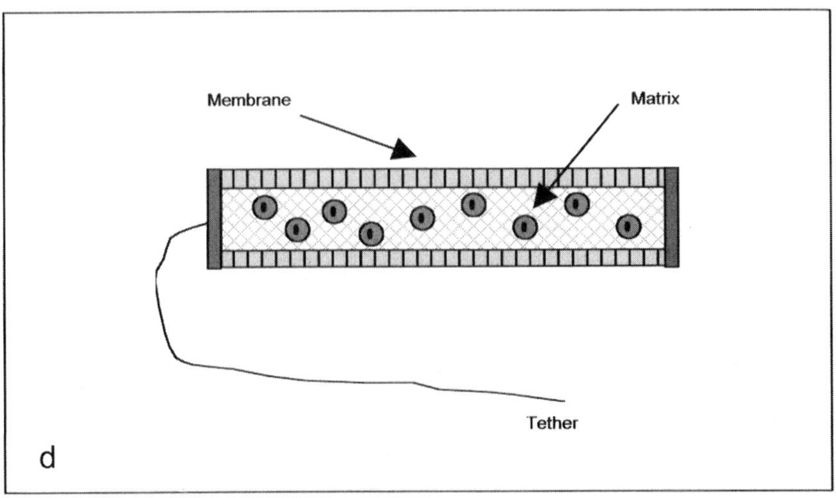

Figure 32.11. Continued.

postprandial injection of insulin. The discontinuous administration of insulin, unrelated to the actual glycemia, leads to fluctuating insulin and glucose plasmatic levels which result in severe complications and eventually lead to the patient's death. Bioartificial devices have been proposed where cells capable of sensing the plasmatic glucose concentration and producing insulin in amounts related to the actual glycemia are entrapped by means of synthetic membranes to protect them against immune rejection. Living human or porcine islets of Langerhans (or pancreatic beta cells), the functional units in the pancreas that regulate glucose homeostasis, insulinomas (pancreatic tumor cells), or genetically engineered cells have been used. Both extravascular (EV) and intravascular (IV) implantable devices have been proposed. In EV devices, tissue immunoisolation has been achieved by entrapment in microcapsules made of hydrogels (Figure 32.11c) or in the lumen of semipermeable hollow fiber membranes sealed at the ends (or else in between two flat sheet membranes sealed at the perifery), and embedded in a gel (Figure 32.11d). The implantation site was intraperitoneal, intrahepatic, intrasplenic, or subcutaneous. In IV devices, cells have been cultured outside hollow fiber membranes arranged in a housing in a "shell-and-tube" configuration (Figure 32.11a) or in a gel matrix placed around a wide-bore semipermeable membrane. Devices were generally implanted as arterovenous shunts. Some devices successfully maintained glucose homeostasis in small diabetic animals. Long-term survival of cells in a functional state, aggravated by blood clotting in IV devices and the formation of a fibrous capsule around EV devices, have so far doomed any scale-up attempt.

c. Bioartificial Devices Delivering Bioactive Species. Macroencapsulation in the lumen of hollow fiber membranes (Figure 32.11d) of living cells embedded in a gel may provide a long-term supply of bioactive species. PC12 cells, a catecholaminergic cell line capable of secreting dopamine, macroencapsulated and implanted in the striatum reportedly ameliorated motor functions of guinea pig models of Parkinsons' disease. Bovine adrenal chromaffin cells, capable of secreting pain-reducing neuroactive substances, entrapped in tethered macrocapsules and implanted into human cerebrospinal fluid are being clinically tested as a means to alleviate chronic pain in terminal cancer patients.

32.4.2. Materials in Bioartificial Devices

The living tissue incorporated in bioartificial devices ensures their functional efficacy. When blood components come into contact with allogeneic or xenogeneic tissue, they sense it as "foreign" and try to reject it.

Thus, in addition to being nontoxic and biocompatible, biomaterials used in bioartificial devices have to fulfil two further requirements:

- They have to protect the graft from rejection, while allowing unhindered transport of nutrients, metabolites (and also toxins) from the blood to cells, and of synthetic products back into the blood.
- They have to provide cells with a physical structure where they can arrange (and possibly grow) similar to that the extracellular matrix (ECM) provides *in vivo*, so that cells stay viable and functional for the expected duration of therapy.

Depending on the intended use, biomaterials used in bioartificial devices can be divided into immunoisolation materials and scaffold, or matrix, materials. The polymeric materials generally used are commodity plastics adapted for medical applications or materials derived from tissue culture or other medical applications.

32.4.3. Matrices and Scaffolds

In bioartificial devices, biomaterials in the form of scaffolds or matrices are used to provide cells with a physical structure providing the mechanical support and the biological interactions that the ECM provides in the natural organ, or to permit physical separation of single cells or cell aggregates.

Matrix materials typically used are hydrogels made of cross-linked polyelectrolytes (e.g., alginate), collagen, ECM derivatives (e.g., Matrigel^{TM}), and synthetically modified natural gels (e.g., esters of the hyaluronic acid). Matrices are often used in combination with synthetic membranes (Figures 32.11a,d) to accomplish multiple tasks. They may keep cells (or small cell aggregates) apart and well distributed in the device, thus preventing formation of bulky cellular aggregates at whose core cells would starve and die for the insufficient supply of oxygen and nutrients. They may provide anchorage-dependent cells (e.g., hepatocytes) with an adhesion support. They may favor cell polarization, i.e., the recovery of cell asymmetric morphology generally lost during isolation. A matrix can also be cross-linked to be mechanically self-supporting. Microcapsules ($\phi = 0.4$–2 mm) can be prepared by extruding droplets of a mixture of alginate (a negatively charged polyelectrolyte obtained from seaweed) and cells into a calcium-containing solution which ionically cross-links alginate. However, immunosolation of the graft requires coating the microcapsules with a more selective membrane.

If we limit our attention to the bioartificial devices considered in this chapter, we notice that scaffolds are used heavily in BALs incorporating primary hepatocytes. In the natural liver, these cells are polyhedral and polarized, with basolateral sides bordering the ducts through which bile is excreted and apical sides facing the sinusoids through which oxygen and metabolites are exchanged with the blood. In some types of BALs, scaffolds are used to favor organization of the isolated hepatocytes in three-dimensional structures resembling that in the natural liver as well as cell polarization. Nonwoven fabrics made of polyester fibers and three-dimensional membrane networks have been used as scaffolds in the BALs we have considered. Nonwoven fabrics are made by crimping and carding fibers 10–40 μm in diameter which are then formed in a nonwoven fabric by means of barbed needles that entangle the fiber and lock them together (see Chapter 3 for further details). In the BAL, oxygenation membranes are often longitudinally inserted in the mesh to supply cells with oxygen (Figure 32.11b). The three-dimensional membrane network is formed by spatially arranging three bundles of different hollow fiber membranes stacked on parallel planes, but orthogonal to one another. In each repeating stack consisting of three membrane mats, plasma flows from the lumen of the TP membranes in the first mat to the extracapillary space, where it bathes the cells and contacts membranes in the second mat. These are generally made of microporous PP for blood oxygenation. They supply cells and plasma with oxygen. Then, plasma permeates into the lumen of the third mat of TP membranes and is returned to the patient. Porcine hepatocytes cultured on these scaffolds generally exhibit liver-specific functions and remain viable and functional for relatively long times.

32.4.4. Immunoisolation Materials

In both extracorporeal and macroencapsulated implantable devices, synthetic membranes are generally used to localize the xeno(allo-)grafts and minimize immune recognition and rejection. They are semipermeable, self-supporting barriers prepared by the phase-inversion technique, whose properties have been discussed in previous parts of this chapter. Many extracorporeal devices (e.g., BALs) are fed with the patient's plasma which is continuously removed from the blood by means of hydrophobic, plasmapheresis membranes as a means to protect xenogeneic cells against immunocompetent cells. In some devices, membranes for hemo(dia)filtration or plasma fractionation are interposed between the plasma and the xeno(allo-)grafts as a means to protect them against immunocompetent plasmatic proteins. In devices fed with whole blood, immunoisolation of the graft is generally accomplished with membranes of the latter type. The membranes used are mostly asymmetric and hydrophobic made of PAN,

PS, polyvinyl copolymers, and mixtures thereof. Occasionally, cellulose derivatives have also been used. *In vivo* and *ex vivo* experiments suggest that membranes with 50,000–100,000 MWCO provide adequate immunoprotection of the graft, although further investigation is still needed.

Immunoisolation of cells or tissues incorporated in microcapsules has been accomplished by coating the inner alginate or cellulose core with a layer of a cationic polyaminoacid, such as polylysine or polyornithine. Although rather thin, the additional layer reportedly provides the required immunoisolation. Occasionally, a third alginate layer would be coated on top of the others to prevent the formation of a fibrous capsule around the microcapsule.

32.4.5. Biocompatibility Issues

Biomaterials used in bioartificial devices should meet all biocompatibility requirements set forward for those used in artificial devices. In addition to what is required of synthetic materials, careful consideration should also be given to the cells or tissues that are used in the device. There is today great concern that there exists a possibility that animal tissues might pass on to the patients unwanted bioactive species, such as endotoxins, viruses, or carcinogens (as in the case of tumor-derived cell lines) that could be life-threatening. The same proteins and bioactive species that we wish tissue to release might induce the patient to produce antibodies against them. Repeated exposure to the device could thus pose a risk of hypersensitivity reactions. Further studies are still needed to evaluate the existing risk and the strategy to minimize it.

Acknowledgment

All figures were published with kind permission of Acordis, Wuppertal, Germany.

Suggested Reading

Bronzino, J.D. (ed.). 1995. *The Biomedical Engineering Handbook*, CRC Press Inc., Boca Raton.

Mulder, M. 1991. *Basic Principles of Membrane Technology*, Kluwer Academic Publishers, London.

Consensus Conference on Biocompatibility, 1994. *Nephrol. Dial. Transplant.* **9** (Suppl. 2).

Ward, R.A., Feldoff, P.W., Klein, E. 1985. Membrane materials for therapeutic applications in medicine, in: *Materials Science of Synthetic Membranes*, ACS.

Nomenclature

C	concentration, ML^{-3}
C_{avg}	mean logarithmic concentration, ML^{-3}
CL	clearance, L^3T
D_M	diffusion coefficient × partition coefficient, L^2T^{-1}
J_s	permeate solute flux, $ML^{-2}T^{-1}$
J_v	permeate solvent flux, $ML^{-2}T^{-1}$
L_p	membrane hydraulic permeability, TL^{-1}
P	pressure, $ML^{-1}T^{-2}$
P_M	membrane diffusive permeability, LT^{-1}
Q	flow rate, L^3T^{-1}
R	rejection coefficient, -
R_g	universal gas constant
S	sieving coefficient, -
T	temperature

Greek letters

δ	membrane wall thickness, L
Δ	transmembrane difference
η	viscosity, $ML^{-1}T^{-1}$
μ	chemical potential
μ'	reference chemical potential
Π	osmotic pressure, $ML^{-1}T^{-2}$
σ	Stavermann's coefficient, -

Subscripts

B	blood side
D	dialysate side
i	inlet
o	outlet
p	permeate

33

Standards on Biomaterials

Maria Vittoria Primiceri and Sandro Paci

33.1. Introduction

The first norms appeared, somehow, to satisfy military demands. Round about the year 1400 some built weapons (rifles and guns) while others made bullets, so that there was much confusion between the diameter of the gun and the ammunition.

Since then much has been done. Nowadays we are aware that regulations must be harmonized in order to preserve man's health and safety. We hope that this will act as the small hole to demolish the huge dike of indifference and human ignorance that has made us slaves of barons and conventions imposed by private interest rather than by love for one's neighbor. The contents of this book should testify about the will to communicate with and consider human beings as part of one race, clan, and family.

33.1.1. The Need for Standards

Since the European Nations felt the need to form an economic union, social and political problems were also considered almost automatically. After the ratification of the Treaty of Rome in 1970, the European Committee realized that the legislative system being created from the experience of the "First approach," dated 1973 (Directive 73/23/CEE concerning low tension), would be long and difficult. The task of the European legislator was mainly hindered by the different interpretations of the Member States on production and application.

Maria Vittoria Primiceri • Notarbartolo & Gervasi SpA, Via Savoia, 82, 00198 Roma, Italy. **Sandro Paci** • ENEA, Via Anguillarese, 306, 00100 Roma, Italy.

Integrated Biomaterials Science, edited by R. Barbucci. Kluwer Academic/Plenum Publishers, New York, 2002.

Thus the European Committee decentralized the production phase to the Member Countries charged with developing the most suitable technical standards in order to develop the topics under discussion in connection with directives concerning safeguarding human health as well as domestic animals. Each Member State became aware of the benefits brought about by harmonizing technical standards in order to avoid complete industrial chaos, and felt the need to create bodies that would control and promote standards that were suitable for the European Community.

Actually these bodies already existed in Europe as well as in the rest of the world; in fact the CEN (European Committee of Regulations) and ISO (International Organisation for Standardisation) were born long before the Community addressed the problem. They were getting organized in order to operate extensively so that the partners in these organizations would comprise for the CEN all the European standardization bodies, and for the ISO the same ones outside of the U.S.A., Canada, Japan, and elsewhere, except for Australia and New Zealand.

33.1.2. National, EN, and ISO Standards

One cannot speak of technical standards without giving background information about the standardization bodies. They were mainly created to standardize the mechanical needs of war requests, especially since the First World War.

In Italy the standardization body is divided in two parts: the CEI (Italian Electrotechnical Committee), which processes all requests in the electromechanical field, and the UNI (National Body of Unification), which processes all requests of the other industrial sectors.

The CEI was created in 1909 at the initiative of the General Council of the Italian Electrotechnical and Electronics Association (AEI) and its jurisdiction was recognized in 1967. Now, it forms part of the CENELEC at a European level and of the IEC (International Electrotechnical Commission) at an international level. The CEI takes an interest in standards pertaining to electrotechnical subjects, and in Italy its publications have become technical standards for electric installations and their safety.

The UNI has more recent roots; it was founded in 1921 and its jurisdiction was acknowledged in 1955. Besides being a standardization body, the UNI has a social and economical role in promoting security, quality of life, and environmental preservation through the regulation of products, processes, and services.

Italian standards are marked via the promulgating body, UNI or CEI, followed by a number that represents the list to which the standard belongs. The CEI is a partner and member of the CENELEC organization which, in the European context, represents all the standardization bodies of the Member States applicable to electrotechnical matters and electronics.

CENELEC is a Belgian law association (it has its seat in Bruxelles) created in 1975 together with the CEN and all its members are European standardization bodies associated with electrotechnical bodies. The main task of CENELEC is to issue European standards recognized by all the Member States, and to attune those national standards that are accepted, with suitable modifications by the other Member States, by putting its own mark "EN" and incorporating the resulting standard into other similar standards in force in the Member Countries.

CEN has its seat in Bruxelles, too, and has CENELEC's same standardization task, so attuned standards issued by the Member States acquire the inscription EN.

The attuned standards issued by CEN and by CENELEC and used by the Member States are recognizable by the European inscription. In Italy it is for example,

UNI EN xxxx [xxxxx] = decimal number

The most recent European standardization body is ETSI, founded in 1988 after the European Conference of Postal and Telecommunication Services (CEPIT), and it now has its seat in France in Sophia Antipolis. The ETSI's field of standardization deals with the transmission branch.

The "Joint President Group" (JPS) is charged with coordinating all the European standards and is involved in the whole range of activities of the CEN, CENELEC, and ETSI.

The structure of the European standards bodies is shown as a chart in Figure 33.1.

The ISO and IEC are international bodies. The former assembles the standardization concerning industrial activities with the exception of electrotechnical and transmission matters, which form part of the IEC's range of activities.

33.1.3. Standard of Quality System

In 1985 the European policy, termed "Nouvelle Approche," decided to link security at work, security of machinery and products, and protection of the environment to quality. This would be achieved by issuing laws (compulsory) as well as fostering methodological and practice systems (voluntary).

The UE has adopted a common policy and left the State members to develop national laws. Each Member State acknowledges the directives of

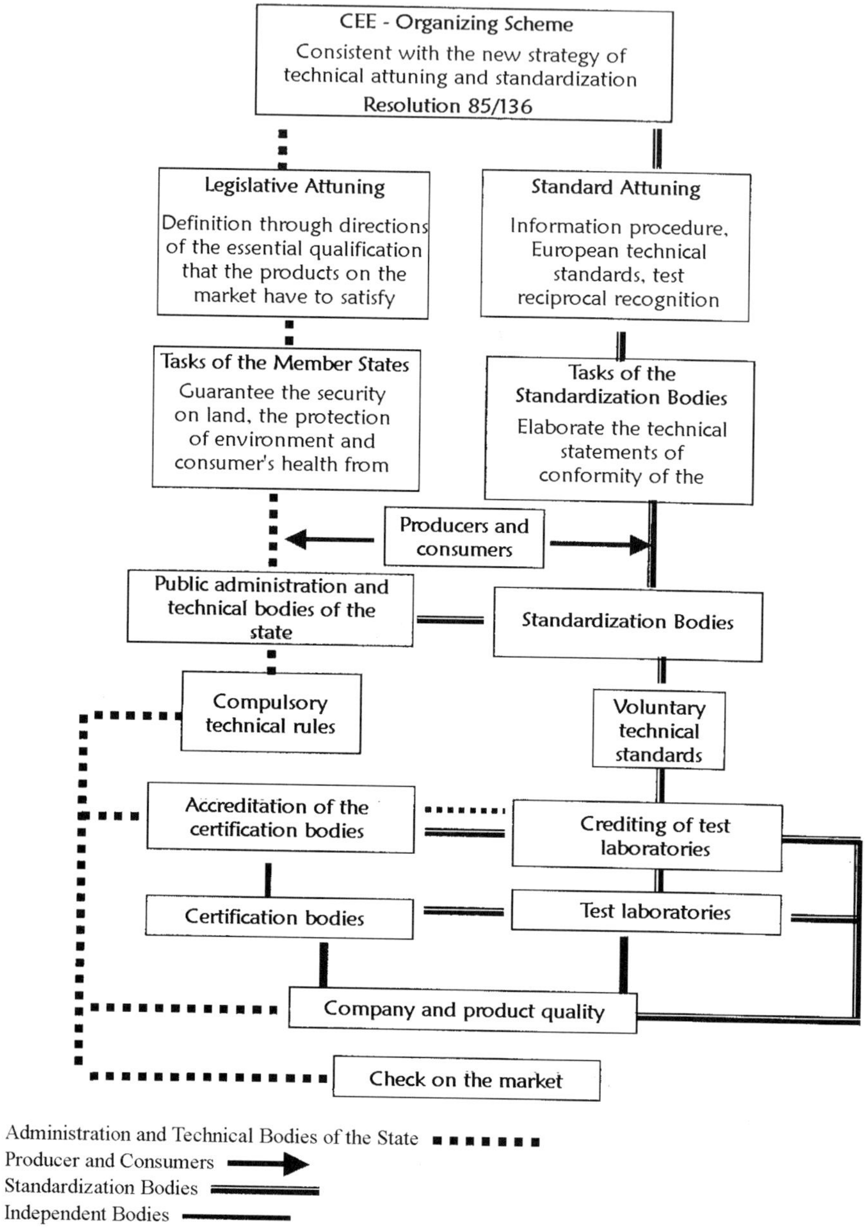

Figure 33.1. Structure of European standards.

the European Union and empowers the relevant bodies with the task of writing the rules and ensuring they are applied by enterprises and citizens. Enterprises follow the rules by continually training and so improving their employees. Ultimately, citizens will live in a country that has public and private services that protect them from accidents and illness. This leads to improving the "quality of life" compatible with a "sustainable development," according to which environmental and economic development will be attuned without either taking over from the other. The combined care of the State, of the standardization and control bodies, and of the enterprises and citizens will allow quality of life through continuous improvement of products, services, the environment, and of our jobs.

The quality, which produced the ISO 9000 series, is regarded as the ability to achieve customer satisfaction through a product and/or service that satisfies contractual requirements and is seen to live up to its expectations. A quality system referred to ISO 9000 possesses the following:

- preparing targets, planning, and training,
- documentation and recording,
- fixing rules through instructions, standards, and specifications,
- establishing completion dates of the audits.

This means optimizing the processes to obtain benefits in terms of the enterprise's process rationalization; organizational clarity as concerns roles, authorities, and responsibilities; reduction in costs pertaining to "bad quality" goods; growth and development of human resources.

33.2. ISO Standards and Overview

In 1979 the Technical International Committee ISO/TC 176 was constituted with the task of preparing plans for international standards on "Quality Management and Quality Insurance," in order to face the increasing number of requests in the nuclear field. During the same period (1983), in fact, the BSI and UNI issued 5750 and 8450 standards, respectively, both concerning nuclear quality systems.

In 1987 the ISO began with the first standards series 9000, the range of which is:

- enterprise management for quality and quality assurance,
- value analysis and functional analysis,
- trustworthiness, including reliability, maintenance, and availability.

The CEN and ISO reached agreement about the nonproliferation of contractual standards and sectorial certification because Member Sates also have standard schemes and sectorial guidelines to facilitate application, without modification, of ISO series 9000, and also standard schemes to integrate, at the request of sectorial interests, the same contractual and certified ISO 9000 standards. (For example, EN 46001 and EN 46002 standards on medical devices respectively integrate ISO 9001 and 9002.)

Such policy is aimed at primarily limiting the integration of ISO 9000 in national standards in order not to cause obstacles to the free exchange of goods and services.

The strategic aims of the ISO are:

- to keep the international standard coherent, updated, and complete with norms and general guides requested by international demands;
- to keep the international standard updated to the European one;
- to actively participate in the continuous improvement of the standards series 9000 according to the "VISION 2000" program.

The CEE considers ISO 9000 a means for attuning international voluntary certification systems. EN series 29000 standard (which is the same as ISO 9000 of the year 1987) was updated by the CEN on order of the third Commission of the CEE. Besides, the decision of the CEE's Counsel of Ministers on 29 July 1993, concerning schemes of procedure for several evaluation steps of product conformity for CE marking, of which more later, prescribes quality systems conformable to EN 29001, 29002, and 29003 (currently EN ISO 9001, 9002, and 9003).

In accordance with European standardization activity, the CEN thought it was not a good idea to create their own standards, because the 18 Partner Countries saw fit to adopt standards laid out by ISO/TC 175.

Some Clarification Regarding Series ISO 9000. The following account illustrates a functional classification of the whole family of ISO 9000, while the next prospectus gives the normative and programmatic outline of ISO/TC 176 up to March 1998.

The content of each standard is instead synthesised in norm EN ISO 900-1 which illustrates the main quality concepts. It is important to point out that ISO 9000 establishes management principles for quality and insurance requisites for quality for the following four aspects linked to the quality of a product or the service supplied by a firm or organization:

- definition and update of the product in order that it keeps tuned to market demands,
- product planning,
- conformity of the product to the plan,
- product support during its life cycle.

Moreover, it must be remembered that ISO 9000 (Figure 33.2) is oriented toward customer satisfaction as well as interested parties (ISO 9000-1), and looks also at processes and their continuous improvement.

These outlines will soon change with the arrival of "VISION 2000," which will incorporate the most meaningful standards, that is to say there will be a numerical and a substantial variation in the standards referred to the quality of a system and of a product.

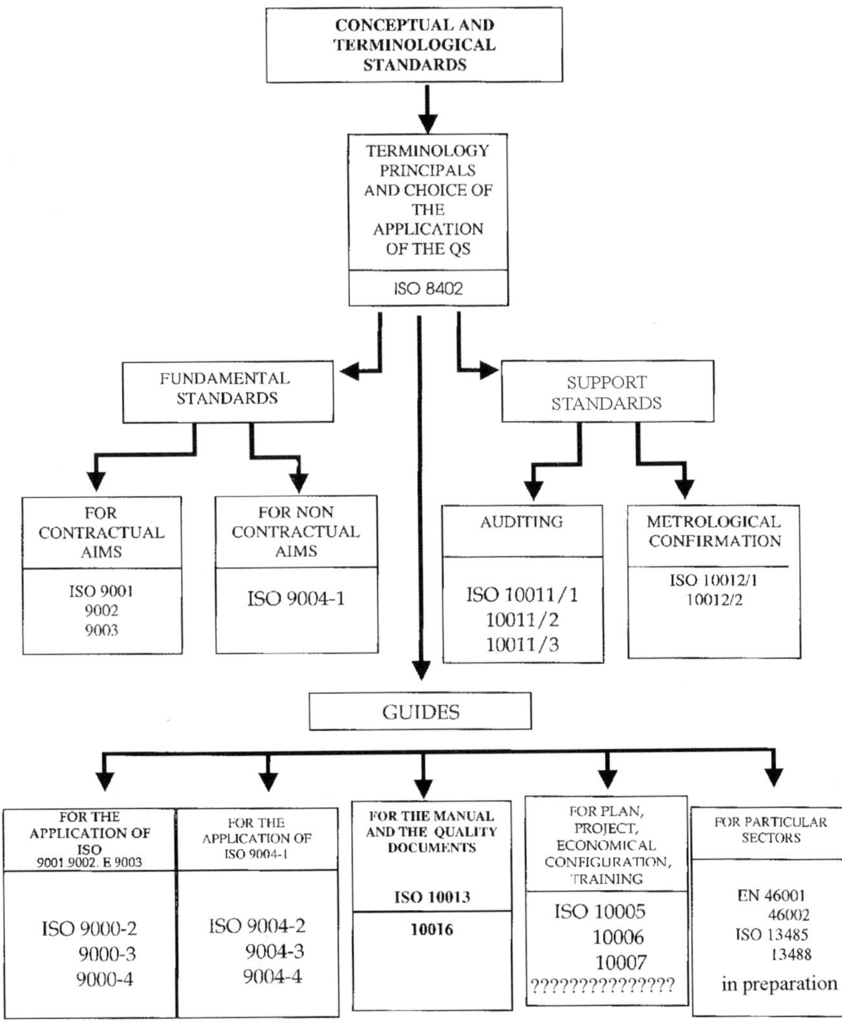

Figure 33.2. The ISO 9000 family.

33.3. European System

33.3.1. EC Directive on Medical Devices

Directive 93/42/CEE of the Counsel of June 14, 1993 regarding medical devices appeared in the GUCE L. n° 169 of 12/07/93 and has been in force since January 1, 1995, and will continue until June 30, 2004. The directive modifications are as follows:

- 65/65/CEE for reconciling the legislation prescribed and administrative dispositions concerning medicines.
- 73/318/CEE for reconciling Member State legislation concerning standards and analytical toxipharmacological and clinical protocols in the field of medical experimentation.
- 76/764/CEE for including Member States legislation in the field of glass clinical thermometers made of mercury of the maximum type.
- 80/181/CEE for unity of measures by measuring devices.
- 80/836/EURATOM for modifying directives that fix fundamental standards concerning sanitary protection of the population and worker protection against risks arising from ionogenic radiation.
- 84/593/CEE for reconciling Member State legislation concerning electrical devices used in human and veterinary medicine.
- 84/466/EURATOM for establishing fundamental measures for radiological protection of people undergoing medical examination and treatment.
- 89/366/CEE for reproaching Member State legislation in the field of electromagnetic compatibility.
- 89/39/CEE for providing measures to foster the improvement of worker safety and health while on duty.
- 89/686/CEE for the reproaching Member State legislation in the field of individual protection devices.
- 90/385/CEE for reproaching Member State legislation in the field of transplantable medical devices.

Directive 93/42/CEE is applicable to medical devices and accessories. In this directive accessories are regarded as medical devices. From now on medical devices and their accessories will be termed "devices." For better interpretation of directive 93/42/CEE we provide some interpretations of its terminology

(a) *Medical device:* any tool, instrument, implant, substance, or any other product, used alone or in combination, including software used for the correct operation and destined to be used on man in order to:

- make a diagnosis, prevention, control, therapy, or attenuation of illness;
- make a diagnosis, control, therapy, attenuation, or compensation of a wound or handicap;
- study, substitute, or modify anatomy or a physiological process;
- intervene on conceiving that these devices should be the only assisted function in and on the human body, and not to be achieved through pharmacological or immunological means, or by means of metabolism.

(b) *Accessory:* a product that, even if not a device, has been destined by the producer to be used with a device in order to allow foreseen use.
(c) *Device for in vitro diagnosis:* any device composed of a reagent, a reactive product, an instrument, an apparatus, or by a system used alone or in combination, destined by the producer to be used *in vitro* for the examination of human body samples in order to give information on physiological conditions or sanitary conditions or illness or congenital anomaly.
(d) *Device made to measure:* any device constructed subject to the written prescription of a qualified doctor who, on his responsibility, points out its planning characteristics in order to be used only by a patient. This prescription could be written also by another person who is professionally qualified and has been charged with doing it. Devices built by methods of continuous manufacture or in series, and that must be subsequently adapted in order to satisfy any specific demand of the doctor or of any other professional user, are not considered devices made to measure.
(e) *Devices for clinical investigation:* a device used by a duly qualified doctor in order to investigate a clinical environment. Clinical investigations may be conducted by a duly qualified doctor or another person who, thanks to his professional qualifications, is authorized to undertake such investigations.

Directive 93/42/CEE is not applied in the following exceptions:

(a) devices assigned to *in vitro* diagnosis;
(b) active plantable devices regulated by directive 90/385/CEE;
(c) medicines subject to directive 65/65/CEE;
(d) cosmetic products considered by directive 76/768/CEE;
(e) human blood, products deriving from human blood, human plasma, ematic cells of human origin, or devices that, once on the market, contain such products deriving from blood, plasma, or cells;

(f) organs, tissues, or cells of human origin, neither contractual or certification products, that include or derive from tissues or cells of human origin;
(g) organs, tissues, or cells of animal origin, unless a device is produced by using not vital animal tissue or not vital products deriving from animal tissue.

This directive is not applied to individual protection devices subject to directive 89/686/CEE. To establish if a certain product is subject to the directive mentioned before or to the present directive, we must consider primarily to whom the product is addressed.

33.3.2. Conformity Assessment and CE Mark

Directive 93/42/CEE distinguishes procedures according to classes of affiliation of the devices. Therefore, we give some classification criteria of the devices:

33.3.2.1. Glossary

Definitions Concerning the Rules of Classification

Duration

- *Temporary:* devices assigned to be used for a continuous duration that lasts less than 60 minutes.
- *Short term:* devices assigned to be used for a continuous duration that lasts less than 30 days.
- *Long term:* devices assigned to be used for a continuous duration that lasts more than 30 days.

Invasive Devices

- *Invasive device:* one that partially or entirely penetrates into the body through an orifice or through a surface of the body.
- *Orifice of the body:* any natural opening of the body, included the external surface of the ocular globe, or any artificial and permanent opening such as a stoma.
- *Surgical invasive device:* an invasive tool that penetrates into the body through its surface by means of or in the context of a surgical intervention. For this directive, devices that differ from those included in the preceding paragraph and penetrate into the body, but not through a certain orifice, are considered surgical invasive devices.

- *Plantable device:* any device assigned to: (1) be entirely installed into human body, or (2) replace an epithelial or ocular surface by means of surgical intervention and remain in that position after the intervention. A plantable device is considered as any device assigned to be partially introduced into the human body by means of surgical intervention and to remain in that place after the intervention for a period of at least 30 days.

Surgical Reusable Instrument. This is an instrument assigned to be used, with no relation to an active medical device, in a surgical context to cut, pierce, saw, scratch, scrape off, curette, seize, staple, or to be used in similar procedures and that can be reused after performing the correct procedures.

Active Medical Device. This is a medical device the use of which depends on electric energy or some other type of energy, different from that directly given by the human body or by gravity and that works converting this energy. A medical device assigned to transmit, without great modification, the energy, the substances, or other elements between an active medical device and the patient, is not considered an active medical device.

Active Therapeutic Device. An active medical device used alone or in combination with other medical devices to support, modify, replace, or restore the functions or biological structures in the context of a treatment or assigned to ease an illness, a wound, or a handicap.

Active Device Assigned to Diagnosis. An active medical device used alone or in combination with other medical devices, assigned to give information about diagnosis, precocious diagnosis, control or treatment of physiological states, of health states, of illness or congenital deformity.

Circulatory Central System. This directive considers vessels of the "circulatory central system," pulmonales arteriae, ascendens aorta, arteriae coronariae, artery comunis carotis, artery externa carotis, artery inside carotis, artery cerebralis, truncus brachicephalicus, venae cordis, pulmonares venae, vein extracts superior, and vein extracts inferior.

Nervous Central System. This directive considers brain, spinal cord, and bone marrow as the nervous central system.

33.3.2.2. Applying Rules

Applying the rules of classification means considering the assignment of each device. If a device is assigned to be used in combination with another device, the rules of classification will be applied for each device separately. The accessories are classified separately from the device with which they are assigned to be used.

Software employed to make a device work, or to influence its use, is automatically part of the same class. If a device is not assigned to be used exclusively or mainly on a certain part of the body, it will be considered and classified according to the most critical specified use.

If a device is applied to which more rules than the performances that the producers assign it apply, then the rules to be applied will be the most rigorous rules that lead to a more elevated classification.

33.3.2.3. Classification

Noninvasive Devices

- All noninvasive devices are included in the I° class, except those to which one of the rules is applied.
- All noninvasive devices addressed to canalization or to maintenance of blood, liquid, or body tissues, liquid or gas employed in a transfusion, provision or introduction in the body, are included in the II° class when:

  (a) they can be connected with an active medical device included in the II° class or in a higher class;
  (b) they are assigned to be used for the maintenance or canalization of blood or other liquid or the maintenance of organs or body tissues. In all other cases they are included in the I° class.

- All devices assigned to modify the biological or chemical composition of blood, or of other body liquids or other liquid assigned to transfusion into the body, are included in the II° b class, unless the treatment does not consist of filtration, centrifugation, or gas exchanges of heat; in this case they are included in the II° a class.
- All noninvasive devices in connection with injured skin:

  (a) are included in the I° class if they are assigned to be used as a mechanical barrier for the compression and absorption of the exudates;
  (b) are included in the II° b class if they are assigned to be mainly used with wounds that have injured the derma and that can scar only for secondary intention;
  (c) all other cases are included in the II° a class including devices mainly assigned to keep under control the micro-ambient of a wound.

Invasive Devices

- All invasive devices in relation to orifices of the body, which are different from surgical invasive devices and are not related to an active medical device:

  (a) are included in the I° class if they are assigned a temporary use;
  (b) are included in the II° class if they are assigned to be used at a short term, unless they are used in the oral chamber up to the pharynx, in a channel of the ear up to the eardrum, or in a nasal chamber, and that do not run the risk of being absorbed by the mucous, in which case they are included in the II° a class.

- All invasive devices connected with orifices of the body, which are different from surgical invasive devices and are assigned to be connected to an active medical device included in the II° a class or in a superior class, are included in the II° a class.
- All surgical invasive devices assigned a temporary use are included in the II° a class, unless they are not:

  (a) specifically assigned to diagnose, guard, or correct defects of the heart or of the circulatory central system through direct contact with these parts of the body, in which case they are included in the III° class;
  (b) surgical reusable tools, in which case they are included in the I° class;
  (c) assigned to release energy set in the form of ionogenic radiation, in which case they are included in the II° b class;
  (d) assigned to have a biological effect or to be entirely or mainly absorbed, in which case they are included in the II° b class;
  (e) assigned to administer medicinal specialities by means of a transmission system, if that happens subject to potential risk considered in the way of application, in which case they are included in the II° b class.

- All surgical invasive devices assigned to be used at a short term are included in the II° a class, unless they are not assigned to:

  (a) specifically diagnose, guard, or correct a defect of the heart or of the circulatory central system through direct contact with these parts of the body, in which case they are included in the III° class;
  (b) specifically be used in direct contact with the central nervous system, in which case they are included in the III° class;

(c) release energy set in the form of ionogenic radiation, in which case they are included in the II° b class;
(d) have a biological effect or to be entirely or mainly absorbed, in which case they are included in the III° class;
(e) undergo a chemical modification of the body, unless they are not set in the teeth, or give medicinal specialities, in which case they are included in the II° b class.

- All plantable devices and all long-term surgical invasive devices are included in the II° b class unless they are not assigned to:

  (a) be put in teeth, in which case they are included in the II° a class;
  (b) be used in direct contact with the heart, the circulatory central system, or the nervous central system, in which case they are in the III° class;
  (c) have a biological effect or be entirely or mainly absorbed, in which case they are included in the III° class;
  (d) undergo a chemical modification in the body, unless they are not set in the teeth, or give medicinal specialities, in which case they are included in the III° class.

Additional Rules to Be Applied to the Active Devices

- All therapeutic devices assigned to release or change energy are included in the II° a class unless their characteristics allow them to release energy to the human body or exchange energy with the human body in a potentially dangerous way, considering the nature, the density, and the part in which energy is applied, in which case they are included in the II° b class.
- All active devices assigned to check or guard performances regulating therapeutic active devices included in the II° b class, or assigned to directly influence the performance of such devices, are included in the II° b class.
- Active devices employed for diagnosis are included in the II° a class if:

  (a) they are assigned to release energy that will be absorbed by the human body, with the exception of devices used to illuminate the patient's body in the visible spectrum;
  (b) they are employed for a live visualization of the distribution of radiomedicals;
  (c) they are assigned to allow direct diagnosis or control of the physiological vital processes, unless they are specifically assigned to check the physiological vital parameters in

which the variations are such as to create immediate danger for the patient, or cause, for example, variations in the cardiac functions, in the respiration, or in the activity of the central nervous system, in which case they are included in the II° b class.

- All active devices assigned to administer and/or subtract medicinal liquids of the body or other substances of the body are included in the II° a class, unless this is done in a potentially dangerous way, considering the nature of the substances in question, and the part of the body, and the method of application, in which case they are included in the II° b class.
- All other devices are included in the I° a class.

Special Rules

- All devices that include as an integral part a substance that, when used separately, can be considered a medicine according to article 1 of directive 65/65/CEE and that can have an effect on the human body with an accessory action to that of the device, are included in the III° class.
- All devices used for contraception or used for the prevention of sexual transmissible illness are included in the II° b class, unless they are plantable devices or long-term invasive devices, in which case they are included in the III° class.
- All devices specifically assigned to be used to disinfect, clean, rinse, or if necessary, hydrate contact lenses are included in the II° b class.
- All devices specifically assigned to be used to disinfect medical devices are included in the II° a class. This rule is not applicable to products assigned to clean by means of physical action medical devices that are not contact lenses.
- Nonactive devices specifically assigned to record X-ray diagnostic images are included in the II° a class.
- All devices made with animal tissues or with by-products that are not vital are included in the III° class, unless these devices have not been assigned to be in contact with intact skin.
- As an exception to the other rules, knapsacks for blood are included in the II° b class.

33.3.3. Procedure to Obtain CEE Marking

1. If the producer wants to put the CE mark on devices included in the III° class, with the exclusion of measuring devices and devices assigned to clinical investigations, he has to:

(a) follow the procedure for the CE conformity declaration (system with quality assurance included), or
(b) follow the relevant procedure of CE conformity declaration of the type with:
   - the procedure concerning CE verification, or
   - the procedure concerning CE conformity declaration (production quality guarantee).

2. If the producer wants to put the CE mark on devices included in the II° a class, with the exclusion of measuring devices and devices assigned to clinical investigations, he has to follow the procedure of the CE conformity declaration. Moreover, he has to follow:

   (a) the procedure concerning CE verification, or,
   (b) the procedure concerning CE conformity declaration (production quality guarantee), or
   (c) the procedure concerning CE conformity declaration (product quality guarantee).

   As an alternative to such procedures, the producer could follow the procedure foreseen in paragraph 3 subsection (a).
3. If the producer wants to put the CE mark on devices included in the II° b class, with the exclusion of measuring devices and the devices assigned to clinical investigations, he has to follow:

   (a) the procedure concerning CE conformity declaration (system with quality guarantee); in this case the point concerning control of product planning is not applied, or
   (b) the procedure concerning CE certification together with:
      - the procedure concerning CE verification;
      - the procedure concerning CE conformity declaration (product quality guarantee).

4. If the producer wants to put the CE mark on devices included in the II° a class, with the exclusion of measuring devices and devices assigned to clinical investigations, he has to follow the procedure according to which he compiles the CE conformity declaration before he puts the products on the market.
5. For measuring devices, the producer must follow the procedure that requires a particular declaration for some devices that have a particular destination and he must compile the declaration in point G, before he puts the devices on the market. The Member States can establish that the producer shows the competent authority a list of devices that work in their territory.

Particular Procedure for Systems and a Complete Kit for the Operating Field.

1. With the exception of the provisions mentioned earlier, the present procedures are applied to the systems and to the complete kit for the operating field.
2. Any physical or juridical person that assembles devices carrying the CE mark must compile a declaration based on the assignment of the devices and the application limits established by the producer when putting them on the market as a system or complete kit for the operating field. The declaration must state that:

   (a) he has checked the mutual compatibility of the devices according to the producer's instructions and that he has operated according to the instructions;
   (b) he has packed the system or the complete kit for the operating field and that he has given users the information containing the producer's instructions;
   (c) the whole activity is subject to adequate checking methods and to internal controls.

   If the above conditions are not satisfied, like in the case in which the system or operating kit contains devices that do not have CE marking or in which the combination of devices chosen is not compatible with the use to which they were originally assigned, then the system or complete operating kit is considered a device in itself and as such is subject to the procedure previously expounded.
3. Any physical or juridical person that, with a view to marketing these devices, sterilizes the systems or complete operating kit referred to in paragraph 2 or other medical devices that have CE marking CE and that are said to be sterilized before use by the producers themselves. The application of this procedure and the intervention of the notified body are limited to the aspects that concern the sterilization procedure. The person declares that the sterilization has been carried out according to the instructions of the producer.
4. The products mentioned in paragraphs 2 and 3 must not have a new CE marking, but must be equipped with all the information furnished by the manufacturer including, where necessary, indications as to the constituent devices from the manufacturer. The declaration foreseen in paragraphs 2 and 3 are held by the competent authorities for 5 years.

33.3.4. Attuned Technical Standards

Since 1993 the CEN has issued a considerable quantity of standards concerning medical products of any kind, especially concerning biomedical products. This is quite a new subject to be approached cautiously owing to the vastness and delicacy of the subject. Working groups are being organized to tackle the relevant problems. Notwithstanding, some standards have already been issued and others are being prepared for general application:

- EN 10993-10: Biological evaluation of medical devices—Part 10: Irritation and sensitization test (ISO 10993-10/1995).
- EN 30993-3: Biological evaluation of medical devices—Part 3: Toxicus, carcinomatus, and toxicity on the reproduction test (ISO 10993-3/1992).
- EN 30993-4: Biological evaluation of medical devices—Part 4: Choice of tests concerning interaction with blood (ISO 10993-4/1992).
- EN 30993-5: Biological evaluation of medical devices—Part 5: Toxicity test—*in vitro* methods (ISO 10993-5/1992).
- EN 30993-6: Biological evaluation of medical devices—Part 6: Tests on local effects after the plant (ISO 10993-6/1994).
- EN 46001: Quality systems—medical devices—particular prescriptions for the application of EN ISO 29001.
- EN 46002: Quality system—medical devices—particular prescriptions for the application of EN ISO 29002.
- EN 50103: Guide for the application of EN ISO 29001 and EN ISO 29002 and EN 46002 for factories that produce active medical devices (including active implantables).

Bibliography

Marino, L., De Girolamo, A. 1996. *Un'Europa di qualità*, Buffetti.

Nicola Airoldi, N. 1997. *Guida alle direttive CE nuovo approccio*, Nuovo Studio Tecna.

Elias, G. 1993. *Europa 1993—libera circolazione delle merci*, UNI.

European Errant, 1993. GUCE L nr. 169 of 12/07/93, European Community.

34

Biomaterials and Patents

Maria Vittoria Primiceri

34.1. Introduction

34.1.1. Historical Overview

Biomaterials are concerned with human health, so it is essential to promote progress and research in this field which is devoted to the improvement of conditions surrounding the life of human beings. Patent protection contributes to ensure progress and innovation on the part of those (companies, universities, etc.) that invest in biomaterials mainly because the cost of research on modern efficacious and safe biomaterials is so considerable that nobody would be able to take the risk of investing the necessary money if anyone—possibly a company without the necessary experience—could afterward freely copy the newly invented biomaterial. The most reasonable insurance is that investors are fairly reimbursed, the incentive to invent in this field should be very high, and the potential cost of the new materials for consumers should be low.

The purpose of patents is therefore to protect inventions. This involves granting a legal title which allows the owner the exclusive right to use the invention for *a limited period of time in a defined geographical area* (see Figure 34.1). This right to use the invention prevents others from exploiting (e.g., manufacturing and selling) the invention without prior authorization of the owner of the patent.

It was in Italy that the first real Patent Law appeared, in Venice, in 1474. The so-called "Parte Veneziana" established that: *"Anyone, who will make in Venice something new and inventive, not present before in this territory, and this invention will be put in practice in order to be exploited, will have to notify what was invented to the Municipal Offices. It is prohibited for*

Maria Vittoria Primiceri • Notarbartolo & Gervasi SpA, Via Savoia, 82, 00198 Roma, Italy.

Integrated Biomaterials Science, edited by R. Barbucci. Kluwer Academic/Plenum Publishers, New York, 2002.

THE PATENT

The patent document is a title granted on demand by a State service (or regional office acting for more than one State).

The patent describes an invention and creates a legal situation according to which the patented invention can not be exploited (manufactured, used, sold, imported) without the authorization of the patent owner.

The right conferred by a patent is **limited in time** (generally a 20 years period) and **limited geographically**.

Figure 34.1

others to reproduce the invention without the inventor's authorization for 10 years."

This is the first example of an exclusive right on which the basic concepts of modern patent laws are based:

- novelty of the invention;
- definition of exclusive right;
- time and territorial limits of the right;
- filing of the application with a public administration.

At this early stage it was still unclear how inventors would gain their reward from exploitation of the invention. Subsequent evolution of laws relating to inventions clarified this fundamental concept. In this sense the Statute of Monopolies, an English law of 1623, allowed inventors to benefit from exclusive rights by exploiting the invention, and the Patent Act, United States law of April 1790, granted inventors the possibility of applying for a Patent to obtain, the exclusive right of producing, using, and selling the object of the Patent for a limited period of time (14 years).

All these laws have in common the same fundamental principles: the inventor describes his invention and obtains a corresponding exclusive and temporary right of exploiting his invention by a granted patent, at the same time denying any third party exploitation of the described invention. That is, what has been invented is divulged, but at the same time removed from competition by a third party. When the monopoly expires, what was invented becomes public property and can be put into practice and enjoyed by everyone. In this manner public knowledge of the invention promotes research and innovation, which leads to technological development for the benefit of society.

However, the effective rights conferred by a patent would be strongly restricted and there could arise conflicting situations unless there exist international and mutual agreements between foreign countries to recognize patent protection and the advantages granted the nationals of each country.

This was the sense of the Paris Convention (1883), which resulted in the "International Union for the Protection of Industrial Property" which, among others, laid the basis for one of the most important principles of the patent system: the provision under which "anybody who has duly applied for a patent in a Convention Country is entitled, when filing a corresponding application in any other Convention country, to claim the filing (priority) date of said first application, provided that such further application is filed within a certain period (12 months), running from the filing date of the first application."

Nowadays, the inventor or the proprietor of an invention files an application for a patent, in general, in his country. Afterward he enjoys a one-year priority (according to the provisions of the Paris Convention) during which time he must design a strategy for an extension of the patent and decide to which countries he is interested in extending it. But what policy should he follow? Sometimes one year is a too short period in which to decide the countries in which it would be worthwhile to extend the patent. In fact, although the theory underlying the patent system is straightforward and virtually universal, the practical details of its operation can vary substantially from country to country. Consider, for example, the case where a given invention is made more or less simultaneously by different inventors working independently. This kind of situation occurs quite frequently in fields of rapidly advancing techology. Who wins the patent race in such circumstances? In almost all countries he who files his application first in the Patent Office wins. In the United States of America, it is, in contrast, the first to invent who succeeds.

Another important aspect to be taken into consideration when extending a patent is connected with the differences existing from country to country in the patent protection policy, such as examination procedure, amendment of patents after grant, employee rights, shop rights, grace periods, renewal fees, criteria for assessment of infringment, intervention of third parties, compulsory licences—to name just a few of the topics discussed in further detail in "Manual for the handling of applications for patents, designs and trade marks throughout the world."

The results of such differences are equally problematic: for example, in some countries the applicant would merely receive a registered patent, i.e., there would be no substantive examination for patentability, while in other countries the examination procedure could result in patents of differing scope.

Filing a Patent Application

☆ NATIONAL LEVEL

- ◆ example: French patent application at the French Patent Office
  - ✓ finality of any filing
  - ✓ sometimes obliged
  - ✓ low cost

☆ INTERNATIONAL LEVEL

- ◆ Separate applications of a patent in each foreign country
- ◆ European patent application at the European Patent Office (EPO)
  - ✓ simplified formalities
  - ✓ one language (GB, DE, FR)
  - ✓ single search
  - ✓ single examination
  - ✓ value of a national filing
- ◆ International application called PCT application
  - ✓ only a patent application
  - ✓ similar to European filing
  - ✓ simultaneous filing for many states
  - ✓ delay of national proceedings
  - ✓ possibility of common examination

Figure 34.2

Generally, there is a trend toward harmonization of patent law on a global scale. Such standardization of the basic principles of patent law and simplification and speeding up of procedures relating to Intellectual Property (IP) protection have led to the creation of most important national institutions, among which the Patent Cooperation Treaty and the European Patent Convention should be mentioned.

Figure 34.2 is a schematic view of some alternatives in extending a patent application.

34.1.2. The European Patent Convention

The European Patent Convention, or EPC, came into force in 1977 and gives the possibility of obtaining a patent in more than one country in Western Europe.

"The aim of EPC is to make the protection of inventions in the Contracting States easier, cheaper and more reliable by creating a single European procedure for the grant of patents on the basis of a uniform body of substantive patent law." A handbook explaining how to manage a European filing is entitled: "How to Get a European Patent," an edition of the European Patent Office.

The EPC enables whoever wishes to seek patent protection in many European countries to file, instead of many national patent applications, one single application covering all the Contracting States designated by the applicant, in only one language (the language of the procedure can be English, French, or German). The application will be subjected to only one procedure of grant instead of many parallel procedures, and a single patent will be granted that will be valid in the various Convention Countries of interest, leading to single patents subjected to the law of each country involved.

A short view of the major single steps of the European granting procedure is shown in Figure 34.3.

34.1.3. The Patent Cooperation Treaty

The Patent Cooperation Treaty, or PCT, is a multilateral treaty that entered into force in 1978. It facilitates the obtaining of protection for inventions in that it gives the possibility to file one single patent application with effect in several states, instead of filing several separate national and/or regional patent applications. Regional patent treaties are the following: the African Regional Industrial Property Organisation (ARIPO), the Eurasian Patent Convention, the above mentioned European Patent Convention, and the Agreement establishing the African Intellectual Property Organization (OAPI).

The PCT does not eliminate the necessity of prosecuting the international application in the national/regional phases but, in its most advantageous aspect, it gives the applicant more time and a better basis for deciding whether and in which countries to further prosecute the application.

Under the PCT provisions there is a possibility, with a single filing in a single language, to designate all the contracting states (more than 100), the election of single states being deferred by 20 or 30 months from the priority. A guide on how to file a PCT application is: "PCT Applicant's Guide" edited by the World Intellectual Property Organisation.

A few of the many advantages in applying for the PCT procedure are shown in Figure 34.4.

The European Patent Grant Procedure

- **Filing the application**
  - ✓ a single application can be filed with the EPO or a national office
  - ✓ in just a language
- **Examination on filing and formalities examination**
- **Search**
  - ✓ a search is carried out to identify the relevant prior art to the invention
- **Publication of application and search report**
  - ✓ the application is published 18 months after priority date, the search report is either published with the application or later on, the applicant has then nine months to decide whether or not to pursue application by requesting substantive examination
- **Substantive examination (grant of patent or refusal of application)**
  - ✓ during the substantive examination it is verified whether or not the invention satisfies the three patentability criteria:
    1. **novelty**
    2. **inventive step**
    3. **industrial applicability**
- **Opposition (in some cases)**
  - ✓ within nine months of the date of grant any third party may oppose a patent that he believes should not have been granted
- **Appeal (in some cases)**
  - ✓ appeals may be lodged against the decisions of :
    1. the Receiving Section
    2. the Examination Division
    3. the Opposition Division
- **Nationalization in:**
  - ✓ AT, BE, CH, CY, DE, DK, ES, FI, FR, GB, GR, IE, IT, LI, LU, MC, NL, PT, SE, TR (situation at the beginning of 2001)

Figure 34.3

Strategies under PCT Procedure

- Gain time to better identify possible markets
- Gain time to find partners
- Gain time to better evaluate the technical value of the invention
- Increased chance of foreign filing
- The final version of the claims is drafted when the commercial value of the invention is better known
- Only one version of description, claims and drawings
- Better information about possible conflicting applications by competitors prior to national entry, enabling adjustment of filing strategy and negotiating position

Figure 34.4

34.1.4. The Patent Application — General Remarks and Patentability Criteria

The essential parts comprising a patent application are set forth in Figure 34.5.

The patent application is filed by the applicant before a Public Administration. The application is subjected to a formal and/or substantive examination and is then granted for a limited period of time, generally 20 years. The applicant must pay maintenance fees for the patent.

34.2. Patentable Inventions

After this historical overview, and the legal aspects and formalities of patents, we go "inside the invention" and find that it is difficult to define what an "invention" is. We could define an "invention" as an intellectual creation consisting in (or such as to permit) the solution of a technical problem. That is, an "invention" is the creation of something not existing before, in contrast to a discovery of something already existing in nature (according to the US patent law Title 35 § 101 — see Figure 34.6).

The Patent Application

- **Title**
- **Introduction**
  - ✓ technological background
  - ✓ prior art
  - ✓ drawbacks of prior art
- **Description (Examples)**
  - ✓ non-characterizing part of Claim 1
  - ✓ object of the invention
  - ✓ characterizing part of Claim 1
  - ✓ explanations
  - ✓ other features (other claims)
- **Claims**
  - ✓ Claim 1 (indipendent)
    - non-characterizing part
    - characterizing part
  - ✓ Claim 2 (dependent)
    - additional features
  - ✓ Claim 3 (dependent)
    - additional features
- **Abstracts**
- **Drawings** (if any)

Figure 34.5

European law does not define "invention"; it only gives a nonexhaustive list of what is to be considered an invention, and what can or cannot be protected with a patent (see Figure 34.6).

For Europe we can identify three basic categories of invention: the invention of a *product*, i.e. the invention of a material and concrete entity, which can be a substance or composition (chemical compound or a mixture of compounds) as well as a physical entity (object, article, apparatus); the invention of a *process* (the process for making a product); and the invention of a *use* (the use of a product).

Title 35 § 101 USC
Inventions patentable
Whoever invents or discovers any new and useful process, machine, manufacture or composition of matter, or any new and useful improvement thereof, may obtain a patent thereof, subject to the conditions and requirements of this title.

Art. 52 EPC
Patentable inventions
(1) European patents shall be granted for any inventions which are susceptible of industrial application, which are new and which involve an inventive step.

(2) The following in particular shall not be regarded as inventions within the meaning of paragraph 1:

(a) discoveries, scientific theories and mathematical methods;
(b) aesthetic creations;
(c) schemes, rules and methods for performing mental acts, playing games or doing business, and programs for computers;
(d) presentation of information.

(3) ...

(4) Methods for treatment of the human or animal body by surgery or therapy and diagnostic methods practised on the human or animal body shall not be regarded as inventions which are susceptible of industrial application within the meaning of paragraph 1. This provision shall not apply to products, in particular substances or compositions, for use in any of these methods.

Figure 34.6

However, any kind of invention must satisfy all the following three requisites:

(a) *Novelty*. The invention shall be considered new if it does not form part of the state of the art. The state of the art comprises everything made available to the public by means of a written or oral disclosure, by use, or in any other way all over the world before the date of filing the patent application (Art. 54 EPC—European Patent Convention).

(b) *Nonobviousness*. The invention shall be considered obvious if it originates from the direct combination of the teachings of prior art and does not involve any skillfulness or ability beyond that to be expected of the person skilled in the art (Guidelines for examination in the European Patent Office, part C, 1994).

(c) *Industrial applicability*, or *utility*. The invention shall have a "technical character" and shall be useful, that is, it shall belong to the useful or practical arts as distinct from the esthetic arts (Guidelines for examination in the European Patent Office, part C, 1994).

34.3. Patentability of Biomaterials

Biomaterials can be chemical compounds, polymers, blends, composites, etc., so they can be protected like other products and, in principle, do not present difficulties in patenting, at least in those countries which accept the patentability of chemical products and, above all, if the already-mentioned patentability criteria are satisfied.

A biomaterial can be claimed:

(a) by its chemical formula,
(b) as a product of a process "Product X obtained by process Y,"
(c) by its parameters (e.g., melting point, flexural strength, conductivity, etc.). The parameters should be "clearly and reliably determined either by indications in the description or by objective procedures which are usual in the art" (Guidelines for examination in the European Patent Office, part C, 1994).

However, some problem could arise for products or materials that are known in different fields of application and, after further research, prove to be characterized by a specific behavior which renders them particularly suitable as a biomaterial. In this case use claims can be widely accepted.

Relevant decisions of the Technical Boards of Appeal published in the Official Journal EPO

T 36/83 OJ 9/86

T 144/83 OJ 9/86

T 245/87 OJ 5/89

T 24/91 OJ 8/95

T 74/93 OJ 10/95

T 329/94 OJ 5/98

Figure 34.7

Different wordings under EP and US laws

The invention: a biocompatible synthetic polymer matrix made of a biocompatible material and cells of various nature attached to said matrix, the matrix being apt for implantation.

EP Claim:
Use of a biocompatible synthetic polymer matrix made of a biocompatible material and cells of various nature attached to said matrix, for manufacturing structures apt for implantation.

US Claim:
Method for implanting in a living body a biocompatible synthetic polymer matrix made of a biocompatible material and cells of various nature attached to said matrix.

Figure 34.8

Nonetheless, care should be taken that a corresponding claim for a particular biomaterial or medical device made to come in contact with the human body could be excepted to be considered a therapeutic treatment and hence the industrial applicability denied.

Figure 34.7 identifies the most relevant decisions issued by the Technical Boards of Appeal of the European Patent Office (EPO) and relating to therapeutic treatments.

In complete contrast, the US Patent Law, which does not accept "use" claims, allows patenting of therapeutic treatments for the reason that Title 35 § 101 USC does not expressely deny their patentability.

Thus, for the same invention two different claims in EP and USA could be possible and, in principle, their wording could be that in Figure 34.8.

In conclusion, when applying for a patent for a biomaterial, care should be taken to obtain the best and widest protection. The most pernicious activity is the "do it yourself," the best being to contact an expert in Industrial Property.

Bibliography

Manual for the handling of applications for patents, designs and trade marks throughout the world, Manual Industrial Property BV ed.

How to get a European Patent, European Patent Office.

European Patent Convention, European Patent Office.

Guidelines for examination in the European Patent Office, European Patent Office.

PCT Applicants Guide, WIPO — World Intellectual Property Organization.

Index

B

D

U